AAOS
Comprehensive
Orthopaedic Review

Volume 1

Editor
Martin I. Boyer, MD, MSc, FRCS(C)

Carol B. and Jerome T. Loeb Professor
Department of Orthopedic Surgery
Washington University School of Medicine
St. Louis, Missouri

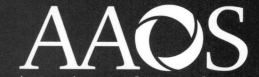

AAOS
AMERICAN ACADEMY OF ORTHOPAEDIC SURGEONS

The material presented in the *AAOS Comprehensive Orthopaedic Review, Second Edition* has been made available by the American Academy of Orthopaedic Surgeons for educational purposes only. This material is not intended to present the only, or necessarily best, methods or procedures for the medical situations discussed, but rather is intended to represent an approach, view, statement, or opinion of the author(s) or producer(s), which may be helpful to others who face similar situations.

Some drugs or medical devices demonstrated in Academy courses or described in Academy print or electronic publications have not been cleared by the Food and Drug Administration (FDA) or have been cleared for specific uses only. The FDA has stated that it is the responsibility of the physician to determine the FDA clearance status of each drug or device he or she wishes to use in clinical practice.

Furthermore, any statements about commercial products are solely the opinion(s) of the author(s) and do not represent an Academy endorsement or evaluation of these products. These statements may not be used in advertising or for any commercial purpose.

Published 2014 by the
American Academy of Orthopaedic Surgeons
300 North River Road
Rosemont, IL 60018
Copyright 2014
by the American Academy of Orthopaedic Surgeons

ISBN: 978-0-89203-845-9

Library of Congress Control Number: 2014938528

Printed in the USA

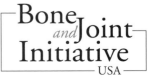
Bone *and* Joint Initiative USA

Acknowledgments

Richard C. Mather III, MD *(General Knowledge)*
Assistant Professor
Department of Orthopaedic Surgery
Duke University Medical Center
Durham, North Carolina

Ryan M. Nunley, MD *(Preservation, Arthroplasty, and Salvage Surgery of the Hip and Knee)*
Assistant Professor of Orthopedic Surgery
Department of Orthopedic Surgery
Washington University School of Medicine
St. Louis, Missouri

Kurt P. Spindler, MD *(Sports Injuries of the Knee and Sports Medicine)*
Professor of Orthopaedics
Director of Sports Medicine
Department of Orthopaedic Surgery and Rehabilitation
Vanderbilt University Medical Center
Nashville, Tennessee

Andrew Brian Thomson, MD *(Foot and Ankle)*
Director, Division of Foot and Ankle Surgery
Department of Orthopaedics and Rehabilitation
Vanderbilt University
Nashville, Tennessee

Kristy Weber, MD *(Orthopaedic Oncology/ Systemic Disease)*
Professor of Orthopaedic Surgery
Director of Sarcoma Program – Abramson Cancer Center
Department of Orthopaedic Surgery
University of Pennsylvania
Philadelphia, Pennsylvania

Rick W. Wright, MD *(Sports Injuries of the Knee and Sports Medicine)*
Professor
Residency Director
Co-Chief Sports Medicine
Department of Orthopedic Surgery
Washington University School of Medicine
St. Louis, Missouri

Contributors

Yousef Abu-Amer, PhD
Professor
Department of Orthopedic Surgery
Washington University School of Medicine
St. Louis, Missouri

Christopher S. Ahmad, MD
Associate Professor
Department of Orthopaedic Surgery
Columbia University Medical Center
New York, New York

Jay C. Albright, MD
Surgical Director of Sports Medicine
Department of Pediatric Orthopedics
Orthopedic Institute
Children's Hospital Colorado/University
  of Colorado
Aurora, Colorado

Annunziato Amendola, MD
Professor and Director of Sports Medicine
Orthopedic Department
University of Iowa
Iowa City, Iowa

John G. Anderson, MD
Professor
Michigan State University College of Human
  Medicine
Assistant Program Director
Grand Rapids Medical Education Partners
  Orthopaedic Residency
Associate Director
Grand Rapids Orthopaedic Foot and Ankle
  Fellowship
Chairman
Spectrum Health Department of Orthopaedics
Foot and Ankle Specialties
Orthopaedic Associates of Michigan, PC
Grand Rapids, Michigan

Jack Andrish, MD
Retired Consultant
Department of Orthopaedic Surgery
Cleveland Clinic
Cleveland, Ohio

Robert A. Arciero, MD
Professor of Orthopaedics
Department of Orthopaedics
University of Connecticut Health Center
Farmington, Connecticut

Elizabeth A. Arendt, MD
Professor and Vice Chair
Department of Orthopaedic Surgery
University of Minnesota
Minneapolis, Minnesota

April D. Armstrong, MD, BSc, FRCSC
Associate Professor
Department of Orthopaedics
Penn State Milton S. Hershey Medical Center
Hershey, Pennsylvania

George S. Athwal, MD, FRCSC
Associate Professor
Hand and Upper Limb Centre
Western University
London, Ontario, Canada

Reed Ayers, MS, PhD
Assistant Professor
Metallurgical and Materials Engineering
Colorado School of Mines
Golden, Colorado

Donald S. Bae, MD
Assistant Professor of Orthopaedic Surgery
Department of Orthopaedic Surgery
Boston Children's Hospital
Harvard Medical School
Boston, Massachusetts

Hyun Bae, MD
Director of Education
Co-Director of Fellowship Program
Division of Orthopedics
Department of Surgery
Cedars-Sinai Medical Center
Los Angeles, California

Keith Baldwin, MD, MSPT, MPH
Assistant Professor
Department of Orthopedic Surgery
Children's Hospital of Philadelphia
Philadelphia, Pennsylvania

Paul Beaulé, MD, FRCSC
Head, Adult Reconstruction
Division of Orthopaedic Surgery
The Ottawa Hospital
Ottawa, Ontario, Canada

Kathleen Beebe, MD
Associate Professor
Department of Orthopaedics
New Jersey Medical School
Rutgers
The State University of New Jersey
Newark, New Jersey

John-Erik Bell, MD, MS
Assistant Professor
Department of Orthopaedic Surgery
Dartmouth-Hitchcock Medical Center
Lebanon, New Hampshire

Gregory C. Berlet, MD
Orthopedic Surgeon
Department of Orthopedic Foot and Ankle
Orthopedic Foot and Ankle Center
Westerville, Ohio

Bruce Beynnon, PhD
Professor of Orthopedics and Director of
 Research
Department of Orthopedics and Rehabilitation
University of Vermont
Burlington, Vermont

Neil Bhamb, MD
Physician
Department of Orthopaedic Surgery
Cedars-Sinai Medical Center
Los Angeles, California

Mohit Bhandari, MD, PhD, FRCSC
Professor and Academic Head
Department of Surgery
Division of Orthopaedic Surgery
McMaster University
Hamilton, Ontario, Canada

Jesse E. Bible, MD, MHS
Orthopaedic Surgery
Vanderbilt Orthopaedic Institute
Vanderbilt University
Nashville, Tennessee

Ryan T. Bickell, MD, MSc, FRCSC
Assistant Professor
Division of Orthopaedic Surgery
Queen's University
Kingston, Ontario, Canada

Allen T. Bishop, MD
Professor of Orthopaedics
Department of Orthopaedic Surgery
Mayo Clinic
Rochester, Minnesota

Debdut Biswas, MD
Department of Orthopaedic Surgery
Rush University Medical Center
Chicago, Illinois

Donald R. Bohay, MD, FACS
Director
Grand Rapids Orthopaedic Foot and Ankle
 Fellowship
Associate Professor
Michigan State University College of Human
 Medicine
Foot and Ankle Specialties
Orthopaedic Associates of Michigan, PC
Grand Rapids, Michigan

Frank C. Bohnenkamp, MD
Department of Orthopaedic Surgery
University of Illinois at Chicago
Chicago, Illinois

Michael P. Bolognesi, MD
Associate Professor
Division Chief – Adult Reconstruction
Department of Orthopaedic Surgery
Duke University Medical Center
Durham, North Carolina

Martin I. Boyer, MD
Carol B. and Jerome T. Loeb Professor
Department of Orthopedic Surgery
Washington University School of Medicine
St. Louis, Missouri

Deanna M. Boyette, MD
Orthopaedic Surgeon
Department of Orthopaedic Surgery
East Carolina University
VIDANT Medical Center
Greenville, North Carolina

Robert H. Brophy, MD
Assistant Professor
Department of Orthopedic Surgery
Washington University School of Medicine
St. Louis, Missouri

Lance M. Brunton, MD
Assistant Professor
Department of Orthopaedic Surgery
University of Pittsburgh
Pittsburgh, Pennsylvania

William Bugbee, MD
Attending Physician
Division of Orthopaedic Surgery
Scripps Clinic
La Jolla, California

M. Tyrrell Burrus, MD
Department of Orthopaedic Surgery
University of Virginia Health System
Charlottesville, Virginia

Lisa K. Cannada, MD
Associate Professor
Department of Orthopaedic Surgery
Saint Louis University
St. Louis, Missouri

Kevin M. Casey, MD
Department of Orthopaedic Surgery
Kaiser Permanente
Riverside, California

Thomas D. Cha, MD, MBA
Spine Surgeon
Department of Orthopaedic Surgery
Massachusetts General Hospital
Boston, Massachusetts

Paul D. Choi, MD
Assistant Professor of Clinical Orthopaedic
  Surgery
Department of Orthopaedic Surgery
Children's Hospital Los Angeles
Los Angeles, California

Thomas J. Christensen, MD
Hand and Microvascular Surgery Fellow
Department of Orthopaedic Surgery
Mayo Clinic
Rochester, Minnesota

John C. Clohisy, MD
Daniel C. and Betty B. Viehmann Distinguished
  Professor of Orthopedic Surgery
Department of Orthopedic Surgery
Washington University School of Medicine
St. Louis, Missouri

Peter Cole, MD
Chief of Orthopaedic Surgery
Department of Orthopaedic Surgery
Regions Hospital
Professor
University of Minnesota
St. Paul, Minnesota

A. Rashard Dacus, MD
Assistant Professor
Department of Orthopaedic Surgery
University of Virginia
Charlottesville, Virginia

Charles Day, MD, MBA
Orthopedic Surgeon
Department of Orthopedics
Beth Israel Deaconess Medical Center
Boston, Massachusetts

D. Nicole Deal, MD
Assistant Professor
Department of Orthopaedic Surgery
University of Virginia
Charlottesville, Virginia

Niloofar Dehghan, BSc, MD
Department of Surgery
Division of Orthopaedics
University of Toronto
Toronto, Ontario, Canada

Alejandro Gonzalez Della Valle, MD
Associate Attending Orthopaedic Surgeon
Hospital for Special Surgery
New York, New York

Craig J. Della Valle, MD
Associate Professor
  Adult Reconstructive Fellowship Director
Department of Orthopaedics
Rush University Medical Center
Chicago, Illinois

Benedict F. DiGiovanni, MD
Professor
Department of Orthopaedics
University of Rochester Medical Center
Rochester, New York

Jon Divine, MD, MS
Associate Professor of Orthopedics and Sports
  Medicine
Department of Orthopedics
University of Cincinnati Medical Center
Cincinnati, Ohio

Seth D. Dodds, MD
Associate Professor of Hand and Upper
  Extremity Surgery
Associate Program Director, Orthopaedic
  Surgery
Department of Orthopaedics and Rehabilitation
Yale University School of Medicine
New Haven, Connecticut

Warren R. Dunn, MD, MPH
Assistant Professor, Orthopaedics and
  Rehabilitation
Assistant Professor, General Internal Medicine
  and Public Health
Vanderbilt Orthopaedic Institute
Vanderbilt University Medical Center
Nashville, Tennessee

Mark E. Easley, MD
Associate Professor
Department of Orthopaedic Surgery
Duke University Medical Center
Durham, North Carolina

Kenneth A. Egol, MD
Professor and Vice Chair
Department of Orthopaedic Surgery
Hospital for Joint Diseases
Langone Medical Center
New York, New York

Howard R. Epps, MD
Associate Professor of Orthopaedic Surgery
Baylor College of Medicine
Texas Children's Hospital
Houston, Texas

Greg Erens, MD
Assistant Professor
Department of Orthopaedic Surgery
Emory University
Atlanta, Georgia

Justin S. Field, MD
Orthopedic Spine Surgery
Desert Institute for Spine Care, PC
Phoenix, Arizona

Robert Warne Fitch, MD
Assistant Professor
Vanderbilt Sports Medicine
Vanderbilt University Medical Center
Nashville, Tennessee

Jared Foran, MD
Orthopaedic Surgeon
Panorama Orthopaedics and Spine Center
Golden, Colorado

Frank J. Frassica, MD
Professor of Orthopaedics and Oncology
Department of Orthopaedics
Johns Hopkins
Baltimore, Maryland

Nathan L. Frost, MD
Pediatric Orthopaedic Surgeon
Madigan Army Medical Center
Tacoma, Washington

Braden Gammon, MD, FRCSC
Assistant Professor
Division of Orthopaedic Surgery
University of Ottawa
Ottawa, Ontario, Canada

Steven R. Gammon, MD
Orthopaedic Traumatology Fellow
Department of Orthopaedic Surgery
University of Minnesota
St. Paul, Minnesota

Charles L. Getz, MD
Associate Professor
Department of Orthopaedic Surgery
Thomas Jefferson University
Philadelphia, Pennsylvania

Vijay K. Goel, MD
Professor
Department of Bioengineering
University of Toledo
Toledo, Ohio

Charles A. Goldfarb, MD
Associate Professor
Department of Orthopedic Surgery
Washington University School of Medicine
St. Louis, Missouri

Guillem Gonzalez-Lomas, MD
Assistant Professor
Department of Orthopaedics
University of Medicine and Dentistry of New
  Jersey
Newark, New Jersey

Gregory Gramstad, MD
Rebound Orthopedics
Portland, Oregon

Jonathan N. Grauer, MD
Associate Professor
Department of Orthopaedics and Rehabilitation
Yale University School of Medicine
New Haven, Connecticut

Tenner J. Guillaume, MD
Staff Spine Surgeon
Twin Cities Spine Center
Minneapolis, Minnesota

Amitava Gupta, MD, FRCS
Clinical Associate Professor
Department of Orthopedic Surgery
Louisville Arm & Hand
University of Louisville
Louisville, Kentucky

Ranjan Gupta, MD
Professor and Chair
Department of Orthopaedic Surgery
University of California, Irvine
Irvine, California

Rajnish K. Gupta, MD
Assistant Professor
Department of Anesthesiology
Vanderbilt University
Nashville, Tennessee

George J. Haidukewych, MD
Chairman
Department of Orthopaedics
Level One Orthopaedics
Orlando Regional Medical Center
Orlando, Florida

David A. Halsey, MD
Associate Professor
Department of Orthopaedics and Rehabilitation
University of Vermont College of Medicine
Burlington, Vermont

Mark Halstead, MD
Assistant Professor
Department of Orthopedics and Pediatrics
Washington University
St. Louis, Missouri

Nady Hamid, MD
Orthopaedic Surgeon
Shoulder and Elbow Center
OrthoCarolina
Charlotte, North Carolina

Erik N. Hansen, MD
Assistant Professor
Department of Orthopaedic Surgery
University of California, San Francisco
San Francisco, California

Peyton L. Hays, MD
Orthopaedic Hand Fellow
Department of Orthopaedic Surgery
Beth Israel Deaconess Medical Center
Harvard Medical School
Boston, Massachusetts

Carolyn M. Hettrich, MD, MPH
Assistant Professor
Department of Sports Medicine
University of Iowa
Department of Orthopaedics and Rehabilitation
Iowa City, Iowa

Timothy E. Hewett, PhD
Director of Research
Department of Sports Health and Performance
  Instruction
The Ohio State University
Columbus, Ohio

Alan S. Hilibrand, MD
Joseph and Marie Field Professor of Spinal
  Surgery
The Rothman Institute
Jefferson Medical College
Philadelphia, Pennsylvania

Anny Hsu, MD
Department of Orthopaedic Surgery
Columbia Orthopaedics
Columbia University Medical Center
New York, New York

Jason E. Hsu, MD
Clinical Fellow
Department of Orthopaedic Surgery
Washington University
St. Louis, Missouri

Clifford B. Jones, MD, FACS
Clinical Professor
Michigan State University College of Human
*   Medicine*
Orthopaedic Associates of Michigan
Spectrum Health, Butterworth Hospital
Grand Rapids, Michigan

Morgan H. Jones, MD, MPH
Staff Physician
Department of Orthopaedic Surgery
Cleveland Clinic
Cleveland, Ohio

Christopher C. Kaeding, MD
Professor of Orthopaedics
Ohio State University Sports Medicine
Ohio State University
Columbus, Ohio

Linda E.A. Kanim, MA
Translation and Clinical Research
Spine Center
Cedars-Sinai
Los Angeles, California

Robert M. Kay, MD
Vice Chief
Children's Orthopaedic Center
Children's Hospital Los Angeles
Los Angeles, California

Mary Ann Keenan, MD
Professor
Department of Orthopaedic Surgery
University of Pennsylvania
Philadelphia, Pennsylvania

Jay D. Keener, MD
Assistant Professor
Department of Orthopedic Surgery
Washington University
St. Louis, Missouri

James A. Keeney, MD
Assistant Professor
Department of Orthopedic Surgery
Washington University School of Medicine
St. Louis, Missouri

Michael P. Kelly, MD
Assistant Professor
Department of Orthopedic Surgery
Washington University School of Medicine
St. Louis, Missouri

Safdar N. Khan, MD
Assistant Professor
Department of Orthopaedics
The Ohio State University
Columbus, Ohio

Vickas Khanna, MD, FRCSC
Orthopaedic Fellow
Department of Adult Reconstruction
University of Ottawa
Ottawa, Ontario, Canada

Kenneth J. Koval, MD
Attending
Department of Orthopaedics
Orlando Health
Orlando, Florida

Marc S. Kowalsky, MD
Clinical Assistant Professor
Lenox Hill Hospital
Hofstra North Shore – LIJ School of Medicine
New York, New York

Erik N. Kubiak, MD
Assistant Professor
Department of Orthopaedics
University of Utah
Salt Lake City, Utah

John E. Kuhn, MD
Director
Division of Sports Medicine
Vanderbilt University Medical Center
Nashville, Tennessee

Nikhil Kulkarni, MS
Research and Development Engineer
Department of Product Development
Medtronic Spine & Biologics
Memphis, Tennessee

Sharat K. Kusuma, MD, MBA
Associate Director
Department of Adult Reconstruction
Grand Medical Center
Columbus, Ohio

Young W. Kwon, MD, PhD
Associate Professor
Department of Orthopaedic Surgery
NYU – Hospital for Joint Diseases
New York, New York

Adam J. La Bore, MD
Associate Professor
Department of Orthopedic Surgery
Washington University in St. Louis
St. Louis, Missouri

Mario Lamontagne, PhD
Professor
Department of Human Kinetics and Mechanical
  Engineering
University of Ottawa
Ottawa, Ontario, Canada

Joshua Langford, MD
Director
Limb Deformity Service
Orlando Health Orthopedic Residency Program
Orlando Health
Orlando, Florida

Christian Latterman, MD
Associate Professor
Director
Center for Cartilage Repair and Restoration
Department of Orthopaedic Surgery
University of Kentucky
Lexington, Kentucky

Francis Y. Lee, MD, PhD
Professor with Tenure
Director, Center for Orthopaedic Research
Chief of Tumor Service
Vice Chair of Research
Department of Orthopaedic Surgery
Columbia University
New York, New York

Simon Lee, MD
Assistant Professor
Department of Orthopaedic Surgery
Rush University Medical Center – Midwest
  Orthopaedics
Chicago, Illinois

Yu-Po Lee, MD
Associate Clinical Professor
Department of Orthopedic Surgery
UCSD Medical Center
San Diego, California

James P. Leonard, MD
Sports Medicine and Shoulder Surgery Fellow
Department of Orthopaedic Surgery
Vanderbilt University
Nashville, Tennessee

Fraser J. Leversedge, MD
Associate Professor
Department of Orthopaedic Surgery
Duke University
Durham, North Carolina

David G. Liddle, MD
Assistant Professor
Vanderbilt Sports Medicine
Vanderbilt University Medical Center
Nashville, Tennessee

Jay R. Lieberman, MD
Professor and Chairman
Department of Orthopaedic Surgery
Keck School of Medicine of the University of
  Southern California
Los Angeles, California

Johnny Lin, MD
Assistant Professor
Department of Orthopedic Surgery
Rush University Medical Center
Chicago, Illinois

Michael Y. Lin, MD, PhD
Clinical Instructor
Department of Orthopedic Surgery
University of California, Irvine
Irvine, California

Sheldon S. Lin, MD
Associate Professor
Department of Orthopedics
New Jersey Medical School
Rutgers, the State University of New Jersey
Newark, New Jersey

Dieter M. Lindskog, MD
Associate Professor
Department of Orthopaedics and Rehabilitation
Yale University School of Medicine
New Haven, Connecticut

Frank A. Liporace, MD
Associate Professor
Director, Trauma and Reconstructive Fellowship
Department of Orthopaedics
University of Medicine and Dentistry of New Jersey/New Jersey Medical School
Newark, New Jersey

David W. Lowenberg, MD
Clinical Professor
Chief, Orthopaedic Trauma Service
Department of Orthopaedic Surgery
Stanford University School of Medicine
Palo Alto, California

Scott Luhmann, MD
Associate Professor
Department of Orthopedic Surgery
Washington University
St. Louis, Missouri

C. Benjamin Ma, MD
Associate Professor
Chief, Sports Medicine and Shoulder Service
Department of Orthopaedic Surgery
University of California, San Francisco
San Francisco, California

Robert A. Magnussen, MD
Assistant Professor
Department of Orthopaedic Surgery
The Ohio State University Medical Center
Columbus, Ohio

Andrew P. Mahoney, MD
Orthopedic Surgeon
Tucson Orthopedic Institute
Tucson, Arizona

David R. Maish, MD
Assistant Professor
Department of Orthopaedics and Rehabilitation
Penn State Hersey Bone & Joint Institute
Hershey, Pennsylvania

Randall J. Malchow, MD
Program Director, Regional Anesthesiology and Acute Pain Fellowship
Department of Anesthesiology
Vanderbilt University Medical Center
Nashville, Tennessee

Peter J. Mandell, MD
Assistant Clinical Professor
Department of Orthopaedic Surgery
University of California, San Francisco
San Francisco, California

Robert G. Marx, MD, MSc, FRCSC
Professor of Orthopedic Surgery and Public Health
Department of Orthopaedic Surgery
Hospital for Special Surgery
Weill Cornell Medical College
New York, New York

Matthew J. Matava, MD
Professor
Department of Orthopedics
Washington University
St. Louis, Missouri

Augustus D. Mazzocca, MS, MD
Associate Professor
Department of Orthopaedic Surgery
University of Connecticut Health Center
Farmington, Connecticut

David R. McAllister, MD
Professor and Chief
Sports Medicine Service
Department of Orthopaedic Surgery
David Geffen School of Medicine at UCLA
Los Angeles, California

Christopher McAndrew, MD
Assistant Professor
Department of Orthopedic Surgery
Washington University School of Medicine
St. Louis, Missouri

Eric C. McCarty, MD
Chief of Sports Medicine & Shoulder Surgery
Associate Professor
Department of Orthopedic Surgery
University of Colorado School of Medicine
Boulder, Colorado

Michael D. McKee, MD, FRCSC
Professor
Division of Orthopaedics
Department of Surgery
*St. Michaels Hospital and the University of
  Toronto*
Toronto, Ontario, Canada

Ross E. McKinney Jr, MD
Professor
Department of Pediatrics
Duke University School of Medicine
Durham, North Carolina

Michael J. Medvecky, MD
Associate Professor
Department of Orthopaedics and Rehabilitation
Yale University School of Medicine
New Haven, Connecticut

Steve Melton, MD
Assistant Professor
Department of Anesthesiology
Duke University Medical Center
Durham, North Carolina

Gary A. Miller, MD
Associate Professor, Clinical
Department of Orthopedic Surgery
Washington University School of Medicine
St. Louis, Missouri

William Min, MD, MS, MBA
Assistant Professor of Orthopaedic Surgery
Department of Surgery
University of Alabama at Birmingham
Birmingham, Alabama

Richard E. Moon, MD
Professor of Anesthesiology
Professor of Medicine
Department of Anesthesiology
Duke University Medical Center
Durham, North Carolina

Steven L. Moran, MD
Division Chair
Division of Plastic Surgery
Mayo Clinic
Rochester, Minnesota

Steven J. Morgan, MD
Orthopaedic Traumatologist
Mountain Orthopaedic Trauma Surgeons
Swedish Medical Center
Englewood, Colorado

Thomas E. Mroz, MD
Director, Spine Fellowship
Center for Spine Health
Department of Orthopaedic Surgery
Cleveland Clinic
Cleveland, Ohio

M. Siobhan Murphy Zane, MD
Assistant Professor
Department of Orthopaedics
Children's Hospital Colorado
Aurora, Colorado

Anand M. Murthi, MD
Department of Orthopaedic Surgery
Union Memorial Hospital
Baltimore, Maryland

Jeffrey J. Nepple, MD
Department of Orthopedic Surgery
Washington University of St. Louis
St. Louis, Missouri

Saqib A. Nizami, BS
Research Associate
Center for Orthopaedic Surgery
Columbia University
New York, New York

Wendy M. Novicoff, PhD
Assistant Professor
Department of Public Health Sciences
University of Virginia
Charlottesville, Virginia

Ryan M. Nunley, MD
Assistant Professor of Orthopedic Surgery
Department of Orthopedic Surgery
Washington University School of Medicine
St. Louis, Missouri

Reza Omid, MD
Assistant Professor
Department of Orthopaedic Surgery
University of Southern California
Los Angeles, California

Robert F. Ostrum, MD
Professor
Department of Orthopaedic Surgery
University of North Carolina
Chapel Hill, North Carolina

Thomas Padanilam, MD
Toledo Orthopaedic Surgeons
Toledo, Ohio

Richard D. Parker, MD
Professor and Chairman
Department of Orthopaedics
Cleveland Clinic Foundation
Cleveland, Ohio

Michael L. Parks, MD
Assistant Professor
Hospital for Special Surgery
Cornell Weill College of Medicine
New York, New York

Javad Parvizi, MD, FRCS
Orthopedic Surgeon
Department of Orthopedics/Reconstructive
* Surgery*
Rothman Institute
Philadelphia, Pennsylvania

Terrence Philbin, DO
Attending Physician
Orthopedic Foot & Ankle Center
Westerville, Ohio

Gregory J. Pinkowsky
Department of Orthopaedics
Penn State Hershey Medical Center
Hershey, Pennsylvania

Kornelis Poelstra, MD, PhD
President
The Spine Institute
Destin – Fort Walton Beach, Florida

Gregory G. Polkowski, MD
Assistant Professor
Department of Orthopaedic Surgery
University of Connecticut Health Center
Farmington, Connecticut

Ben B. Pradhan, MD, MSE
Orthopaedic Spine Surgeon
Risser Orthopaedic Group
Pasadena, California

Steven M. Raikin, MD
Professor, Orthopaedic Surgery
Director, Foot and Ankle Service
Rothman Institute at Thomas Jefferson
* University Hospital*
Philadelphia, Pennsylvania

Gannon B. Randolph, MD
Orthopedic Surgeon
Mercy Clinic Orthopedics
Mercy Hospital Northwest Arkansas
Rogers, Arkansas

Joshua Ratner, MD
Hand and Upper Extremity Center of Georgia
Atlanta, Georgia

David R. Richardson, MD
Associate Professor
Department of Orthopaedic Surgery
University of Tennessee – Campbell Clinic
Memphis, Tennessee

E. Greer Richardson, MD
Professor of Orthopaedic Surgery
Department of Orthopaedics
University of Tennessee – Campbell Clinic
Memphis, Tennessee

John T. Riehl, MD
Orthopaedic Trauma Fellow
Level One Orthopaedics
Orlando Regional Medical Center
Orlando, Florida

Michael D. Ries, MD
Fellowship Director
Tahoe Fracture & Orthopaedic Clinic
Carson City, Nevada
Professor Emeritus
University of California, San Francisco
San Francisco, California

K. Daniel Riew, MD
Orthopaedic Surgeon
Department of Orthopedics
Washington University
St. Louis, Missouri

David Ring, MD, PhD
Chief, Orthopaedic Hand & Upper Extremity
  Service
Department of Orthopaedic Surgery
Massachusetts General Hospital
Boston, Massachusetts

Marco Rizzo, MD
Associate Professor
Department of Orthopedic Surgery
Mayo Clinic
Rochester, Minnesota

Scott B. Rosenfeld, MD
Assistant Professor
Department of Orthopaedic Surgery
Texas Childrens Hospital
Baylor College of Medicine
Houston, Texas

Tamara D. Rozental, MD
Associate Professor
Harvard Medical School
Department of Orthopaedic Surgery
Beth Israel Deaconess Medical Center
Boston, Massachusetts

Khaled J. Saleh, MD, MSc, FRCSC, MHCM
Professor and Chairman
Division of Orthopaedic Surgery
Southern Illinois University School of Medicine
Springfield, Illinois

Vincent James Sammarco, MD
Reconstructive Orthopaedics
Cincinnati, Ohio

David W. Sanders, MD, FRCSC
Associate Professor
Department of Orthopedic Surgery
Western University
London, Ontario, Canada

Anthony A. Scaduto, MD
Lowman Professor & Chief of Pediatric
  Orthopaedic Surgery
Department of Orthopaedic Surgery
UCLA and Los Angeles Orthopaedic Hospital
Los Angeles, California

Perry L. Schoenecker, MD
Professor of Orthopaedic Surgery
Department of Orthopaedic Surgery
Shriner's Hospital for Children
St. Louis, Missouri

Thomas Scioscia, MD
Spine Surgeon
Department of Orthopaedics
OrthoVirginia
Richmond, Virginia

Jon K. Sekiya, MD
Professor
Department of Orthopaedic Surgery
University of Michigan
Ann Arbor, Michigan

Sung Wook Seo, MD, PhD
Associate Professor
Department of Orthopaedic Surgery
Samsung Medical Center
Sungkyunkwan University College of Medicine
Seoul, Korea

Ritesh R. Shah, MD
Orthopaedic Surgeon
Clinical Assistant Professor
Illinois Bone and Joint Institute
University of Illinois Chicago
Morton Grove, Illinois

Arya Nick Shamie, MD, QME
Chief, Orthopaedic Spine Surgery
Department of Orthopaedic Surgery and
  Neurosurgery
UCLA David Geffen School of Medicine
Los Angeles, California

Alexander Y. Shin, MD
Professor of Orthopaedics
Department of Orthopaedic Surgery
Division of Hand Surgery
Mayo Clinic
Rochester, Minnesota

Allen K. Sills, MD, FACS
Associate Professor
Department of Neurosurgery
Vanderbilt University
Nashville, Tennessee

Kern Singh, MD
Associate Professor
Department of Orthopaedic Surgery
Rush University Medical Center
Chicago, Illinois

David L. Skaggs, MD, MMM
Chief of Orthopaedic Surgery
Director, Scoliosis and Spine Deformity
 Program
Professor of Orthopaedic Surgery
Division of Orthopaedic Surgery
Children's Hospital Los Angeles
Los Angeles, California

Matthew V. Smith, MD
Assistant Professor
Department of Sports Medicine
Department of Orthopedics
Washington University in St. Louis
St. Louis, Missouri

Michael D. Smith, MD
Department of Orthopaedic Surgery
Emory University
Atlanta, Georgia

Nelson Fong SooHoo, MD
Associate Professor
Department of Orthopaedic Surgery
UCLA School of Medicine
Los Angeles, California

Jeffrey T. Spang, MD
Assistant Professor
Department of Orthopaedics
University of North Carolina
Chapel Hill, North Carolina

Samantha Spencer, MD
Orthopaedic Surgeon
Department of Orthopaedics
Boston Childrens Hospital
Boston, Massachusetts

Robert J. Spinner, MD
Burton M. Onofrio Professor of Neurosurgery
Professor of Anatomy and Orthopaedics
Department of Neurologic Surgery
Mayo Clinic
Rochester, Minnesota

Lynne S. Steinbach, MD
Professor of Clinical Radiology and
 Orthopaedic Surgery
University of California, San Francisco
San Francisco, California

Michael P. Steinmetz, MD
Chairman
Department of Neurological Surgery
Case Western Reserve University/MetroHealth
 Medical Center
Cleveland, Ohio

Karen M. Sutton, MD
Assistant Professor
Department of Orthopaedic Surgery
Yale University School of Medicine
New Haven, Connecticut

John S. Taras, MD
Associate Professor
Department of Orthopaedic Surgery
Thomas Jefferson University
Chief
Division of Hand Surgery
Drexel University
Philadelphia, Pennsylvania

Robert Z. Tashjian, MD
Associate Professor
Department of Orthopaedics
University of Utah School of Medicine
Salt Lake City, Utah

Ross Taylor, MD
Orthopedic Surgeon, Foot and Ankle
Coastal Orthopedics
Conway Medical Center
Conway, South Carolina

Nirmal C. Tejwani, MD
Professor
Department of Orthopaedics
NYU Hospital for Joint Diseases
New York, New York

Stavros Thomopoulos, PhD
Associate Professor
Department of Orthopedic Surgery
Washington University
St. Louis, Missouri

Andrew Brian Thomson, MD
Director
Division of Foot and Ankle Surgery
Department of Orthopaedics and Rehabilitation
Vanderbilt University
Nashville, Tennessee

Armando F. Vidal, MD
Assistant Professor
Sports Medicine & Shoulder Service
Department of Orthopaedic Surgery
University of Colorado School of Medicine
Denver, Colorado

Jeffrey C. Wang, MD
Chief, Orthopaedic Spine Service
Professor of Orthopaedics and Neurosurgery
USC Spine Center
University of Southern California Keck School
  of Medicine
Los Angeles, California

Jeffry T. Watson, MD
Assistant Professor
Department of Orthopaedic Surgery
Vanderbilt University
Nashville, Tennessee

Kristy Weber, MD
Professor of Orthopaedic Surgery
Director of Sarcoma Program – Abramson
  Cancer Center
Department of Orthopaedic Surgery
University of Pennsylvania
Philadelphia, Pennsylvania

Samuel S. Wellman, MD
Assistant Professor
Department of Orthopaedics
Duke University Medical Center
Durham, North Carolina

Peter G. Whang, MD, FACS
Associate Professor
Department of Orthopaedics and Rehabilitation
Yale University School of Medicine
New Haven, Connecticut

Glenn N. Williams, PT, PhD, ATC
Associate Professor
Department of Physical Therapy and
  Rehabilitation Science
University of Iowa
Iowa City, Iowa

Brian R. Wolf, MD, MS
Associate Professor
Department of Orthopaedics and Rehabiliation
University of Iowa
Iowa City, Iowa

Philip Wolinsky, MD
Professor of Orthopaedic Surgery
Department of Orthopaedic Surgery
University of California, Davis Medical Center
Sacramento, California

Raymond D. Wright Jr, MD
Assistant Professor, Orthopaedic Traumatology
Department of Orthopaedic Surgery and Sports
  Medicine
University of Kentucky Chandler Medical
  Center
Lexington, Kentucky

Rick W. Wright, MD
Professor
Residency Director
Co-Chief Sports Medicine
Department of Orthopedic Surgery
Washington University School of Medicine
St. Louis, Missouri

Dane K. Wukich, MD
Professor of Orthopaedic Surgery
Department of Orthopaedic Surgery
University of Pittsburgh Medical Center
Pittsburgh, Pennsylvania

S. Tim Yoon, MD, PhD
Associate Professor
Department of Orthopaedic Surgery
Emory University
Atlanta, Georgia

Jim Youssef, MD
Spine Surgeon
Orthopedic Department
Spine Colorado
Durango, Colorado

Elizabeth Yu, MD
Assistant Professor
Department of Orthopaedics
The Ohio State University
Columbus, Ohio

Warren Yu, MD
Associate Professor
Department of Orthopaedic Surgery
George Washington University
Washington, DC

Preface

A project such as the AAOS Comprehensive Orthopaedic Review 2 is Herculean in scope and could not possibly have been completed without the dedication and excellent work of the section editors: Lisa Berglund, MD; Kevin J. Bozic, MD, MBA; Jacob M. Buchowski, MD, MS; A. Bobby Chhabra, MD; John Clohisy, MD; D. Nicole Deal, MD; Kenneth A. Egol, MD; Steven L. Frick, MD; Leesa Galatz, MD; Bethany Gallagher, MD; Michael J. Gardner, MD; Jonathan N. Grauer, MD; Jay D. Keener, MD; Michael P. Kelly, MD; R. Chad Mather III, MD; Ryan M. Nunley, MD; Kurt P. Spindler, MD; Andrew Brian Thomson, MD; Kristy Weber, MD; and Rick W. Wright, MD. These editors, along with the chapter authors, deserve full and complete credit for all materials contained in this important educational publication.

It is our collective hope that students, residents, and fellows who use this compendium for education and in preparing for Board examinations will find it concise, broad-based, and representative of the knowledge that orthopaedic surgeons need in their practices. Best of luck to all of you in your studies and careers.

I dedicate this book to the greatest of all orthopaedic educators, Richard H. Gelberman, MD, whose commitment to excellence in resident and fellow education is a lasting legacy.

Martin I. Boyer, MD, MSc, FRCS(C)
Carol B. and Jerome T. Loeb Professor
Department of Orthopedic Surgery
Washington University School of Medicine
St. Louis, Missouri

Table of Contents

VOLUME 1

Section 1

Basic Science

Section Editors:
Leesa Galatz, MD
Jonathan N. Grauer, MD

Chapter 1

Cellular and Molecular Biology, Immunology, and Genetics Terminology

Francis Y. Lee, MD, PhD   Sung Wook Seo, MD, PhD   Saqib A. Nizami, BS   Anny Hsu, MD

I. Cellular Components—Terminology and Definitions

A. Nucleus—An organelle found in eukaryotic cells and enclosed by a double membrane. It contains the chromosomes of the cell, which contain the genes of the cell, as well as various nuclear proteins that communicate with the surrounding cytosol via transportation through numerous pores in the nucleus. The nucleus is clinically important in karyotyping, or characterization of the number and appearance of a cell's chromosomes; flow cytometry, in which large numbers of various types of cells are classified and defined according to their physical and other characteristics; and the mitotic characteristics of the cells of various types of cancers, including the rate at which these cells divide.

B. Nucleolus—A prominent organelle in the nucleus of a cell that contains the structures known as ribosomes, which translate the genetic codes that messenger RNA (mRNA) carries from the chromosomes of a cell, into peptides that are transformed into proteins. Pathologies with clinical relevance to the nucleolus include Rothmund-Thompson syndrome, Bloom syndrome, and Treacher Collins syndrome. Rothmund-Thompson, Bloom, and Treacher Collins syndromes are caused by genetic mutations that produce protein abnormalities via the nucleolus mechanism. Mutations in the *RECQL4* gene are heavily involved in Rothmund-Thompson syndrome. This gene provides instructions on producing a member of a protein family called RecQ helicases, which play a large role in replicating and repairing DNA.

Dr. Hsu or an immediate family member serves as a paid consultant to or is an employee of Hoffmann-La Roche. None of the following authors nor any immediate family member has received anything of value from or has stock or stock options held in a commercial company or institution related directly or indirectly to the subject of this chapter: Dr. Lee, Dr. Seo, and Mr. Nizami.

Rothmund-Thompson syndrome is characterized by sparse hair, eyebrows, and eyelashes, as well as slow growth and small stature. There are many related skeletal abnormalities such as malformed bones, fused bones, and low bone mineral density. There is also a greater risk for developing osteosarcoma. Bloom syndrome is caused by mutations in the *BLM* gene, which are also responsible for producing RecQ helicases. Individuals with Bloom syndrome usually have short stature, sun-sensitive skin changes, a high-pitched voice, a small lower jaw, a large nose, and prominent ears. They are also more susceptible to cancers. Mutations in *TCOF1*, *POLR1C*, and *POLR1D* are responsible for Treacher Collins syndrome. These mutations reduce the production of ribosomal RNA, which is heavily involved in protein production. This syndrome affects the development of the bones of the face resulting in a small jaw, chin, and cheek bones.

C. Cytosol/cytoplasm—The cytosol is the fluid contained by the membrane of a cell and is the component in which most of the cell's metabolism occurs. It surrounds the cell nucleus, the nucleolus, and various other intracellular organelles. The cytoplasm is the component in which proteins and other substances are synthesized, and contains a wide range of soluble substances including salts and many proteins and peptides, as well as serving as a medium of suspension for fats and other water-insoluble substances and larger molecules of carbohydrates. The cytoplasm is the site of many signal transduction pathways and of the glycolysis by which complex carbohydrates are digested chemically into simpler carbohydrates and other substances.

D. Golgi body—A structure surrounded by a single membrane, in which enzymes and hormones are produced, packaged, and released into membrane-bound vesicles that then pass into the cytoplasm of the cell.

E. Lysosome—An organelle containing the enzymes known as acid hydrolases. These enzymes are responsible for the intracellular digestion of aged organelles, cellular waste, and phagocytosed pathogens, including viruses and bacteria. The lysosomes are clinically relevant as the cellular foci of lysosomal storage disorders (LSDs). LSDs are a group of about 50 metabolic disorders that arise from defective lysosomal function. Most commonly, these are the result of a deficiency of an enzyme needed for the metabolism of lipids, glycoproteins, and mucopolysaccharides. This results in excess products being stored in the cells. Tay-Sachs disease and Gaucher disease are examples of this. Niemann-Pick disease is also considered an LSD because it is characterized by sphingomyelin accumulation in cells. Dysfunctional metabolism of cell membrane components such as sphingolipids can result in enlargement of the liver and spleen, pain, unsteady gait, dysphagia, dystonia, and seizures. It can also result in an enlargement of bone marrow cavity and thinning cortical bone.

F. Cell membrane—A double layer of phospholipids, or lipid bilayer, that encloses the cytosol, nucleus, and other internal structures of a cell and acts as a protective barrier against the external environment of the cell. The cell membrane is clinically relevant in Duchenne-type muscular dystrophy (a mutation in dystrophin causes increased cell membrane fragility and permeability), long QT syndrome (disruption of ion channels in cell membrane), hemolytic uremic anemia (red cell membrane abnormality), and a range of other pathologies.

G. Peroxisome—A membrane-bound packet of oxidative enzymes involved in metabolic processes such as the oxidation of fatty acids and the production of cholesterol and bile acids. The peroxisomes of cells are clinically relevant in brain storage diseases, adrenoleukodystrophy, infantile Refsum disease, and cerebrohepatorenal syndrome, among other diseases.

H. Mitochondria—Organelles with a double membrane that provide energy for the movement, division, and other functions of a eukaryotic cell. Mitochondria provide most of this energy in the form of adenosine triphosphate (ATP), which they generate through the action of enzymes. The mitochondria of cells are also involved in synthesizing the amino acids that are the building blocks of proteins, and are involved in signaling within a cell, in the differentiation of cells into specific cell types, and in cell death. Mitochondrial abnormalities are clinically relevant in being involved in myopathies, diabetes, deafness, ataxia epilepsy, optic neuropathy, and various other disorders.

I. Smooth endoplasmic reticulum (SER)/rough endoplasmic reticulum (RER)—The SER is a structure that extends throughout the cytoplasm of plant and animals cells and appears as a smooth membrane when visualized with electron microscopy. It is the site of synthesis of lipids and steroid hormones. The SER of liver cells also degrades lipid-soluble toxins, and the SER of muscle cells stores calcium and controls calcium release, thereby affecting muscle contraction and relaxation. RER has numerous ribosomes on its surface that are sites of protein synthesis. Among various conditions in which the endoplasmic reticulum is clinically relevant is liver endoplasmic reticulum storage disease, which affects various proteins that are critical to normal intracellular and intercellular function.

J. Ribosome—An intracellular structure that makes peptides/proteins by reading the nucleotide sequence of mRNA molecules and assembling the amino acids that correspond to specific triple-nucleotide sequences in the mRNA into proteins and peptides. Disorders of the ribosomes of eukaryotic cells are clinically relevant in causing diseases, including macrocytic anemia and cartilage-hair hypoplasia. Improper amino acid assembly results in faulty peptide configurations for proteins, which will not fold correctly to be active. This results in ribosomal diseases.

K. Cytoskeleton—An intracellular network of microtubules, actin filaments (microfilaments), and intermediate fibers that plays a critical role in maintaining the shapes and motility of cells and the intracellular movements of cell organelles and in cell motility. The cytoskeleton is also responsible for the contraction and relaxation of muscle fibers. Abnormalities of the cytoskeleton are clinically relevant in cardiomyopathies, congenital myopathies, defects in phagocytosis and the motility of osteoclasts, and some types of deafness, as well as other disorders. Because the cytoskeleton provides structure, phagocytic actions, and motility; any defect in the arrangement of the actin filaments, either by disruption as a result of stress, or faulty fiber production, can result in loss of cell function and normal activity.

II. Extracellular Matrix

A. Extracellular matrix (ECM)—The noncellular portion of a tissue that provides structural support for cells and affects their development and biochemical and physiologic function (**Table 1**).

B. Collagen—The chief structural protein in the body's connective tissues. It consists of a triple-helix composed of three interwoven strands or chains of proteins, known as $\alpha1$, $\alpha2$, and $\alpha3$ chains, and constitutes most of the fibrils in the ECM (**Table 1**). Collagen typically has both great strength and flexibility.

C. Glycosaminoglycans (GAGs)—Structural polysaccharides in the ECM. A GAG is composed of repeating molecules of a disaccharide. The disaccharides that constitute GAGs include hyaluronic acid,

Table 1

Types of Collagen

Type	Tissues
I	Skin, tendon, bone, annulus of intervertebral disk
II	Articular cartilage, vitreous humor, nucleus pulposus of intervertebral disk
III	Skin, muscle, blood vessels
IX	Articular cartilage
X	Articular cartilage, mineralization of cartilage in growth plate
XI	Articular cartilage

dermatan sulfate, chondroitin sulfate, heparin, heparan sulfate, and keratan sulfate. Most GAGs become covalently linked to a protein core, resulting in the substances known as proteoglycans. Hyaluronic acid, a nonsulfated GAG, does not attach to proteins, but becomes linked to various proteoglycans to form giant molecules that, through their presence in joint fluid and other locations within the body, provide lubrication or shock absorption for various tissues.

D. Fibronectin—A high-molecular-weight glycoprotein that is part of the ECM and binds to other components of the ECM such as fibrin and collagen, and which therefore plays a role in both the structure and function of cells and tissues. Fibronectin also contains tripeptide (arg-gly-asp) sequences known as RGD domains, which are sites at which integrin binds to fibronectin. Fibronectin has been known to regulate cell migration and differentiation.

E. Laminin—An important component of the basal lamina. Laminin and type IV collagen form a network for the basement membrane, an ECM that consists of a thin layer of connective tissue that acts as a scaffold underlying the epithelial tissue of many of the body's organs that supports and facilitates the growth of epithelial-cell populations.

III. Intracellular Signaling

A. Cell response—Cells express specific genes in response to extracellular influences such as biochemical signaling through ligand molecules that bind to receptors on the surfaces of cells, mechanical forces, extracellular matrices, and contact with other cells, hormones, and cytokines (**Figures 1** and **2**).

B. Signal transduction—The process by which an extracellular signal is transformed into an intracellular message that elicits a specific response from a cell.

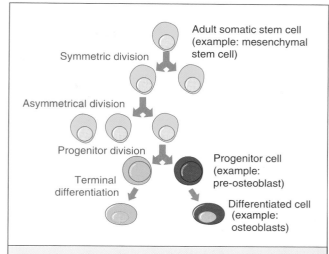

Figure 1   Adult somatic stem cells. (Reproduced from Lee FY, Zuscik MJ, Nizami S, et al: Molecular and cell biology in orthopaedics, in O'Keefe RJ, Jacobs JJ, Chu CR, Einhorn TA, eds: *Orthopaedic Basic Science*, ed 4. Rosemont, IL, American Academy Orthopaedic Surgeons, 2013, pp 3-42.)

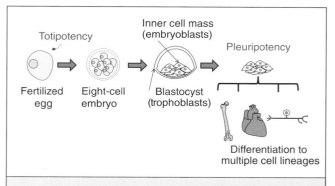

Figure 2   Embryonic stem cells. (Reproduced from Lee FY, Zuscik MJ, Nizami S, et al: Molecular and cell biology in orthopaedics, in O'Keefe RJ, Jacobs JJ, Chu CR, Einhorn TA, eds: *Orthopaedic Basic Science*, ed 4. Rosemont, IL, American Academy Orthopaedic Surgeons, 2013, pp 3-42.)

C. Initiation of signal transduction—The binding of a specific ligand to a specific receptor on the cell surface initiates signal transduction in various ways, depending on the type of receptor.

1. Guanosine nucleotide-binding (G)-protein-coupled receptors—The binding of a ligand to this type of receptor activates a G protein, which functions as a molecular switch that hydrolyzes guanosine triphosphate to guanosine diphosphate releasing a phosphate group and energy. The G protein modulates a specific second messenger or an ion channel.

2. Ion channel receptors—Binding of a ligand to this type of receptor alters the conformation of a specific ion channel. The resultant movement of ions

1: Basic Science

through this channel and across the cell membrane activates a specific intracellular molecule.

3. Tyrosine kinase–linked receptors—Binding of a ligand to this type of receptor activates cytosolic protein–tyrosine kinase, an enzyme that transfers a phosphate group from ATP to tyrosine residues on proteins within the cell.

4. Receptors with intrinsic enzyme activity—Some receptors have intrinsic catalytic activity. Some have guanine cyclase activity, which converts guanosine triphosphate to cyclic guanosine monophosphate (cGMP). Other receptors, with intrinsic tyrosine kinase activity, act to phosphorylate various protein substrates.

D. Second messengers—Intracellular signaling molecules whose concentration is controlled by the binding of a specific ligand or "first messenger" to a particular type of receptor on the membrane of a cell. An increased concentration of a second messenger, brought about the effects of enzymes and other substances generated by the first messenger, activates other signaling molecules. These include cyclic adenosine monophosphate, cyclic guanosine monophosphate, diacylglycerol, inositol triphosphate, phosphoinositides, and Ca^{2+}

IV. DNA-Related Terminology and Definitions

A. DNA—A double-stranded polymer in which each strand consists of deoxyribonucleotides that are bound covalently to one another, and whose nucleic acid components are paired, through hydrogen bonds, with their corresponding nucleic acids in the deoxyribonucleotides in the opposite strand of the polymer. Deoxyribonucleotides consist of deoxyribose, a phosphate group, and one of the four bases named adenine, guanine, cytosine, and thymine. DNA constitutes each of the genes in a eukaryotic cell, and contains biologic information vital for the synthesis of proteins and other substances that are critical to cell replication and cell growth, to the nature of the various types of cells that constitute tissues, and to many other cell and tissue functions, including regulation of the expression of different genes. The nucleotide sequence of DNA determines the specific biologic information that is contained and conveyed by each of the genes of a eukaryotic cell. DNA is clinically relevant to studies of genetic inheritance, the individual risk for various diseases, the development of DNA vaccines, and a range of other applications.

B. Chromosome—A nuclear structure that contains linear strands of DNA. Humans have 46 chromosomes (23 pairs). Chromosomes are clinically relevant in that abnormalities in chromosome number, structure, or both are responsible for a wide variety of diseases, including Down syndrome, DiGeorge syn-

drome, and various types of dwarfism.

C. Gene promoter—The region of a DNA molecule that controls the initiation of transcription of genes. The clinical relevance of gene promoters is that mutations in them are responsible for a number of diseases, such as Alzheimer disease.

D. Chromatin—Genetic material composed of DNA and proteins. It is located within the nucleus of the cell and condenses to form chromosomes. The clinical relevance of chromatin is that defects in it are responsible for chromatin remodeling diseases, including a number of types of cancer.

E. Gene—A specific DNA segment that contains all of the information required for the synthesis of a protein. The gene includes both base sequences that participate in encoding a protein, and noncoding sequences that do not participate in this but have other functions, such as determining when the gene is expressed. Genes are clinically relevant in that mutations that alter their normal structure have been linked to a wide range of pathologies, including various cancers, metabolic disorders, and anatomic and structural deformities of the body.

F. Genome—The full array of genes of an organism, encoding the structure of all of its proteins and other genetic information, and therefore the fundamental structure and function of the organism. The genome is clinically relevant in being the subject of genome-wide screening with gene microarrays to identify known and possible genetic defects that may result in disease.

G. Mitochondrial DNA (mtDNA)—A circular form of DNA that is found in the mitochondria of cells. mtDNA encodes proteins that are essential for the function of mitochondria. Mammalian mtDNA are 16 kb long and contain no introns and very little noncoding DNA. mtDNA is clinically relevant in that mutations in it cause diseases such as thyroid disease, cataracts, and diabetes.

H. DNA polymerase—An enzyme that synthesizes new strands of DNA by linking individual deoxyribonucleotides into polymers. Deoxyribonucleotide polymerase is clinically relevant in that mutations in this enzyme can cause cancers and other diseases.

I. Exon—The portion of a gene that encodes for mRNA

J. Intron—The portion of a gene that does not encodes for mRNA

K. Gene enhancer—A short region of a gene that enhances the level of its transcription. Gene enhancers are clinically relevant in that mutations in them are responsible for certain diseases, such as Hirschsprung disease.

L. Recombinant DNA—DNA that is artificially made by recombining, through splicing DNA segments that do not usually adjoin one another, or which are parts of different DNA molecules.

M. Transgene—A gene that is artificially inserted into a single-celled embryo. An organism that develops from this embryo will have the transgene present in all of its cells.

N. Single nucleotide polymorphism (SNP)—An alteration in the nucleotide sequence of a DNA molecule caused by a change in a single nucleotide. SNPs are found among different members of a particular species of plant or animal. SNPs are clinically relevant in the diagnostic and other investigation of the genomes of individual patients for an association of these polymorphisms with various diseases and traits.

O. Central dogma of molecular biology—A framework or "map" that shows how genetic information is sequentially processed in a cell. It is commonly depicted as: DNA→RNA→Protein.

P. Epigenetics—The study of the way in which environmental factors affect gene expression without changing the base sequence of DNA. Medical epigenetics is clinically relevant in cancer research.

Q. Genomics—The study of genomes and the functions of different genes. It is clinically relevant in genome-wide screening for the presence of particular alleles or variants of different genes, and in gene imprinting, in which various genes within an individual's genome are expressed and others are silenced.

V. Basic Genetics

A. Genomic DNA

1. Human chromosomes contain 6 billion base pairs, which constitute approximately 50,000 to 100,000 individual genes. All of the genetic information present in a single haploid set of chromosomes, consisting of one-half of one of the paired sets of chromosomes normally present in the nucleus of a eukaryotic cell, constitutes the genome of an individual human being. A variety of orthopaedic disorders are caused by mutations in genomic DNA (**Tables 2** through **6**).

2. Only 5% to 10% of genomic DNA in humans is transcribed. The genes consisting of this genomic DNA are organized into introns, or noncoding sequences, and exons, which contain the code for the particular mRNA that is needed to transcribe the genetic code carried by an individual gene into a specific protein.

3. The noncoding sequences of DNA contain promoter regions, regulatory elements, and enhancers. About one-half of the coding genes in human genomic DNA are solitary genes, which are present in sequences that occur only once in the haploid genome.

4. Directionality—Single-stranded nucleic acid is synthesized in vivo in a 5'-to-3' direction, or in an orientation that begins with the fifth and passes sequentially to the third carbon of the cyclic sugar molecule that is a part of each nucleotide in a strand of DNA (**Figure 3**).

5. mtDNA encodes ribosomal RNA (rRNA), transfer RNA (tRNA), and the proteins needed for electron transport and the synthesis of ATP within the mitochondria of a cell. mtDNA originates only from the maternal egg cells of an individual, and is not found in the paternal sperm cells. Mutations in mtDNA can cause neuromuscular disorders.

B. Control of gene expression

1. Transcription—Transcriptional control is the primary step in gene regulation (**Figure 3**). The process of transcription involves the synthesis, from the "template" provided by one of the two strands of a DNA molecule, of a complementary strand of RNA whose nucleotide sequences are paired with and correspond to the base sequences of the DNA from which the RNA is transcribed. The nucleotides in the strand of RNA that is assembled in this way are joined to one another by the enzyme RNA polymerase.

2. Translation (**Figure 3**)—In the process of translation, a ribosome binds to the initiation or "start" site of translation of an mRNA molecule and initiates the synthesis of the protein or peptide molecule whose specific sequence of amino acids is encoded by the mRNA molecule. Transfer RNA interprets the code that is carried by the mRNA and delivers the appropriate amino acids, in the proper sequence of their assembly, to the ribosome for creation of the protein or peptide encoded by the mRNA.

C. Inheritance patterns of genetic disease

1. Autosomal mutation—A gene mutation located on a chromosome other than the X or Y chromosome.

2. Sex-linked mutation—A gene mutation located on the X or Y chromosome.

3. Dominant mutation—A mutation of a single allele of a gene that is sufficient to cause an abnormal phenotype of the organism carrying that allele.

4. Recessive mutation—A mutation that must occur in both alleles of a gene to cause an abnormal phenotype of the organism carrying the two alleles.

D. Musculoskeletal genetic disorders are listed in **Tables 2** through **5**.

Table 2

Skeletal Dysplasias

Type	Genetic Mutation	Functional Defect	Characteristic Phenotypes
Achondroplasia	FGF receptor 3	Inhibition of chondrocyte proliferation	Short stature (skeletal dysplasia), normal- to large-sized head, rhizomelic shortening of the limbs, shortened arms and legs (especially the upper arm and thigh), a normal-sized trunk
Thanatophoric dysplasia	FGF receptor 3	Inhibition of chondrocyte proliferation	Severe dwarfism (marked limb shortening, a small chest, and a relatively large head; lethal after birth because of respiratory compromise
Hypochondroplasia	FGF receptor 3	Inhibition of chondrocyte proliferation	Milder dwarfism than achondroplasia
Pseudoachondroplasia	COMP	Abnormality of cartilage formation	Short stature (skeletal dysplasia), rhizomelic limb shortening, similar body proportions to those in achondroplasia, lack of distinct facial features, characteristic of achondroplasia, early-onset osteoarthritis
Multiple epiphyseal dysplasia	COMP or type IX collagen-encoding gene (*COL9A2*)	Abnormality of cartilage formation	Short stature (skeletal dysplasia); early-onset osteoarthritis
Spondyloepiphyseal dysplasia	Type II collagen-encoding gene (*COL2A1*)	Defect in cartilage matrix formation	Short stature (skeletal dysplasia), short trunk, malformation of spine, coxa vara, myopia, and retinal degeneration
Diastrophic dysplasia	Sulfate transporter (DTDS gene)	Defect in sulfation of proteoglycan	Fraccato-type achondroplasia, dwarfism, fetal hydrops
Schmid metaphyseal chondrodysplasia	Type X collagen (COL10A1)	Defect in cartilage matrix formation	Short stature, coxa vara, genu varum, involvement of metaphyses of the long bones but not in the spine; less severe than in Jansen metaphyseal chondrodysplasia; none of the disorganized metaphyseal calcification that occurs in Jansen type metaphyseal chondrodysplasia
Jansen metaphyseal chondrodysplasia	PTH/PTH-related peptide receptor	Functional defect of parathyroid hormone	Short limb, characteristic facial abnormalities, and additional skeletal malformations; sclerotic bones in the back cranial bones, which may lead to blindness or deafness; hypercalcemia
Cleidocranial dysplasia	RUNX2 (CBF-alpha-1)	Impaired intramembranous ossification	Hypoplasia or aplasia of the clavicles, open skull suture, mild facial hypoplasia, wide symphysis pubis, mild short stature, dental abnormality, vertebral abnormality

CBF = core-binding factor, COMP = cartilage oligometric matrix protein, DTDS = diastrophic dysplasia, FGF = fibroblast growth factor, PTH = parathyroid hormone, RUNX2 = runt-related transcription factor-2.

VI. RNA-Related Terminology and Definitions

A. RNA—A polymer composed of ribonucleotide monomers that are covalently linked to one another. The ribonucleotides in this polymer have ribose (rather than deoxyribose, as in DNA) as their cyclic sugar component, a phosphate group, and a base consisting of adenine, guanine, cytosine, or uracil. RNA is essential for protein synthesis, biologic reactions, and cellular communication.

B. mRNA—An RNA molecule that encodes the specific amino acid sequence of a protein or peptide. mRNA is transcribed from DNA and travels to the ribosomes of cells, where its sequence of nucleic acids is translated into an appropriately corresponding protein or peptide.

C. Microribonucleic acid (miRNA)—Small segments (approximately 22 nts) of RNA that regulate the expression of mRNA molecules by interacting with them to inhibit their translation into proteins or peptides.

Table 3

Metabolic Diseases of Bone

Type	Genetic Mutation	Functional Defect	Characteristic Phenotypes
X-linked hypophosphatemic rickets	PEX (a cellular endopeptidase)	Vitamin D–resistant rickets	Rickets, short stature, and impaired renal phosphate reabsorption and vitamin D metabolism
Hypophosphatasia	Tissue nonspecific alkaline phosphatase gene (alkaline phosphatase gene)	Generalized impairment of skeletal mineralization	Rickets, bow legs, loss of teeth, short stature
Familial osteolysis	Tumor necrosis factor receptor superfamily member 11A gene (osteoprotegerin ligand; receptor activator of nuclear factor-κB)	Idiopathic multicentric osteolysis	Typical facies with a slender nose, maxillary hypoplasia, and micrognathia; rheumatoid arthritis-like hand deformities
MPS I	Iduronidase gene	Deficiency of α-ʟ-iduronidase (lysosomal enzymes for cleavage of glycosaminoglycans)	Hurler syndrome; progressive cellular damage that affects the development of neurologic and musculoskeletal system (short stature and bone dysplasia)
MPS II	Iduronate sulfatase gene; X-linked recessive	Deficiency of iduronate sulfatase	Hunter syndrome; mild to moderate features of MPS
MPS III	Heparan N-sulfatase (IIIA); N-acetylglucosaminidase [NAGLU] gene (IIIB); GNAT gene (IIIC); N-acetylglucosamine 6-sulfatase (IIID)	Deficiency of heparan N-sulfatase (IIIA); α-N-acetylglucosaminidase (IIIB) ; acetyl-coenzyme A:α-glucosaminide-N-acetyltransferase (IIIC); N-acetylglucosamine 6-sulfatase (IIID)	Sanfilippo syndrome; severe neurologic syndrome with mild progressive musculoskeletal syndrome
MPS IV	Deficient enzymes N-acetylgalactosamine 6-sulfatase (Type A) or β-galactosidase (Type B)	Deficiency of lysosomal enzymes for breaking keratan sulfate	Morquio syndrome; bell-shaped chest, anomaly of spine, shortened long bones, and dysplasia of the hips, knees, ankles, and wrists; odontoid hypoplasia

GNAT = glucosaminide N-acetyltransferase, MPS = mucopolysaccharidosis.

Table 4

Connective Tissue Disorders

Type	Genetic Mutation	Functional Defect	Characteristic Phenotypes
Osteogenesis imperfecta	Type I collagen (COL1A1 or COL1A2) genes	Decreased amount and poorer quality of collagen than normal	Common charicteristics: Fragile bone, low muscle tone, possible hearing loss, dentinogenesis imperfecta Type I: Most common and mildest form; blue sclera Type II: Most severe form; lethal after birth because of respiratory problem Type III: Significantly shorter stature than normal; blue sclera Type IV: Normal sclera
Ehlers-Danlos syndrome	Fibrillar collagen gene (collagen V or III)	Laxity and weakness of connective tissue	Lax joints, hyperextensible skin
Marfan syndrome	Fibrillin	Abnormality of connective tissue	Tall stature, scoliosis, myopia, lens dislocation, aortic aneurysm, mitral valve prolapse

1: Basic Science

Table 5

Musculoskeletal Tumors

Type	Genetic Mutation	Functional Defect	Characteristic Phenotypes
Bloom syndrome	Mutation in Bloom syndrome-protein–encoding (*BLM*) gene located on chromosome 15, in band q26.1.	Helicase dysfunction (unwinding of double strands of DNA and RNA from one another)	Short stature and predisposition to sarcoma and various other types of cancer
Rothmund-Thompson syndrome	RecQ helicase gene (*RECQ4*)	Defect in DNA replication and cell proliferation	Short stature; cataracts; patchy changes in pigmentation of skin; baldness; abnormalities of bones, nails; and teeth; high incidence of sarcoma
Li-Fraumeni syndrome	p53 tumor-suppressor gene	Increased susceptibility to cancer	Various cancers, including osteosarcoma and liposarcoma at an early age
Fibrous dysplasia	Gsα (receptor-coupled signaling protein); guanine nucleotide-binding protein (G protein) alpha-stimulating activity polypeptide 1 (*GNAS1*) gene	Inappropriate stimulation of adenyl cyclase	McCune-Albright syndrome: fibrous dysplasia; abnormalities in skin pigmentation and endocrine function
Multiple hereditary exostoses	Exostosin-1 and -2 (*EXT1, EXT2*) genes	Dysfunction of tumor-suppressor gene	Noticeable exostoses
Ewing sarcoma	t(11;22): Ewing sarcoma (*EWS*) gene of chromosome 22 fuses Friend leukemia integration (*FLI*) gene on chromosome	Primitive neuroectodermal tumor in bone and soft tissue	Commonly occurs in diaphyses of long bones
Synovial sarcoma	T(X;18): synaptotagmin-synovial sarcoma X (*SYT-SSX*) fusion gene	Dysregulation of gene expression (SYT-SSX fusion protein)	A sarcoma adjacent to joints
Myxoid liposarcoma	T(12;16)(q13:p11): fused in sarcoma-DNA damage inducible transcript-3 (*FUS-DDIT3*) chimeric gene	Cytogenic abnormality	A lipogenic tumor occurring in soft tissue

Table 6

Other Musculoskeletal Disorders

Type	Affected Site or Substance	Functional Defect	Characteristic Phenotypes
Duchenne muscular dystrophy	Dystrophin	Absence of dystrophin in muscle	Progressive weakness and degeneration of muscle, short life expectancy
Osteopetrosis	Carbonic anhydrase type II; proton pump (human) c-src, M-CSF, β3 integrin (mouse)	Osteoclast dysfunction	Fragile bone, anemia, immune deficiencies because of bone marrow deficiency
Fibrodysplasia ossificans progressiva	Mutation of the noggin (*NOG*) gene BMP-1 receptor	Heterotopic ossification	Heterotopic ossification and rigidity of joints

BMP = bone morphogenetic protein, M-CSF = macrophage colony-stimulating factor.

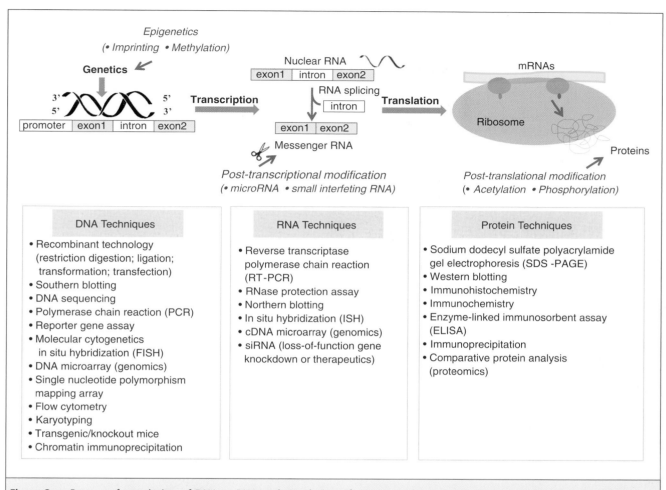

Figure 3 Process of translation of DNA to RNA and translation of protein and peptide codes in RNA into proteins, and research techniques using various aspects of this process. (Reproduced from Lee FY, Zuscik MJ, Nizami S, et al: Molecular and cell biology in orthopaedics, in O'Keefe RJ, Jacobs JJ, Chu CR, Einhorn TA, eds: *Orthopaedic Basic Science*, ed 4. Rosemont, IL, American Academy Orthopaedic Surgeons, 2013, pp 3-42.)

D. Ribosomal RNA (rRNA)—RNA that is part of the ribosome and is involved in protein synthesis. The clinical relevance of rRNA is in the ability to use it for detecting bacterial pathogens. This is conducted by amplification and sequence analysis of the 16S rRNA gene. By using sequences from this gene of varying lengths, bacteria can be detected in clinical samples using a polymerase chain reaction (PCR).

VII. Terminology Related to Gene Expression and Protein Synthesis

A. Gene expression: Transcription: DNA→mRNA

1. Transcription—A process in which the information contained in the nucleotide sequences of DNA is encoded in RNA through the assembly of corresponding, complementary sequences of RNA by the enzyme RNA polymerase. Transcription is clinically relevant to orthopaedics in that it

must be correct for accurate protein synthesis and cellular function. Aberrations in transcription can result in diseases and structural pathologies.

2. Splicing—The removal of intronic sequences from newly transcribed RNA, resulting in the production of mRNA. Splicing is clinically relevant to orthopaedics in that variations in splicing can alter the functions of genes and may cause disease.

3. Transcription factor—A protein that can initiate the transcription of DNA by binding to its regulatory elements. Transcription factors of orthopaedic importance are runt-related transcription factor-2 (RUNX2; CBF-alpha-1), which is essential for the differentiation of osteoblasts and for skeletal morphogenesis; osterix, which is also essential for osteoblast differentiation; SOX-9, which is essential for cartilage differentiation; and protein proliferator-activated receptors (PPARs), which function as transcription factors that regulate gene expression, and one of which, PPAR-γ,

is essential for the differentiation of adipose tissue.

B. Protein expression: Translation: mRNA→Proteins

1. Translation—The process in which a nucleotide sequence in mRNA acts as the code for a series of amino acids that are assembled in the ribosome into a specific protein or peptide. The assembly process requires tRNAs that bring the necessary amino acids to the ribosome, where they are assembled according to the base sequence of the mRNA to yield the requisite protein or peptide. The correct translation of mRNA into the protein or peptide that it encodes is essential for cell survival. Antibiotics such as tetracycline inhibit tRNA from binding to the ribosome.

2. Post-translational modification—The enzymatic processing of a newly formed peptide. This enzymatic processing can occur in numerous ways, such as disulfide-bridge formation, acetylation, glycosylation, and phosphorylation. Posttranslational modifications of certain proteins, such as various enzymes, are essential to their proper final functions.

3. Proteomics—The study of all proteins encoded in the genome of a cell, also known as the proteome.

VIII. Molecular Biology Methods Related to DNA or mRNA

A. Molecular cytogenetics—Techniques that combine molecular biology and cytogenetics for the analysis of a specific DNA within the genome of a cell. These techniques include fluorescence in situ hybridization (FISH) and comparative genomic hybridization (CGH). In orthopaedics, these cytogenetic techniques have been used for the detection of bone tumors, the genetic study of anatomic deformities, and in orthopaedic research.

B. In situ hybridization—A technique that involves the use of a short, labeled strand of DNA or RNA (a probe) that is complementary to the section of DNA or RNA in a cell or tissue specimen to localize and detect a specific nucleic acid or sequence of nucleic acids in the cell or tissue specimen. In the FISH technique, a fluorescent substance is linked chemically to the DNA or RNA probe, permitting the individual nucleic acid or sequence of nucleic acids to which the probe becomes bound to be identified by fluorescence microscopy. In orthopaedics, FISH is used to detect oncogenes (mRNA) or mutated genes in pathologic specimens.

C. Flow cytometry—A technique used to sort, analyze, or count biologic components, usually cells, by passing them through a detection device. In orthopaedics, flow cytometry has been used to identify bone

tumors. For example, Ewing sarcoma cells have been detected via flow cytometry by using the expression of CD99 antigen and lack of CD45 antigen on the cancerous cells.

D. Reporter gene assay—A method that uses a specific gene as a marker or signal for studying the expression and localization of other, neighboring or associated genes in cells. Among such signal-producing genes are the genes for green fluorescence protein, luciferase, and LacZ, the gene that encodes the enzyme β-galactosidase. Reporter gene assays are commonly used in orthopaedic research for assessing the expression of a specific gene in a cell or tissue. *BGLAP*, which codes for osteocalcin, is one such reporter gene used to identify bone anabolism or formation.

E. PCR—A method of replicating, or amplifying, a specific region of interest in the DNA of a cell to a concentration that can be detected using one of several analytic methods. The amplification is performed using an appropriate primer for initiating transcription of the relevant DNA region, with the complementary nucleotides needed to replicate the region of interest, with a thermostable DNA polymerase, and with other requisite components for the procedure. To expose the region of interest that is to be amplified, the double-stranded DNA that contains this region within a cell is denatured into a single strand by heating. The primer needed to initiate transcription of this DNA is allowed to bind to the region of DNA that is to be amplified, and this region of DNA is repeatedly transcribed, in the presence of the needed bases and DNA polymerase, to yield a measurable amount of the region of DNA that is of interest. In orthopaedics and other clinical specializations, as well as research, PCR is used for the diagnosis of infection when culture of the causative pathogen is not feasible (for example, tuberculosis or HIV infection).

F. Reverse transcriptase (RT)–RT-PCR—A sensitive technique that uses both reverse transcription (generating cDNA from an RNA template) and PCR to generate multiple copies of the mRNA of a particular gene in the genome of a cell. This mRNA is used as a template, in the presence of the appropriate nucleotides and DNA polymerase, for generating copies of the gene of interest. Products of RT-PCR are detected on a real-time basis using a technique known as real-time RT-PCR or quantitative real-time PCR (Q-PCR).

G. Northern blotting—A technique used to identify and quantitate specific RNA molecules. In this technique, RNA is subjected to agarose gel electrophoresis, which separates RNAs of different size and electric charge according to their ability to migrate through a gel on a flat plate to which an electrical field is applied. Probes that hybridize specifically to the RNA molecule(s) of interest are applied to the plate to identify these RNA molecules, or the RNA molecules are extracted from the plate and analyzed using other methods. In orthopaedics, Northern blotting has been used to detect the expression of various mRNAs in cells, tissues, and fluids. The osteoclast-associated receptor and its ligand were discovered using Northern blot analysis of osteo-clastogenic RAW264.7 cells.

H. Complementary DNA (cDNA) microarray—A process in which a small surface or chip of a solid material, containing microquantities of various genes or segments of DNA or the mRNA that is complementary to this DNA, is used to determine whether a cell or tissue specimen contains the DNA segments that complement and correspond to any of the DNA or mRNA segments on the chip. If so, the corresponding DNA or mRNA segments bind to and hybridize with those on the chip. The genes or DNA segments on the chip are labeled with fluorescent substances that act as probes to facilitate identification of the genes or DNA segments of interest. In orthopaedics, cDNA microarrays are used for comparing the expression of genes in normal and malignant cells (such as pathologically resorbing bone cells, as in osteosarcoma) and for examining the gene-expression profile of macrophages that have been exposed to biomaterials to determine the release of inflammatory cytokines and chemokines in an implant wear particle (metal/polyethylene) scenario.

I. DNA sequencing—Identification of the sequences in which specific nucleotides occur within a gene or region of DNA.

J. Southern blotting—A technique for detecting a specific sequence of DNA in a sample of DNA. In Southern blotting, an endonuclease enzyme is used to digest the sample of DNA into fragments, which are applied to an agarose gel on a flat plate to which an electrical field is applied. The fragments of DNA migrate across the plate according to their size and electrical charge, after which they are blotted up onto either a sheet of nitrocellulose or a nylon membrane. The nitrocellulose sheet or nylon membrane is then heated in an oven and exposed to ultraviolet radiation to bind the DNA fragments to the sheet or membrane, after which the sheet or membrane is exposed to a solution containing DNA or RNA that is complementary to the specific DNA fragments of interest, and which is labeled with a fluorescent or chromogenic substance that permits any such DNA in the original sample to be visualized and recognized as being present in the original sample. Southern blotting has been used in orthopaedic research to identify specific genes of bone specimens. Southern blotting was used to determine that there were multiple copies of the osteocalcin gene in mice instead of just one, as was previously thought. Bone morphogenic protein receptor type 2 (*BMPR2*) gene rearrangements were also uncovered by using Southern blotting.

K. Recombinant technology—A series of procedures used to produce a desired protein. In recombinant technology, a specific sequence of DNA that encodes the desired protein is synthesized from its nucleic acids and inserted into the DNA of a cell, which generates the desired protein, or the DNA or mRNA for the desired protein is subjected to RT-PCR, which synthesizes the protein in vitro. Recombinant technology has been used for the production of numerous proteins of interest in orthopaedics, including recombinant human bone morphogenetic protein-2 (rhBMP-2), which stimulates the generation of bone to replace bone defects and expedite bone union in fractures; rhBMP-7; erythropoietin; receptor activator of nuclear factor-κ B ligand (RANKL) blocker, which blocks the proliferation of osteoclasts; tumor necrosis factor (TNF) blocker; and interleukin-6 (IL-6) blocker, which blocks the generation of osteoclasts. It is also used for functional studies of genes.

L. Manipulation of DNA—A series of procedures involving the enzymatic cutting of DNA or RNA, the combination with or insertion of segments of DNA or RNA into other segments of DNA or RNA, or the copying of DNA or RNA to produce specific proteins or peptides or to correct defects in genes.

M. Restriction digestion of DNA—A technique that involves the use of restriction endonuclease enzymes that cut double-stranded DNA at specific locations determined by the nature of the restriction enzyme. Restriction digestion is a widely used molecular technique for removing specific fragments of DNA from larger strands of DNA.

N. Ligation or pasting of DNA fragments—A technique involving the use of an enzyme called a ligase, which makes covalent phosphate bonds between nucleotides, and which is used to link nucleotides to one another. In orthopaedic research, ligation is used in research for inserting fragments of DNA into longer sequences of DNA, including genes.

O. Transformation—The insertion of a gene or other fragment of DNA into the genome of a cell, resulting in genetic modification of that cell. Transformation can occur naturally, through the passage of a fragment of DNA through the membrane of a cell and incorporation of the fragment into the genome of the cell, or intentionally, through the insertion, into the genome of a cell, of a fragment of naturally occurring or synthetic DNA, made by RT-PCR. For example, a gene fragment for a bioluminescent protein can be introduced to an osteogenic cell, essentially tagging the cell and making its progress detectable via molecular imaging.

P. Transfection—A method of introducing exogenous nucleic acids into a eukaryotic cell in such a way that these nucleic acids are incorporated into the chromosomal DNA of the cell. The nucleic acids can be introduced to a cell using several methods, including electroporation, which renders the membrane of the cell permeable to entry of the desired DNA fragment, and the use of substances such as calcium phosphate, which acts chemically to render the cell membrane permeable.

IX. Molecular Biologic Methods Related to Proteins (Cytokines, Enzymes, Transcription Factors, Disease Markers)

A. Immunohistochemistry/immunocytochemistry—A method for detecting and localizing a target protein in a cell or tissue. The method involves the use of an antibody that is specific for the protein of interest and binds to that protein in a tissue or a cell. Typically, a fluorescent or other substance that serves as a label is linked to the antibody, permitting identification of the target protein after the antibody has become bound to it. Some common target proteins in the use of immunohistochemistry and immunocytochemistry are tumor markers and cytokines. In orthopaedics, immunohistochemistry and immunocytochemistry are used for the diagnosis of musculoskeletal and hematopoietic tumors.

B. Enzyme-linked immunosorbent assay (ELISA)—A biochemical method for detecting and quantifying a specific soluble protein. In the ELISA technique, an enzyme is linked chemically to an antibody that recognizes and binds to a specific protein. After this binding has occurred, the enzyme that is bound to the antibody is exposed to a substrate, and transforms this substrate into a colored and therefore visible product that acts as a marker for identifying the presence of the protein that is being sought. In orthopaedics, ELISA is used to identify and quantify alkaline phosphatase, amylase, and other substances of clinical interest in body fluids, cells, and tissues.

C. Bicinchoninic acid assay—A biochemical test used for determining the total concentration of protein in a body-fluid specimen. In this method, the peptide bonds in a protein reduce the bivalent copper ions (Cu^{2+}) a fluid specimen to monovalent copper ions (Cu^+), which form a purple combination product with a bicinchoninic acid reagent. The color intensity of the purple combination product is proportional to the concentration of protein in the original fluid specimen, and can be quantitated photometrically. In clinical and research orthopaedics, the bicinchoninic acid assay is used to determine the concentrations of various proteins in fluid specimens.

D. Tartrate-resistant acid phosphatase (TRAP) assay—A staining technique for identifying TRAP, an enzyme that is a common marker of osteoclast cells (**Figure 4**). In orthopaedic research, the TRAP assay is used to identify and quantify osteoclasts in bone specimens.

E. Sodium dodecyl sulfate–polyacrylamide gel electrophoresis (SDS-PAGE)—A technique that separates proteins according to their molecular weight and electric charge. In this technique, a fluid containing dissolved proteins is applied to one end of a gel medium on a flat plate, and an electric current is applied to the plate. When the current is applied, the proteins applied to the plate travel to different points on the plate according to their molecular weight and charge. In orthopaedics, SDS-PAGE is used to identify, isolate, and investigate a wide range of proteins.

F. Coomassie Blue staining—A method of visualizing, using the dye Coomassie Brilliant Blue, bands of proteins that have been separated by SDS-PAGE. The dye binds nonspecifically to proteins. This technique is used in biomedical research to observe proteins in SDS-PAGE gels. This can be used to separate and identify proteins by size (such as bone matrix proteins or bone morphogenic proteins) in a tissue sample for further investigation and identification.

G. Western blotting—A technique commonly used to identify a specific protein of interest in a homogenate or extract of tissue extract. The technique involves the separation of proteins by SDS–PAGE, followed by transfer or blotting of the proteins on the polyacrylamide gel to a membrane. After this transfer, the protein of interest is detected on the membrane by the application of an enzyme-linked antibody that binds specifically to the protein of interest, and which is then exposed to a substance from which the linked enzyme generates a colored "marker" product to identify the protein. In orthopaedics, Western blotting is used to investigate the expression of specific proteins in tissue specimens. With Western blotting, it is possible to identify proteins that might be unregulated in a pathologic situation, or elucidate mechanistic pathways of bone functions such as osteoclastogenesis.

H. Immunoprecipitation—A method of precipitating a protein from a solution through the use of a specific antibody that binds specifically to the protein. Immunoprecipitation is used in orthopaedic research to isolate proteins and establishing the presence of a protein that could be used for elucidating bone biologic mechanisms.

I. Chromatin immunoprecipitation (ChIP) assay—A type of immunoprecipitation assay used to examine the interactions and localizations of proteins to DNA in a cell. This assay is used in research for the analysis of proteins, such as transcription factors, that are associated with specific regions of DNA.

J. Comparative proteomic analysis—A method that uses a computer and a peptide sequencing machine for the comprehensive and rapid analysis of entire proteins in tissues or cells. This method of analysis would enable an orthopaedic researcher to create a profile of protein activity in a normal, malignant, or

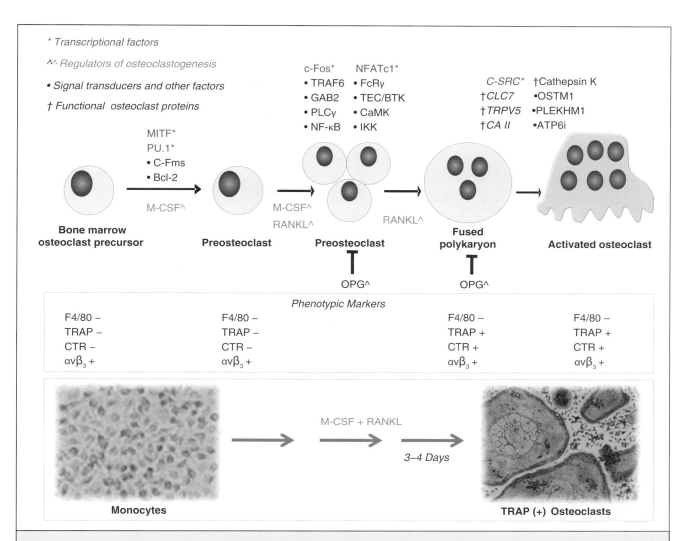

Figure 4 Transcriptional factors in osteoclastogenesis. ATP = adenosine triphosphate, BTK = Bruton tyrosine kinase, CaMK = Ca²⁺/calmodulin–dependent kinase, CTR = calcitonin receptor, FcR = Fc receptor, GAB2 = GRB2-associated-binding protein 2, IKK = IκB kinase, M-CSF = macrophage colony-stimulating factor, NF-κB = nuclear factor kappa-light-chain-enhancer of activated B cells, NFATc1 = nuclear factor of activated T cells, cytoplasmic 1, OPG = osteoprotegerin, OSTM = osteopetrosis-associated transmembrane, PLC = phospholipase C, PLEKHM1 = pleckstrin homology domain-containing family M member 1, RANKL = receptor activator of nuclear factor-κ B ligand, TEC = tyrosine-protein kinase, TRAF = tumor necrosis factor receptor–associated factor, TRAP = tartrate-resistant acid phosphate. (Reproduced from Lee FY, Zuscik MJ, Nizami S, et al: Molecular and cell biology in orthopaedics, in O'Keefe RJ, Jacobs JJ, Chu CR, Einhorn TA, eds: *Orthopaedic Basic Science*, ed 4. Rosemont, IL, American Academy Orthopaedic Surgeons, 2013, pp 3-42.)

treated bone specimen that would be highly advantageous for drug research.

X. Immunology

A. Innate and adaptive immunity—The body's defense against substances and proteins that are foreign or alien to it, and against various pathogens, is mediated early in life by innate or intrinsic immunity and later in life by adaptive immunity.

1. Intrinsic or innate immunity, which provides the body's early defense against alien substances and pathogens, is stimulated by a certain structure shared by a group of microbes. It responds rapidly to infection, and will respond in the same way to repeated infections. Physical barriers: epidermis, dermis, mucosa; cellular barriers: phagocytotic cells and natural killer cells; chemical barriers: antimicrobial substances, blood proteins (complement system), and cytokines.

2. In adaptive immunity, exposure to a specific antigen initiates a process that prompts the development of a group of immune cells that recognize and "recall" that antigen, and which are ready to respond to it should it ever again enter the body.

Table 7

Disease-Modifying Antirheumatic Drugs Commonly Used for Treating Rheumatoid Arthritis

Drug	Drug Type	Target	Mechanism of Action
Abatacept	Recombinant fusion protein	MHC receptors	Binds to MHC receptors on antigen-presenting cells to block T cell activation
Anakinra	Receptor antagonist	IL-1 receptors	Binds to IL-1 receptors to block IL-1 proinflammatory signaling pathway
Canakinumab	Monoclonal IgG antibody	IL-1β	Binds to IL-1β with high affinity to inhibit IL-1β and receptor association
Infliximab	Recombinant chimeric human-murine monoclonal antibody	TNF-α	Binds to TNF-α. The drug has higher affinity to TNF-α than the receptor, so TNF-α could dissociate from its receptor.
Adalimumab	Recombinant monoclonal antibody	TNF-α	Binds to TNF-α and inhibits the interactions of this cytokine to p55 and p75 receptors
Etanercept	Recombinant fusion protein	TNF-α	Competes with TNF-α receptor for the binding of TNF-α
Tocilizumab	Humanized monoclonal antibody	IL-6 receptors	Binds to IL-6 receptors to inhibit the association between the receptor and IL-6
Sulfasalazine	Combination of sulfapyridine and 5-salicylic acid	Unknown	Modulates B cell response and angiogenesis
Methotrexate	Folate antagonist	Dihydrofolate reductase	Inhibits dihydrofolate reductase activity, resulting in adenosine-dependent inhibition of inflammation

IgG = immunoglobulin, IL = interleukin, MHC = major histocompatibility complex, TNF = tumor necrosis factor.

Through adaptive immunity, the body, after first encounters with diverse and specific antigens, is able to recognize and combat them. Successive exposure to antigens increases the magnitude of the immune reaction to them. Adaptive immunity includes two types of responses, known as humoral immune responses and cell-mediated immune responses.

a. Humoral immunity—Mediated by antibodies, produced by B lymphocytes, and directed against specific antigens belonging to a foreign substance or to a pathogen such as a virus or infectious bacterium.

b. Cell-mediated immunity—Mediated by T lymphocytes (T cells). T cells can activate macrophages to kill phagocytosed antigens or can destroy infected cells directly. An individual who has contracted chicken pox has immunity against the varicella virus. If the virus again attempts to enter the body, it will be engulfed by the white blood cells known as macrophages, which will secrete protein substances that signal other cells of the immune system to rapidly destroy the cells that have engulfed the virus and the virus within them.

B. Immune mediators and regulation of bone mass (**Table 7**)

1. Inflammatory bone destruction or osteolysis is seen clinically in rheumatoid arthritis (disease-modifying antirheumatic drugs), chronic inflammatory disease, periodontitis, and wear particle-induced osteolysis. Osteoblasts and osteoclasts communicate in the regulation of bone mass.

2. Inflammatory stimuli may stimulate osteoblasts to express RANKL, a member of the TNF superfamily of proteins, and the key molecule that induces osteoclastogenesis.

3. Anabolic factors such as transforming growth factor beta (TGF-β) and BMPs may stimulate the precursor cells of osteoblasts to differentiate into osteoblasts.

XI. Stem Cells

A. Adult somatic stem cells (**Figure 5**)

1. Undifferentiated cells in the body that are capable of self-renewal and multipotency

2. Adult somatic stem cells can divide indefinitely and are also capable of generating various different types of cells, which is accomplished through two types of cell division:

a. Symmetric division, in which somatic stem

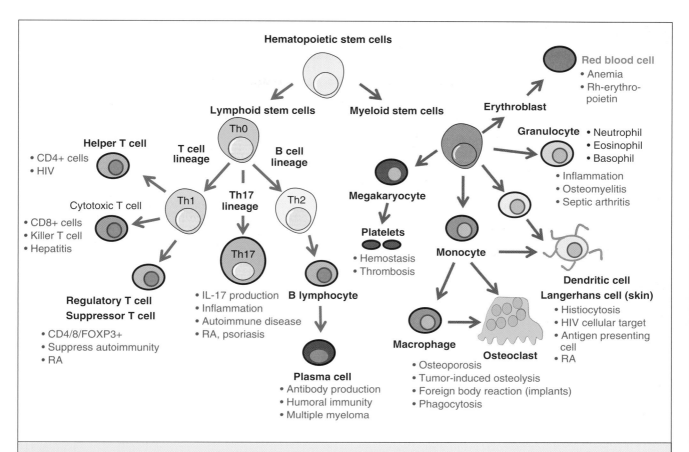

Figure 5 Orthopaedic implications of hematopoietic stem cell differentiation. JL = interleukin, RA = rheumatoid arthritis. (Reproduced from Lee FY, Zuscik MJ, Nizami S, et al: Molecular and cell biology in orthopaedics, in O'Keefe RJ, Jacobs JJ, Chu CR, Einhorn TA, eds: *Orthopaedic Basic Science*, ed 4. Rosemont, IL, American Academy Orthopaedic Surgeons, 2013, pp 3-42.)

1: Basic Science

cells replicate and create more somatic stem cells

   b. Asymmetric division, which produces a stem cell and a progenitor cell, which differentiates into a particular type of cell

3. Mesenchymal stem cells (MSCs) are adult somatic stem cells that can differentiate into chondrocytes, osteoblasts, fibroblasts, tenocytes and adipocytes.

B. Embryonic stem (ES) cells

1. Are harvested from the inner cell mass of a blastocyst (**Figure 1**)

2. Are characterized by two important properties:

   a. Pluripotency, the ability of ES cells to differentiate into cells of any of the three germ layers: mesoderm, endoderm, or ectoderm

   b. Self-renewal, by which ES cells can replicate and remain in an undifferentiated study, thereby propagating more ES cells

3. Can be afflicted with host-versus-graft rejection.

C. Induced pluripotent stem cells

1. Induced pluripotent stem cells are an artificially derived form of pluripotent stem cells (**Figure 2**).

2. Viral transduction is used to induce differentiated adult cells to undergo retrograde evolution into stem cells through stem cell–associated genes.

   a. Stem cell–associated genes include *SOX2*, *Oct3/4*, *c-Myc*, *KLF4*, and others. These genes are important for the self-renewal aspects of pluripotent stem cells. They are important for inducing pluripotency.

3. Similarities between induced pluripotent stem cells and ES cells are currently being investigated. A few parallels that have already been observed for these two types of cells are cell doubling time, embryoid body formation, teratoma formation, and chromatin methylation patterns.

Top Testing Facts

1. Signal transduction is the process by which extracellular signals, in the form of substances that bind to receptors on a cell membrane or via other means act to generate a specific response in a cell.

2. mRNA carries the genetic information contained in DNA to the ribosomes of a cell, where this information is transformed into proteins and peptides.

3. DNA is a double-stranded polymer in which each strand consists of deoxyribonucleotides that are bound covalently to one another.

4. The genome of a cell or organism is the full array of its genes, encoding the structure of all proteins and other genetic information.

5. A transgene is a gene that is artificially inserted into a single-celled embryo.

6. All genetic information present in a single haploid set of chromosomes, consisting of one-half of one of the paired sets of chromosomes normally present in the nucleus of a eukaryotic cell, constitutes the genome of an individual human being.

7. An autosomal mutation is a gene mutation located on a chromosome other than the X or Y chromosome.

8. In situ hybridization is a technique that involves the use of a short, labeled strand of DNA or RNA (a probe) that is complementary to a section of DNA or RNA in a cell or tissue specimen to localize and detect a specific nucleic acid or sequence of nucleic acids in the cell or tissue specimen.

9. Recombinant technology involves the linking with DNA or RNA segments with other such segments, or the insertion of such segments into larger segments of DNA or RNA, to produce specific proteins or peptides.

10. Infliximab is a monoclonal antibody that prevents the binding of TNF-α to its receptors on cells.

11. Inflammatory stimuli may stimulate osteoblasts to express RANKL, a key molecule in the proliferation of osteoclasts.

Bibliography

Alberts B, Bray D, Lewis J, Raff M, Roberts K, Watson JD: *Molecular Biology of the Cell*, ed 4. New York, NY, Garland Publishing, 2002.

Shore EM, Kaplan FS: Tutorial: Molecular biology for the clinician. Part II: Tools of molecular biology. *Clin Orthop Relat Res* 1995;320:247-278.

Zuscik MJ, Drissi MH, Chen D, Rosier RN: Molecular and cell biology in orthopaedics, in Einhorn TA, O'Keefe RJ, Buckwalter JA, eds: *Orthopaedic Basic Science*, ed 3. Rosemont, IL, American Academy of Orthopaedic Surgeons, 2000, pp 3-23.

Chapter 2
Skeletal Development

Kornelis Poelstra, MD, PhD

I. Cartilage and Bone Development

A. Formation of the bony skeleton

1. Intramembranous bone formation is achieved through the formation of a calcified osteoid matrix by osteoblasts inside a cartilage framework. This type of bone formation can be found at the periosteal surfaces of bone as well as in parts of the pelvis, the scapula, the clavicles, and the skull.

2. Endochondral ossification occurs at the growth plates and within fracture callus and is characterized by osteoblast production of osteoid on, not within, a cartilaginous framework. The cartilage framework ultimately is resorbed.

B. Vertebral and limb bud development (**Table 1**)

1. Four weeks of gestation

   a. The vertebrate limb begins as an outpouching of the lateral body wall.

   b. Formation of the limb is controlled along three cardinal axes of the limb bud: proximal-distal, anterior-posterior, and dorsal-ventral.

   c. Interactions between the ectoderm and mesoderm characterize development along each axis and are governed by the interaction of fibroblast growth factors, bone morphogenetic proteins, and several homeobox genes.

2. Six weeks of gestation

   a. The mesenchymal condensations that represent the limbs and digits chondrify.

   b. The mesenchymal cells differentiate into chondrocytes.

3. Seven weeks of gestation

   a. The chondrocytes hypertrophy and the local matrix begins to calcify.

   b. A periosteal sleeve of bone forms in a circum-

ferential fashion around the midshaft of each anlage, and intramembranous bone formation begins to occur via direct ossification.

4. Eight weeks of gestation

   a. Vascular invasion into the cartilaginous anlage occurs as capillary buds expand through the periosteal sleeve.

   b. The capillaries deliver the bloodborne precursors of osteoblasts and osteoclasts and thus create a primary center of ossification. This process occurs first at the humerus, and signals the transition from the embryonic to the fetal period.

C. Formation of endochondral bone and ossification centers

1. As development continues, the osteoblasts produce an osteoid matrix on the surface of the calcified cartilaginous bars and form the primary trabeculae of endochondral bone.

2. The osteoclasts help create the medullary canal by removing the primary trabecular bone. This

Table 1

Limb Bud Development

Weeks of Gestation	Major Biologic Events
4	Limb begins as outpouching from lateral body wall
6	Mesenchymal condensations that represent limbs and digits develop Mesenchymal cells differentiate into chondrocytes
7	Chondrocytes become hypertrophic; local matrix begins to calcify Periosteal sleeve of bone forms around midshaft of each anlage Intramembranous bone formation begins via direct ossification
8	Vascular invasion into the cartilaginous anlage Capillaries deliver precursor cells; primary center of ossification develops

Dr. Poelstra or an immediate family member has received royalties from DePuy; is a member of a speakers' bureau or has made paid presentations on behalf of DePuy; and serves as a paid consultant to or is an employee of DePuy.

1: Basic Science

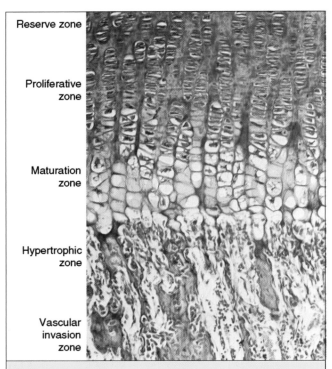

Reserve zone

Proliferative zone

Maturation zone

Hypertrophic zone

Vascular invasion zone

Figure 1 Photomicrograph shows the structure and zones of the growth plate (×220). (©Science Source, New York, NY.)

process of formation and absorption enlarges the primary center of ossification so that it becomes the growth region.

3. These growth regions differentiate further and become well-defined growth plates.

4. Division within the growth plate is coupled with the deposition of bone at the metaphyseal side of the bud, and long bone growth begins.

5. At a specific time in the development of each long bone, a secondary center of ossification develops within the chondroepiphysis.

6. The secondary center of ossification typically grows in a spherical fashion and accounts for the centripetal growth of the long bone.

7. The rates of division within the centers of ossification ultimately determine the overall contour of each joint.

II. Normal Growth Plate

A. Structure, organization, and function

1. The function of the growth plate is related to its structure. In its simplest form, the growth plate comprises three histologically distinct zones surrounded by a fibrous component and bounded by a bony metaphyseal component.

2. The three cellular zones of the growth plate are the reserve zone, proliferative zone, and hypertrophic zone (**Figure 1**).

a. The reserve zone is adjacent to the secondary center of ossification and is characterized by a sparse distribution of cells in a vast matrix.

- Cellular proliferation in this zone is sporadic, and the chondrocytes in this region do not contribute to longitudinal growth.

- Type II collagen content is highest here.

- Blood is supplied to this zone via the terminal branches of the epiphyseal artery, which enter the secondary center of ossification.

b. The proliferative zone is characterized by longitudinal columns of flattened cells. The uppermost cell in each column is the progenitor cell, which is responsible for longitudinal growth.

- The total longitudinal growth of the growth plate depends on the number of cell divisions of the progenitor cell.

- The rate at which the cells divide is influenced by mechanical and hormonal factors.

- The matrix of the proliferative zone comprises a nonuniform array of collagen fibrils and matrix vesicles.

- Proliferative zone chondrocytes are also supplied by the terminal branches of the epiphyseal artery; however, these vessels do not penetrate the proliferative zone but rather terminate at the uppermost cell. These vessels deliver the oxygen and nutrients that facilitate the cellular division and matrix production that occur within this zone.

c. The cells in the hypertrophic zone are 5 to 10 times the size of those in the proliferative zone. Because of growth in the columns, this is the weakest layer. Fractures in the growth plate occur through this layer.

- The role of the chondrocytes in the hypertrophic zone is the synthesis of novel matrix proteins.

- The hypertrophic zone has the highest content of glycolytic enzymes, and the chondrocytes participate in matrix mineralization through the synthesis of alkaline phosphatase, neutral proteases, and type X collagen.

- The hypertrophic zone is avascular.

3. Metaphysis

a. The metaphysis begins distal to the hypertrophic zone and removes the mineralized cartilaginous matrix of the hypertrophic zone.

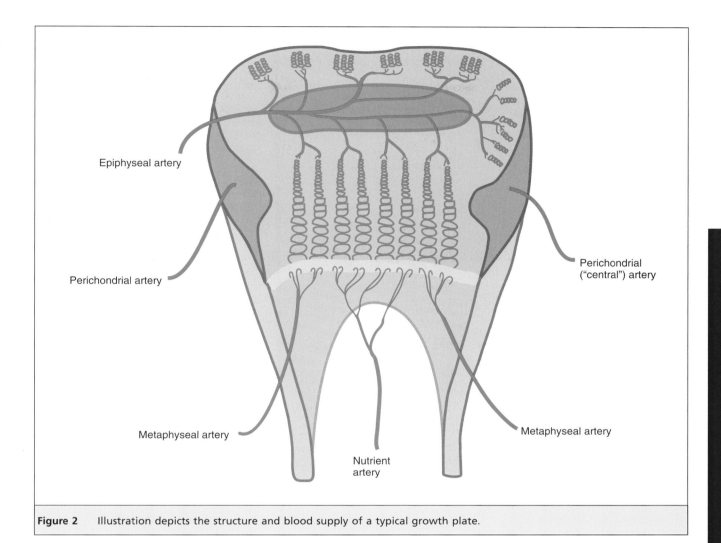

Figure 2   Illustration depicts the structure and blood supply of a typical growth plate.

b. The metaphysis is also involved in bone formation and the histologic remodeling of cancellous trabeculae.

c. The main nutrient artery of the long bone enters at the middiaphysis, then bifurcates and sends a branch within the medullary canal to each metaphysis.

d. The capillary loops of these arteries terminate at the bone-cartilage interface of the growth plate (**Figure 2**).

4. The periphery of the growth plate is surrounded by the groove of Ranvier and the perichondrial ring of LaCroix.

a. Three cell types are found in the groove of Ranvier: an osteoblast-type cell, a chondrocyte-type cell, and a fibroblast-type cell.

b. These cells are active in cell division and contribute to bone formation, latitudinal growth, and anchorage to the perichondrium.

c. The ring of LaCroix is a fibrous collagenous

network that is continuous with both the groove of Ranvier and the metaphysis. It functions as mechanical support at the bone-cartilage junction.

B. Biochemistry

1. Reserve zone

a. The reserve zone has the lowest intracellular and ionized calcium content

b. Oxygen tension is low in this zone.

2. Proliferative zone

a. Oxygen tension is highest in this zone, secondary to its rich vascular supply.

b. Abundant glycogen stores and a high oxygen tension support aerobic metabolism in the proliferative chondrocyte.

3. Hypertrophic zone

a. Oxygen tension in the hypertrophic zone is low, secondary to the avascular nature of the

1: Basic Science

Table 2

Skeletal Dysplasias Associated With Genetic Defects

Genetic Disorder	Genetic Mutation	Functional Defect	Characteristic Phenotypes
Achondroplasia	FGFR-3	Inhibition of chondrocyte proliferation	Short stature (skeletal dysplasia), normal- to large-size head, rhizomelic shortening of the limbs (especially the upper arm and thigh), a normal-size trunk
Thanatophoric dysplasia	FGFR-3	Inhibition of chondrocyte proliferation	Severe dwarfism (marked limb shortening, a small chest, and a relatively large head) Lethal after birth because of respiratory compromise
Hypochondroplasia	FGFR-3	Inhibition of chondrocyte proliferation	Milder dwarfism than achondroplasia
Pseudoachondroplasia	COMP	Abnormality of cartilage formation	Short stature (skeletal dysplasia) Rhizomelic limb shortening, similar body proportion as achondroplasia; lacks the distinct facial features characteristic of achondroplasia Early-onset osteoarthritis
Multiple epiphyseal dysplasia	COMP or type IX collagen	Abnormality of cartilage formation	Short stature (skeletal dysplasia) Early-onset osteoarthritis
Spondyloepiphyseal dysplasia	Type II collagen	Defect in cartilage matrix formation	Short stature (skeletal dysplasia), short trunk Spine malformation, coxa vara, myopia, and retinal degeneration
Diatrophic dysplasia	Sulfate transporter	Defect in sulfation of proteoglycan	Fraccato-type achondroplasia, dwarfism, hydrops fetalis
Schmid metaphyseal chondrodysplasia	Type X collagen	Defect in cartilage matrix formation	Short stature, coxa vara, genu varum, involvement in metaphyses of the long bones but not in the spine Less severe than in the Jansen type—none of the disorganized metaphyseal calcification that occurs in the Jansen type
Jansen metaphyseal chondrodysplasia	PTH/PTHrP receptor	Functional defect of PTH	Short limbs, characteristic facial abnormalities, and additional skeletal malformations Sclerotic bones in the back cranial bones, which may lead to blindness or deafness Hypercalcemia
Cleidocranial dysplasia	Runx2 (cbfa-1)	Impaired intramembranous ossification	Hypoplasia or aplasia of the clavicles, open skull suture, mild facial hypoplasia, wide symphysis pubis, mild short stature, dental abnormality, vertebral abnormality

COMP = cartilage oligomeric matrix protein; FGFR-3 = fibroblast growth factor receptor 3; PTH = parathyroid hormone; PTHrP = parathyroid hormone–related protein.

region. Because of this low oxygen tension, energy production in the hypertrophic zone occurs via anaerobic glycolysis of the glycogen stored in the proliferative zone.

b. In the upper hypertrophic zone, a switch from adenosine triphosphate production to calcium production occurs. After the glycogen stores have been depleted, calcium is released. This is the mechanism by which the matrix is calcified.

c. The region of the hypertrophic zone where mineralization occurs is known as the zone of provisional calcification.

d. Slipped capital femoral epiphysis (SCFE) involves hypertrophic zone abnormality.

4. Cartilage matrix turnover

a. Several enzymes are involved in cartilage matrix turnover, including metalloproteinases, which depend on the presence of calcium and zinc for activity. Collagenase, gelatinase, and stromelysin are produced by the growth plate chondrocytes in an inactive form and then activated by interleukin-1, plasmin, or tissue inhibitor of metalloproteinases.

b. The metaphysis (which is characterized by anaerobic metabolism, vascular stasis, and low oxygen tension, secondary to the limited blood supply to the region) removes the mineralized cartilage matrix as well as the unmineralized last transverse septum of the hypertrophic zone.

c. The unmineralized portion is removed via lysosomal enzymes, and the cartilaginous lacunae are invaded by endothelial and perivascular cells.

d. After the removal process is complete, osteoblasts begin the remodeling process, in which the osteoblasts progressively lay down bone on the cartilage template, creating an area of woven bone on a central core that is known as primary trabecular bone. The primary trabecular bone is resorbed via osteoclastic activity and replaced by lamellar bone, which represents the secondary bony trabeculae.

e. This remodeling process occurs around the periphery and subperiosteal regions of the metaphysis and results in funnelization, a narrowing of the diameter of the metaphysis to meet the diaphysis.

C. Pathophysiology

1. Overview

a. Most growth plate abnormalities can be attributed to a defect within a specific zone or to a particular malfunction in the system.

b. Most growth plate abnormalities affect the reserve zone; however, no evidence currently available suggests that any disease state originates from cytopathology unique to the reserve zone.

c. Any disease state that affects the matrix will have an impact on the proliferative zone.

2. Achondroplasia (**Table 2** and **Figure 3**)

a. Achondroplasia originates in the chondrocytes of the proliferative zone.

b. The disorder usually results from a single amino acid substitution, which causes a defect in fibroblast growth factor receptor 3 (FGFR-3).

3. Jansen metaphyseal chondrodysplasia

a. A mutation in the parathyroid hormone (PTH)–related protein (PTHrP) receptor affects the negative feedback loop in which PTHrP slows the conversion of proliferating chondrocytes to hypertrophic chondrocytes.

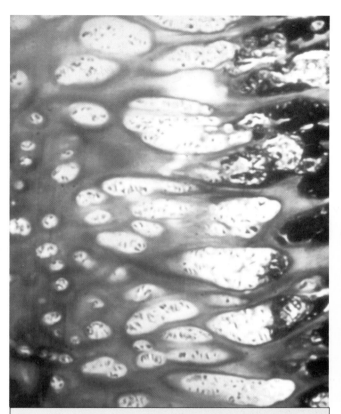

Figure 3   Histologic image shows the disorganized arrangement seen in achondroplasia. Compare this with the organized structure in **Figure 1**. (Reproduced from Iannotti JP, Goldstein S, Kuhn J, Lipiello L, Kaplan FS, Zaleske DJ: The formation and growth of skeletal tissues, in Buckwalter JA, Einhorn TA, Simon SR, eds: *Orthopaedic Basic Science: Biology and Biomechanics of the Musculoskeletal System*, ed 2. Rosemont, IL, American Academy of Orthopaedic Surgeons, 2000, p 103.)

b. The mutation in the receptor results in a continuously active state that is the molecular basis for Jansen metaphyseal chondrodysplasia. Because this receptor is the shared receptor for PTH, hypercalcemia and hypophosphatemia can occur.

D. Growth plate mineralization

1. Growth plate mineralization is a unique process because of the specialized blood supply to the growth plate, its unique energy metabolism, and its handling of intracellular calcium stores.

2. The major factors that affect growth plate mineralization are intracellular calcium homeostasis and the extracellular matrix vesicles and extracellular macromolecules. Various microenvironmental factors and systemic hormones also modulate this process.

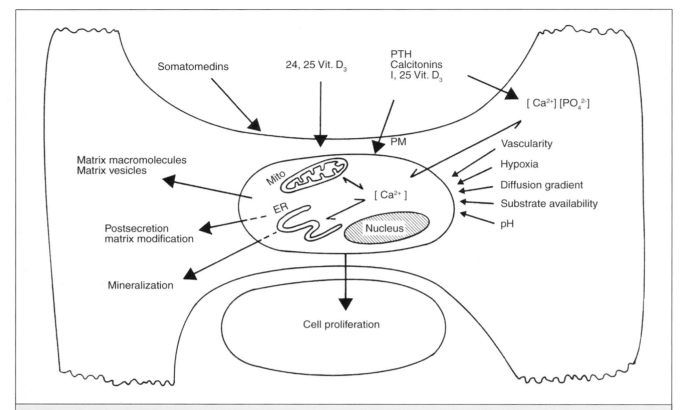

Figure 4   Illustration shows the factors influencing growth plate chondrocyte function and matrix mineralization. PTH = parathyroid hormone, ER = endoplasmic reticulum, PM = plasma membrane, Mito = mitochondria. (Adapted with permission from Iannotti JP: Growth plate physiology and pathology. *Orthop Clin North Am* 1990;21:1-17.)

a. Intracellular calcium

- The role of intracellular calcium in matrix mineralization is so important that the mitochondria in the chondrocytes are specialized for calcium transport.

- Compared with nonmineralizing cells, the chondrocyte mitochondria have a greater capacity for calcium accumulation and can store calcium in a labile form so that it can be used for release.

- Histologic studies have demonstrated that mitochondrial calcium accumulates in the upper two thirds of the hypertrophic zone and is depleted in the lower chondrocytes.

- When the mitochondrial calcium is released in the lower cells, matrix mineralization occurs (**Figure 4**).

b. Extracellular matrix vesicles

- The initial site for matrix calcification is unclear, although data exist to support the role of the matrix vesicle in this process.

- The matrix vesicles are rich in alkaline phosphatase and neutral proteases, which are critical in promoting mineralization.

c. Extracellular macromolecules

- Most of the collagen in the hypertrophic zone is type II; however, the terminal hypertrophic chondrocytes also produce and secrete type X collagen.

- The appearance of this collagen in the matrix initiates the onset of endochondral ossification.

III. Effects of Hormones and Growth Factors on the Growth Plate

A. Influence on growth plate mechanics

1. Hormones, growth factors, and vitamins have been shown to influence the growth plate through mechanisms such as chondrocyte proliferation and maturation, macromolecule synthesis, intracellular calcium homeostasis, and matrix mineralization.

2. Each growth plate zone may be targeted by one or more factors that help to mediate the cytologic characteristics unique to that zone. These factors

may be exogenous or endogenous to the growth plate.

 a. Paracrine factors are produced by the cell within the growth plate and act within the growth plate, but on another cell type.

 b. Autocrine factors act on the cells that produced them.

B. Thyroid hormones and PTH

 1. The thyroid hormones thyroxine (T4) and triiodothyronine (T3) act on the proliferative and upper hypertrophic zone chondrocytes through a systemic endocrine effect.

  a. T4 is essential for cartilage growth. It increases DNA synthesis in the cells of the proliferative zone and affects cell maturation by increasing glycosaminoglycan synthesis, collagen synthesis, and alkaline phosphatase activity.

  b. Excess T4 results in protein catabolism; a deficiency of T4 results in growth retardation, cretinism, and abnormal degradation of mucopolysaccharides.

 2. PTH also acts on the proliferative and upper hypertrophic zone chondrocytes.

  a. PTH has a direct mitogenic effect on epiphyseal chondrocytes. Furthermore, PTH stimulates proteoglycan synthesis through an increase in intracellular ionized calcium and the stimulation of protein kinase C.

  b. PTHrP is a cytokine with autocrine or paracrine action.

  c. The common PTHrP-PTH receptor has a role in the conversion of the small cell chondrocyte to the hypertrophic phenotype.

 3. Calcitonin is a peptide hormone that is produced by the parafollicular cells of the thyroid. It acts primarily in the lower hypertrophic zone to accelerate growth plate calcification and cell maturation.

C. Adrenal corticoids

 1. Adrenal corticoids, or glucocorticoids, are steroid hormones primarily produced by the adrenal cortex. These hormones primarily affect the zones of cellular differentiation and proliferation.

  a. The primary influence of the glucocorticoids is a decrease in proliferation of the chondroprogenitor cells in the zone of differentiation.

  b. Supraphysiologic amounts of these hormones result in growth retardation through a depression of glycolysis and a reduction of energy stores.

 2. Sex steroids (androgens) function as anabolic factors.

  a. The primary active androgen metabolite is postulated to be dihydrotestosterone, based on the presence of this receptor in both male and female growth plate tissue.

  b. The role of the androgens is to regulate mineralization in the lower part of the growth plate, increase the deposition of glycogen and lipids in cells, and increase the number of proteoglycans in the cartilage matrix.

D. Growth hormone (GH) and vitamins

 1. Growth hormone

  a. GH is produced by the pituitary gland and is essential for growth plate function. The effects of GH are mediated by the somatomedins, a group of peptide factors.

  b. When GH binds to epiphyseal chondrocytes, insulin-like growth factor 1 (IGF-1) is released locally. Therefore, GH regulates not only the number of cells containing the IGF receptor, but also the synthesis of IGF-1 in all zones of the growth plate.

 2. Vitamin D

  a. The active metabolites of vitamin D are the 1,25- and 24,25-dihydroxylated forms, both of which are produced by the liver and kidneys.

  b. A direct mitogenic effect has been reported with 24,25-dihydroxyvitamin D.

  c. The metabolite significantly increases DNA synthesis and inhibits proteoglycan synthesis.

  d. The level of vitamin D metabolites is highest in the proliferative zone; no metabolites are found in the hypertrophic zone.

 3. Vitamin A

  a. Vitamin A (carotenes) is essential for the metabolism of epiphyseal cartilage.

  b. A deficiency of vitamin A results in impairment of cell maturation, which ultimately causes abnormal bone shape.

  c. Excessive vitamin A leads to bone weakness secondary to increases in lysosomal body membrane fragility.

 4. Vitamin C is a cofactor in the enzymatic synthesis of collagen, and therefore it is necessary for the development of the growth plate.

IV. Biomechanics of the Growth Plate

A. Growth plate injury

 1. The weakest structure in the ends of the long bones is the growth plate, and the weakest region

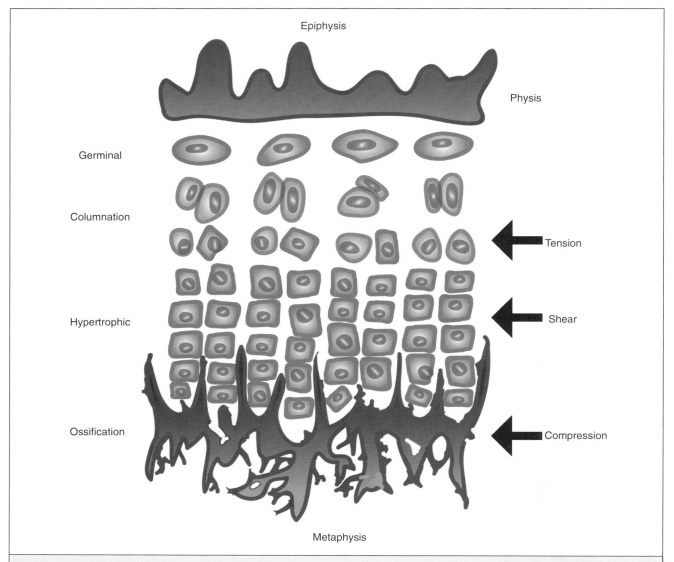

Epiphysis

Physis

Germinal

Columnation

Tension

Hypertrophic

Shear

Ossification

Compression

Metaphysis

Figure 5   Illustration shows how the histologic zone of failure varies with the type of load applied to the specimen.

within the growth plate itself is the hypertrophic zone. Although the perichondral ring provides some stability, shear forces are frequently high and can lead to fractures at the end of a long lever arm (thin, long extremities).

2. Growth plate injuries occur when the mechanical demands exceed the mechanical strength of the epiphysis–growth plate metaphysis complex.

3. The mechanical properties of the growth plate are described by the Hueter-Volkmann law, which states that increasing compression across a growth plate leads to decreasing growth (**Figure 5**).

B. Growth plate properties

1. The morphology of the growth plate allows it to adapt its form to follow the contours of principal

tensile stresses. The contours allow the growth plate to be subjected to compressive stress.

2. The tensile properties of the growth plate have been determined by controlled uniaxial tension tests in the bovine femur. The ultimate strain at failure has been shown to be uniform throughout the growth plate. The anterior and inferior regions of the growth plate are the strongest.

3. Mechanical forces can influence the shape and length of the growing bone, and studies have demonstrated that mechanical forces are present and can influence bone development during the earliest stages of endochondral ossification.

4. The biologic interface between the metaphyseal ossification front and the adjacent proliferative cartilage is partially determined by mechanical

Table 3

Genetic Abnormalities With Musculoskeletal Manifestations

Disease	Subtype	Inheritance Pattern	Affected Gene/Gene Product
Achondroplasia		AD	*FGRC-3*
Apert syndrome		AD	*FGRC-2*
Chondrodysplasia punctata		XLD	Unknown
Cleidocranial dysplasia		AD	Unknown
Diastrophic dysplasia		AR	Diastrophic dysplasia sulfate transporter
Hypochondroplasia		AD	*FGRC-3*
Kniest syndrome		AD	Type II collagen
Metaphyseal chondrodysplasia			
	Jansen type	AD	Parathyroid hormone–related peptide receptor
	McKusick type	AR	Unknown
	Schmid type	AD	Type X collagen
McCune-Albright syndrome		Unknown	Guanine nucleotide-binding protein alpha
Mucopolysaccharidosis			
	Type I (Hurler)	AR	α-L-iduronidase
	Type II (Hunter)	XLR	Sulfoiduronate sulfatase
	Type IV (Morquio)	AR	Galactosamine-6-sulfate sulfatase, β-galactosidase
Multiple epiphyseal dysplasia			
	Type I	AD	Cartilage oligomeric matrix protein
	Type II	AD	Type IX collagen
Nail-patella syndrome		AD	Unknown
Osteopetrosis		AR	Macrophage colony–stimulating factor
Pseudoachondroplasia		AD	Cartilage oligomeric matrix protein
Stickler syndrome		AD	Type II collagen
Spondyloepiphyseal dysplasia			
	Congenital	AD	Type II collagen
	Tarda	AR	Type II collagen
	X-linked	XLD	Unknown
Angelman syndrome		AR	Unknown
Dystrophinopathies			
	Duchenne muscular dystrophy	XLR	Dystrophin
	Becker muscular dystrophy	XLR	Dystrophin

(continued on next page)

1: Basic Science

Table 3

Genetic Abnormalities With Musculoskeletal Manifestations (*continued*)

Disease	Subtype	Inheritance Pattern	Affected Gene/Gene Product
Charcot-Marie-Tooth disease			
	Type IA	AD	Peripheral myelin protein 22
	Type IB	AD	Myelin protein zero
	Type IIA	AD	Unknown
	Type IVA	AR	Unknown
	X-linked	XL	Connexin 32
Friedreich ataxia		AR	Frataxin
Myotonic dystrophy		AD	Myotonin-protein kinase
Myotonia congenita		AD	Muscle chloride channel-1
Prader-Willi syndrome		AR	Unknown
Spinocerebellar ataxia			
	Type I	AD	Ataxin-1
	Type II	AD	*MJD/SCA1*
Spinal muscular atrophy		AR	Survival motor neuron
Ehlers-Danlos syndrome			
	Type IVA	AD	Type III collagen
	Type VI	AR	Lysine hydroxylase
	Type X	AR	Fibronectin-1
Marfan syndrome		AD	Fibrillin-1
Osteogenesis imperfecta			
	Type I	AD	Type I collagen (COL1A1, COL1A2)
	Type II	AR	Type I collagen (COL1A1, COL1A2)
	Type III	AR	Type I collagen (COL1A1, COL1A2)
	Type IVA	AD	Type I collagen (COL1A1, COL1A2)

AD = autosomal dominant, XLD = X-linked dominant, AR = autosomal recessive, XLR = X-linked recessive.

A portion of this table was adapted with permission from Dietz FR, Matthews KD: Update on the genetic bases of disorders with orthopaedic manifestations. *J Bone Joint Surg Am* 1996;78:1583-1598.

forces, initially in the form of muscle contractions.

5. The function of the growth plate and its mechanical properties appear to be influenced by both the internal structure and external mechanical factors.

V. Pathologic States Affecting the Growth Plate

A. Genetic disorders (**Tables 3** and **4**)

1. Cartilage matrix defects

a. All cartilage matrix defects produce some form of skeletal dysplasia, with varied degrees of ef-

Table 4

Genetic Defects Associated With Metabolic Bone Diseases

Genetic Disorder	Genetic Mutation	Functional Defect	Characteristic Phenotypes
X-linked hypophosphatemic rickets	Acellular endopeptidase	Vitamin D–resistant rickets	Rickets, short stature, and impaired renal phosphate reabsorption and vitamin D metabolism
Hypophosphatasia	Alkaline phosphatase gene	Generalized impairment of skeletal mineralization	Rickets, bowed leg, loss of teeth, short stature
MPS type I	α-L-iduronidase	Deficiency of α-L-iduronidase (lysosomal enzymes for breaking glycosaminoglycans)	Hurler syndrome; progressive cellular damage that affects the development of neurologic and musculoskeletal system (short stature and bone dysplasia)
MPS type II	Iduronate sulfatase; X-linked recessive	Deficiency of iduronate sulfatase	Hunter syndrome; mild to moderate features of MPS
MPS type III	Heparan N-sulfatase or N-acetylglucosamine 6-sulfatase	Deficiency of heparan N-sulfatase (IIIA); α-N-acetylglucosaminidase (IIIB); acetyl coenzyme A: α-glucosaminide N-acetyltransferase (IIIC); N-acetylglucosamine 6-sulfatase (IIID)	Sanfilippo syndrome; severe neurologic syndrome with mild progressive musculoskeletal syndrome
MPS type IV	Deficient enzymes N-acetylgalactosamine 6-sulfatase (type A) or β-galactosidase (type B)	Deficiency of lysosomal enzymes for breaking keratin sulfate	Morquio syndrome: bell-shaped chest, anomaly of spine, shortened long bones, and dysplasia of the hips, knees, ankles, and wrists Odontoid hypoplasia

MPS = mucopolysaccharidosis.

fect on articular and growth plate cartilage.

  b. Abnormalities of type II collagen cause Kniest dysplasia and some types of Stickler syndrome and spondyloepiphyseal dysplasia.

  c. Abnormalities of type IX collagen cause some forms of multiple epiphyseal dysplasia.

  d. Defects in type X collagen cause the Schmidt-type metaphyseal chondrodysplasia.

2. Diastrophic dysplasia

  a. Diastrophic dysplasia is a classic example of a defect in proteoglycan metabolism.

  b. The disorder is caused by a mutation in the sulfate transporter molecule, which results in undersulfation of the proteoglycan matrix.

  c. The phenotype is short stature and characteristic severe equinovarus feet.

3. Mucopolysaccharidoses

  a. Mucopolysaccharidoses are six disorders that result from defects in the proteoglycan metabolism (**Table 3**).

  b. These disorders are caused by a defect in the enzymes involved in proteoglycan metabolism with a resultant accumulation of undegraded glycosaminoglycans (**Table 4**).

  c. The clinical presentation of each mucopolysaccharidosis depends on the specific enzyme defect and the resultant glycoprotein accumulation.

  d. Common to all six disease states is a toxic effect on the central nervous system, the skeleton, or the ocular or visceral system.

4. Metabolic mineralization disorders

  a. Hypophosphatasia is an autosomal recessive defect in alkaline phosphatase (characteristic laboratory finding) with resultant normal serum levels of calcium and phosphate but an inability of the matrix to calcify. The hypertrophic zone widens, but no mineralization occurs in the osteoid that is laid down. The zone of provisional calcification never forms. The histologic appearance and effect are similar to nutritional rickets, with a resultant inhibition of growth.

1: Basic Science

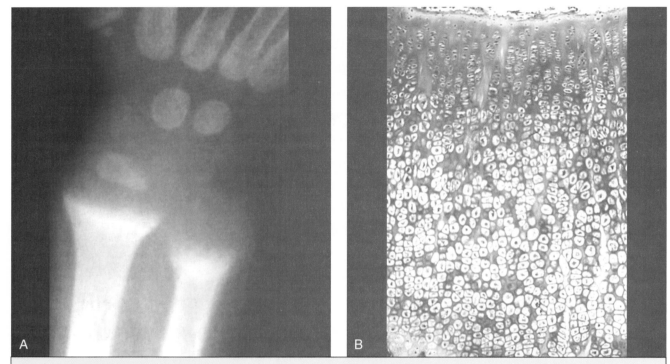

Figure 6   **A,** PA view of the wrist of a child demonstrates radiographic features of rickets in the distal radius and ulna. Note the widened growth plates and flaring of the metaphyses. **B,** The histologic features of rickets are seen in this specimen. Note that the zone of proliferation is largely unaffected, but the hypertrophic zone is markedly widened. (Courtesy of Dr. Henry J. Mankin, Brookline, MA.)

   b. Hypophosphatemic familial rickets is a sex-linked dominant disorder characterized by low serum calcium and phosphorus. Alkaline phosphatase activity is high, with resultant abnormal conversion of vitamin D to its metabolites. The skeletal changes seen are those typical of nutritional rickets, which is discussed below.

B. Environmental factors

  1. Infection

    a. Bacterial infection typically affects the metaphyseal portion of the growth plate. This is due to the slow circulation, low oxygen tension, and deficiency of the reticuloendothelial system in this area.

    b. Bacteria become lodged in the vascular sinusoids, resulting in the production of small abscesses in the area.

    c. If the infection extends into the Haversian canals, osteomyelitis of the cortical bone ensues, with associated subperiosteal abscess.

    d. In the first year of life, cartilage canals may persist across growth plates and serve as an additional conduit for the spread of infection. Severe infection may cause local or total cessation of growth; in most instances, inhibited or angular growth results.

  2. Irradiation—Depending on the dose, irradiation can result in shortened bones with increased width as a result of the preferential effect of irradiation on longitudinal chondroblastic proliferation, with sparing of latitudinal bone growth.

C. Nutritional disorders

  1. Nutritional rickets

    a. Nutritional rickets results from the abnormal processing of calcium, phosphorus, and vitamin D.

    b. The common result is failure to mineralize the matrix in the zone of provisional calcification.

    c. The hypertrophic zone is expanded greatly, with widening of the growth plate and flaring of the metaphysis noted on plain radiographs (**Figure 6**).

  2. Scurvy

    a. Caused by vitamin C deficiency, scurvy results in a decrease in chondroitin sulfate and collagen synthesis.

    b. The greatest deficiency in collagen synthesis is seen in the metaphysis, where the demand for type I collagen is highest during new bone formation.

c. Characteristic radiographic findings of scurvy are the Frankel line (a transverse dense white line that represents the zone of provisional calcification) and osteopenia of the metaphysis.

d. Clinical findings include microfractures, hemorrhages, and collapse of the metaphysis.

Top Testing Facts

1. Formation of the bony skeleton occurs via either intramembranous bone formation or endochondral bone formation. Intramembranous bone formation occurs through osteoblast activity; endochondral ossification occurs at the growth plates and within fracture callus.

2. In the primary center of ossification, bloodborne precursors of osteoblasts and osteoclasts are delivered by the capillaries. This process signals the transition from the embryonic to the fetal period and first occurs at the humerus.

3. The total length of the growth plate depends on the number of cell divisions of the progenitor cell.

4. The region of the hypertrophic zone, where mineralization occurs, is known as the zone of provisional calcification.

5. SCFE and fractures through the growth plate typically occur in the hypertrophic zone.

6. The genetic mutation in achondroplasia is a defect in FGFR-3.

7. Growth plate injuries occur when the mechanical demands of bone exceed the strength of the epiphysis–growth plate metaphysis complex. The Hueter-Volkmann law states that increasing compression across the growth plate leads to decreased growth (eg, Blount disease).

8. Diastrophic dysplasia is a defect in proteoglycan sulfation.

9. Bacterial infection affects the metaphyseal portion of the growth plate.

10. Scurvy is caused by a vitamin C deficiency with a resultant decrease in chondroitin sulfate and collagen synthesis.

Acknowledgments

The author wishes to recognize the work of Drs. Kelley Banagan and Thorsten Kirsch for their contribution to the *AAOS Comprehensive Orthopaedic Review* and this chapter.

Bibliography

Blair HC, Robinson LJ, Huang CL, et al: Calcium and bone disease. *Biofactors* 2011;37(3):159-167.

Colnot C: Cellular and molecular interactions regulating skeletogenesis. *J Cell Biochem* 2005;95(4):688-697.

DiGirolamo DJ, Kiel DP, Esser KA: Bone and skeletal muscle: Neighbors with close ties. *J Bone Miner Res* 2013;28(7):1509-1518.

Lazar L, Phillip M: Pubertal disorders and bone maturation. *Endocrinol Metab Clin North Am* 2012;41(4):805-825.

Mäkitie O: Molecular defects causing skeletal dysplasias. *Endocr Dev* 2011;21:78-84.

Pacifici M : The development and growth of the skeleton, in O'Keefe RJ, Jacobs JJ, Chu CR, Einhorn TA, eds: *Orthopaedic Basic Science: Foundations of Clinical Practice*, ed 4. Rosemont, IL, American Academy of Orthopaedic Surgeons, 2013, pp 135-148.

Provot S, Schipani E: Molecular mechanisms of endochondral bone development. *Biochem Biophys Res Commun* 2005; 328(3):658-665.

Schmitt CP, Mehls O: Mineral and bone disorders in children with chronic kidney disease. *Nat Rev Nephrol* 2011;7(11): 624-634.

Shimizu H, Yokoyama S, Asahara H: Growth and differentiation of the developing limb bud from the perspective of chondrogenesis. *Dev Growth Differ* 2007;49(6):449-454.

Staines KA, Pollard AS, McGonnell IM, Farquharson C, Pitsillides AA: Cartilage to bone transitions in health and disease. *J Endocrinol* 2013;219(1):R1-R12.

White KK: Orthopaedic aspects of mucopolysaccharidoses. *Rheumatology (Oxford)* 2011;50(Suppl 5):v26-v33.

1: Basic Science

Chapter 3

Musculoskeletal Infections and Microbiology

Gary Miller, MD

1: Basic Science

I. Infection Burden: Epidemiology

A. Microbiology of musculoskeletal infection

1. The most common pathogens in musculoskeletal infections and their suggested empiric therapies are outlined in **Table 1**.

2. *Staphylococcus aureus* is the organism responsible for most musculoskeletal infections, followed by *Staphylococcus epidermidis* and related coagulase-negative *Staphylococcus* species. *Enterococcus* species and *Escherichia coli* are less prevalent.

3. Differences in genetic strain and virulence are demonstrable between community-acquired methicillin-resistant *S aureus* (MRSA) and hospital-acquired MRSA. The line between the two is becoming indistinct.

4. Septic arthritis

   a. Pathogens in septic arthritis vary with patient age. *S aureus*, *Streptococcus* species, and *Neisseria gonorrhoeae* show a high affinity for synovium. Aerobic gram-negative bacilli such as *E coli* rarely infect synovium.

   b. Among all ages and risk categories, with the exception of children younger than 4 years, *S aureus* is the most frequent pathogen.

   c. *Streptococcus* species are the next most common pathogens in adults.

   • *Streptococcus pyogenes* (Group A) is most often isolated.

   • Group B *Streptococcus* (*Streptococcus agalactiae*) has a predilection for infirm, elderly, particularly diabetic patients.

   • Group D *Streptococcus* species have been reclassified as *Enterococcus*. *Enterococcus* species uncommonly cause septic arthritis.

   d. Gram-negative cocci

   • Account for 20% of septic arthritis

   • *N gonorrhoeae* and *Neisseria meningitidis* are the most common.

   • *N gonorrhoeae* is the most frequent causative organism of septic knee arthritis in young, sexually active patients.

   • Gonococcal arthritis manifests as a bacteremic infection (arthritis-dermatitis syndrome; 60% of cases) or as a localized septic arthritis (40%).

   • Arthritis-dermatitis syndrome includes the triad of dermatitis, tenosynovitis, and migratory or additive polyarthritis. Skin lesions, found in 75% of cases, are small erythematous papules that may progress to pustules.

   • Urethral specimens demonstrating polymorphonuclear (PMN) leukocytes with intracellular gram-negative diplococci are diagnostic for infection with *N gonorrhoeae* in symptomatic men.

   • *N meningitides* is underestimated as a cause of septic arthritis. Concomitant septic arthritis occurs in 11% of meningococcemia cases.

   e. Gram-negative bacilli

   • Account for 10% to 20% of septic arthritis

   • Common pathogens include *E coli, Proteus, Klebsiella*, and *Enterobacter*.

   • Most often affect neonates, intravenous (IV) drug abusers, and elderly, immunocompromised patients with diabetes

   f. Although *S aureus* is the most common infectious agent in IV drug users, such patients are highly susceptible to *Pseudomonas, Serratia*, mixed bacterial, and fungal infections.

Neither Dr. Miller nor any immediate family member has received anything of value from or has stock or stock options held in a commercial company or institution related directly or indirectly to the subject of this chapter.

Table 1

Most Common Pathogens and Suggested Empiric Antibiotic Therapy in Musculoskeletal Infections

Infection and Clinical Setting	Most Common Pathogens	Empiric Antibiotic Therapy
Osteomyelitis and septic arthritis		
Infant	Staphylococcus aureus Streptococcus pyogenes Streptococcus pneumoniae Streptococcus agalactiae Gram-negative organisms	Penicillinase-resistant penicillin and aminoglycoside or ceftriaxone
Child < 3 years	S aureus S pneumoniae S pyogenes Kingella kingae	Ceftriaxone
Older child	S aureus	Cefazolin or penicillinase-resistant penicillin
Child with sickle cell disease	Salmonella species S aureus	Ceftriaxone
Adult	S aureus Suspected MRSA	Penicillinase-resistant penicillin Vancomycin plus ceftriazone
Immunocompromised adult or child	Gram-positive cocci Gram-negative organisms	Penicillinase-resistant penicillin and aminoglycoside
Septic arthritis in sexually active patients	S aureus Neisseria gonorrhoeae	Ceftriaxone
Diskitis	S aureus	Penicillinase-resistant penicillin
Lyme disease	Borrelia burgdorferi	Amoxicillin-doxycycline
Clenched-fist bite wounds	Eikenella corrodens Staphylococcus species Streptococcus viridans Anaerobes	Ampicillin-sulbactam or piperacillin-tazobactam
Nail puncture wounds	S aureus Pseudomonas aeruginosa	Penicillinase-resistant penicillin and aminoglycoside or piperacillin-tazobactam
Necrotizing fasciitis	Streptococcus group A beta-hemolytic MRSA Gram-positive cocci, anaerobes ± gram-negative organisms	Penicillin or Ampicillin-sulbactum plus clindamycin ± Ciprofloxacin OR Vancomycin plus Clindamycin ± aminoglycoside

MRSA = methicillin-resistant *Staphylococcus aureus*.

Reproduced from Patzakis MJ, Zalavras C: Infection, in Vaccaro AR, ed: *Orthopaedic Knowledge Update*, ed 8. Rosemont, IL, American Academy of Orthopaedic Surgeons, 2005, pp 217-228.

g. *Kingella kingae*

- *K kingae* is a slow-growing gram-negative coccobacillus normally colonizing the oropharynx of many children.

- *K kingae* causes infection in children between 6 months and 4 years of age. *K kingae* is the single most common bacterial cause of osteoarticular infections in children younger than age 4 years, causing far more cases of septic arthritis than osteomyelitis.

- Clinical presentation is subtle and may be associated with normal levels of acute-phase reactants.

- Gram stains of joint aspirates often fail to reveal *K kingae*, and the organism is difficult to grow on standard media.

- Empiric selection of clindamycin for the treatment of the young child with acute hematogenous osteomyelitis (AHO) would cover most gram-positive organisms, but offer no activity against *K kingae*.

h. For decades, *Haemophilus influenzae* was the

Table 2

Microoganisms Isolated From Patients With Bacterial Osteomyelitis

Microorganism	Most Common Clinical Association
Staphylococcus aureus (susceptible or resistant to methicillin)	Most frequent microorganism in any type of osteomyelitis
Coagulase-negative staphylococci or propionibacterium	Foreign-body–associated infection
Enterobacteriaceae or *Pseudomonas aeruginosa*	Nosocomial infections, injection drug users
Streptococci or anaerobic bacteria	Animal and human bites, diabetic foot lesions, and decubitus ulcers
Salmonella or *Streptococcus pneumoniae*	Sickle cell disease
Bartonella henselae	HIV infection
Pasteurella multocida	Cat/dog bites
Eikenella corrodens	Human bites
Aspergillus, Mycobacterium avium complex, or *Candida albicans*	Immunocompromised patients
Mycobacterium tuberculosis	Populations in which tuberculosis is prevalent
Brucella, Coxiella burnetii (chronic Q fever), or other fungi found in specific geographic areas	Populations in which these pathogens are endemic

Adapted from Gross JM, Schwarz EM: Infections in orthopaedics, in Einhorn TA, O'Keefe RJ, Buckwalter JA, eds: *Orthopaedic Basic Science*, ed 3. Rosemont, IL, American Academy of Orthopaedic Surgeons, 2007, pp 299-314.

predominant cause of septic arthritis in children younger than 3 years. Since the advent of *Haemophilus influenzae* type B vaccine, this pathogen has been superseded by *Kingella*.

5. Osteomyelitis (**Table 2**)

   a. Across all age groups, the most common cause of osteomyelitis is *S aureus*.

   b. Community-aquired MRSA is associated with a longer treatment course and an increased risk of subperiosteal and deep abscess formation, deep vein thrombosis (DVT), and septic pulmonary emboli than is methicillin-sensitive *S aureus* (MSSA).

   c. *Salmonellae* are the most prevalent bacterial pathogens of osteomyelitis in patients with sickling hemoglobinopathies in the United States. The worldwide prevalence of *Salmonellae* in this population may be waning, whereas that of *S aureus* is increasing.

6. Shoulder surgery poses an increased risk of infection with *Propionibacterium acnes*, a slow-growing gram-positive rod.

7. Foot puncture wounds are predisposed to infection by *Pseudomonas*.

II. Pathophysiology of Musculoskeletal Infection

A. Pathogenesis

   1. Inoculation of the microorganism

      a. Synovium has no limiting basement membrane, allowing microorganisms to more readily enter synovial fluid.

      b. Surgical site infection (SSI) risk increases when a surgical site is contaminated with more than 10^5 microorganisms per gram of tissue. The size of the inoculum may be considerably smaller in the presence of foreign material such as sutures or implants.

   2. Virulence—*S aureus* may be protected from host immune defenses by several mechanisms.

      a. Excretion of protein A, which inactivates immunoglobulin G antibodies

      b. Production of a capsular polysaccharide, which reduces opsonization and phagocytosis

      c. A biofilm secluding the organisms from host defenses; a biofilm is a community of bacterial cells (15%) embedded in a self-generated protein-polysaccharide complex (85%) referred to as extracellular polymeric substance (**Figure 1**).

      d. Panton-Valentine leukocidin (PVL) is a cytotoxin that lyses white blood cells (WBCs)

1: Basic Science

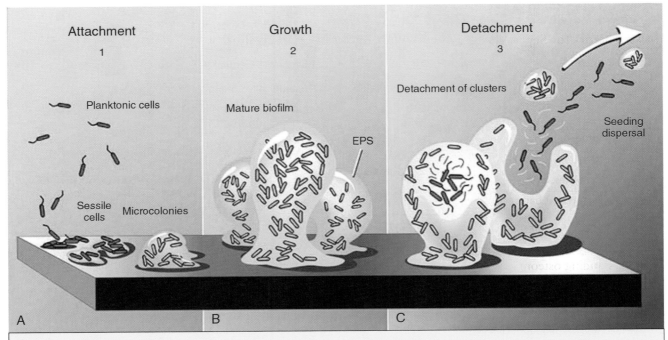

Figure 1   Illustration depicts the development of a biofilm. Bacteria in a biofilm produce a complex matrix of extracellular polymers that promote surface attachment and provide protection for the colony. Biofilm evolution entails three stages: attachment (**A**), growth of colonies (**B**), and periodic dispersal of planktonic (floating) cells (**C**). EPS = extracellular polymeric substance. (Copyright Peg Dirckx, Montana State University, Center for Biofilm Engineering, Bozeman, MT.)

and causes tissue necrosis. The presence of Panton-Valentine leukocidin may be associated with an increased virulence of certain strains of *S aureus*. PVL is produced far more commonly by community-acquired than by hospital-acquired MRSA.

B. Biofilm infections

1. Most bacterial infections are caused by organisms growing in biofilms. The formation of adherent, multilayered biofilms is central to the pathogenesis of medical device–associated infections.

2. A biofilm strongly adheres to an inert or biologic surface. The biofilm is remarkably resistant to shear, hence difficult to dislodge. Because extracellular polymeric substance is not water soluble, irrigation is inadequate to remove biofilm.

3. Bacteria in biofilms may display resistance to antibiotic concentrations two to three orders of magnitude higher than the minimum inhibitory concentration for planktonic bacteria.

4. Biofilms display mechanisms for spreading along colonized surfaces.

5. Biofilm infections may be indolent, displaying few signs of inflammation.

6. Fluid aspirates of biofilm diseases often yield negative cultures.

7. Infected biomaterials and their adherent biofilms must be completely removed by surgery before infection can be eradicated.

III. Clinical Presentation

A. History and physical examination—The clinical presentation of musculoskeletal infection varies based on patient age, chronicity, virulence, variability among bacterial strains, biofilm formation, host viability and immune status, site, previous treatment, and circulation.

B. Septic arthritis in adults

1. Risk factors for septic arthritis are listed in **Table 3**.

2. Septic arthritis is most often monoarticular. The knee is affected in 50% of cases, followed by, in decreasing order, the hip, shoulder, and elbow.

3. Unusual locations, such as sacroiliac and sternoclavicular joints, are affected more often in parenteral drug users.

4. Symptoms suggestive of systemic infection may be lacking. Only 60% of patients are febrile at presentation.

C. Osteomyelitis in adults—Malignant squamous cell carcinoma transformation of chronic osteomyelitis

Table 3

Risk Factors for Septic Arthritis

Age > 80 years
Medical conditions: diabetes mellitus, rheumatoid arthritis, cirrhosis
Recent joint surgery
Parenteral drug abuse
HIV-1 infection
Prior joint problems: crystal disease
Endocarditis or recent bactermia

in sinus tracts is rare. Degeneration develops in long-standing osteomyelitis, usually between 20 and 40 years into disease. Onset of new bleeding or other changes in a sinus tract warrant biopsy. A radical surgical approach to the treatment of squamous cell carcinoma arising within a sinus tract is advised.

D. Pediatric patients

1. Septic arthritis

   a. Consequences of the delayed diagnosis of septic arthritis are profound; extensive cartilage damage can develop within hours.

   b. Neonates and infants with septic arthritis present a more deceptive clinical picture than children. Features such as irritability and failure to thrive are nonspecific.

   c. In infants, septic arthritis of the hip produces a flexed, abducted, externally rotated position to accommodate increased joint volume.

   d. Transient synovitis is the most common cause of acute hip pain in children aged 3 to 10 years. Distinction between septic arthritis and transient synovitis in a child with an acutely irritable hip is challenging. A clinical prediction rule based on four independent factors for hip septic arthritis has been validated.

   - History of fever

   - Refusal to bear weight

   - Erythrocyte sedimentation rate (ESR) greater than 40

   - Peripheral WBC count greater than 12,000

   - Diagnostic accuracy ranges between 73% and 93% if three predictors are present.

2. Osteomyelitis

   a. *S aureus* is the most common pathogen in pediatric AHO.

   b. An algorithm for distinguishing between

MRSA and MSSA osteomyelitis in children has identified four important independent multivariate predictors.

- Temperature higher than 38°C

- Hematocrit less than 34%

- Peripheral WBC count greater than 12,000 cells/µL

- C-reactive protein (CRP) level greater than 13 mg/L.

   c. The probability of MRSA osteomyelitis was 92% for all four predictors, 45% for three, 10% for two, 1% for one, and 0% for zero predictors.

   d. Hematogenous osteomyelitis is far more common in children than adults. The initial site of infection is metaphyseal, owing to an abundant vascular supply and the presence of large sinusoids at the epiphyseal-metaphyseal junction.

   e. The physis serves a protective function, impeding infection from entering the epiphysis and (in nonarticular physes) the joint until physeal closure. In the proximal femur, proximal humerus, distal lateral tibia, distal fibula, and proximal radius, the joint capsule attaches to the metaphysis. In these joints, hematogenous osteomyelitis may decompress directly into the articulation.

   f. Because transphyseal vessels persist until about 12 to 18 months of age, osteomyelitis in the infant can spread rapidly into the epiphysis and adjacent articulation. Osteomyelitis in the neonate is multifocal in 40% of patients.

   g. Musculoskeletal infection in children predisposes to the development of DVT and septic pulmonary emboli. Children older than 8 years who have MRSA osteomyelitis and in whom CRP at presentation exceeds 6 mg/dL exhibit a 40% incidence of DVT.

IV. Diagnostic Evaluation

A. Radiographic findings

1. Joint space changes occur early in pyogenic arthritis; late with more indolent infections such as tuberculous arthritis.

2. Radiologic findings in early septic arthritis are joint effusion, soft-tissue swelling, and periarticular osteopenia. The joint space may appear widened in young children because of joint laxity. As cartilage destruction ensues, the space becomes uniformly narrow. The absence of sclerosis and osteophytes distinguish infection from degenerative arthropathy.

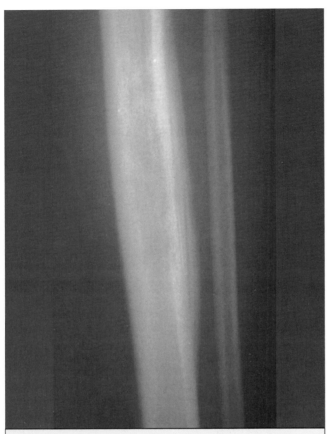

Figure 2   AP radiograph shows a lamellated or "onion skin" periosteal reaction along the tibial diaphysis in a 23-year-old woman with osteomyelitis. Rapidly growing processes may exceed the capacity of periosteum to respond. Rather than produce solid new bone, the periosteum may generate a series of concentric shells in an interrupted pattern. (Reproduced with permission from Roche CJ, O'Keeffe DP, Lee WK, Duddalwar VA, Torreggiani WC, Curtis JM: Selections from the buffet of food signs in radiology. *Radiographics* 2002;22[6]:1369-1384.)

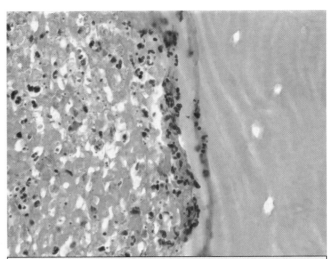

Figure 3   Hematoxylin-eosin stain shows histology of acute suppurative osteomyelitis. At right, necrotic trabecular bone features lacunae devoid of osteocytes. The adjoining fatty marrow has been replaced by a polymorphous infiltrate of fibrin and leukocytes, predominantly neutrophils. (Reproduced with permission from Pathorama, Zurich, Switzerland. http://alf3.urz.unibas.ch/pathopic/e/getpic-fra.cfm?id=8234. Accessed December 2, 2013.)

3. Tuberculous arthritis features the Phemister triad.

   a. Prominent periarticular osteoporosis

   b. Gradual narrowing of joint space

   c. Ill-defined peripheral erosions

4. Plain radiographic features of osteomyelitis, such as periosteal elevation, typically are not visible before 10 to 14 days of illness. Changes in flat bones and the spine may take longer to appear.

5. Bone loss of 30% to 40% is required before bone destruction becomes visible on plain radiographs.

6. Acute osteomyelitis may produce a periosteal reaction (**Figure 2**).

   a. Presentations of eosinophilic granuloma, Ewing sarcoma, and acute osteomyelitis in appropriately aged patients (first 2 decades of life) mimic one another. All three diseases may present with pain, fever, local tenderness, leukocytosis, and elevated ESR. Both osteomyelitis and Ewing sarcoma may exhibit a lamellated periosteal reaction. CT or MRI of these lesions may reveal a soft-tissue mass.

   b. Histopathology differentiates among these diagnoses.

   • Acute osteomyelitis—Replacement of fatty marrow by a polymorphous field of PMNs, lymphocytes, and plasma cells (**Figure 3**).

   • Eosinophilic granuloma (EOG)—Mixed inflammatory infiltrate featuring Langerhans histiocytes (**Figure 4**).

   • Ewing sarcoma—Monomorphous (**Figure 5**) lesion composed of small, round, blue tumor cells. In contrast to EOG, Ewing typically has a soft-tissue extension from the bony lesion. Osteomyelitis may be accompanied by a soft-tissue mass (abscess).

7. Osteomyelitis may display a Codman triangle (**Figure 6**).

8. Subacute osteomyelitis

   a. Subacute disease features an insidious onset with mild symptoms. The ESR and WBC count are variable, and blood cultures are often negative.

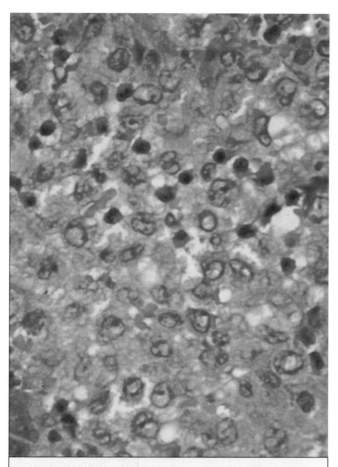

Figure 4 Hematoxylin-eosin stain shows eosinophilic granuloma histology. Fatty marrow is replaced by a polymorphous proliferation of Langerhans histiocytes accompanied by eosinophils, lymphocytes, and scattered plasma cells. (Copyright Bonetumor.org, Newton, MA. http://www. bonetumor.org/eosinophilic-granuloma-pathology-40x. Accessed December 2, 2013.)

b. Subacute osteomyelitis may mimic various benign and malignant conditions, resulting in delayed diagnosis and treatment.

9. Brodie abscess

a. Brodie abscess is a form of subacute osteomyelitis. The disease has an insidious onset, mild symptoms, and no systemic reaction.

b. Radiographic features are protean but often feature a radiolucent area with a thick rim of sclerotic-appearing bone. The distal tibial metaphysis is the most common location. A lucent tortuous channel extending toward the growth plate before physeal closure is characteristic (**Figure 7**).

c. The appearance of a cortical Brodie abscess may mimic that of osteoid osteoma. Also in the differential are intracortical hemangioma and stress fracture. The presence of a sinus tract distinguishes a Brodie abscess.

B. CT

1. CT may reveal gas adjacent to fascial planes, decreased density of infected bone, and soft-tissue masses.

2. An abscess appears on CT as a heterogeneous fluid collection with thick margins that enhance after administration of IV contrast.

C. MRI

1. MRI can detect subtle marrow changes associated with very early osteomyelitis with almost 100% sensitivity. Standard sequences may include a combination of T1-weighted, T2-weighted, and/or short tau inversion recovery or T2-weighted sequences with chemical fat suppression.

1: Basic Science

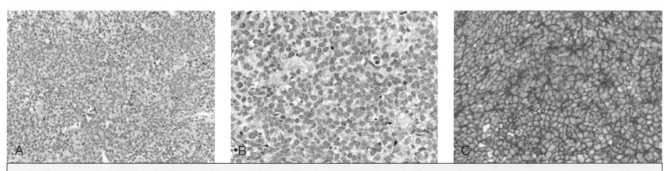

Figure 5 Hematoxylin-eosin stain shows the histologic and immunohistochemical features of Ewing sarcoma. **A,** Ewing sarcoma appears as a monomorphous infiltrate of small, round, blue cells. **B,** Tumor cells have scant cytoplasm and round nuclei with evenly distributed chromatin and inconspicuous nucleoli. **C,** Strong, diffuse membrane staining is seen, with O13 monoclonal antibody to p30/32MIC2 (CD99). O13 detects a cell surface antigen expressed in 95% of Ewing sarcomas. (Reproduced with permission from Bernstein M, Kovar H, Paulussen M, et al: Ewing sarcoma family of tumors: Current management. *Oncologist* 2006;11[5]:503-519.)

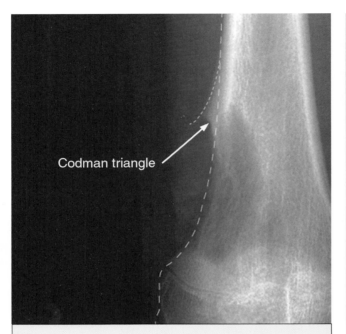

Figure 6 AP radiograph shows a Codman triangle. Some lesions grow too rapidly for the periosteum to respond with even thin shells of new bone; only the edges of the raised periosteum have time to ossify. Seen tangentially on radiographs, the reactive bone forms an angle with the bone surface. This layer of reactive bone at the lesion's margin is termed the Codman triangle. (Courtesy of Andrew Dixon, MD and Behrang Amini, MD. http://radiopaedia.org/articles/codman_triangle_periosteal_reaction. Accessed December 2, 2013.)

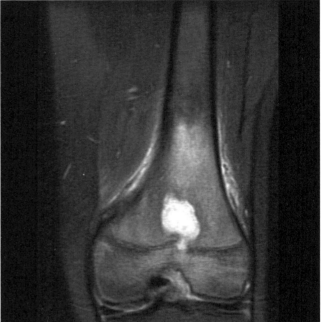

Figure 7 T2-weighted MRI depicts a Brodie abscess. Radiographic features of this form of subacute osteomyelitis vary. When found, a tortuous channel extending toward the growth plate before physeal closure is characteristic. On plain radiographs, this is referred to as the "serpentine sign," described by Letts. (Courtesy of John C. Hunter, MD, Henry Knipe, MD, and Frank Gaillard, MD, UC Davis Department of Radiology. http://radiopaedia.org/articles/brodie-abscess-1. Accessed December 2, 2013.)

2. Classic findings

   a. Signal intensity change due to increased edema and water content

   b. Reduction in T1 marrow signal intensity is a primary sign of osteomyelitis. This is accompanied by an increase in T2 signal intensity. T2-weighted and short tau inversion recovery images have an increased signal intensity because fatty marrow has been replaced by inflammation.

   c. MRI features of septic arthritis include effusion, synovial thickening, bone erosions, marrow edema, and, most typically, synovial enhancement after administration of contrast.

   d. Rim enhancement after administration of IV gadolinium is typical, although not pathognomonic, of infection. MRI shows an area of decreased density surrounded by a bright rim from enhancing contrast.

3. The "penumbra sign" on unenhanced T1-weighted images is characteristic, although not pathognomonic, of subacute osteomyelitis. The zone rimming a bone abscess exhibits intermedi-

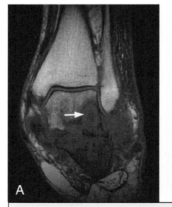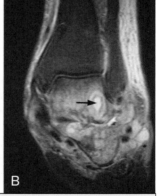

Figure 8 Coronal MRIs show the penumbra sign in subacute osteomyelitis. **A,** T1-weighted hindfoot image shows an intermediate signal rim (arrow) around a central area of lower signal intensity, suggesting an intraosseous abscess in the talus. **B,** Short tau inversion recovery image demonstrates the talar abscess (arrow). (Reproduced with permission from Tan PL, Teh J: The MRI of the diabetic foot: Differentiation of infection from neuropathic change. *Br J Radiol* 2007; 80[959]:939-948.)

ate signal intensity compared with the cavity itself and the surrounding lower-intensity reactive bone (**Figure 8**).

D. Blood tests

1. CRP and ESR measure acute-phase response markers elevated in infection and/or inflammation.

   a. ESR is an indirect measure and is affected by a variety of factors. Normal ESR values increase with age and vary among laboratories; however, an ESR of 30 mm/h is generally accepted as the upper limit of normal.

   b. CRP is a direct measure of acute-phase reaction, is age-independent, and displays a more rapid response. CRP of 10 mg/L is generally accepted as the upper limit of normal.

   c. Absence of an acute-phase response does not exclude septic arthritis.

   d. ESR remains elevated 6 weeks or longer after surgery; CRP normalizes within 2 to 3 weeks.

   e. Within hours of infection, CRP values increase up to 400 mg/L and peak within 48 hours. CRP may normalize within 1 week of treatment.

   f. ESR rises within 2 days of the onset of infection, increases for 3 to 5 days after treatment begins, and normalizes after 3 to 4 weeks.

   g. CRP and ESR trends are useful in monitoring the response to infection treatment.

2. An elevated peripheral WBC count with an increased number and percentage of PMNs suggests infection, but these results are highly variable in patients with septic arthritis. A normal peripheral WBC count does not exclude septic arthritis.

E. Gram stain

1. Sensitivity of synovial fluid Gram stain is poor, with 45% to 71% false-negative rates. A negative Gram stain does not rule out septic arthritis.

2. Synovial fluid should be assessed for uric acid and calcium pyrophosphate crystals because the differential includes crystalline disease. Septic arthritis occurs concurrently with gout or pseudogout in less than 5% of cases, but neither diagnosis excludes the other.

3. Synovial fluid Gram stain in gonococcal arthritis is positive in less than 10% of cases.

F. Synovial leukocytosis

1. A WBC count greater than 50,000/mm³ is found in the synovial fluid aspirate of up to 50% of patients with septic arthritis.

2. A WBC count less than 25,000/ mm³ reduces, but

does not eliminate, the possibility of septic arthritis.

3. A synovial fluid PMN cell count differential of at least 90% suggests septic arthritis.

4. Crystalline arthropathy also can yield WBC counts between 15,000 and 30,000/mm³ (ranging above 100,000/mm³) and differentials with greater than 90% PMNs.

G. Cultures

1. Synovial fluid culture in gonococcal arthritis is often negative.

2. Blood cultures should be obtained before antibiotic treatment. Blood cultures yield a pathogen in more than 40% of pediatric patients with AHO.

3. When indicated by the history, obtaining a culture of other sites (skin, urine, throat, genitourinary tract) may be appropriate.

4. The rate of positive cultures in histologically proven cases of osteomyelitis obtained from image-guided bone biopsies is low. Sampling error and the localized nature of biofilm colonization explain the low yield.

V. Antibiotics

A. The mechanism of action, ribosomal subunit binding, clinical use, side effect profiles, and pertinent pearls for antibiotics most frequently prescribed to treat musculoskeletal infections are summarized in **Table 4**.

B. The mechanisms of antibiotic resistance are outlined in **Table 5**.

C. Duration and route of treatment

1. The recommended duration of treatment varies: osteomyelitis (range, 4 to 6 weeks); MRSA osteomyelitis (minimum, 6 weeks); septic arthritis (range, 3 to 4 weeks).

2. A trend toward foreshortening length of parenteral therapy in patients with suitable organisms has been seen because the bioavailability of some oral agents is comparable to that of IV treatment. Although 6 weeks of IV antibiotic administration is widely advocated, evidence to support the long-term antibiotic treatment of chronic osteomyelitis is lacking.

D. Antibiotic selection for osteomyelitis and septic arthritis

1. The most common pathogens and their suggested empiric antibiotic therapies in musculoskeletal infections are outlined in **Table 1**.

2. Treatment should include coverage for *S aureus*

Table 4

Summary of Antimicrobial Agents and Mechanism of Action

Antibiotic	Category	Mode of Action	Clinical Use	Side Effects/Toxicity	Notes of Interest
Penicillins	Bactericidal	Inhibition of cell wall synthesis by blocking cross-linking	DOC for gram-positive bacteria, *Streptococcus pyogenes Streptococcus agalactiae*, and *Clostridium perfringens* Ampicillin/amoxicillin: DOC for *Enterococcus faecalis*, *Escherichia coli* Ticarcillin: DOC-antipseudomonal	Hypersensitivity reaction, hemolytic anemia All penicillins can cause interstitial nephritis	Probenecid inhibits renal tubular secretion of penicillin, carboxy-penicillins, and ureidopenicillins
β-lactamase inhibitors (clavulanic acid, sulbactam, tazobactam)	Bactericidal	Inhibition of cell wall synthesis by blocking cross-linking	DOC against gram-positive (*Staphylococcus aureus*, *Staphylococcus epidermidis*) and gram-negative (*E coli*, *Klebsiella*) bacteria	Hypersensitivity, hemolytic anemia Interstitial nephritis	
Cephalosporins First generation (cephalothin, cephapirin, cefazolin) Second generation (cefoxitin, cefotetan) Third generation (cefotaxime, ceftriaxone, ceftazidime) Fourth generation (cefepime)	Bactericidal	Inhibition of cell wall sythesis by blocking cross-linking	Effective against *S aureus*, *S epidermidis*, and some gram-negative activity (*E coli*, *Klebsiella*, *Proteus mirabilis*) More active against gram-positive bacteria Less active against gram-positive bacteria, but more active against Enterobacteriaceae Ceftazidime highly effective against *Pseudomonas* High activity against gram-positive bacteria	Allergic reactions (3% to 7% cross-reactivity with penicillin) Coombs-positive anemia in 3% Second- and third-generation drugs may cause a disulfiram reaction with alcohol	Cefazolin has the longest half-life of the first-generation cephalosporins All cephalosporins lack activity against *Enterococcus*
Vancomycin	Bactericidal	Inhibition of cell wall synthesis Disrupts peptidoglycan cross-linkage	DOC for MRSA DOC for patients with penicillin and cephalosporin allergies Excellent activity against *S aureus*, *S epidermidis*	Red man syndrome (5% to 13% of patients), nephrotoxicity/ototoxicity, neutropenia, thrombocytopenia	
Aminoglycosides (gentamicin, tobramycin, streptomycin, amikacin)	Bactericidal	Inhibition of protein synthesis, irreversibly binding to 30S ribosomal subunit	Effective against aerobic gram-negative organisms and Enterobacteriaceae, *Pseudomonas*	Nephrotoxicity/ototoxicity increased with multiple drug interactions	
Lincosamide (clindamycin)	Bacteriostatic	Inhibition of protein synthesis, binds 50S ribosomal subunit, inhibits peptidyl transferase by interfering with binding amino acyl-tRNA complex	Effective against *Bacteroides fragilis*, *S aureus*, coagulase-negative *Staphylococcus*, *Streptococcus*	Pseudomembranous colitis (*Clostridium difficile*), hypersensitivity reaction	Excellent penetration into bone. Potentiates neuro-muscular blocking agents

(continued on next page)

Table 4

Summary of Antimicrobial Agents and Mechanism of Action (*continued*)

Antibiotic	Category	Mode of Action	Clinical Use	Side Effects/Toxicity	Notes of Interest
Tetracycline/doxycline	Bacteriostatic	Blocks tRNA binding to 50S ribosome	Effective against mycoplasma, rickettsia, Lyme disease	Anorexia, nausea, diarrhea Interacts with divalent metal agents (antacids), inhibiting antibiotic absorption. May cause hepatotoxicity, photosensitivity	Not used in children younger than 12 years because of discoloration of teeth and impairment of bone growth
Macrolides (erythromycin, clarithromycin, azithromycin)	Bacteriostatic	Reversibly binds to 50S ribosomal subunit	Effective against *Haemophilus influenzae, Moraxella catarrhalis, Mycoplasma pneumonia, Legionella, Chlamydia*	Nausea, vomiting. Drug interaction with coumadin and other drugs due to stimulated cytochrome P450	
Rifampin	Bactericidal	Binds to DNA-dependent RNA polymerase inhibits RNA transcription	Used in combination with semisynthetic penicillin, for *S aureus* infection Effective against *Mycobacterium* species	Orange discoloration of body fluids, GI symptoms, hepatitis Multiple drug interactions inducing hepatic microsomal pathway and altering drug metabolism Interaction with INH can result in hepatotoxicity Interaction with ketoconazole may decrease the effectiveness of both drugs	Resistant organisms rapidly develop if used alone.
Fluoroquinolones Second generation (ciprofloxacin, ofloxacin) Third generation (levofloxin) Fourth generation (trovafloxacin)	Bactericidal	Inhibits DNA gyrase, required for DNA synthesis	Effective against gram-negative *Streptococcus, Mycoplasma, Legionella, Chlamydia* Aerobic gram-positive Anaerobic coverage	GI symptoms (nausea, vomiting), phototoxicity, tendinitis, predisposition to Achilles tendon rupture. Drug interactions	Poor *Enterococcus* coverage Later-generation fluoroquinolones have better gram-positive coverage
Trimethoprim/sulfamethoxazole	Bacteriostatic	Inhibits folic acid synthesis	Aerobic gram-negative, GI and UTI organisms. Some gram-positive, such as *Staphylococcus*, in addition to *Enterobacter, Proteus, H influenzae*	GI, hemolytic anemia, agranulocytopenia, thrombocytopenia, urticaria, erythema nodosum. Serum sickness. Drug interactions Renal failure Hyperkalemia	Not to be used in third trimester of pregnancy
Metronidazole (Flagyl)	Bactericidal	Metabolic by-products disrupt DNA	Anaerobic organisms	Seizures, cerebellar dysfunction, disulfram reaction with alcohol	
Chloramphenicol	Bacteriostatic	Inhibits 50S ribosomal subunit/inhibits protein synthesis	*H influenzae* Drug resistant *Enterococcus* gram-negative rods	Aplastic anemia, gray baby syndrome	

DOC = drug of choice, GI = gastrointestinal, INH = isonicotinic acid hydracide, MRSA = methicillin-resistant *S aureus*, PABA = p-aminobenzoic acid, UTI = urinary tract infection.

1: Basic Science

Table 5

Mechanisms of Antibiotic Resistance

Antibiotic Class and Type of Resistance	Specific Resistance Mechanism
Altered Target	
β-lactam antibiotics	Altered penicillin-binding proteins
Vancomycin	Altered peptidoglycan subunits
Aminoglycosides	Altered ribosomal proteins
Macrolides	Ribosomal RNA methylation
Quinolones	Altered DNA gyrase
Sulfonamides	Altered DNA dihydropteroate
Trimethoprim	Altered dihydrofolate reductase
Rifampin	Altered RNA polymerase
Detoxifying Enzymes	
Aminoglycosides	Phosphotransferase, acetylotransferase, nucleotidyltransferase
β-lactam antibiotics	β-lactamase
Chloramphenicol	HIV inhibits chloramphenicol transacetylate, reducing the resistance of chloramphenicol in HIV.
Decreased Cellular Concentration	
Tetracycline, fluoroquinolones, trimethoprim, erythromycin	Active efflux pumps

Adapted with permission from the Centers for Disease Control and Prevention, Atlanta, GA.

in all cases. Empiric therapy in adult osteomyelitis/septic arthritis might consist of vancomycin plus ceftriaxone.

3. For children with acute hematogenous MRSA osteomyelitis and septic arthritis, IV vancomycin is recommended, dosed at 15 mg/kg every 6 hours.

4. For adults with acute osteomyelitis or septic arthritis, parenteral antibiotic choices include vancomycin, daptomycin, or linezolid.

5. Vancomycin

   a. Cornerstone of therapy for serious MRSA infections despite poor bone penetration and limited activity against biofilm organisms

   b. Efficacy against MSSA infections is less than that of antistaphylococcal β-lactams.

6. Rifampin is never used alone, but its synergistic activity with a host of other antibiotics makes it a useful addition for serious MRSA and MSSA infections. Rifampin offers excellent bone penetration and is rapidly bactericidal. It is often used to treat foreign body infections.

E. *Clostridium difficile* infection (CDI)

1. *C difficile* is a gram-positive, anaerobic, spore-forming bacillus.

2. CDI may develop when antibiotic administration leads to an overgrowth of toxin-producing strains of *C difficile*. CDI symptoms range in severity from mild diarrhea to pseudomembranous colitis to toxic megacolon.

3. Alcohol-based hand cleansers do not kill *C difficile* spores.

4. Unexplained postoperative leukocytosis, fever, and/or watery diarrhea should prompt an investigation for CDI.

5. CDI is treated with the cessation of the inciting antibiotic and the addition of oral metronidazole or vancomycin.

VI. Antibiotic Prophylaxis

A. Routine antibiotic prophylaxis is not currently recommended for elective orthopaedic surgery that does not involve a prosthetic device.

B. Timing of antibiotic prophylaxis

1. Prophylactic IV antibiotics should be administered within 1 hour of skin incision.

   a. Because of its extended infusion time, vancomycin should be started within 2 hours of skin incision.

2. Additional antibiotic doses are administered if surgical time exceeds one to two times the antibiotic half-life or if substantial blood loss occurs.

3. The duration of prophylactic antibiotic administration should not exceed the 24-hour postoperative period. The literature does not support continuation of antibiotics until drains or catheters are removed.

C. Selection of antibiotic prophylaxis

1. Cephalosporins (cefazolin, cefuroxime) are the perioperative prophylactic antibiotics of choice. These agents provide coverage against most bacteria and are relatively nontoxic (<10% cross-reactivity with penicillin allergy) and inexpensive.

2. Clindamycin or vancomycin are selected for confirmed β-lactam allergy.

a. Clindamycin can be given intravenously or orally and offers rapid bone absorption. It causes *C difficile* colitis in up to 8% of patients

3. Vancomycin

a. Vancomycin is used alone or in addition to a cephalosporin in institutions with a significant incidence of MRSA SSIs.

b. Compared with cephalosporins and penicillinase-resistant penicillins, vancomycin is an inferior antistaphylococcal agent for MSSA.

VII. Prevention of SSI

A. SSI is defined as superficial or deep infection developing within 30 days of surgery or within 1 year of surgical implant insertion. SSIs are the most common form of nosocomial infection.

B. Patient factors

1. Patient factors play less of a role in SSI than intraoperative ones. Risk factors include diabetes, tobacco use, steroids, vascular insufficiency, malnutrition, and nasal MRSA colonization.

2. Diabetes is an independent risk factor for SSI and delayed wound healing.

3. A history of SSI greatly increases the risk of subsequent infection.

4. History of MRSA colonization

a. More than one half of orthopaedic SSIs are caused by *S aureus*.

b. *S aureus* is carried in the nares of as many as 30% of patients; 85% of *S aureus* SSIs are caused by strains found in the patient's own nares.

c. Higher rates of SSI are found in patients colonized with MRSA.

d. Preoperative skin preparation using chlorhexidine wipes before knee and hip arthroplasty has been shown to reduce SSI.

5. Obesity is a risk factor for SSI.

6. Data support a relationship between malnutrition and SSI.

a. Malnutrition is common in elderly patients irrespective of body habitus.

b. Markers of malnutrition include serum albumin less than 3.5 mg/dL; serum transferrin less than 200 mg/dL; and total lymphocyte count less than 1,500/mm^3.

7. Tobacco use increases SSI risk. Tobacco abstinence for at least 30 days before elective surgery

---

Table 6

Patients at Increased Risk for Hematogenous Total Joint Arthroplasty Infection

All patients during the first two years after prosthetic joint replacement
Immunocompromised/immunosuppressed patients
Inflammatory arthropathies (rheumatoid arthritis, systemic lupus erythematosus)
Patients with comorbidities such as previous prosthetic joint infections, malnourishment, hemophilia, HIV infection, diabetes, malignancy, endocarditis

Adapted from Clark CR: Perioperative medical management, in Barrack RL, Booth RE Jr, Lonner JH, McCarthy JC, Mont MA, Rubash HE eds: *Orthopaedic Knowledge Update: Hip and Knee Reconstruction*, ed 3. Rosemont, IL, American Academy of Orthopaedic Surgeons, 2006, pp 205-216.

---

has been advocated.

8. Dentition

a. Bacteremia associated with dental pathology can lead to postoperative joint infection in total joint arthroplasty (TJA) patients, both in the postoperative interval and subsequently.

b. The prevalence of untreated dental conditions in arthroplasty candidates is disturbingly high.

9. Urinary tract infection—Preoperative urinalysis and urine culture may be indicated for patients exhibiting urinary tract symptoms and those at greater risk for urinary tract infection. Indications to consider postponing surgery include dysuria and frequency in the setting of a count greater than 10^3/mL.

10. Rheumatoid arthritis patients undergoing TJA have a two to three times greater risk of SSI than patients with osteoarthritis. Other immunocompromised patients are also at increased risk (**Table 6**).

11. Medications—Disease-modifying antirheumatic drugs

a. Methotrexate need not be discontinued perioperatively.

b. Severe infection is a known complication of tumor necrosis factor inhibitor therapy. Patients undergoing major surgery should have these agents withheld preoperatively for at least one dosing cycle and postoperatively until wound healing is ensured.

c. Corticosteroids increase the infection rate and impair wound healing. Patients on chronic therapy should receive their maintenance dose perioperatively.

C. Perioperative strategies

1: Basic Science

1. Perioperative antibiotic prophylaxis is the only intervention that qualifies as a standard of treatment.

2. Selection of antiseptic agent

   a. Alcohol-based solutions with iodophor or chlorhexidine appear to be the most effective antiseptic agents.

   b. Chlorhexidine may be more effective against gram-positive organisms than aqueous-based iodophors such as povidone-iodine. Chlorhexidine has residual antimicrobial properties owing to its ability to bind to skin.

3. Materials

   a. Gloves are uniformly punctured after 3 hours of surgery. Double gloving is highly recommended.

   b. Among absorbable synthetic sutures, monofilament carries a lower risk of infection than braided material. Both are superior to nonabsorbable braided or natural sutures.

   c. Occlusive dressings are associated with a lower rate of infection.

   d. Retention of postsurgical drains for more than 24 hours is associated with an increased risk of contamination from resistant nosocomial organisms.

4. Surgical duration longer than 2 hours is an independent risk factor for SSI.

5. Hypothermia during surgery is an independent risk factor for SSI.

6. Glycemic control

   a. Postoperative hyperglycemia is an independent risk factor for SSI.

   b. Diabetes mellitus and morning postoperative hyperglycemia are predictors for postoperative infection following TJA.

   c. HemoglobinA_{1C} concentration in excess of 7% raises SSI risk.

7. Prolonged wound drainage—Drainage exceeding 5 postoperative days is correlated with a several-fold increased risk of deep SSI.

8. Transfusion—Allogeneic blood transfusion may be an overlooked risk factor for the development of postoperative bacterial infection. Each unit of intraoperative or postoperative allogeneic blood may increase the risk of SSI up to 9%.

VIII. Periprosthetic Infection

A. Synovial fluid WBC count greater than 2,500/mm^3 or more than 90% PMN leukocytes is strongly indicative of chronic infection in a total knee arthroplasty.

B. Gram stains have poor predictive value and are not useful in diagnosing periprosthetic infection.

IX. Atypical Infections

A. Necrotizing fasciitis

1. Necrotizing fasciitis is any necrotizing soft-tissue infection spreading along fascial planes, with or without overlying cellulitis.

2. Necrotizing fasciitis may be caused by a single organism (*S pyogenes*) or a combination. Anaerobic or microaerophilic streptococci are believed to be the most common pathogens, but are difficult to culture. CA-MRSA is an increasingly frequent pathogen in endemic areas.

3. Clinical signs

   a. Severe pain and systemic findings (hyperpyrexia, tachycardia, and chills) are common but nonspecific.

   b. The infection typically begins as a localized abscess, particularly among at-risk groups such as IV drug users, patients with diabetes, those who abuse alcohol, patients who have undergone abdominal surgery, obese patients, or patients with peripheral vascular disease.

   c. Initial findings are localized pain and minimal swelling, often with no visible trauma or skin discoloration. Unexplained, rapidly increasing pain may be the first manifestation.

   d. Dermal induration and erythema eventually appear; skin blistering develops late.

   e. High elevations of body temperature help differentiate necrotizing fasciitis from anaerobic cellulitis and clostridial myonecrosis, which produce modest, if any, changes in temperature.

   f. Suspected cases demand immediate surgery. Awaiting results of imaging or cultures should be avoided if the clinical picture is compelling. In equivocal cases, fascial biopsy reveals the diagnosis.

B. Clostridial myonecrosis (gas gangrene)

1. A triad of symptoms suggests clostridial myonecrosis: progressively severe and out-of-proportion pain, tachycardia unexplained by fever, and crepitus.

2. Spore-forming clostridial species (for example, *Clostridium perfringens, Clostridium septicum,* and *Clostridium novyi*) account for most cases.

3. Clinical presentation usually includes progressive pain, edema (distant from wound), foul-smelling serosanguinous discharge, and a feeling of impending doom. Late findings include ecchymosis, necrosis, dark red serous exudate, and numerous gas-filled vesicles and bullae.

4. Intense out-of-proportion pain is characteristic; within hours, signs of systemic toxicity appear, including confusion, tachycardia, and diaphoresis.

5. Radiographs typically show widespread gas in tissues.

6. Treatment is immediate surgical débridement. Adjuvant therapy with high-dose penicillin and clindamycin is widely used. Hyperbaric oxygen treatment warrants strong consideration but should never delay surgical débridement.

7. *C septicum* gas gangrene is associated with colorectal malignancy.

C. Tuberculosis

1. The prevalence of HIV has been a leading factor in the reactivation of latent tuberculosis infections and in the progression of active disease.

2. Orthopaedic manifestations of tuberculosis may involve the entire skeletal system. The spine is the major site of infection, involved in 50% of cases.

3. Radiographic evaluation

a. Common findings—Cyst formation and subchondral erosions around joints, soft-tissue swelling, and mild periosteal reactions. With spine involvement, skip lesions, thinning of end plates, loss of disk height, and possible late fusion are present.

4. *Mycobacterium tuberculosis* is an acid-fast bacillus and may take 6 weeks to grow.

5. Treatment

a. Therapy begins with four drugs (isoniazid, rifampin, pyrazinamide, and ethambutol). Duration of therapy is a minimum of 6 months

b. Spine—Absolute indications for surgical intervention of the spine are marked neurologic involvement related to a kyphotic deformity or herniation, worsening neurologic condition despite chemotherapy, an abscess with respiratory obstruction, and worsening kyphosis with instability.

D. Nontuberculous mycobacteria

1. Nontuberculous mycobacteria infection has in-

creased as the prevalence of tuberculosis has declined.

2. Nontuberculous myeobacteria may cause skin and soft-tissue infection after a skin abrasion or inoculation. *Mycobacterium marinum* is an atypical species capable of producing subacute and chronic hand infections in patients exposed to aquatic environments.

E. *Vibrio* infection—*Vibrio vulnificus*, a gram-negative bacterium, may cause severe soft-tissue infections of the upper extremity.

1. Gains access to soft tissues by direct inoculation through a penetrating (for example, finning) injury or through abraded skin exposed to contaminated water.

2. Infections begin with swelling, erythema, and intense pain around the infected site. Fluid-filled blisters form and may progress to tissue necrosis in an aggressive process resembling gas gangrene.

F. *Propionibacterium* infection—Shoulder surgery has an increased risk of infection with *P acnes*, a gram-positive anaerobic bacillus.

1. Isolated on culture, this bacterium should not be dismissed as a contaminant.

2. The organism may require more than 6 days to grow and requires anaerobic conditions. Cultures should be observed for at least 10 days.

G. Fungal infections

1. The most common location for musculoskeletal fungal infections is the hand.

2. Periprosthetic TJA infections may be associated with fungal organisms.

a. The most common pathogen is *Candida albicans.*

b. Deep periprosthetic infection with fungal organisms is rare and is associated with an immunocompromised host.

c. Adjuvant treatment of periprosthetic infections, in addition to IV amphotericin, may involve the use of oral fluconazole.

H. Lyme disease

1. Multisystem spirochetal disorder caused by *Borrelia burgdorferi* and transmitted by the bite of an infected tick

2. Geographic predominance—Northeast, Midwest, and Northwest United States

3. Lyme disease occurs in three clinical stages.

a. Early/localized disease—Pathognomonic skin lesion of erythema migrans ("bull's-eye" rash) (**Figure 9**).

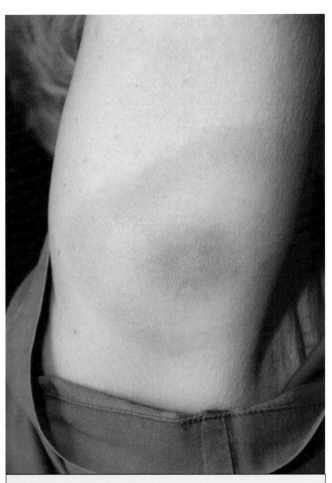

Figure 9 Photograph shows erythema chronicum migrans (the "bull's-eye" rash), which is associated with Lyme disease. The rash is sufficiently distinctive to allow an early diagnosis of Lyme disease. (Courtesy of the Centers for Disease Control and Prevention: Public Health Image Library Image 9875. Atlanta, GA, 2009. http://phil.cdc.gov/phil/details.asp?pid=9875. Accessed May 27, 2014.)

b. Early disseminated disease—Neurologic and cardiac manifestations.

c. Late disease—Musculoskeletal symptoms (arthralgia, intermittent arthritis, and chronic monoarthritis, often in the knee) develop in 80% of untreated patients.

4. Acute form of monoarthritis may resemble septic arthritis; however, the synovial fluid cell count (10,000 to 25,000 WBC/mm^3) is typically lower than that observed with bacterial septic arthritis and shows a predominance of PMN leukocytes.

5. Enzyme-linked immunosorbent assay testing detects antibodies to *B burgdorferi*, but false-positive results are common. The diagnosis may be confirmed using Western blot analysis.

I. HIV/AIDS

1. The risk of transmission after a percutaneous exposure to HIV-infected blood has been estimated to be approximately 0.3%; after mucous membrane exposure, 0.09%. Seroconversion is more likely if the injury was deep and the needle visibly contaminated with the source patient's blood.

2. AIDS patients have a potential for higher infection rates and longer healing times because of impaired cellular and humoral immunity. Patients with CD4 counts less than 200 or a viral load in excess of 10,000 copies/mL were found to have a tenfold higher rate of infection than individuals without AIDS.

3. Recommendations for reducing the risk of infection during elective orthopaedic surgery include

a. Absolute PMN count greater than 1,000

b. Platelet count greater than 60,000

c. Serum albumin greater than 2.5 g/dL

d. Reduction of viral loads to undetectable levels, which increases the lymphocyte count

Top Testing Facts

1. *K kingae* is the most common bacterial cause of osteoarticular infection in children younger than 4 years, giving rise to far more cases of septic arthritis than osteomyelitis.

2. Shoulder surgery poses an increased risk of infection with *P acnes*, a slow-growing gram-positive rod.

3. Most bacterial infections are caused by organisms growing in biofilms. Formation of adherent biofilms is central to the pathogenesis of implant-associated infection. Bacteria proliferating in biofilms are resistant to host defenses and antibiotic therapy. Infected implants and their adherent biofilms must be removed surgically before infection can be resolved.

4. A clinical prediction rule has been validated for the distinction between septic arthritis and transient synovitis of the hip.
   - History of fever
   - Refusal to bear weight
   - ESR greater than 40
   - Peripheral WBC greater than 12,000
   - Diagnostic accuracy ranges between 73% and 93% if three predictors are present
   - Accuracy rises to 93% to 99% in the presence of four predictors

5. Musculoskeletal infection in children predisposes to the development of DVT and septic pulmonary emboli. Children older than 8 years who have MRSA osteomyelitis and in whom CRP at presentation exceeds 6 mg/dL exhibit a 40% incidence of DVT.

6. Radiographic features of osteomyelitis, such as periosteal elevation, typically are not visible before 10 to 14 days of illness. Changes in flat bones and the spine may take longer to appear. Bone loss of 30% to 40% is required before bone resorption can be seen on radiographs.

7. The presentations of EOG, Ewing sarcoma, and acute osteomyelitis in appropriately aged patients can mimic one another. All three diseases may present with fever, pain, local tenderness, leukocytosis, elevated ESR, and a lamellated periosteal reaction.

8. Brodie abscess is a form of subacute osteomyelitis characterized by insidious onset. Cortical lesions may mimic osteoid osteoma, intracortical hemangioma, and stress fracture. Presence of a sinus tract distinguishes a cortical Brodie abscess.

9. Unexplained postoperative leukocytosis, fever, and/or watery diarrhea should prompt a search for CDI and, in some instances, empiric treatment with oral metronidazole.

10. More than half of orthopaedic SSIs are caused by *S aureus*; the proportion from MRSA is increasing. Of *S aureus* SSIs, 85% are caused by strains found in the patient's own nares. Nasal colonization is a prime risk factor for the development of SSI with *S aureus* after arthroplasty.

1: Basic Science

Bibliography

Barrack RL, Jennings RW, Wolfe MW, Bertot AJ: The Coventry Award: The value of preoperative aspiration before total knee revision. *Clin Orthop Relat Res* 1997;345:8-16.

Bozic KJ, Lau E, Kurtz S, Ong K, Berry DJ: Patient-related risk factors for postoperative mortality and periprosthetic joint infection in medicare patients undergoing TKA. *Clin Orthop Relat Res* 2012;470(1):130-137.

Cierny G III, DiPasquale D: Treatment of chronic infection. *J Am Acad Orthop Surg* 2006;14(10 Spec No.):S105-S110.

Copley LA: Pediatric musculoskeletal infection: trends and antibiotic recommendations. *J Am Acad Orthop Surg* 2009; 17(10):618-626.

Kocher MS, Mandiga R, Zurakowski D, Barnewolt C, Kasser JR: Validation of a clinical prediction rule for the differentiation between septic arthritis and transient synovitis of the hip in children. *J Bone Joint Surg Am* 2004;86(8):1629-1635.

Matar WY, Jafari SM, Restrepo C, Austin M, Purtill JJ, Parvizi J: Preventing infection in total joint arthroplasty. *J Bone Joint Surg Am* 2010;92(suppl 2):36-46.

Moucha CS, Clyburn TA, Evans RP, Prokuski L: Modifiable risk factors for surgical site infection. *Instr Course Lect* 2011; 60:557-564.

Olsen MA, Nepple JJ, Riew KD, et al: Risk factors for surgical site infection following orthopaedic spinal operations. *J Bone Joint Surg Am* 2008;90(1):62-69.

Spellberg B, Lipsky BA: Systemic antibiotic therapy for chronic osteomyelitis in adults. *Clin Infect Dis* 2012;54(3): 393-407.

Chapter 4
Biomechanics

Vijay K. Goel, PhD   Nikhil Kulkarni, MS   Jonathan N. Grauer, MD

1: Basic Science

I. Introduction

A. Biomechanics combines fundamental principles of physics, engineering, and biology to describe and predict the effects of energy and various types of forces on biologic systems.

1. It relies on external and internal factors to characterize the static and/or dynamic response of a body to the application of different forces.

2. The principles of biomechanics can help in understanding the forces that act on and in the human body and their effects under normal conditions and in unusual and pathologic circumstances such as injury or surgery. In orthopaedics, these principles can be used in the design of instruments, implants, and prostheses.

B. Definitions and basic concepts

1. Scalars—Quantities that are fully described by a numerical value alone, such as the speed of a car.

2. Vectors—Quantities whose full description requires a direction in addition to a numerical value of magnitude, as in the case of velocity, which is the rate of change in the position of an object, and which includes both direction and magnitude.

3. Mass—A measure of the amount of inertia or resistance to movement of a physical object to which a force is applied. Mass is a scalar quantity and does not change with the position or shape of an object unless matter is added to or removed from the object. The unit of mass in the International System of Units (SI) is the kilogram (kg).

   a. The weight of an object is the force with which it is attracted toward earth through the action of gravity, and it is used to calculate the mass of the object. The mass of an object does not depend on its location or position and is the same everywhere, whereas the weight of an object may differ in relation to its location. Thus, an object weights less on the moon than on earth, and weighs almost nothing in outer space, because of the relative force of gravity in each of these locations.

   b. For simplification of calculations of mass and weight, the entire mass of an object may be considered as being concentrated at a point called the center of mass (COM) of the object, with the center of gravity (COG) of the object being a point within it and from which its weight is considered to act.

   c. In most applications on earth, including engineering and medicine, COM and COG are assumed to be located at a single, identical point, and the gravitational force of the earth is assumed to be uniform everywhere.

4. Displacement—The shortest distance between the initial and final position of an object that moves with the application of a force. Displacement is a vector quantity and is linear or angular, depending on the path of an object to which one or more forces are applied. In SI units, linear displacement is measured in meters and angular displacement is measured in radians.

5. Velocity—The rate of change of the linear or angular displacement of an object with time. It is a vector quantity, and the SI units for linear velocity and angular velocity are meters per second (m/s) and radians per second (rad/s), respectively. Velocity is similar to speed, except that speed is a scalar quantity whereas velocity is a vector quantity in having both direction and magnitude.

6. Acceleration—The rate at which the velocity of an object changes with time. Like velocity, acceleration can be either linear or angular. The SI units for linear acceleration and angular

Dr. Goel or an immediate family member has received royalties from X-Spine, Inc.; and has received research or institutional support from DePuy, a Johnson & Johnson company. Mr. Kulkarni or an immediate family member serves as a paid consultant to or is an employee of Medtronic Sofamor Danek and Osteomed. Dr. Grauer or an immediate family member is a member of a speakers' bureau or has made paid presentations on behalf of Alphatec Spine, Smith & Nephew, and Stryker; serves as a paid consultant to or is an employee of Affinergy, Alphatech Spine, DePuy, a Johnson & Johnson company, KCI, Smith & Nephew, Stryker, and Venture MD; has received research or institutional support from Medtronic Sofamor Danek and Smith & Nephew; and serves as a board member, owner, officer, or committee member of the American Academy of Orthopaedic Surgeons and the Cervical Spine Research Society.

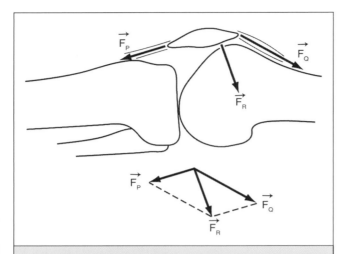

Figure 1 The forces applied on the patella by the quadriceps muscle ($\vec{F}_Q$) and patellar tendon ($\vec{F}_P$), and the resultant force ($\vec{F}_R$). (Adapted from Mow VC, Flatow EL, Ateshian GA: Biomechanics, in Buckwalter JA, Einhorn TA, Simon SR, eds: *Orthopaedic Basic Science: Biology and Biomechanics of the Musculoskeletal System*, ed 2. Rosemont, IL, American Academy of Orthopaedic Surgeons, 2000, p 134.)

acceleration are m/s² and rad/s², respectively.

7. Force—A physical quantity that changes the state of rest or state of uniform motion of an object and/or deforms its shape.

   a. Forces result from interactions and are not necessarily associated with motion; for example, a person sitting on a chair exerts a force on the chair but the chair does not move.

   b. A force is a vector quantity, and has both magnitude and direction. The SI unit for force is the newton (N), with 1 N being the force required to give a 1-kg mass an acceleration of 1 m/s².

8. Resultant force—The vector sum of all of the forces applied to an object.

   a. A force vector can be represented graphically by an arrow, with the orientation of the arrow indicating the direction of action of the force, the base of the arrow representing the origin of the force, the head of the arrow identifying the direction in which the force is acting, and the length of the arrow being proportional to the magnitude of the force that the arrow represents.

   b. Graphic and trigonometric methods can be used to add or sum the forces acting on an object, with the sum of multiple forces being known as a resultant (**Figure 1**).

9. Moment— A measure of the ability of a force to generate rotational motion.

   a. The axis about which an object rotates as the result of a force exerted on the object is called the instantaneous axis of rotation (IAR).

   b. The shortest distance between the IAR of an object and the point at which the force causing rotation is applied to the rotating object is called the moment arm.

   c. The magnitude of the moment generated by a force is the magnitude of the force multiplied by its moment arm. The SI unit for moment is the newton-meter (N·m).

10. Torque—A rotational moment. In general, torque is associated with the rotational or twisting effect of applied forces, whereas moment is related to a bending effect of such forces.

11. Equilibrium—A state of rest or balance of an object resulting from the equivalence of forces acting in opposite directions on the object.

   a. Static equilibrium—A state that exits when all of the objects in a system of objects are at rest as the result of the net equivalence of all of the forces acting on each object in the system.

   b. Mechanical equilibrium—The state of a system that exists when the sums of all the external forces and moments acting on objects in the system are zero. An object in mechanical equilibrium can be undergoing translation or rotation at a constant velocity without linear or rotational acceleration.

12. Statics—A topic in applied mechanics that is concerned with the forces that produce a state of equilibrium in a system of objects.

13. Dynamics—A topic in physics that is concerned with the study of forces and torques and their effects on the motion of objects.

14. Rigid body—A body that maintains the relative position of any two particles within it when the body itself is subjected to external forces. All objects deform to some degree in response to forces to them, but in the case of a rigid body these deformations are so small in comparison with the size of the rigid body itself that they can be ignored. Thus, for example, the small deformations of bones that occur under normal conditions of loading are ignored, with the bones themselves considered to be rigid bodies.

15. Deformable body—A body that undergoes significant changes in shape or volume when external forces are applied to it. For example, intervertebral disks are considered to be deformable bodies. Deformable body mechanics is concerned with the internal forces (stresses) that act within the body and the deformations (strains) of the body that they produce. These terms are described in detail in the chapter on biomaterials,

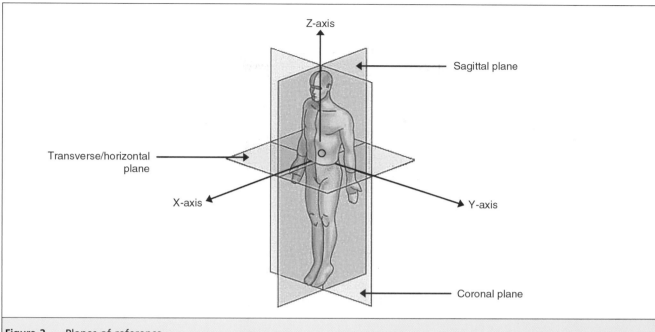

Figure 2   Planes of reference.

Chapter 5 in *AAOS Comprehensive Orthopaedic Review 2.*

16. Newton's laws of motion—The foundation of classical mechanics.

    a. Newton's first law—A body remains at rest, or the velocity of the body remains constant, unless an unbalanced external force acts on the body.

    b. Newton's second law—The acceleration of a body is parallel to and directly proportional to the summary vector, or resultant, of the forces acting on the body, and is inversely proportional to the mass of the body.

    c. Newton's third law—For every action there is an equal and opposite reaction. In other words, the mutual forces of action and reaction of two bodies on one another are equal, opposite, and collinear.

17. Free-body diagrams—Drawings used to show the location and direction of all known forces and moments acting on an object in a given situation. Free-body diagrams are useful for identifying and evaluating unknown forces and moments acting on individual parts of a system in equilibrium.

18. Degrees of freedom (DOF)—The number of parameters that are required to uniquely specify the position and movement of a point or body in space.

    a. A point or object moving in two-dimensional space has three DOF, of which two DOF are translational, within the plane of the space,

and one DOF is rotational.

    b. A body moving in three-dimensional space has six DOFs, of which three are translational and three are rotational.

    c. Clinical examples of DOF

    • A hinge joint has one DOF; the geometric constraints of the joint permit only one rotational motion, about the axis of rotation of the joint, as in the case of the elbow or interphalangeal joints.

    • A ball-and-socket joint, such as the shoulder joint or the hip joint, has three rotational DOF.

19. In biomechanics, the three-dimensional motion of a body segment is generally expressed with a Cartesian coordinate system having X, Y, and Z axes. These axes compose the following planes (**Figure 2**):

    a. Sagittal plane, which divides the body vertically into right and left sections.

    b. Coronal or frontal plane, which divides the body vertically into anterior and posterior sections.

    c. Transverse or horizontal plane, which divides the body horizontally into upper and lower sections.

Table 1

Joint Reaction and Muscle Forces for Various Activities

Joint	Activity	Joint Reaction Force/Contact Force	Muscle Force
Elbow	Elbow flexed at right angle holding an object weighing approximately 0.06 times the body weight	Force at elbow joint: 0.5 times body weight	Biceps muscle force: approximately 0.6 times body weight
Shoulder	Arm abducted to horizontal position and holding a dumbbell of 0.08 times body weight to exercise shoulder muscles	Force at shoulder joint: approximately 1.5 times body weight	Deltoid muscle force: approximately 1.5 times body weight
Spinal column	Weight lifter bent forward by 45° and lifting a weight equal to his or her body weight	Compressive force generated at the union of L5–S1: approximately 10 times body weight	Erector spinae muscle (supporting the trunk) force: approximately 12 times body weight
Hip	Single-leg stance during walking	Force at hip joint: approximately 3 times body weight	Hip abductor muscle force: approximately 3 times body weight
Knee	Person wearing a weight boot and doing a leg raise from a sitting position	Force at tibiofemoral joint: approximately 1 times body weight	Quadriceps muscle force: approximately 1 times body weight

II. Kinematics and Kinetics

A. Kinematics is the field within classic mechanics that describes the motion of objects without regard to their mass or how their motion is brought about.

1. In general, kinematics is concerned with the geometric and time-dependent aspects of motion, without considering the forces or moments responsible for the motion.

2. Kinematics principally involves the relationships to one another of position, velocity, and acceleration.

3. In orthopaedics, the knowledge of joint kinematics helps in understanding an articulation. As an example, this is important for designing prosthetic implants that restore the function of a particular joint, and for understanding joint wear, stability, and degeneration.

B. Kinetics is the study of motion and its causes. In othopaedics, this involves analysis of the effects of the forces or moments that produce or modify the motion of the body. Newton's first and third laws of motion are particularly applicable to kinetics.

C. Kinematics and kinetics involve categorizing motion into translational components, rotational components, or both.

III. Joint Mechanics

A. Each joint of the body provides various degrees of mobility and stability based on specific structural considerations (**Table 1**). Each joint is subject to the action of internal and external loads.

B. Mechanics of the elbow joint—**Figure 3** shows a free-body diagram in the two-dimensional X–Y plane for the forearm at 90° of flexion and with a weight held in the hand.

1. The forces acting on the forearm are the total weight of the forearm (W_f), the weight of the object in the hand (W_o), the magnitude of the force exerted by the biceps muscle on the forearm (F_{muscle}), and the magnitude of the joint reaction force at the elbow (F_{joint}).

2. Point O is the IAR of the elbow joint, point P is the point of attachment of the biceps on the radius, point Q represents the COG of the forearm, and point R lies on the vertical line passing through the COG of the weight held in the hand.

3. The distances from these points to the center of rotation (moment arms) are shown in **Figure 3** and are assumed to be known from the anatomy of the particular arm being considered. The direction of the muscle force (F_{muscle}) is also known; in this problem, it is assumed to be vertical.

4. Considering the rotational equilibrium of the forearm about IAR, summation of moments ($\Sigma \vec{M}$) about O would be zero.

$$\Sigma \vec{M} = 0 \rightarrow pF_{muscle} = qW_f + rW_o.$$

Where O → IAR

F_{muscle} → Muscle force

W_f → Total weight of the forearm

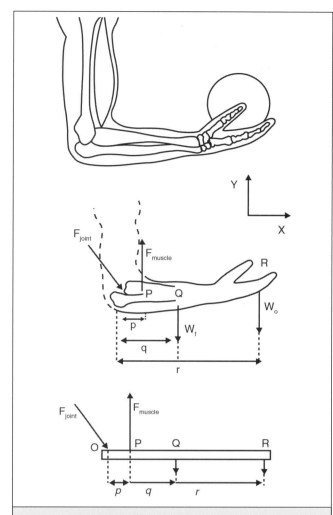

Figure 3   Free-body diagram for an arm holding weight in the hand.

$W_o \rightarrow$ Muscle force—Weight of the object in hand

$p \rightarrow$ Muscle force—Distance between point O of the elbow joint and point P (the point of attachment of the biceps on the radius)

$q \rightarrow$ Muscle force—Distance between point O of the elbow joint and point Q (the **COG** of the forearm)

$r \rightarrow$ Muscle force—Distance between point O of the elbow joint and point R, which lies on the vertical line passing through the **COG** of the weight held in the hand

5. Because the forearm is in translational equilibrium, the sum of the forces ($\sum \overrightarrow{F}$) acting on it is zero:

$$\sum \overrightarrow{F} = 0$$

6. Splitting the above vector $\sum \overrightarrow{F}$ into its components along the Cartesian axes X

$$(\sum F_x) \text{ and Y}(\sum F_y)$$

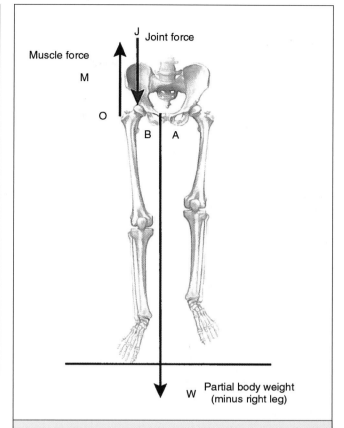

Figure 4   Forces acting across the limb joint during single-limb stance.

$$\sum F_x = 0 \rightarrow F_{Xjoint} = 0$$

(There is no joint reaction force along the X-axis.)

$$\sum F_y = 0 \rightarrow F_{Yjoint} = F_{joint} = F_{muscle} - (W_f + W_o).$$

$F_{muscle} \rightarrow$ The magnitude of the force exerted by the biceps muscle on the forearm

$F_{joint} \rightarrow$ The magnitude of the joint reaction force at the elbow

$F_{Xjoint} \rightarrow$ The magnitude of the joint reaction force at the elbow along the X axis

$F_{Yjoint} \rightarrow$ The magnitude of the joint reaction force at the elbow along the Y axis

7. The foregoing equations can be solved for the muscle force and the joint reaction force for given geometric parameters and weights. By assuming that W_f = 30 N, W_o = 95 N, P = 5 cm, q = 10 cm, and r = 42 cm, the muscle force and joint reaction force can be calculated as follows:

$$F_{muscle} = (1/0.05)[(0.12 \times 25) + (0.4 \times 100)]$$
$$= 860 \text{ N}\uparrow$$

$$F_{joint} = (860 - 25) - 100 = 735 \text{ N}\downarrow$$

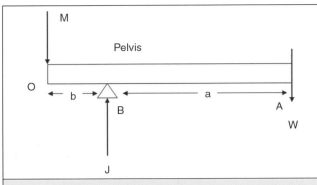

Figure 5 The free-body diagram for the problem defined in Figure 4.

C. Mechanics of the hip joint—**Figures 4** and **5** show the forces acting across the hip joint during single-limb stance (a two-dimensional problem). During walking and running, the full weight of the body is momentarily applied to one leg.

1. The forces acting on the leg carrying the total weight of the body during such a single-leg stance are shown in **Figure 4**, where M is the magnitude of the resultant force exerted by the hip abductor muscles and is assumed to act in a vertical direction; J is the magnitude of the joint reaction force applied by the pelvis on the femur and is also assumed to act in a vertical direction; and W is the partial body weight (body weight minus the weight of the right leg).

2. The free-body diagram of the body without the supported leg is shown in **Figure 5**, where O is the point at which the hip abductor muscles insert on the femur; B is a point along the IAR of the hip joint; and A is the COG of the body without the supported leg.

3. The distances between O and B and between A and B are specified as b and a, respectively.

4. To find the magnitude of the force, M, exerted by the hip abductor muscles, the condition of the rotational equilibrium of the leg about B can be applied. (Assumption: Clockwise moments are positive.)

$$(W \cdot a) - (M \cdot b) = 0$$
$$M = (W \cdot a)/b$$

For W = 500 N, b = 5 cm, and a = 10 cm:

$$M = (500 \cdot 10)/(5)$$
$$M = 1000 \text{ N} \downarrow$$

5. To calculate the joint reaction force, J, consider force equilibrium along the Y-axis. (Assumption: Forces acting downward are negative.)

$$\Sigma F_y = 0$$
$$J - M - W = 0$$
$$J = M + W = 1000 + 500$$
$$J = 1500 \text{ N} \uparrow$$

Glossary of Terms

Acceleration—The rate at which the velocity of an object changes with time

Biomechanics—The use of fundamental principles of physics, engineering, and biology to describe and predict the effects of energy and various types of forces on biologic systems

Deformable body—A body that undergoes significant changes in shape or volume when external forces are applied to it

Degrees of freedom (DOF)—The number of parameters that are required to uniquely specify the position and movement of a point or body in space

Displacement—The shortest distance between the initial and final position of an object that moves with the application of a force

Dynamics—A topic in physics that is concerned with the study of forces and torques and their effects on the motion of objects

Equilibrium—A state of rest or balance of an object resulting from the equivalence of forces acting in opposite directions on the object

Free-body diagrams—Drawings used to show the location and direction of all known forces and moments acting on an object in a given situation

Instantaneous axis of rotation (IAR)—The axis about which an object rotates as the result of a force exerted on the object

Kinematics—The field within classical mechanics that describes the motion of objects without regard to their mass or how their motion is brought about

Mass—A measure of the amount of inertia or resistance to movement of a physical object to which a force is applied. Mass is a scalar quantity and does not change with the position or shape of an object.

Mechanical equilibrium—The state of a system that exists when the sums of all the external forces and moments acting on objects in the system are zero

Moment—A measure of the ability of a force to generate rotational motion of an object

Newton's laws of motion—The foundation of classical mechanics. Newton's first law states that a body remains at rest, or the velocity of the body remains constant, unless an unbalanced external force acts on the body; Newton's second law states that the acceleration of a body is parallel to and directly proportional to the summary vector, or resultant, of the forces acting on the body, and is inversely proportional to the mass of the body; and Newton's third law states that for every action there is an equal and opposite reaction.

Resultant force—The vector sum of all of the forces applied to an object

Rigid body—A body that maintains the relative position of any two particles within it when the body itself is subjected to external forces

Scalar—A quantity that is fully described by a numerical value alone, without a specific direction or other component, such as the speed of a car

Static equilibrium—A state that exists when all of the objects in a system of objects are at rest as the result of the net equivalence of all of the forces acting on each object in the system

Statics—A topic in applied mechanics that is concerned with the forces that produce a state of equilibrium in a system of objects

Torque—A rotational moment, generally associated with the rotational or twisting effect of applied forces

Vector— A quantity whose full description requires both a direction and a numerical value of magnitude

Velocity—The rate of change of the linear or angular displacement of an object with time. Velocity is a consequence of the application of a force to an object, and is a vector quantity in having both direction and magnitude.

Weight—The force with which an object is attracted toward a much large object such as the Earth or Moon through the action of gravity

Top Testing Facts

1. Mechanical equilibrium exists when the sums of all forces and moments are zero.

2. Torque is associated with the rotational or twisting effect of applied forces, whereas moment is related to their bending effect.

3. Newton's laws of motion are the basis of the principles used in biomechanics.

4. The expression "What goes up, must come down!" refers to Newton's first law of motion.

5. Free-body diagrams show the locations and directions of all forces and moments acting on a body.

6. For simplification of calculations, the entire mass of the body may be considered to be concentrated at its COM.

7. The hip joint has three rotational DOF.

8. Kinematics describes the motion of objects without regard to their mass or how their motion is brought about.

9. Kinetics involves analysis of the effects of forces and/or moments that are responsible for motion.

10. Each joint has specific load interactions because of the particular characteristics of the joint and the actions of the muscles that cross the joint.

Bibliography

Ashton-Miller JA, Schultz AB: Basic orthopaedic biomechanics, in Mow VC, Hayes WC, eds: *Biomechanics of the Human Spine*, ed 2. Philadelphia, PA, Lippincott-Raven, 1997, pp 353-385.

Caffrey JP, Sah RL: Biomechanics of musculoskeletal tissues, in O'Keefe RJ, Jacobs JJ, Chu CR, Einhorn TA, eds: *Ortho-paedic Basic Science: Foundations of Clinical Practice*, ed 4. Rosemont, IL, American Academy of Orthopaedic Surgeons, 2013, pp 55-68.

Panjabi MM, White AA, eds: *Biomechanics in the Musculo-skeletal System*. New York, NY, Churchill Livingstone, 2001.

Chapter 5
Biomaterials

Reed Ayers, MS, PhD   Kern Singh, MD

I. General Information

A biomaterial is a synthetic material derived from organic or inorganic components and intended to interact with biologic systems. The properties and performance of any biomaterial are dictated by its structure (elemental composition, atomic bonding, atomic organization, or crystallinity) and processing (any one of hundreds of manufacturing techniques, including but not limited to casting, forging, extrusion or injection molding, sintering, welding, solid-state bonding, or filament winding) **Figure 1**.

A. Classes of biomaterials

1. Metals—Typically hard, durable, and often shiny materials, many of which consist of a single element, such as copper or silver, and others of which are alloys of more than one metallic element, such as stainless steel, and many of which are good conductors of heat and electricity.

2. Ceramics—Strong, brittle, and corrosion-resistant materials consisting of elements linked to one another by covalent or ionic bonds, and many of which are oxides of metallic elements, such as alumina (Al_2O_3) and zirconia (ZrO_2), or oxides of silicon (such as SiO_2) or of silicon in combination with metallic or other elements.

3. Polymers—Materials made of atoms of carbon and other elements that are covalently bound to one another to form identical subunits, known as monomers, with the subunits themselves also bound one another, often in repeating sequences, to form chains or sheets. Polymers are typically corrosion resistant, and many are flexible. Examples are polyethylene, polypropylene, polytetrafluoroethylene (PTFE, Teflon), silicones, and hydrogels.

4. Composites—Materials made of mixtures of different constituent materials (a "resin" and a "matrix") that are bound together, although physical interference or weak chemical bonds and not necessarily strong covalent, metal, or ionic bonds, and which have widely varying properties according to their composition. Many engineered polymer and ceramic composite materials are strongly corrosion resistant, and many are made specifically to have desired, tailored material properties. Plywood and concrete are examples of the most common composite materials. Other examples are steel (metal/ceramic composite), fiberglass (polymer/ceramic composite), carbon/kevlar fiber reinforced composites (polymer/polymer composite), adobe (polymer/ceramic composite)—the key is that each has at least two distinct, chemically different phases that together create a new material with a blending of properties (for example, modulus, strength, conductivity). Composite constituents are joined in numerous ways. In metals, it may be done using casting or forging methods. Fiber-reinforced composites may use fiber layup or winding followed by polymer impregnation via vacuum molding or autoclave molding. Ceramic composites may be created using sintering processes.

5. Natural biomaterials—Plant and animal tissues, proteins, polysaccharides, and lipids.

Dr. Ayers or an immediate family member has received research or institutional support from Lanx Spine and DePuy, a Johnson & Johnson company; and has received nonincome support (such as equipment or services), commercially derived honoraria, or other non–research-related funding (such as paid travel) from Lanx Spine. Dr. Singh or an immediate family member has received royalties from Pioneer, Zimmer, and Stryker; and serves as a paid consultant to or is an employee of DePuy, a Johnson & Johnson company, Stryker, and Zimmer.

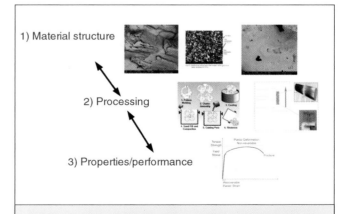

Figure 1   The relationship between properties and performance are related to microscopic structure, chemical constituents and how the material is synthesized (processed).

1: Basic Science

B. Orthopaedic uses—Biomaterials are used in orthopaedics for the internal fixation of fractures, in osteotomies and arthrodeses, in wound closure, as tissue substitutes, and in prostheses and total joint replacements.

C. Orthopaedic requirements—Biomaterials used in orthopaedics must be biocompatible with the anatomic sites and tissues in which they are to be used, with the ability to function in vivo without eliciting detrimental local or systemic responses; must be resistant to corrosion and degradation and able to withstand their in vivo environment; and must have adequate mechanical and wear properties for the applications and settings in which they are to be used.

II. Biocompatibility

Biocompatibility is defined as an acceptable host response for a specific application of a natural or synthetic biomaterial or device. It is neither an intrinsic property nor a single state of a material or device, but rather a series of responses that allow the material or device to fulfill its intended function.

A. Inert biomaterials—Elicit little or no host response.

B. Interactive biomaterials—Designed to elicit specific beneficial responses from the host into which they are implanted, such as tissue ingrowth into the material (for example, in the case of porous metals such as titanium and tantalum).

C. Viable biomaterials—Implanted biomaterials that incorporate and attract cells and are then absorbed and/or remodeled by the host (for example, biodegradable ceramic or polymeric scaffolds for functional tissue engineering).

D. Replanted biomaterials—Native tissues that have been obtained from a donor and cultured in vitro before being implanted in a host (for example, chondroplasts harvested from a host and used for chondroplasty).

E. Biologically incompatible materials—Materials that elicit unacceptable biologic reactions in a host (for example, implant or tissue rejection).

III. Corrosion and Degradation Resistance

Corrosion is defined as an electrochemical process, typically occurring in a metallic substance, that cleaves its chemical bonds and destroys it. Degradation is the same type of process occurring in ceramics and polymers.

A. The in vivo environment of the human body can be highly corrosive.

B. Corrosion can weaken metal implants and release products that can adversely affect their biocompatibility and cause pain, swelling, and the destruction of nearby tissue.

C. Metallic orthopaedic devices are susceptible to several modes of corrosion. The most generally recognized such modes in medical devices are:

1. Pitting corrosion, the most severe form of corrosion of metals, resulting in damage to a metal-containing orthopaedic device and the often toxic release of metal ions. Such corrosion begins in defects in the thin protective oxide layer on a metallic prosthetic component or metal-containing implant.

   a. Stainless steel (A316L) and other alloys of iron are subject to pitting corrosion. Titanium and its alloys, as well as cobalt/chromium/molybdenum/carbon (CoCrMoC) alloys, do not generally exhibit pitting corrosion.

2. Crevice corrosion is a localized attack that can occur when a crevice geometry is created. This type of corrosion can occur in metals that would otherwise resist pitting and other types of corrosion.

   a. Often occurs in the threads of stress and other types of junctions such as weldments, bolted parts, or where two parts are interference fit (for example, a hip stem pressed into a femur). The parts do not necessarily need to be metal-on-metal; however, that is the most common with metal-on-metal surfaces. A crevice geometry can potentially create ionic gradients such that the pH can reach as low as 1, as evidenced in retrieval studies of tapered hip stems.

   b. Damaging ions accumulate in the crevice in which corrosion begins, leading to the development of an environment similar to that in which pitting develops.

   c. Can be eliminated by redesign of the part or device that becomes corroded.

3. Corrosion fatigue and stress corrosion cracking are forms of corrosion caused by the combined effects of the environment around a metal or metallic alloy and mechanical forces on the metal or alloy, such as the regions around screws inserted into metal or metal-alloy plates and rods.

   a. Both corrosion fatigue and stress corrosion cracking can result from cracks, notches, surface imperfections, and damage during wear or handling of a metal or metal-alloy component of an orthopaedic device.

   b. Corrosion fatigue depends on the cyclic loading of a metal or metal-alloy part or device.

   c. Stress crack corrosion depends on the tensile

loading of a metal or metal-alloy part or device.

   d. Stress crack corrosion is a common corrosion mechanism in titanium, its alloys, and CoCrMoC.

4. Galvanic corrosion results from a difference in the electrochemical potential of two metals or metal alloys that are in electrical contact with one another because both are in an electrically conductive medium such as serum or interstitial fluid.

   a. Galvanic corrosion is seen in fracture fixation plates, at the interface between a plate made of one metal or metal alloy and screws or constructs made of a different metal or metal alloy.

   b. Galvanic corrosion is best avoided through the use of similar metals or metal alloys that are in contact with one another in a construct or device, such as titanium screws in a titanium bone plate. The use of dissimilar metals that are to be in contact with each other in such a construct or device, such as platinum and titanium, can enhance corrosion protection but the composition of the metals or alloys being used, and their compatibility, must be determined in advance.

5. Fretting corrosion occurs at contact sites between materials that are subject to micromotion in relation to one another when a load is imposed on them.

   a. Fretting corrosion can be seen in devices that use tapered junctions or movable mechanical interfaces between components, such as a calcar replacement or a modular hip prosthesis.

   b. Fretting corrosion is best prevented by avoiding junctions of different metals or alloys with one another in an implant, or by preventing the micromotion, relative to one another, of parts made of such different metals or alloys.

6. Degradation of orthopaedic biomaterials such as polymers

   a. The degradation of biomaterials made of polymers and other substances can occur through depolymerization; the cross-linking to one another of atoms in different parts of the polymer; oxidative degradation (most common); the leaching of additives; hydrolysis; and crazing or stress cracking.

IV. Mechanical Properties

A. Performance factors—The mechanical performance of an orthopaedic device depends on several factors:

1. The forces to which it is subjected.

2. The mechanical burdens imposed by those forces.

3. The ability of the materials in the device to withstand those burdens over the lifetime of the device.

B. Definitions

1. Compression/tension—Forces perpendicular to the surface of application of a device or other object.

2. Shear—Forces acting in parallel or tangentially to the surface of application of a device or other object.

3. Torsion—A force that causes an object to rotate about an axis.

4. Stress—Force applied over a unit of area

   a. Stress (ς) = force (F)/area (A).

   b. The Standard International (SI) unit for stress is newtons/meter^2 (N/m^2), or Pascals (Pa).

   c. A force that acts perpendicularly to a surface results in a normal stress.

   d. A force that acts tangentially to a surface results in a shear stress.

   e. A stress is tensile if it stretches the material on which it acts, and is compressive if it compresses the material on which it acts.

5. Strain—The deformation of a material by a force acting on the material.

   a. Strain (ε) = change in length (ΔL)/original length (L). Strain is unitless and is generally reported as a percent (%) or unit length of change per unit length of an object (mm/mm).

   b. The types of strain associated with normal and shear stress are called normal strain and shear strain, respectively.

   c. Like stress, strain can be either tensile or compressive.

6. Strength—The load-carrying capacity of a material. A plot of the deformation of a material or object versus the stress acting on the material or object, or stress-strain curve, can be used to describe the strength of the material or object independently of its cross-sectional area. Material properties are generally reported using the term strength, not stress.

7. Toughness—The area under the stress-strain curve of a material or object. It describes the energy needed to cause the material or object to break or fail.

   a. A typical stress-strain diagram for a material is shown in **Figure 2**.

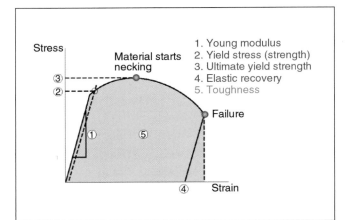

1. Young modulus
2. Yield stress (strength)
3. Ultimate yield strength
4. Elastic recovery
5. Toughness

Figure 2 The various components and relationships in the stress-strain diagram. Note that the slope of elastic recovery is the same as the Young modulus.

Material	Modulus of Elasticity (E) (GPa)	Tensile Strength (MPa)
PMMA	3	70–120
Cancellous bone[a]	10–13	
Cortical bone[a]	18–20	
Titanium (Ti6Al4V ELI)	138	1150
Tantalum	186	285 annealed/650 cold-worked
Stainless steel (A316L)	200	580–650
CoCrMoC	220–234	600
Alumina (Al$_2$O$_3$)	300	NA

Table 1

How the Young Modulus of Elasticity Correlates With Tensile Strength

[a]Cancellous and cortical bone are structural terms and as such the modulus is a structural modulus and not a material modulus. Structural modulus and strength depend on the anatomic location and orientation.

CoCrMoC = cobalt/chromium/molybdenum/carbon, NA = not applicable, PMMA = polymethyl methacrylate.

b. The slope of the linear portions of the curve in **Figure 2** (Item 1 in **Figure 2**) denotes the modulus of elasticity (E) or Young modulus. This is a unique property of a particular material. The modulus of elasticity is a measure of the atomic bonds in a material to resist deformation and return the material to its original shape. The modulus of elasticity (Young modulus) does not correlate with the strength of a material (**Table 1**).

c. A higher modulus of elasticity indicates that a material is stiffer and more resistant to elastic deformation than a material with a lower modulus of elasticity.

d. As the stress on a material or object increases, the slope of the stress-strain curve changes at a point called yield stress (Item 2 in **Figure 2**). Up to this point, the material or object is operating elastically, which means that if the stress is gradually removed, the strain on the material or object decreases until it returns to its original shape.

e. The yield stress is the transition point between elastic and plastic deformation. When the stress on a material or object reaches the yield point, the material or object begins to demonstrate plastic behavior and is permanently deformed. Beyond the yield point, the stress on a material or object either does not increase or increases only slightly, but the material or object undergoes considerable elongation as the result of atomic movement.

f. The maximum stress that a material or object can support is called its ultimate strength. Beyond this ultimate strength, the stress on the material or object decreases while the material or object deforms (necks) until it fractures or fails.

g. A material can be classified as either brittle or ductile, on the basis of the characteristics of its stress-strain curve (**Figure 3**).

- A brittle material exhibits very little plastic deformation before fracture, and when tension is applied to it, it fails at a relatively low strain (**Figure 3**). Examples of brittle materials are ceramics such as alumina (Al$_2$O$_3$), hydroxyapatite and other calcium phosphates, commercially pure titanium, concrete, cast irons, glasses such as silica, and thermoset polymers such as Bakelite.

- In contrast, ductile materials undergo large strains during plastic deformation before they fracture or otherwise fail. Stainless steel (A316L), cobalt-chromium alloys (CoCrMoC), titanium alloys (Ti6Al4V, TNTZ), copper, magnesium, nylon, and PTFE (Teflon) are examples of ductile materials.

h. Fatigue failure is failure related to the cyclic loading of a material or object.

- This is the most common mode of failure in orthopaedic applications.

- When a metal or other material is subjected

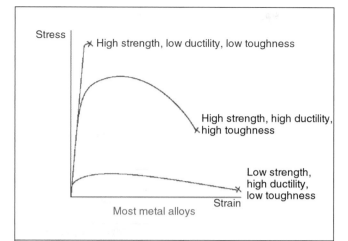

Stress

✕ High strength, low ductility, low toughness

High strength, high ductility,
✕ high toughness

Low strength,
high ductility,
✕ low toughness

Strain

Most metal alloys

Figure 3   The various stress-strain relationships. High strength with low ductility is indicative of a ceramic. High strength and high ductility is typical of steels, certain polymers, and viscoelastic responses of materials. Low strength and high ductility is typical of most polymers such as rubber, silicone, elastin, and collagen.

to a dynamic load with a large number of loading cycles, failure will occur at loads below the yield stress point of the metal or other material. The failure strength of a metal or other material decreases with an increasing number of loading cycles.

- Fatigue failure consists of three steps: the initiation of a crack in a metal or other material, the propagation of the crack, and catastrophic failure of the metal or other material.

- The endurance limit (fatigue strength) is a characteristic only of ferrous alloys such as stainless steel. Nonferrous alloys, such as aluminum or titanium alloys, ceramics, and polymers, do not exhibit endurance limits. The endurance limit is defined as the strength of a ferrous alloy after 10^6 loading cycles.

i. When subject to loads or other forces, isotropic materials (for example, stainless steel, titanium alloys) have the same mechanical properties along all axes or in all directions within these materials.

j. In contrast to isotropic materials, anisotropic materials (for example, bone, cartilage, muscle, ligament, carbon-fiber composites) exhibit varying mechanical properties along different axes or in different directions within these materials under loading. This anisotropic behavior is a result of specifically oriented constituent parts of these materials, such as collagen fibrils or crystals.

k. All materials except for very brittle materials can be considered viscoelastic, exhibiting viscosity in that they resist both shear flow and strain when subjected to stress, and exhibiting elasticity in that they undergo distortion when subjected to stress and return rapidly to their original state when the stress is removed. Viscoelastic properties are time or rate dependent.

- Stress and/or strain depend on time.

- Hysteresis is the dependence of a system on both its present and past environments because the system can be in more than one internal state. Hysteresis is represented by the area between the loaded and unloaded regions of a stress-strain curve.

- Creep is the increased deformation of a material over time in response to the application of a constant force. An example of creep occurs in a rubber band wrapped around a book for an extended period.

- Stress relaxation is a decrease in the stress on a material or object over time as the result of a constant displacement within the material or object.

- The polar moment of inertia is a quantity determined by the cross-sectional area and distribution of an object around a neutral axis upon torsional loading of the object. The greater the polar moment of inertia, the stiffer and stronger the object. Accordingly, a thicker or larger part of a device is more resistant to increased loads and deformations than would be a similar thinner or smaller part. For example, a spine surgeon may select a 6.5-mm spine rod over a 5.5-mm spine rod to create a stiffer construct to more rigidly fix the spine.

V. Properties of Specific Biologic and Medical Materials

A. Host tissue

1. Bone

   a. Bone is a composite of inorganic mineral salts (consisting mainly of calcium and phosphate) and an organic matrix (mainly type I collagen and ground substance). The inorganic component of bone is what makes it hard and rigid, whereas the organic component gives bone its flexibility.

   b. Bone is anisotropic as a result of the orientation of its components.

   c. The stiffness and strength of bone and its storage of energy increase with the rate at which it

1: Basic Science

is loaded (for example, it is viscoelastic).

   d. Macroscopically, skeletal tissue is composed of cortical and cancellous (trabecular) bone. Bone of both types can be considered as a single material with widely varying porosity, density, and other properties.

   e. The apparent density of bone is determined by the mass of a specimen of bone divided by the volume of the specimen.

- The apparent density of cortical bone is approximately 1.8 g/cm^3.

- The apparent density of trabecular bone ranges from 0.1 g/cm^3 to 1.0 g/cm^3.

   f. With aging, a progressive net loss of bone mass occurs, beginning in the fifth decade and proceeding at a faster rate in women than in men. The loss of bone mass results in reduced bone strength, a reduced modulus of elasticity of bone, and an increased likelihood of fractures.

   g. Several radiographic studies have suggested that aging is associated with bone remodeling that affects the force distribution within bone (the Wolff Law).

- Subperiosteal apposition of bone occurs along with endosteal absorption in tubular bones, transforming these bones into cylinders of larger diameter.

- This remodeling of the diaphysis of long bones is hypothesized to serve a mechanical "compensatory" function for environmental changes to the individual (for example, individual aging, increased limb loading because of athletics, reduced loading because of space flight). Stated simply, the bone is reshaped in terms of cross-sectional geometry and wall thickness to best match the load environment imposed upon it. For example, in older individuals, the cross-sectional moment of inertia of long bones is remodeled so that where the cortical wall thins, the load-bearing capacity is not lost. Essentially, the reshaping of the bone compensates for the lost load-bearing capacity of a thin cortical wall so that load-bearing capacity is not lost.

- The increase in outer diameter of a long bone as the result of bone apposition is much smaller in women than in men, potentially predisposing women to an increased rate of fracture.

2. Tendons

   a. Tendons consist predominantly of type I collagen.

   b. Tendons transmit muscle forces to bone.

- Tendons center the action of several muscles into a single line of pull (such as with the Achilles tendon).

- Tendons distribute the contractile force of a single muscle (such as the posterior tibialis) to several bones, such as metatarsal and cuneiform bones.

- Tendons allow the direction of pull on bones to be changed in conjunction with an anatomic pulley (for example, posterior tibialis tendon around the medial malleolus).

   c. Tendons are anisotropic as a result of the orientation of their components. The alignment of tendon fibers along a specific axis creates a structure that has one set of properties, strength, and modulus, in one direction and a different set of properties perpendicular to that direction.

   d. Tendons are viscoelastic.

- Under conditions of low loading, tendons are relatively compliant.

- With increasing loads, tendons become increasingly stiff until they reach a range in which they exhibit nearly linear stiffness.

   e. Many tendons have components of varying orientation that may experience variable loads with any action. Loads applied obliquely during eccentric contractions pose the highest risk of tendon ruptures.

   f. The ultimate tensile load on a tendon is rarely more than 5% of that ultimate load and as such, muscle ruptures and tendon avulsions are more common than ruptures of tendons themselves. Midsubstance disruptions of tendons usually occur only in tendons that are diseased before being subjected to a tensile overload (for example, in an Achilles tendon with tendinosis).

3. Ligaments

   a. Ligaments are composed predominantly of type I collagen.

   b. Ligaments connect bones to other bones.

- The bony attachments of ligaments are very important to their structural strength.

- Forces directed perpendicularly to the insertions of ligaments have been shown to cause the shear failure of ligaments at their bone interfaces under relatively low loads.

   c. Like tendons, ligaments are viscoelastic, with properties that depend on the rate at which loads are applied to them.

B. Metals

1. Metals are crystalline arrays. Within each crystal,

Table 2		

Metals Used in Orthopaedic Applications

Metal	Properties	Applications
Stainless steel	Predominantly an iron-nickel-chromium-carbon alloy. Carbon in the iron matrix imparts strength. Chromium forms a tenacious oxide on the surface (passivation). Susceptible to pitting and crevice corrosion.	Fracture plates and screws.
Cobalt alloys	Composed of cobalt, chromium, molybdenum, and carbon. Chromium increases strength and corrosion resistance (passivation). Molybdenum combines with carbon to increase strength. Among the strongest metals used for orthopaedic implants.	High-load applications that require longevity such as joint arthroplasty devices.
Titanium and titanium alloys	Biocompatibility is imparted by the formation of a titanium oxide film that spontaneously forms on the surface (passivation). Uniform corrosion is limited. Susceptible to stress crack corrosion, especially if the surface is notched or damaged. Titaniums are notch sensitive (sharp corners, holes, scratches, dents, and other stress concentrators that lower the strength of the metal).	Commercially pure titanium is used for low-load fracture fixation (for example, phalangeal fractures). Higher-strength applications (hip and knee implants) must use alloys (Ti6Al4V, TNTZ).
Tantalum	Highly biocompatible, corrosion resistant, and osteoconductive.	Porous forms of tantalum deposited on pyrolytic carbon backbones have been promoted as superior structures for bone ingrowth. Applications include coatings for joint arthroplasty components (acetabular cups)

1: Basic Science

the atoms of the metal are regularly spaced and packed in specific configurations, allowing them to share their outer valence electrons, which are responsible for the excellent heat and electrical conductivity of metals.

2. Alloys are mixtures of different metals or of metals and nonmetallic elements.

3. Metals are typically fabricated by casting, forging, or extrusion.

   a. Casting—Molten metal is poured into a mold. Objects or parts formed in this way tend to be weaker and require further processing to gain strength.

   b. Forging—Hot mechanical forming of metal using hammers, presses, or forging machines is used to form a metal object or part by compressing, bending, or otherwise shaping a mass of heated, malleable metal. Forged metal objects tend to be stronger than cast metal objects.

   c. Extrusion—Metal is heated and forced through a die to obtain a continuous object with a specifically shaped cross section, such as a duct or tube.

4. Several alloys are commonly used in orthopaedics (**Table 2**).

   a. Stainless steel (the most commonly used alloy

of which is 316L, in which iron is alloyed with substantial amounts of chromium and nickel to enhance its corrosion resistance). Note because they contain potentially allergenic metals, notably nickel, chromium, and molybdenum, 316L and other steels can induce an allergenic response.

- The ductility of stainless steel is important in applications such as bone screws, in which a definite yield point of bone allows the surgeon to feel the beginning of plastic deformation. Because the steel has a single yield point where the metal begins to deform, the surgeon can feel if the bone begins to yield prior to the screw yielding, unlike titanium, which has a range of yield points.

- Carbon is added to impart strength to steel, but it must remain in solution with molten iron to do so. If the carbon concentration of the molten iron–carbon mixture is too high, iron carbides (Fe_3C) segregate, forming a brittle ceramic phase and substantially weakening the resulting steel by making it prone to corrosion-related fracture.

- Stainless steel is susceptible to pitting and crevice corrosion, although its corrosion resistance can be improved by increased nitrogen alloying.

b. Cobalt alloys—Are among the strongest orthopaedic implant materials and are suitable for high-load applications that require longevity.

- Consist of approximately 70% cobalt and 27% chromium by atomic content, with small percentages of molybderum and carbon included to enhance strength and ductility.

- The predominant fabrication technique for cobalt alloys is casting.

c. Titanium and its alloys

- Pure titanium is typically used for fracture fixation at anatomic sites at which large loads are not expected (for example, maxilla, wrist, phalanges). Pure titanium is less ductile than stainless steel and is highly susceptible to notch hardening and stress corrosion cracking, explaining the screw and rod breakage often noted with titanium prostheses.

- For higher-strength applications, titanium alloys must be used (for example, Ti6Al4V, which consists of titanium with atomic contents of 6% aluminum for increased strength and 4% vanadium for increased ductility).

d. Tantalum

- A transitional metal that is highly corrosion resistant.

- Facilitates bone ingrowth into a prosthetic device.

C. Polymers

1. Polymers are large molecules consisting of combinations of smaller molecules. The properties of a polymer are dictated by:

a. Its chemical structure (the monomer of which multiple units are linked together to create the polymer).

b. Its molecular weight. Determined by the number of monomers in the polymer.

c. Its physical structure (the way in which the monomers are attached to each other within the polymer).

d. Isomerism (the different orientations of atoms in some polymers).

e. Crystallinity (the packing of polymer chains into ordered atomic arrays).

2. Polymethyl methacrylate (PMMA, also known as Lucite or Plexiglas) is the most commonly used polymer in orthopaedics. It is a member of the same family of methacrylate polymers used in contact lenses.

a. PMMA is produced through an addition reaction in which molecules of methyl methacrylate, the methyl ester of methacrylic acid, become chemically bound to one another to generate PMMA, with the resulting solid polymer then being machined into a final configuration or used as bone cement. PMMA can also be molded into specific shapes. Cementing in situ follows the same reaction process described below. In situ temperature control is maintained via appropriate balance between resin and hardener.

- The liquid component in the formation of PMMA is predominantly a methyl methacrylate monomer.

- The powder in the formation of PMMA is composed mainly of polymerized PMMA or a blend of PMMA with a copolymer consisting either of PMMA and polystyrene or of PMMA and methacrylic acid. The powder also contains dibenzoyl peroxide, which intiates the polymerization reaction.

- Mixing of the liquid and solid two components for the generation of PMMA results in an exothermic reaction (with a temperature of approximately 82°C).

b. Antibiotics can be added to PMMA bone cement to provide prophylaxis or aid in the treatment of infection. However, the addition of antibiotics during the mixing process used in producing PMMA can adversely affect the properties of PMMA bone cement by interfering with the crystallinity of the polymer.

c. The performance of PMMA bone cement has been enhanced through improved protocols in its handling, in bone preparation, and in delivery of the cement to the site at which it acts.

d. Vacuum mixing or centrifugation may decrease the porosity of PMMA cement, increasing its ultimate tensile strength by about 40%.

3. Ultra-high–molecular-weight polyethylene (UHMWPE) is another polymer commonly used in orthopaedics.

a. This long polyethylene polymer has a very high molecular weight, providing substantially greater impact strength, toughness, and better abrasive wear characteristics to the devices in which it is used than do polyethylenes of lower molecular weights.

b. Three methods are used to fabricate orthopaedic components from UHMWPE:

- Ram extrusion—The semisolid resin of UHMWPE is extruded through a die under heat and pressure to form a cylindrical bar that is then machined into a final shape.

- Compression molding—The resin of UHMWPE is modeled into a large sheet that is cut into smaller pieces to use in machining of the final components of a prosthesis or other device.

- Direct molding—The resin of UHMWPE is directly molded into a finished part.

c. The most common method for sterilizing components of an orthopaedic device that are made of UHMWPE is by exposing them to gamma radiation.

d. Postirradiation oxidation adversely affects the material properties of UHMWPE by increasing its modulus of elasticity, decreasing its elongation to the point at which it breaks, and decreasing its toughness. Free radicals generated by the irradiation of UHMWPE may have one of several ends:

- Recombination—The bonds that were broken to create the free radicals are simply reformed, regenerating the UHMWPE without a net change in its chemistry.

- Chain scission—The free radicals generated from UHMWPE may react with oxygen, fragmenting the polymer. The resulting polyethylene polymer will have a lower molecular weight and greater density than the original polymer.

- Cross-linking—Free radicals generated from different UHMWPE polymer strands can combine with one another, forming chemical bonds between the strands. The resulting cross-linked polymer strands may constitute a harder and more abrasion-resistant material than the original polymer strands that were cross-linked to form the material. Extremely high numbers of cross-links between two or more polymer strands may result in a brittle material susceptible to cracking. Increased cross-linking, resulting from the generation of free radicals by either gamma or electron-beam irradiation of UHMWPE, improves the wear resistance of polyethylene components used in total joint arthroplasty. However, the irradiation process increases the susceptibility of these components to fracture and wear.

- Degradation—Breakdown of the polymer chain. This may be avoided or minimized by:

  ○ Sterilization that does not involve irradiation, such as through exposure to ethylene oxide or gas plasma, which does not generate free radicals and therefore does not cause the cross-linking of UHMWPE chains. However, recent clinical studies of total hip arthroplasty have demonstrated substantially less wear of these prostheses with radiation sterilization than with sterilization using ethylene oxide or gas plasma.

  ○ Irradiation with nitrogen or argon, in the absence of oxygen, minimizes free-radical formation.

4. Biodegradable polymers that degrade chemically and/or physically in a controlled manner over time can be synthesized.

   a. Examples of such polymers include variations of polylactic acid (PLA), polyglycolic acid (PGA), polydioxanone, and polycaprolactone. Polylactic acid has been a desirable choice because its degradation product is lactic acid, a natural constituent of the Krebs cycle.

   b. The biodegradable polymers of PLA, PGA, polydioxanone, and polycaprolactine are resorbed at different rates.

   - PLA is more rapidly resorbed than PGA.

   - Products that are composites of these polymers may have properties intermediate to those of any of the pure polymers.

   c. Resorption of the components of polymer as it degrades allows the host tissue to assume its original biologic role as a prosthesis or other device made from the polymer gradually loses is load-sharing capabilities. This must be balanced with the need to maintain the mechanical properties of an anatomic structure through the use of a supportive device while the tissues of the structure undergo healing.

   d. A resorbable polymer can also be used in drug delivery by releasing a drug as the polymer degrades.

5. Hydrogels—Networks of water-swollen polymer chains whose classification depends on the way in which they are prepared, their ionic charge, or their physical structure. Hydrogels have been considered for use in a wide range of applications, including contact lenses (polyhydroxyethylmethacrylate, drug delivery, and tissue engineering.

   a. Hydrogels are soft, porous, and permeable polymers that absorb water readily.

   b. Hydrogels have low coefficients of friction and time-dependent mechanical properties that can be varied by altering their composition and structure.

D. Ceramics

1. Ceramics are solid, inorganic compounds consisting of metallic and nonmetallic elements bound

1: Basic Science

by ionic or covalent bonds.

2. Ceramics include compounds such as silica (SiO_2) and alumina (Al_2O_3).

3. Structural ceramics of the type used in orthopaedic applications are typically three-dimensional crystalline arrays of positively charged metal ions and negatively charged nonmetal ions such as oxygen (in oxides), carbon (in carbides), and nitrogen (in nitrides).

4. When processed to high purity, ceramics have excellent biocompatibility because of their insolubility and chemical inertness.

5. Ceramic materials are stiff and brittle but very strong under compressive loads.

6. Ceramics have gained favor in two types of orthopaedic applications: as components of total joint arthroplasty procedures and as bone-graft substitutes.

   a. Bearings—Ceramic-on-polyethylene and ceramic-on-ceramic bearings are becoming more widely used in total joint arthroplasty.

   • Ceramics have high hardness and high lubricity, allowing them to be polished to a very smooth finish and to resist wear when used as bearing surfaces.

   • Ceramics also have good wettability, suggesting that lubricating layers can be used between ceramic surfaces to reduce adhesive wear (for example, fretting) of these surfaces.

   • Alumina, in the form of aluminum oxide, has shown lower rates of wear when used for prosthetic bearings than have conventional metal-on-polyethylene bearings. Although early clinical experience found that the fracture of femoral heads made of alumina was a substantial problem, this problem appears to be design related, not material related. Newer device designs have shown significantly lower fracture rates.

   • Zirconia, in the form of zirconium oxide (ZrO_2), has shown less clinical success than alumina when used as a bearing surface in contact with polyethylene. Zirconia has less toughness (lower energy absorbance to surface failure, called fretting) than alumina, which makes it more susceptible to roughening and increased wear.

   b. Bone substitutes

   • Certain ceramics have been found to be osteoconductive, supporting the attachment of osteogenic precursor cells, and have accordingly been developed as bone-graft materials.

• Hydroxyapatite (HA)

   ○ HA ($Ca_5(PO4)_3(OH)$) is a hydrated calcium phosphate that is similar in crystalline structure to the HA that is the major mineral component of bone.

   ○ Because of its low solubility, HA is very slowly resorbed by the body.

• β-Tricalcium phosphate, α-tricalcium phosphate, and calcium sulfate are alternatives to HA as bone-graft materials. These alternative materials have less strength and faster resorption than HA, but appear to have greater bioactivity.

• Other molecules, such as the ceramic silica (SiO_2), have been shown to induce bone formation when combined with other ceramics such as calcium phosphates.

Glossary of Terms

Biomaterial—A synthetic material derived from organic or inorganic components and intended to interact with biologic systems

Brittle material—A material that exhibits very little plastic deformation before fracture, and when tension is applied to it, it fails at a relatively low strain

Ceramics—Strong, brittle, and corrosion-resistant materials consisting of elements linked to one another by covalent or ionic bonds, and many of which are oxides of metallic elements, such as alumina (Al_2O_3) and zirconia (ZrO_2)

Corrosion—An electrochemical process, typically occurring in a metallic substance, that cleaves its chemical bonds and destroys it

Creep—The increased deformation of a material over time in response to the application of a constant force

Ductile material—A material that can undergo large strains during plastic deformation before it fractures or otherwise fails

Extrusion—The heating and forcing of a metal through a die to obtain a continuous object with a specifically shaped cross section, such as a duct or tube

Fatigue failure—Failure of a material or object related to its cyclic loading

Hysteresis—The dependence of a system on both its present and past environments because the system can be in more than one internal state

Interactive biomaterial—A biomaterial designed to elicit specific beneficial responses from the host into which it is implanted, such as tissue ingrowth into the material (for example, in the case of porous metals such as titanium and tantalum)

Isotropic material—A material that has the same mechanical properties along all of its internal axes or directions when subjected to loads or other forces

Load—The force that acts on an object

Metals—Typically hard, durable, and often shiny materials, many of which consist of a single element, such as copper or silver, and others of which are alloys of more than one metallic element

Modulus of elasticity—A measure of the atomic bonds in a material to resist deformation and return the material to its original shape

Polymer—A material made of atoms of carbon and other elements that are covalently bound to one another to form identical subunits, known as monomers, with the subunits themselves also bound one another, often in repeating sequences, to form chains or sheets

Polymethyl methacrylate (PMMA)—The most commonly used polymer in orthopaedics

Strain—The deformation of a material by a force acting on the material

Toughness—The area under the stress-strain curve of a material or object, describing the energy needed to cause the material or object to break or fail

Top Testing Facts

General Information

1. Ceramics are strong, brittle, and corrosion-resistant materials consisting of elements linked to one another by covalent or ionic bonds, and many of which are oxides of metallic elements, such as alumina (Al_2O_3) and zirconia (ZrO_2), or oxides of silicon (such as SiO_2) or of silicon in combination with metallic or other elements.

2. Polymers are materials made of atoms of carbon and other elements that are covalently bound to one another to form identical subunits, known as monomers, with the subunits themselves also bound to one another, often in repeating sequences, to form chains or sheets.

3. Biomaterials used in orthopaedics must be biocompatible with the anatomic sites and tissues in which they are to be used, with the ability to function in vivo without eliciting detrimental local or systemic responses; must be resistant to corrosion and degradation and able to withstand their in vivo environment; and must have adequate mechanical and wear properties for the applications and settings in which they are to be used.

Biocompatibility

1. Interactive biomaterials are designed to elicit specific beneficial responses from the host into which they are implanted, such as tissue ingrowth into the material (for example, in the case of porous metals such as titanium and tantalum).

2. Viable biomaterials are implanted biomaterials that incorporate and attract cells and are then absorbed and/or remodeled by the host (for example, biode-gradable ceramic or polymeric scaffolds for functional tissue engineering).

3. Biologically incompatible materials are materials that elicit unacceptable biologic reactions in a host (for example, implant or tissue rejection).

Corrosion and Degradation Resistance

1. Corrosion is an electrochemical process, typically occurring in a metallic substance, that cleaves its chemical bonds and destroys it.

2. Corrosion can weaken metal implants and release products that can adversely affect their biocompatibility and cause pain, swelling, and the destruction of nearby tissue.

3. Both corrosion fatigue and stress corrosion cracking can result from cracks, notches, surface imperfections, and damage during wear or handling of a metal or metal alloy component of an orthopaedic device.

4. Galvanic corrosion results from a difference in the electrochemical potential of two metals or metal alloys that are in electrical contact with one another because both are in an electrically conductive medium such as serum or interstitial fluid.

5. The degradation of biomaterials made of polymers and other substances can occur through depolymerization; the cross-linking to one another of atoms in different parts of the polymer; oxidative degradation (most common); the leaching of additives; hydrolysis; and crazing or stress cracking.

Top Testing Facts

Mechanical Properties

1. Load is the force that acts on an object.

2. Compression and tension are forces perpendicular to the surface of application of a device or other object.

3. Shear forces are forces that act in parallel or tangentially to the surface of application of a device or other object.

4. Torsion is a force that causes an object to rotate about an axis.

5. Strain is the deformation of a material by a force acting on the material.

6. Strength is the load-carrying capacity of a material.

7. The modulus of elasticity measures the ability of a material to maintain its shape under the application of an external load. The higher the modulus of elasticity, the stiffer the material.

8. A viscoelastic material has properties that are rate-dependent or have time-dependent responses to applied forces.

9. An isotropic material has the same mechanical properties in all directions. In general, ceramics and metals are isotropic.

10. An anisotropic material has properties that differ depending on the direction of load. Bone, muscle, ligament, and tendon all are anisotropic.

Properties of Specific Biologic and Medical Materials

1. The stiffness and strength of bone and its storage of energy increase with the rate at which it is loaded.

2. Forces directed perpendicularly to the insertions of ligaments have been shown to cause the shear failure of ligaments at their bone interfaces under relatively low loads.

3. Alloys are metals composed of mixtures or solutions of metallic and nonmetallic elements that are varied to influence their biomechanical properties, including strength, stiffness, corrosion resistance, and ductility.

4. The properties of a polymer are dictated by its chemical structure (the monomer), the molecular weight (the number of monomers), the physical structure (the way monomers are attached to each other), isomerism (the different orientation of atoms in some polymers), and crystallinity (the packing of polymer chains into ordered atomic arrays).

5. Ceramics are solid, inorganic compounds consisting of metallic and nonmetallic elements held together by ionic or covalent bonds.

6. Cobalt alloys are among the strongest orthopaedic implant materials and are suitable for high-load applications that require longevity.

7. Pure titanium is typically used for fracture fixation at anatomic sites at which large loads are not expected (for example, maxilla, wrist, phalanges).

8. PMMA is the most commonly used polymer in orthopaedics.

9. In the process of cross-linking, free radicals generated from different UHMWPE polymer strands can combine with one another, forming chemical bonds between the strands. The resulting cross-linked polymer strands may constitute a harder and more abrasion-resistant material than the original polymer strands that were cross-linked to form the material.

10. Hydrogels are soft, porous, and permeable polymers that absorb water readily.

11. Ceramics also have good wettability, suggesting that lubricating layers can be used between ceramic surfaces to reduce adhesive wear (for example, fretting) of these surfaces.

12. β-Tricalcium phosphate, α-tricalcium phosphate, and calcium sulfate are alternatives to HA as bone graft materials.

Bibliography

Black J: *Biologic Performance of Materials: Fundamentals of Biocompatibility.* New York, NY, Taylor & Francis, 2006.

Behravesh E, Yasko AW, Engel PS, Mikos AG: Synthetic biodegradable polymers for orthopaedic applications. *Clin Orthop Relat Res* 1999;367, suppl:S118-S129.

Davis JR, ed: *Handbook of Materials for Medical Devices.* Materials Park, OH, ASM International, 2003.

Einhorn TA, O'Keefe RJ, Buckwalter JA, eds: *Orthopaedic Basic Science: Foundations of Clinical Practice,* ed 3. Rosemont, IL, American Academy of Orthopaedic Surgeons, 2007.

Gerdau MACSTEEL: *Metallurgical Data,* ed 4. Lansing, MI, Gerdau MACSTEEL, 1998, pp 79, 104-109, 128-144.

Hamadouche M, Sedel L: Ceramics in orthopaedics. *J Bone Joint Surg Br* 2000;82(8):1095-1099.

Jacobs JJ, Gilbert JL, Urban RM: Corrosion of metal orthopaedic implants. *J Bone Joint Surg Am* 1998;80(2):268-282.

Laurencin CT, ed: *Bone Graft Substitutes.* West Conshohocken, PA, ASTM International, 2003.

Lewis G: Properties of acrylic bone cement: State of the art review. *J Biomed Mater Res* 1997;38(2):155-182.

Ratner BD, Hoffman FJ, Schoen FJ, Lemons JE, eds: *Biomaterials Science: An Introduction to Materials in Medicine*, ed 2. San Diego, CA, Elsevier Academic Press, 2004.

Shackelford J: *Introduction to Materials Science for Engineers*, ed 7. Upper Saddle River, NJ, Pearson Prentice Hall, 2010.

Shalaby SW, Burg KJL, eds: *Absorbable and Biodegradable Polymers*. New York, NY, CRC Press, 2004.

1: Basic Science

Chapter 6

Bone Grafts, Bone Morphogenetic Proteins, and Bone Substitutes

Hyun Bae, MD   Neil Bhamb, MD   Linda E.A. Kanim, MA   Justin S. Field, MD

I. Bone Healing

A. Primary bone healing—Occurs with constructs that provide absolute stability. When open reduction and internal fixation is performed, the initial fracture hematoma is disrupted, possibly slowing repair via removal of the fibrin scaffold and loss of early infiltrating cells and cytokines.

1. Fixation of bony surfaces enables primary healing by creating a low-strain environment.

2. Bone heals directly by cortical remodeling.

3. Areas not in direct apposition may be filled by woven bone that is subsequently remodeled to lamellar bone.

B. Secondary bone healing—Involves responses in the periosteum and surrounding soft tissues. Two types of secondary healing occur: endochondral and intramembranous. Typically, both types occur concurrently at a fracture site.

C. Fracture healing is classically described in three phases.

1. Inflammation (early phase)

a. Hematoma formation and inflammation occur rapidly in the early phases of bone repair.

b. Surface osteocytes may survive and are important in synthesizing new bone.

c. Inflammatory cells migrate to the fracture site, followed by fibroblasts and chondrocytes.

d. Vasodilation increases local flow and angiogenesis is stimulated, with capillary ingrowth primarily from the periosteum.

e. Bone morphogenetic proteins (BMPs) are thought to play an important role in inducing host mesenchymal stem cell migration and differentiation at the repair site.

2. Reparative (middle phase) (**Figure 1**)

a. New bone formation takes the form of immature woven bone (soft callus).

b. Seams of osteoid surround the core of necrotic

Dr. Bae or an immediate family member has received royalties from Biomet, Stryker, Zimmer, and Nuvasive; is a member of a speakers' bureau or has made paid presentations on behalf of Medtronic and Synthes; serves as a paid consultant to or is an employee of Medtronic, Zimmer, and Synthes; has stock or stock options held in Medtronic, Stryker, Orthovita, Spinal Restoration, and Difusion; has received research or institutional support from Stryker, LDR, J&J, Orthovita, and Medtronic; and serves as a board member, owner, officer, or committee member of KASS. Ms. Kanim or an immediate family member has stock or stock options held in Medtronic. Dr. Field or an immediate family member has received royalties from Globus Medical and Nuvasive; is a member of a speakers' bureau or has made paid presentations on behalf of Biomet, Globus Medical, and Precision Spine; serves as a paid consultant to or is an employee of Advanced Biologics, Alphatec Spine, Biomet, Globus Medical, Paradigm Spine, and Precision Spine; and has received research or institutional support from Globus Medical and Relievant. Neither Dr. Bhamb nor any immediate family member has received anything of value from or has stock or stock options held in a commercial company or institution related directly or indirectly to the subject of this chapter.

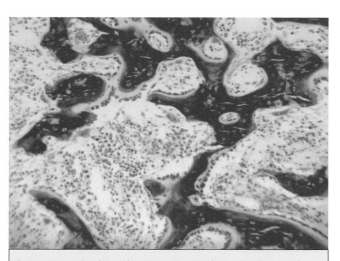

Figure 1   Histology shows reparative bone healing with osteoblasts lining new trabecular bone spicules.

1: Basic Science

bone and form viable new bone (hard callus).

   c. During endochondral ossification, hyaline cartilage provides a framework bridging fracture fragments.

   d. Cartilage is subsequently calcified by osteoblasts.

3. Remodeling (late phase)

   a. Coupled resorption and formation occur.

   b. Remodeling is influenced by the Wolff law and is usually complete by 1 year.

D. Endochondral versus intramembranous bone healing

1. Healing occurs via endochondral ossification, which directly bridges the fracture gap, and intramembranous bone formation subperiosteally adjacent to the fracture.

2. Factors that impair bone healing

   a. Excessive instability at the fracture site or nonapposition of bone

   b. Lack of blood supply because of the local vascular anatomy or periosteal stripping from injury/dissection

   c. Anti-inflammatory medications (NSAIDs, steroids)

   d. Smoking

   e. Systemic disease: metabolic bone conditions

II. Role of Bone Grafts

A. Multiple clinical problems may indicate the use of bone graft.

1. Fracture healing, treatment of delayed unions or nonunions

2. Arthrodesis (**Figure 2**)

3. Replacement of osseous defects occurring as a result of trauma, tumor, or wear

B. Bone grafts perform one or more physiologic mechanisms.

1. Osteogenesis

   a. Osteogenic graft material directly provides cells that are capable of in vivo bone formation.

   b. Osteoprogenitor cells can proliferate and differentiate to osteoblasts and eventually to osteocytes. Mesenchymal stem cells are multipotent and may be induced to differentiate into bone-forming cells by the local environment.

   c. Examples: Autologous bone graft, bone marrow aspirate

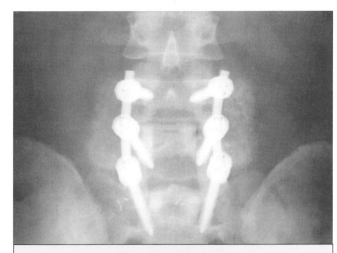

Figure 2   AP radiograph shows L4-S1 instrumented posterior fusion with bone graft placed in the posterolateral gutters.

2. Osteoinduction

   a. Osteoinductive graft material has factors that induce progenitor cells down a bone-forming lineage via cytokines acting as chemoattractants and differentiation factors.

   b. Example: BMPs

3. Osteoconduction

   a. Osteoconductive materials serve as a mechanical scaffold into which new bone can form.

   b. The three-dimensional configuration and building-block material dictates osteoconductive properties.

   c. Cancellous bone has greater bone-forming potential than cortical bone because of its greater surface area, increased porosity for cellular infiltration, and space for angiogenesis; however, it provides less immediate structural support.

   d. Examples: Acellular cancellous chips

III. Bone Graft Materials

A. Bone graft materials come from a variety of sources and exhibit heterogenous properties (**Table 1**). Different materials can be combined into a composite graft.

B. Autograft is tissue transferred from one site to another in the same individual and has classically been the gold standard of bone graft material. It is still the gold standard by which other grafting materials are measured. Often, the supply may be limited, and procurement can result in donor site morbidity.

1. Autograft is osteogenic, osteoinductive, and osteoconductive.

2. Autograft may be cortical, cancellous, or corticocancellous; it also may be nonvascularized or vascularized.

   a. Cortical autograft provides structural support, but its high inorganic density means it provides fewer cells and factors for osteogenesis.

   b. Cancellous autograft provides less structural support but greater osteoconduction and greater osteogenesis and osteoinduction because of its greater cellular and organic density.

3. Iliac crest bone graft (ICBG) is the most frequent autograft.

   a. It has the potential to provide abundant cancellous and/or cortical graft.

   b. Studies have shown complications associated with ICBG, including chronic pain, hematoma formation, injuries to the lateral femoral cutaneous or cluneal nerves, infection, fracture, and scars. The rate of complications is contested in the literature, with studies conducted before 2000 demonstrating major complication rates between 0.76% and 25.0% and minor complication rates, including pain, between 9.4% and 24.0%. More recent studies have shown variable complications rates but seem to suggest lower rates with current techniques (not harvesting the full outer iliac table).

4. Local autograft may be found at the surgical site. In spinal surgery, bone from the lamina is often a source of local autograft after a laminectomy; however, the quantity available may be limited.

5. Other bone graft sources include the ribs, fibula, and tibial metaphysis. The fibula and rib are the most common potentially vascularized options considered.

C. Allograft is tissue harvested from a cadaver, processed, and then implanted into another individual of the same species. Because of its availability, it is the most frequently used bone-graft alternative in the United States.

1. Allograft can be cortical, cancellous, or corticocancellous.

2. Most allograft lacks viable cells and therefore does not provide osteogenic properties. Osteoinductive factors are reduced because of the sterilization needed to reduce the risk of disease transmission and avoid host immune responses.

3. Allograft products containing viable cells or enhanced with viable cells are new to the market and may offer another grafting option. Tissues selected from a highly screened donor pool are cryopreserved in a process that maintains cellular viability. Few independent published clinical studies on efficacy exist. This class of allograft remains primarily osteoconductive but may have osteogenic and osteoinductive properties.

4. Disease transmission is exceedingly rare in bone allografts. Precise incidence data are not available. However, with recommended donor screening the estimated chance of obtaining a graft from an HIV-positive individual is less than 1 in 1.67 million. The last reports of viral transmission are of hepatitis C in 2002, and human T-cell lymphocytic virus in 1991.

5. The extent of osteoconductive properties, as well as mechanical strength, depends in part on the method of graft processing (fresh, frozen, or freeze-dried form) and whether it is cortical or cancellous.

6. Several different types of allograft may be considered.

   a. Fresh allograft

   • Rarely used because of the potential for an immune response and disease transmission

   • Fresh allograft may be processed to remove cells and reduce host immune reaction. This process has been shown to improve incorporation.

   b. Frozen allograft

   • Reduces immunogenicity; frozen allograft requires cold storage logistics and rewarming before implantation to avoid brittleness, which could result in longitudinal fractures.

   • Maintains the osteoconductive properties and potentially some limited osteoinductive capabilities

   • The shelf life of fresh-frozen bone maintained at −20°C is 1 year; 5 years if kept at −70°C.

   c. Freeze-dried allograft has properties similar to frozen allograft, with a few exceptions.

   • Prepared by freeze-drying

   • Stored at room temperature

   • The shelf life of freeze-dried bone is indefinite but the sterilization of the packaging may expire.

   • Biomechanical studies in the 1980s demonstrated a similar compressive and tensile strength as frozen but reduced torsional/bending strength.

   d. Demineralized bone matrix (DBM)

Table 1

Characteristics of Bone Grafts and Grafting Substitutes

Grafting Modality	Substance/Implant	Osteogenic	Osteoinductive	Osteoconductive
Autografts	Cancellous bone Morcellized iliac crest Metaphyseal long bone	+++	++	+++
	Cortical bone Local bone Iliac crest Fibula	+	+/−	+/−
	Cellular Bone marrow aspirate	++	+/−	−
Allografts	Fresh	−	+/−	++
	Frozen	−	+/−	+
	Freeze-dried Cortical cancellous chips	−	+/−	+
	Demineralized bone matrix Various preparations	−	+/−	+
Growth factors	rhBMP-2 rhBMP-7	−	+++	−
Ceramics	Hydroxyapatite Tricalcium phosphate	−	−	+
Collagen	Absorbable collagen hemostatic sponge	−	−	−

- DBM is allograft processed with a mild acid extraction to remove the mineral content of bone but leave behind the collagenous structure (mostly type I, with some types IV and X) and noncollagenous proteins.

- DBMs are combined with carriers such as collagen, gelatin, hyaluronic acid, and glycerol into DBM-based products.

- The antigenic potential is low because of sterilization and other processing.

- Theoretically, DBMs have osteoinductive activity, but the level of activity depends on the sterilization process, processing methods, particle size/surface area, and geometry. Significant interproduct (between products) and interlot (between lots) variability exists because each production lot is derived from a single patient.

- DBM-based products are osteoconductive and serve as a scaffold for new bone, but they lack structural support.

- The most popular format is a moldable putty containing a DBM base powder mixed with a carrier. The proportion of the DBM base compared with that of the carriers tends to be low in some products.

D. Autologous bone marrow aspirate

1. Bone marrow aspirate is a potential source of mesenchymal stem cells and osteoprogenitors.

2. It may be aspirated percutaneously from the iliac crest, vertebral body, or other sources. Bone marrow aspirate can then be mixed with other bone graft extenders and ceramics to create a composite graft material.

3. The number of cells varies depending on host

Table 1

Characteristics of Bone Grafts and Grafting Substitutes (*continued*)

Donor Site Morbidity	Immunogenicity	Absorption/ Remodeling Rate	Immediate Structure/ Torque Strength	Typical Orthopaedic Applications
++++	–	+++	–	Lumbar spine Cervical spine Long bones
++++	–	++	++	Spine Tibial nonunion
+/–	–	–	–	Augmentation of other grafting materials Spine Long-bone fracture
–	++	+	++	Spine Long-bone fracture
–	+	–	++	Spine Long-bone fracture
–	+/–	–	+	Spine Long-bone fracture
–	+	–	–	Spine Long-bone fracture
–	–	–	–	Spine Long-bone fracture Nonunions
–	–	–	+/–	Spine Coating for fixation/arthroplasty devices
–	+	–	+/–	Functions poorly alone but functions well coupled with BMPs

BMP = bone morphogenetic protein, rh = recombinant human, – = not present, +/– = variable, +, ++, +++ = is present, qualitative importance.

characteristics such as age and sex.

4. It has been suggested that the potency of marrow aspirates could be increased via selective precursor selection, centrifugation, or clonal expansion.

E. Collagen

1. Collagen contributes to mineral deposition, vascular ingrowth, and growth factor binding, providing a favorable environment for bone regeneration. It does not provide structural support but may carry immunogenic potential.

2. Collagen functions poorly alone but is used as a nonstructural carrier for BMPs, DBMs, or other graft materials.

F. Inorganic compounds and synthetic bioceramics

1. Bioceramics are ionically or covalently bonded calcium phosphate compounds composed of metallic and nonmetallic elements. The most commonly used are alumina, zirconia, bioactive glass, hydroxyapatite (HA), and tricalcium phosphate (TCP). Bioceramics are relatively inert. They demonstrate material properties that are strong in compression but weak in tension. Bioceramics easily bond with living tissues. They may provide good scaffolds for the addition of potentially osteogenic cells in skeletal tissue engineering applications.

2. Several classes of ceramic materials are available.

a. Synthetic HA has the chemical composition $Ca_{10}(PO_4)_6(OH)_2$. It typically is used in its crystalline form and is slow to resorb or remodel. For orthopaedic implants, HA usually is coated onto a metal core or incorporated into polymers as composites. HA provides a substrate for bony apposition and ongrowth.

b. β-TCP has the chemical composition $Ca_3(PO_4)_2$. Because of its porous nature and chemical composition, it is faster. It is typically developed for orthopaedic implants as a porous biphasic calcium phosphate scaffold with 60% HA and 40% β-TCP.

c. Other materials, such as bioactive glass, contain silicone salt combinations. These materials typically interact with the body fluids and, through a salt exchange, form an amorphous layer of HA, which provides the scaffold for bony apposition.

3. Bioceramics alone possess no osteogenic or osteoinductive properties, and they have variable immediate structural support secondary to resorption. They provide an osteoconductive effect or scaffold, which varies based on the pore size of the synthesized material. Larger pore sizes (>50 μm) provide more space for the migration and ingrowth of osteogenic cells and vascular supply. A typical preparation is HA and TCP, sometimes mixed with autograft.

IV. Bone Morphogenetic Proteins

A. This family of proteins (**Table 2**) contains at least 20 unique peptides that have now been identified and include members of the transforming growth factor-β (TGF-β) superfamily. Only certain BMPs are osteoinductive; others are unrelated to bone formation or have alternative functions. BMPs play a key role in normal embryonic development.

B. Recombinant human forms of these two types of BMPs are currently available: recombinant human BMP-2 (rhBMP-2) and rhBMP-7. These rhBMPs are highly water soluble; without a carrier, they will rapidly diffuse from a wound bed and may be washed away by irrigation. rhBMP-2 is indicated for use in spinal fusion and tibial shaft fractures. It is delivered in a purified absorbable collagen sponge. rhBMP-7 is available only under a humanitarian device exemption and may be indicated for use in recalcitrant long-bone nonunions.

C. The current use of BMPs in spinal fusion is controversial. Multiple studies from 2011 to 2013 have debated the safety of rhBMPs for spinal fusion; rhBMP-2 is considered equivalent to ICBG in the formation of bone.

D. Because of the controversies surrounding safety and the possible bias in the reporting of adverse advents during the approval of rhBMP-2, two independent studies reviewed the available data on the safety and effectiveness of rhBMP-2.

1. Studies indicated that clinical outcomes or success scores were not clinically different between patients treated with rhBMP-2 and those treated with ICBG. However, one of the studies showed that radiographic fusion was 12% more common in patients treated with rhBMP-2 than in those treated with ICBG.

2. ICBG and rhBMP-2 are associated with similar complication rates when used as a graft material for anterior lumbar interbody fusions, including the rates for retrograde ejaculation.

3. RhBMP-2 is associated with higher complication rates in anterior cervical fusion and higher ectopic bone formation in posterior lumbar interbody fusions.

4. Posterior lateral lumbar fusions using rhBMP-2 are associated with increased transient leg/back pain.

5. A risk of local swelling exists in anterior cervical fusions in which rhBMP-2 is used.

E. Bone graft materials may be used together to combine required properties or because of limited availability of one component.

1. A combination of bone graft materials allows products having different properties to be obtained (for example, structural cortical allografts augmented by DBM and local bone graft).

2. Available grafts such as ICBG or local bone graft that is in limited supply may be augmented by other grafting materials. Example: The supply of autogenous local bone graft or ICBG providing osteogenesis, osteoinduction, and osteoconduction may be limited; therefore, augmentation by osteoconductive DBM may be performed to obtain sufficient volume.

V. Other Modalities to Enhance Bone Healing

A. Electromagnetic stimulation

1. Bone tissue has bioelectric potential.

a. Bioelectric potential is electronegative in areas of growth or healing. The area returns to neutral or electropositive as healing progresses.

b. Bioelectric potential is electronegative in areas of compression and electropositive in areas of tension.

2. Efficacy

a. Trials have shown significant variability in outcomes, with overall efficacy unclear. Benefits have been seen in single studies for some fracture types. Because of the low morbidity of the treatment, the clinical use of electromagnetic

Table 2

A Comparative Overview of Bone Morphogenetic Proteins

BMP	Synonyms	Function	Knockout Phenotype in Mice	Chromosomal Location in Humans	Chromosomal Location in Mice
BMP-1	hTld1	Induction of cartilage, metalloprotease	Reduced ossification	8p21.3	14 32.5 cM
BMP-2	BMP2A	Cartilage and bone formation	Embryonic lethal, heart defect and lack of amnion	20p12	2 76.1 cM
BMP-3	Osteogenin	Negative regulator of bone development	Increased bone mass, bone volume	4q21	5 55.0 cM
BMP-4	BMP2B	Bone and teeth	Embryonic lethal, heart defect, lack of allantois	14q22-q23	14 15.0 cM
BMP-5		Cartilage development	Loss of one pair of ribs in rib cage, short ear	6p12.1	9 42.0 cM
BMP-6	Vgr-1	Liver and joint development	Delayed sternum ossification	6p24-p23	13 20.0 cM
BMP-7	OP-1	Kidney development	Renal defects	20q13	2 102.0 cM
BMP-8	OP-2	Cartilage and bone formation	Spermatogenesis defects	1p35-p32	Not known
BMP-9	Gdf-2	CNS and liver development and angiogenesis	Postnatal retinal vascular remodeling	10q11.22	Chromosome 14
BMP-10		Heart development	Proliferation defects in embryonic cardiomyocytes	2p13.3	6 D2
BMP-11	Gdf-11	CNS development	Skeletal *A–P* axis growth pattern abnormalities	12q13.2	Chromosome 10
BMP-12	Gdf-7, Cdmp3	Tendon and cartilage development	Abnormal skull development	2p24.1	Chromosome 12
BMP-13	Gdf-12, Cdmp2	BMP inhibitor in tendon development	Abnormal skull, bone fusions at wrist and ankle	8q22.	Chromosome 4
BMP-14	GDF-5, CDMP1	Cartilage development	Delay in fracture healing	20q11.2	11 50.5 cM
BMP-15	Gdf-9	Oocyte development	Decreased ovulation and fertilization	Xp11.2	X 0.5 cM

BMP = bone morphogenetic protein, CNS = central nervous system.

Adapted with permission from Bandyopadhyay A, Yadav PS, Prashar, P: BMP signaling in development and diseases: A pharmacological perspective. *Biochemical Pharmacology* 2013;85(7):857-864.

stimulation is common despite its unclear efficacy.

3. Types

   a. Pulsed electromagnetic field—Alternating current is delivered through an external coil used intermittently during the treatment period.

   b. Capacitively coupled electrical stimulation—

Current is delivered between two plates that form a magnetic field over the site of healing.

   c. Direct current electrical stimulation— Direct current is delivered through implanted electrodes.

B. Low-intensity ultrasound may affect bone healing, but it is not in widespread clinical use.

Top Testing Facts

1. Bone healing progresses through three stages: early (inflammation), middle (reparative), and late (remodeling).

2. Bone grafts may be osteogenic, osteoinductive, and/or osteoconductive.

3. Autograft is the gold standard of bone graft materials.

4. Disease transmission is exceedingly rare in bone allografts. It is estimated that with donor screening protocols there is less than a 1 in 1.6 million chance of a false-negative result for HIV status.

5. DBM-based products have been shown to have significant interproduct (between products) and interlot (between lots) donor-specific variability. DBMs are predominantly osteoconductive.

6. Bone marrow aspirates provide potential access to osteogenic mesenchymal precursor cells.

7. Bioceramics are inorganic compounds consisting of metallic and nonmetallic elements held together by ionic or covalent bonds.

8. BMPs (BMP-2, -4, -6, and -7) are potent osteoinductive factors of the TGF-β superfamily.

9. Hyaline cartilage serves as the precursor for bone formation via endochondral ossification.

Bibliography

Arrington ED, Smith WJ, Chambers HG, Bucknell AL, Davino NA: Complications of iliac crest bone graft harvesting. *Clin Orthop Relat Res* 1996;329:300-309.

Bandyopadhyay A, Yadav PS, Prashar P: BMP signaling in development and diseases: A pharmacological perspective. *Biochem Pharmacol* 2013;85(7):857-864.

Bauer TW, Muschler GF: Bone graft materials: An overview of the basic science. *Clin Orthop Relat Res* 2000;371:10-27.

Brighton CT, Hunt RM: Early histological and ultrastructural changes in medullary fracture callus. *J Bone Joint Surg Am* 1991;73(6):832-847.

Buck BE, Malinin T, Brown MD: Bone transplantation and human immunodeficiency virus: An estimate of risk of acquired immunodeficiency syndrome (AIDS). *Clin Orthop Relat Res* 1989;240:129-136.

Carragee EJ, Hurwitz EL, Weiner BK: A critical review of recombinant human bone morphogenetic protein-2 trials in spinal surgery: Emerging safety concerns and lessons learned. *Spine J* 2011;11(6):471-491.

Cooper GS, Kou TD: Risk of cancer after lumbar fusion surgery with recombinant human bone morphogenic protein-2 (rh-BMP-2). *Spine (Phila Pa 1976)* 2013;38(21):1862-1868.

Department of Health and Human Services: Technology Assessment: Bone Morphogenetic Protein. The State of the Evidence of On-Label and Off-Label Use. Original, August 6, 2010. www.cms.gov/Medicare/Coverage/Determination Process/downloads/id75ta.pdf. Accessed December 11, 2013. Correction, December 13, 2010. www.ahrq.gov/clinic/ta/comments/boneprotein/bmpetab2.htm. Accessed December 11, 2013.

Dimitriou R, Mataliotakis GI, Angoules AG, Kanakaris NK, Giannoudis PV: Complications following autologous bone graft harvesting from the iliac crest and using the RIA: A systematic review. *Injury* 2011;42(suppl 2):S3-S15.

Dinopoulos H, Dimitriou R, Giannoudis PV: Bone graft substitutes: What are the options? *Surgeon* 2012;10(4):230-239. Retraction in *Surgeon* 2013;11(2):115.

Even J, Eskander M, Kang J: Bone morphogenetic protein in spine surgery: Current and future uses. *J Am Acad Orthop Surg* 2012;20(9):547-552.

Howard JM, Glassman SD, Carreon LY: Posterior iliac crest pain after posterolateral fusion with or without iliac crest graft harvest. *Spine J* 2011;11(6):534-537.

Laine C, Guallar E, Mulrow C, et al: Closing in on the truth about recombinant human bone morphogenetic protein-2: Evidence synthesis, data sharing, peer review, and reproducible research. *Ann Intern Med* 2013;158(12):916-918.

Miclau T III, Bozic KJ, Tay B, et al: Bone injury, regeneration, and repair, in Einhorn TA, O'Keefe RJ, Buckwalter JA, eds: *Orthopaedic Basic Science*, ed 3. Rosemont, IL, American Academy of Orthopaedic Surgeons, 2007, pp 331-348.

Ng VY: Risk of disease transmission with bone allograft. *Orthopedics* 2012;35(8):679-681.

Rodgers MA, Brown JV, Heirs MK, et al: Reporting of industry funded study outcome data: Comparison of confidential and published data on the safety and effectiveness of rhBMP-2 for spinal fusion. *BMJ* 2013;346:f3981.

Seeherman H, Wozney J, Li R: Bone morphogenetic protein delivery systems. *Spine (Phila Pa 1976)* 2002;27(16, suppl 1)S16-S23.

Younger EM, Chapman MW: Morbidity at bone graft donor sites. *J Orthop Trauma* 1989;3(3):192-195.

Chapter 7

Bone and Joint Biology

John C. Clohisy, MD   Dieter M. Lindskog, MD   Yousef Abu-Amer, PhD

I. Bone

A. Overview

  1. Functions of bone

    a. Provides mechanical support

    b. Regulates mineral homeostasis

    c. Houses the marrow elements

  2. Types of bones—long, short, and flat

  3. Formation of bones

    a. Long bones are formed via endochondral ossification, the formation of bone from a cartilage model.

    b. Flat bones are formed by intramembranous bone formation, the formation of bone through loose condensations of mesenchymal tissue.

B. Anatomy

  1. Long bones are composed of three anatomic regions: the diaphysis, the metaphysis, and the epiphysis (**Figure 1**).

    a. Diaphysis—The shaft of a long bone, consisting of a tube of thick cortical bone surrounding a central canal of trabecular bone, the intramedullary (IM) canal

      • The inner aspect of the cortical bone is called the endosteal surface.

      • The outer region is called the periosteal surface. It is covered by the periosteal membrane, which is composed of an outer layer of fibrous connective tissue and an inner layer of undifferentiated, osteogenic progen-

itor cells.

    b. Metaphysis—Transition zone from epiphysis to diaphysis; composed of loose trabecular bone surrounded by a thin layer of cortical bone

    c. Epiphysis—Specialized end of bone that forms the joint articulation

      • The growth plate (physis or physeal scar) divides the epiphysis from the metaphysis.

      • The epiphysis is composed of loose trabecular bone surrounded by a thin layer of cortical bone.

      • The articular portion of the bone has a specialized subchondral region underlying the articular cartilage.

  2. Flat bones

    a. Flat bones include the pelvis, scapula, skull, and mandible.

    b. The composition of these bones varies from purely cortical to cortical with a thin inner region of trabecular bone.

  3. Neurovascular anatomy of bone

    a. Innervation—The nerves that innervate bone derive from the periosteum and enter the bone in tandem with blood vessels. Nerves are found in the haversian canals and Volkmann canals (**Figure 2**).

    b. Blood supply

      • Nutrient arteries pass through the diaphyseal cortex and enter the IM canal. These vessels supply blood to the inner two-thirds of the cortical bone and are at risk during IM reaming.

      • The outer one-third of the cortical bone derives its blood supply from the periosteal membrane vessels, which are at risk from periosteal stripping during surgery.

C. Structure

  1. Macroscopic level

    a. Cortical bone—Dense, compact bone with low

Dr. Clohisy or an immediate family member serves as a paid consultant to or is an employee of Biomet and Pivot Medical; and has received research or institutional support from Wright Medical Technology and Zimmer. Dr. Lindskog or an immediate family member serves as a paid consultant to or is an employee of Merck. Neither Dr. Abu-Amer nor any immediate family member has received anything of value from or has stock or stock options held in a commercial company or institution related directly or indirectly to the subject of this chapter.

1: Basic Science

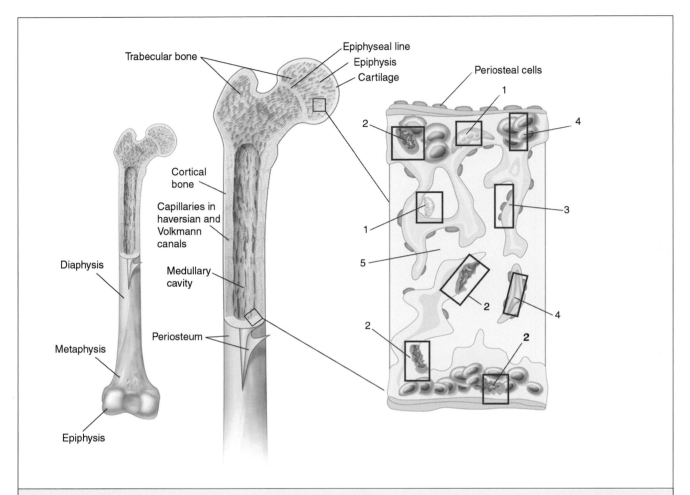

Figure 1   Illustrations of cortical and trabecular bone show the different structures and cell types. 1 = osteoclasts, 2 = osteo-blasts, 3 = bone-lining cells, 4 = osteocytes, 5 = marrow space. (Adapted from Hayes WC: Biomechanics of cortical and trabecular bone: Implications for assessment of fracture risk, in *Basic Orthopaedic Biomechanics*. New York, NY, Raven Press, 1991, pp 93-142 and Bostrom MPG, Boskey A, Kaufma JK, Einhorn TA: Form and function of bone, in Buckwalter JA, Einhorn TA, Simon SR, eds: *Orthopaedic Basic Science: Biology and Biomechanics of the Musculoskeletal System*, ed 2. Rosemont, IL, American Academy of Orthopaedic Surgeons, 2000, pp 320-369.)

porosity and no macroscopic spaces

- In the diaphyseal region, cortical bone is load bearing.

- In the metaphysis and epiphysis, cortical bone serves as a border to trabecular bone. It supports only a portion of the load, which is primarily carried by the trabecular bone in these regions.

b. Trabecular bone—Composed of a loose network of bony struts (rods and plates), which have a maximum thickness of approximately 200 μm.

- Trabecular bone is porous, with a macroscopic porosity ranging from 30% to 90%; it houses the bone marrow contents.

- In osteoporosis, the macroscopic porosity is increased because of thinning of the trabec-

ular struts.

2. Microscopic level

a. Woven bone is primary bone characterized by a random orientation of collagen and mineral.

b. Lamellar bone is secondary bone that results from the remodeling of woven bone into an organized bone tissue.

c. Lacunae are ellipsoidal spaces in bone occupied by osteocytes. Small channels through the bone called canaliculi connect the lacunae and contain osteocyte cell processes that interact with other cells.

D. Composition of the extracellular matrix (ECM) is 60% to 70% mineral components and 20% to 25% organic components.

1. Mineral matrix

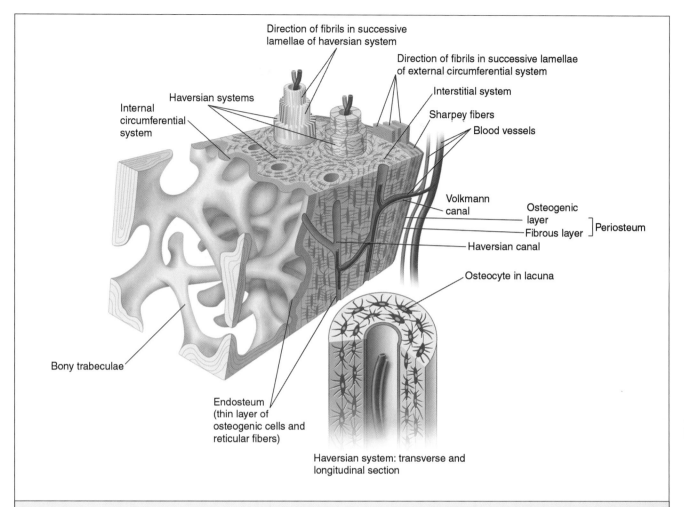

Figure 2 Illustration of the structure of cortical bone shows the types of cortical lamellar bone: the internal circumferential system, interstitial system, osteonal lamellae, and outer circumferential system. The illustration also shows the intraosseous vascular system that serves the osteocytes and connects the periosteal and medullary blood vessels. The haversian canals run primarily longitudinally through the cortex, whereas the Volkmann canals create oblique connections between the haversian canals. Cement lines separate each osteon from the surrounding bone. Periosteum covers the external surface of the bone and consists of two layers: an osteogenic inner cellular layer and a fibrous outer layer. (Adapted from Kessel RG, Kardon RH: *Tissues and Organs: A Text-Atlas of Scanning and Microscopy*. New York, NY, WH Freeman, 1979, p 25.)

a. Responsible for the compression strength of bone

b. Composed primarily of calcium and phosphate (and some sodium, magnesium, and carbonate) in the form of hydroxyapatite and tricalcium phosphate

c. The mineral component of bone is closely associated with collagen fibrils.

d. Tropocollagen helices in the fibrils are organized in a quarter-staggered arrangement, with empty regions (hole zones) between the ends and pores running lengthwise between collagen fibrils (**Figure 3**).

e. Mineral crystals form in the hole zones and pores.

f. Provides mineral homeostasis as a source for calcium, phosphate, and magnesium ions

2. Organic matrix is 90% type I collagen; 5% other collagen types (III and IV), noncollagenous proteins, and growth factors; the remaining tissue volume is occupied by water.

a. Collagen

- Type I collagen is the primary ECM protein of bone.

- Type I collagen is fibril forming, with a triple helical structure (three α chains) that contributes tensile strength to the ECM.

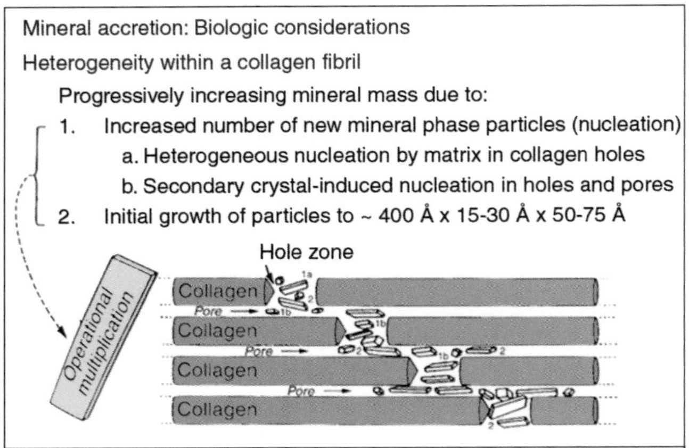
Mineral accretion: Biologic considerations
Heterogeneity within a collagen fibril
Progressively increasing mineral mass due to:
1. Increased number of new mineral phase particles (nucleation)
a. Heterogeneous nucleation by matrix in collagen holes
b. Secondary crystal-induced nucleation in holes and pores
2. Initial growth of particles to ~ 400 Å x 15-30 Å x 50-75 Å
Hole zone
Collagen
Pore
Collagen
Pore
Collagen
Pore
Collagen
Operational multiplication

Figure 3 Diagram describes mineral accretion. (Adapted from Bostrom MPG, Boskey A, Kaufman JK, Einhorn TA: Form and function of bone, in Buckwalter JA, Einhorn TA, Simon SR, eds: *Orthopaedic Basic Science: Biology and Biomechanics of the Musculoskeletal System*, ed 2. Rosemont, IL, American Academy of Orthopaedic Surgeons, 2000, pp 320-369.)

- Fibrils are intrinsically stable because of noncovalent interconnections and covalent cross-links between lysine residues.
- Small amounts of types III and IV collagen also are present in bone.
- Collagen α chains form bone-unique intramolecular and intermolecular cross-links that can be secreted in urine and are used as diagnostic biomarkers of bone resorption.

b. Noncollagenous ECM proteins

- Vitamin K–dependent proteins—Osteocalcin is the most common vitamin K–dependent, noncollagenous protein in bone; a marker of osteoblast differentiation; undergoes carboxylation in a vitamin K–dependent manner
- Adhesive proteins—Facilitate the interaction of cells (attachment and detachment) with the ECM via cell surface receptors called integrins. Fibronectin and vitronectin are common adhesive proteins of bone.
- Matricellular proteins—Mediate cell-matrix interactions by modulating signaling from the matrix to the cell
- Phosphoproteins—Phosphorylated (negatively charged) extracellular proteins; interact with calcium; thought to play a role in mineralization
- Growth factors and cytokines—Biologically active proteins; potent regulators of differentiation and activation. They include bone morphogenetic proteins (BMPs) (**Table 1**), transforming growth factor-β (TGF-β), basic fibroblast growth factor (bFGF), insulin growth factors (IGFs), and interleukins (ILs).
- Proteoglycans—Macromolecules composed of protein core and glycosaminoglycan side chains; provide tissue structure, bind to growth factors, regulate proliferation, act as cell surface receptors

E. Composition of bone cells—Cells associated with the bone ECM include osteoblasts, osteocytes, and osteoclasts. Cells of the marrow and periosteum also contribute greatly to the process of bone remodeling.

1. Osteoblasts—Bone surface cells that form bone matrix and regulate osteoclast activity

a. Marker proteins include alkaline phosphatase, osteocalcin, osteonectin, and osteopontin

b. Osteoblasts have parathyroid hormone (PTH) receptors and secrete type I collagen.

c. Differentiation

- Osteoblasts arise from mesenchymal marrow stromal cells and periosteal membrane cells. A series of cellular regulators serve as differentiation cues for osteoblast development from stem cell to mature osteoblast/osteocyte (**Figure 4**).
- Cells committed to osteoblastic differentiation are called osteoprogenitor cells.
- Each stage of differentiation has characteristic molecular markers, transcription factors, and secreted proteins.
- Runx2 and osterix are essential transcription factors required for osteoblast cell function.
- The mature osteoblast has a lifespan of 100 days. It can then become a bone-lining cell or an osteocyte, or it can undergo apoptosis. Bone-lining cells are relatively inactive cells that cover the surfaces of bone. They likely can become reactivated as functional osteoblasts.

d. Osteoblast differentiation is regulated by several cytokines, including BMPs, hedgehog proteins, PTH, TGF-β, and Wnts.

2. Osteocytes

a. Active osteoblasts become embedded in the mineralized matrix and become osteocytes.

b. Osteocytes reside in the lacunar spaces of trabecular and cortical bone. They are nonmitotic and are not highly synthetic.

c. Distinct from the osteoblast, they do not ex-

Table 1

A Comparative Overview of Different Bone Morphogenetic Proteins

S. no.	BMPs	Synonyms	Function	Knockout Phenotype in Mice
1	BMP1	hTld1	Induction of cartilage, metalloprotease	Reduced ossification
2	BMP2	bmp2a	Cartilage and bone formation	Embryonic lethal, heart defects, lack of amnion
3	BMP3	Osteogenin	Negative regulator of bone development	Increased bone mass, bone volume
4	BMP4	bmp2b	Bone and teeth	Embryonic lethal, heart defects, lack of allantois
5	BMP5		Cartilage development	Loss of one pair of ribs in ribcage, short ear
6	BMP6	VgR-1	Liver and joint development	Delayed sternum ossification
7	BMP7	OP-1	Kidney development	Renal defects
8	BMP8	OP-2	Cartilage and bone formation	Spermatogenesis defects
9	BMP9	GDF2	CNS and liver development and angiogenesis	Postnatal retinal vascular remodeling
10	BMP10	None	Heart development	Proliferation defects in embryonic cardiomyocytes
11	BMP11	GDF11	CNS development	Abnormality in anterior-posterior axis of skeleton
12	BMP12	GDF7, CDMP-3	Tendon and cartilage development	Abnormal skull development
13	BMP13	GDF12, CDMP-2	BMP inhibitor in tendon development	Abnormal skull, bone fusions at wrist and ankle
14	BMP14	GDF5, CDMP-1	Cartilage development	Delay in fracture healing
15	BMP15	GDF9	Oocyte development	Decreased ovulation and fertilization

BMP = bone morphogenetic protein, CDMP = cartilage-derived morphogenetic protein, CNS = central nervous system, GDF = growth differentiation factor, OP = osteogenic protein, VgR = decapentaplegic-Vg–related protein.

Adapted from Bandyopadhyay A, Yadav PS, Prashar P: BMP signaling in development and diseases: A pharmacological perspective. *Biochem Pharmacol* 2013;85:857-864.

press alkaline phosphatase.

   d. Osteocytes have numerous cell processes that communicate with other cells via the canaliculi.

   e. Signaling between osteocytes is mediated by protein complexes called gap junctions.

   f. Osteocytes contribute to the regulation of bone homeostasis.

   g. Osteocytes are mechanosensing, load-sensing cells, secrete receptor activator for nuclear factor-κ B ligand (RANKL), and regulate adult bone remodeling directly.

3. Osteoclasts—Multinucleated bone-resorbing cells.

   a. Marker proteins include tartrate-resistant acid phosphatase (TRAP), calcitonin receptor, and cathepsin K.

   b. Differentiation—Osteoclasts are hematopoietic cells, members of the monocyte/macrophage lineage. The multinuclear osteoclast polykaryons form by fusion of mononuclear precursors, a process that requires RANKL and macrophage-colony stimulating factor (M-CSF).

   c. Activity and important features—Mature osteoclasts attach to bone/mineral surfaces and form a sealing zone underneath the cells. The plasma membrane underneath the cell forms the resorptive domain of the cell, which features a highly convoluted ruffled border. Proteases and ions are secreted through this domain to dissolve both organic and nonorganic material.

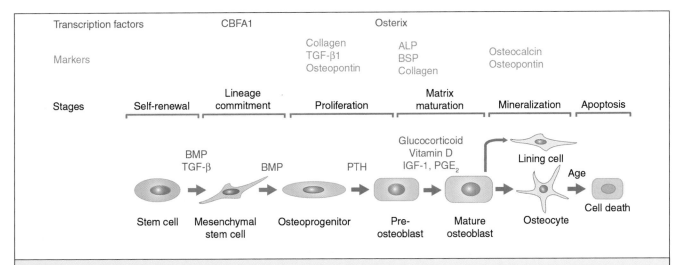

Figure 4   This idealized depiction of the osteoblast developmental lineage illustrates the key concepts of early proliferation versus terminal phenotypic differentiation, the temporal onset of molecular markers, and important regulators of this process, as well as the different fates possible for cells of the osteoblastic lineage. CBFA1 = core binding factor α 1, TGF = transforming growth factor, ALP = alkaline phosphatase, BSP = bone sialoprotein, BMP = bone morphogenetic protein, PTH = parathyroid hormone, IGF-1 = insulin-like growth factor 1, PGE$_2$ = prostaglandin E$_2$. (Adapted with permission from Lian JB, Stein GS, Aubin JE: Bone formation: Maturation and functional activities of osteoblast lineage cells, in Favus MJ, ed: *Primer on the Metabolic Bone Diseases and Disorders of Mineral Metabolism*, ed 5. Washington, DC, American Society for Bone and Mineral Research, 2003, pp 13-28.)

d. Regulation—The differentiation and activity of osteoclasts are regulated primarily by RANKL and osteoprotegerin (OPG). RANKL binds to its cognate receptor, RANK, on the membrane of monocyte/macrophage. OPG is a decoy receptor, a member of the tumor necrosis factor (TNF) receptor family, that binds to and sequesters RANKL, thus inhibiting osteoclast differentiation and activity (**Figure 5**).

F. Bone homeostasis—Balanced bone formation and resorption

1. Remodeling

   a. Bone is a dynamic tissue that constantly undergoes remodeling, primarily through osteoblasts (bone-forming cells) and osteoclasts (resorptive cells) (**Figure 5**).

   b. The regulatory mechanisms of remodeling are critical to understanding bone homeostasis and disease states.

   c. Bone mass "turns over" completely every 4 to 20 years, depending on age. At adulthood, the rate of turnover is 5% per year. This process replaces potentially compromised bone with structurally sound bone.

2. Trabecular bone remodeling (**Figure 6**)

   a. Osteoclastic activation results in the development of a resorption pit called a Howship lacuna.

   b. After pit formation, osteoclasts are replaced by

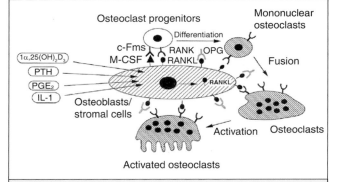

Figure 5   Illustration shows osteoclast differentiation and function regulated by receptor activator for nuclear factor-κ B (RANK) ligand (RANKL) and macrophage-colony stimulating factor (M-CSF). Osteoclast progenitors and mature osteoclasts express RANK, the receptor for RANKL. Osteotropic factors such as 1α,25(OH)$_2$D$_3$, parathyroid hormone (PTH), and interleukin 1 (IL-1) stimulate expression of RANKL in osteoblasts/stromal cells. Membrane-associated or matrix-associated forms of both M-CSF and RANKL expressed by osteoblasts/stromal cells are responsible for the induction of osteoclast differentiation in the coculture. RANKL also directly stimulates fusion and activation of osteoclasts. Mainly osteoblasts/stromal cells produce osteoprotegerin (OPG), a soluble decoy receptor of RANKL. OPG strongly inhibits the entire differentiation, fusion, and activation processes of osteoclast induced by RANKL. c-Fms = CSF-1 receptor, PGE$_2$ = prostaglandin E$_2$. (Reproduced with permission from Takahashi N, Udagawa N, Takami M, Suda T: Osteoclast generation, in Bilezikian HP, Raisz LG, Rodan GA, eds: *Principles of Bone Biology*, ed 2. San Diego, CA, Academic Press, 2002, pp 109-126.)

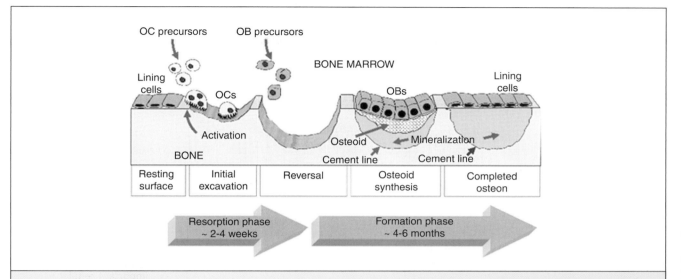

Figure 6 Illustration of a bone marrow unit shows the various stages of cellular activity from the resorption of old bone by osteoclasts to the subsequent formation of new bone by osteoblasts. For simplicity, the illustration shows remodeling in only two dimensions, whereas in vivo it occurs in three dimensions, with osteoclasts continually enlarging the cavity at one end and osteoblasts filling it in at the other end. OB = osteoblast, OC = osteoclast. (Adapted with permission from Riggs BL, Parfitt AM: Drugs used to treat osteoporosis: The critical need for a uniform nomenclature based on their action on bone remodeling. *J Bone Miner Res* 2005;20:177-184.)

osteoblasts that form new bone matrix.

c. The cement line is the region where bone resorption has stopped and new bone formation begins.

d. After new bone formation is complete, bone lining cells cover the surface.

3. Cortical bone remodeling (**Figure 7**)

a. Osteoclasts tunnel through bone to form a cutting cone of resorption.

b. Blood vessel formation occurs in the cutting cone.

c. Osteoblast recruitment and new bone formation occur in the resorbed space of the cutting cone.

d. This results in circumferential new bone formation around a blood vessel. This structure is called an osteon, and the vessel space is the haversian canal (**Figure 8**).

4. Mechanisms of osteoblast/osteoclast coupling

a. The biologic activity of osteoblasts is closely associated with that of osteoclasts; intercellular signaling mechanisms are being studied.

b. Osteoblastic regulation of osteoclast function has been well documented. PTH is a pro-osteoclastogenic cytokine that acts through osteoblast cell-surface receptors. These receptors stimulate the synthesis of factors, including RANKL and M-CSF, critical to osteoclast development.

c. In addition to secreting pro-osteoclastogenic RANKL, osteoblasts also can produce OPG, a potent antiosteoclastogenic protein. Therefore, osteoblasts have positive and negative regulatory effects on osteoclast activity.

d. Osteoclast activity also is regulated by systemic factors like serum calcium levels and circulating hormones.

• Vitamin D and PTH stimulate osteoclastic activity.

• Calcitonin reduces osteoclastic activity.

e. Osteoclast regulation of osteoblast differentiation and activity is less understood. One hypothesis is that osteoclastic bone resorption releases bioactive factors (BMP, TGF-β, IGF-1) that stimulate osteoblast differentiation and new bone formation.

f. The process of bone remodeling is abnormal in disease states (for example, osteoporosis and osteopetrosis); therapies are directed at correcting the remodeling abnormalities.

G. Disease states

1. Characteristics (**Table 2**)

2. Therapies

a. Bisphosphonates—Inhibit osteoclastic bone resorption; used to treat osteoporosis, bone metastasis, and Paget disease. Complications of long-term use include osteonecrosis of the jaw

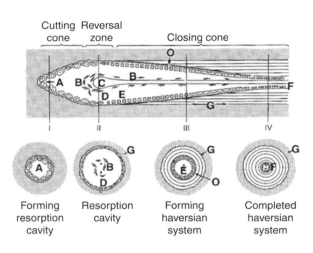

Figure 7 Illustration shows a longitudinal section through a cortical remodeling unit with corresponding transverse sections below. A, Multinucleated osteoclasts in a Howship lacuna advancing longitudinally from right to left and radially to enlarge a resorption cavity. B, Perivascular spindle-shaped precursor cells. C, Capillary loop delivering osteoclast precursors and pericytes. D, Mononuclear cells (osteoblast progenitors) lining reversal zone. E, Osteoblasts apposing bone centripetally in radial closure and its perivascular precursor cells. F, Flattened cells lining the haversian canal of completed haversian system or osteon. Transverse sections at different stages of development: (I) resorptive cavities lined with osteoclasts; (II) completed resorption cavities lined by mononuclear cells, the reversal zone; (III) forming haversian system or osteons lined with osteoblasts that had recently apposed three lamellae; and (IV) completed haversian system or osteon with flattened bone cells lining canal. Cement line (G); osteoid (stippled) between osteoblast (O) and mineralized bone. (Reproduced with permission from Parfitt AM: The actions of parathyroid hormone on bone: Relation to bone remodeling and turnover, calcium homeostasis, and metabolic bone diseases. II: PTH and bone cells. Bone turnover and plasma calcium regulation. *Metabolism* 1976;25;909-955.)

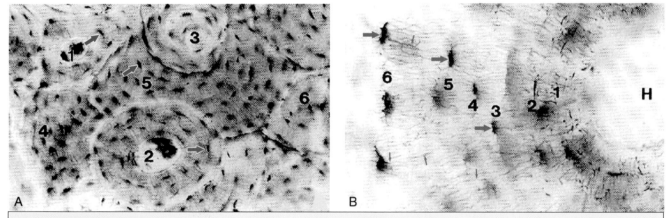

Figure 8 Electron photomicrographs show cortical bone. **A,** A thin-ground cross section of human cortical bone in which osteocyte lacunae (arrows) and canaliculi have been stained with India ink. Osteocytes are arranged around a central vascular channel to constitute haversian systems. Active haversian systems (1, 2, and 3) have concentric lamellae in this plane. Older haversian systems (4, 5, and 6) have had parts of their original territories invaded and remodeled. This is seen clearly where 2 and 3 have invaded the territory originally occupied by 5. (Original magnification: ×185.) **B,** Higher magnification of part of a haversian system shows the successive layering (numbers) of osteocytes (large arrows) from the central core (H) that contains the vasculature. Small arrows identify the canaliculi that connect osteocyte lacunae in different layers. (Original magnification: ×718.) (Adapted with permission from Marks SC, Odgren PR: Structure and development of the skeleton, in Bilezikian JP, Raisz LG, Rodan GA, eds: *Principles of Bone Biology*, ed 2. San Diego, CA, Academic Press, 2002, pp 3-15.)

Table 2

Characteristics of Various Disease States

Disease	Characteristics
Osteoporosis	Decreased bone formation with age, leading to loss of bone mass
Osteopetrosis	Decreased bone resorption from loss of osteoclast function
Fibrodysplasia ossificans	Excess bone formation
Paget disease	Increased formation and resorption
Metastatic bone disease	Local tumor secretion of PTH and IL-1 stimulates osteoclast differentiation
Rheumatoid arthritis	Synovial fibroblasts secrete RANKL, which stimulates formation of periarticular erosions
Periprosthetic osteolysis	RANKL production in periprosthetic membrane stimulates local bone resorption

IL-1 = interleukin 1, PTH = parathyroid hormone, RANKL = receptor activator for nuclear factor-κ B ligand.

and poor bone quality due to defective remodeling.

b. Intermittent PTH dosing stimulates bone formation; continuous dosing stimulates bone resorption.

c. OPG and anti-RANKL antibodies—Potential use as antiresorptive agents for various bone loss disorders (currently at various stages of clinical trials)

d. Corticosteroids decrease bone formation and increase bone resorption; osteopenia is a common side effect of chronic steroid use.

H. Injury and repair (fracture)

1. Injury

    a. Bone injury can be caused by trauma or surgical osteotomy.

    b. Injury disrupts the vascular supply to the affected tissue, resulting in mechanical instability, hypoxia, depletion of nutrients, and an elevated inflammatory response.

2. Repair

    a. Unlike tissues that repair by developing scar tissue, bone heals by forming new bone that is indistinguishable from the original tissue.

    b. Motion at the fracture site (cast, external fixator, IM rod) results in healing, primarily through endochondral ossification, whereas rigidity at the fracture site (plate fixation) enables direct intramembranous ossification. Most fractures heal with a combination of these processes.

3. Repair stages

    a. Hematoma and inflammatory response—Macrophages and degranulating platelets infiltrate the fracture site and secrete various inflammatory cytokines, including platelet-derived growth factor, TGF-β, IL-1 and IL-6, prostaglandin E_2, and TNF-α. These factors affect various cells in the microenvironment of fracture hematoma.

    b. Early postfracture period

       • Periosteal preosteoblasts and local osteoblasts form new bone.

       • Mesenchymal cells and fibroblasts proliferate and are associated with the expression of basic and acidic fibroblast growth factors. Primitive mesenchymal and osteoprogenitor cells are associated with the expression of the BMPs and TGF-β family of proteins.

    c. Fracture hematoma maturation

       • The fracture hematoma produces a collagenous matrix and a network of new blood vessels. Neovascularization provides progenitor cells and growth factors for mesenchymal cell differentiation.

       • Cartilage formation (endochondral ossification), identified by the expression of collagen types I and II, stabilizes the fracture site. Chondrocytes proliferate, undergo hypertrophy, and express factors that stimulate ossification.

    d. Conversion of hypertrophic cartilage to bone—A complex process in which hypertrophic chondrocytes undergo terminal differentiation, cartilage calcifies, and new woven bone is formed

       • Various factors are expressed as hypertrophic cartilage is replaced by bone, including BMPs, TGF-β, IGFs, osteocalcin, and collagen types I, V, and XI.

       • Hypertrophic chondrocyte apoptosis and vascular invasion ensue.

    e. Bone remodeling

       • The newly formed woven bone is remodeled through coordinated osteoblast and osteoclast functions.

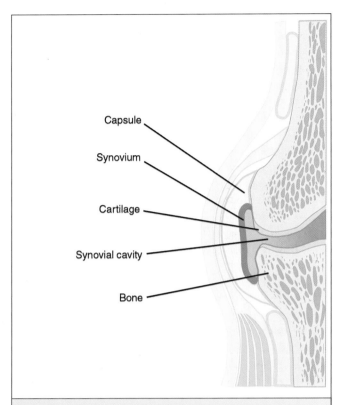

Figure 9 Illustration shows a synovial joint. (Adapted from Recklies AD, Poole AR, Banerjee S, et al: Pathophysiologic aspects of inflammation in diarthrodial joints, in Buckwalter JA, Einhorn TA, Simon SR, eds: *Orthopaedic Basic Science: Biology and Biomechanics of the Musculoskeletal System*, ed 2. Rosemont, IL, American Academy of Orthopaedic Surgeons, 2000, p 490.)

- Mature bone is eventually established and is indistinguishable from the surrounding bone. Mature bone contains a host of growth factors, including TGF-β, BMPs, and IGFs.

II. Synovial Joints

A. Overview—Synovial joints are specialized structures that allow movement at bony articulations.

  1. Composed of a joint cavity lined by synovium containing bones lined with articular cartilage

  2. Joints are stabilized by ligaments and motored by tendon attachments from adjacent musculature (**Figure 9**).

B. Formation and development of synovial joints is poorly understood.

  1. Limb skeletogenesis starts with long, uninterrupted condensations of mesenchymal tissue.

  2. Condensations of mesenchymal cells form at spe-

cific locations. This process appears to be controlled by the homeobox family of genes.

  3. Apoptosis then occurs within the so-called interzone, and the tissues separate through cavitation.

  4. Joint-specific development then ensues through a control mechanism not yet understood.

C. Structure

  1. The anatomy of each joint varies according to the location and demands of motion placed on the joint. Joint structure ranges from highly matched bony surfaces, such as the ball-and-socket hip joint, to the less congruent shoulder joint, which allows greater range of motion but provides less stability.

  2. Structural components

   a. Articular cartilage—Highly specialized tissue enabling low-friction movement

   b. Ligament—Collagenous structure connecting articulating bones; provides stability and restraint to nonphysiologic motion

   c. Joint capsule—Tough, fibrous tissue surrounding the joint cavity

   d. Synovium—Tissue that lines the noncartilaginous portions of the joint cavity; composed of two layers, the intimal lining and the connective tissue sublining

    - The intimal lining is only a few cells thick; in direct contact with the joint cavity; produces synovial fluid. Functions as a porous barrier and lacks tight junctions between cells; has no true basement membrane. Composed of type A and type B cells. Type A cells make up only 10% to 20% of the synovial cells, derive from bone marrow precursors, and function as tissue macrophages. Type B cells are from the fibroblast lineage, produce hyaluronan, and contain a unique enzyme, uridine diphosphoglucose dehydrogenase, which is critical to the pathway for hyaluronan synthesis.

    - The relatively acellular sublining is composed of fibroblasts, fat, blood vessels, and lymphoid cells. A rich vascular network supplies the sublining and enables the high solute and gas exchange that supplies the cartilage with nutrition

   e. Synovial fluid

    - Produced and regulated by the synovium

    - An ultrafiltrate of plasma with a low albumin concentration (45% compared with plasma) and a high concentration of hyaluronic acid and lubricin

D. Sensory innervation—Composed of two systems

1. Fast-conducting myelinated type A fibers, found in the joint capsule and surrounding musculature, produce information on joint positions and motion

2. Slow-conducting unmyelinated type C fibers are found along blood vessels in the synovium and transmit diffuse pain sensations.

E. Function

1. The synovial joint allows extremely low-friction motion between articulating bones.

2. Its function depends on the nature of the anatomic makeup of the joints as well as the characteristics of the tissue.

III. Nonsynovial Joints

A. Lack a synovial lining bordering the joint cavity; do not allow low-friction or large-range movements. The body contains different kinds of nonsynovial joints, including the symphyses, synchondroses, and syndesmoses.

B. Symphyses

1. In this type, bone ends are separated by a fibro-cartilaginous disk and are attached with well-developed ligamentous structures that control movement.

2. Intervertebral disks form a symphysis between vertebral bodies.

3. The pubic symphysis occurs at the anterior articulation between each hemipelvis and is composed of articular cartilage–covered rami separated by a fibrocartilage disk with firm ligamentous support. This joint is optimized for stability and load transmission but allows only limited motion.

C. Synchondroses

1. In this type, bone ends are covered with articular cartilage, but no synovium is present, and no substantial motion occurs.

2. Examples include the sternomanubrial joint, rib costal cartilage, and several articulations within the skull base.

D. Syndesmoses

1. This type consists of two bones that articulate without a cartilaginous interface and have strong ligamentous restraints that allow limited motion.

2. The distal tibia-fibula syndesmosis is the only extracranial syndesmosis.

1: Basic Science

Top Testing Facts

1. Endochondral bone formation (long and short bones) occurs through a cartilage model; intramembranous bone formation (flat bones) results from condensations of mesenchymal tissue.

2. The inner two-thirds of cortical bone are vascularized by nutrient arteries that pass through the diaphyseal cortex and enter the IM canal; they are at risk during IM reaming. The outer one-third of the cortical bone derives blood from the periosteal membrane vessels, which are at risk from periosteal stripping during surgery.

3. The extracellular matrix of bone is composed of 60% to 70% mineral components and 20% to 25% organic components. The organic matrix is 90% type I collagen and 5% noncollagenous proteins.

4. Type I collagen is fibril forming and has a triple helical structure (three α chains). The fibrils are intrinsically stable because of noncovalent interconnections and covalent cross-links between lysine residues.

5. Mature osteoblast marker proteins include alkaline phosphatase, osteocalcin, osteonectin, and osteopontin. The potential fates of a mature osteoblast include differentiation into an osteocyte or bone-lining cell, or apoptosis.

6. The marker proteins for osteoclasts include TRAP, calcitonin receptor, and cathepsin K. Osteoclast differentiation and activity are regulated largely by the bioactive factors RANKL (positive regulator) and OPG (negative regulator).

7. Osteoblast and osteoclast functions are coupled via various systemic and local factors. Regulatory proteins (RANKL and OPG) secreted by osteoblasts and osteocytes provide direct coupling in bone remodeling.

8. Fractures commonly heal with a combination of endochondral and intramembranous bone formation. Motion at the fracture site results in healing primarily through endochondral ossification, whereas stability at the fracture site enables direct intramembranous ossification.

9. Fracture healing occurs in a sequence of biologic stages including injury, inflammation, hematoma maturation, hypertrophic cartilage formation, new bone formation, and remodeling to mature bone.

10. Articular joint synovium is composed of two layers: the intimal lining, which contains tissue macrophage-like cells and fibroblast-like cells that produce hyaluronan, and the connective tissue sublining.

Bibliography

Deeks ED, Perry CM: Zoledronic acid: A review of its use in the treatment of osteoporosis. *Drugs Aging* 2008;25(11): 963-986.

Gamble JG, Simmons SC, Freedman M: The symphysis pubis: Anatomic and pathologic considerations. *Clin Orthop Relat Res* 1986;203:261-272.

Karsenty G, Kronenberg HM, Settembre C: Genetic control of bone formation. *Annu Rev Cell Dev Biol* 2009;25: 629-648.

Ke HZ, Richards WG, Li X, Ominsky MS: Sclerostin and Dickkopf-1 as therapeutic targets in bone diseases. *Endocr Rev* 2012;33(5):747-783.

Khosla S: Minireview: The OPG/RANKL/RANK system. *Endocrinology* 2001;142(12):5050-5055.

Khosla S, Burr D, Cauley J, et al: Bisphosphonate-associated osteonecrosis of the jaw: Report of a task force of the American Society for Bone and Mineral Research. *J Bone Miner Res* 2007;22(10):1479-1491.

Miller JD, McCreadie BR, Alford AI, Hankenson KD, Goldstein SA: Form and function of bone, in Einhorn TA, O'Keefe RJ, Buckwalter JA, eds: *Orthopaedic Basic Science*, ed 3. Rosemont, IL, American Academy of Orthopaedic Surgeons, 2007, pp 129-160.

Pacifici M, Koyama E, Iwamoto M: Mechanisms of synovial joint and articular cartilage formation: Recent advances, but many lingering mysteries. *Birth Defects Res C Embryo Today* 2005;75(3):237-248.

Rosen CJ, Compston JE, Lian JB: *Primer on the Metabolic Bone Diseases and Disorders of Mineral Metabolism*, ed 7. Washington, DC, American Society for Bone and Mineral Research, 2008.

Chapter 8

Articular Cartilage and Osteoarthritis

Karen M. Sutton, MD   Jonathan N. Grauer, MD
Debdut Biswas, MD   Jesse E. Bible, MD, MHS

I. Overview

A. Articular cartilage consists mainly of extracellular matrix (ECM, 95%) and a sparse population of chondrocytes (5%), which maintain the ECM throughout life.

B. The major components of the ECM are water, collagen, and proteoglycans.

II. Components

A. Water

1. Water makes up 65% to 80% of articular cartilage; this allows for a deformation response to stress.

2. The distribution is 80% at the superficial layers and 65% at the deep layers.

3. Most water is contained in the ECM and is moved through the matrix by applying a pressure gradient across the tissue.

4. The frictional resistance of the water through the pores of the ECM and the pressurization of the water within the ECM are the basic mechanisms

by which articular cartilage derives its ability to support very high joint loads.

5. Alteration of the water content affects the permeability, strength, and Young modulus of elasticity of the cartilage.

6. The flow of water through the tissue also promotes the transport of nutrients and other factors through cartilage.

B. Collagen

1. Collagen makes up more than 50% of the dry weight of articular cartilage and 10% to 20% of the wet weight.

2. Collagen provides shear and tensile strength.

3. Type II collagen comprises 90% to 95% of the total collagen weight in hyaline cartilage.

   a. Other minor types of collagen in articular cartilage include types V, VI, IX, X, and XI (**Table 1**).

   b. Type VI—Significant increase seen in early stages of osteoarthritis.

   c. Type X—Produced only in endochondral ossification by hypertrophic chondrocytes; associated with cartilage calcification. Examples include the growth plates, fracture sites, calcifying cartilage tumors, and the calcified deep zone of cartilage.

4. The specialized amino acid composition of increased amounts of glycine, proline, hydroxyproline, and hydroxylysine help form the triple helix collagen molecules, which line up in a staggered fashion resulting in banded fibrils (**Figure 1**).

   a. Intramolecular and intermolecular covalent cross-linking occurs between fibrils to help provide strength and form the resulting collagen fiber.

   b. Types V, VI, and XI help mediate collagen-collagen and collagen-proteoglycan interactions.

Dr. Sutton or an immediate family member serves as an unpaid consultant to Advanced Orthopaedic Technologies and SportsMD. Dr. Grauer or an immediate family member is a member of a speakers' bureau or has made paid presentations on behalf of Alphatec Spine, Smith & Nephew, and Stryker; serves as a paid consultant to or is an employee of Affinergy, Alphatec Spine, DePuy, KCI, Medtronic, Smith & Nephew, Stryker, and VentureMD; has received research or institutional support from Medtronic, Sofamor Danek, and Smith & Nephew; and serves as a board member, owner, officer, or committee member of the American Academy of Orthopaedic Surgeons and the Cervical Spine Research Society. Neither of the following authors nor any immediate family member has recieved anything of value from or has stock or stock options held in a commercial company or institution related directly or indirectly to the subject of this chapter: Dr. Biswas and Dr. Bible.

Table 1

Types of Collagen

Type	Location
I	Bone Skin Tendon Anulus fibrosus of intervertebral disk Meniscus
II	Articular cartilage Nucleus pulposus of intervertebral disk
III	Skin Blood vessels
IV	Basement membrane (basal lamina)
V	Articular cartilage with type I (in small amounts)
VI	Articular cartilage (in small amounts) Tethers the chondrocyte to pericellular matrix
VII	Basement membrane (epithelial, endothelial)
VIII	Basement membrane (epithelial)
IX	Articular cartilage with type II (in small amounts)
X	Hypertrophic cartilage Associated with calcification of cartilage (matrix mineralization)
XI	Articular cartilage with type II (in small amounts)
XII	Tendon
XIII	Endothelial cells

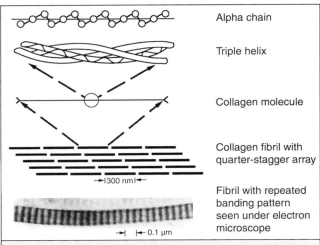

Alpha chain

Triple helix

Collagen molecule

Collagen fibril with quarter-stagger array

Fibril with repeated banding pattern seen under electron microscope

Figure 1 Illustration shows a scheme for the formation of collagen fibrils. The triple helix is made from three α chains, forming a procollagen molecule. Outside the cell, the N- and C-terminal globular domains of the α chains are cleaved off to allow fibril formation, which occurs in a specific quarter-stagger array that ultimately results in the typical banded fibrils seen under electron microscopy. (Reproduced with permission from Mow VC, Zhu W, Ratcliffe A: Structure and function of articular cartilage and meniscus, in Mow VC, Hayes WC, eds: *Basic Orthopaedic Biomechanics.* New York, NY, Raven Press, 1991, pp 143-198.)

5. Cartilage disorders linked to defects or deficiencies in type II collagen

   a. Achondrogenesis

   b. Type II achondrogenesis-hypochondrogenesis

   c. Spondyloepiphyseal dysplasia

   d. Kniest dysplasia

6. Cartilage disorder linked to defects in type X collagen–Schmid metaphyseal chondrodysplasia.

C. Proteoglycans

1. Represent 10% to 15% of dry weight

2. Provide compression strength to cartilage

3. Are produced and secreted into the ECM by chondrocytes

4. Consist of repeating disaccharide subunits, glycosaminoglycans (GAGs); two subtypes are found in cartilage: chondroitin sulfate and keratan sulfate.

   a. Chondroitin sulfate is the most prevalent GAG. With increasing age, chondroitin-4-sulfate decreases and chondroitin-6-sulfate remains constant.

   b. Keratan sulfate increases with age.

5. Sugar bonds link GAG to a long protein core to form a proteoglycan aggrecan molecule (**Figure 2**).

6. Aggrecan molecules bind to hyaluronic acid molecules via link proteins to form a macromolecule complex known as a proteoglycan aggregate (**Figure 3**).

7. Proteoglycans entangle between collagen fibers to create the fiber-reinforced solid matrix that helps determine the movement of water in the ECM (**Figure 4**).

8. Proteoglycans also help trap water in the ECM by way of their negative charge, regulating matrix hydration.

D. Chondrocytes

1. Chondrocytes represent 5% of the wet weight of articular cartilage.

2. Chondrocytes are the only cells found in articular cartilage and are responsible for the production, organization, and maintenance of the ECM.

3. Mesenchymal cells aggregate and differentiate into chondroblasts, which remain in lacunae to become chondrocytes.

4. Chondrocytes produce collagen, proteoglycans, and other proteins found in the ECM.

5. Compared with the more superficial levels of cartilage, chondrocytes in the deeper levels are less active and contain less rough endoplasmic reticulum and more intracellular degenerative products.

E. Other matrix molecules

1. Noncollagenous proteins—These molecules (including chondronectin, fibronectin, and anchorin) play a role in the interactions between the ECM and chondrocytes.

2. Lipids and phospholipids

III. Structure

A. Overview

1. Articular cartilage can be divided into different layers, or zones, at various depths.

2. The division is based on descriptive information such as collagen orientation, chondrocyte organization, and proteoglycan distribution.

B. Layers/zones (**Figures 5** and **6**)

1. Superficial (tangential, or zone I)

a. The superficial zone lies adjacent to the joint cavity and forms the gliding surface.

b. This zone is characterized by collagen fibers and disk-shaped chondrocytes uniformly aligned parallel to the articular surface along with a low proteoglycan concentration.

c. High collagen and water concentrations are found in this zone.

d. Fibers are arranged tangentially and resist shear forces.

2. Middle (transitional, or zone II)

a. The middle zone is characterized by thicker, obliquely oriented collagen fibers, round chondrocytes, and marked proteoglycan content.

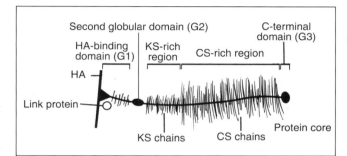

Figure 2 Illustration shows the proteoglycan aggrecan molecule and its binding to hyaluronic acid (HA). The protein core has several globular domains (G1, G2, and G3), with other regions containing the keratan sulfate (KS) and chondroitin sulfate (CS) glycosaminoglycan chains. The N-terminal G1 domain is able to bind specifically to HA. This binding is stabilized by link protein. (Adapted from Mankin HJ, Mow VC, Buckwalter JA, Iannotti JP, Ratcliffe A: Articular cartilage structure, composition, and function, in Buckwalter JA, Einhorn TA, Simon SR, eds: *Orthopaedic Basic Science: Biology and Biomechanics of the Musculoskeletal System*, ed 2. Rosemont, IL, American Academy of Orthopaedic Surgeons, 2000, p 449.)

1: Basic Science

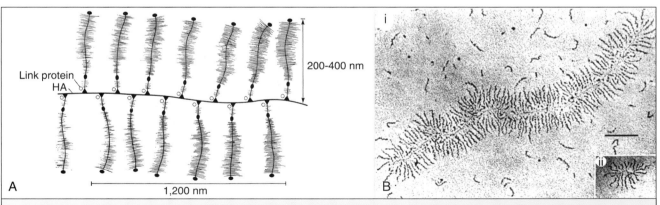

Figure 3 **A,** Illustration shows aggrecan molecules arranged as a proteoglycan aggregate. Many aggrecan molecules can bind to a chain of hyaluronic acid (HA), forming macromolecular complexes that effectively are immobilized within the collagen network. **B,** Electron micrographs of bovine articular cartilage proteoglycan aggregates from (i) skeletally immature calf and (ii) skeletally mature steer. These show the aggregates to consist of a central HA filament and multiple attached monomers (bar = 500 μm). (Adapted with permission from Buckwalter JA, Kuettner KE, Thonar EJ: Age-related changes in articular cartilage proteoglycans: Electron microscopic studies. *J Orthop Res* 1985;3:251-257.)

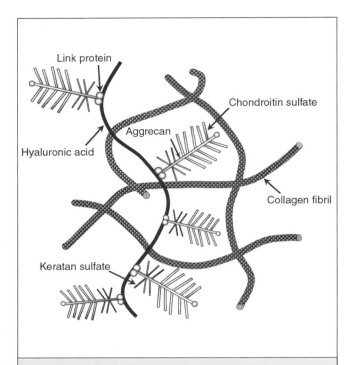

Figure 4 Illustration shows the matrix of hyaline cartilage, emphasizing its major matrix components. The proteoglycan aggregates and collagen fibers form a large, space-filling complex that binds large amounts of water and anions. (Courtesy of Dr. Andrew Thompson.)

b. This zone constitutes most of the cartilage depth.

c. It resists compression forces.

3. Deep (radial, or zone III)

a. This zone is characterized by collagen fibers oriented perpendicular to the articular surface (vertically), round chondrocytes arranged in columns, and high proteoglycan content.

b. It functions to resist shear stress during movement of the cartilage.

4. Calcified (zone IV)

a. The calcified zone is characterized by radially aligned collagen fibers and round chondrocytes buried in a calcified matrix that has a high concentration of calcium salts and hydroxyapatite crystals and a very low concentration of proteoglycans.

b. Hypertrophic chondrocytes in this layer produce type X collagen and alkaline phosphatase, helping to mineralize the ECM.

c. The borders of the calcified cartilage layer include the tidemark layer as the upper border and the cement line, which formed during growth plate ossification at skeletal maturity, as the lower border.

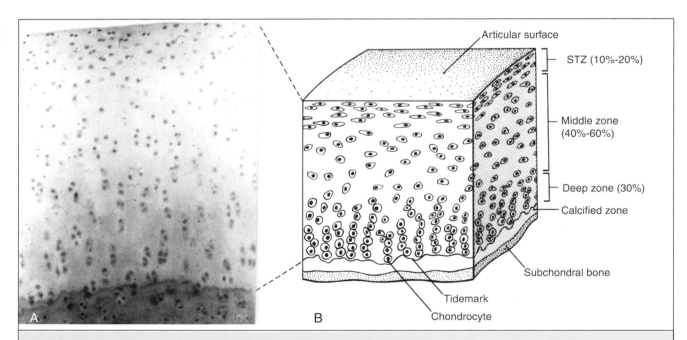

Figure 5 **A,** Histologic section of normal adult articular cartilage shows even Safranin 0 staining and distribution of chondrocytes. **B,** Illustration shows chondrocyte organization in the three major zones of the uncalcified cartilage. The tidemark and the subchondral bone are also shown. STZ = superficial tangential zone. (Reproduced with permission from Mow VC, Proctor CS, Kelly MA: Biomechanics of articular cartilage, in Nordin M, Frankel VH, eds: *Basic Biomechanics of the Musculoskeletal System*, ed 2. Philadelphia, PA, Lea & Febiger, 1989, pp 31-57.)

C. Extracellular matrix

1. The ECM can also be characterized based on its proximity to the surrounding chondrocytes.

2. Each region has a different biochemical composition.

   a. Pericellular matrix—Thin layer that completely surrounds the chondrocytes and helps control cell matrix interactions.

   b. Territorial matrix—Thin layer of collagen fibrils surrounding the pericellular matrix.

   c. Interterritorial matrix—The largest region, it contains larger collagen fibrils and a large number of proteoglycans.

IV. Metabolism

A. Nutrition

1. Cartilage is an avascular, alymphatic, and aneural structure in the adult.

2. It is believed that nutrients diffuse through the matrix from the surrounding synovial fluid, the synovium, or the underlying bone.

B. Chondrocytes

1. Chondrocytes synthesize and assemble cartilaginous matrix components and direct their distribution within tissue.

2. The processes include the synthesis of matrix proteins and GAG chains and their secretion into the ECM.

3. Each chondrocyte is responsible for the metabolism and maintenance of the ECM under avascular and, at times, anaerobic conditions.

4. The maintenance of the ECM depends on the proper incorporation of components into the matrix as well as the balance between the synthesis and the degradation of matrix components.

5. Chondrocytes respond to both their chemical environment (growth factors, cytokines) and physical environment (mechanical load, hydrostatic pressure changes).

C. Collagen

1. Collagen synthesis (**Figure 7**)

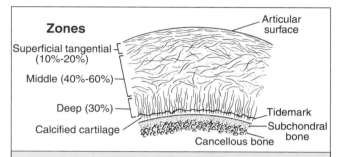

Figure 6 Illustration of collagen fiber architecture in a sagittal cross section shows the three salient zones of articular cartilage. (Reproduced with permission from Mow VC, Proctor CS, Kelly MA: Biomechanics of articular cartilage, in Nordin M, Frankel VH, eds: *Basic Biomechanics of the Musculoskeletal System*, ed 2. Philadelphia, PA, Lea & Febiger, 1989, pp 31-57.)

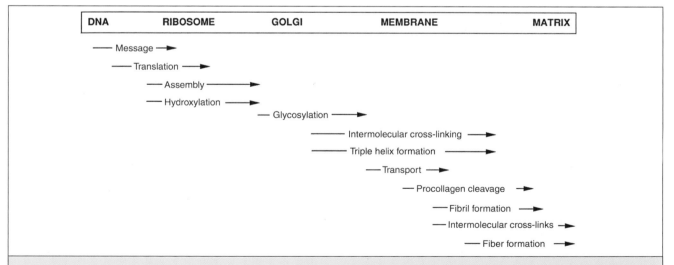

Figure 7 The events involved in the synthesis of collagen, along with the intracellular site where each step occurs. (Reproduced with permission from Mankin HJ, Brandt KD: Biochemistry and metabolism of articular cartilage in osteoarthritis, in Moskowitz RW, Howell DS, Goldberg VM, et al, eds: *Osteoarthritis: Diagnosis and Medical/Surgical Management*, ed 2. Philadelphia, PA, WB Saunders, 1992, pp 109-154.)

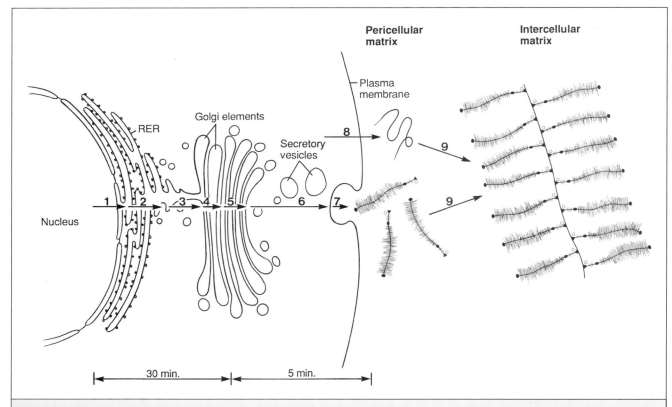

Figure 8   Illustration depicts the various stages involved in the synthesis and secretion of aggrecan and link protein by a chondrocyte. (1) The transcription of the aggrecan and link protein genes to mRNA. (2) The translation of the mRNA in the rough endoplasmic reticulum (RER) to form the protein core of the aggrecan. (3) The newly formed protein is transported from the RER to the (4) cis and (5) medial trans-Golgi compartments, where the glycosaminoglycan chains are added to the protein core. (6) On completion of the glycosylation and sulfation, the molecules are transported via secretory vesicles to the plasma membrane, where (7) they are released into the extracellular matrix. (8) Hyaluronate is synthesized separately at the plasma membrane. (9) Only in the extracellular matrix can aggrecan, link protein, and hyaluronate come together to form proteoglycan aggregates. (Reproduced from Mankin HJ, Mow VC, Buckwalter JA, Iannotti JP, Ratcliffe A: Articular cartilage structure, composition, and function, in Buckwalter JA, Einhorn TA, Simon SR, eds: *Orthopaedic Basic Science: Biology and Biomechanics of the Musculoskeletal System*, ed 2. Rosemont, IL, American Academy of Orthopaedic Surgeons, 2000, p 452.)

a. Most knowledge about collagen synthesis has originated from studies of major fibrillar types (types I through III).

b. Hydroxylation requires vitamin C; deficiencies (for example, scurvy) can result in altered collagen synthesis.

2. Collagen catabolism

   a. The exact mechanism is unclear.

   b. Breakdown occurs at a slow rate in normal cartilage.

   c. In degenerative cartilage and cartilage undergoing repair (for example, during skeletal growth), evidence of accelerated breakdown is seen.

   d. Enzymatic processes have been proposed, such as the cleaving of metalloproteinases to the triple helix.

D. Proteoglycan

1. Proteoglycan synthesis

   a. A series of molecular events—beginning with gene expression, messenger RNA transcription, translation, and aggregate formation—is involved in proteoglycan synthesis (**Figure 8**).

   b. The chondrocyte is responsible for the synthesis, assembly, and sulfation of the proteoglycan molecule.

   c. The addition of GAG and other posttranslational modifications can result in tremendous variation in the final molecule.

   d. The control mechanisms for proteoglycan synthesis are very sensitive to biochemical, mechanical, and physical stimuli (for example, lacerative injury, osteoarthritis, NSAIDs).

2. Proteoglycan catabolism (**Figure 9**)

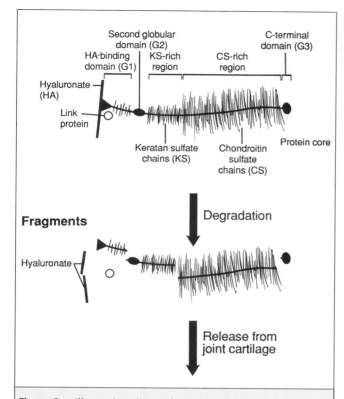

Figure 9 Illustration shows the mechanism of degradation of proteoglycan aggregates in articular cartilage. The major proteolytic cleavage site is between the G1 and G2 domains, making the glycosaminoglycan-containing portion of the aggrecan molecule nonaggregating. This fragment can now be released from the cartilage. Other proteolytic events also can cause the G1 domain and link protein to disaggregate and leave the cartilage. (Reproduced from Mankin HJ, Mow VC, Buckwalter JA, Iannotti JP, Ratcliffe A: Articular cartilage structure, composition, and function, in Buckwalter JA, Einhorn TA, Simon SR, eds: *Orthopaedic Basic Science: Biology and Biomechanics of the Musculoskeletal System*, ed 2. Rosemont, IL, American Academy of Orthopaedic Surgeons, 2000, p 454.)

a. Proteoglycans are being broken down continually; this is a normal event in the maintenance of cartilage.

b. Catabolism occurs during remodeling in repair processes and appears to be accelerated during degenerative processes.

c. Catabolism can be affected by soluble mediators (interleukin [IL]-1) and joint loading (loss of proteoglycans during joint immobilization).

d. The GAG chains and other proteoglycan chains are released into synovial fluid during degradation. These may be quantified and could provide a diagnostic measure of catabolic activity in the joint.

E. Growth factors

1. Polypeptide growth factors regulate synthetic processes in normal cartilage and have been implicated in the development of osteoarthritis.

2. Platelet-derived growth factor (PDGF)—In osteoarthritis, and especially in lacerative injury, PDGF may play an increased role in healing.

3. Fibroblast growth factor-2 (FGF-2)

   a. Decreases aggrecanase activity

   b. Upregulates matrix metalloproteinases (MMPs)

4. Transforming growth factor-β1 (TGF-β1)

   a. TGF-β1 appears to potentiate DNA synthesis stimulated by FGF-2, epidermal growth factor, and insulinlike growth factor (IGF)-I.

   b. TGF-β1 also appears to suppress type II collagen synthesis.

   c. TGF-β1 stimulates the formation of plasminogen activator inhibitor-1 and tissue inhibitor of metalloproteinase (TIMP), preventing the degradative action of plasmin and stromelysin.

   d. TGF-β1 decreases the catabolic activity of IL-1 and MMPs.

5. IGF-I and IGF-II

   a. IGF-I has been demonstrated to stimulate DNA and matrix synthesis in the immature cartilage of the growth plate as well as in adult articular cartilage.

   b. IGF-I decreases matrix catabolism, except in aged and osteoarthritic cartilage.

6. Bone morphogenetic protein 2 (BMP-2)

   a. BMP-2 stimulates ECM synthesis.

   b. It also partially reverses dedifferentiated phenotype in osteoarthritis.

7. BMP-7/osteogenic protein-1 (OP-1)

   a. BMP-7/OP-1 stimulates cartilage matrix synthesis.

   b. It decreases the catabolic activity of numerous catabolic cytokines, including IL-1 and MMPs.

   c. Effects are not affected by age or osteoarthritis.

F. Degradation

1. The breakdown of the cartilage matrix in normal turnover and in degeneration appears to occur by the action of proteolytic enzymes (proteinases).

2. The overactivity of proteinases may play a role in the pathogenesis of osteoarthritis.

1: Basic Science

Table 2

Changes in Articular Cartilage Properties With Aging and Osteoarthritis

Property	Aging	Osteoarthritis
Water content (hydration, permeability)	↓	↑
Collagen	Remains relatively unchanged (some increase in type VI)	Relative concentration ↑ Content ↓ in severe cases Matrix becomes disordered
Proteoglycan content (concentration)	↓	↓
Proteoglycan synthesis	Unchanged	↑
Proteoglycan degradation	↓	↑
Total chondroitin sulfate concentration	↓	↑
Chondroitin-4-sulfate concentration	↓	↑
Keratan sulfate concentration	↑	↓
Chondrocyte size	↑	Unchanged
Chondrocyte number	↓	Unchanged
Modulus of elasticity	↑	↓

3. Metalloproteinases

a. The metalloproteinases include collagenase, stromelysin, and gelatinase.

b. They are synthesized as latent enzymes (proenzymes) and require activation via enzymatic action.

c. The active enzymes can be inhibited irreversibly by TIMP. The molar ratios of metalloproteinases and TIMP determine whether net metalloproteinase activity is present.

G. Aging and articular cartilage (**Table 2**)

1. Immature articular cartilage varies considerably from adult articular cartilage.

2. With aging, chondrocytes become larger, acquire increased lysosomal enzymes, and no longer reproduce.

3. Cartilage becomes relatively hypocellular in comparison with immature articular cartilage.

4. Proteoglycan mass and size decrease with aging in articular cartilage, with decreased concentration of chondroitin sulfate and increased concentration of keratan sulfate.

5. Protein content increases with aging, whereas water content decreases.

6. As age advances, cartilage loses its elasticity, developing increased stiffness and decreased solubility.

V. Lubrication and Wear

A. Synovium

1. Synovial tissue is vascularized tissue that mediates the diffusion of nutrients between blood and synovial fluid.

2. Synovium is composed of two cell types.

a. Type A is important in phagocytosis.

b. Type B comprises fibroblast-like cells that produce synovial fluid.

3. Synovial fluid lubricates articular cartilage.

a. Synovial fluid is composed of an ultrafiltrate of blood plasma and fluid produced by the synovial membrane.

b. Synovial fluid is composed of hyaluronic acid, lubricin, proteinase, collagenases, and prostaglandins. Lubricin is the key lubricant of synovial fluid.

c. The viscosity coefficient of synovial fluid is not a constant; its viscosity increases as the shear rate decreases.

d. Hyaluronic acid molecules behave like an elastic solid during high-strain activities.

e. Synovial fluid contains no red blood cells, hemoglobin, or clotting factors.

B. Elastohydrodynamic lubrication is the major mode of lubrication of articular cartilage.

C. The coefficient of friction of human joints is 0.002 to 0.04.

1. Fluid film formation, elastic deformation of articular cartilage, and synovial fluid decrease the coefficient of friction.

2. Fibrillation of articular cartilage increases friction.

D. Two forms of movement occur during joint range of motion: rolling and sliding. Almost all joints undergo both types of movement during range of motion.

1. Pure rolling occurs when the instant center of rotation is at rolling surfaces.

2. Pure sliding occurs when there is pure translational movement without an instant center of rotation.

E. Types of lubrication

1. Elastohydrodynamic lubrication is the major mode of lubrication during dynamic joint motion. In this type of lubrication, deformation of articular surfaces occurs and thin films of joint lubricant separate surfaces.

2. Boundary (also called "slippery surfaces") lubrication—The load-bearing surface is largely nondeformable, and the lubricant only partially separates articular surfaces.

3. Boosted lubrication— Lubricating fluid pools in regions contained by articular surfaces in contact with one another. The coefficient of friction is generally higher in boosted lubrication than in elastohydrodynamic lubrication.

4. Hydrodynamic lubrication—Fluid separates the articular surfaces.

5. Weeping lubrication—Lubricating fluid shifts toward load-bearing regions of the articular surface.

VI. Mechanisms of Cartilage Repair

A. The repair of significant defects in articular cartilage is limited by a lack of vascularity and a lack of cells that can migrate to injured sites.

B. Cartilage also lacks undifferentiated cells that can migrate, proliferate, and participate in the repair response.

C. Repair of superficial lacerations

1. Superficial lacerations that do not cross the tidemark (the region between uncalcified and calcified cartilage) generally do not heal.

2. Chondrocytes proliferate near the site of injury and may synthesize new matrix, but they do not

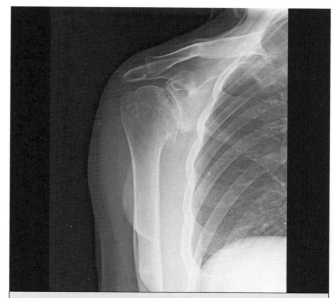

Figure 10 AP radiograph demonstrates glenohumeral osteoarthritis with advanced joint space narrowing, osteophyte formation, subchondral cysts, and subchondral sclerosis.

migrate toward the lesion and do not repair the defects.

3. The poor healing response is believed to be partly due to the lack of hemorrhage and the lack of an inflammatory response necessary for proper healing.

D. Repair of deep lacerations

1. Cartilage defects that penetrate past the tidemark into underlying subchondral bone may heal with fibrocartilage.

2. Fibrocartilage is produced by undifferentiated marrow mesenchymal stem cells that later differentiate into cells capable of producing fibrocartilage.

3. In most situations, the repair tissue does not resemble the normal structure, composition, or mechanical properties of an articular surface and is not as durable as hyaline cartilage.

E. Factors affecting cartilage repair

1. Continuous passive motion is believed to have a beneficial effect on cartilage healing; immobilization of a joint leads to atrophy and/or degeneration.

2. Joint instability (for example, anterior cruciate ligament transection) leads to an initial decrease in the ratio of proteoglycan to collagen (at 4 weeks) but a late elevation (at 12 weeks) in the ratio of proteoglycan to collagen and an increase in hydration.

1: Basic Science

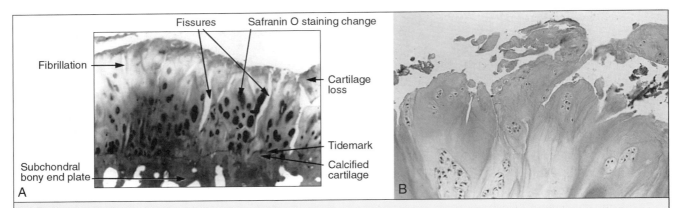

Figure 11 Histologic findings in osteoarthritis. **A,** Low-power magnification of a section of a glenohumeral head of osteoarthritic cartilage removed at surgery for total shoulder arthroplasty. Note the significant fibrillation, the vertical cleft formation, the tidemark, and the subchondral bony end plate. **B,** A higher power magnification of surface fibrillation shows vertical cleft formation and widespread large necrotic regions of the tissue devoid of cells. Clusters of cells, common in osteoarthritic tissues, also are seen. (Reproduced from Mankin HJ, Mow VC, Buckwalter, JA: Articular cartilage repair and osteoarthritis, in Buckwalter JA, Einhorn TA, Simon SR, eds: *Orthopaedic Basic Science: Biology and Biomechanics of the Musculoskeletal System*, ed 2. Rosemont, IL, American Academy of Orthopaedic Surgeons, 2000, p 478.)

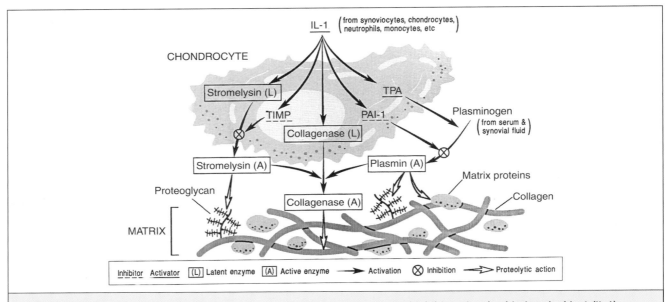

Figure 12 Illustration depicts the cascade of enzymes and their activators and inhibitors involved in interleukin-1 (IL-1)–stimulated degradation of articular cartilage. PAI-1 = plasminogen activator inhibitor-1, TIMP = tissue inhibitor of metalloproteinase, TPA = tissue plasminogen activator. (Reproduced from Mankin HJ, Mow VC, Buckwalter, JA: Articular cartilage repair and osteoarthritis, in Buckwalter JA, Einhorn TA, Simon SR, eds: *Orthopaedic Basic Science: Biology and Biomechanics of the Musculoskeletal System*, ed 2. Rosemont, IL, American Academy of Orthopaedic Surgeons, 2000, p 486.)

   3. Joint instability leads to a marked decrease in hyaluronan, but disuse does not.

VII. Osteoarthritis

A. Overview

   1. Osteoarthritis, which eventually results in the destruction and loss of articular cartilage, is the most prevalent disorder of the musculoskeletal system.

   2. The disease process leads to limitation of joint movement, joint deformity, tenderness, inflammation, and severe pain.

B. Radiographic findings (**Figure 10**)

   1. Joint space narrowing

   2. Subchondral sclerosis and cyst formation

3. Osteophyte formation

C. Macroscopic findings

1. Articular cartilage may show areas of softening (chondromalacia), fibrillation, and erosions.

2. With severe degeneration, focal areas of ulceration may be present, with exposure of sclerotic, eburnated subchondral bone.

D. Histologic findings (**Figure 11**)

1. Early alterations include surface erosion and irregularities.

2. Secondary centers of ossification are reactivated, leading to endochondral ossification.

3. Other changes include the replication and deterioration of the tidemark, fissuring, and cartilage destruction, with eburnation of subchondral bone.

E. Biochemical changes

1. Osteoarthritis is directly linked to a loss of proteoglycan content and composition, with increased water content (90%).

2. Proteoglycans exist in shorter chains with an increased chondroitin sulfate–keratan sulfate ratio.

3. Proteoglycans are largely unbound to hyaluronic acid because of proteolytic enzymes and a decreased number of link proteins.

4. Collagen content is maintained, but its organization and orientation are severely disturbed, presumably due to collagenase.

5. The modulus of elasticity decreases.

6. The keratan sulfate concentration decreases.

7. Mechanical overloading of articular cartilage results in chondrocyte necrosis and apoptosis.

F. Molecular mechanisms of osteoarthritis (**Figure 12**)

1. Levels of the following proteolytic enzymes are found to be elevated in osteoarthritic cartilage.

   a. Metalloproteinases (collagenase, gelatinase, stromelysin)

   b. Cathepsins B and D

   c. Nitric oxide synthase

2. Inflammatory cytokines may exacerbate the degeneration seen in osteoarthritis.

3. IL-1β, tumor necrosis factor-α (TNF-α), and other cytokines may further disrupt cartilage homeostasis and amplify the destructive actions of proteolytic enzymes.

Top Testing Facts

1. Articular cartilage consists mainly of ECM, with only a small percentage of chondrocytes, which are responsible for the synthesis, maintenance, and homeostasis of cartilage.

2. The major components of the ECM are water, proteoglycans, and collagen.

3. Articular cartilage is classified into four layers (superficial, middle, deep, and calcified) according to collagen orientation, chondrocyte organization, and proteoglycan distribution.

4. Cartilage is an avascular structure in the adult; this has implications for repair and healing.

5. The breakdown of the cartilage matrix in normal turnover and in degeneration appears to be the action of proteinases; their overactivity is implicated in osteoarthritis.

6. The water content of cartilage decreases with aging and increases in osteoarthritis.

7. Proteoglycan content and keratan sulfate concentrations decrease with osteoarthritis; proteoglycan degradation and chondroitin-4-sulfate concentration increase.

8. Elastohydrodynamic lubrication is the principal mode of lubrication of articular cartilage.

9. Superficial lacerations to cartilage rarely heal; deeper lacerations may heal with fibrocartilage.

10. Inflammatory cytokine and metalloproteinases are responsible for the macroscopic and histologic changes seen in osteoarthritis.

Bibliography

Buckwalter JA, Mankin HJ, Grodzinsky AJ: Articular cartilage and osteoarthritis. *Instr Course Lect* 2005;54:465-480.

Carter DR, Beaupré GS, Wong M, Smith RL, Andriacchi TP, Schurman DJ: The mechanobiology of articular cartilage development and degeneration. *Clin Orthop Relat Res* 2004;(427, Suppl)S69-S77.

Chubinskaya S, Malait AM, Wimmer M: Form and function of articular cartilage, in O'Keefe RJ, Jacobs JJ, Chu CR, Einhorn TA, eds: *Orthopaedic Basic Science*, ed 4. Rosemont, IL, American Academy of Orthopaedic Surgeons, 2013, pp 183-197.

Fortier LA, Barker JU, Strauss EJ, McCarrel TM, Cole BJ: The role of growth factors in cartilage repair. *Clin Orthop Relat Res* 2011;469(10):2706-2715.

Madry H, Luyten FP, Facchini A: Biological aspects of early osteoarthritis. *Knee Surg Sports Traumatol Arthrosc* 2012;20(3):407-422.

Mortazavi SMJ, Parvizi J: Arthritis, in Flynn JM, ed: *Orthopaedic Knowledge Update*, ed 10. Rosemont, IL, American Academy of Orthopaedic Surgeons, 2011, pp 213-224.

Pearle AD, Warren RF, Rodeo SA: Basic science of articular cartilage and osteoarthritis. *Clin Sports Med* 2005;24(1):1-12.

Ulrich-Vinther M, Maloney MD, Schwarz EM, Rosier R, O'Keefe RJ: Articular cartilage biology. *J Am Acad Orthop Surg* 2003;11(6):421-430.

1: Basic Science

Chapter 9

Tendons and Ligaments

Stavros Thomopoulos, PhD

1: Basic Science

I. Tendons

A. Anatomy and function

1. Function—Tendons transfer force from muscle to bone to produce joint motion.

2. Composition and structure

   a. Tendon is made up of densely packed collagen fibers and water, with trace amounts of proteoglycans and elastin. The tissue is paucicellular.

   b. The fibroblast is the predominant cell type in tendon. In longitudinal histologic sections, fibroblasts appear spindle shaped, with a preferred orientation in the direction of collagen fibers. In cross section, fibroblasts are star shaped, with long cytoplasmic processes.

   c. Tendon has a hierarchical structure (**Figure 1**). Collagen molecules are arranged in quarter-stagger arrays. Five collagen molecules form an ordered microfibril unit. Microfibrils combine to form subfibrils, which further combine to form fibrils. Fibril units then form highly ordered parallel bundles oriented in the direction of muscle force. Fibrils accumulate to form fascicle units, which in turn combine to form the tendon.

   d. Type I collagen is the major constituent of tendon, making up 86% of its dry weight. The primary structure of collagen consists of glycine (33%), proline (15%), and hydroxyproline (15%). The collagen molecule is fibrillar in structure, with a length of 300 nm and a diameter of 1.5 nm.

   e. Proteoglycans make up 1% to 5% of the dry weight of a tendon. Proteoglycans are hydrophilic and bind tightly to water.

   f. Decorin is the predominant proteoglycan in tendon.

      • The role of decorin during development and healing is to regulate collagen fiber diameter. The presence of decorin inhibits lateral fusion of collagen fibers.

      • The function of decorin in adult tendon is debated. Decorin molecules form cross-links between collagen fibers. It was therefore hypothesized that the molecules transfer loads between collagen fibers, thereby increasing the stiffness of the tendon. Recent experimental evidence has disputed this hypothesis, however.

   g. Aggrecan (a proteoglycan abundant in articular cartilage) is found in areas of tendon that are under compression (eg, regions of hand flexor tendons that wrap around bone).

   h. The vascularity of tendon varies. Sheathed tendons (eg, flexor tendons of the hand) have regions that are relatively avascular. These regions get nutrition through diffusion from the synovium. Tendons not enclosed by a sheath receive their blood supply from vessels entering from the tendon surface or from the tendon enthesis (the tendon-to-bone insertion).

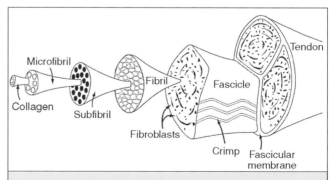

| **Figure 1** | Illustration shows the highly ordered hierarchical structure of tendon tissue. (Adapted with permission from Kastelic J, Baer E: Deformation in tendon collagen, in Vincent JFV, Currey JD, eds: *The Mechanical Properties of Biologic Materials.* Cambridge, United Kingdom, Cambridge University Press, 1980, pp 397-435.) |

Neither Dr. Thomopoulos nor any immediate family member has received anything of value from or has stock or stock options held in a commercial company or institution related directly or indirectly to the subject of this chapter.

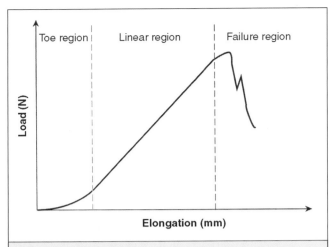

Figure 2 Graph represents the tensile behavior of tendon and ligament tissue, which includes a nonlinear toe region at low loads, a linear region at intermediate loads, and a failure region at high loads.

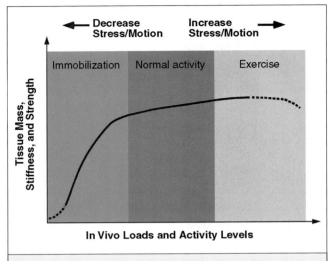

Figure 3 Graph demonstrates that immobilization leads to a dramatic drop in mechanical properties and that exercise has a positive effect on mechanical properties. (Reproduced with permission from Woo SL-Y, Chan SS, Yamaji T: Biomechanics of knee ligament healing, repair and reconstruction. *J Biomech* 1997;30:431-439.)

3. Biomechanics

   a. Tendons have high tensile properties and buckle under compression (ie, they behave like ropes). A typical load-elongation curve for tendon includes a toe region, a linear region, and a failure region (**Figure 2**).

   b. Tendon biomechanics can be characterized by structural properties (load-elongation behavior) or material properties (stress-strain behavior, where stress is calculated by dividing load by cross-sectional area, and strain is calculated by dividing change in elongation by initial length).

      - Structural properties describe the overall load-bearing capacity of the tissue and include the contribution of the muscle and bone attachments as well as the geometry of the tissue (cross-sectional area and length). Structural properties include stiffness (the slope of the linear portion of the curve in **Figure 2** and failure load.

      - Material properties (also referred to as mechanical properties) describe the quality of the tissue. Material properties are calculated by normalizing structural properties to account for tissue geometry. Material properties include the modulus of elasticity (the slope of the linear portion of the stress-strain curve) and failure stress (ie, strength).

   c. Tendons exhibit viscoelastic behavior; the mechanical properties of the tissue depend on loading history and time. Time dependence is best illustrated by the phenomena of creep and stress relaxation.

      - Creep is the increase in strain for a constant applied stress.

      - Stress relaxation is the decrease in stress for a constant applied strain.

   d. Several factors influence the biomechanical properties of tendons.

      - Anatomic location—Tendons from different anatomic locations have different structural properties; eg, digital flexor tendons have twice the ultimate strength of digital extensor tendons.

      - Exercise and immobilization—Exercise has a positive effect and immobilization has a detrimental effect on the biomechanical properties of tendons (**Figure 3**).

      - Age—The material and structural properties of tendons increase from birth through maturity. The properties then decrease from maturity through old age.

      - Laser/heat treatment causes tendons to shrink. This denatures the collagen fibers, resulting in a detrimental effect on the biomechanical properties of the tissue.

   e. The following factors should be considered when mechanically testing tendons.

      - The mechanical properties of tendons vary with hydration, temperature, and pH, so tendons should be tested under physiologically relevant hydration, temperature, and pH conditions.

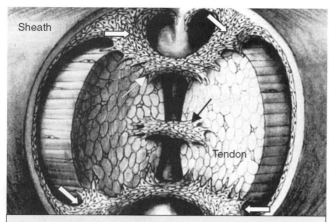

Figure 4 Illustration shows a sheathed tendon. Sheathed tendons heal primarily through infiltration of fibroblasts from the outer and inner surfaces of the tendon (black arrow). Adhesions between the outer surface of the tendon and the sheath (white arrows) can be prevented with passive motion rehabilitation. (Courtesy of Dr. R.H. Gelberman, Boston, MA.)

- The high strength of tendons results in difficulty in gripping the tissue during mechanical testing. Specialized grips (eg, freeze clamps) often are necessary to prevent the tendon from slipping out of the grip.

- Measurement of tissue cross-sectional area is necessary for the calculation of stress (recall that stress = load/cross-sectional area). Care must be taken when measuring the cross-sectional area of tendon because the tissue will deform if contact methods (eg, calipers) are used.

- Because tendons are viscoelastic (ie, their properties are time dependent), the rate at which the tendon is pulled can influence the mechanical properties. Higher strain rates result in a higher elastic modulus.

- Specimens should be stored frozen and hydrated. Improper storage may affect the mechanical properties of the tendon.

- The orientation of a tendon during testing will influence the mechanical properties measured; eg, the structural properties of the supraspinatus tendon depend on the angle of the humeral head relative to the glenoid.

B. Injury, repair, and healing

1. Tendon injury occurs because of direct trauma (eg, laceration of a flexor tendon) or indirect tensile overload (eg, Achilles tendon rupture). Several tendinopathies (eg, rotator cuff degeneration) predispose tendons to injury.

2. Three phases of healing

    a. Hemostasis/inflammation—After injury, the wound site is infiltrated by inflammatory cells. Platelets aggregate at the wound and create a fibrin clot to stabilize the torn tendon edges. The length of this phase is on the order of days.

    b. Cell proliferation and extracellular matrix production—Fibroblasts infiltrate the wound site and proliferate. They produce extracellular matrix, including large amounts of type I and III collagen. The injury response in adult tendon is scar mediated (ie, large amounts of disorganized collagen are deposited at the repair site) rather than regenerative. The length of this phase is on the order of weeks.

    c. Remodeling/maturation—Matrix metalloproteinases degrade the collagen matrix, replacing type III collagen with type I collagen. Collagen fibers are reorganized so that they are aligned in the direction of muscle loading. The length of this phase is on the order of months to years.

3. Long-term effects—The structural properties of repaired tendons typically reach only two thirds of normal, even years after repair. Material property differences are even higher.

4. Sheathed tendons—Flexor tendons of the hand are often injured through direct trauma (eg, laceration). The two critical considerations for sheathed tendon healing are prevention of adhesion formation and accrual of mechanical strength (**Figure 4**).

5. Tendons not enclosed in sheaths fail because of trauma (eg, an acute sports injury) or preexisting pathology (eg, a rotator cuff tear after years of chronic tendon degeneration). Nonsheathed tendons have a greater capacity to heal than sheathed tendons. Injury often occurs at the attachments of the tendon (ie, at the tendon-to-bone insertion or at the musculotendinous junction).

6. The role of rehabilitation during healing is complex.

    a. Protective immobilization in the early period after tendon repair is beneficial in many scenarios (eg, after rotator cuff repair).

    b. Active loading, including exercise, can be detrimental if started too early in the rehabilitation period, but is beneficial during the remodeling phase of healing.

    c. Early passive motion is beneficial for flexor tendon healing. Early motion suppresses adhesion formation between the tendon and the sheath, preventing the typical range-of-motion losses seen with immobilized tendons.

II. Ligaments

A. Anatomy and function

1. The function of ligaments is to restrict joint motion (ie, to stabilize joints).

2. Composition and structure

   a. Ligaments are composed of densely packed type I collagen, proteoglycans, elastin, and water.

   b. Ligaments are similar in composition and structure to tendons, but there are several important differences.

      • Ligaments are shorter and wider than tendons.

      • Ligaments have a lower percentage of collagen and a higher percentage of proteoglycans and water.

      • The collagen fibers in ligaments are less organized.

   c. Ligaments have a highly ordered hierarchical structure, similar to tendons.

   d. Type I collagen makes up 70% of the dry weight of ligaments.

   e. Like tendons, the main cell type in ligaments is the fibroblast, but ligament fibroblasts appear rounder than tendon fibroblasts.

   f. Ligaments have relatively low vascularity and cellularity.

3. Biomechanics

   a. The biomechanical properties of ligaments are expressed as the structural properties of the bone-ligament-bone complex or the material properties of the ligament midsubstance itself.

   b. Ligaments exhibit viscoelastic behavior similar to that of tendons.

   c. Several factors that influence the mechanical properties of ligaments are the same as those described earlier for tendons (I.A.3.d).

   d. Factors that must be considered when mechanically testing ligaments are the same as those listed earlier for tendons (I.A.3.e).

B. Injury, repair, and healing

1. Ligament injuries are generally classified into three grades: I, II, and III. Grade I corresponds to a mild sprain, grade II corresponds to a moderate sprain/partial tear, and grade III corresponds to a complete ligament tear. An additional type of injury is avulsion of the ligament from its bony insertion.

2. Ligament healing occurs through the same phases as tendon healing: hemostasis/inflammation, matrix and cell proliferation, and remodeling/maturation.

3. Extra-articular ligaments (eg, the medial collateral ligament [MCL] of the knee) have a greater capacity to heal than do intra-articular ligaments (eg, the anterior cruciate ligament [ACL] of the knee).

   a. MCL of the knee

      • Grade I and II injuries to the MCL heal without surgical treatment.

      • The optimal treatment of grade III MCL injuries is controversial. Up to 25% of patients with these injuries continue to have clinical problems whether or not the tear is repaired surgically.

   b. ACL of the knee—Midsubstance ACL injuries typically do not heal. Surgical reconstruction of the ACL often is necessary to restore stability in the injured knee. Several graft materials have been used to reconstruct the ACL, including autografts and allografts.

      • Autografts, including bone–patellar tendon–bone, semitendinosus, quadriceps, and gracilis, are commonly used. The structural properties of the reconstructed graft attain only 50% of normal properties at the longest follow-up studied. The major disadvantage of autograft use is donor site morbidity.

      • ACL allografts, typically taken from cadavers, are also used for ACL reconstruction. Disadvantages of these grafts include the potential for disease transmission and the loss of mechanical properties due to graft sterilization processing.

      • A process described as "ligamentization" occurs in both autografts and allografts after ACL reconstruction. Autograft fibroblasts die soon after reconstruction and are replaced by local fibroblasts. Similarly, allografts are infiltrated by local fibroblasts in the early period after implantation.

III. Enthesis (Tendon/Ligament–Bone Junction)

A. Anatomy and function

1. Tendons and ligaments insert into bone across a complex transitional tissue, the enthesis.

2. Composition and structure

   a. In indirect insertions (eg, the femoral insertion of the MCL), the superficial layer connects with the periosteum, and the deep layer anchors to bone via Sharpey fibers.

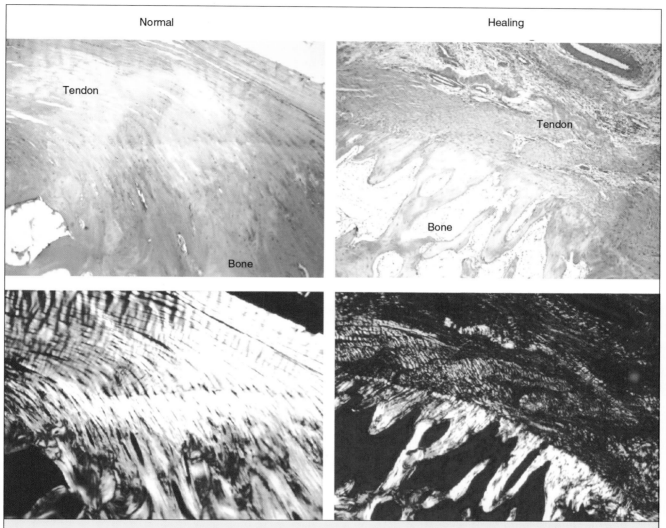

Figure 5 Bright field microscopic images (top row) and polarized light images (bottom row) show canine flexor tendon-to-bone enthesis. Note that the transitional tissue between tendon and bone is not regenerated at the healing interface.

1: Basic Science

b. Direct insertions (eg, the supraspinatus insertion of the rotator cuff) classically have been categorized into four zones.

- First zone: tendon proper. The properties in this zone are similar to those found at the tendon midsubstance. It consists of well-aligned type I collagen fibers with small amounts of the proteoglycan decorin. The cell type in this zone is the fibroblast.

- Second zone: fibrocartilage. This zone marks the beginning of the transition from tendinous material to bony material. It is composed of type II and III collagen, with small amounts of type I, IX, and X collagen, and small amounts of the proteoglycans aggrecan and decorin. The cell type in this zone is the fibrochondrocyte.

- Third zone: mineralized fibrocartilage. This zone is characterized by a marked transition toward bony tissue. The predominant collagen is type II, with significant amounts of type X collagen and aggrecan. The cell types in this zone are the fibrochondrocyte and the hypertrophic chondrocyte.

- Fourth zone: bone. This zone is made up predominantly of type I collagen with a high mineral content. The cell types in this zone are the osteoblast, the osteocyte, and the osteoclast.

c. Although the insertion site is typically categorized into four zones, changes in the tissue are graded, without distinct borders between zones (**Figure 5**). This graded transition in tissue composition is presumed to aid in the efficient transfer of load between tendon and bone.

3. Biomechanics

   a. A functionally graded transition between tendon and bone is necessary to reduce stress concentrations at the interface of two very different materials (tendon/ligament and bone). Composition grading is evident in mineral content and proteoglycan content, structural grading is evident in collagen fiber organization, and mechanical grading is evident in elastic and viscoelastic properties.

   b. The enthesis typically has lower mechanical properties in tension than does the tendon or ligament midsubstance. This compliant region between tendon/ligament and bone reduces stress concentrations that would otherwise arise between the dissimilar materials.

B. Injury, repair, and healing

   1. Tendon-to-bone and ligament-to-bone healing is necessary in several scenarios.

      a. Rotator cuff injuries, which comprise most of the soft-tissue injuries to the upper extremity, commonly require surgical repair of the tendon(s) to the humeral head.

      b. Most ACL reconstruction techniques use tendon grafts that must heal in tibial and femoral bone tunnels.

      c. Avulsion injuries to the flexor tendons of the hand require tendon-to-bone repair.

   2. In most cases of tendon-to-bone healing, clinical outcomes are disappointing. The most dramatic feature of the failed healing response is the lack of a transitional tissue between the healing tendon and bone (**Figure 5**). Regeneration of the natural functionally graded interface between tendon and bone is critical for the restoration of joint function and the prevention of reinjury.

IV. Tissue Engineering

A. Overview

   1. Definition—Tissue engineering is the regeneration of injured tissue through the merging of three areas: scaffold microenvironment, responding cells, and signaling biofactors.

   2. Tissue engineering approaches hold great promise for improving tendon and ligament repair, but they have not yet succeeded clinically.

B. Scaffold microenvironment

   1. The scaffold can serve as a delivery system for biofactors, an environment to attract or immobilize cells, and/or a mechanical stabilizer.

   2. Scaffold matrices commonly are made of collagen, fibrin, polymer, or silk.

C. Responding cells

   1. Responding cells may include tendon/ligament fibroblasts or mesenchymal stem cells (commonly derived from bone marrow or adipose tissue).

   2. Responding cells may be seeded onto the scaffold before implantation or may infiltrate the acellular scaffold after it is implanted.

D. Signaling biofactors

   1. Growth factors

      a. Platelet-derived growth factor-BB (PDGF-BB) promotes cell proliferation and matrix synthesis.

      b. Transforming growth factor-β (TGF-β) promotes matrix synthesis.

      c. Basic fibroblast growth factor (bFGF) promotes cell proliferation and matrix synthesis.

      d. Bone morphogenetic proteins (BMPs) 12, 13, and 14 (also known as growth and differentiation factors 7, 6, and 5, respectively) promote matrix synthesis and the differentiation of mesenchymal stem cells into tendon/ligament fibroblasts.

   2. Mechanical signals

      a. Cyclic tensile loads promote matrix synthesis.

      b. Compressive loads promote proteoglycan production.

Top Testing Facts

1. Tendons and ligaments are materials with a highly ordered hierarchical structure.

2. The composition of tendons and ligaments is primarily type I collagen, aligned in the direction of loading.

3. Structural properties describe the capacity of the tissue to bear load; material properties describe the quality of the tissue.

4. Tendons and ligaments are viscoelastic; that is, their mechanical properties are time dependent.

5. The physical environment influences uninjured tissue maintenance. Immobilization is detrimental and exercise is beneficial to the biomechanical properties of tendon and ligament.

6. Several biologic (eg, age) and environmental (eg, temperature) factors influence the mechanical properties of tendons and ligaments.

7. Tendon/ligament healing progresses through clearly defined phases: hemostasis/inflammation, matrix and cell proliferation, and remodeling/maturation.

8. Nonsheathed tendons and extra-articular ligaments have a greater capacity to heal than do sheathed tendons and intra-articular ligaments.

9. For tendon and ligament healing, increased loading can be beneficial or detrimental depending on the anatomic location and type of injury.

10. The tendon/ligament enthesis is a specialized transitional tissue between tendon or ligament and bone that is necessary to minimize stress concentrations at the interface of two dissimilar materials.

Bibliography

Amiel D, Kleiner JB, Roux RD, Harwood FL, Akeson WH: The phenomenon of "ligamentization": Anterior cruciate ligament reconstruction with autogenous patellar tendon. *J Orthop Res* 1986;4(2):162-172.

Reuther KE, Gray CF, Soslowsky LJ: Form and function of tendon and ligament, in O'Keefe RJ, Jacobs JJ, Chu CE, Einhorn TA, eds: *Orthopaedic Basic Science*, ed 4. Rosemont, IL, American Academy of Orthopaedic Surgeons, 2013, pp 213-228.

Gelberman RH, Woo SL, Lothringer K, Akeson WH, Amiel D: Effects of early intermittent passive mobilization on healing canine flexor tendons. *J Hand Surg Am* 1982;7(2):170-175.

Lu HH, Thomopoulos S: Functional attachment of soft tissues to bone: Development, healing, and tissue engineering. *Annu Rev Biomed Eng* 2013;15:201-226.

Thomopoulos S, Genin GM: Tendon and ligament biomechanics, in Winkelstein BA, ed: *Orthopaedic Biomechanics*. Boca Raton, FL, CRC/Taylor and Francis, 2013, pp 49-74.

1: Basic Science

Chapter 10

Peripheral Nervous System

Seth D. Dodds, MD

I. Function

A. Peripheral nerves connect the central nervous system (CNS) with tissues such as bone, joints, muscles, tendons, and skin.

B. Nerves that supply the musculoskeletal system provide both motor and sensory function.

II. Structure and Composition

A. Neuron anatomy

1. Every neuron contains a cell body, which is its metabolic center.

2. The cell bodies of most neurons also give rise to one long branch, known as an axon, and to several short branches, known as dendrites (**Figure 1, A**).

3. Dendrites are thin nerve processes that receive input from other nerves.

4. The axon is the primary distal projection of the cell body of the neuron.

   a. The neuron conveys signals to tissues and to other nerve cells via the axon, which conveys action potentials to the other cells.

   b. The neuron receives messages from other neurons via its dendrites, which convey action potentials from the axons of the other neurons.

   c. The axon of a neuron meets the dendrites of one or more adjoining neurons at a junction called the synapse, where action potentials from the axon pass into the dendrites of the other neurons.

   d. Axons typically measure 0.2 to 20.0 μm in diameter and arise from an axon hillock, which initiates the action potentials of neurons.

5. Myelin, which is composed of fatty substances

and proteins, forms an insulating sheath around the axons of neurons in the peripheral nervous system. The myelin that forms this sheath is produced by Schwann cells, which belong to a larger family of nonneuronal cells known as glial cells. One function of myelin is to speed the conduction of action potentials along the axons of nerve cells.

   a. In unmyelinated nerve fibers, a single Schwann cell envelops multiple axons, and conduction proceeds more slowly than in myelinated nerve fibers, in which each axon is circumferentially laminated by a Schwann cell. In both unmyelinated and myelinated nerve fibers, the Schwann cells neighbor one another along the length of the fiber.

   b. The nodes of Ranvier are interruptions or gaps between segments of the myelin sheath; they permit the propagation of action potentials.

6. As an axon reaches its end organ, it divides into fine terminal branches with specialized endings called presynaptic terminals, which are responsible for transmitting a signal to postsynaptic receptors (**Figure 1**).

B. Nerve anatomy

1. Nerve fibers are collections of axons with Schwann cell sheaths surrounding them.

2. Afferent nerve fibers convey information from sensory receptors to the CNS.

3. Efferent nerve fibers transmit signals from the CNS to muscle and other tissue in the periphery of the body, that is, outside the brain and spinal cord.

4. Nerve fibers have been classified on the basis of their size and conduction velocity (**Table 1**).

C. Composition—A nerve consists of collections of nerve fibers called fascicles and of neural connective tissue, which both surrounds and lies within each fascicle (**Figure 2**).

1. The axons within a fascicle are surrounded by a connective tissue layer called endoneurium. Endoneurium is primarily composed of a collagenous matrix with fibroblasts, mast cells, and capillaries,

---

Dr. Dodds or an immediate family member is a member of a speakers' bureau or has made paid presentations on behalf of Integra and Medartis.

1: Basic Science

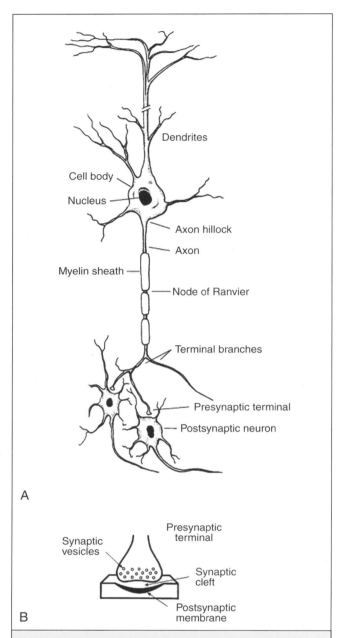

Figure 1   **A,** The primary morphologic features of a peripheral nerve cell are the dendrites, cell body, axon, and presynaptic terminals. **B,** Communication between the terminal end of a nerve axon and an end organ occurs through the release of neurotransmitter molecules from the synaptic vesicle of presynaptic nerve terminal. The neurotransmitter molecules travel across the synaptic cleft to receptors on the postsynaptic membrane of the end organ. (Reproduced from Bodine SC, Lieber RL: Peripheral nerve physiology, anatomy, and pathology, in Buckwalter JA, Einhorn TA, Simon SR, eds: *Orthopaedic Basic Science*, ed 2. Rosemont, IL, American Academy of Orthopaedic Surgeons, 2000, p 618.)

and forms a bilaminar sheath around the axon, Schwann cells, and myelin of a nerve fiber.

2. Perineurium is a thin, dense connective tissue layer that surrounds the fascicles of a nerve.

   a. It has a high tensile strength and maintains interfascicular pressure, providing a barrier to perineurial diffusion. This barrier limits injury to nerve fibers by limiting diffusion of the epineurial edema fluid that occurs in stretch and compression injuries. The barrier created by the perineurium also limits the diffusion of endoneurial edema fluid that can occur when a nerve is compressed.

   b. Spinal nerve roots have less perineurium than peripheral nerves and are more susceptible to stretch and compression injury.

3. Epineurium is a supportive sheath that contains multiple groups of fascicles. It also contains a well-developed network of extrinsic, interconnected blood vessels that run parallel to the fascicles.

4. The structural organization of fascicles changes throughout the length of a nerve. Fascicles do not run as isolated, parallel strands from the spinal cord to a presynaptic terminal or end organ. The number and size of fascicles changes as fascicular plexuses unite and divide within a nerve (**Figure 3**).

   a. At the joint level, the fascicles of a nerve are numerous and are smaller to accommodate nerve deformation as the joint goes through a range of motion. For example, the ulnar nerve at the elbow contains many small fascicles, which minimize injury to this nerve with elbow flexion and extension.

   b. In contrast to the ulnar nerve, the radial nerve at the level of the spiral groove has a small number of large fascicles, which do not tolerate stretch well. This level-specific internal anatomy places the radial nerve at greater risk for neurapraxia when it is mobilized and retracted from the spiral groove.

D. Blood supply—A peripheral nerve has both intrinsic and extrinsic vessels, with multiple anastomoses between one another throughout the length of the nerve.

   1. At the epineural level, no blood-nerve barrier exists.

   2. At the capillary level within the endoneurium, however, a blood-nerve barrier exists, similar to the blood-brain barrier. This barrier prevents the diffusion of many different macromolecules into the nerve, maintaining neural integrity. The blood-nerve diffusion barrier can be damaged by infection, radiation, or metabolic disease.

E. Nerve endings—Afferent nerve fibers use specific primary receptors to collect sensory information

Table 1

Classification of Peripheral Nerve Fibers

Fiber Type	Example of Function	Fiber Characteristic	Fiber Diameter (μm)	Conduction Velocity (m/s)
Aα	Motor axon	Myelinated—Large	12–20	72–120
Aβ	Cutaneous touch and pressure	Myelinated—Medium	6–12	36–72
Aδ	Pain and temperature	Myelinated—Small	1–6	4–36
B	Sympathetic preganglionic	Myelinated—Small	1–6	3–15
C	Cutaneous pain, sympathetic postganglionic	Unmyelinated	0.2–1.5	0.4–2.0

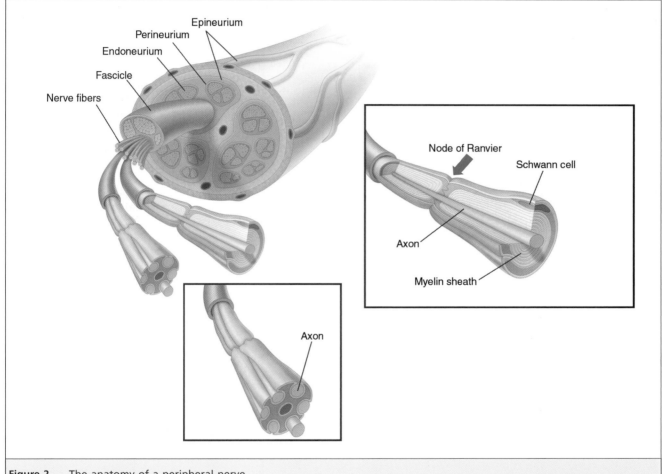

Figure 2 The anatomy of a peripheral nerve.

from the periphery. There are three types of sensory information and four attributes of the sensory information conveyed by afferent nerve fibers (mechanoreceptors) (**Table 2**).

1. Types of sensory information

   a. Mechanical stimulation (touch, proprioception, pressure)

   b. Painful stimulation (noxious, tissue-damaging stimuli)

   c. Thermal stimulation (heat, cold)

2. Attributes: location, intensity, quality, and duration

3. Nociceptors and thermoceptors consist of bare nerve endings.

4. Mechanoreceptors—Three types

  a. Cutaneous (superficial) skin mechanoreceptors: Small

  • Meissner corpuscle: a rapidly adapting sensory receptor that is very sensitive to touch

  • Merkel disk receptors: adapt slowly and sense sustained pressure, texture, and low-frequency vibrations

  b. Subcutaneous mechanoreceptors: Larger and fewer in number

  • Pacini (or pacinian) corpuscles: ovoid in shape, measuring approximately 1 mm in length. They react to high-frequency vibration and rapid indentations of the skin.

  • Ruffini corpuscles, slowly adapting receptors that respond to stretching of the skin, such as occurs with the flexing of a finger.

  c. Intramuscular and skeletal mechanoreceptors: Muscle, tendon, and joint capsular receptors that guide proprioception

F. Nerve metabolism

  1. Axoplasmic transport (that is, intracellular transport of substances along an axon) is made possible by the polarization of the neuron.

  2. Proteins, which are created only in the cell body of a neuron, travel via antegrade transport through the axon and dendrites of the neuron to support neural functions, such as action potential propagation and neurotransmitter release.

  3. Degradation products travel back to the cell body via retrograde transport. Several other factors also travel to the cell body in retrograde fashion, including nerve-growth factors, some viruses (for example, herpes simplex, rabies, polio), tetanus toxin, and horseradish peroxidase (used in the laboratory to identify the location of a cell body in a dorsal root ganglion or in the spinal cord).

  4. The rate of axonal transport decreases with decreasing temperature and anoxia.

G. Embryology of the nervous system

  1. The nervous system (and skin) is formed by the ectoderm, which, with the mesoderm and endoderm, is one of the three germ layers of embryonic tissue.

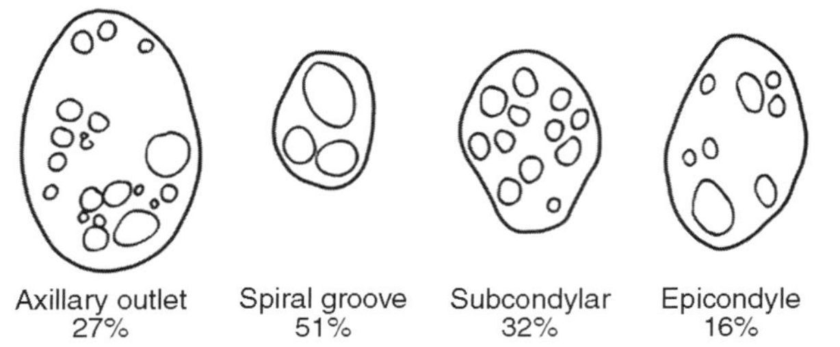

Axillary outlet 27%	Spiral groove 51%
Subcondylar 32%	Epicondyle 16%

Figure 3 The size, number, and arrangement of fascicles within a nerve vary along the course of the nerve. This figure depicts the percentage of the cross-sectional area of nerve devoted to fasciculi (given as a percentage of total cross-sectional area) in the radial nerve at different points along the nerve from the shoulder to the elbow. (Reproduced with permission from Lundborg G: *Nerve Injury and Repair.* New York, NY, Churchill Livingstone, 1988, p 198.)

Table 2

Types of Receptors

	Receptor Type	Quality	Fiber Type
Nociceptors	Mechanical	Sharp, pricking pain	$A\delta$
	Polymodal	Slow, burning pain	C
Cutaneous mechanoreceptors	Meissner corpuscle	Touch	$A\beta$
	Merkel receptor	Steady skin indentation	$A\beta$
Subcutaneous mechanoreceptors	Pacini corpuscle	Vibration	$A\beta$
	Ruffini corpuscle	Skin stretch	$A\beta$
Muscle and skeletal mechanoreceptors	Muscle spindle, primary	Limb proprioception	$A\alpha$
	Muscle spindle, secondary	Limb proprioception	$A\beta$
	Golgi tendon organ	Limb proprioception	$A\alpha$
	Joint capsule mechanoreceptor	Limb proprioception	$A\beta$

Adapted with permission from Kandel ER, Schwartz JH, Jessel TM, eds: *Principles of Neural Science*, ed 3. Norwalk, CT, Appleton & Lange, 1991, p 342.

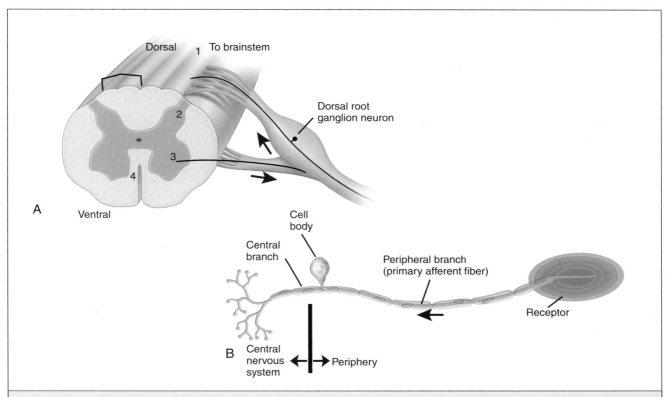

Dorsal   To brainstem

Dorsal root
ganglion neuron

2

3

4

A   Ventral

Cell
body

Central
branch

Peripheral branch
(primary afferent fiber)

Receptor

B   Central
nervous
system

Central
nervous
system ← → Periphery

Figure 4   Illustrations show the cell body of a sensory nerve resides in the dorsal root ganglion, far from its distal nerve ending. The dorsal root ganglion is located proximally and near the spinal cord, where the spinal nerve exits the thecal sac or dura. **A,** Spinal cord with dorsal and ventral markings demonstrating the formation of the dorsal root ganglion. **B,** Projections of the central branch.

2. The ectoderm divides to form the neural tube, which gives rise to the brain, spinal cord, and motor neurons; the neural crest, which evolves into afferent neurons; and the epidermal layer of the skin.

3. The peripheral nervous system is divided into the autonomic nervous system, a purely motor visceral system, and a mixed sensory and motor somatic system, which helps control voluntary motion.

H. Axonal growth and development are initially guided by different nerve growth factors.

1. N-cadherin and neural cell adhesion molecule are adhesive membrane glycoproteins that are expressed on neural ectoderm and help guide growing axons.

2. Laminin and fibronectin are glycoproteins of the extracellular matrix that promote the directional growth of nerve fibers.

3. Other factors thought to enhance nerve regeneration include nerve-growth factor, fibroblast growth factor, ciliary neuronotrophic factor, and insulin-like growth factor.

I. Spinal nerves

1. Spinal nerves are collections of axons that exit the spinal cord at distinct levels (8 cervical, 12 thoracic, 5 lumbar, 5 sacral, 1 coccygeal).

2. The efferent ventral root of a spinal nerve transmits information from the brain to muscle; the afferent dorsal root carries signals from the periphery back to the CNS.

a. The cell bodies of afferent sensory nerves are located in the dorsal root ganglion, which lies near the point at which the spinal nerve exits the spinal cord (**Figure 4**).

b. The cell bodies of efferent motor nerves are located in the anterior horn of the spinal cord.

3. Spinal nerves frequently collect into plexuses (cervical, brachial, lumbar) before branching.

III. Nerve Conduction and Biomechanics

A. Propagation of a nerve signal

1. The axon membrane of a neuron consists of a selectively permeable lipid bilayer that contains gated ion channels and transmembrane pumps.

These pumps derive their energy from sodium/potassium adenosine triphosphate (Na^+/K^+–ATP). The control of gated ion channels (Na^+ and K^+) is governed primarily by electrical, chemical, and mechanical stimuli. The Na^+/K^+–ATP–dependent pumps create an accumulation of sodium ions outside the membrane, which is responsible for the negative resting potential that exists within the axon membrane. When a stimulus causes the gated ion channels to open, sodium flows rapidly into the axon, causing its depolarization.

2. Conduction of signals along an axon begins with action potentials, which are generated when the axon membrane is depolarized beyond a critical threshold.

3. The rate at which an action potential is conducted along an axon depends on the size of the axon and the presence of myelin; larger axons and myelinated axons carry action potentials more rapidly than do smaller or unmyelinated axons.

4. Within the nodes of Ranvier along the axon, dense collections of sodium channels propagate the action potential, allowing saltatory (pulse-like) conduction between one node and the next.

5. Most peripheral motor and sensory nerves are myelinated; the axons of efferent motor nerves are the most heavily myelinated. Autonomic nerve fibers and slow pain fibers are examples of unmyelinated nerves.

6. Multiple sclerosis (MS) and Guillain-Barré syndrome are examples of nervous system diseases that cause demyelination and slowed nerve-conduction velocities.

   a. MS is a chronic (and occasionally remitting) neurologic disorder characterized by the perivascular infiltration of inflammatory cells, followed by damage to the myelin sheaths of nerves as well as to nerve fibers themselves. Problems with motor control (for example, vision, strength, balance) and cognition develop in patients with MS.

   b. Guillain-Barré syndrome is an acute, inflammatory condition affecting nerves and spinal nerve roots (that is, a polyradiculoneuropathy). It is presumed to be an autoimmune condition, typically triggered by a viral or bacterial infection, that causes the production of antibodies that attack the myelin sheath. The loss of myelin leads to an acute impairment of sensory and motor nerve function, ranging in severity from paresthesias and weakness to complete loss of sensation and paralysis.

7. Neuromuscular junction—A highly specialized region between the distal nerve terminal and a skeletal muscle fiber. It consists of the presynaptic terminal, or distalmost end of a nerve fiber; a synaptic cleft, into which the nerve terminal releases neurotransmitter substance; and a postsynaptic membrane, a part of the cell membrane of a neuron or muscle fiber on which the neurotransmitter released by the nerve terminal acts to produce a response (**Figure 1, B**).

   a. The arrival of an action potential at the presynaptic terminal triggers the release of acetylcholine from vesicles in the terminal.

   b. Acetylcholine travels across the synaptic cleft and, once bound to receptors on the postsynaptic membrane, causes depolarization of the motor end plate and stimulation of the muscle fiber.

B. Biomechanics

1. Nerves are viscoelastic structures that respond to stress in a nonlinear manner.

2. When a nerve is stretched, it becomes ischemic before disrupting; for example, a nerve may undergo ischemia at 15% strain and rupture at 20% strain.

3. The ultimate strain that can be endured by a nerve ranges from 20% to 60%.

IV. Nerve Injury, Repair, and Healing

A. Response to injury

1. Peripheral nerves respond to injury with an initial inflammatory response.

   a. This response typically results in increased epineurial permeability and edema because the vessels within the epineurium lack a blood-nerve barrier.

   b. An injury that involves disruption (for example, crush, transection) that exposes the endoneurium disrupts the blood-nerve barrier, thus increasing the permeability of the endoneurial capillaries.

2. Injury from ischemia and compression can increase endoneurial pressure, fluid edema, and capillary permeability without affecting the perineurial vascular system.

   a. In these cases, the positive fluid pressure inside the endoneurium affects blood flow, decreasing nutrition and oxygen delivery to nerve cells and the removal of waste products from them.

   b. Persistent intraneural edema can diminish nerve function, as seen in chronic compressive neuropathies.

B. Seddon classification of nerve injury (**Table 3**)

Table 3			

Nerve Injury Classification

Seddon	Sunderland	Pathoanatomy	Prognosis
Neurapraxia	Type 1	Temporary conduction block with local myelin damage	Typically full recovery
Axonotmesis	Type 2	Axons disrupted; endoneurium, perineurium, and epineurium intact	Reasonable recovery of function
	Type 3	Axons and endoneurium disrupted; perineurium and epineurium intact	Incomplete recovery due to intrafascicular fibrosis
	Type 4	Axons, endoneurium, and perineurium disrupted; epineurium intact	Negligible recovery due to axonal misdirection
Neurotmesis	Type 5	Complete disruption of nerve	No spontaneous recovery

Adapted from Lee SK, Wolfe SW: Peripheral nerve injury and repair. *J Am Acad Orthop Surg* 2000;8:245.

1. Neurapraxia

   a. Neurapraxia is an immediate, localized blocking of neural conduction, with normal conduction above and below the injury site.

   b. Neurapraxias are typically reversible. Axon continuity is maintained, but local demyelination and ischemia occur.

   c. Mechanisms of injury causing neurapraxia include compression, traction, and contusion.

2. Axonotmesis

   a. Axonotmesis involves axon disruption without the destruction of Schwann cells, the perineurium, or the epineurium. The axon distal to the point of injury degenerates (wallerian degeneration).

   b. Some nerve function may be recovered because nerve fiber regeneration is guided by an intact neural connective tissue layer (for example, intact endoneurium).

   c. Mechanisms of injury causing axonotmesis include crush and forceful stretch.

3. Neurotmesis

   a. Neurotmesis is complete disruption of a nerve.

   b. No spontaneous recovery of the affected nerve can be expected.

   c. Mechanisms of injury include open crush, violent stretch, and laceration.

4. Sunderland revised the Seddon classification of nerve injuries into the categories of neurapraxia, axonotmesis, and neurotmesis by defining three subtypes of axontmesis.

C. Pathoanatomy of injury

   1. Laceration (**Figure 5, A** and **B**)

   a. When the continuity of a nerve is disrupted, the two nerve ends retract, the cell body of the neuron swells, the nucleus is displaced peripherally, and chromatolysis (dispersion of basophilic Nissl granules with relative eosinophilia of the cell body) occurs.

   b. The nerve cell stops producing neurotransmitters and begins synthesizing proteins required for axonal regeneration.

   c. Wallerian degeneration distal to the site of injury begins within hours and is characterized by axonal disorganization caused by proteolysis, followed by the breakdown of myelin.

   d. Schwann cells become active in clearing myelin and axonal debris from the site of injury.

   2. Compression

   a. When a nerve is compressed, nerve fibers are deformed, local ischemia occurs, and vascular permeability is increased.

   b. Edema then affects the endoneurial environment, resulting in poor axonal transport and nerve dysfunction.

   c. If compression continues, the edema and dysfunction persist and fibroblasts invade the nerve, producing scar tissue, which impairs the gliding of nerve fascicles over one another in joint flexion.

   d. Tissue pressures of up to 30 mm Hg can cause paresthesias and increase the latency of nerve conduction. A tissue pressure of 60 mm Hg can completely block nerve conduction.

   3. Ischemia

   a. After 15 minutes of anoxia, axonal transport stops.

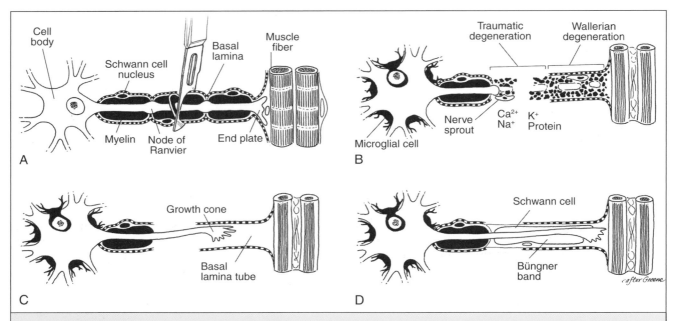

Figure 5   Illustrations show peripheral nerve injury, degeneration, and regeneration. **A,** Laceration of the nerve fiber. **B,** Degeneration of the proximal stump to the nearest node of Ranvier and wallerian degeneration of the distal stump. **C,** Axonal sprouting of the growth cone into a basal lamina tube. **D,** The Schwann cell forms a column (Büngner band) to assist directed axonal growth. (Adapted with permission from Seckel BR: Enhancement of peripheral nerve regeneration. *Muscle Nerve* 1990;13:785-800.)

b. Axonal transport can recover if reperfusion occurs within 12 to 24 hours.

D. Nerve regeneration after injury

1. With or without suture reapproximation of disrupted nerve ends, nerve regeneration begins with axonal elongation across the zone of injury (**Figure 5, C and D**).

    a. The zone of injury undergoes an ingrowth of both capillaries and Schwann cells.

    b. The Schwann cells migrate from both the proximal and distal stumps of a disrupted axon or nerve fiber into the gap created by the disruption and attempt to form columns (Büngner bands) to guide the tip or growth cone of the axon or fiber.

    c. The growth cone is sensitive to neurotrophic growth factors, such as nerve growth factor, and to factors that promote the formation of neurites (axons or dendrites), such as laminin.

2. Distal reinnervation of muscle occurs only when the muscle has viable motor end plates that a regenerating nerve can stimulate.

    a. In the acute period after a nerve injury, muscle innervated by the injured nerve increases the number of its motor end plates, seeking stimulation by the nerve.

    b. With the occurrence and continuation of fibro-

sis, the number of motor end plates diminishes.

    c. Typically, a muscle is no longer receptive to reinnervation beyond 12 months after injury to the motor nerve that serves it.

V. Treatment of Peripheral Nerve Injuries

A. Nonsurgical treatment

1. Nonsurgical treatment is appropriate for all neurapraxias and most axonotmeses.

2. During the recovery of a motor nerve serving a limb muscle, great care should be taken to maintain the functionality and viability of the limb. Specifically, distal joints should be mobilized and distal muscle groups stretched or protectively splinted to avoid contractures.

3. Neglect of the affect limb can result in osteopenia, joint stiffness, and muscle atrophy.

B. Recovery of an injured sensory nerve occurs in the following sequence:

1. Pressure sense

2. Protective pain

3. Moving touch

4. Moving two-point discrimination

5. Static two-point discrimination

6. Threshold sensation (measured with Semmes-Weinstein monofilaments and exposure to vibration).

C. Surgical repair

1. Prerequisites to nerve repair (neurorrhaphy) include a clean wound, a well-vascularized repair bed, skeletal stability, and viable soft-tissue coverage.

2. Nerve ends are sharply débrided of injured or devitalized nerve, scar tissue, and fibrotic tissue to expose healthy nerve fascicles.

3. A repair performed within the first few days after injury has distinct advantages because disrupted nerves retract and scar tissue and neuromas develop rapidly after injury.

4. Immobilization for 2 to 3 weeks postoperatively prevents stress at the repair site in a limb or extremity with a repaired nerve injury.

5. The most effective repair technique for an injured nerve is an epineurial repair (that is, a sutured repair of the epineurium only) performed with a fine monofilament nylon suture (such as 9-0), using microsurgical instrumentation and technique.

   a. In reapproximating the ends of an injured nerve in an epineurial repair, care should be taken to orient the nerve ends to match fascicles as accurately as possible. This technique typically minimizes scar formation.

   b. The repair can be performed with fine microsuture or with fibrin glue.

   c. The repair should be done with minimal tension on the nerve.

6. A group fascicular repair involves reapproximating fascicular groups by perineurial repair. This technique is more precise than epineurial repair, but it typically requires intraneural dissection, which results in greater scar-tissue formation and intraneural fibrosis.

7. Muscular neurotization involves implanting the end of an injured nerve directly into the belly of the muscle served by the nerve.

8. Nerve grafting is used when segmental defects in a nerve cannot be overcome through joint flexion or nerve transposition. A nerve repair only made possible with a flexed joint will not tolerate joint extension well after healing, potentially resulting in permanent joint stiffness.

   a. Autografts are implanted in the same manner as that used in the primary repair of a nerve, although it is recommended that these grafts be reversed to decrease axonal dispersion through the graft. Nerve grafts may be cabled to increase their diameter to match the size of the injured nerve; they should also be reversed to minimize the early arborization of regenerating nerve fibers.

   b. The sural nerve is a common source of autograft and can be cut into parallel sections to create a cable graft of greater diameter.

   c. Fresh allografts require immunosuppression and are infrequently used.

   d. Cleansed or processed allografts do not require immunosuppression and have the advantage of not involving a donor site. However, cleansed allografts do not currently have a track record sufficiently consistent to permit recommendations of their use. In animal studies, these grafts have been shown to promote nerve-fiber regeneration more densely across gaps than do nerve conduits. In lieu of bridging with an autograft, nerve gaps can be bridged with either biologic (vein graft) or bioabsorbable nerve conduits (polyglycolic acid, collagen).

9. Nerve transfers are an effective means of treating severe nerve injuries that are not amenable to nerve grafting, such as cervical nerve–root avulsions or large segmental nerve injuries.

   a. To transfer a nerve from a site of its healthy functioning to a nonfunctioning nerve, an intrafascicular dissection must be performed. In this procedure, a single fascicle without critical end-organ/muscle function is isolated with a nerve stimulator. The healthy donor fascicle is released and is then sutured to the cut end of the nonfunctioning recipient nerve.

   b. An example of a nerve transfer is the transfer of a fascicle of a functioning ulnar nerve that innervates the flexor carpi ulnaris to the musculocutaneous nerve branch to the biceps muscle in a patient with a brachial plexus palsy, to restore active elbow flexion.

10. Results of peripheral nerve repair vary.

   a. Young patients with early repairs of distal single-function nerves performed with short nerve grafts or as direct repairs have better outcomes than do older patients with late repairs of proximal, mixed nerves performed with long nerve grafts.

   b. The rate of nerve regeneration after repair also varies; historically, it has been estimated to be 1 mm per day, which is approximately equal to the rate of axonal transport of neurofilament proteins essential to nerve growth.

1: Basic Science

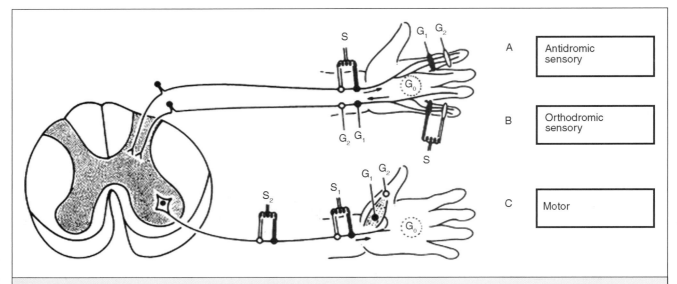

Figure 6   Illustration shows electrode placement for three types of nerve conduction velocity studies: antidromic sensory study (**A**), orthodromic sensory study (**B**), and motor nerve conduction velocity study (**C**). G1 = active recording electrode, G2 = reference recording electrode, G0 = ground electrode, S1 = distal stimulation site, S2 = proximal stimulation site. The cathode is black and the anode is white. (Reproduced with permission from Sethi RD, Thompson LL: *The Electromyographer's Handbook*, ed 2. Boston, MA, Little, Brown and Co, 1989, p 4.)

VI. Diagnostic Studies

A. Overview

1. The primary tests used to evaluate the integrity of the peripheral nervous system are electromyography and nerve conduction velocity studies.

2. These tests assess the function of sensory nerves, motor nerves, and muscles to confirm diagnoses of neuropathies and myopathies.

3. They also can differentiate causes of weakness, identify the level and severity of nerve injuries or abnormalities of conduction, and demonstrate the existence of denervated muscle and its reinnervation.

B. Nerve conduction velocity studies

1. Sensation

   a. The signal produced by stimulation of a mixed (motor and sensory) nerve is called a compound nerve action potential.

   b. A signal specifically related to the sensory function of a nerve is called a sensory nerve action potential (SNAP).

   c. The nerve being examined in a conduction velocity study can be stimulated in an antidromic manner, in which the nerve impulse travels in a proximal-to-distal direction, or in an orthodromic manner, in which the nerve impulse travels in a distal-to-proximal direction (**Figure 6**). The speed of conduction of the impulse is similar in the two directions.

   d. Quantification of the speed of conduction of an action potential requires knowledge of both the distance (in millimeters) across which the action potential travels and the time (in milliseconds) required for it to travel across that distance.

   e. Nerve conduction velocity (distance/time) or latency (time between the stimulus that induces an action potential and the onset of the potential) is typically recorded (**Figure 7**). Both nerve conduction velocity and latency are typically increased by temperature, age, demyelination, and loss of axons because these factors decrease the rate of impulse transmission through nerves.

   f. The amplitude of a SNAP also can be measured. Reductions in temperature increase SNAP amplitude; increasing age decreases it.

2. Motor nerve function

   a. A motor nerve action potential is recorded in a muscle, in which multiple muscle fibers are innervated by a single nerve. The information recorded is therefore called a compound muscle action potential (CMAP).

   b. The CMAP measures not only the speed over the course of a nerve of an impulse produced by stimulation but also the transmission of the impulse through the neuromuscular junction and its conduction through muscle fibers.

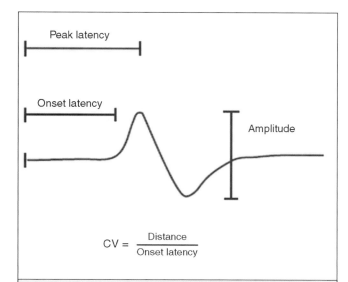

Figure 7   Conduction velocity (CV) is the distance from the stimulating electrode to the receiving electrode of an electromyograph divided by the time from a stimulus to either the onset of the action potential (onset latency) or the peak of the action potential (peak latency). (Reproduced from Robinson LR: Role of neurophysiologic evaluation in diagnosis. *J Am Acad Orthop Surg* 2000;8[3]:191.)

c. An F-wave is the recorded signal of a late response from distal muscles during CMAP testing.

- When a stimulus is applied to a nerve innervating a muscle, the signal travels in the typical proximal-to-distal fashion along the nerve, toward the muscle. However, the nerve may also conduct a separate and immediately sequential signal in a distal-to-proximal direction, toward the cells of the anterior horn of the spinal cord.

- With sufficient stimulation, cells of the anterior horn may discharge another proximal-to-distal impulse (such as an F-wave), which is recorded after the initial CMAP.

C. Electromyography

1. Electromyographic studies cover an entire motor unit (for example, anterior horn cell of the spinal cord, motor neuron, and muscle) and involve measuring insertional activity, which is the activity of a muscle when the needle electrode of an electromyograph is inserted into it; spontaneous activity of the muscle; motor unit action potentials (MUAPs) of the muscle, which are characterized by their duration, amplitude, and shape; and recruitment, which is the successive activation of additional motor units upon stimulation of a single motor unit. These studies do not measure or assess sensory information.

2. Insertional activity is measured as the needle electrode is passed into the muscle belly.

a. Decreased insertional activity results from poor muscle viability, muscle fibrosis, or muscle atrophy.

b. Increased insertional activity may be a sign of denervation or of a primary muscle disorder (for example, polymyositis, myopathy).

3. Spontaneous activity involves electrical discharges in muscle that occur without muscle contraction and without movement of the testing needle.

a. Fibrillations are an example of abnormal spontaneous activity; they occur in denervated muscle fibers and in some myopathies. The density of fibrillations is graded from 1+ to 4+, but it is their amplitude that helps in understanding the time of occurrence of denervation of a muscle. Large-amplitude fibrillations frequently occur acutely (within 3 to 12 months after denervation), and smaller amplitude fibrillations occur later in the process of denervation (after the muscle has atrophied).

b. Positive sharp waves are abnormal electrical discharges of single muscle fibers that can be seen in association with fibrillations. They also can be seen without fibrillations when a muscle is traumatized but not denervated. Fibrillations and positive sharp waves typically appear 2 to 3 weeks after the onset of denervation.

c. Fasciculations are spontaneous discharges of a single motor unit. They can be detected clinically by placing an electrode on the skin. They occur in various neuromuscular disorders, including the syndrome of benign fasciculations, chronic radiculopathies, peripheral polyneuropathies, thyrotoxicosis, and overdose of anticholinesterase medications.

4. Motor unit action potentials can measure voluntary muscle activity.

a. The amplitude of a MUAP characterizes the density of the muscle fibers within the motor unit in which the MUAP is measured.

b. The duration and shape of the wave produced by the MUAP are affected by the quality of conduction. For example, the MUAP of a partly denervated motor unit will be prolonged in duration and polyphasic in shape as the motor unit is reinnervated with axonal sprouting (**Figure 8**). If no reinnervation occurs, no MUAP will be generated.

5. Recruitment is also measured through rate of MUAP generation and can be used to understand whether muscle weakness is the result of a

1: Basic Science

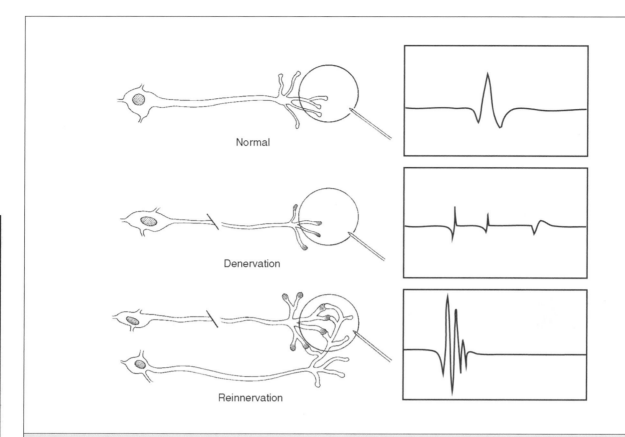

Figure 8   **Top,** Normal motor unit action potential (MUAP), recorded using a needle electrode from muscle fibers within its recording area. **Middle,** After denervation, single muscle fibers spontaneously discharge, producing fibrillations and positive sharp waves. **Bottom,** When reinnervation by axon sprouting has occurred, the newly formed sprouts will conduct slowly, producing temporal dispersion (that is, prolonged MUAP duration) and MUAP polyphasicity. The higher density of muscle fibers within the recording area of the needle belonging to the enlarging second motor unit results in an increased-amplitude MUAP. (Reproduced from Robinson LR: Role of neurophysiologic evaluation in diagnosis. *J Am Acad Orthop Surg* 2000;8[3]:194.)

decrease in numbers of peripheral motor neurons and motor units or the result of a central problem in recruitment as the result of a CNS lesion, pain, or poor voluntary effort.

D. MRI

1. MRI can be a useful adjunct to electrodiagnostic studies for assessing various disorders of the peripheral nervous system.

2. MRI can show changes in muscle from denervation. For example, chronic denervation will show evidence of fatty atrophy.

3. High-resolution images with sufficient contrast are required to emphasize peripheral nerve anatomy and nerve morphology.

4. The studies that provide these images take advantage of differences in the MRI signal of distinct intraneural tissues, resulting from differences in the water content and physical structure of fascicles, perineurium, and epineurium.

VII. Peripheral Nerve Pharmacology

A. Local anesthetic agents

1. These agents create a sensorimotor nerve block, causing transient numbness and paralysis by temporarily disrupting the transmission of action potentials along axons.

2. Lidocaine, mepivacaine, and bupivacaine (amide-type agents) have different durations of action based on their specific biochemistries, with lidocaine having the shortest duration of action and bupivacaine the longest.

3. C nerve fibers (for example, cutaneous pain fibers) are the most susceptible to the effects of local anesthetics, and A fibers (for example, motor axons and deep pressure sense) are the least susceptible.

4. Local anesthetics of the amide type are processed by the liver via cytochrome P450 enzyme into metabolites that are more water soluble than

their parent compounds; these metabolites are then excreted in the urine.

5. Epinephrine may be combined with these anesthetics for vasoconstriction.

   a. This combination reduces the systemic absorption of local anesthetics from the injection site by decreasing blood flow in the area around the site.

   b. Epinephrine reduces the systemic blood levels of local anesthetic agents by up to 30%.

   c. Because epinephrine-induced local vasoconstriction causes less of a local anesthetic to be absorbed systemically, it increases the local neuronal uptake of the anesthetic in the region in which it is injected.

B. Botulinum toxin

1. Botulinum toxin, produced by the bacterium *Clostridium botulinum*, can be injected into muscle to treat muscular spasticity.

2. The toxin works at the level of the neuromuscular junction. When injected into muscle, it blocks the release of acetylcholine from axon terminals at the presynaptic clefts of the neuromuscular junction, thus preventing acetylcholine from reaching the motor end plate and triggering muscle contraction. It therefore causes chemical denervation and muscle paralysis.

3. When used to treat muscle spasticity, the beneficial effect of botulinum toxin begins at approximately 7 to 14 days after injection and typically lasts 3 months.

Top Testing Facts

1. Schwann cell myelination accelerates the transmission of action potentials by saltatory conduction occurring at nodes of Ranvier.

2. A nerve consists of collections of nerve fibers called fascicles and of neural connective tissue, which both surrounds and lies within each fascicle.

3. Temperature, age, demyelination, and loss of axons decrease the rate of impulse transmission through nerves.

4. Nerve injury causes loss of distal function in the following sequence: motor, proprioception, touch, temperature, pain, and sympathetic activity. Nerve function recovers in the inverse order.

5. Neurapraxia is a reversible blocking of nerve conduction caused by traction or compression of a nerve; axonotmesis involves axon disruption, with preserved neural connective tissue, from a stretch or crush injury; neurotmesis is complete disruption of a nerve as the result of an open crushing injury or laceration.

6. Tissue pressures of up to 30 mm Hg can cause paresthesias and increased nerve conduction latencies.

7. Fibrillations are an electromyographic finding of abnormal spontaneous activity that occurs in muscle fibers 2 to 3 weeks after their denervation.

8. Nerve repair (neurorrhaphy) involves reapproximation of the ends of a damaged or transected nerve, with the fascicles appropriately oriented and under minimal tension. It is accomplished with a fine monofilament epineurial suture.

9. Nerve grafts may be cabled to increase their diameter; they should also be reversed to minimize the early arborization of regenerating nerve fibers.

10. Nerve transfer involves releasing a nerve fascicle from a functioning nerve and transferring it to a nerve that has lost function.

Bibliography

Freedman M, Helber G, Pothast J, Shahwan TG, Simon J, Sher L: Electrodiagnostic evaluation of compressive nerve injuries of the upper extremities. *Orthop Clin North Am* 2012; 43(4):409-416.

Jackson WM, Diao E: Peripheral nerves: Form and function, in O'Keefe RJ, Jacobs JJ, Chu CR, Einhorn TA, eds: *Orthopaedic Basic Science: Foundations of Clinical Practice*, ed 4. Rosemont, IL, American Academy of Orthopaedic Surgeons, 2013, pp 239–251.

Lundborg G: A 25-year perspective of peripheral nerve surgery: Evolving neuroscientific concepts and clinical significance. *J Hand Surg Am* 2000;25(3):391-414.

Robinson LR: Role of neurophysiologic evaluation in diagnosis. *J Am Acad Orthop Surg* 2000;8(3):190-199.

Scholz T, Krichevsky A, Sumarto A, et al: Peripheral nerve injuries: An international survey of current treatments and future perspectives. *J Reconstr Microsurg* 2009;25(6):339-344.

Terenghi G, Hart A, Wiberg M: The nerve injury and the dying neurons: Diagnosis and prevention. *J Hand Surg Eur Vol* 2011;36(9):730-734.

Chapter 11
Skeletal Muscle

Michael J. Medvecky, MD

I. General Information

A. The skeletal muscles receive innervation from the peripheral nervous system.

B. The skeletal muscles affect volitional control of the axial and appendicular skeleton.

II. Muscle Structure

A. Skeletal muscle fibers and connective tissue

1. Skeletal muscle fibers (**Figure 1**) are highly specialized multinucleated cells characterized by a collection of contractile filaments called

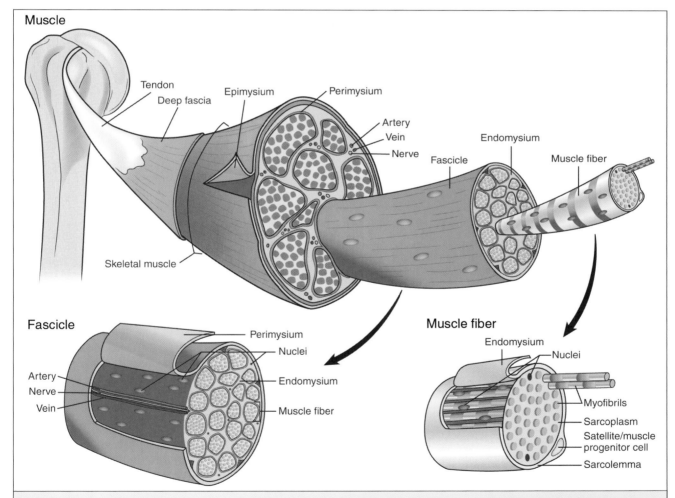

Muscle

Tendon
Deep fascia
Epimysium
Perimysium
Artery
Vein
Nerve
Fascicle
Endomysium
Muscle fiber
Skeletal muscle

Fascicle

Perimysium
Nuclei
Artery
Nerve
Vein
Endomysium
Muscle fiber

Muscle fiber

Endomysium
Nuclei
Myofibrils
Sarcoplasm
Satellite/muscle progenitor cell
Sarcolemma

Figure 1   Structure of the skeletal muscle. (Reproduced from Wright A, Gharaibeh B, Huard J: Form and function of skeletal muscle, in O'Keefe RJ, Jacobs JJ, Chu CR, Einhorn TA, eds: *Orthopaedic Basic Science: Foundations of Clinical Practice*, ed 4. Rosemont, IL, American Academy of Orthopaedic Surgeons, 2013, p. 230.)

Dr. Medvecky or an immediate family member is a member of a speakers' bureau or has made paid presentations on behalf of Smith & Nephew and has received research or institutional support from Wyeth.

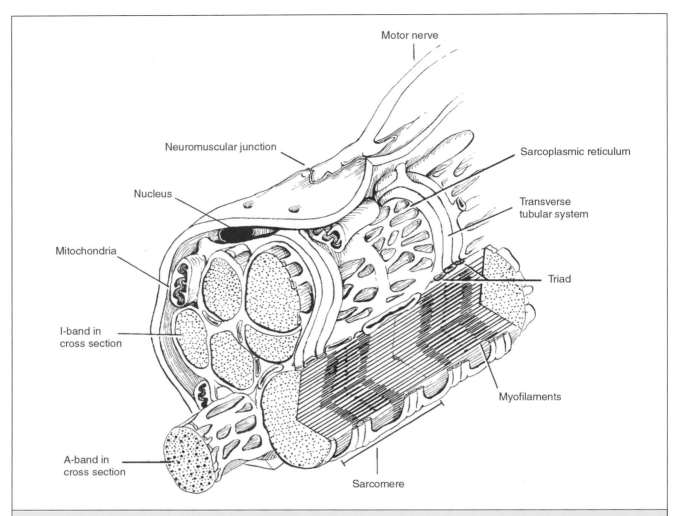

Figure 2   Illustration shows the structure of a muscle cell. The muscle cell, which is specialized for the production of force and movement, contains an array of filamentous proteins as well as other subcellular organelles such as mitochondria, nuclei, satellite cells, the sarcoplasmic reticulum, and the transverse tubular system. Note the formation of triads, which represent the T-tubules flanked by the terminal cisternae of the sarcoplasmic reticulum. Also note that when the myofilaments are sectioned longitudinally, the stereotypic striated appearance is seen. When myofilaments are sectioned transversely at the level of the A- or I-bands, the hexagonal array of the appropriate filaments is seen. (Reproduced with permission from Lieber R, ed: *Skeletal Muscle Structure, Function, and Plasticity: The Physiological Basis of Rehabilitation*, ed 2. Philadelphia, PA, Lippincott Williams & Wilkins, 2002, p 15.)

myofilaments. Filaments are organized in a defined hierarchy, with the basic functional unit of muscle contraction being the sarcomere.

2. The largest functional unit is the myofibril, which is a string of sarcomeres arranged in series. Adjacent myofibrils are connected by a set of specialized proteins called intermediate filaments. They allow for mechanical coupling between myofibrils.

3. Endomysium is the connective tissue surrounding individual fibers.

4. Perimysium is the connective tissue surrounding collections of muscle fibers, or fascicles.

5. Epimysium is the connective tissue covering the entire muscle.

B. Cell membrane systems—A specially designed membrane system exists within the cell that assists in activating the contractile properties of the muscle cell. The system consists of two main components: the transverse tubular system and the sarcoplasmic reticulum (**Figure 2**).

1. The transverse tubular system begins as invaginations of the cell membrane and extends into the cell, perpendicular to its long axis. It relays the activation signal from the motor neuron to the myofibrils.

2. The sarcoplasmic reticulum is a system of membrane-bound sacs that collect, release, and reuptake calcium stores to regulate the muscle contractile process.

a. Calcium channels and pumps are contained within the sarcoplasmic reticulum and are regulated by a complex enzymatic system.

b. The portion of the sarcoplasmic reticulum that abuts the transverse tubules is called the junctional sarcoplasmic reticulum.

c. The transverse tubule and the two adjacent sacs of the junctional reticulum together are called a triad.

C. Sarcomere composition

1. Sarcomeres are composed of two major types of contractile filaments:

   a. Myosin (thick filaments)

   b. Actin (thin filaments)

2. The two sets of filaments interdigitate; the active interdigitation of these filaments produces muscle contraction via a shortening translation of the filaments.

3. The arrangement of these filaments also creates the characteristic pattern of alternating bands of light and dark seen under microscopy.

   a. Tropomyosin, another protein, is situated between two actin strands in its double-helix configuration. In the resting state, tropomyosin blocks the myosin binding sites on actin (**Figure 3**).

   b. Troponin is a complex of three separate proteins that is intimately associated with tropomyosin.

• When troponin binds calcium, a conformational change in the troponin complex ensues.

• This in turn results in a conformational change in tropomyosin, exposing the myosin-binding sites on actin.

• A resultant contractile protein interaction occurs, and muscle contraction is initiated.

D. Sarcomere organization

1. The structure of the sarcomere is shown in **Figure 4**.

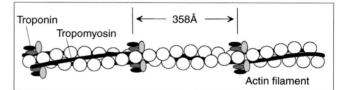

Figure 3   Illustration shows the features of regulation of muscle contraction. The structure of actin is represented by two chains of beads in a double helix. The troponin complex consists of calcium-binding protein (TN-C, black); inhibitory protein (TN-I, red); and protein binding to tropomyosin (TN-T, yellow). The tropomyosin (dark line) lies in each groove of the actin filament. (Reproduced from Garrett WE Jr, Best TM: Anatomy, physiology, and mechanics of skeletal muscle, in Buckwalter JA, Einhorn TA, Simon SR, eds: *Orthopaedic Basic Science: Biology and Biomechanics of the Musculoskeletal System*, ed 2. Rosemont, IL, American Academy of Orthopaedic Surgeons, 2000, p 690.)

1: Basic Science

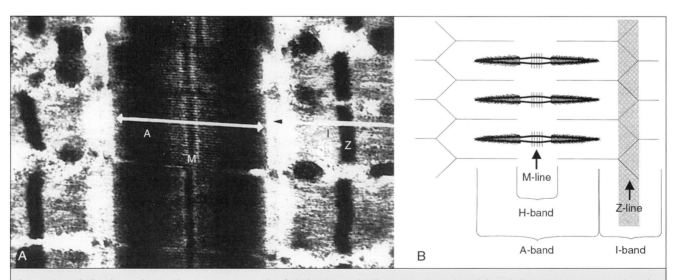

Figure 4   Skeletal muscle. **A,** Electron micrograph of skeletal muscle illustrates the striated, banded appearance. A = A-band; M = M-line; I = I-band; Z = Z-line. **B,** Illustration shows the basic functional unit of skeletal muscle, the sarcomere. (Reproduced from Garrett WE, Best TM: Anatomy, physiology, and mechanics of skeletal muscle, in Buckwalter JA, Einhorn TA, Simon SR, eds: *Orthopaedic Basic Science: Biology and Biomechanics of the Musculoskeletal System*, ed 2. Rosemont, IL, American Academy of Orthopaedic Surgeons, 2000, p 688.)

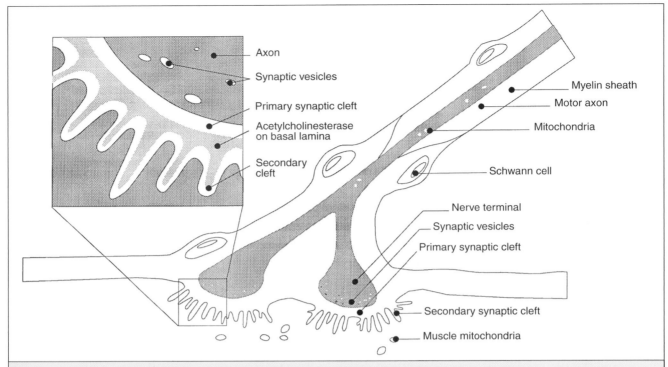

Figure 5   Illustration depicts the structure of the motor end plate. (Reproduced from Garrett WE, Best TM: Anatomy, physiology, and mechanics of skeletal muscle, in Buckwalter JA, Einhorn TA, Simon SR, eds: *Orthopaedic Basic Science: Biology and Biomechanics of the Musculoskeletal System*, ed 2. Rosemont, IL, American Academy of Orthopaedic Surgeons, 2000, p 686.)

a. The A-band is composed of both actin and myosin.

b. The M-line is a central set of interconnecting filaments for myosin.

c. The H-band contains only myosin.

d. The I-band is composed of actin filaments only, which are joined together at the interconnecting Z-line.

2. During muscle contraction, the sarcomere length decreases but the length of individual thick and thin filaments remains the same. During contraction, the thick and thin filaments bypass one another, resulting in increased overlap.

E. Nerve-muscle interaction

1. A motor unit consists of a single motor neuron and all of the muscle fibers it contacts.

a. Every muscle fiber is contacted by a single nerve terminal at a site called the motor end plate (**Figure 5**).

b. The number of muscle fibers within a motor unit varies widely.

2. Chemical transmission of the electrical impulse passing down the cell membrane of the axon occurs at the motor end plate or neuromuscular junction (NMJ). The primary and secondary synaptic folds or invaginations of the cell membrane increase the surface area for communication.

3. Acetylcholine (ACh) is the neurotransmitter released into the synaptic cleft.

a. The electrical impulse reaches the terminal axon, and calcium ions are allowed to flow into the neural cell.

b. This increase in intracellular calcium causes the neurotransmitter vesicles to fuse with the axon membrane, and the ACh is released into the synaptic cleft.

c. ACh then binds to receptors on the muscle membrane, triggering depolarization of the cell, which in turn triggers an action potential.

d. This action potential is passed along through the sarcoplasmatic reticulum network.

e. The ACh is enzymatically deactivated by acetylcholinesterase located within the extracellular space.

4. Pharmacologic and physiologic alteration of neuromuscular transmission

a. Myasthenia gravis is a disorder resulting in a shortage of ACh receptors; it is characterized by severe muscle weakness.

b. Nondepolarizing drugs (eg, pancuronium, vecuronium, and curare)

- Competitively bind to the ACh receptor, blocking transmission.

- Site of action is the NMJ.

c. Polarizing drugs (eg, succinylcholine)

- Bind to the ACh receptor, causing temporary depolarization followed by failure of the impulse transmission.

- Site of action is the NMJ.

d. Reversible acetylcholinesterase inhibitors (eg, neostigmine, edrophonium)

- Prevent the breakdown of ACh.

- Allow for prolonged interaction with the ACh receptor.

e. Irreversible acetylcholinesterase inhibitors (eg, nerve gases and certain insecticides)

- Similarly prevent the breakdown of ACh.

- Result in sustained muscle contraction.

III. Muscle Function

A. Nerve activation of muscle contraction

1. A muscle twitch (**Figure 6, A**) is the muscle tension response to a single nerve stimulus.

    a. If a second nerve stimulus arrives after the muscle tension has returned to baseline resting tension, no increase in muscle tension development occurs.

    b. Absolute refractory period—The period during which no stimulus will produce a muscle contraction.

    c. Relative refractory period—The period during which the stimulus required for muscle activation is greater than the typical threshold stimulus level.

2. Paired twitch (**Figure 6, B**)—If a successive nerve stimulus arrives before the resting tension reaches baseline, the tension rises above the level of a single twitch.

    a. This phenomenon is called summation (wave summation or temporal summation).

    b. As the frequency of gross muscle stimulation increases, higher peak tensions develop (**Figure 6, C**).

    c. A plateau of maximal tension eventually is reached (**Figure 6, D**) at which no relaxation of muscle tension between successive stimuli occurs (tetany).

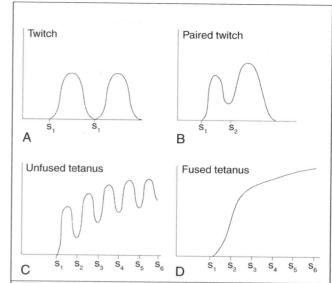

Figure 6 Graphs show the nerve activation of muscle contraction, including twitch (**A** and **B**) and tetanus (**C** and **D**). As the frequency of stimulation is increased, muscle force rises to an eventual plateau level known as fused tetanus. (Reproduced from Garrett WE, Best TM: Anatomy, physiology, and mechanics of skeletal muscle, in Buckwalter JA, Einhorn TA, Simon SR, eds: *Orthopaedic Basic Science: Biology and Biomechanics of the Musculoskeletal System*, ed 2. Rosemont, IL, American Academy of Orthopaedic Surgeons, 2000, p 691.)

B. Skeletal muscle can develop varying levels of muscle force, even though each individual motor unit contracts in an all-or-none fashion. This graded response is controlled by different mechanisms.

1. Spatial summation—Different motor units have different thresholds of stimulation; therefore, more motor units are activated with increased stimulus intensity.

2. Temporal summation—Increasing stimulus frequency results in increased tension development by each individual motor unit (eg, tetany).

3. Maximal force production is proportional to muscle physiologic cross-sectional area (PCSA); however, force production is not directly related to anatomic cross-sectional area.

    a. Other factors that contribute to PCSA are surface pennation angle (fiber angle relative to the force-generating axis of the muscle), muscle density, and fiber length.

    b. Longer fiber lengths allow long excursions with less force production.

C. Types of muscle contraction

1. Isotonic—Muscle shortens against a constant load. Muscle tension remains constant.

1: Basic Science

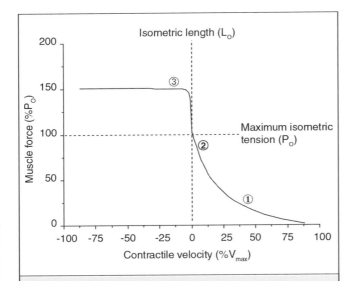

Figure 7 Graph depicts the muscle force–velocity curve for skeletal muscle obtained using sequential isotonic contractions. Note that the force increases dramatically upon forced muscle lengthening and drops precipitously upon muscle shortening. (Reproduced with permission from Lieber R, ed: *Skeletal Muscle Structure, Function, and Plasticity: The Physiological Basis of Rehabilitation*, ed 2. Philadelphia, PA, Lippincott Williams & Wilkins, 2002, p. 62.)

2. Isokinetic—Muscle contracts at a constant velocity.

3. Isometric—Muscle length remains static as tension is generated.

4. Concentric—Muscular contraction results in a decrease in muscle length. This occurs when the resisting load is less than the muscle force generated.

5. Eccentric—Muscular contraction accommodates an increase in muscle length. This occurs when the resisting load is greater than the muscle force generated.

6. Isotonic and isokinetic contractions can demonstrate either concentric action or eccentric action; isometric contractions, however, do not fit the definition of concentric or eccentric action.

D. Force-velocity relationship (**Figure 7**)—Under experimental conditions, a load is applied to a contracting muscle until no change in length is seen (isometric length). As higher external load is applied, the muscle begins to lengthen, and tension increases rapidly (eccentric contraction). If load is decreased from the isometrically contracting muscle, the muscle force will rapidly decrease and the muscle will shorten in length (concentric contraction). Progressively decreased loads result in increased contraction.

1. Concentric contractions—The force generated by the muscle is always less than the muscle's maximum force. As seen from the force-velocity curve, the force drops off rapidly as velocity increases. For example, when the muscle velocity increases to only 17% of maximum, the muscle force has decreased to 50% of maximum.

2. Eccentric contractions—The absolute tension quickly becomes very high relative to the maximum isometric tension. Eccentric contraction generates the highest tension and greatest risk for musculotendinous injury. The absolute tension is relatively independent of the velocity.

E. Fiber types

1. The muscle fibers of each motor unit share the same contractile and metabolic properties.

2. These muscle fibers may be one of three primary types (I, IIA, or IIB), characterized according to their structural, biochemical, and physiologic characteristics (**Table 1**).

   a. Type I fibers (slow-contracting, oxidative)

   - High aerobic capacity

   - Resistant to fatigue

   - Contain more mitochondria and more capillaries per fiber than other types

   - Slower contraction and relaxation times than other types

   b. Type IIA (fast-contracting, oxidative and glycolytic)—Intermediate fiber type between the slow oxidative type I fiber and the fast glycolytic type IIB fiber.

   c. Type IIB (fast-contracting, glycolytic)

   - Primarily anaerobic

   - Least resistant to fatigue

   - Most rapid contraction time

   - Largest motor unit size

   d. Strength training may result in an increased percentage of type IIB fibers, whereas endurance training may increase the percentage of type IIA fibers.

   e. Speed and duration of contraction are most dependent upon fiber type.

IV. Energetics

A. Three main energy systems provide fuel for muscular contractions.

1. The phosphagen system (**Figure 8**)

   a. The adenosine triphosphate (ATP) molecule is hydrolyzed and converted directly to adenosine diphosphate (ADP), inorganic phosphate, and

Table 1

Characteristics of Human Skeletal Muscle Fiber Types

	Type I	Type IIA	Type IIB
Other names	Red, slow twitch (ST) Slow oxidative (SO)	White, fast twitch (FT) Fast oxidative glycolytic (FOG)	Fast glycolytic (FG)
Speed of contraction	Slow	Fast	Fast
Strength of contraction	Low	High	High
Fatigability	Fatigue resistant	Fatigable	Most fatigable
Aerobic capacity	High	Medium	Low
Anaerobic capacity	Low	Medium	High
Motor unit size	Small	Larger	Largest
Capillary density	High	High	Low

(Reproduced from Garrett WE, Best TM: Anatomy, physiology, and mechanics of skeletal muscle, in Buckwalter JA, Einhorn TA, Simon SR, eds: *Orthopaedic Basic Science: Biology and Biomechanics of the Musculoskeletal System*, ed 2. Rosemont, IL, American Academy of Orthopaedic Surgeons, 2000, p 692.)

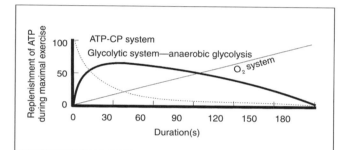

Figure 8   Graph demonstrates the energy sources for anaerobic activity. CP = creatine phosphate. (Reproduced from Garrett WE, Best TM: Anatomy, physiology, and mechanics of skeletal muscle, in Buckwalter JA, Einhorn TA, Simon SR, eds: *Orthopaedic Basic Science: Biology and Biomechanics of the Musculoskeletal System*, ed 2. Rosemont, IL, American Academy of Orthopaedic Surgeons, 2000, p 694.)

energy. ADP also may be hydrolyzed further to create adenosine monophosphate (AMP), again releasing inorganic phosphate and energy.

b. Creatine phosphate is another source of high-energy phosphate bonds; however, its high-energy phosphate bond is used by creatine kinase to synthesize ATP from ADP.

c. Myokinase is used to combine two ADP molecules to create one ATP molecule and one AMP molecule.

d. Total energy from the entire phosphagen system is enough to fuel the body to run approximately 200 yards.

e. No lactate is produced via this pathway; also, no oxygen is used.

2. Anaerobic metabolism (glycolytic or lactic acid metabolism) (**Figure 9**)

a. Glucose is transformed into two molecules of lactic acid, creating enough energy to convert two molecules of ADP to ATP.

b. This system provides metabolic energy for approximately 20 to 120 seconds of intense activity.

c. Oxygen is not used in this pathway.

3. Aerobic metabolism (**Figure 10**)

a. Glucose is broken into two molecules of pyruvic acid, which then enter the Krebs cycle, resulting in a net gain of 34 ATP per glucose molecule.

b. Glucose exists in the cell in a limited quantity of glucose-6-phosphate. Additional sources of energy include stored muscle glycogen.

c. Fats and proteins also can be converted to energy via aerobic metabolism.

d. Oxygen is used in this pathway.

B. Training effects on muscle

1. Strength training usually consists of high-load, low-repetition exercise and results in increased muscle cross-sectional area. This is more likely due to muscle hypertrophy (increased size of muscle fibers) rather than hyperplasia (increased number of muscle fibers).

a. Increased motor unit recruitment or improved synchronization of muscle activation is another way weight training contributes to strength gains.

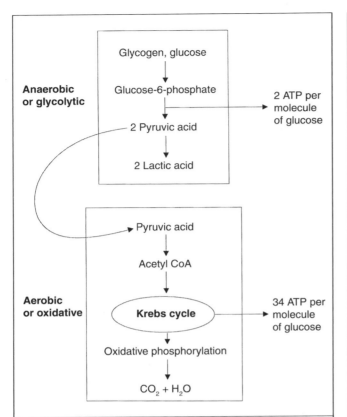

Figure 9 Diagram summarizes the ATP yield in the anaerobic and aerobic breakdown of carbohydrates. Glycolysis and anaerobic metabolism occur in the cytoplasm; oxidative phosphorylation occurs in the mitochondria. (Reproduced from Garrett WE, Best TM: Anatomy, physiology, and mechanics of skeletal muscle, in Buckwalter JA, Einhorn TA, Simon SR, eds: *Orthopaedic Basic Science: Biology and Biomechanics of the Musculoskeletal System*, ed 2. Rosemont, IL, American Academy of Orthopaedic Surgeons, 2000, p 696.)

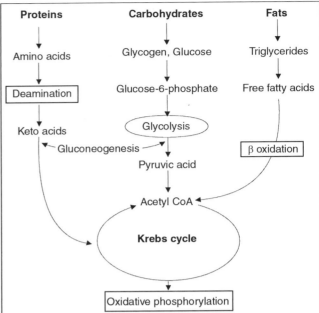

Figure 10 Diagram demonstrates food (fats, carbohydrates, proteins) containing carbon and hydrogen for glycolysis, fatty acid oxidation, and the Krebs cycle in a muscle cell. (Reproduced from Garrett WE, Best TM: Anatomy, physiology, and mechanics of skeletal muscle, in Buckwalter JA, Einhorn TA, Simon SR, eds: *Orthopaedic Basic Science: Biology and Biomechanics of the Musculoskeletal System*, ed 2. Rosemont, IL, American Academy of Orthopaedic Surgeons, 2000, p 695.)

   c. The oxidative capacity of all three fiber types increases. In addition, the percentage of the more highly oxygenated type IIA fibers increases.

V. Muscle Injury and Repair

A. Cytokines and growth factors regulate the repair processes after muscle injury. Sources of cytokines include infiltrating neutrophils, monocytes, and macrophages; activated fibroblasts; and stimulated endothelial cells.

   1. Necrotic muscle fibers are removed by macrophages. New muscle cells are thought to arise from satellite cells, which are undifferentiated cells that exist in a quiescent state until needed for a reparative response.

   2. The simultaneous formation of fibrotic connective tissue or scar may interfere with a full recovery of muscle tissue after injury.

B. Delayed-onset muscle soreness (DOMS) is muscle ache and pain that typically occurs 24 to 72 hours after intense exercise.

   b. Strength training results in adaptation of all fiber types.

   c. Little evidence exists at a microscopic, cellular level that muscle cell injury is required to generate muscle strengthening or hypertrophy.

  2. Endurance training

    a. Aerobic training results in changes in both central and peripheral circulation as well as muscle metabolism. Energy efficiency is the primary adaptation seen in contractile muscle.

    b. Mitochondrial size, number, and density increase. Enzyme systems of the Krebs cycle and respiratory chain and those involved with the supply and processing of fatty acids by mitochondria all increase markedly. Metabolic adaptations occur that result in an increased use of fatty acids rather than glycogen.

1. DOMS is primarily associated with eccentric loading–type exercise.

2. Several theories have been proposed to explain DOMS; the most popular states that structural muscle injury occurs and leads to progressive edema formation and resultant increased intramuscular pressure.

3. These changes seem to occur primarily in type IIB fibers.

C. Muscle contusion is a nonpenetrating blunt injury to muscle resulting in hematoma and inflammation. Characteristics include:

1. Later development of scar formation and variable amount of muscle regeneration.

2. New synthesis of extracellular connective tissue within 2 days of the injury, peaking at 5 to 21 days.

3. Myositis ossificans (bone formation within muscle) secondary to blunt trauma. This sometimes mimics osteogenic sarcoma on radiographs and biopsy. Myositis ossificans becomes apparent approximately 2 to 4 weeks after injury.

4. Muscle strain

   a. Both complete and incomplete muscle tears usually occur by passive stretch of an activated muscle.

   b. Muscles at greatest risk are those that cross two joints; eg, the rectus femoris and gastrocnemius.

   c. Incomplete muscle tears typically occur at the myotendinous junction, with hemorrhage and fiber disruption. A cellular inflammatory response occurs for the first few days, with the muscle demonstrating decreasing ability to generate active tension. In an animal model, force production normalized after 7 days.

   d. Complete muscle tears also typically occur near the myotendinous junction. They are characterized by muscle contour abnormality.

5. Muscle laceration

   a. After complete laceration of muscle, fragments heal by dense connective scar tissue. Regeneration of muscle tissue across the laceration or reinnervation is not predictable, and only partial recovery is likely.

   b. Muscle activation does not cross the scar.

   c. Unstimulated muscle segment shows histologic characteristics of denervated muscle.

   d. Denervation injury leads to an increased sensitivity to acetylcholine and fibrillations occur 2 to 4 weeks after injury.

D. Immobilization and disuse

1. Immobilization and disuse result in muscle atrophy, with associated loss of strength and increased fatigability.

2. A nonlinear rate of atrophy occurs, with changes occurring primarily during the initial days. Atrophy is seen at a cellular level, with loss of myofibrils within the muscle fibers.

3. Atrophic changes are related to the length at which muscle is immobilized. Atrophy and strength loss are more prominent when muscle is immobilized under no tension; eg, when the knee is immobilized in extension, quadriceps atrophy is greater than hamstring atrophy.

4. Muscle fiber held under stretch creates new contractile proteins with sarcomeres added onto existing fibrils. This slightly offsets the atrophy of cross-sectional muscle mass.

1: Basic Science

Top Testing Facts

1. Muscle fiber is a collection of myofibrils.

2. Fascicles are collections of muscle fibers.

3. Tropomyosin blocks the myosin binding sites on actin.

4. The sarcomere is organized into bands and lines as described in section II.D and shown in Figure 4.

5. The site of action of both depolarizing and non-depolarizing drugs is the NMJ.

6. Maximal force production is proportional to muscle PCSA.

7. The phosphagen energy system has enough ATP for approximately 20 seconds of activity.

8. Eccentric contraction generates the highest tension and greatest risk of musculotendinous injury.

9. DOMS peaks at 24 to 72 hours after exercise, is most common in type IIB fibers, and is associated primarily with eccentric exercise.

10. Muscle strain is most likely in muscles that cross two joints.

Bibliography

Best TM, Kirkendall DT, Almekinders LC, Garrett WE Jr: Basic science of soft tissue, in DeLee J, Drez D, Miller MD, eds: *Orthopaedic Sports Medicine: Principles and Practice.* Philadelphia, PA, Saunders, 2002, pp 1-19.

Garrett WE Jr, Best TM: Anatomy, physiology, and mechanics of skeletal muscle, in Buckwalter JA, Einhorn TA, Simon SR, eds: *Orthopaedic Basic Science: Biology and Biomechanics of the Musculoskeletal System*, ed 2. Rosemont, IL, American Academy of Orthopaedic Surgeons, 2000, pp 683-716.

Wright A, Gharaibeh B, Huard J: Form and function of skeletal muscle, in O'Keefe RJ, Jacobs JJ, Chu CR, Einhorn TA, eds: *Orthopaedic Basic Science: Foundations of Clinical Practice*, ed 4. Rosemont, IL, American Academy of Orthopaedic Surgeons, 2013, pp 229-237.

Chapter 12

Intervertebral Disk

S. Tim Yoon, MD, PhD   Michael D. Smith, MD

I. Function

A. The intervertebral disk connects adjacent vertebral bodies.

B. The adjacent vertebral bodies, the disk, and the facet joints constitute the functional spinal unit that provides mechanical stability and allows physiologic motion.

C. The nucleus pulposus is centrally located and confined by the end plates and the anulus fibrosus (**Figure 1**). The nucleus pulposus resists compressive loads, dampens mechanical loads, and evenly distributes forces onto the end plates.

D. The anulus fibrosus of the disk is designed to resist tensile loads, allow spinal motion, provide mechanical connection between the vertebrae, and confine the nucleus pulposus. The anulus fibrosus is peripheral to the nucleus pulposus and confines the nucleus pulposus.

II. Anatomy

A. Embryology

1. The axial skeleton is derived from the sclerotome of the somites.

2. The nucleus pulposus cells are initially of notochordal origin, but by adulthood they are replaced by chondrocyte-like cells that are thought to arise from the cartilaginous end plate.

3. Chordomas are rare tumors that are thought to arise from notochordal residua.

B. Nucleus pulposus (**Figure 1**)

Dr. Yoon or an immediate family member serves as a paid consultant to Meditech; serves as an unpaid consultant to Biomet and Stryker; has stock or stock options held in Phygen, Meditech Advisors, and Medyssey; has received research or institutional support from Biomet and SpineNet; and serves as a board member, owner, officer, or committee member of the International Society for the Study of the Lumbar Spine, the North American Spine Society, and Korean American Spine Society. Dr. Smith or an immediate family member has received royalties from Biomet and serves as a paid consultant to Bioment.

1. The nucleus pulposus is the central portion of the disk.

2. It is composed primarily of type II collagen.

3. The nucleus pulposus is hypoxic and relatively acidic; nucleus pulposus cells are more synthetically active in this type of environment.

4. In a normal healthy lumbar disk, large aggregating proteoglycans (aggrecan and versican) constitute a high percentage of the dry weight in the nucleus.

   a. The glycosaminoglycan molecules (keratan sulfate and chondroitin sulfate) decorate the aggrecan and versican core protein and are highly negatively charged. This creates a highly hydrophilic matrix that attracts H_2O molecules, which provides swelling pressure that counteracts the axial loads encountered by the disk.

   b. The matrix is viscoelastic and therefore dissipates mechanical energy and is subject to creep (disk height is less at the end of each day).

C. Anulus fibrosus

1. The anulus fibrosus is located more peripherally and surrounds the nucleus pulposus. Defects in the anulus fibrosus lead to herniated disks that could cause radiculopathy.

2. The anulus fibrosus is composed primarily of concentric layers of type I collagen. The collagen fibers are obliquely orientated within each layer, and the orientation of the fibers alternates between layers.

3. The alternating, oblique orientation of collagen fibers gives the anulus fibrosus high tensile strength and helps resist intervertebral distraction but also keeps the anulus fibrosus flexible enough to deform and allow intervertebral motion.

4. As the nucleus pulposus degenerates, the anulus fibrosus takes proportionately more axial load.

D. End plates

1. The end plates form the interface between the vertebrae and the disk and define the upper and lower boundaries of the disk.

1: Basic Science

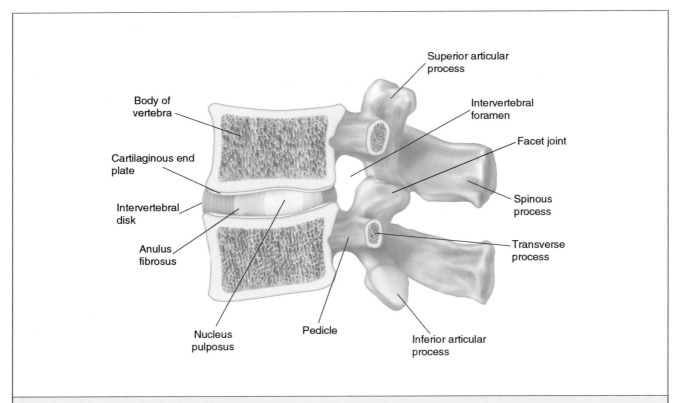

Figure 1 Illustration shows a sagittal cross section of a motion segment comprising two vertebral bodies and the intervertebral disk, which forms a strong connection between the bones. The four regions of the disk are shown: cartilaginous end plate, outer anulus fibrosus, inner anulus fibrosus, and nucleus pulposus. The posterior articular and spinous processes and the articular surface of a facet joint are also shown.

2. The central portion of the end plate provides a major pathway for nutrients from the vertebral bodies to diffuse into the disk.

E. Vascular supply

1. In the adult, the disk is avascular.

   a. The blood supply ends at the bony end plate of the vertebral body and the outer anulus fibrosus. Therefore, most of the disk is considered immunologically isolated.

   b. Because of this avascularity, nutrients are supplied to the disk cells primarily through diffusion (**Figure 2**).

2. As the disk gets larger during development, the distances that nutrition must diffuse across become larger, further impeding nutritional supply to the disk cells. This decrease in nutritional transport is thought to contribute to disk degeneration.

F. Innervation

1. Innervation is confined to the peripheral anulus fibrosus.

2. The sinuvertebral nerve, which arises from the dorsal root ganglion, innervates the outer anulus

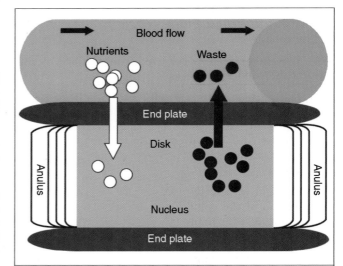

Figure 2 Illustration represents intervertebral disk nutrition. The blood supply reaches the bony end plate but does not cross into the disk. The nutrients diffuse across the end plate to reach disk cells. The metabolic waste products leave the disk tissue by diffusing across the end plate and are carried away by blood flow.

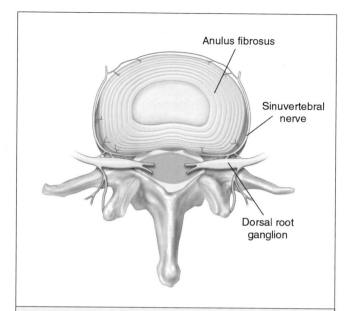

Figure 3 Illustration shows a lumbar intervertebral disk and its nerve supply in transverse cross section. Branches of the sinuvertebral nerve also supply the anterior aspect of the dural sac and dural sleeve.

fibrosus (**Figure 3**). In some degenerated disks with fissures, nerve fibers may be found deeper in the anulus fibrosus.

3. The normal nucleus pulposus is not innervated.

4. Pain sensation from the disk arises only from the anulus fibrosus, but the nucleus pulposus can generate molecules such as cytokines and proteinases that can lead to pain.

III. Biologic Activity

A. Homeostasis

1. Disk cells are metabolically active, synthesizing disk matrix, catabolic enzymes, and growth factors (eg, bone morphogenetic protein [BMP]-2, BMP-7, transforming growth factor beta [TGF-β]).

2. Although disk cells constitute only a small proportion of the volume of the adult disk, they are responsible for maintaining the volume and composition of the disk matrix.

3. The normal turnover rate of the disk matrix is slow, but even a small deviation in the balance of disk homeostasis can result in disk degeneration over a period of years.

B. Cell characteristics by region

1. Nucleus pulposus cells are chondrocyte-like. They exist in a hypoxic environment and characteristi-

cally synthesize proteoglycans (aggrecan, versican, and small leucine-rich proteoglycans), collagen type II, and other matrix molecules.

2. Anulus fibrosus cells are fibroblast-like. They characteristically produce type I collagen, but they also produce other matrix molecules, including proteoglycans. Inner anulus fibrosus cells produce relatively more proteoglycans than outer anulus fibrosus cells.

IV. Disk Degeneration

A. Aging

1. Disks undergo a natural degenerative process during aging that does not implicate a disease process.

2. In the young child, the nucleus pulposus cells are mostly notochordal cells.

3. By age 10 years, notochordal cells in the nucleus pulposus have disappeared and are replaced by chondrocyte-like cells.

4. In the young person, the disk is tall and the nucleus pulposus has a high water content. The anulus fibrosus is intact and well organized.

5. With increasing age, the disk undergoes several changes:

   a. Disk cells produce less aggrecan and type II collagen, leading to decreases in proteoglycan and water content.

   b. Biosynthetic function decreases, and the concentration of viable cells in the central region is lower.

   c. Degradative enzyme activity increases.

   d. As the nucleus pulposus desiccates, disk height is lost and the anulus fibrosus develops fissures.

6. Ninety percent of asymptomatic individuals older than 60 years have MRI evidence of disk degeneration.

B. Genetics

1. Strong evidence suggests that genetics plays an important role in disk degeneration.

2. Twins studies have indicated that genetic factors are more important determinants of disk degeneration than factors such as lifetime occupation and leisure activities.

3. Additional genetic studies have shown that disk degeneration inheritance is nonmendelian and involves multiple genes (**Table 1**).

   a. Mutations in the genes for vitamin D receptor (*VDR*), interleukin-1 (*IL-1*), collagen I (*COL1A1*), and collagen IX (*COL9A2* and

1: Basic Science

Table 1

Genes Associated With Intervertebral Disk Degeneration

Gene	Function
COL1A1	Collagen I
COL9A2 and COL9A3	Collagen IX
COL11A2	Collagen XI
IL-1	Interleukin 1; inflammatory modulation
IL-6	Interleukin 6; inflammatory modulation
MMP-3	Matrix metalloproteinase
VDR	Vitamin D receptor
CILP	Cartilage intermediate layer protein
Aggrecan (encoded by the ACAN gene)	Aggregates hyaluronan (certain polymorphisms associated with disk degeneration)

CILP = cartilage intermediate layer protein, COL = collagen, IL = interleukin, MMP = matrix metalloproteinase, VDR = vitamin D receptor.

COL9A3) have been implicated in disk degeneration.

   b. A mutation in the cartilage intermediate layer protein gene (CILP) has been associated with an increased need for surgery to treat sciatica resulting from lumbar disk herniation.

C. Pain

   1. Disk degeneration is associated with a higher incidence of low back pain, but the presence of one or more degenerated disks does not correlate directly with low back pain.

   2. Despite improvements in imaging modalities such as MRI and CT, imaging studies remain unreliable in identifying a painful disk.

   3. Diskography, which involves introducing a needle into the disk and injecting fluid under pressure, has been used to assess disk morphology and in attempts to identify the pain-generating disk.

      a. Elicitation of the familiar, or concordant, pain is considered a positive test.

      b. Diskography has been shown to have a high false-positive rate, especially in patients with chronic pain and abnormal psychometric testing results.

      c. Diskography was recently shown to be correlated with a higher incidence of disk degeneration and herniation in research participants followed for 10 years after undergoing diskography compared with the control group.

      d. The limitations and risks of diskography have led to decreased use of the procedure.

D. Toxic substances—in vitro studies have shown that several substances can be cytotoxic to intervertebral disk cells. These include bupivacaine, radiocontrast solution, and nicotine.

V. Repair

A. Natural repair process—Perhaps because the disk is avascular, spontaneous biologic repair processes are quite limited and are thought to be ineffective.

B. Biologic therapy disk repair has been successful in some experiments in small animals, but no credible report of success in humans has yet been published.

Top Testing Facts

1. The nucleus pulposus resists primarily compressive loads, whereas the anulus fibrosus resists primarily tensile loads.

2. The intervertebral disk allows motion and provides mechanical stability of the functional spinal unit.

3. Nucleus pulposus cells are more synthetically active in a hypoxic environment.

4. The nucleus pulposus is normally rich in aggregating proteoglycans (aggrecan and versican), which attract water and help maintain disk height. The nucleus pulposus is composed primarily of type II collagen.

5. The anulus fibrosus is a well-organized laminated fibrous tissue composed primarily of type I collagen.

6. With increasing age, the disk cells produce less aggrecan and type II collagen, leading to decreases in proteoglycan and water content. As the nucleus pulposus desiccates, disk height is lost and the anulus fibrosus develops fissures.

7. Ninety percent of asymptomatic individuals older than 60 years have MRI evidence of disk degeneration.

8. Genetics plays a stronger role in disk degeneration than occupation, but this seems to involve a multifactorial process that does not fit a Mendelian pattern.

9. Diskography has a high false-positive rate in patients with abnormal psychometric testing results and can increase disk degeneration.

Bibliography

Akmal M, Kesani A, Anand B, Singh A, Wiseman M, Goodship A: Effect of nicotine on spinal disc cells: A cellular mechanism for disc degeneration. *Spine (Phila Pa 1976)* 2004; 29(5):568-575.

Anderson DG, Tannoury C: Molecular pathogenic factors in symptomatic disc degeneration. *Spine J* 2005;5(6, suppl): 260S-266S.

Battié MC, Videman T: Lumbar disc degeneration: Epidemiology and genetics. *J Bone Joint Surg Am* 2006;88(suppl 2): 3-9.

Battié MC, Videman T, Gibbons LE, Fisher LD, Manninen H, Gill K: 1995 Volvo Award in clinical sciences: Determinants of lumbar disc degeneration. A study relating lifetime exposures and magnetic resonance imaging findings in identical twins. *Spine (Phila Pa 1976)* 1995;20(24):2601-2612.

Carragee EJ, Don AS, Hurwitz EL, Cuellar JM, Carrino JA, Herzog R: 2009 ISSLS Prize Winner: Does discography cause accelerated progression of degeneration changes in the lumbar disc. A ten-year matched cohort study. *Spine (Phila Pa 1976)* 2009;34(21):2338-2345.

Gruber HE, Rhyne AL III, Hansen KJ, et al: Deleterious effects of discography radiocontrast solution on human annulus cell in vitro: Changes in cell viability, proliferation, and apoptosis in exposed cells. *Spine J* 2012;12(4):329-335.

Jünger S, Gantenbein-Ritter B, Lezuo P, Alini M, Ferguson SJ, Ito K: Effect of limited nutrition on in situ intervertebral disc cells under simulated-physiological loading. *Spine (Phila Pa 1976)* 2009;34(12):1264-1271.

Kalichman L, Hunter DJ: The genetics of intervertebral disc degeneration: Associated genes. *Joint Bone Spine* 2008;75(4): 388-396.

Moss IL, An HS: Form and function of the intervertebral disk, in O'Keefe RJ, Jacobs JJ, Chu CR, Einhorn TA, eds: *Orthopaedic Basic Science: Foundations of Clinical Practice*, ed 4. Rosemont, IL, American Academy of Orthopaedic Surgeons, 2013, pp 253-260

Patel AA, Spiker WR, Daubs M, Brodke D, Cannon-Albright LA: Evidence for an inherited predisposition to lumbar disc disease. *J Bone Joint Surg Am* 2011;93(3):225-229.

Quero L, Klawitter M, Nerlich AG, Leonardi M, Boos N, Wuertz K: Bupivacaine: The deadly friend of intervertebral disc cells? *Spine J* 2011;11(1):46-53.

Virtanen IM, Karppinen J, Taimela S, et al: Occupational and genetic risk factors associated with intervertebral disc disease. *Spine (Phila Pa 1976)* 2007;32(10):1129-1134.

1: Basic Science

Chapter 13

Statistics: Practical Applications for Orthopaedics

Mohit Bhandari, MD, PhD, FRCSC   Khaled J. Saleh, MD, MSc, FRCSC, MHCM

Wendy M. Novicoff, PhD

1: Basic Science

I. Presentation of Study Results

A. Terminology

1. Absolute risk increase—The difference in absolute risk (as a percentage or proportion of patients with a specific outcome) between patients exposed and those unexposed to a specific treatment or other factor, or between the patients in the experimental and control groups in a study. It is typically used with regard to a harmful exposure.

2. Absolute risk reduction—The difference in absolute risk (as a percentage or proportion of patients with a specific outcome) between patients exposed (experimental event rate) and those unexposed (control event rate) to a specific treatment or other factor. It is typically used only regarding a beneficial exposure or intervention.

3. Bayesian analysis—An analysis that begins with a particular probability of an event (the prior probability) and incorporates new information to generate a revised probability (a posterior probability).

4. Blind (or blinded or masked)—A type of study/ assessment in which participants in the conduction of the study are unaware of whether members of the study population have been assigned to an experimental group or a control group within the study. Patients, clinicians, persons monitoring outcomes, persons assessing outcomes, data analysts, and the authors of a study report can all be blinded or masked. To avoid confusion, the term "masked" is preferred in studies in which loss of vision is an outcome of interest.

5. Dichotomous outcome—A direct positive or negative outcome that does not include gradations (that is, an outcome that either happens or does not happen), such as reoperation, infection, or death.

6. Dichotomous variable—A variable that can have only one of two characteristics or values, such as male or female, dead or alive, infection present or absent.

7. Effect size—The difference in outcome in the intervention group and the control group in a study, divided by some measure of variability, typically the standard deviation (SD).

8. Hawthorne effect—A change in human behavior generated by participants' awareness that their behavior is being observed. In a clinical study, the Hawthorne effect might result in a treatment being deemed effective when it is actually ineffective. In a diagnostic study, the Hawthorne effect might result in a patient's belief that he or she has the condition being investigated in the study purely on the basis of undergoing a test for this condition.

9. Intention-to-treat principle, or intention-to-treat analysis—The analysis of patient outcomes

Dr. Bhandari or an immediate family member is a member of a speakers' bureau or has made paid presentations on behalf of Stryker; serves as a paid consultant to or is an employee of Eli Lilly, Smith & Nephew, and Stryker; and has received research or institutional support from Johnson & Johnson and Stryker. Dr. Saleh or an immediate family member serves as a paid consultant to or is an employee of the Southern Illinois University School of Medicine, Division of Orthopaedics, Chairman and Professor; serves as a paid consultant to or is an employee of Aesculap and Blue Cross Blue Shield Blue Distinction Panel for Knee and Hip Replacement; has received research or institutional support from Smith & Nephew, the Orthopaedic Research and Education Foundation (OREF), and the National Institutes of Health; and serves as a board member, owner, officer, or committee member of the American Orthopaedic Association Finance Committee, OREF, and the American Board of Orthopaedic Surgeons Examiner. Neither Dr. Novicoff nor any immediate family member has received anything of value from or has stock or stock options held in a commercial company or institution related directly or indirectly to the subject of this chapter.

	Infection		No Infection
Treatment Group	10	**A** | **B**	90
Control Group	50	**C** | **D**	50

Treatment event rate (TER): A/A+B = 10/100 = 10%
    The incidence of infection in the treatment group

Control event rate (CER): C/(C+D) = 50/100 = 50%
    The CER is the incidence of infection in the
    control group.

Relative risk (RR): TER/CER = 10/50 = 0.2
    The RR is the relative risk of infection in the
    treatment group relative to the control group.

Relative risk reduction (RRR): 1 − RR = 1 − 0.2 = 0.8, or 80%
    An RRR of 80% means that treatment reduces
    the risk of infection by 80% compared to controls.

Absolute risk reduction (ARR): CER − TER = 50% − 10% = 40%
    The ARR is the actual numerical difference in infection
    rates between treatment and controls.

Number needed to treat (NNT): 1/ARR = 1/0.40 = 2.5
    An NNT of 2.5 means that for every 2.5 patients who
    receive the treatment, 1 infection can be prevented.

Odds ratio (OR): AD/BC = (10)(50)/(90)(50) = 500/4500 = 0.11
    An OR of 0.11 means that the odds of infection in
    treatment compared to controls is 0.11.

Figure 1   Presentation of study results. A hypothetical example of a study evaluating infection rates in 200 patients with a treatment and control group is presented. A 2 × 2 table is constructed, and multiple approaches to describing the results are presented. (Reproduced with permission from Bhandari M, Devereaux PJ, Swiontkowski M, et al: Internal fixation compared with arthroplasty for displaced fractures of the femoral neck. *J Bone Joint Surg Am* 2003; 85:1673-1681.)

according to the group into which patients are randomized, regardless of whether they actually receive a planned treatment or other intervention. This type of analysis preserves the power of randomization so that important unknown factors that influence outcome are likely to be equally distributed among the comparison groups in a study.

10. Meta-analysis—An overview that incorporates a quantitative strategy for combining the results of multiple studies into a single pooled or summary estimate.

11. Null hypothesis—The initial or baseline hypothesis that is to be accepted or rejected on the basis of a statistical test.

12. Number needed to harm—The number of patients who would have to be treated over a spe-

cific period of time before a specific adverse effect of the treatment would be expected to occur. The number needed to harm is the inverse of the absolute risk increase.

13. Number needed to treat—The number of patients who would have to be treated over a specific period of time to prevent one bad outcome. When discussing the number needed to treat, it is important to specify the treatment, its duration, and the bad outcome being prevented. The number needed to treat is the inverse of the absolute risk reduction.

14. Odds—The ratio of the probability of occurrence of an event to the probability of its nonoccurrence.

15. Odds ratio—The ratio of the odds of an event occurring in a group exposed to a specific factor to the odds of the same event occurring in a group not exposed to that factor.

16. Relative risk—The ratio of the risk of an event occurring among an exposed population to the risk of its occurring among an unexposed population.

17. Relative risk reduction—An estimate of the proportion of the baseline risk of an event that is removed by a particular treatment or other intervention. The relative risk reduction is calculated by dividing the absolute reduction in the risk of the event in a treatment or other intervention group by the absolute risk of occurrence of the event in a control group.

18. Reliability—The consistency or reproducibility of data.

19. Treatment effect—The magnitude of the difference, or a measure of difference other than magnitude, in the effect of a treatment or in the outcome of a treated group as compared to an untreated control group, such as in a comparative clinical study. Examples are absolute risk reduction, relative risk reduction, odds ratio, number needed to treat, and effect size. The appropriate measure for expressing a treatment effect and the appropriate calculation to use for determining it, whether a probability, mean, or median, depends on the type of outcome variable used to measure the effect. For example, relative risk reduction is used for dichotomous variables, whereas effect sizes are normally used for continuous variables.

20. Continuous variable—A variable with a potentially infinite number of possible values. Examples include range of motion and blood pressure.

21. Categorical variable—A variable whose values occur within several different and discrete categories. An example would be types of fractures.

B. **Figure 1** illustrates a typical presentation of study results.

C. Bias in research

1. Definition—Bias is a systematic tendency to produce an outcome that differs from the true outcome.

   a. Channeling effect, or channeling bias—The tendency of clinicians to prescribe a treatment on the basis of prognosis. The result of this in a clinical study is that comparisons of treated and untreated patients' outcomes will yield a biased estimate of treatment effect.

   b. Data completeness bias—A bias that may occur when an information system (for example, a hospital database) is used to enter data directly for the treatment group in a study, whereas the data for the control group are entered manually.

   c. Detection bias, or surveillance bias—The tendency to look more carefully for a particular outcome in only one of two or more groups that are being compared in a randomized clinical trial or other comparative study.

   d. Incorporation bias—The study of a diagnostic test that incorporates features of the target outcome.

   e. Interviewer bias—More intense or extensive probing of one or more variables in one of two or more treatment or other groups than in the other groups, or any selective subjectivity that can affect the findings in such a comparative investigation.

   f. Publication bias—Reporting of research results according to the apparent trend or other apparent outcome of the results of a study without determination of whether they are statistically significant.

   g. Recall bias—A difference in the likelihood of accurate recall of an event among patients who experience an adverse outcome of that event as opposed to patients in whom the event does not have an adverse outcome, independent of the true nature or extent of the event.

   h. Surveillance bias—See detection bias, section I.C.1.c.

   i. Verification bias—A nonobjective effect of the results of a diagnostic test on whether patients are assigned to a treatment group.

2. Limiting bias—The limiting of bias in a clinical research study through randomization, concealment of treatment allocation, and blinding.

   a. Random allocation (randomization)

      • The allocation by chance of individual subjects in a study to groups, usually through use of a table of random numbers. A sample derived by selecting sampling units (for example, individual patients) in such a way that each unit has an independent and fixed (generally equal) chance of being selected.

      • Random allocation should not be confused with systematic allocation (for example, on even and odd days of the month) or allocation at the convenience or discretion of the investigator.

   b. Concealment of treatment allocation

      • Allocation is concealed when the investigators conducting a study cannot determine the treatment group or other group to which the next patient enrolled in the study will be allocated.

      • The use of even/odd days or hospital chart numbers to allocate patients to a group within a study is not considered concealed allocation.

   c. Blinding (see definition in section I.A.4).

II. Basic Statistical Concepts

A. A statistician should be consulted when a study or analysis of a study is planned.

B. Hypothesis testing—Null hypothesis

1. Typically, the null hypothesis is that there is no difference in the effect of two or more treatments or other independent or interventional variables being compared in a study. The investigators begin the study with such a null hypothesis and use statistical testing to determine whether there is a significant difference in this effect, which would disprove the null hypothesis.

2. In a randomized trial in which investigators compare an experimental treatment with a placebo control, the null hypothesis can be stated as follows: "There is no true difference in effect of the experimental and control treatments on the outcome of interest."

C. Errors in hypothesis testing—Any comparative study can have one of the following four possible outcomes (**Figure 2**):

1. A true-positive result (the study correctly identifies a true difference between treatments or other independent variables).

2. A true-negative result (the study correctly identifies no difference between treatments or other independent variables).

3. A false-negative result, called a type II (β) error (the study incorrectly concludes that there is no difference between treatments when a difference really exists). By convention, the error rate is set

at 0.20 (20% false-negative rate). Study power (see section II.D.) is derived from the 1–β error rate (1–0.2 = 0.80, or 80%).

4. A false-positive result, called a type I (α) error (the study incorrectly concludes that there is a difference between treatments when any such difference is really to the result of chance). By convention, most studies in orthopaedics adopt an α error rate of 0.05. Thus, investigators can expect a false-positive error about 5% of the time.

D. Study power—The ability of a study to detect the difference between two interventions if such a difference in fact exists. The power of a statistical test is typically a function of the magnitude of the treatment effect, the designated type I (α) and type II (β) error rates, and the sample size, n.

	Truth	
Results of Study	Difference Exists in Actuality	No Difference Exists in Actuality
Study Shows a Difference	Correct conclusion (1 – β)	False-positive (α, or type I, error)
Study Shows No Difference	False-negative (β, or type II, error)	Correct conclusion (1 – α)

Figure 2   Errors in hypothesis testing. A 2 × 2 table is used to depict the results of a study comparing two treatments (difference, no difference) and the "truth" (whether or not there is a difference in actuality). Common errors are presented, including type I and II errors. (Reproduced with permission from Bhandari M, Devereaux PJ, Swiontkowski M, et al: Internal fixation compared with arthroplasty for displaced fractures of the femoral neck. *J Bone Joint Surg Am* 2003;85:1673-1681.)

E. *P* value—Defined as the probability, under the assumption of no difference (null hypothesis), of obtaining a result equal to or more extreme than what was actually observed if the experiment were repeated any number of times. The *P* value threshold for significance has arbitrarily been set at 0.05 by convention. A significant result is therefore a result that is so unlikely to be caused by chance alone that it leads to rejection of the null hypothesis.

F. Confidence interval (CI)—A range of numerical values of a variable defined by two values within which it is probable (to a specified percentage) that the true value lies for an entire population of patients or other subjects being investigated in a study. Various percentages can be used for the degree of confidence with which the range of values of the variable is likely to include the true value, but by convention, 95% (95% CI) is the value of confidence typically used for this in clinical research.

III. Basic Statistical Inference

A. Normal distribution (**Table 1**)

1. Definition—A normal distribution is a distribution of continuous data that forms a bell-shaped plot or curve; that is, a plot or curve with many values near the mean and progressively fewer values toward the extremes.

2. Several statistical tests are based on the assumption that the variables to which these tests are applied will have a normal distribution. If a sample is not normally distributed, a separate set of statistical tests should be applied to the sample. These tests are referred to as nonparametric tests because they do not rely on parameters such as the mean and SD.

Table 1

Common Statistical Tests

		Data Type and Distribution		
		Categorical	**Ordered Categorical or Continuous and Non-normal**	**Continuous and Normal**
Two samples	Different individuals	χ^2 test Fisher exact test	Mann-Whitney test Wilcoxon rank sum test	Unpaired *t* test
	Related or matched samples	McNemar test	Wilcoxon signed rank test	Paired *t* test
Three or more samples	Different individuals	χ^2 test Fisher exact test	Kruskal-Wallis test	ANOVA
	Related samples	Cochran *Q* test	Friedman test	Repeated measures ANOVA

ANOVA = analysis of variance.

Reproduced with permission from Bhandari M, Devereaux PJ, Swiontkowski M, et al: Internal fixation compared with arthroplasty for displaced fractures of the femoral neck. *J Bone Joint Surg Am* 2003;85:1673-1681.

B. Descriptive statistics

1. Measures of central tendency

a. Mean—The sum of the values of all of these variables divided by the number of observations used in the sample; it is identical with the average numerical value of the numbers in the sample.

b. Median—The measurement whose numerical value falls in the middle of the set.

c. Mode—The most frequently occurring number in a set of numerical measurements.

d. Use of measures of central tendency

• Continuous variables (such as blood pressure or body weight) that can be measured quantitatively or numerically can be summarized with a mean number if the numerical values of the variables are normally distributed.

• For quantitative data that are not normally distributed, the median may be a better summary statistic than the mean or average.

• Categorical variables (for example, pain grade [0,1,2,3,4,5]) can be summarized with a median.

2. Measures of spread

a. Standard deviation—A measure that shows the variation from the mean, or dispersion, of a set of quantitatively or numerically measurable values. It is derived from the square root of the sample variance, which is calculated as the average of the squares of the deviations, or differences of the measurements from their mean value. To calculate the SD, the square of each of these differences is calculated, the squared values are added and the resulting sum is divided by the number of measurements in the set of measurable values, and the square root of the sum if calculated.

b. Range—The smallest to the largest numbers in the set, is usually expressed only by stating these two numbers.

C. Comparing means

1. Comparing two means

a. When two independent samples of normally distributed continuous variables are compared, the Student t test (often called "Student's t test," leading to the common misattribution of this test to students) is used.

b. When the data within a set of data are not normally distributed, a nonparametric test such as the Mann-Whitney U test or Wilcoxon rank-sum test can be used to calculate their mean

value. When the means of two sets of data are paired, such as left and right knees (as with a KT-1000 test), a paired Student t test is most appropriate. The nonparametric correlate of this test is the Wilcoxon signed rank test.

2. Comparing three or more means—When three or more different means are compared (for example, hospital stay among patients treated for tibial fracture with plate fixation, intramedullary nailing, and external fixation), the procedure of choice for evaluating a significant difference is single-factor analysis of variance (ANOVA).

D. Comparing proportions

1. Independent proportions—The chi-square (χ^2) test is a simple method of comparing two proportions, such as a difference in infection rates (%) between two groups. A Yates correction factor is sometimes used to adjust for small sample sizes, but when measured values are very small (for example, fewer than five events in any of a set of treatment or control groups), the χ^2 test is unreliable and the Fisher exact test is the test of choice.

2. Paired proportions—When proportions are paired (for example, as in the proportions of patients showing a specific characteristic in a before- and after-treatment study of the same patients), a McNemar test is used to examine the differences between groups.

E. Regression and correlation

1. Regression analysis—Used to predict (or estimate) the association between a response variable (dependent variable) and a series of known explanatory (independent) variables.

a. Simple regression—Used to predict the association between a response variable and a single independent variable is used.

b. Multiple regression—Used to predict the association between a response variable and multiple independent variables.

c. Logistic regression—Used to predict the association between a response variable and one or more independent variables when the response variable is dichotomous (for example, yes or no; infection present or absent).

d. Cox proportional hazards regression—Used in survival analysis to assess the relationship between two or more variables and a single dependent variable (the time to an event).

2. Correlation—The strength of the relationship between two variables (for example, age versus hospital stay in patients with ankle fractures) can be summarized in a single number, the correlation coefficient, denoted by the letter r. The correlation coefficient can range from −1.0 to 1.0.

1: Basic Science

a. A correlation coefficient of −1.0 represents a completely negative or inverse correlation of one variable with another.

b. A correlation coefficient of 1.0 represents absolute or complete correlation of one variable with another.

c. A correlation coefficient of 0 denotes a complete lack of relationship between two variables.

d. The Pearson correlation r is used to assess the relationship between two normally distributed continuous variables. If one of the variables is not normally distributed, it is better to use the Spearman correlation.

F. Survival analysis

1. Time-to-event analysis involves estimating the probability that an event will occur at various time.

2. Survival analysis estimates the probability of survival as a function of time from a discrete starting point (time of injury, time of surgery).

3. Survival curves, also called Kaplan–Meier curves, are often used to report the survival of one or more groups of patients over time.

IV. Determining Sample Size for a Comparative Study

A. Difference in means—The anticipated sample size, N, for a continuous outcome measure is calculated with the following equation:

$$N = 2 \left\{ \frac{(Z\alpha + Z\beta)\sigma}{\delta} \right\}^2$$

where $Z\alpha$ = type I error, $Z\beta$ = type II error, σ = SD, and δ = mean difference between groups.

B. Difference in proportions—For dichotomous variables, the following calculation is used for determining sample size, N:

$$N = \left\{ \frac{PA(100 - PA) + PB(100 - PB)}{(PB - PA)^2} \right\} f(\alpha,\beta)$$

where PA and PB = % successes in A and B, and $f(\alpha,\beta)$ = function of type I and II errors.

V. Reliability

A. Test-retest reliability measures the extent to which the same observer, assessing a subject for one or more variables on multiple occasions, achieves similar results. Because time elapses between the assess-

ments, the characteristics being assessed may also change. For example, the range of motion (ROM) of a hip may change substantially over a 4-week period.

B. Intraobserver reliability is the same as test-retest reliability except that the characteristics being assessed are fixed and unchanging. Because time is the only factor that varies between assessments, a study with this type of design will typically yield a higher estimate of reliability than will test-retest or interobserver reliability studies.

C. Interobserver reliability measures the extent to which two or more observers obtain similar scores when assessing the same subject. Interobserver reliability is the greatest and, when observer-related error is highly relevant, the most clinically useful measure of reliability.

1. The κ coefficient, or κ statistic, is the most commonly reported statistic in reliability studies and can be thought of as a measure of agreement beyond chance.

2. The κ coefficient has a maximum value of 1.0 (indicating perfect agreement). A value of κ = 0.0 indicates no agreement beyond chance; negative values of κ indicate poorer agreement than by chance alone.

3. The κ coefficient can be used when data are categorical (categories of answers such as definitely healed, possibly healed, or not healed) or binary (a yes or no answer, such as infection or absence of infection).

D. Intraclass correlation coefficients (ICCs) are a set of related measures of reliability that yield a value that is closest to the formal definition of reliability. One ICC measures the proportion of total variability that comes from true between-subject variability. ICCs are used when data are continuous.

VI. Diagnostic Tests

A. Definition of terms

1. Specificity—The proportion of individuals who are truly free of a designated disorder and who are so identified by a diagnostic test for the disorder.

2. Sensitivity—The proportion of individuals who truly have a designated disorder and who are so identified by a diagnostic test.

3. Positive predictive value—The proportion of individuals who test positively for a disease and who have that disease.

4. Negative predictive value—The proportion of individuals who test negatively for a disease and who are free of that disease.

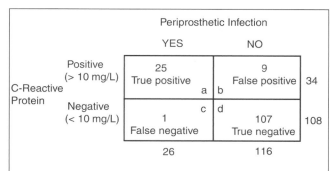

Likelihood ratio = (a/a + c)/(b/b + d) = sensitivity/(1 − specificity)
(for positive test) = (25/26)/(9/116) = 0.96/0.077 = 12.5

Likelihood ratio = (c/a + c)/(d/b + d) = (1 −t sensitivity/specificity)
(for negative test) = (1/26)/(107/116) = 0.038/0.92 = 0.041

Sensitivity: a/(a + c) = 25/26 = 96%

Specificity: d/(b + d) = 107/116 = 92%

Positive predictive value: a/(a + b) = 25/34 = 74%

Negative predictive value: d/(c + d) = 107/108 = 99%

Accuracy: a + d/(a + b + c + d) = 132/142 = 93%

Prevalence: (a + c)/(a + b + c +d) = 26/142 = 18%

Figure 3   Diagnostic tests. A 2 × 2 table depicts C-reactive protein thresholds for diagnosing infection. Several test characteristics are presented, including sensitivity, specificity, and likelihood ratios. (Reproduced with permission from Bhandari M, Devereaux PJ, Swiontkowski M, et al: Internal fixation compared with arthroplasty for displaced fractures of the femoral neck. *J Bone Joint Surg Am* 2003;85:1673-1681.)

5. Likelihood ratio—For a screening or diagnostic test (including the presence of clinical signs or symptoms of a disorder), the likelihood ratio expresses the relative likelihood that a given test result would be expected in a patient with (as opposed to one without) the disorder of interest.

6. Accuracy—The accuracy of a screening or diagnostic test for a disease is its overall ability to identify patients with the disease (true positives) and those without the disease (true negatives) in a study population.

B. **Figure 3** illustrates the application of these concepts to threshold values of the serum concentration of C-reactive protein in the diagnosis of infection.

Top Testing Facts

1. Bias in clinical research is best defined as a systematic deviation from the true outcome.

2. Randomization, concealment of allocation, and blinding are key methodologic principles to limit bias in clinical research.

3. The power of a study is its ability to find a difference between treatments when a true difference exists.

4. The *P* value is defined as the probability, under the assumption of no difference in the result of an intervention (null hypothesis), of obtaining a result equal to or more extreme than the result observed without the intervention.

5. The CI is a quantification of the uncertainty of measurement of a variable. Typically, a 95% CI consists of the range of values of a variable that is 95% certain to contain the true value of the variable.

6. A 95% CI is the interval or range of a value within which the true value of the variable can be found in 95% of instances.

7. Two means can be compared with a Student *t* test.

8. Two proportions can be compared statistically with a χ^2 test.

9. The specificity of a test is the proportion of individuals who are truly free of a designated disorder and who are so identified by a diagnostic test for the disorder.

10. The sensitivity of a test is the proportion of individuals who have a designated disorder and who are identified by a test as having that disorder.

11. A type II error is the probability of determining that there is no difference in the effects of a treatment or other intervention or variable in a treatment group and in an untreated control group when there is a difference. Type II errors often occur when the sample size of a treatment group is too small to yield a statistically valid result and leads to a false-negative result.

12. A type I error is a false-positive conclusion that occurs when one rejects a null hypothesis that is actually true.

1: Basic Science

Bibliography

Dorrey F, Swiontkowski MF: Statistical tests: What they tell us and what they don't. *Ad Orthop Surg* 1997;21:81-85.

Griffin D, Audige L: Common statistical methods in orthopaedic clinical studies. *Clin Orthop Relat Res* 2003;413: 70-79.

Guyatt GH, Jaeschke R, Heddle N, Cook DJ, Shannon H, Walter SD: Basic statistics for clinicians: 1. Hypothesis testing. *CMAJ* 1995;152(1):27-32.

Guyatt GH, Jaeschke R, Heddle N, Cook DJ, Shannon H, Walter SD: Basic statistics for clinicians: 2. Interpreting study results: Confidence intervals. *CMAJ* 1995;152(2):169-173.

Moher D, Dulberg CS, Wells GA: Statistical power, sample size, and their reporting in randomized controlled trials. *JAMA* 1994;272(2):122-124.

Chapter 14
Evidence-Based Medicine

Khaled J. Saleh, MD, MSc, FRCSC, MHCM   Wendy M. Novicoff, PhD

I. Basics of Evidence-Based Medicine

A. Definition—Evidence-based medicine is the practice of integrating individual clinical expertise with the best available clinical evidence from systematic research to maximize the quality and quantity of life for individual patients.

B. Goal—To achieve the best possible patient management and patient outcomes through the combination of empirical evidence, clinical expertise, and patient values.

C. Steps in evidence-based medicine

   1. Formulate an answerable question

   2. Identify and locate the best available evidence of outcomes

   3. Appraise the evidence

   4. Apply the evidence in practice (integrate it with clinical expertise)

   5. Evaluate the efficacy and efficiency of the evidence-based process in direct clinical practice

D. Assessing evidence

   1. Assessment of evidence is not restricted to randomized trials and meta-analyses.

   2. Collect evidence of studies with similar results and provide indications of this similarity in different aspects of clinical practice (such as prognosis or diagnosis)

Dr. Saleh or an immediate family member serves as a paid consultant to or is an employee of the Southern Illinois University School of Medicine, Division of Orthopaedics; serves as a paid consultant to or is an employee of Aesculap and Blue Cross Blue Shield Blue Distinction Panel for Knee and Hip Replacement; has received research or institutional support from Smith & Nephew, the Orthopaedic Research and Education Foundation (OREF), and the NIH; and serves as a board member, owner, officer, or committee member of the American Orthopaedic Association, OREF, and the American Board of Orthopaedic Surgeons. Neither Dr. Novicoff nor any immediate family member has received anything of value from or has stock or stock options held in a commercial company or institution related directly or indirectly to the subject of this chapter.

   3. Develop a grade by matching directly the level of evidence and quality of study. (for example, low, intermediate, and high)

II. Types of Studies

A. Therapeutic studies—Investigate the results of a particular treatment.

   1. Level I

      a. High-quality randomized controlled trial with a significant difference in the results of two treatments or of a specific treatment and lack of any treatment, or the absence of such a significant difference but a narrow confidence interval indicating a positive effect of a treatment

      b. Systematic review of level I randomized controlled trials (in which study results are homogeneous)

   2. Level II

      a. Lesser-quality randomized controlled trial (for example, <80% follow-up, no blinding, or improper randomization of participants in the trial)

      b. Prospective comparative study

      c. Systematic review of level II studies or level I studies, yielding inconsistent results

   3. Level III

      a. Case-control study

      b. Retrospective comparative study

      c. Systematic review of level III studies

   4. Level IV—Case series, or cohort and case-control studies of poor quality.

   5. Level V—Expert opinion.

B. Prognostic studies—Investigate the effect of a patient characteristic on the outcome of a disease.

   1. Level I

      a. High-quality prospective study (for example, all patients enrolled at the same point in their disease, with ≥80% follow-up)

  b. Systematic review of level I studies

2. Level II

  a. Retrospective study

  b. Untreated controls from a randomized controlled trial

  c. Lesser-quality prospective study (for example, patients enrolled at different points in their disease or <80% follow-up)

  d. Systematic review of level II studies

3. Level III—Case-control study

4. Level IV—Case series

5. Level V—Expert opinion

C. Diagnostic studies—Investigate a diagnostic test

1. Level I

  a. Testing of previously developed diagnostic criteria in series of consecutive patients (using a universally applied reference standard of established validity [gold standard])

  b. Systematic review of level I studies

2. Level II

  a. Development of diagnostic criteria on the basis of consecutive patients (using a gold standard)

  b. Systematic review of level II studies

3. Level III

  a. Study of nonconsecutive patients (without using a gold standard)

  b. Systematic review of level III studies

4. Level IV

  a. Case-control study

  b. Poor reference standard

5. Level V—Expert opinion

D. Economic and decision analyses—Develop an economic or decision model.

1. Level I

  a. Sensible costs and alternatives; values obtained from many studies; multimodal analyses of sensitivity

  b. Systematic review of level I studies

2. Level II

  a. Sensible costs and alternatives; values obtained from limited studies; audits and chart reviews

  b. Systematic review of level II studies

3. Level III

  a. Analyses based on limited alternatives and costs; poor estimates

  b. Systematic review of level III studies

4. Level IV—No sensitivity analyses

5. Level V—Expert opinion

III. Examples of Study Types Used in Orthopaedics

Therapeutic study, evidence level I
Ritting AW, Leger R, O'Malley MP, Mogielnicki H, Tucker R, Rodner CM: Duration of postoperative dressing after mini-open carpal tunnel release: A prospective, randomized trial. *J Hand Surg Am* 2012;37: 3-8.

Therapeutic study, evidence level II
Shin SJ: A comparison of 2 repair techniques for partial-thickness articular-sided rotator cuff tears. *Arthroscopy* 2012;28:25-33.

Therapeutic study, evidence level III
Yaszay B, O'Brien M, Shufflebarger HL, et al: Efficacy of hemivertebra resection for congenital scoliosis: A multicenter retrospective comparison of three surgical techniques. *Spine (Phila Pa 1976)* 2011;36:2052-2060.

Therapeutic study, evidence level IV
Lenarz C, Shishani Y, McCrum C, Nowinski RJ, Edwards TB, Gobezie R: Is reverse shoulder arthroplasty appropriate for the treatment of fractures in the older patient? Early observations. *Clin Orthop Relat Res* 2011;469:3324-3331.

Prognostic study, evidence level IV
Frobell RB: Change in cartilage thickness, posttraumatic bone marrow lesions, and joint fluid volumes after acute ACL disruption: A two-year prospective MRI study of sixty-one subjects. *J Bone Joint Surg Am* 2011; 93(12):1096-1103.

Diagnostic study, evidence level II
Harris MB, Sethi RK: The initial assessment and management of the multiple-trauma patient with an associated spine injury. *Spine (Phila Pa 1976)* 2006; 31(suppl 11):S9-S15.

Diagnostic study, evidence level III
Vaccaro AR, Kreidel KO, Pan W, et al: Usefulness of MRI in isolated upper cervical spine fractures in adults. *J Spinal Disord* 1998;11:289-294.

Economic and decision analysis study, evidence level II
Slobogean GP, Marra CA, Sadatsafavi M, Sanders DW; Canadian Orthopedic Trauma Society: Is surgical fixation for stress-positive unstable ankle fractures cost effective? Results of a multicenter randomized control trial. *J Orthop Trauma* 2012;26:652-658.

Economic and decision analysis study, evidence level IV
Hurwitz SR, Tornetta P III, Wright JG: An AOA critical issue: How to read the literature to change your practice. An evidence-based medicine approach. *J Bone Joint Surg Am* 2006;88:1873-1879.

Glossary of Evidence-Based Medicine Terms

Absolute risk reduction (ARR)—Difference in the event rate in a control group (control event rate, CER) and in a treated group (experimental event rate, EER): ARR = CER – EER.

Blinded study—A study in which any or all of the clinicians, patients, participants, outcome assessors, or statisticians are unaware of which patients received which study intervention. A double-blinded study usually signifies that the patients and clinicians involved in the study are blinded, but because this term is ambiguous in terms of who is blinded, it is better to specify who in such a study is blinded.

Case-control study—A study that identifies both a group of patients who have an outcome of interest (cases) on exposure to a treatment or other independent variable and a group of patients who do not have this same outcome (controls) following the same exposure.

Case series—A series of patients with an outcome of interest. No control group is involved in this type of study.

Clinical practice guideline—A systematically developed statement designed to assist practitioners and patients in making decisions about appropriate healthcare measures to be followed under specific clinical circumstances or to achieve a desired clinical outcome.

Cohort study—A study performed with two groups (cohorts) of patients, one that has an exposure or treatment of interest and the other that does not, and which follows these cohorts in a progressive manner to identify which group manifests an outcome of interest.

Confidence interval (CI)—A quantification of the uncertainty in the measurement of a variable; usually reported as the 95% CI, which is the range of values that is 95% certain to contain the true value of the measured variable.

Control event rate (CER)—see Event rate.

Cost-benefit analysis—An analysis that converts the benefits of a clinical procedure or other healthcare intervention into the same monetary terms as the costs of the procedure or intervention and compares the monetary values of the costs with those of the benefits.

Cost-effectiveness analysis—An analysis that converts effects into health-specific terms and describes the costs for some additional health gain (for example, cost per

additional adverse event prevented), as in the cost of a vaccination program in comparison with the population-care costs of the disease that the vaccination prevents.

Cost-utility analysis—An analysis that converts effects into personal preferences (for example, desired goals of an intervention, or utilities) and determines the cost for some additional gain in quality (for example, cost per additional quality-adjusted life-year).

Crossover study design—A study designed to provide two or more experimental therapies, one at a time, to be given in a specified sequential order or in random order, to the same group of patients.

Cross-sectional study—Observation of a defined population at a single time point or within a specific interval. Exposure and outcome are determined simultaneously.

Decision analysis—Application of explicit, quantitative methods to analyze decisions under conditions of uncertainty, with the goal of identifying which decisions will provide a desired or optimum outcome.

Ecological survey—A survey based on aggregated data for a population at some point or points in time for the purpose of investigating the relationship of an exposure to a known or presumed risk factor to a specified outcome.

Event rate—The proportion of patients in a group in whom a particular event is observed. Thus, the event rate for an event that is observed in 27 of 100 patients is 0.27. The CER and EER refer to the event rate in control and experimental groups of patients, respectively.

Evidence-based health care—Extension of application of the principles of evidence-based medicine to all aspects of professional health care, including the purchasing of equipment and supplies and patient management.

Evidence-based medicine—The conscientious, explicit, and judicious use of current best evidence in making decisions about the care of individual patients. The practice of evidence-based medicine involves integrating individual clinical expertise with the best available external clinical evidence for a specific care-related intervention or other practice on the basis of findings made in systematic research.

Experimental event rate (EER)—see Event rate.

Likelihood ratio—The likelihood of a given test result in a patient with a specific target disorder compared with the likelihood of that same result in a patient without the disorder.

Meta-analysis—The systematic use of quantitative methods to summarize the results for each of one or more specific outcomes or other measures through analysis of the data for those outcomes or measures in a group of studies.

N-of-1 trials—A study in which patients undergo pairs of treatment periods organized so that one period involves the use of the experimental treatment and a next, paired period involves the use of an alternate or placebo therapy. The patients and physicians in such a trial are blinded, if possible, and outcomes are monitored. Treatment periods are replicated until the study data clearly indicate that the treatment has a definitely different effect or no apparent effect.

Negative predictive value (NPV)—The proportion of patients in whom a diagnostic test for a disease indicates absence of the disease and who are actually free of the disease.

Number needed to treat (NNT)—The number of patients who need to be treated to prevent all from having an adverse outcome of a disease; the inverse of the absolute risk reduction.

Odds—The ratio of an event to its nonoccurrence. If the event rate for a disease is 0.2 (20%), its nonevent rate is 0.8 (80%), and its odds are 0.2/0.8 = 0.25. See also Odds ratio.

Odds ratio—The ratio of the occurrence to the nonoccurrence of a particular study result under a given set of controlled circumstances, such as of a study patient experiencing a treatment-related or disease-related event relative to the odds of a control patient experiencing the same event.

Overview—A systematic review and summary of the medical literature.

P value—The numeric probability of obtaining a particular or specific result under a given set of circumstances; *P* values are generally (but arbitrarily) considered significant if $P < 0.05$.

Positive predictive value (PPV)—The proportion of patients with a positive test result for a particular disease who actually have the disease.

Posttest probability—The proportion of patients with a particular test result for a disease who actually have the disease (posttest odds/[1 + posttest odds]).

Power—The probability that the mean value of a sample of values resulting from a clinical intervention or other known effect will differ sufficiently from the mean value under the null hypothesis as to allow rejection of the null hypothesis.

Randomized controlled clinical trial—A clinical trial in which a group of patients is separated randomly into an experimental group of patients and a control group of patients. These groups are followed up to determine whether, after a specific intervention, they manifest a particular outcome of interest (**Figure 1**).

Relative risk reduction (RRR)—The percent reduction in the number or frequency of specific events in a treatment group (EER) subtracted from the number or frequency of the same events in a control group (CER).

Sample size—The calculated number of subjects who must participate in a clinical trial or other study to avoid a type I or type II error. See **Table 1**.

Type I error—The probability of rejecting a null hypothesis when it is true. The probability of making a type I error is denoted by the Greek letter α.

Type II error—The probability of failing to reject a null hypothesis that is false. The probability of making a type II error is denoted by the Greek letter β.

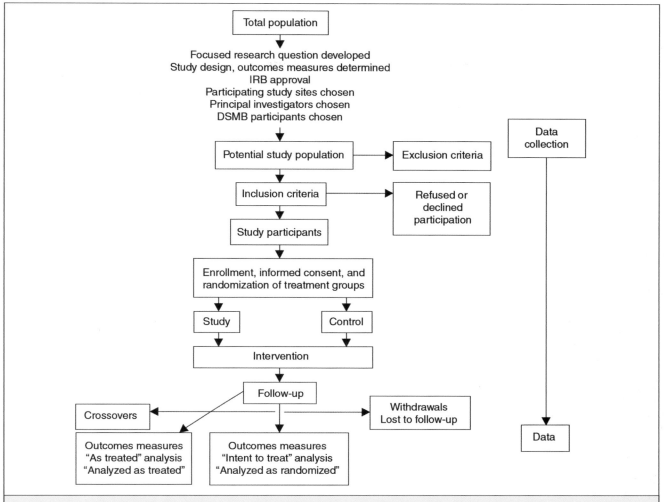

Figure 1   Basic design of a randomized controlled clinical trial. DSMB = Data and Safety Monitoring Board, IRB = Institutional Review Board. (Adapted from Abdu WA: Outcomes assessment and evidence-based practice guidelines in orthopaedic surgery, in Vaccaro AR, ed: *Orthopaedic Knowledge Update*, ed 8. Rosemont, IL, American Academy of Orthopaedic Surgeons, 2005, pp 99-107.)

Table 1

Common Formulas for the Determination of Sample Size

Study Design and Type of Error	Sample Size Formula
Studies using the paired *t* test (before and after studies) with α (type I) error only	$N = \dfrac{(z_a)^2 \cdot (s)^2}{(d)^2}$ = total number of subjects
Studies using the *t* test (randomized controlled trials with one experimental and one control group, considering α error only)	$N = \dfrac{(z_a)^2 \cdot 2 \cdot (s)^2}{(d)^2}$ = number of subjects/group
Studies using the *t* test considering α and β errors	$N = \dfrac{(z_a + z_b)^2 \cdot 2 \cdot (s)^2}{(d)^2}$ = number of subjects/group
Tests of difference in proportions considering α and β errors	$N = \dfrac{(z_a + z_b)^2 \cdot 2 \cdot p(1-p)}{(d)^2}$ = number of subjects/group

N = sample size, z_a = value for α error (equals 1.96 for *P* = 0.05 in two-tailed test), z_b = value for β error (equals 0.84 for 20% β error = 80% power in one-tailed test), $(s)^2$ = variance, p = mean proportion of success, d = smallest clinically important difference to be detected.

Reproduced from Abdu WA: Outcomes assessment and evidence-based practice guidelines in orthopaedic surgery, in Vaccaro AR, ed: *Orthopaedic Knowledge Update*, ed 8. Rosemont, IL, American Academy of Orthopaedic Surgeons, 2005, pp 99-107.

1: Basic Science

Top Testing Facts

1. Evidence-based medicine is the practice of integrating individual clinical expertise with the best available clinical evidence, based on systematic research, for the procedures used in medical practice.

2. Evidence-based practice guidelines serve to assist the practicing orthopaedic surgeon in his or her quest to improve patient care by consolidating the relevant evidence favoring a treatment option and using it to guide a clinical intervention or other procedure.

Bibliography

Bhandari M, Guyatt GH, Swiontkowski MF: User's guide to the orthopaedic literature: how to use an article about a surgical therapy. *J Bone Joint Surg Am* 2001;83(6):916-926.

Bhandari M, Montori VM, Swiontkowski MF, Guyatt GH: User's guide to the surgical literature: How to use an article about a diagnostic test. *J Bone Joint Surg Am* 2003;85(6):1133-1140.

The Cochrane Collaboration: www.cochrane.org.

Evidence JA: Using Evidence to Improve Care. www.jamaevidence.com.

Evidence-Based Medicine Working Group: Evidence-based medicine: A new aproach to teaching the practice of medicine. *JAMA* 1992;268(17):2420-2425.

Greenhalgh T: *How to Read a Paper: The Basics of Evidence-Based Medicine*, ed 3. Malden, MA, Blackwell Publishing, 2006.

Guyatt GH, Haynes RB, Jaeschke RZ, et al: Users' Guides to the Medical Literature: XXV. Evidence-based medicine: Principles for applying Users' Guides to patient care. Evidence-Based Medicine Working Group *JAMA* 2000;284(10):1290-1296.

Guyatt GH, Rennie D, eds: *User's Guides to the Medical Literature: A Manual for Evidence-Based Clinical Practice*, ed 2. Chicago, IL, American Medical Association Press, 2008.

Sackett DL, Richardson WS, Rosenberg WS, Haynes RB, eds: *Evidence-Based Medicine*. London, United Kingdom, Churchill-Livingstone, 1996.

Sackett DL, Rosenberg WM, Gray JA, Haynes RB, Richardson WS: Evidence based medicine: What it is and what it isn't. *BMJ* 1996;312(7023):71-72.

University of Oxford: Center for Evidence Based Medicine. www.cebm.net.

Section 2

General Knowledge

Section Editors:
Kevin J. Bozic, MD, MBA
Richard C. Mather III, MD

Chapter 15
Musculoskeletal Imaging

C. Benjamin Ma, MD   Lynne S. Steinbach, MD

I. Radiography

A. Principles of radiography

1. Radiographic images are obtained by projecting x-ray beams through an object onto an image detector.

2. The image produced is a projectional map of the amount of radiation absorbed by the object along the course of the x-ray beam.

3. The amount of whiteness of the image is a function of the radiodensity and thickness of the object.

4. The denser the object, the more radiation is absorbed, and hence the object appears lighter or whiter. Metal objects and bone are very radiodense and appear white on radiographs.

B. Digital radiography

1. Commonly used now

2. Image processing and distribution are achieved through a picture archiving and communication system.

3. The process allows the images to be portable and transferable via computers or compact discs.

4. Tradeoffs of digital radiography versus conventional film screen radiography

   a. Film screen radiography has higher spatial resolution.

   b. Improved contrast resolution for digital radiography means the technique is comparable in terms of diagnostic efficiency.

Dr. Ma or an immediate family member serves as a paid consultant to or is an employee of Zimmer and Moximed; has received research or institutional support from Wyeth, Histogenics, and Zimmer; and serves as a board member, owner, officer, or committee member of the American Orthopaedic Society for Sports Medicine, the Arthroscopy Association of North America, and the International Society of Arthroscopy, Knee Surgery, and Orthopaedic Sports Medicine. Dr. Steinbach or an immediate family member serves as a board member, owner, officer, or committee member of the International Skeletal Society, the International Society for Magnetic Resonance in Medicine, the Society of Skeletal Radiology, and the Association of University Radiologists.

C. Radiation dose measurements

1. The scientific unit of measurement of radiation dose, commonly referred to as "effective dose," is the millisievert (mSv).

2. Other radiation dose measurement units include the rad, rem, roentgen, and sievert.

D. Radiation exposure

1. Continual from natural sources

2. The average person in the United States receives an effective dose of 3 mSv/y from naturally occurring radioactive materials and cosmic radiation.

3. The mean radiation dose from a standard chest radiograph is 0.1 mSv.

E. Advantages of radiography

1. Most commonly used medical imaging modality

2. Relatively inexpensive

3. Real-time radiographic imaging, or fluoroscopy, allows instantaneous feedback on stress radiographs, angiography, and orthopaedic interventions.

F. Disadvantages of radiography

1. Radiation is transmitted to the patient.

2. It is not effective for soft-tissue imaging because of poor contrast resolution.

3. The images are always magnified. Measurement "standards" can be placed with the object to calculate the magnification.

4. Although most medical x-ray beams do not pose a risk to a fetus, there is a small likelihood that serious illness and developmental problems will occur. The actual risk depends on the type of imaging study and the trimester of pregnancy.

II. Computed Tomography

A. Principles of CT

1. CT uses x-ray beams to produce tomographic images, or slices, of an object.

2: General Knowledge

2. Multiple images are obtained and can be reassembled to generate a three-dimensional image.

3. X-ray densities are measured in Hounsfield units (HUs) or CT numbers.

   a. Water is assigned a value of 0 HU.

   b. Air is assigned a value of –1,000 HU.

4. Images are displayed as grayscale; denser objects are lighter.

5. CT is good for soft-tissue imaging; grayscale can be modified ("windowed") to show data that fall within a fixed range of densities, such as bone windows or lung windows.

B. Advantages of CT

1. The tomographic nature of the images is an advantage.

2. CT has higher contrast resolution than plain radiography

3. The latest generation of CT scanners uses multiple-detector row arrays, which leads to improved resolution and shorter acquisition times.

4. Images are processed digitally; images obtained in planes other than the one in which the original images were obtained can be reconstructed to give a different perspective of the object/tissue of interest.

5. The magnification artifact that occurs in plain radiography is absent in CT, so direct measurements can be performed on the scans.

6. CT imaging can be combined with arthrography or myelography to evaluate specific joint or spinal abnormalities.

7. CT is useful for guiding injections, biopsies, and aspirations.

8. It provides better detail of cortical and trabecular bone structures than does MRI.

C. Disadvantages of CT

1. Subject to motion artifact—This is a possibility because most CT slices require approximately 1 second, which is longer than the time required for a plain radiographic image.

2. Subject to artifact with metal objects

   a. Metal has high x-ray density, which prevents sufficient x-ray beams from being transmitted through the body part.

   b. This results in an artifact called "beam hardening." Beam hardening appears as streaks of white or black that can obscure the anatomy adjacent to the metal object. The kilovolt peak (kVp) and amperage (mA) can be increased to decrease beam hardening, but this creates a greater radiation dose.

3. Impractical for obese patients

   a. Most scanners have a weight limit.

   b. Above the limit, the table that carries the patient through the scanner may not move or may break.

4. CT produces higher radiation exposure than plain radiography. To minimize this, lower dose CT should be used when possible, and unnecessary CT imaging should be avoided.

5. CT is generally contraindicated for pregnant patients, except in life-threatening circumstances.

III. Magnetic Resonance–Based Imaging

A. General principles of MRI

1. MRI is similar to CT in that images are produced by reconstruction of a data set.

2. MRI does not use radiation or have the tissue-damaging properties of radiation-based imaging modalities.

3. MRI uses a strong magnet that generates a magnetic field in which protons line up like compasses. Multiple coils send and/or receive radio-frequency (RF) signals.

4. The strength of the magnet is expressed in tesla (T) units. The stronger the magnet, the higher the intrinsic signal-to-noise ratio, which can improve imaging speed and resolution.

5. All clinical MRI images the protons in hydrogen.

6. A brief RF pulse is applied to the tissue, deflecting the protons. When the pulse is terminated, the protons realign, or relax, along the strong magnetic field, emitting a weak signal. The protons relax at different rates depending on their atomic environment.

7. The signal emitted during relaxation allows the detector to detect the properties within the tissue.

8. Contrast on MRI can be manipulated by changing the pulse sequence parameters. Two important parameters are the repetition time (TR) and the echo time (TE). The most common pulse sequences are T1-weighted and T2-weighted sequences. The T1-weighted sequence uses a short TR and short TE; the T2-weighted sequence uses a long TR and long TE. Different structures are identified more easily on each sequence (**Figure 1** and **Table 1**).

B. Types of MRI machines

1. Conventional

   a. Requires a large room and a small bore

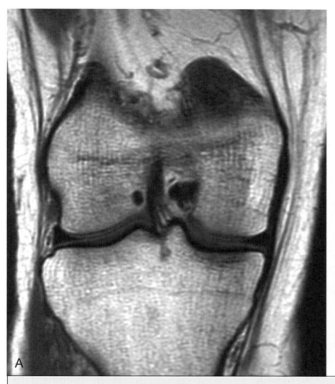 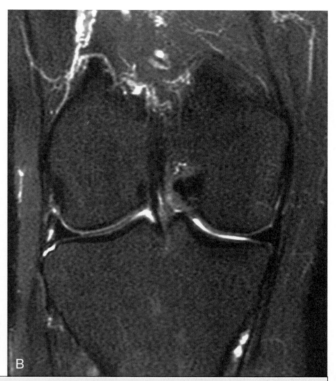

Figure 1 The appearance of different anatomic structures on T1- and T2-weighted coronal MRIs of the knee. **A,** On the T1-weighted image, fat and bone marrow are bright and the menisci and tendon are dark. **B,** On the T2-weighted image, joint fluid and blood vessels are bright in contrast to other structures.

Table 1		

Relative Signal Intensities of Selected Structures on MRI

Structure	T1-Weighted Image	T2-Weighted Image
Fat	Bright	Intermediate
Fluid	Dark	Bright
Bone	Dark	Dark
Ligament	Dark	Dark
Muscle	Intermediate	Dark
Bone marrow edema	Dark	Bright
Fibrocartilage	Dark	Dark
Osteomyelitis	Dark	Bright

b. Has a weight limit for patients

c. Takes longer than CT

d. Patients with claustrophobia may not tolerate the scan well.

2. Open

a. Usually has lower field strength

b. More comfortable for claustrophobic patients

c. Images are of lower quality and provide less resolution than images from conventional closed machines. Open MRI should be used only for larger joints and masses that do not require detail.

3. Extremity MRI machines

a. Image extremities distal to the shoulder and hip

b. Image quality acceptable at 1.0 T and above

c. Useful for patients with claustrophobia and adolescents

C. Magnetic resonance arthrography—Commonly used to augment MRI to diagnose soft-tissue conditions.

1. Two techniques

a. Direct—A dilute gadolinium-containing solution is percutaneously injected into the joint.

b. Indirect—Gadolinium is administered intravenously and allowed to travel through the vascular system to the region of interest.

2. Commonly used for the following:

   a. Diagnosis of labral tears in the shoulder and hip joints

   b. Diagnosis of triangular fibrocartilage complex and ligament tears of the wrist

   c. Evaluation of the collateral ligament in the elbow

   d. Postoperative evaluation of a repaired meniscus

D. Advantages of MRI

   1. Provides superior images of soft tissues such as ligaments, tendons, fibrocartilage, cartilage, muscle, bone marrow, and fat (**Figure 1** and **Table 1**)

   2. Provides tomographic images of the object of interest

   3. Can be more effective than CT at detecting changes in intensity within the bone marrow to diagnose osteomyelitis, malignancy, contusions, occult fractures, and stress fractures

   4. MRI contrast (gadolinium) is safer than iodine-based media.

   5. No radiation to patient

E. Disadvantages of MRI

   1. Prone to large and severe types of artifact

      a. Metal screws, pellets, prostheses, and foreign bodies can produce significant artifact, obscuring anatomic structures.

      b. Metal suppression sequences can be used, but with loss of resolution.

   2. Patient motion can cause significant artifact.

   3. Imaging time is much longer than with CT.

   4. Sedation often is needed for pediatric patients younger than 7 years.

F. Dangers associated with MRI

   1. Because of the strong magnet in the machine, extreme caution is needed when any person (patient, physician, nurse, technician) enters the room. Electrical appliances such as pacemakers and mechanical pumps can malfunction.

   2. Metal objects brought into the scanner can turn into dangerous projectiles.

   3. Metal foreign bodies within the eye or brain can migrate and cause blindness and brain damage. To avoid this, plain radiographs or CT scans of the skull can be obtained prior to MRI.

   4. Patients with metal implants in their joints or body can undergo MRI if the implant is secured in bone or is stable, but discussion with the physician and technician before the scan is important to avoid a potentially disastrous outcome.

   5. MRI is contraindicated in patients with implanted objects such as pacemakers, cochlear implants, and some stents and filters because these devices can malfunction in the magnetic field. It is important to determine which devices can be scanned with MRI and at what field strength. A good resource is MRIsafety.com.

G. Considerations in pregnant women

   1. Although MRI does not use radiation, the effect of RF and magnetic field on the fetus is unknown.

   2. It is usually recommended that a pregnant woman not undergo MRI.

H. Use of gadolinium as contrast

   1. Gadolinium behaves like iodinated contrast media, accumulating in highly vascular and metabolically active tissues.

   2. Gadolinium contrast medium is contraindicated in patients with renal insufficiency because of the risk of irreversible renal damage, known as nephrogenic systemic fibrosis (NSF).

      a. Intravenous gadolinium should not be administered to patients on dialysis or those with an estimated glomerular filtration rate less than 30 mg/dL.

      b. Patients with hepatorenal syndrome and those in the perioperative liver transplantation period are also at high risk for NSF after gadolinium administration.

IV. Ultrasonography

A. Principles of ultrasonography

   1. Ultrasonography uses high-frequency sound waves to produce images, analogous to using sonar waves to obtain images of the ocean. A transducer produces sound waves that travel through the patient; the tissues deflect echo waves back to the same transducer. The echo waves are then analyzed according to the time traveled and amplitude, and the information is converted into an image.

   2. Image resolution and beam attenuation depend on the wavelength and frequency.

   3. A lower frequency ultrasonographic beam has a longer wavelength and less resolution but deeper penetration.

   4. A higher frequency ultrasonographic beam can provide higher resolution images of superficial structures such as tendons and ligaments.

   5. Doppler ultrasonography can be used to image blood vessels for flow velocity and direction.

Color maps can be generated for color Doppler ultrasonography.

B. Advantages of ultrasonography

1. Noninvasive at the frequencies used for diagnostic imaging

2. Commonly used in the imaging of children and pregnant women

3. Shows nonossified structures such as the femoral head; useful to diagnose hip dysplasia and dislocation

4. Equipment is portable and inexpensive compared with MRI and CT equipment.

5. Highly echogenic structures, such as a foreign body that may not be visible on radiographs, can be easily detected using ultrasonography.

6. It can be used to guide targeted therapy, such as injections and ablations. It also is useful to guide injections and aspirations.

7. Provides dynamic assessment of structures (eg, tendon and nerve subluxation)

C. Disadvantages of ultrasonography

1. Image quality and interpretation depend on the experience of the ultrasound technician and the radiologist.

2. Ultrasonography cannot image inside bone because bone cortex reflects almost all sound waves.

3. Internal joint structures are not well visualized unless they are in a superficial location.

V. Nuclear Medicine

A. Principles of nuclear medicine

1. Uses radioisotope-labeled, biologically active drugs

2. The radioactive tracer is administered to the patient to serve as a marker of biologic activity.

3. The images produced by scintigraphy are a collection of the radiation emissions from the isotopes.

B. Bone scintigraphy (bone scan)

1. Generally performed using bisphosphonates labeled with radioactive technetium Tc 99m

2. Phases

a. The initial (transient) phase is characterized by tracer delivery to the tissue, which represents the perfusion images.

b. The second (blood pool) phase follows the initial phase.

c. The final (delayed) phase shows tracer accumulation in tissues with active turnover of phosphates, mostly in bone undergoing growth and turnover.

C. Positron emission tomography (PET)

1. PET using the metabolic tracer fluorodeoxyglucose (FDG) is used widely in clinical oncology.

2. FDG accumulation reflects the rate of glucose utilization in tissue.

a. FDG is transported into tissue by the same mechanisms as glucose transport and is trapped in the tissue as FDG-6-phosphate.

b. Use of FDG in evaluating the musculoskeletal system is based on the increased glycolytic rate observed in pathologic tissues. High-grade malignancies tend to have higher rates of glycolysis than do low-grade malignancies and have greater uptake of FDG than do low-grade or benign lesions.

D. Advantages of nuclear medicine imaging

1. Scintigraphy allows imaging of metabolic activity.

2. Most metabolic processes involving bone have slow metabolic activity compared with soft-tissue organs, such as the kidney and liver. Fortunately, most radioisotopes are relatively long lived.

3. White blood cell scintigraphy can be used to diagnose osteomyelitis.

4. Scintigraphy can be used to diagnose metastasis, stress fracture, or occult fracture.

E. Disadvantages of nuclear medicine imaging

1. Lack of detail and spatial resolution

2. Limited early sensitivity to detect acute fractures in patients with slow bone metabolism; eg, with occult femoral neck fracture, the result of the bone scan may not be positive for several days.

3. May have low sensitivity for lytic bone lesions such as those seen in multiple myeloma and some metastases.

4. Contraindicated in breastfeeding mothers because the nuclear agent can pass from the mother's milk to the child.

VI. Radiation Safety

A. Children and fetuses are especially susceptible to ionizing radiation.

B. Plain radiography, CT, and bone scintigraphy produce ions that can deposit energy in organs and tissues that can damage DNA.

C. Radiation from radioactive-labeled tracers primarily

affects the patient. Some tracers (for example, iodine-131) have a half-life of several days and can concentrate in excreted body fluid and breast milk.

D. Rapidly dividing cells are the most susceptible to radiation-induced neoplasia (**Table 2**). These include cells of the bone marrow, breast tissue, gastrointestinal mucosa, gonads, and lymphatic tissue.

E. The risk of cancer is approximately 4% per sievert (100 rem).

F. Effect on fetus

1. The risk of fetal malformation is greatest in the first trimester and with doses higher than 0.1 Gy (10 rad).

2. Late in pregnancy (≥150 days postconception), the greatest risk is an increase in childhood malignancies such as leukemia. A 10-mGy (1-rad) dose increases childhood leukemia risk as much as 40% (**Table 2**).

3. It is important to ascertain that the patient is not pregnant when obtaining any imaging examinations other than ultrasonography.

G. Protection

1. Sensitive organs such as gonads should be shielded.

2. The principle of "as low as reasonably achievable" (ALARA) dosing is recommended for children and pregnant women.

3. Radiation exposure decreases as an inverse square of the distance from the source.

4. Medical personnel should wear lead aprons and should be monitored using devices such as film badges.

Table 2

Threshold Acute Exposure Doses for Effects in Humans

Organ Exposed	Dose (in Gy)	Effect
Ocular lens	2	Cataracts
Bone marrow	2-7	Marrow failure with infection, death
Skin	3	Temporary hair loss
Skin	5	Erythema
Testes	5-6	Permanent decrease in sperm count
Skin	7	Permanent hair loss
Intestines	7-50	Gastrointestinal failure, death
Brain	50-100	Cerebral edema, death

Adapted from Radiation safety, in Johnson TR, Steinbach LS, eds: *Essentials of Musculoskeletal Imaging.* Rosemont, IL, American Academy of Orthopaedic Surgeons, 2004, p 28.

5. CT delivers the highest radiation dose of all medical imaging procedures (5 to 15 mSv versus 0.1 to 2.0 mSv for plain radiography). CT should not be ordered unless necessary. Caution should be exercised when ordering multiple CTs at different times for the same patient.

Top Testing Facts

1. All clinical MRIs image the protons in hydrogen atoms.

2. Patients must be screened for metallic objects before entering the MRI machine. Ferromagnetic objects in or on the body can be pulled toward the magnet and cause serious injuries.

3. Patients with advanced kidney failure should not receive gadolinium-containing contrast agents because exposure to the agent can cause NSF.

4. Lower frequency ultrasonography beam has a longer wavelength and less resolution but deeper penetration.

5. A higher frequency ultrasonography beam can give higher resolution for superficial structures such as tendons and ligaments.

6. Caution is advised when ordering nuclear medicine tests for women who are breastfeeding; some of the pharmaceuticals can pass into the mother's milk and subsequently into the child.

7. Risk of cancer from radiation is approximately 4% per sievert (100 rem). It is important to practice ALARA.

8. Exposure to radiation decreases as an inverse square of the distance from the source.

9. CT delivers the highest radiation dosage of all imaging modalities.

10. It is important to ensure that the patient is not pregnant when obtaining any imaging examinations other than ultrasonography. The decision to order other imaging modalities should be made in consultation with the radiologist and physician.

Bibliography

Brent RL, Gorson RO: Radiation exposure in pregnancy, in *Current Problems in Radiology: Technic of Pneumoencephalography.* Chicago, IL, Year Book Medical, 1972.

Committee on the Biological Effects of Ionizing Radiations, Board on Radiation Effects Research, Commission on Life Sciences, National Research Council: *Health Effects of Exposure to Low Levels of Ionizing Radiation: BEIR V.* Washington, DC, National Academy Press, 1990.

Johnson TR, Steinbach LS, eds: Imaging modalities, in *Essentials of Musculoskeletal Imaging.* Rosemont, IL, American Academy of Orthopaedic Surgeons, 2003, pp 3-30.

Ohashi K, El-Khoury GY, Menda Y: Musculoskeletal imaging, in Flynn JM, ed: *Orthopaedic Knowledge Update*, ed 10. Rosemont, IL, American Academy of Orthopaedic Surgeons, 2011, pp 85-107.

2: General Knowledge

Chapter 16

Coagulation and Thromboembolism

Jared Foran, MD   Craig J. Della Valle, MD

I. Coagulopathies

A. Coagulation cascade

1. The coagulation cascade is a series of enzymatic reactions that lead to the eventual formation of fibrin.

2. Fibrin forms a lattice that traps platelets to form a clot and stem bleeding (**Figure 1**).

3. Each step in the cascade involves the activation of a clotting factor that, in turn, activates the next step in the cascade.

4. There are two pathways for the initiation of clot formation, the intrinsic and extrinsic pathways.

   a. Intrinsic pathway

      • Activated by the exposure of collagen from the subendothelium of damaged blood vessels to factor XII

      • Measured using the partial thromboplastin time (PTT)

   b. Extrinsic pathway

      • Activated by the release of thromboplastin (via cell damage) into the circulatory system

      • Measured by prothrombin time (PT)

   c. Platelet dysfunction can be identified by prolongation of the bleeding time.

Dr. Della Valle or an immediate family member serves as a paid consultant to or is an employee of Biomet, Convatec, and Smith & Nephew; or an immediate family member has stock or stock options held in CD Diagnostics; or an immediate family member has received research or institutional support from Smith & Nephew and Stryker; and or an immediate family member serves as a board member, owner, officer, or committee member of the American Association of Hip and Knee Surgeons, the Arthritis Foundation, and the Knee Society. Neither Dr. Foran nor any immediate family member has received anything of value from or has stock or stock options held in a commercial company or institution related directly or indirectly to the subject of this chapter.

B. Fibrinolytic system

1. The fibrinolytic system acts to stem clot formation and maintain vascular patency.

2. The key step is the formation of active plasmin from plasminogen.

3. Plasminogen dissolves fibrin.

4. Tranexamic acid

   a. Synthetic derivative of the amino acid lysine

   b. Competitive inhibitor of plasminogen

   c. Interferes with fibrinolysis

      • Decreases postoperative bleeding in total knee arthroplasty (TKA) and total hip arthroplasty (THA)

      • Decreases postoperative transfusion rates

      • Does not appear to increase risk of deep vein thrombosis (DVT) or pulmonary embolism (PE)

      • No effect on PTT or PT

C. Hemophilia

1. Hereditary deficiency that leads to abnormal bleeding (**Table 1**)

2. Recurrent hemarthrosis and resultant synovitis of the large joints can lead to joint destruction (the knee is the most commonly affected joint).

3. Treatment options

   a. Initial treatment consists of factor replacement, aspiration, initial splinting, and physical therapy.

   b. If bleeding continues despite prophylactic factor infusion, radioisotope or arthroscopic synovectomy is indicated if the cartilaginous surfaces are relatively preserved.

   c. TKA in patients with hemophilia can be complex secondary to severe preoperative stiffness and contracture.

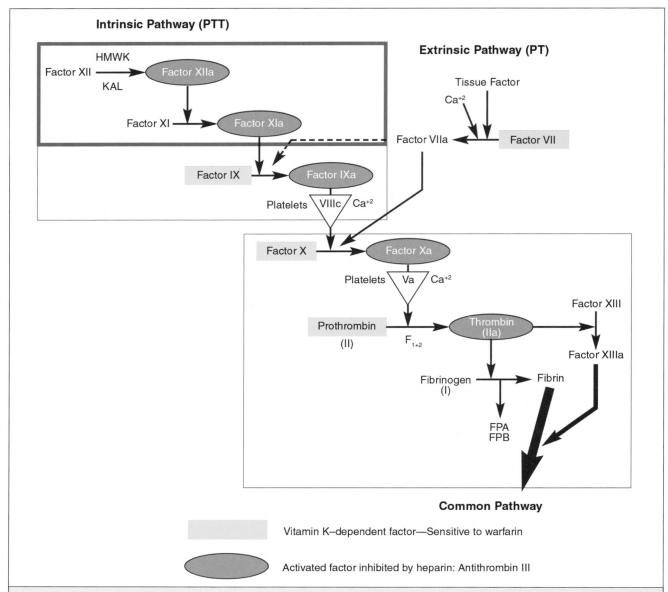

Figure 1   The coagulation pathways. PT measures the function of the extrinsic and common pathways, whereas PTT measures the function of the intrinsic and common pathways. HMWK = high-molecular-weight kininogen; KAL = kallikrein; FPA = fibrinopeptide A; FPB = fibrinopeptide B. (Adapted with permission from Stead RB: Regulation of hemostasis, in Goldhaber SZ, ed: *Pulmonary Embolism and Deep Venous Thrombosis*. Philadelphia, PA, WB Saunders, 1985, p 32.)

4. These patients are at high risk for infection because of:

  a. Insufficient hemostasis

  b. High incidence of HIV positivity

  c. Increased use of central venous catheters

5. Use of factor replacement

  a. If surgical intervention is planned, intravenous factor replacement is required to maintain factor levels of 100% immediately preoperatively, for 3 to 5 days postoperatively for soft-tissue

procedures, and for 3 to 4 weeks postoperatively for bony procedures such as THA and TKA.

  b. Although plasma derivatives were commonly used for factor replacement in the past (associated with a high risk of infection with blood-borne pathogens such as hepatitis and HIV), recombinant derived factor currently is used.

6. Inhibitors-circulating antibodies that neutralize factor VIII or IX

Table 1

Factor Deficiencies Causing Bleeding Disorders

Factor	Disease	Frequency	Inheritance
VII	Hemophilia A	1:5,000 males	X-linked recessive
IX	Hemophilia B (Christmas disease)	1:30,000 males	X-linked recessive
XI	Hemophilia C	1:100,000 males	Autosomal dominant
I	Fibrinogen deficiency	1-2:1,000,000	Autosomal recessive
II	Prothrombin deficiency	1:2,000,000	Autosomal recessive
V	Parahemophilia	1:1,000,000	Autosomal recessive
VII	Alexander disease	1:500,000	Autosomal recessive
X	Factor X deficiency	1:500,000	Autosomal recessive
XII	Hageman factor deficiency	1:1,000,000	Autosomal recessive
XIII	Fibrin stabilizing factor deficiency	1:5,000,000	Autosomal recessive

a. These antibodies are suspected when a patient fails to respond to increasing doses of factor replacement.

b. Diagnosis is confirmed via an in vitro assay, whereby the addition of normal plasma or factor concentrate fails to correct a prolonged PTT.

c. Although they previously were considered a contraindication to elective surgery, presently they can be overwhelmed to counteract the effect of the inhibitor.

D. von Willebrand disease

1. von Willebrand disease is a collection of genetic coagulopathies secondary to a deficiency of von Willebrand factor (vWF).

2. Role of vWF

   a. Integral to normal platelet adhesion and to the functioning of factor VIII

   b. Normally found in platelets and in the vascular endothelium

3. Types of deficiencies

   a. Type 1 (quantitative; decreased vWF levels)—A milder form that presents as heavy menstrual bleeding or excessive bleeding from the gums, easy bruising, or excessive surgical bleeding

   b. Type 2 (qualitative; abnormal vWF)

   c. Type 3 (quantitative; no vWF produced)—The most severe form of the disease, which is very rare (1 in 500,000)

4. Diagnosis is made via measuring the bleeding time, factor VIII activity, and both quantitative and qualitative tests for vWF.

5. Treatment

   a. Desmopressin, usually administered via a nasal spray, works via increased endogenous release of vWF from vascular endothelium.

   b. Factor VIII concentrates combined with vWF may be required in patients with more severe deficiencies (types 2 and 3).

E. Coagulopathies

1. Coagulopathies are caused by high blood loss secondary to major trauma or extended surgical procedures.

2. Fluid volume and packed red blood cells must be replaced.

3. The need for platelet and fresh frozen plasma transfusion must be assessed by monitoring platelet counts and coagulation parameters.

II. Venous Thromboembolic Disease

A. Pathophysiology—DVT is the end result of a complex interaction of events including activation of the clotting cascade and platelet aggregation.

B. Virchow triad (predisposing factors)

1. Venous stasis

   a. Impaired mobility

   b. Intraoperative vascular congestion

2. Endothelial damage secondary to injury or surgical trauma

3. Hypercoagulability

   a. Release of tissue factors and procoagulants

2: General Knowledge

Table 2

Risk Factors for Thromboembolic Disease

History of prior thromboembolic event
Advanced age
Obesity
Malignant disease
Genetic hypercoagulable state
Oral contraceptive use
Pregnancy
Extended immobilization
Major orthopaedic surgery
History of myocardial infarction/stroke/congestive heart failure

(such as collagen fragments, fibrinogen, and tissue thromboplastin)

b. Large release of thrombogenic factors during preparation of the femur during THA, particularly if a cemented femoral component is used

C. Epidemiology and risk factors

1. Without prophylaxis, patients with a proximal femur fracture have a reported prevalence of fatal PE of as high as 7%.

2. Patients undergoing elective THA and TKA have historically been described as having rates of symptomatic PE without prophylaxis of up to 20% and 8%, respectively; it is unclear what the risk is with contemporary surgical techniques and perioperative pathways.

3. Patients undergoing TKA seem to be at higher risk for the development of venographically identified DVT, but at lower risk of symptomatic PE than patients with THA.

4. Risk factors for venous thromboembolism (VTE) (Table 2)

   a. May have a cumulative effect; a combination of risk factors present in a given patient may greatly increase the risk.

   b. Patients with a prior history of a thromboembolic event deserve special attention, given the numerous inherited hypercoagulable states (such as factor V Leiden) that have recently been identified. Preoperative consultation with a hematologist may be appropriate.

III. Prophylaxis

A. Given the high risk of VTE in patients undergoing major orthopaedic surgery, the difficulty in diagnosing these events, and their potential for morbidity and mortality (approximately two thirds of patients who sustain a fatal PE die within 60 minutes of the development of symptoms), some form of prophylaxis is often necessary.

B. The optimal duration of prophylaxis is unclear; however, patients may be at risk for VTE for several weeks postoperatively.

C. CHEST Guidelines for patients undergoing major orthopaedic surgery (THA, TKA, and hip fracture surgery) (Table 3)

1. The latest version of the American College of Chest Physicians clinical practice guidelines were published in 2012 and are now more similar to the American Academy of Orthopaedic Surgeons (AAOS) guidelines with more of an emphasis on agent safety.

2. Low-dose aspirin is now considered an acceptable form of prophylaxis, although there still is a preference for low-molecular-weight heparin (LMWH) as prophylaxis (however, this is a weaker recommendation).

3. Many of the changes made because the committee did not base its recommendations on venographic screening of asymptomatic patients (which had been used heavily in the past).

D. AAOS guidelines for patients undergoing TKA or THA (2011)

1. There is no specific recommendation for any particular agent or dosing regimen for prophylaxis because it was thought that the current literature could not support one regimen over any other with the network meta-analysis that was used to examine the literature.

2. Strong recommendation

   a. Recommend against routine postoperative duplex ultrasonography screening

3. Moderate recommendation

   a. Suggest the use of pharmacologic and/or mechanical compression devices for patients who are not at risk for VTE or bleeding beyond that of the surgery itself. There is no specific recommendation for any one agent because the available evidence was thought to be inadequate to distinguish among agents.

4. Weak recommendation

   a. Patients undergoing elective TKA and THA are already at high risk for VTE. The practitioner might further assess the risk of VTE by de-

Table 3

Highlights: Prevention of Venous Thromboembolism in Orthopaedic Surgery. American College of Chest Physicians Evidence-based Clinical Practice Guidelines, Ninth Edition

2.1.1	In patients undergoing THA or TKA we recommend use of one of the following for a minimum of 10 to 14 days rather than no antithrombotic prophylaxis: LMWH, fondaparinux, apixaban, dabigatran, rivaroxaban, LDUH, adjusted-dose VKA, aspirin (all grade 1B), or an IPCD (grade 1C)
2.2	For patients undergoing major orthopaedic surgery (THA, TKA, HFS) and receiving LMWH as thromboprophylaxis, we recommend starting either 12 h or more preoperatively or 12 h or more postoperatively rather than within 4 h or less preoperatively or 4 h or less postoperatively (grade 1B)
2.3.1	In patients undergoing THA or TKA, irrespective of the concomitant use of an IPCD or length of treatment, we suggest the use of LMWH in reference to the other agents we have recommended as alternatives: fondaparinux, apixaban, dabigatran, rivaroxaban, LDUH (all grade 2B), adjusted-dose VKA, or aspirin (all grade 2C)
2.4	For patients undergoing major orthopaedic surgery, we suggest extending thromboprophylaxis in the outpatient period for up to 35 days from the day of surgery rather than for only 10 to 14 days (grade 2B)
2.5	In patients undergoing major orthopaedic surgery, we suggest using dual prophylaxis with an antithrombotic agent and an IPCD during the hospital stay (grade 2C)
2.6	In patients undergoing major orthopaedic surgery and increased risk of bleeding, we suggest using an IPCD or no prophylaxis rather than pharmacologic treatment (grade 2C)
2.8	In patients undergoing major orthopaedic surgery, we suggest against using filter placement for primary prevention over no thromboprophylaxis in patients with an increased bleeding risk or contraindications to both pharmacologic and mechanical thromboprophylaxis (grade 2C)
2.9	For asymptomatic patients following major orthopaedic surgery, we recommend against Doppler (or duplex) ultrasound screening before hospital discharge (grade 1B)

HFS = hip fracture surgery, IPCD = intermittent pneumatic compression device, IVC = inferior vena cava, LDUH = low-dose unfractionated heparin, LMWH = low-molecular-weight heparin, THA = total hip arthroplasty, TKA = total knee arthroplasty, VKA = vitamin K antagonist.

Lieberman JR: Guest editorial: American College of Chest Physicians evidence-based guidelines for venous thromboembolic prophylaxis. The guideline wars are over. *J Am Acad Orthop Surg* 2012;20(6):333-335.

terming whether patients had a previous VTE.

5. Consensus recommendations ("absence of reliable evidence")

a. Assess patients undergoing elective TKA or THA for known bleeding disorders and for the presence of active liver disease.

b. Physicians and patients should discuss the duration of prophylaxis.

c. Patients undergoing elective TKA or THA who have had previous VTE should receive pharmacologic and mechanical prophylaxis.

d. Patients undergoing elective TKA or THA who have a known bleeding disorder or active liver disease should receive mechanical prophylaxis only.

e. Patients undergoing elective TKA or THA should undergo early mobilization.

6. Inconclusive recommendations ("current evidence not clear")

a. Do not recommend for or against assessing for VTE risk factors other than a history of previ-

ous VTE for elective TKA or THA.

b. Do not recommend for or against assessing for bleeding risk factors other than known bleeding disorder or active liver disease for elective TKA or THA.

c. Do not recommend for or against specific prophylactic strategy in patients undergoing elective TKA or THA and who are not at elevated risk for VTE or bleeding beyond that of the surgery itself.

d. Do not recommend for or against inferior vena cava (IVC) filters in patients undergoing elective TKA or THA who also have a contraindication to chemoprophylaxis and/or known residual venous thromboembolic disease.

E. Mechanical approaches

1. Sequential compression devices

a. Act via increasing peak venous flow to decrease venous stasis

b. Stimulate the fibrinolytic system

c. Present no risk of bleeding

Table 4

Pharmacologic Agents for Thromboembolic Prophylaxis

Agent	Site of Action	Metabolism	Reversal Agent
UFH	Antithrombin III, IIA, XA	Hepatic	Protamine sulfate
LMWH	Antithrombin III, Xa>IIa	Renal	Protamine sulfate (partial)
Fondaparinux	Xa	Renal	None
Warfarin	II,VII,IX,X (vitamin K antagonist)	Hepatic	Vitamin K, FFP
Aspirin	Platelets (COX inhibitor)	Hepatic	Platelets
Rivaroxaban	Xa	Hepatic	Prothrombin complex concentrate (Under study)

UFH = unfractionated heparin, LMWH = low molecular-weight heparin, FFP = Fresh frozen plasma, COX = cyclo-oxygenase.

d. Poor patient compliance and/or inappropriate application are common.

e. Good efficacy has been shown in patients who undergo TKA.

2. Plantar compression devices

a. Compression of the venous plexus of the foot produces pulsatile flow in the deep venous system of the leg (simulates walking).

b. Inadequate data are available to recommend these devices alone.

3. Graduated compression stockings

a. These stockings produce a pressure differential between the distal and proximal portions of the lower extremity, decreasing venous stasis.

b. These stockings should be a useful adjunct only and not as the sole means of prophylaxis.

4. Prophylactic IVC filters

a. IVC filters are retrievable devices that are typically placed before surgery and then electively removed 10 to 14 days later.

b. Indications

• Patients who require surgery in the context of a recent thromboembolic event

• Critically ill multiple-trauma patients (relative indication)

• May be considered in patients at high risk for VTE (for example, those with a hereditary hypercoagulable state). Consultation with a hematologist is useful for these patients.

F. Pharmacologic approaches (**Table 4**)

1. Unfractionated heparin (UFH)

a. Binds to antithrombin III, potentiating its in-hibitory effect on thrombin (factor IIa) and factor Xa

b. Higher risk of bleeding and lower efficacy than low-molecular-weight heparin (LMWH)

c. Increased risk of heparin-induced thrombocytopenia (HIT), which is secondary to heparin-dependent antibodies that activate platelets

d. Fixed, low-dose heparin (5,000 U administered subcutaneously twice daily) generally is not effective in orthopaedic patients.

e. Reversed using protamine sulfate

2. Low-molecular-weight heparin

a. LMWH is derived from the fractionation of UFH into smaller, more homogenous molecules.

b. LMWH is unable to bind both antithrombin III and thrombin simultaneously and thus have a greater inhibitory effect on factor Xa than factor IIa (thrombin).

c. Provides superior protection against DVT and does not inhibit hemostasis as vigorously at surgical sites as compared to UFH

d. Less inhibition of platelet function and less vascular permeability than UFH

e. Improved bioavailability (90% versus 35% for UFH)

f. Longer half-life (less frequent dosing)

g. Laboratory monitoring is not required.

h. First full dose 12 to 24 hours postoperatively or until hemostasis obtained at the operative site

i. Should not be used in conjunction with an indwelling epidural catheter or in patients who have had a traumatic neuraxial anesthetic placed (secondary to a risk of epidural bleed-

Table 5

Common Drug Interactions With Warfarin

Trimethoprim-sulfamethoxazole (Bactrim or Septra)
Rifampin
Macrolide antibiotics (such as erythromycin)
Quinolone antibiotics (such as ciprofloxacin)
Metronidazole (Flagyl)
Certain cephalosporins (such as cefamandole)
Thyroid hormones (such as levothyroxine)
Phenytoin (Dilantin)
Cimetidine (Tagamet)
Antiarrhythmic drugs (such as amiodarone)
Herbal medications (such as garlic)

ing). Neuraxial anesthesia can be performed 12 hours after administration of LMWH.

    j. Compared to warfarin, LMWH is associated with a decreased risk of venographically identified DVT, but a higher risk of bleeding complications.

    k. Excretion is primarily renal and thus dosing needs to be adjusted in patients with chronic renal failure.

    l. Several agents are presently available, and pharmacokinetics, dosing, and outcomes differ among agents.

3. Fondaparinux

    a. Synthetic pentasaccharide and an indirect factor Xa inhibitor

    b. Dosing is 2.5 mg/d subcutaneously; first dose is given 6 to 12 hours postoperatively.

    c. Decreased incidence of venographically identified DVT compared with enoxaparin in patients with hip fracture and TKA

    d. Trend toward an increased risk of bleeding complications

    e. Not recommended for patients who weigh less than 50 kg or those with renal insufficiency; has not been used in conjunction with indwelling epidural catheters

4. Warfarin

    a. Antagonizes vitamin K, which prevents the γ-carboxylation of glutamic acid required for the synthesis of factors II, VII, IX, and X and proteins C and S.

    b. Typical dosing regimens start on the night of surgery, as soon as the patient can tolerate oral pain medication.

    c. The anticoagulant effect is delayed for 24 to 36 hours after the initiation of therapy, and the target International Normalized Ratio (INR) is often not achieved until 3 days postoperatively.

    d. The target level of anticoagulation has been controversial; however, a target INR of 2.0 is appropriate for orthopaedic patients.

    e. Warfarin interacts with many other medications that can augment its effect (**Table 5**).

    f. Not recommended for use in conjunction with NSAIDs, secondary to a higher risk of bleeding at the surgical and nonsurgical sites (particularly gastrointestinal bleeding)

    g. Patients who ingest large amounts of vitamin K-rich foods (for example, green, leafy vegetables) may require increased doses to achieve the target INR.

    h. Reversible with vitamin K administration; complete reversal can take several days. Fresh frozen plasma is given if immediate reversal is required.

5. Aspirin

    a. Aspirin irreversibly binds to and inactivates cyclo-oxygenase (COX) in both developing and circulating platelets, which blocks the production of thromboxane A2, the necessary prostaglandin for platelet aggregation.

    b. The role of aspirin when used alone as a prophylactic agent is controversial given lower efficacy compared with other agents when venographic evidence of DVT is used as an end point, but is now considered acceptable by both AAOS and CHEST guidelines.

    c. Pulmonary Embolism Prevention Trial. A randomized, double-blind study of aspirin versus placebo in hip fracture and elective TKA and THA (more than 17,000 patients), which showed that aspirin reduced the risk of fatal PE and symptomatic nonfatal DVT and PE.

    d. When combined with neuraxial anesthetics and particularly hypotensive epidural techniques, aspirin seems to be associated with a lower risk of postoperative thromboembolic events secondary to enhanced blood flow in the lower extremities.

    e. Data exist to support prolonged prophylaxis (up to 35 days) in patients who have had THA but prolonged prophylaxis has not been shown to have an effect in patients who have had TKA.

6. Rivaroxaban

    a. Factor Xa inhibitor

b. Daily dosing starting 12 to 24 hours postoperatively

- 12 days for TKA, 35 days for THA

c. Prothrombin complex concentrate as a reversal agent is under study. It appears to be effective; however, more data are needed.

d. Advantages—oral administration, fixed daily dosing, monitoring not required

e. Disadvantages—bleeding risks, reversal agent poorly defined, cost (moderate)

7. Apixaban

a. Factor Xa inhibitor

b. Twice daily dosing starting 12 to 24 hours postoperatively. 12 ± 3 days for TKA and 35 ± 3 days for THA.

c. Advantages: Oral administration, fixed oral dosing (bid), monitoring not required

d. Disadvantages: Bleeding risks, reversal agent poorly defined, cost

8. Dabigatran

a. Direct thrombin inhibitor

b. Oral administration

c. Not currently FDA approved for orthopaedic use

IV. Diagnosis of Thromboembolic Events

A. Approach to diagnosing thromboembolism

1. No clinical signs are specific for diagnosis of DVT or PE.

2. Calf pain, swelling, and pain on forced dorsiflexion of the foot (Homan sign) are common in the perioperative period secondary to postoperative pain, swelling, and abnormal gait patterns leading to muscular strain.

B. Initial patient evaluation

1. Chest radiograph to rule out alternative causes of hypoxia such as pneumonia, congestive heart failure, and atelectasis

2. Electrocardiogram (ECG) to rule out cardiac pathology; tachycardia is the most common ECG finding in PE, although a right ventricular strain pattern can be seen.

3. Arterial blood gas measurements on room air

4. Assessing oxygenation

a. Most patients are hypoxic (P_{AO2} <80mm Hg), hypocapnic (P_{ACO2} <35 mm Hg) and have a high A-a gradient (>20 mm Hg).

b. The A-a gradient (pulmonary alveolar-arterial oxygen gradient; indicative of poor gas exchange between the alveolus and arterial blood supply) can be calculated as (150–1.25[P_{ACO2}])–P_{AO2}.

c. Pulse oximetry is not an adequate alternative to arterial blood gas measurements on room air; patients can hyperventilate to maintain adequate oxygenation.

5. Ventilation/perfusion (V/Q) scanning

a. V/Q scanning has been the standard of care for diagnosing PE for many years.

b. Scans are compared to identify "mismatch defects," which are areas that are ventilated without associated perfusion.

c. Graded as normal, low, intermediate, or high probability based on criteria determined from prior studies that compared V/Q scans and pulmonary angiograms

- Patients with normal or low-probability scans should be evaluated for alternative sources of hypoxemia (particularly if a search for lower extremity DVT is negative).

- Patients with high-probability scans require treatment.

- If the scan is intermediate and clinical suspicion is high, the lower extremities should be assessed for DVT; if negative, a high resolution chest CT or pulmonary angiogram is indicated to rule out PE.

6. High-resolution (helical or spiral) chest CT angiography

a. Recently widely adopted as the first-line study for diagnosing PE, given the high rate of indeterminate V/Q scans and the accuracy of this technique compared to other imaging modalities

b. Advantage—Ability to identify alternative diagnosis if no PE is identified

c. Requires contrast

d. Radiation dose can be a concern in certain patient populations (for example, pregnant women).

e. Sensitivity may be such that high rates of smaller, peripheral emboli are identified that are not clinically relevant, leading to overtreatment.

7. Pulmonary angiography

a. Pulmonary angiography is considered the "gold standard" for diagnosing PE.

b. It is both expensive and invasive and therefore

is rarely used in clinical practice.

8. Duplex ultrasonography

a. Noninvasive, simple, and inexpensive

b. Accuracy has been shown to be operator dependent.

c. Accurate in diagnosis of symptomatic proximal clots. Ability to visualize veins in the calf and pelvis is limited.

d. Routine screening for DVT before hospital discharge has not been shown to be cost-effective.

9. Lower extremity contrast venography

a. Still considered the gold standard for diagnosing lower extremity DVT

b. Expensive and invasive; therefore, rarely used in clinical practice

10. D-dimer testing

a. D-dimer testing can be used as an adjunct to diagnosing thromboembolic events.

b. Elevated D-dimer levels indicate a high level of fibrin degradation products (which also can be seen following a recent surgery).

c. A low D-dimer level indicates a low risk for DVT (high negative predictive value).

C. Approach to diagnosing PE

1. PE is difficult to diagnose based on classic symptoms of dyspnea and pleuritic chest pain, because these are rarely seen.

2. Vague symptoms such as cough, palpitations, and apprehension or confusion are common.

3. The most common sign seen in diagnosed PE is tachypnea followed by tachycardia and fever; therefore, even vague signs and symptoms require a thorough evaluation.

4. If chest radiograph and ECG do not point to an alternative diagnosis, a D-dimer level can be obtained; if it is negative, the likelihood of PE is low.

5. Depending on availability, chest CT or ventilation/perfusion scan is obtained.

6. If the ventilation/perfusion scan is low or intermediate probability and clinical suspicion is high, duplex ultrasonography of the lower extremities can be used.

7. If the ultrasound is negative and suspicion is still high, pulmonary angiography can be used to determine the presence or absence of PE.

D. Treatment of a thromboembolic event

1. Continuous intravenous heparin for at least 5 days, followed by oral warfarin. LMWH is now

commonly used because it is easy to administer and the patient may not need to be admitted to the hospital.

a. It prevents clot propagation while allowing the fibrinolytic system to dissolve clots that have already formed.

b. It decreases mortality in these patients compared to patients who have no anticoagulation.

c. Risk of bleeding at the surgical site has been related to supratherapeutic levels of anticoagulation and initiation of therapy within 48 hours after surgery.

d. Intravenous heparin therapy is adjusted to maintain a goal PTT of 1.5 to 2.5 times the control value for 5 days.

e. Avoiding the use of a bolus dose of intravenous heparin in the early postoperative period can reduce bleeding.

f. Warfarin is initiated with a target INR of 2.0 to 3.0 maintained for a minimum of 3 months, but oftentimes it is administered for 6 months. Further extended therapy may be required in patients with recurrent PE or a heritable coagulopathy.

2. In patients who have sustained a PE, elective surgery should not be considered for at least 3 months after the event, and a thorough evaluation is needed to ensure that the clot has resorbed and that residual effects (such as pulmonary hypertension) are not present.

3. LMWH is an alternative to intravenous UFH therapy (dosed at 1mg/kg administered subcutaneously twice daily).

a. LMWH has more predictable onset, but is associated with the potential for a higher risk of bleeding at the surgical site.

b. Although commonly used to treat orthopaedic patients, no studies to date have specifically examined the use of LMWH for the treatment of diagnosed thromboembolic events in patients who have had orthopaedic surgery.

4. IVC filters

a. Indications (controversial; see aforementioned CHEST and AAOS recommendations)

• Patients who have sustained a thromboembolic event despite adequate prophylactic anticoagulation

• Patients with poor cardiopulmonary reserve and at high risk for further morbidity and mortality if clot extension or recurrence occurs.

b. Emboli can recur as small emboli that pass through the filter, as collateral circulation develops, or as propagation of a large thrombus above the filter.

c. Complications include insertional problems, distal migration or tilting, vena cava occlusion (which can lead to severe lower extremity swelling and rarely complete venous outflow obstruction), and vena cava or aortic perforation.

d. In current practice, the IVC filter is often retrieved within 3 weeks, but certain designs allow for retrieval up to 1 year postinsertion.

5. DVT isolated to the calf is rarely associated with PE; proximal extension can occur in 10% to 20% of patients. In isolated calf vein thrombosis, serial ultrasonography can be performed and anticoagulant treatment withheld unless proximal extension is identified.

Top Testing Facts

1. Tranexamic acid, a synthetic derivative of the amino acid lysine, acts as a competitive inhibitor of plasminogen and interferes with fibrinolysis.

2. LMWH and rivaroxaban inhibit factor Xa activity.

3. Fondaparinux is a synthetic pentasaccharide and an indirect inhibitor of factor X activity.

4. Both LMWH and fondaparinux are metabolized in the kidneys, and warfarin and rivaroxaban are metabolized primarily in the liver.

5. Patients undergoing major elective orthopaedic surgery such as hip and knee arthroplasty and those who have sustained multiple trauma and proximal femoral fractures are at high risk for thromboembolic events.

6. The diagnosis of thromboembolic events can be difficult to make postoperatively; clinical signs and symptoms are unreliable.

7. Initial evaluation of the patient suspected of PE includes an arterial blood gas on room air, a chest radiograph, and ECG to rule out an alternative diagnosis.

8. Pulse oximetry is not an adequate alternative to arterial blood gas measurements on room air because patient hyperventilation can maintain adequate oxygenation.

9. Treatment of thromboembolic events with intravenous heparin or LMWH followed by oral warfarin is effective at reducing morbidity and mortality.

Bibliography

Alshryda S, Sarda P, Sukeik M, Nargol A, Blenkinsopp J, Mason JM: Tranexamic acid in total knee replacement: A systematic review and meta-analysis. *J Bone Joint Surg Br* 2011; 93(12):1577-1585.

Colwell CW, Hardwick ME: Venous thromboembolic disease and prophylaxis in total joint arthroplasty, in Barrack RL, Booth RE, Lonner JH, McCarthy JC, Mont MA, Rubash HE, eds: *Orthopaedic Knowledge Update: Hip & Knee Reconstruction*, ed 3. Rosemont, IL, American Academy of Orthopaedic Surgeons, 2006, pp 233-240.

Conduah AH, Lieberman JR: Thromboembolism and pulmonary distress in the setting of orthopaedic surgery, in Einhorn TA, O'Keefe RJ, Buckwalter JA, eds: *Orthopaedic Basic Science: Foundations of Clinical Practice*, ed 3. Rosemont, IL, American Academy of Orthopaedic Surgeons, 2007, pp 105-113.

Della Valle CJ, Mirzabeigi E, Zuckerman JD, Koval KJ: Thromboembolic prophylaxis for patients with a fracture of the proximal femur. *Am J Orthop (Belle Mead NJ)* 2002; 31(1):16-24.

Falck-Ytter Y, Francis CW, Johanson NA, et al: Prevention of VTE in orthopedic surgery patients: Antithrombotic Therapy and Prevention of Thrombosis, 9th ed. American College of Chest Physicians Evidence-Based Clinical Practice Guidelines. *Chest* 2012;141(2 Suppl):e278S-e325S.

Friedman RJ: Novel oral anticoagulants for VTE prevention in orthopedic surgery: Overview of phase 3 trials. *Orthopedics* 2011;34(10):795-804.

Geerts WH, Pineo GF, Heit JA, et al: Prevention of venous thromboembolism: The seventh ACCP conference on antithrombotic and thrombolytic therapy. *Chest* 2004;126(3, Suppl):338S-400S.

Jacobs JJ, Mont MA, Bozic KJ, et al: American Academy of Orthopaedic Surgeons clinical practice guideline on: Preventing venous thromboembolic disease in patients undergoing elective hip and knee arthroplasty. *J Bone Joint Surg Am* 2012;94(8):746-747.

Luck JV Jr, Silva M, Rodriguez-Merchan EC, Ghalambor N, Zahiri CA, Finn RS: Hemophilic arthropathy. *J Am Acad Orthop Surg* 2004;12(4):234-245.

Morris CD, Creevy WS, Einhorn TA: Pulmonary distress and thromboembolic conditions affecting orthopaedic practice, in Buckwalter JA, Einhorn TA, Simon SR, eds: *Orthopaedic Ba-*

sic Science: Biology and Biomechanics of the Musculoskeletal System, ed 2. Rosemont, IL, American Academy of Orthopaedic Surgeons, 2000, pp 307-316.

Prevention of pulmonary embolism and deep vein thrombosis with low dose aspirin: Pulmonary Embolism Prevention (PEP) trial. Lancet 2000;355(9212):1295-1302.

Rodriguez-Merchan EC: Preventing surgical site infection in haemophilia patients undergoing total knee arthroplasty. Blood Coagul Fibrinolysis 2012;23(6):477-481.

Shen FH, Samartzis D, De Wald CJ: Coagulation and thromboembolism in orthopaedic surgery, in Vaccaro AR, ed: Orthopaedic Knowledge Update, ed 8. Rosemont, IL, American Academy of Orthopaedic Surgeons, 2005, pp 169-176.

Turpie AG, Eriksson BI, Bauer KA, Lassen MR: Fondaparinux. J Am Acad Orthop Surg 2004;12(6):371-375.

Whang PG, Lieberman JR: Low-molecular-weight herapin. J Am Acad Orthop Surg 2002;10(5):299-302.

Zimlich RH, Fulbright BM, Friedman RJ: Current status of anticoagulation therapy after total hip and knee arthroplasty. J Am Acad Orthop Surg 1996;4(2):54-62.

2: General Knowledge

Chapter 17
Normal and Pathologic Gait

Keith Baldwin, MD, MSPT, MPH   Mary Ann Keenan, MD

I. Normal Gait

A. Walking is the process by which the body moves forward while maintaining stance stability. During the gait cycle, agonist and antagonist muscle groups work in concert to advance the limb.

 1. Most muscle groups undergo eccentric (lengthening with contraction) contractions.

 2. The quadriceps undergoes concentric contraction (muscle shortening) during midstance.

 3. Alternatively, some muscle groups undergo isocentric contracture (muscle length stays constant). An example of this is the hip abductors during midstance.

B. The gait cycle, or stride (**Figure 1**)

 1. The gait cycle is the complete sequence of all of the functions of a single limb during walking, from initial contact to initial contact. The phases of the gait cycle are often expressed as a percentage, beginning with initial contact (0%) and ending with the most terminal portion of swing (100%).

 2. During running, no double-limb support occurs; rather, neither foot is on the ground. This is sometimes referred to as "double float."

 3. The gait cycle comprises two periods: stance and swing.

  a. Stance—The period when the foot is in contact with the ground. At normal walking speed, stance constitutes approximately 60% of the gait cycle.

  b. Swing—The period when the foot is off the ground and the leg is moving forward. Swing constitutes 40% of the gait cycle.

  c. The percentage relationship between the stance and swing periods is velocity dependent.

4. The gait cycle also can be described as step and stride.

  a. Stride is the distance between consecutive initial contacts of the same foot with the ground.

  b. Step is the distance between the initial contacts of alternating feet.

5. Three tasks are required during gait. During stance, the leg must accept body weight and provide single-limb support. During swing, the limb must be advanced.

6. Eight phases of the gait cycle

  a. Weight acceptance (stance): initial contact, limb-loading response

  b. Single-limb support (stance): midstance, terminal stance, preswing

  c. Limb advancement (swing): initial swing, midswing, terminal swing

7. Characteristic joint positions and muscle activity during each phase of gait

  a. Initial contact begins as the foot contacts the ground.

   • In normal gait, the heel is the first part of the foot to touch the ground.

   • The hip is flexed, the knee is extended, and the ankle is dorsiflexed to neutral.

   • The hip extensor muscles contract to stabilize the hip because the body's mass is behind the hip joint.

  b. Loading response

   • Loading response marks the beginning of the initial double-limb stance period. During loading response in normal gait, the heel contacts the floor first, which begins the "first rocker" or "heel rocker."

   • Loading response begins when the heel contacts the floor, and it continues until the opposite foot is lifted for swing.

   • Body weight is transferred onto the supporting leg.

2: General Knowledge

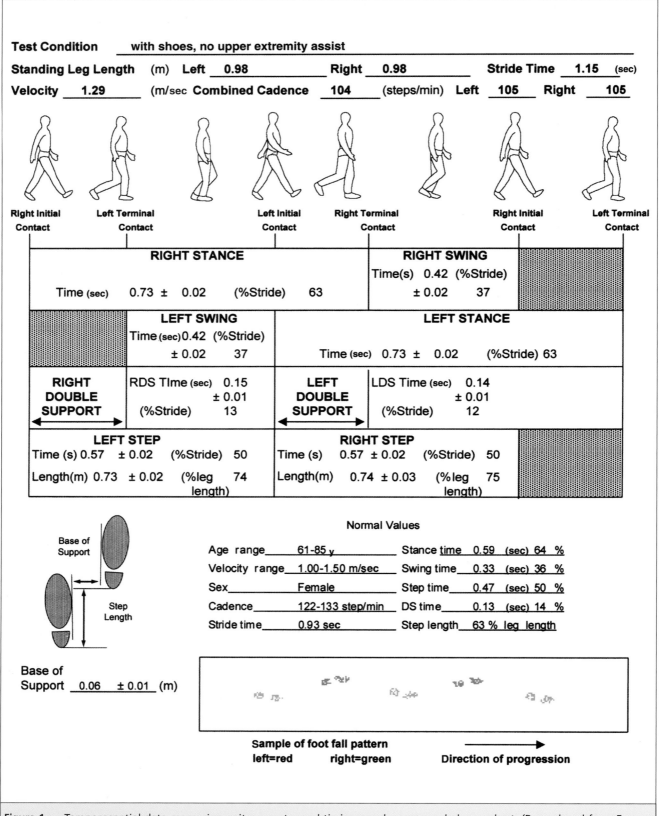

Test Condition _____with shoes, no upper extremity assist_____

Standing Leg Length (m) **Left** __0.98__ **Right** __0.98__ **Stride Time** __1.15__ (sec)

Velocity __1.29__ (m/sec **Combined Cadence** __104__ (steps/min) **Left** __105__ **Right** __105__

Right Initial Contact · Left Terminal Contact · Left Initial Contact · Right Terminal Contact · Right Initial Contact · Left Terminal Contact

RIGHT STANCE		RIGHT SWING
Time (sec) 0.73 ± 0.02 (%Stride) 63		Time(s) 0.42 (%Stride) ± 0.02 37

LEFT SWING		LEFT STANCE
Time(sec) 0.42 (%Stride) ± 0.02 37		Time (sec) 0.73 ± 0.02 (%Stride) 63

RIGHT DOUBLE SUPPORT	RDS TIme (sec) 0.15 ± 0.01 (%Stride) 13	LEFT DOUBLE SUPPORT	LDS Time (sec) 0.14 ± 0.01 (%Stride) 12

LEFT STEP	RIGHT STEP
Time (s) 0.57 ± 0.02 (%Stride) 50	Time (s) 0.57 ± 0.02 (%Stride) 50
Length(m) 0.73 ± 0.02 (%leg length) 74	Length(m) 0.74 ± 0.03 (%leg length) 75

Base of Support

Step Length

Normal Values

Age range	61-85 y	Stance time	0.59 (sec) 64 %
Velocity range	1.00-1.50 m/sec	Swing time	0.33 (sec) 36 %
Sex	Female	Step time	0.47 (sec) 50 %
Cadence	122-133 step/min	DS time	0.13 (sec) 14 %
Stride time	0.93 sec	Step length	63 % leg length

Base of Support __0.06__ ± 0.01 (m)

Sample of foot fall pattern
left=red   right=green   **Direction of progression**

Figure 1   Temporospatial data measuring gait symmetry and timing are shown recorded on a chart. (Reproduced from Esquenazi A: Biomechanics of gait, in Vaccaro AR, ed: *Orthopaedic Knowledge Update*, ed 8. Rosemont, IL, American Academy of Orthopaedic Surgeons, 2005, p 380.)

2: General Knowledge

- During the loading response, the knee flexes to 15°, and the ankle plantar flexes to dampen the downward force.

- The ankle dorsiflexor muscles are active with an eccentric contraction (lengthening contraction) to control the plantar flexion moment.

- As the knee flexes and the stance leg accepts the weight of the body, the quadriceps muscle becomes active to counteract the flexion moment and stabilize the knee.

c. Midstance

- Midstance is the initial period of single-limb support.

- Midstance begins with the lifting of the opposite foot and continues until body weight is aligned over the supporting foot.

- The supporting leg advances over the supporting foot by ankle dorsiflexion while the hip and knee extend. This pattern of ankle motion and shifting of weight has been referred to as the "second rocker" or "ankle rocker."

- The hip extensors and quadriceps undergo concentric contraction (muscle shortening) during midstance.

- As the body's mass moves ahead of the ankle joint, the calf muscles become active to stabilize the tibia and ankle and allow the heel to rise from the floor.

d. Terminal stance

- Terminal stance begins when the supporting heel rises from the ground and continues until the heel of the opposite foot contacts the ground.

- Body weight progresses beyond the supporting foot as increased hip extension puts the leg in a more trailing position.

- The heel leaves the floor, and the knee begins to flex as momentum carries the body forward.

- In the final portion of terminal stance, as the body rolls forward over the forefoot, the toes dorsiflex at the metatarsophalangeal joints (the "third rocker," or "forefoot rocker").

- The toe flexor muscles are most active at this time.

e. Preswing

- Preswing marks the second double-limb stance interval in the gait cycle.

- This phase begins with the initial contact of the previous swing limb and ends with toe-off of the previously supporting leg.

- Ground contact by the opposite leg, making initial contact, causes the knee of the trailing limb to flex to 35° and the ankle to plantar flex to 20°.

- Body weight is transferred to the opposite limb.

- The quadriceps should be inactive at this time to allow the knee to flex.

- The hip flexor muscles provide the power for advancing the limb and are active during the initial two thirds of the swing phase.

- Forward movement of the leg provides the inertial force for knee flexion.

f. Initial swing

- Initial swing marks the period of single-limb support for the opposite limb.

- This phase begins when the foot is lifted from the floor and ends when the swinging foot is opposite the stance foot.

- The swing leg is advanced by concentric contraction of the hip flexor muscles.

- The knee flexes in response to forward inertia provided by the hip flexors.

- The ankle partially dorsiflexes to ensure ground clearance.

g. Midswing

- Midswing begins when the swinging foot is opposite the stance foot and continues until the swinging limb is in front of the body and the tibia is vertical.

- Advancement of the swing leg is accomplished by further hip flexion.

- The knee extends with the momentum provided by hip flexion while the ankle continues dorsiflexion to neutral.

- The ankle dorsiflexors become active during the latter two thirds of the phase to ensure foot clearance as the knee begins to extend.

h. Terminal swing

- Terminal swing begins when the tibia is vertical and ends when the foot contacts the floor.

- Limb advancement is completed by knee extension.

- The hamstring muscles decelerate the forward motion of the thigh during the terminal period of the swing phase.

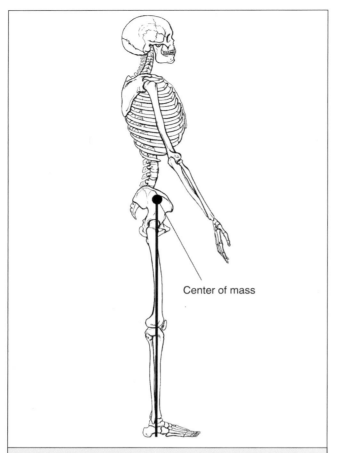

Figure 2   Illustration depicts a sagittal view of a human skeleton, showing the center of mass and weight-bearing line in the standing position.

- The hip maintains its flexed position.

- The ankle dorsiflexors maintain their activity to ensure that the ankle remains dorsiflexed to neutral.

C. Center of mass

1. The center of mass (COM) is located anterior to the second sacral vertebra, midway between the hip joints (**Figure 2**).

2. The body requires the least amount of energy to move along a straight line.

3. During gait, the COM deviates from the straight line in smooth vertical and lateral sinusoidal displacements.

   a. The COM displaces vertically in a rhythmic fashion as it moves forward.

   b. The highest point occurs at midstance, and the lowest point occurs at the time of double-limb support.

   c. The mean vertical displacement is 5 cm, and

the mean lateral displacement is approximately 5 cm.

   d. The speed of movement of the COM decreases at midstance, and the peak vertical displacement is achieved.

   e. The speed of movement of the COM increases as the stance limb is unloaded.

   f. The COM displaces laterally with forward movement.

   g. As weight is transferred from one leg to the other, the pelvis shifts to the weight-bearing side.

   h. The limits of lateral displacement are reached at midstance.

D. Gait analysis—A clinically useful way to assess lower-limb function either by visual observation or with quantitative measurements.

1. Visual analysis

   a. Visual analysis begins with a general assessment, noting symmetry and smoothness of movements of the various body parts.

   b. The cadence (steps per minute), base width, stride length, arm swing, movement of the trunk, and rise of the body should be noted. This is the basis for a useful clinical test, the Timed Up and Go test. For this test, the patient gets up from a chair, walks 3 m, returns to the chair, and sits down. The patient is allowed to use any walking aids normally used, including orthoses. A total time less than 10 seconds is considered normal for an elderly patient. Longer times are correlated with a risk of falls and dependence in activities of daily living.

   c. Because of the speed and complexity of walking, visual analysis does not supply the observer with enough quantitative information to enable precise diagnosis.

   d. Videotaping is useful for supplementing clinical observation.

2. Laboratory analysis

   a. Kinematics is the analysis of the motion produced during the gait cycle (**Figure 3**).

   b. Kinetics is the analysis of forces that produce motion (**Figure 4**).

   c. Dynamic polyelectromyography assesses the activity of multiple muscles during gait (**Figure 5**).

3. Stride can be assessed with gait pressure mats or other timing devices. Characteristics include velocity, cadence (steps per minute), stance and swing times, and single-limb and double-limb support times.

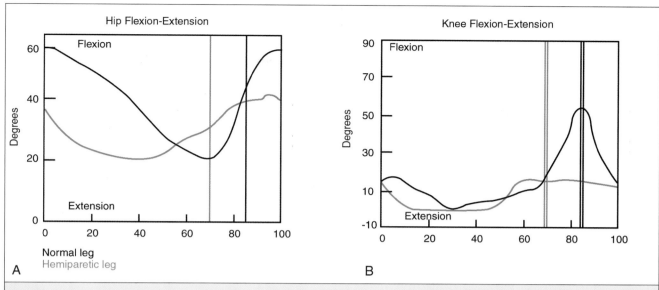

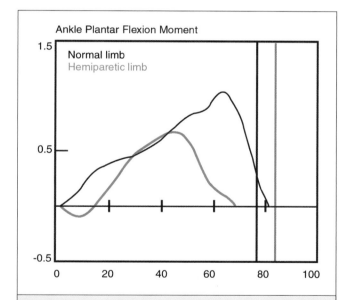

Figure 3 Graphs show three-dimensional sagittal kinematic data for normal and hemiparetic limbs in the same patient for hip flexion-extension (**A**) and knee flexion-extension (**B**). Data were obtained using the CODA MPX motion-tracking system (Charnwood Dynamics, Leicestershire, England). The normalized gait cycle is expressed as a percentage of the gait cycle (x-axis); 0 = initial contact, vertical line indicates the beginning of swing phase, 100 = the next initial contact.

Figure 4 Graph shows kinetic data from the ankle plantar flexion moments of a normal and hemiparetic limb in the same patient.

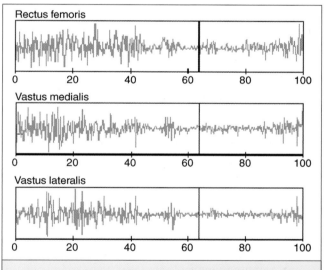

Figure 5 Dynamic polyelectromyography of the quadriceps muscles obtained from the hemiparetic limb of a patient with a stiff-knee gait.

4. Kinematic analysis

   a. Videotaping in two planes is useful for recording motion.

   b. Electrogoniometers or tensiometers are used to record individual joint movement.

   c. Motion analysis uses multiple cameras that detect sensors on a patient. The data from the cameras can be used to recreate a three-dimensional model of the patient's gait pattern.

5. Kinetic analysis

   a. Force plate studies measure ground reaction forces and changes in the center of pressure as a patient walks.

   b. Pedobaric measurements can be used to determine the magnitude and distribution of forces under the foot.

2: General Knowledge

c. Joint moments and powers can be calculated using movement and force data.

6. Dynamic polyelectromyography measures and records the electrical activity in the multiple muscle groups that work during functional activity.

II. Pathologic Gait

A. Antalgic gait—Any gait abnormality resulting from pain. *Antalgic gait* is a nonspecific term. Different pathologies can result in similar compensations during gait.

1. Hip osteoarthritis

   a. Leaning of the trunk laterally over the painful leg during stance brings the COM over the joint.

   b. Compressive forces decrease across the joint as the need for contraction of the hip abductor muscles decreases.

2. Knee pain

   a. The knee is maintained in slight flexion throughout the gait cycle, especially if an effusion is present.

   b. Moderate flexion reduces tension on the knee joint capsule.

   c. Compensation for knee flexion involves toe walking on the affected side.

   d. Weight-bearing time on the painful leg is reduced.

3. Foot and ankle pain

   a. The patient attempts to limit weight bearing through the affected area.

   b. The stride length is shortened.

   c. Normal heel-to-toe motion is absent.

4. Forefoot pain

   a. The patient has a characteristic flatfoot gait.

   b. The patient avoids weight bearing on the metatarsal heads.

5. Ankle or hindfoot pain

   a. The patient avoids heel strike at initial contact.

   b. The patient ambulates on the toes of the affected side.

B. Joint contractures

1. Flexion contracture of the hip

   a. The contracture is compensated for by increased lumbar lordosis.

   b. Compensatory knee flexion is required to maintain the COM over the feet for stability.

c. The characteristic crouched posture is energy inefficient and results in shorter overall walking distances.

2. Flexion contracture of the knee

   a. Flexion contracture of the knee causes a relative limb-length discrepancy.

   b. Compensations for contractures less than 30° become more pronounced at faster walking speeds, whereas contractures greater than 30° are apparent at normal walking speeds.

   c. Gait is characterized by toe walking on the affected side.

   d. Increased hip and knee flexion (steppage gait) of the opposite limb may be required to clear the foot because the affected limb is relatively too long (**Figure 6**).

   e. Fixed-knee flexion contractures of bilateral knees can result in a crouched gait.

   f. This type of gait is most common in the adolescent cerebral palsy population and is thought to be partially the result of incompetent triceps surae.

3. Plantar flexion contracture of the ankle

   a. This contracture results in a knee extension moment (knee extension thrust) at initial contact of the forefoot with the floor.

   b. During swing phase, hip and knee flexion of the affected limb (steppage gait) must be increased to clear the foot because the limb is relatively too long.

C. Joint instability

1. Knee instability can result in variable gait presentations depending on the ligament involved.

2. Knee recurvatum

   a. Knee recurvatum results from weakness of the ankle plantar flexors and quadriceps.

   b. During stance, the patient compensates by leaning the trunk forward to place the COM anterior to the knee.

   c. This leads to degenerative changes of the knee joint over time (**Figure 7**).

3. Injuries of the posterolateral corner of the knee (the posterior cruciate ligament, lateral collateral ligament, posterior joint capsule, and the popliteus tendon) result in a varus thrust gait pattern during stance.

4. Quadriceps avoidance gait

   a. Quadriceps avoidance gait occurs in patients with an anterior cruciate ligament (ACL)–deficient knee

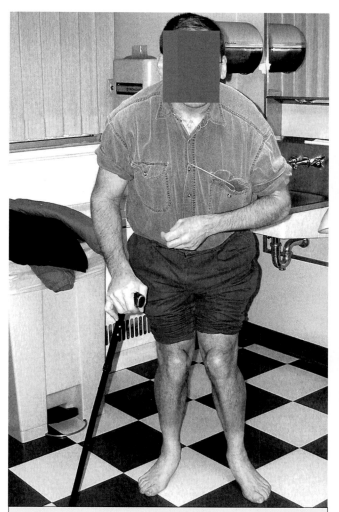

Figure 6   Clinical photograph of a patient with a knee flexion contracture, which often is associated with a concurrent hip flexion contracture. A crouched posture results in high-energy demands because the hip, knee, and ankle extensors must be active continuously to maintain an upright posture. This limits the time and distance a person is able to walk.

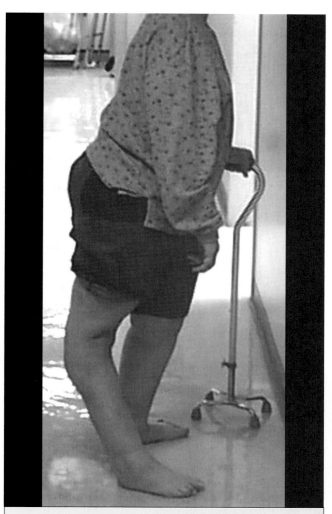

Figure 7   Clinical photograph shows a patient with genu recurvatum. Weakness of the ankle plantar flexors and quadriceps muscles causes the patient to position the center of mass anterior to the flexion axis of the knee to prevent the knee from buckling. Over time, this compensation leads to a recurvatum deformity of the knee.

b. With an ACL-deficient knee, the tibia is prone to anterior subluxation because the contraction of the quadriceps provides an anterior force to the tibia.

c. Attempts to decrease the load response phase on the affected limb are made by decreasing stride length and avoiding knee flexion during the midportion of stance.

5. Ankle instability

a. Ankle instability results in difficulty with supporting body weight during initial contact.

b. An unstable ankle often buckles, resulting in an antalgic gait that limits the load response phase on the affected side.

D. Muscle weakness

1. Weakness of the hip abductors

a. This weakness can result in a Trendelenburg gait.

b. Similar to compensations seen in hip osteoarthritis, the patient shifts the COM over the involved limb, which results in increased lateral trunk lean to the side of the lesion.

c. Additionally, the pelvis dips to the contralateral side as a result of the inability of the hip abductors to maintain joint position.

d. This gait may be treated with a cane in the hand opposite the lesion to prevent collapse to that side.

e. Bilateral Trendelenburg gait results in a waddling gait.

2. Weakness of the hip flexors

   a. Limits limb advancement during swing

   b. Results in a shortened step length

3. Moderate weakness of the hip extensors

   a. Compensated for by forward trunk flexion

   b. This posture places the hip extensors on stretch and in a position of increased mechanical advantage (**Figure 8**).

4. Severe weakness of the hip extensors results in the need for upper-limb assistive devices to maintain an erect posture.

5. Quadriceps weakness

   a. Makes the patient susceptible to falls at initial contact

   b. The patient compensates by leaning the trunk forward to keep the COM anterior to the knee joint.

   c. The gastrocnemius muscle contracts more vigorously to maintain the knee in extension.

   d. The patient may use the hand to push the knee into extension with initial weight bearing.

6. Ankle plantar flexor weakness

   a. Causes instability of the tibia and knee as the COM moves anterior to the knee

   b. Quadriceps activity increases to keep the knee extended.

   c. This compensation limits step length, which predisposes the patient to painful overuse syndromes of the patella and quadriceps.

7. Combined quadriceps and ankle plantar flexor weakness

   a. Causes the patient to hyperextend the knee for stability at initial contact

   b. Over time, this compensation results in a genu recurvatum deformity.

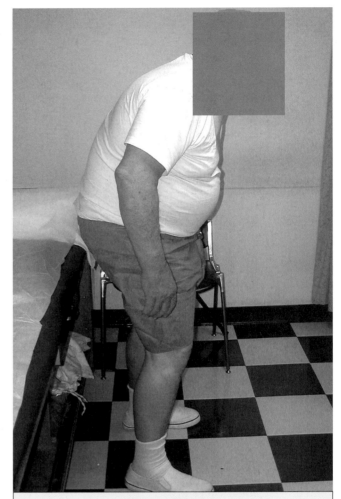

Figure 8   Clinical photograph shows a patient with forward trunk flexion. Assuming a posture of hip flexion places the hip extensor muscles in a position of greater mechanical advantage. This helps to compensate for moderate weakness of the hip extensor muscles (grade 4) during walking.

Top Testing Facts

1. A gait cycle, also known as a stride, is the complete sequence of all the functions of a single limb during walking, from initial contact to initial contact. The phases of the gait cycle describe the events that occur and often are expressed as percentages, beginning with the initial contact of the foot with the floor (0%) and ending with the most terminal portion of swing (100%).

2. The three tasks required during gait are as follows: During stance, the leg must accept body weight and provide single-limb support. During swing, the limb must be advanced.

3. The normal gait cycle has two periods (stance and swing) and eight phases (initial contact, limb-loading response, midstance, terminal stance, preswing, initial swing, midswing, and terminal swing).

4. The COM is located anterior to the second sacral vertebra, midway between the hip joints.

5. Antalgic gait is a nonspecific term that describes any gait abnormality resulting from pain.

6. Weakness of the hip flexors limits limb advancement during swing and results in a shortened step length.

7. Flexion contracture of the hip requires compensatory knee flexion to maintain the COM over the feet for stability, resulting in the characteristic crouched posture.

8. A plantar flexion contracture of the ankle results in a knee extension moment (knee extension thrust) at initial contact of the forefoot with the floor.

9. A patient with a Trendelenburg gait should hold the assistive device on the side opposite the side of weakness.

10. With quadriceps weakness, the patient compensates by leaning the trunk forward to keep the COM anterior to the knee joint.

11. Ankle plantar flexor weakness causes increased quadriceps activity, limiting step length and predisposing the patient to painful overuse syndromes of the patella and quadriceps.

Bibliography

Crosbie J, Green T, Refshauge K: Effects of reduced ankle dorsiflexion following lateral ligament sprain on temporal and spatial gait parameters. *Gait Posture* 1999;9(3):167-172.

Esquenazi A: Biomechanics of gait, in Vaccaro AR, ed: *Orthopaedic Knowledge Update*, ed 8. Rosemont, IL, American Academy of Orthopaedic Surgeons, 2005, pp 377-386.

Gage JR, ed: *The Treatment of Gait Problems in Cerebral Palsy Series: Clinics in Developmental Medicine*. London, England, Mac Keith Press, No. 164.

Keenan MA, Esquenazi A, Mayer N: The use of laboratory gait analysis for surgical decision making in persons with upper motor neuron syndromes. *Phys Med Rehabil* 2002;16:249-261.

Lim MR, Huang RC, Wu A, Girardi FP, Cammisa FP Jr: Evaluation of the elderly patient with an abnormal gait. *J Am Acad Orthop Surg* 2007;15(2):107-117.

Neumann DA: Biomechanical analysis of selected principles of hip joint protection. *Arthritis Care Res* 1989;2(4):146-155.

Perry J: *Gait Analysis: Normal and Pathological Function*. Thorofare, NJ, Slack Publishers, 2010.

Podsiadlo D, Richardson S: The timed "Up & Go": A test of basic functional mobility for frail elderly persons. *J Am Geriatr Soc* 1991;39(2):142-148.

Vuillermin C, Rodda J, Rutz E, Shore BJ, Smith K, Graham HK: Severe crouch gait in spastic diplegia can be prevented: A population-based study. *J Bone Joint Surg Br* 2011;93(12):1670-1675.

2: General Knowledge

Chapter 18

Orthoses, Amputations, and Prostheses

Keith Baldwin, MD, MSPT, MPH   Mary Ann Keenan, MD

I. Lower Limb Orthoses

A. Terminology

1. Orthosis (or orthotic device)—The medical term for a brace or splint. Orthoses generally are named according to body region and can be custom or "off the shelf."

2. The basic types are static and dynamic devices.

   a. Static—Rigid devices used to support the weakened or paralyzed body parts in a particular position

   b. Dynamic—Used to facilitate body motion to allow optimal function

B. Principles

1. Orthoses are used to manage a specific disorder, including a painful joint, muscle weakness, or joint instability or contracture.

2. Orthotic joints should be aligned at the approximate anatomic joints.

3. Orthoses should be simple, lightweight, strong, durable, and aesthetically acceptable.

4. Considerations for orthotic prescription

   a. Three-point pressure control system

   b. Static or dynamic stabilization

   c. Tissue tolerance to compression and shear force

   d. Whether the goal of prescription is to accommodate a rigid deformity or correct a flexible one

   e. Level of function of the patient (Is the goal positional or functional?)

5. Construction materials include metal, plastic (most commonly polypropylene), leather, synthetic fabric, or any combination thereof.

C. Foot orthoses

1. Shoes are a type of foot orthosis and can be modified to accommodate deformities or to provide support to the limb during walking.

   a. A cushioned or negative heel is often used with a rigid ankle to reduce the knee flexion moment (that is, it creates a relative plantar flexion, which encourages knee extension).

   b. Medial and lateral wedges can be added to the heel or sole of a shoe to accommodate fixed varus or valgus foot deformities. These wedges also influence the varus and valgus forces on the knee (that is, a medial heel wedge for posterior tibial tendon dysfunction or a lateral heel wedge to partially unload the medial knee compartment).

   c. Medial and lateral flares can be added to the heel or sole of a shoe to widen the base of support for the foot.

   d. Rocker-bottom shoes help to transfer body weight forward while walking when the rockers described by Perry are dysfunctional, but they destabilize the knee by transferring body weight forward too rapidly. Whether to prescribe these shoes must be considered carefully in patients with balance or proprioception problems.

   e. An extra-deep shoe allows additional room for deformities and inserts.

   f. High-top lace-up sneakers may assist patients with poor distal proprioception, such as those with diabetes, by providing feedback more proximally to help balance.

2. A foot orthosis placed inside the shoe can provide support, control motion, stabilize gait, reduce pain, correct flexible deformities, and prevent the progression of fixed deformities.

Dr. Baldwin or an immediate family member has stock or stock options held in Pfizer. Neither Dr. Keenan nor any immediate family member has received anything of value from or has stock or stock options held in a commercial company or institution related directly or indirectly to the subject of this chapter.

2: General Knowledge

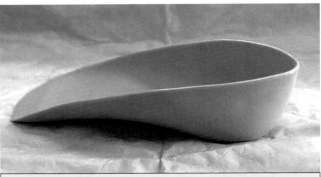

Figure 1   Photograph shows the University of California Biomechanics Laboratory foot orthosis, which encompasses the heel and midfoot. It has medial, lateral, and posterior walls.

Table 1

Types of Ankle Motion Allowed by Orthotic Ankle Joints and the Effect on Gait

Ankle Joint Motion	Effect on Gait
Unrestricted plantar flexion and dorsiflexion	Provides medial-lateral ankle stability
Unrestricted plantar flexion	Allows normal weight acceptance in early stance
Unrestricted dorsiflexion	Allows calf strengthening and stretching of the plantar flexors (Achilles tendon)
Plantar flexion stop	Limits a dynamic equinus deformity and provides a knee flexion moment during weight acceptance
Dorsiflexion assistance	Corrects a flexible footdrop during swing
Limited dorsiflexion (dorsiflexion stop)	Provides a knee extension moment in the later part of stance Useful to stabilize the knee in the presence of quadriceps or plantar flexion weakness
Locked ankle	Limits motion for multiplanar instability or ankle pain

a. Heel cup

- A heel cup is a rigid plastic insert.

- It covers the plantar surface of the heel and extends posteriorly, medially, and laterally up the side of the heel.

- Heel cups are used to prevent lateral calcaneal shift in the flexible flatfoot.

b. University of California Biomechanics Laboratory (UCBL) foot orthosis (**Figure 1**)

- The UCBL foot orthosis is constructed of plastic. It is fabricated over a cast of the foot held in maximal manual correction.

- It encompasses the heel and midfoot with rigid medial, lateral, and posterior walls.

- Designed for flexible flatfoot, the UCBL orthosis holds the heel in a neutral vertical position. If the flatfoot is not flexible, the UCBL will become painful and could lead to skin breakdown.

c. Arizona brace

- The Arizona brace combines the UCBL orthosis with a laced ankle support.

- It provides more rigid hindfoot support.

- This brace is also is used for flexible flatfoot.

D. Ankle-foot orthoses

1. Ankle-foot orthoses (AFOs) are prescribed for weakness or muscle overactivity of ankle dorsiflexion, plantar flexion, inversion, and eversion (**Table 1**).

2. AFOs are used to prevent or correct deformities.

3. The ankle position indirectly affects knee stability, with ankle plantar flexion providing a knee extension force and ankle dorsiflexion providing a knee flexion force.

4. All AFOs consist of a footplate with stirrups, uprights, and a calf band, regardless of the materials used for construction (**Figure 2**).

5. Nonarticulated AFOs

a. Nonarticulated AFOs are more aesthetically acceptable.

b. They place a flexion force on the knee during weight acceptance because they are positioned in neutral dorsiflexion/plantar flexion and do not allow gradual eccentric plantar flexion in early stance.

c. The trim lines of plastic AFOs determine the degree of flexibility during late stance and are described as having maximal, moderate, or minimal resistance to ankle dorsiflexion.

d. Nonarticulated AFOs may be constructed of plastic, composite materials, or leather and metal.

e. Thermoplastic AFOs must be used with care in patients with fluctuating edema or a lack of sensation because they can lead to skin breakdown in these patients.

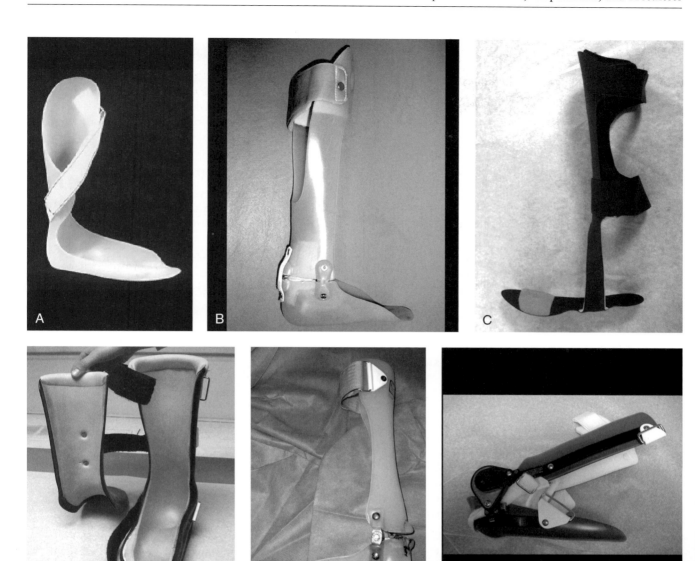

Figure 2   Photographs show examples of ankle-foot orthoses (AFOs). **A,** Posterior leaf spring AFO. **B,** Floor reaction AFO. **C,** Carbon fiber composite AFO. **D,** Clamshell AFO for neuropathic arthropathy. **E,** Articulated AFO with simple joint. **F,** Dynamic dorsiflexion AFO.

f. Nonarticulated AFOs are described according to the amount of rigidity of the brace, which depends on the thickness and composition of the plastic, as well as the trim lines and shape.

6. Articulated AFOs

   a. Articulated AFOs allow a more natural gait pattern and adjustment of plantar flexion and dorsiflexion.

   b. They can be designed to provide dorsiflexion assistance to clear the toes during swing.

   c. Adjustable ankle joints can be set to the desired range of ankle dorsiflexion or plantar flexion.

d. Mechanical ankle joints

   • These joints can control or assist ankle dorsiflexion or plantar flexion by means of stops (pins) or assists (springs).

   • They also control medial-lateral stability of the ankle joint.

   • Limits on ankle motion affect knee stability: Unrestricted plantar flexion allows normal weight acceptance in early stance; plantar flexion stop causes a knee flexion moment during weight acceptance; dorsiflexion stop provides a knee extension moment during the later part of stance.

7. Types of AFO designs

a. Free-motion ankle joints—Allow unrestricted ankle dorsiflexion and plantar flexion motion, provide only medial-lateral stability, and are useful for ligamentous instability.

b. Unrestricted (free) plantar flexion—Allows normal weight acceptance in early stance.

c. Unrestricted (free) dorsiflexion—Allows calf muscle strengthening and stretching of the plantar flexors (Achilles tendon).

d. Limited motion ankle joints—Can be adjusted for use in ankle weakness affecting all muscle groups.

e. Plantar flexion stop ankle joints

- These joints are used in patients with weakness of dorsiflexion during the swing phase.

- The plantar flexion stop limits a dynamic (flexible) equinus deformity.

- These joints provide a knee flexion moment during weight acceptance. They should not be used in patients with quadriceps weakness.

f. Dorsiflexion stop ankle joints

- In the setting of mild equinus, this joint can be used to promote a knee extension moment during the loading response to prevent buckling of the knee.

- Limited ankle dorsiflexion provides a knee extension moment in the later part of stance.

- These joints are useful for stabilizing the knee during the later part of stance in the presence of quadriceps or ankle plantar flexion weakness.

g. Locked ankle joints—Limit motion for multiplanar instability or ankle pain; useful for spina bifida patients with a midlumbar level of function.

h. Dorsiflexion assist spring joints—Provide dynamic ankle dorsiflexion during the swing phase and correct a flexible footdrop during swing.

i. Floor reaction AFOs—Have a distal trim line that extends to the forefoot and plastic that extends proximally over the pretibial area; provide maximal resistance to plantar flexion and encourage knee extension; ideal for patients with cerebral palsy who may have incompetent or overly lengthened triceps surae and mild crouch gait.

j. Supramalleolar orthoses (SMOs)—These AFOs control varus/valgus deformities that are passively correctable. They allow full dorsiflexion–plantar flexion and are appropriate in patients with mild spasticity, with no dorsiflexion–plantar flexion weakness.

k. Cam walkers—A simple off-the-shelf AFO used to provide removable protection to the foot and ankle when an injury such as a sprain or fracture requires immobilization but weight bearing is allowed and casting is not necessary or desired.

8. Varus or valgus correction straps (T-straps)

a. When used for valgus correction, these straps contact the skin medially and circle the ankle until buckled on the outside of the lateral upright.

b. When used for varus correction, the straps contact the skin laterally and buckle around the medial upright.

E. Knee-ankle-foot orthoses

1. Construction

a. Knee-ankle-foot orthoses (KAFOs) consist of an AFO with metal uprights, a mechanical knee joint, and two thigh bands (**Figure 3**).

b. They can be made of metal-leather and metal-plastic or plastic and plastic-metal.

2. Principles of operation

a. KAFOs can be used in quadriceps paralysis or weakness to maintain knee stability and control flexible genu valgum or genu varum.

b. They limit the weight bearing of the thigh, leg, and foot with quadrilateral or ischial containment brim.

c. KAFOs are more difficult to don and doff than are AFOs.

d. KAFOs are not recommended for patients with moderate to severe cognitive dysfunction.

3. Types of KAFO designs

a. Double-upright metal KAFO (most common)

- This type comprises an AFO with two metal uprights extending proximally to the thigh to control knee motion and alignment.

- It consists of a mechanical knee joint and two thigh bands between two uprights.

b. Scott-Craig orthosis

- Includes a cushioned heel with a T-shaped foot plate for mediolateral stability, an ankle joint with anterior and posterior adjustable stops, double uprights, a pretibial band, a posterior thigh band, and a knee joint with pawl locks and bail control

- Hip hyperextension allows the center of gravity to fall behind the hip joint and in

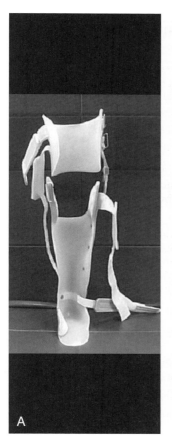
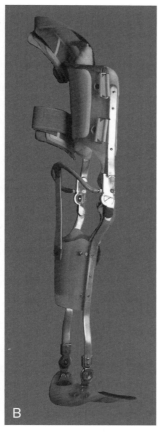
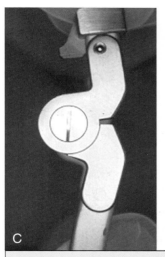
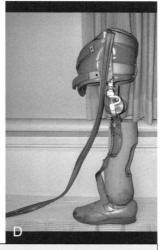

Figure 3 Photographs show examples of knee-ankle-foot orthoses (KAFOs). **A**, KAFO. **B**, KAFO with bail lock knee joint. **C**, Posterior knee joint and drop lock for a KAFO. **D**, Combined prosthesis for ankle disarticulation and KAFO for quadriceps weakness.

front of the locked knee and ankle joint.

- With 10° of ankle dorsiflexion alignment, a swing-to or swing-through gait with crutches is possible.

- The Scott-Craig orthosis is used for standing and ambulation in patients with paraplegia from a spinal cord injury.

c. Supracondylar plastic orthosis

- The ankle is immobilized in slight plantar flexion to produce a knee extension moment in stance to help eliminate the need for a mechanical knee lock.

- This orthosis resists genu recurvatum and provides medial-lateral knee stability.

d. Plastic shell and metal upright orthosis—Posterior leaf spring AFO with double metal uprights that extend up to a plastic shell in the thigh with an intervening knee joint.

4. Knee joints (**Table 2**)

a. Single-axis knee joint—The axis of rotation of the joint is aligned with the rotational axis of the anatomic knee joint.

- The single-axis knee joint is useful for knee stabilization.

- The arc of knee motion can be full or limited.

- A free motion knee joint allows unrestricted knee flexion and extension with a stop to prevent hyperextension; used for patients with recurvatum but good strength of the quadriceps to control knee motion.

b. Posterior offset knee joint—The axis of rotation of the orthotic joint is aligned posterior to the rotational axis of the anatomic knee joint.

- The posterior offset knee shifts the weight-bearing axis provided by the center of mass (COM) more anterior to the anatomic knee joint.

- At initial contact and during weight acceptance, the ground reaction force is anterior to the flexion axis of the anatomic knee. This extends the knee and results in greater stability during early stance.

- It provides a knee extension moment during stance.

- The knee can flex freely during swing phase.

c. Polycentric joint—Allows limited multiplanar motion during flexion and extension; useful for patients with knee arthritis.

d. Dynamic knee extension joint—Provides active knee extension, usually by means of a coiled spring within the joint; helpful for patients with quadriceps weakness but full knee extension.

5. Types of knee joint locking mechanisms—Orthotic knee joints can be modified to allow locking of the joint for stability during stance.

Table 2

Designs of Orthotic Knee Joints and Their Uses

Knee Joint	Design	Use
Single-axis joint	The axis of rotation of the joint is aligned with the rotational axis of the anatomic knee joint	Provides medial-lateral knee stability May allow full knee movement or be locked
Posterior offset joint	The axis of rotation of the joint is aligned posterior to the rotational axis of the anatomic knee joint	Provides additional stability to the extended knee Limits knee recurvatum
Polycentric joint	Allows limited multiplanar motion during flexion and extension	Decreases joint contact forces in a painful arthritic knee
Dynamic extension joint	A spring or coil provides active knee extension force	Provides active knee extension for quadriceps

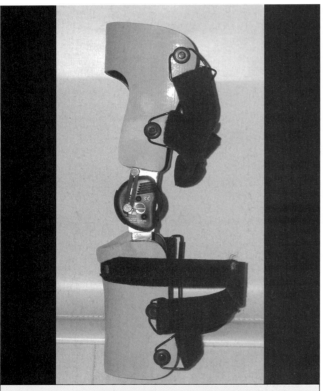

Figure 4   Photograph shows a dynamic knee extension orthosis.

a. Drop ring lock knee joint

- This is the most commonly used knee lock to prevent knee flexion while walking.

- Rings drop over the joint to lock it while the knee is in extension.

- The knee is stable, but gait is stiff without knee motion.

- This type of lock is appropriate for patients with severe quadriceps weakness or gross ligamentous instability.

- Extensions may be added to the rings to allow the patient to unlock the joint for sitting without the need to bend forward.

b. Pawl lock with bail release knee joint

- A semicircular bail attaches to the knee joint posteriorly; the patient can unlock both joints easily by pulling up the bail or backing up to sit down in a chair.

- A major drawback is that the knee can accidentally unlock, such as if bumped on a chair.

c. Adjustable knee lock joint (dial lock)

- This serrated adjustable knee joint allows knee locking at different degrees of flexion.

- This type of lock is used for patients with knee flexion contractures that are improving gradually with stretching.

6. Additional potential modifications of a KAFO

a. Anterior knee pad: can be placed over the patella to prevent knee flexion

b. Medial strap or pad: controls a valgus knee deformity

c. Lateral strap or pad: controls a varus knee deformity

d. For ischial weight bearing, the upper thigh band cuff is brought up above the ischium to provide a weight-bearing surface.

F. Knee orthoses—Provide support or control to the knee only, not the foot and ankle (**Figure 4**).

1. Knee orthoses for patellofemoral disorders—Supply medial-lateral knee stability, control patellar tracking during knee flexion and extension, and generally include an infrapatellar strap (as in Osgood-Schlatter disease).

2. Knee orthoses for knee control in the sagittal plane—Control genu recurvatum with minimal

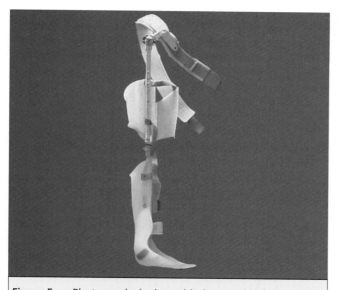

Figure 5 Photograph depicts a hip-knee-ankle-foot orthosis.

medial-lateral stability and include a Swedish knee cage and a three-way knee stabilizer.

3. Knee orthoses for knee control in the frontal plane—Consist of thigh and calf cuffs joined by sidebars with mechanical knee joints, are usually polycentric, and closely mimic anatomic joint motion.

4. Knee orthoses for axial rotation control—Can provide angular control of flexion-extension and medial-lateral planes and control axial rotation; used mostly for managing sports injuries of the knee.

G. Hip-knee-ankle-foot orthoses

1. Hip-knee-ankle-foot orthoses (HKAFOs) consist of an AFO with metal uprights, a mechanical knee joint, thigh uprights, a thigh socket, a hip joint, and a waistband (**Figure 5**).

2. The hip joint can be adjusted in two planes to control flexion/extension and abduction/adduction. These orthoses can be very useful clinically for hip instability in total hip arthroplasty and can be used to maintain the hip in 15° of abduction and limit flexion to a stable arc postoperatively.

   a. Single-axis hip joint with lock

   - This is the most common hip joint with flexion and extension.

   - It may include an adjustable stop to control hyperextension.

   b. Two-position lock hip joint

   - This type of hip joint can be locked at full extension and 90° of flexion.

Table 3

Percentage of Lower Limb Amputations Associated With Specific Causes

Cause	Amputations (%)
Vascular disorders	80
Trauma	15
Tumor, infection, congenital	5

- It is used for hip spasticity control in patients with difficulty maintaining a seated position.

   c. Double-axis hip joint

   - The double-axis hip joint has a flexion/extension axis to control these motions.

   - It also has an abduction/adduction axis to control these motions.

3. The orthotic hip joint is positioned with the patient sitting upright at 90°; the orthotic knee joint is centered over the medial femoral condyle.

4. Pelvic bands

   a. Pelvic bands complicate dressing after toileting unless the orthosis is worn under all clothing.

   b. They also increase energy demands for ambulation.

H. Trunk-hip-knee-ankle-foot orthoses

1. Trunk-hip-knee-ankle-foot orthoses (THKAFOs) consist of a spinal orthosis in addition to an HKAFO to control trunk motion and spinal alignment.

2. THKAFOs are indicated in patients with paraplegia.

3. These orthoses are very difficult to don and doff.

4. Reciprocating gait orthosis—A special type of THKAFO that can be useful for paraplegic individuals or those with thoracic or high lumbar spina bifida. It uses weight shifts to allow gait in these patients.

II. Lower Limb Amputations

A. Demographics

1. Approximately 130,000 new amputations are performed annually in the United States.

2. The causes and levels of amputations performed are listed in **Tables 3** and **4**.

B. Goals of lower limb amputation

Table 4

Percentage of Lower Limb Amputations by Level

Level	Amputations (%)
Foot	50
Transtibial	25
Transfemoral	25

1. General goals

   a. Remove a diseased, injured, or nonfunctioning limb in a reconstructive procedure

   b. Restore function to the level of patient need

   c. Preserve length and strength

   d. Balance the forces of the remaining muscles to provide a stable residual limb

2. Goals for ambulatory patients

   a. Restore a maximum level of independent function

   b. Ablate diseased tissue

   c. Reduce morbidity and mortality

3. Goals for nonambulatory patients

   a. Achieve wound healing while minimizing complications

   b. Improve sitting balance

   c. Facilitate position and transfers

C. Preoperative evaluation

   1. The preoperative evaluation should include an assessment of skin integrity and sensation, joint mobility, and muscle strength.

   2. Vascular status also should be evaluated to determine the viable level of amputation. Several assessment techniques are used.

      a. Doppler ultrasonography

         • Ankle-brachial index greater than 0.45 correlates with 90% healing.

         • Advantages—Readily available, noninvasive.

         • Disadvantages—Arterial wall calcification can give misleadingly elevated readings.

      b. Toe systolic blood pressure

         • The minimum requirement for distal healing is 55 mm Hg.

         • Advantages—Noninvasive, readily available, inexpensive.

   c. Transcutaneous oxygen tension

      • P_{O2} > 35mm Hg is necessary for wound healing.

      • Advantages—Noninvasive, highly accurate in assessing wound healing.

      • Disadvantages—Results may be altered by skin disorders such as edema or cellulitis.

   d. Skin blood flow measurement

      • Xenon 133 clearance has been used in the past.

      • Disadvantages—Expensive and time consuming.

   e. Fluorescence studies have been used but provide unreliable results.

   f. Arteriography

      • Advantage—Visualizes the patency of vessels.

      • Disadvantages—Invasive and unreliable in determining successful wound healing.

D. Assessment of nutritional status and immunocompetence

   1. Nutritional status: Serum albumin should be 3 g/dL or higher.

   2. Immunocompetence: Total lymphocyte count should be at least 1,500/mL.

E. Psychologic preparation

   1. Viewing amputation as a step in recovery, not a failure

   2. Early plan for prosthetic fitting and return to function

   3. Preoperative counseling for the patient and family

   4. Referral to amputee support groups

F. Surgical principles

   1. Blood and soft-tissue considerations

      a. A tourniquet should be used to minimize blood loss if no significant vascular disease is present.

      b. Soft-tissue flaps should be planned for mobile and sensate skin.

      c. Muscle forces should be balanced across the residual joints.

   2. Bone considerations

      a. The bone ends should be beveled to minimize skin pressure and maximize the weight-bearing capacity of the residual limb.

      b. Periosteal stripping should be avoided to preserve bone viability and to minimize the likelihood of heterotopic bone formation.

3. Surgical procedure

   a. Myodesis is the direct suturing of distal muscle to bone or tendon, covering the distal bone end and maximizing the weight-bearing capacity of the residual limb.

   b. Nerves are divided proximally and sharply to avoid painful neuromas.

   c. The wound is closed with minimal tension, and a drain is placed to decompress the underlying tissue.

4. Postoperative management

   a. A compressive dressing is applied to protect the wound and control edema.

   b. A splint or cast also may be applied to limit edema and prevent contractures.

G. Complications

   1. Failure of the wound to heal properly occurs as the result of insufficient blood supply, infection, or errors in surgical technique.

   2. Infection may develop postoperatively without widespread tissue necrosis or flap failure, especially if active distal infection was present at the time of the definitive amputation or the amputation was done near the zone of a traumatic injury.

   3. Postoperative edema is common; rigid dressings help reduce this problem.

   4. Phantom sensation—The feeling that all or a part of the amputated limb is still present.

      a. Occurs in nearly everyone who undergoes amputation

      b. Usually diminishes over time

   5. Phantom pain—A bothersome painful or burning sensation in the part of the limb that is missing

      a. Unrelenting phantom pain occurs in only a minority of patients.

      b. It can usually be treated successfully with neuromodulators like gabapentin.

   6. Joint contractures

      a. Joint contractures usually develop between the time of amputation and prosthetic fitting.

      b. Treatment is difficult and often unsuccessful.

      c. Prevention with adequate pain control and the initial use of casts or splints is paramount.

      d. The classic problem is a knee maintained in flexion following a transtibial amputation.

   7. Dermatologic problems

      a. The residual limb and prosthetic socket must be kept clean. After cleaning, it should be rinsed well to remove all soap residue, and thoroughly dried.

      b. Shaving increases problems with ingrown hairs and folliculitis.

      c. Epidermoid cysts commonly occur at the prosthetic socket brim. The best approach is to modify the socket and relieve pressure over the cyst.

      d. Verrucous hyperplasia is a wartlike overgrowth of skin that can occur on the distal end of the residual limb. It is caused by a lack of distal contact and failure to remove normal keratin.

      e. Contact dermatitis is caused by contact with acids, bases, or caustics and frequently results from the failure to rinse detergents from prosthetic socks.

      f. Candidiasis and other dermatophytoses present with scaly, itchy skin, often with vesicles at the border and clearing centrally. Dermatophytoses are diagnosed with a potassium hydroxide preparation and are treated with topical antifungal agents.

III. Levels of Amputation

A. Foot

   1. Hallux amputation

      a. The base of the proximal phalanx should be saved to preserve push-off strength.

      b. Tenodesis of the flexor hallucis brevis tendon is performed to stabilize the sesamoid bones.

   2. Lesser toes can be amputated through the interphalangeal joint, the metatarsophalangeal joint, or the phalanx.

      a. Side-to-side or plantar dorsal flaps can be used.

      b. The base of the proximal phalanx should be saved to provide better stability and push-off strength.

   3. Ray amputations are best done on the border rays; central ray resections take longer to heal.

   4. Transmetatarsal amputations can be performed through the metatarsals or the Lisfranc joints.

      a. Bone cuts should be beveled on the plantar surface to prevent skin pressure.

      b. A cascade should be created from the medial to the lateral side of the foot.

      c. Achilles lengthening should be considered to prevent equinus.

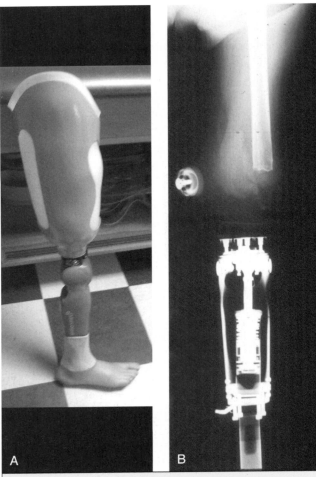

Figure 6 **A,** Photograph shows a transfemoral prosthesis with a microprocessor knee joint. **B,** AP radiograph shows an abducted femur within the socket of a transfemoral prosthesis.

5. Hindfoot

　a. Chopart amputation—Performed through the transverse tarsal joints.

　　• Preserves the talus and calcaneus.

　　• Equinus deformity can result.

　　• The muscle forces are rebalanced by lengthening the Achilles tendon and reattaching the tibialis anterior and extensor hallucis longus tendons to the anterior talus.

　b. Boyd amputation—Combines a talectomy with a calcaneotibial arthrodesis.

　c. Pirogoff amputation—The distal end of the calcaneus is excised, then rotated and fused to the tibia.

　d. Both the Boyd and Pirogoff amputations prevent migration of the heel pad and provide a stable distal weight-bearing surface.

B. Ankle disarticulation (Syme)

1. Provides superior mechanics compared with transtibial amputation.

2. Surgical procedure

　a. A long posterior flap is preferred to sagittal flaps.

　b. The length of the residual tibia should be preserved.

　c. The tibial cut is beveled and a myodesis performed to protect the distal end of the limb.

　d. The distal limb is covered by a heel pad and plantar skin, and the fascia is sutured.

3. Postoperative management includes a rigid dressing or cast to control edema, protect the skin from pressure, and prevent knee flexion contracture.

C. Knee disarticulation

1. Indications

　a. Ambulatory patients who cannot undergo a transtibial amputation

　b. Nonambulatory patients

2. Retains the length of the femur for good sitting balance

3. Prosthetic fitting is challenging because the knee joint is distal to the opposite leg.

4. The longer limb provides better leverage for using the prosthesis.

D. Transfemoral amputation

1. Usually done with equal anterior-posterior flaps

2. Muscle stabilization is critical (**Figure 6**).

3. Abduction and flexion forces must be balanced, even in nonambulatory patients.

4. Without an adductor myodesis, the femur can migrate to a subcutaneous position even within a well-fitted prosthetic socket.

E. Hip disarticulation

1. Rarely performed

2. Ambulation with the prosthesis requires more energy than a swing-through gait with crutches.

3. A lateral approach is preferred for several reasons

　a. The anatomy is more familiar to orthopaedic surgeons.

　b. Dissection is simplified.

　c. Few perforating vessels are encountered.

　d. The procedure is quick, with minimal blood loss.

e. Femoral and gluteal circulation is preserved.

4. Mortality varies with the underlying disease process.

IV. Lower Limb Prostheses

A. Overview

1. Goals of lower limb prostheses—Comfortable to wear, easy to don and doff, lightweight, durable, aesthetically pleasing, good mechanical function, reasonably low maintenance requirements.

2. Major advances

   a. Lightweight structural materials

   b. Elastic-response (energy-storing) designs

   c. Computer-assisted design and computer-assisted manufacturing technology for sockets

   d. Microprocessor control of the prosthetic knee joint

3. Major components

   a. Socket

   b. Suspension mechanism

   c. Knee joint

   d. Pylon

   e. Terminal device

B. Socket—The connection between the residual limb and the prosthesis; the socket must protect the residual limb but also must transmit the forces associated with standing and ambulation.

1. Preparatory (temporary) socket

   a. The preparatory socket must be adjusted several times as the volume of the residual limb stabilizes.

   b. It can be created by using a plaster mold of the residual limb as a template.

2. The most common socket used in a transtibial amputation is a patellar tendon–bearing prosthesis.

C. Suspension mechanism

1. Attaches the prosthesis to the residual limb using belts, wedges, straps, suction, or a combination thereof.

2. The two types of suspension are standard suction and silicone suspension.

   a. Standard suction—Form-fitting rigid or semi-rigid socket into which the residual limb is fitted (**Figure 7**).

   b. Silicone suspension—Uses a silicon-based sock that slips onto the residual limb, which is in-

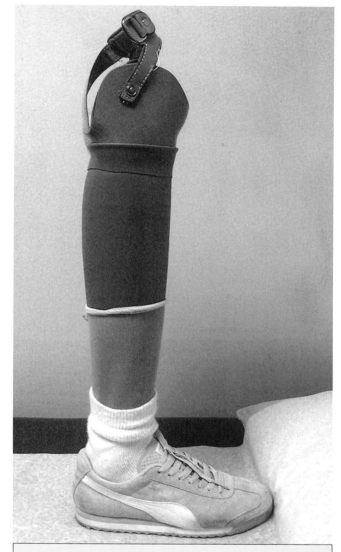

Figure 7   Photograph shows a transtibial prosthesis with a standard socket and a supracondylar suspension strap.

serted into the socket. The silicone helps to form an airtight seal that stabilizes the prosthesis (**Figure 8**).

D. Knee (articulating) joint (if needed)

1. Three principal functions

   a. Provide support during stance phase

   b. Produce smooth control during swing phase

   c. Maintain unrestricted motion for sitting and kneeling

2. Two types of axes

   a. Single axis with a simple hinge and a single pivot point

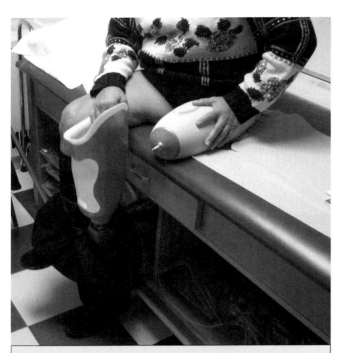

Figure 8 Photograph shows a transfemoral prosthesis with a silicone suspension system.

b. Polycentric axis with multiple centers of rotation

3. Microprocessor control systems have been applied to knee units for transfemoral amputees (**Figure 9**).

   a. The microprocessor alters the resistance of the knee unit to flexion or extension appropriately by sensing the position and velocity of the shank relative to the thigh.

   b. Current microprocessor-controlled knee units do not provide power for active knee extension, which would help the amputee rise from the sitting position or go up stairs and would provide power to the gait.

   c. The new microprocessor-controlled, "intelligent" knee units offer superior control when walking at varied speeds, descending ramps and stairs, and walking on uneven surfaces.

E. Pylon—A simple tube or shell that attaches the socket to the terminal device.

   1. Pylons have progressed from simple static shells to dynamic devices that allow axial rotation and absorb, store, and release energy.

   2. The pylon can be an exoskeleton (soft foam contoured to match the other limb with a hard laminated shell) or an endoskeleton (internal metal frame with aesthetic soft covering).

F. Terminal device—Typically a foot, but other special-

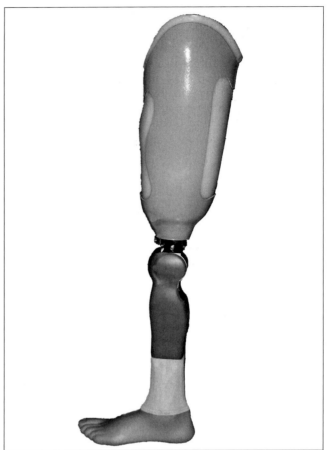

Figure 9 Photograph shows a transfemoral prosthesis with a microprocessor knee joint.

ized forms are available for water sports or other activities.

1. Ankle

   a. Ankle function usually is incorporated into the terminal device.

   b. Separate ankle joints can be beneficial in heavy-duty industrial work or in sports, but the added weight requires more energy expenditure and more limb strength to control the additional motion.

2. Foot—The prosthetic foot has five basic functions: Provide a stable weight-bearing surface, absorb shock, replace lost muscle function, replicate the anatomic joint, and restore aesthetic appearance.

   a. Non–energy-storing feet

   • Solid ankle/cushioned heel (SACH) foot— Mimics ankle plantar flexion, which permits a smooth gait. The SACH foot is a low-cost, low-maintenance foot for a sedentary patient who has had a transtibial or a transfemoral amputation.

- Single-axis foot—Adds passive plantar flexion and dorsiflexion, which increase stability during stance phase.

b. Energy-storing feet

- Multiaxis foot—Adds inversion, eversion, and rotation to plantar flexion and dorsiflexion; handles uneven terrain well and is a good choice for the individual with a minimal to moderate activity level.

- Dynamic-response foot—This top-of-the-line foot is commonly used by young active and athletic individuals with amputations; it is often made of an energy-storing material that can permit higher-level function such as running and sports participation.

G. Prosthetic prescription—Includes the type of prosthesis and its components; considers the patient's functional level.

1. Functional level 1: Has the ability or potential to use a prosthesis for transfers or ambulation on level surfaces at a fixed cadence.

2. Functional level 2: Has the ability or potential to ambulate and traverse low-level environmental barriers such as curbs, stairs, or uneven surfaces,

3. Functional level 3: Has the ability or potential to ambulate with a variable cadence.

4. Functional level 4: Has the ability or potential to perform prosthetic ambulation that exceeds basic ambulation skills and exhibits high impact, stress, or energy levels.

H. Prosthetic training

1. Basics of prosthesis care

a. How to don and doff the prosthesis

b. How to inspect the residual limb for signs of skin breakdown; should be checked daily

c. How to perform safe transfers

2. Skills training—The goal is to ambulate safely on all usual surfaces without adaptive equipment. Training includes the following:

a. Weight bearing with the prosthesis

b. Ambulation on level surfaces with a walker or other assistive device

c. Ambulation on stairs, uneven surfaces, and ramps/inclines

I. Problems with prosthesis use

1. Choke syndrome

a. Venous outflow can be obstructed when the proximal part of the socket fits too snugly on the residual limb. When this occurs and there is an empty space more distally in the socket,

swelling can occur until that empty space is filled.

b. With acute choke syndrome, the skin is red and indurated and may have an orange peel appearance with prominent skin pores.

c. If the constriction is not resolved, chronic skin changes with hemosiderin deposits and venous stasis ulcers can develop.

2. Dermatologic problems

a. Contact dermatitis—The usual culprits are the liner, socks, and suspension mechanism, with the socket a less likely cause. Treatment consists of removal of the offending item and symptomatic treatment with topical diphenhydramine or cortisone creams.

b. Cysts and excessive sweating—Can be signs of excessive shear forces and components that are improperly fitted.

c. Scar management—Focuses on massaging and lubricating the scar to obtain a well-healed result without dog ears or adhesions.

3. Painful residual limb

a. Possible causes of prosthesis-related pain

- Excessive pressure over anatomic bony prominences or heterotopic ossification

- Friction between the skin and the prosthetic socket from a poor fit

b. Possible causes of residual limb–related pain

- Insufficient soft-tissue coverage over bony prominences

- An unstable residual limb from a lack of myodesis to balance muscle forces (for example, no adductor myodesis in a transfemoral amputation leads to unopposed hip abductor force)

- Unstable soft-tissue pad over the distal residual limb

- Neuroma formation in a superficial location

4. Prosthetic gait—The ability to walk with a prosthesis is related to the mechanical quality of the prosthesis and the physiologic quality of the residual limb. The physiologic quality of the residual limb is related to passive joint mobility and muscle strength.

a. Transtibial amputation

- The demands of weight acceptance require heightened muscle control and strength.

- The increased muscle demand results from insufficient knee flexion and persistent ankle dorsiflexion of the prosthesis.

Table 5

Metabolic Cost of Ambulation per Level and Nature of Amputation

Amputation Level	Metabolic Cost
Syme	Increased 15%
Traumatic transtibial	Increased 25%
Vascular transtibial	Increased 40%
Traumatic transfemoral	Increased 68%
Vascular transfemoral	Increased 100%

Reproduced from Munin MC, Galang GF: Limb amputation and prosthetic rehabilitation, in Vaccaro AR, ed: *Orthopaedic Knowledge Update*, ed 8. Rosemont, IL, American Academy of Orthopaedic Surgeons, 2005, p. 652. Data from Czerniecki JM: Rehabilitation in limb deficiency: Gait and motion analysis. *Arch Phys Med Rehabil* 1996;77:S3-S8.

- A knee flexion contracture greater than 10° is the most significant obstacle to walking with a transtibial prosthesis.

  b. Transfemoral amputation

  - Walking is arduous for the transfemoral amputee, requiring significant functional contributions from the trunk and intact limb.

  - Residual limb function is hampered by the loss of musculature, the lack of direct contact between the thigh and the prosthetic knee joint, and limitations of the prosthetic foot, which ideally should provide increased flexibility without loss of stance stability.

J. Energy requirements of prosthetic gait (**Table 5**)

1. The increase in energy requirements can be the limiting factor in ambulation.

2. An individual who has a lower limb amputation and requires a walker or crutches to ambulate uses 65% more energy than an individual with a normal gait.

3. Increased levels of energy consumption (percentage above normal)

   a. Transtibial unilateral amputation: 10% to 20%

   b. Transtibial bilateral amputation: 20% to 40%

   c. Transfemoral unilateral amputation: 60% to 70%

   d. Transfemoral bilateral amputation: greater than 200%

4. Energy consumption actually is less with a transtibial prosthesis than ambulating with crutches. Ambulating with a transfemoral prosthesis re-

quires more energy, however, so the cardiopulmonary status of the patient is more significant.

K. The first year of amputee care

1. The residual limb must mature before the definitive prosthesis is worn.

2. Temporary prostheses allow for residual limb shrinking and maturation.

3. The surgeon must resist the urge to have a definitive prosthesis fashioned too early.

4. Redness and pain must be addressed; most often, the solution is to increase the number or ply of socks at the residual limb/prosthesis interface.

5. Ultimately, the goal of the first year of care is a mature residual limb without contracture or skin breakdown that can accept a prosthesis of the appropriate type for the patient's level of function.

V. Upper Limb Amputations

A. Traumatic amputation

1. Overview

   a. Initial management of traumatic amputations often occurs at centers that lack the expertise needed to replant the amputated body part or appropriately treat the amputee.

   b. The physicians involved in initial care need to understand the indications for replantation and the proper care of the patient, the residual limb, and the amputated limb segment.

2. Replantation

   a. Indications—The decision whether to replant depends on patient factors (such as age, comorbidities) and the condition of the residual limb and amputated body part.

   b. Common replantations—The most commonly replanted parts are the thumb, multiple digits in adults, and amputated digits in children.

   c. Initial treatment of the trauma patient

   - Stabilization of the patient and evaluation for other conditions that may supersede the amputation

   - Life-threatening injuries always take precedence over amputation or replantation.

   - Consultation with a hand center helps to determine whether a replantation is indicated. The goal is to expedite patient transfer to a hand center if a replantation may be needed.

   d. Initial management of the amputated body part

- The amputated part should never be placed directly on ice; direct exposure to ice or ice water will result in tissue damage.

- The amputated part should be wrapped in wet gauze and placed in a plastic bag on ice.

e. Preoperative management for replantation

- The patient should be placed on nothing-by-mouth (NPO) status.

- Tetanus prophylaxis, antibiotic therapy, and intravenous fluids should be administered.

- Other emergent medical conditions should be treated.

- Radiographs of the residual limb and the amputated part should be obtained.

- Delay in treatment should be minimized; the likelihood of successful replantation decreases with prolonged tissue ischemia.

f. Contraindications to replantation

- Replantation of a single digit may result in a stiff, painful, and nonfunctional finger. Ray resection may be more useful.

- Replantation after multiple-level injuries, crush injuries, and injuries in which gross contamination occurs may be less successful.

- In patients with factors or injury characteristics that contraindicate single-digit replantation (for example, advanced age, diabetes mellitus, smoking), revision amputation is indicated.

- Amputations of the distal thumb or fingers can be shortened and closed primarily.

B. Surgical amputation

1. Indications—Irreparable loss of the blood supply or tissue of a diseased or injured upper limb is the only absolute indication for amputation, regardless of all other circumstances.

a. Vascular compromise or occlusion—Patients present very differently, depending on the etiology.

b. Trauma—Most cases involve significant avulsion and crush components.

c. Thermal burns and frostbite—These cases rarely require amputation proximal to the hand.

d. Neglected compartment syndromes

e. Systemic sepsis—Amputations may be necessary to control an otherwise rampant infection.

f. Malignant tumors

2. Incidence

a. Published estimates of the annual incidence of upper limb amputations in the United States vary significantly, from 20,000 to 30,000 new amputations per year.

b. Prevalence—The number of all types of amputations in the United States is 350,000 to 1,000,000.

3. Goals of upper limb amputation surgery

a. Preservation of functional length

b. Durable skin and soft-tissue coverage

c. Preservation of useful sensation

d. Prevention of symptomatic neuromas

e. Prevention of adjacent joint contractures

f. Controlled short-term morbidity

g. Early prosthetic fitting

h. Early return to work and recreation

4. Levels of amputation

a. Ray resection—A digital ray resection (for example, index or little finger) may be preferable to a digital replantation if replantation would result in a stiff, useless, or painful digit.

b. Transcarpal amputation

- Advantages—Preserves supination and pronation of the forearm and limited flexion and extension of the wrist; the long lever arm increases the ease and power of prosthetic use.

- Disadvantages—Prosthetic fitting is more difficult with a transcarpal amputation than with a wrist disarticulation.

- Surgical technique—A long full-thickness palmar flap and a shorter dorsal flap are created in a ratio of 2:1. The finger flexor and extensor tendons are transected. The wrist flexors and extensors are anchored to the remaining carpus in line with their insertions to preserve active wrist motion.

c. Wrist disarticulation

- Indications—Wrist articulation is the procedure of choice in children because it preserves the distal radial and ulnar physes. It also provides a longer lever arm for strength in both adults and children.

- Advantages—It preserves the distal radioulnar joint, allowing pronation and supination.

- Surgical technique—The prominent styloid processes should be rounded off. The radial styloid flare should be preserved to improve prosthetic suspension.

d. Transradial (below-elbow) amputation

- Advantages—Despite resection of the distal radioulnar joint, some pronation and supination are preserved.

- Surgical technique—Amputation at the junction of the distal and middle third of the forearm appears to provide a good compromise between adequate functional length and adequate wound healing. If amputation at this level is impossible, a shorter residual limb still is preferable to a transhumeral amputation. Detaching the biceps tendon and reattaching it proximally to the ulna at a position approximating its resting length is advised to facilitate prosthetic fitting. Distal reattachment may cause a flexion contracture at the elbow.

e. Transhumeral (above-elbow) amputation

- As much of the bone length that has suitable soft-tissue coverage should be retained as possible. Even if no functional length is salvageable, retaining the humeral head results in an improved shoulder contour and aesthetic appearance.

- Myodesis helps preserve biceps and triceps strength, prosthetic control, and myoelectric signals.

f. Shoulder disarticulation

- Indications—Shoulder disarticulation is performed only rarely, usually in cases of cancer or severe trauma.

- Disadvantages—Results in a loss of the normal shoulder contour and causes clothing to fit poorly.

- Surgical considerations—The humeral head should be saved, if possible, to improve the contour of a shoulder disarticulation.

C. Postoperative management of upper limb amputations

1. A soft compressive dressing is applied.

2. An elastic bandage is applied to prevent edema.

3. If a drain is used, it is removed within 24 to 48 hours.

4. If no contraindications exist, anticoagulants may be administered for deep vein thrombosis prophylaxis.

5. Active range of motion of the shoulder, elbow, and wrist is initiated immediately to prevent joint contractures.

D. Immediate or early postoperative prosthetic fitting

1. Advantages include decreased edema, postoperative pain, and phantom pain; accelerated wound healing; improved rehabilitation; and shorter hospital stays.

2. Benefits are less pronounced at amputation levels above the elbow.

VI. Upper Limb Prostheses

A. Overview

1. Terminology

a. Relief—A concavity within the socket designed to accommodate pressure-sensitive bony prominences.

b. Buildup—A convexity designed for areas tolerant to high pressure.

c. Terminal device—The most distal part of the prosthesis used to do work (such as the hand).

d. Myodesis—Direct suturing of muscle or tendon to bone.

e. Myoplasty—Suturing of muscle to the periosteum.

f. Prehensile—Designed for grasping.

2. Considerations for upper limb prostheses

a. Amputation level

b. Expected function of the prosthesis

c. Cognitive function of the patient

d. Vocation of the patient (desk job versus manual labor)

e. Recreational interests of the patient

f. Aesthetic importance of the prosthesis

g. Financial resources of the patient

B. Types of upper limb prostheses

1. Body-powered prostheses

a. Advantages—Moderate cost and weight, most durable prostheses, higher level of sensory feedback.

b. Disadvantages—Less aesthetically pleasing than a myoelectric unit; require more gross limb movement.

2. Myoelectric prostheses function by transmitting electrical activity to the surface electrodes on the residual limb muscles that is then sent to the electric motor.

a. Advantages—Provide more proximal function, better aesthetic appearance.

b. Disadvantages—Heavy and expensive, less sensory feedback, require more maintenance.

c. Types of myoelectric units

- The two-site/two-function devices use separate electrodes for flexion and extension.

- The one-site/two-function devices use one electrode for both flexion and extension. The patient uses muscle contractions of different strengths to differentiate between flexion and extension (a strong contraction opens the device, and a weak contraction closes it).

C. Prosthesis characteristics by amputation level

1. Transradial

    a. Voluntary-opening split hook

    b. Friction wrist

    c. Double-walled plastic laminate socket

    d. Flexible elbow hinge, a single-control cable system

    e. Biceps or triceps cuff

    f. Figure-of-8 harness

2. Transhumeral

    a. Similar to transradial, but has several differences

    b. Substitutes an internal-locking elbow for the flexible elbow hinge

    c. Dual-control instead of single-control cable

    d. No biceps or triceps cuff

D. Components

1. Terminal devices (prehension devices)

    a. Passive terminal devices

    - Advantages—Excellent aesthetic appearance; new advances in materials and design can produce a device that is virtually indistinguishable from a native hand.

    - Disadvantages—Passive terminal devices usually are less functional and more expensive than active terminal devices.

    b. Active terminal devices

    - More functional than aesthetic.

    - Can be divided into two main categories: hooks and prosthetic hands with cables and myoelectric devices.

    c. Grips—Five types are available.

    - Precision grip (pincer grip)

    - Tripod grip (palmar grip, three-jaw chuck pinch)

    - Lateral pinch (key pinch)

- Hook power grip (carrying a briefcase)

- Spherical grip (turning a doorknob)

d. Considerations for choosing terminal devices

- Handlike devices

    ○ Composed of a thumb and an index and long finger

    ○ The thumb and fingers are oriented to provide palmar prehension.

    ○ The fingers are coupled as one unit, with the thumb in a plane perpendicular to the axis of the finger joints.

    ○ May be covered with a silicone glove simulating the appearance of an intact hand

    ○ Often the device of choice for a person working in an office

- Nonhand prehension devices

    ○ Hooks or two-finger pincer designs with parallel surfaces

    ○ Good for work that requires higher prehension force

    ○ May be fitted with quick-release mechanisms to attach task-specific tools for work and recreational activities

    ○ Often used in an environment requiring physical labor

- Externally powered myoelectric devices

    ○ Use force-sensing resistors

    ○ Offer freedom from a control suspension harness

    ○ Provide stronger prehension

    ○ Can be used only in a nonhostile environment, free from dirt, dust, water, grease, or solvents

- Many upper extremity amputees have both a body-powered prosthesis and a myoelectric prosthesis for specific activities.

e. Terminal device mechanisms

- Voluntary opening mechanism

    ○ The device is closed at rest.

    ○ More common than a voluntary closing mechanism

    ○ The proximal muscles are used to open a hook-based device against the resistive force of rubber bands or cables.

    ○ Relaxation of the proximal muscles allows the terminal device to close around the desired object.

- ○ In a myoelectric device, contraction of the proximal muscles activates the electric motor.

- • Voluntary closing mechanism

  - ○ The terminal device is open at rest.

  - ○ The patient uses the residual forearm flexors to grasp the desired object.

  - ○ Usually heavier and less durable than a voluntary opening mechanism

2. Wrist units

   a. Quick-disconnect wrist unit—Allows easy exchange of terminal devices with specialized functions.

   b. Locking wrist unit—Prevents rotation during grasping and lifting.

   c. Wrist flexion unit—In a patient with bilateral upper limb amputations, a wrist flexion unit can be placed on the longer residual limb (regardless of premorbid hand dominance) to allow midline activities such as shaving or buttoning.

3. Elbow units—Chosen based on the level of the amputation and the amount of residual function.

   a. Rigid elbow hinge—When a patient cannot achieve adequate pronation and supination but has adequate native elbow flexion, such as in a short transradial amputation, a rigid elbow hinge provides additional stability.

   b. Flexible elbow hinge—When a patient has sufficient voluntary pronation and supination and elbow flexion and extension, such as in a wrist disarticulation or a long transradial amputation, a flexible elbow hinge usually works well.

4. Prostheses for amputations about the shoulder

   a. When amputation is required at the shoulder or forequarter level, function is very difficult to restore because of the weight of the prosthetic components and the increased energy expenditure necessary to operate the prosthesis.

   b. For this reason, some individuals with this level of amputation choose a purely aesthetic prosthesis to improve body image and the fit of clothes.

E. Problems associated with upper limb prostheses

1. Dermatologic problems

   a. Contact dermatitis—Usually caused by the liner and suspension mechanism; the socket is a less likely cause. Treatment consists of removing the offending item and symptomatic treatment with topical diphenhydramine or cortisone creams.

   b. Cysts and excessive sweating—Can be signs of excessive shear forces and components that are improperly fitted.

   c. Scar management—Focuses on massaging and lubricating the scar to obtain a well-healed result without adhesions.

2. Painful residual limb

   a. Possible causes of prosthesis-related pain include excessive pressure over anatomic bony prominences or heterotopic ossification, or friction between the skin and prosthetic socket from a poor fit.

   b. Possible causes of residual limb–related pain include the following:

      - • Insufficient soft-tissue coverage over bony prominences

      - • An unstable residual limb because no myodesis was done to balance muscle forces

      - • An unstable soft-tissue pad over the distal residual limb

      - • Neuroma formation in a superficial location

Top Testing Facts

1. Articulated AFOs allow a more natural gait pattern and adjustment of plantar flexion and dorsiflexion. They can be designed to provide stability in terminal stance and to provide dorsiflexion assistance to clear the toes during swing.

2. A KAFO can be used in patients with quadriceps paralysis or weakness to maintain knee stability and control flexible recurvatum, valgus, or varus.

3. A polycentric knee joint allows limited multiplanar motion during flexion and extension that decreases specific areas of joint contact forces; this type of joint is helpful for persons with osteoarthritis.

4. Lower limb amputation is a reconstructive procedure designed to preserve length and strength and to balance the forces of the remaining muscles to provide a stable residual limb.

5. Wound healing characteristics—Ankle-brachial index greater than 0.45 correlates with 90% healing; minimum toe systolic blood pressure for distal healing is 55 mm Hg; P_{O2} greater than 35 mm Hg is necessary for wound healing; nutritional competence is indicated by a total lymphocyte count greater than 1,500/mL and a serum albumin level of at least 3 g/dL.

6. The major advances in lower limb prostheses include (a) new lightweight structural materials; (b) elastic-response (energy-storing) designs; (c) computer-assisted design and computer-assisted manufacturing technology in sockets; and (d) microprocessor control of the prosthetic knee joint.

7. Increased levels of energy (percentage above normal) are associated with amputations: unilateral transtibial, 10% to 20%; bilateral trantibial, 20% to 40%; unilateral above-knee, 60% to 70%; bilateral transfemoral, greater than 200%.

8. Preoperative management for replantation: Emergent medical conditions should be treated; radiographs of the residual limb and the amputated part should be obtained; the patient should be placed on NPO status; and tetanus prophylaxis, antibiotic therapy, and intravenous fluids should be administered. The amputated part should be wrapped in wet gauze and placed in a plastic bag on ice.

9. Goals of upper limb amputation surgery include the preservation of functional length, durable skin and soft-tissue coverage, preservation of useful sensation, prevention of symptomatic neuromas, prevention of adjacent-joint contractures, controlled short-term morbidity, early prosthetic fitting, and early patient return to work and recreation.

10. A voluntary opening mechanism is commonly used for the hand.

Acknowledgments

The authors wish to recognize the contributions of Douglas G. Smith, MD, to the *AAOS Comprehensive Orthopaedic Review* and this chapter.

Bibliography

Davids JR, Rowan F, Davis RB: Indications for orthoses to improve gait in children with cerebral palsy. *J Am Acad Orthop Surg* 2007;15(3):178-188.

Fergason JR, Smith DG: Socket considerations for the patient with a transtibial amputation. *Clin Orthop Relat Res* 1999;361:76-84.

Friel K: Componentry for lower extremity prostheses. *J Am Acad Orthop Surg* 2005;13(5):326-335.

Garst RJ: The Krukenberg hand. *J Bone Joint Surg Br* 1991;73(3):385-388.

Legro MW, Reiber GE, del Aguila M, et al: Issues of importance reported by persons with lower limb amputations and prostheses. *J Rehabil Res Dev* 1999;36(3):155-163.

Potter BK, Scoville CR: Amputation is not isolated: An overview of the US Army Amputee Patient Care Program and associated amputee injuries. *J Am Acad Orthop Surg* 2006;14(10 Spec No):S188-S190.

Waters RL, Perry J, Antonelli D, Hislop H: Energy cost of walking of amputees: The influence of level of amputation. *J Bone Joint Surg Am* 1976;58(1):42-46.

Wright TW, Hagen AD, Wood MB: Prosthetic usage in major upper extremity amputations. *J Hand Surg Am* 1995;20(4):619-622.

2: General Knowledge

Chapter 19
Occupational Health/Work-Related Injury and Illness

Peter J. Mandell, MD

I. Workers' Compensation

A. Burden of proof

1. The injured worker does not have to prove the employer was at fault.

2. The injured worker must prove that work at least partially caused the injury or illness.

3. A patient's particular disease or injury must be caused by work-related factors to be compensable under workers' compensation.

   a. Results of the history and physical examination should support the diagnosis and causative factors.

   b. A thorough review of the injured worker's records also is needed to support the conclusions about diagnosis and causation.

   c. A detailed history of the injury may reveal important facts to support the diagnosis and opinions about causation.

B. Assessment of the injured worker

1. Patient history

   a. Specific information regarding how, when, where, and why an accident or injurious exposure occurred should be elicited.

   b. The areas of the body that were involved should be identified.

   c. The extent and onset of symptoms following the accident or injurious exposure should be identified.

   d. The treatment history should be reviewed in detail, with specific emphasis on what has been tried and how effective it was. Failure to respond at all to multiple, usually reliable treatments of common diagnoses suggests a nonorganic response to injury.

   e. The worker's perception of events compared with those depicted in the medical records should be analyzed to assess credibility.

2. Current symptoms should be discussed to document answers to the following questions.

   a. What hurts now?

   b. What can the patient do? What can the patient not do?

   c. How does the injury impact the patient's ability to work, perform activities of daily living, and play?

3. The past medical history and review of systems should focus on other possible causes or contributors.

   a. Prior injuries to the same or related body regions

   b. Prior surgeries

   c. Prior industrial accidents of any type

   d. A family history of similar problems

   e. Diseases and habits that impact the neuromusculoskeletal system

      • Diabetes mellitus

      • Rheumatoid arthritis

      • Obesity

      • Smoking

      • Alcohol abuse

      • High-impact hobbies/sports activities

4. A detailed work history is essential. Knowledge of the patient's work activities and environment can determine possible causative factors and the feasibility of modified work activities. The work history should include

   a. How long the patient has worked at the job

   b. Prior work experience

2: General Knowledge

Table 1

Waddell Nonorganic Physical Signs in Low Back Pain

1. Tenderness	Tenderness related to physical disease should be specific and localized to specific anatomic structures. Superficial—tenderness to pinch or light touch over a wide area of lumbar skin Nonanatomic—deep tenderness over a wide area, not localized to a specific structure
2. Simulation tests	These tests should not be uncomfortable Axial loading—reproduction of low back pain with vertical pressure on the skull Rotation—reproduction of back pain when shoulders and pelvis are passively rotated in the same plane
3. Distraction tests	Findings that are present during physical examination and disappear at other times, particularly while the patient is distracted
4. Regional disturbances	Findings inconsistent with neuroanatomy Motor—nonanatomic voluntary release or unexplained giving way of muscle groups Sensory—nondermatomal sensory abnormalities
5. Overreaction	Disproportionate verbal or physical reactions

Reproduced from Moy OJ, Ablove RH: Work-related illnesses, cumulative trauma and compensation, in Vaccaro AR, ed: *Orthopaedic Knowledge Update, ed 8.* Rosemont, IL, American Academy of Orthopaedic Surgeons, 2005, pp 143-148.

c. Concurrent employment at a second or third job

d. Job satisfaction

- Recent job changes such as increased workload resulting from layoffs

- Conflicts with a supervisor or associates

- A high-demand–low-control (stressful) work environment

5. A musculoskeletal examination of the injured area is critical. Physical findings may form a major portion of the basis for administrative and financial decisions that will substantially affect the patient.

a. The injured body part(s) should be examined.

b. Other, less obvious explanations should be investigated.

- Cervical disk disease as a cause of shoulder pain

- Hip arthritis as a cause of back or knee pain

c. Comments on the reliability of the patient's physical findings and whether the findings support the degree of subjective symptoms reported by the patient

d. For patients with low back pain, the Waddell signs (**Table 1**) should be assessed. Strictly speaking, three of five signs must be present for the pain to be considered nonorganic.

II. Workplace Safety

A. Ergonomics

1. Ergonomics is the science that studies ways to make the workplace more congenial to human capabilities.

2. It considers the realities of human anatomy and the physiology of human muscle strength and fatigue.

3. Ergonomics involves machine and workstation design to improve workplace safety.

B. US Department of Labor Occupational Safety and Health Administration (OSHA)

1. OSHA developed guidelines and programs to improve worker health and safety.

2. Workplace safety measures resulted in a sharp reduction in the incidence of distinct workplace injuries in the late 20th century.

3. The decline of these specific injuries revealed a host of other conditions that may develop in the workplace and can increase in severity over time.

a. Controversy exists about what to call these conditions and whether they are work related. Many call them cumulative trauma disorders (CTDs). This term is cited frequently in both the medical and legal literature.

- The term CTD is problematic because some authors argue that it implies a specific etiology that generally has not been substantiated clearly and scientifically. These authors argue that the cause is multifactorial.

- Not all CTDs become chronic; in fact, many disappear as workers become conditioned to specific work activities. But if rest is not provided or if activities exceed physiologic limits, then no amount of conditioning will prevent tissue damage.

b. OSHA calls CTDs musculoskeletal disorders (MSDs).

- An MSD is an injury of the musculoskeletal and/or nervous system that may be associated with or caused by repetitive tasks, forceful exertions, vibrations, mechanical compression (pressing against hard surfaces), or sustained or awkward positions.

- According to OSHA, MSDs include low back pain, sciatica, bursitis, epicondylitis, and carpal tunnel syndrome.

c. In OSHA parlance, conditions caused by an extended exposure to employment are termed occupational *illnesses*, whereas distinct events cause occupational *injury*.

III. Legal Issues in Occupational Orthopaedics

A. Advantages of workers' compensation

1. For injured workers

   a. Workers' compensation obligates the company to compensate the injured worker for high-quality, timely treatment needed to cure or relieve the worker of the effects of the work injuries.

   b. The employer must also pay lost wages, up to a maximum that varies from state to state.

   c. In addition, the employer is obligated to pay a final disability settlement (analogous to the "damages" awarded in civil cases).

2. For employers

   a. The employer is shielded from being sued for negligence, except in particularly egregious circumstances.

   b. Workers' compensation is usually the "exclusive remedy," precluding claims against employers for pain and suffering, emotional distress, punitive damages, and bad faith.

   c. The system is no-fault.

   d. The employer is required to pay benefits only when work is the cause—at least partially—of the worker's problem(s).

B. Components of the claim

1. Determining causation

2. The need for treatment and, if needed, its type and duration

3. The extent of current disability

4. The ultimate disability settlement

C. Allocating or apportioning causation

1. Some causes may be work related, and some may be preexisting.

2. Legal apportionment varies by state.

   a. Many states require employers to "take their workers as they find them," which makes apportioning to preexisting (but asymptomatic) conditions such as gout, diabetes mellitus, and obesity difficult or illegal.

   b. Other states seemingly allow apportionment to factors beyond the employer's control, such as those listed above. Factors such as sex, race, smoking, and obesity may not survive constitutional challenge.

IV. Assignment of Impairment and Disability

A. Definitions of terms in workers' compensation

1. Different jurisdictions assign somewhat different meanings to the same words.

2. The same word or terms can mean different things in different contexts.

3. The meaning of important terms may vary by state and should be checked.

4. Commonly accepted words and definitions (not universal)

   a. Impairment: a deviation or loss of body structure or of physiologic or psychologic function

   b. Disease: a pathologic condition of a body part

   c. Illness: the total effect of an injury or disease on the entire person

   d. Disability: any restriction or lack of ability to perform an activity in the manner or within the range considered normal for an individual

5. Impairment and disease are purely biologic issues that usually have an objectively measurable effect on the anatomy and/or physiology of the injured organ. An injury leads to an impairment that leads to a disease that may lead to a disability and an illness.

6. Illness and disability are the final complete functional manifestations of impairment and disease, including the social, physiologic, and economic (work) consequences of the employee's injury.

B. Assessment of level of impairment

1. Under the American Medical Association system, only physicians can evaluate for and assign levels of impairment.

2. The assessment must be based on medical probability, also known as medical certainty, which implies that a statement or opinion is correct with greater than 50% certainty.

2: General Knowledge

3. In most states, providing a medically probable opinion about an injured worker's impairment generally requires using the American Medical Association *Guides to the Evaluation of Permanent Impairment.*

    a. This reference provides tables and other standardized methods (depending on the body part or parts involved) for determining impairment.

    b. It also supplies rules for combining the regional impairments into a "whole-person" impairment.

4. Impairments are translated into disability ratings by state workers' compensation boards and other jurisdictions.

5. At the conclusion of an impairment assessment, the physician should include his or her opinions about causation, treatment, light work status, and residual impairments.

V. Malingering, Somatization, and Depression

A. Special considerations

1. Unlike most medical problems, with workers' compensation injury or illness, the patient often thinks she or he knows what is wrong.

2. Skepticism is reasonable when insurance issues are on the line.

B. Malingering

1. Malingering is an act, not a disease. Calling someone a malingerer is an accusation, not a diagnosis.

2. Malingering lies at the far end of a spectrum of explanations about a problem with many names, including

    a. Nonorganic findings

    b. Symptom magnification

    c. Exaggeration

    d. Submaximal, insincere, or low effort

    e. Selling oneself short

    f. Inappropriate pain or illness behavior

C. Somatization (formerly called hysteria or Briquet syndrome)

1. Somatization is an extreme form of body language.

2. Patients who cannot (or whose cultures will not allow them to) express psychologic problems may unconsciously communicate such problems through sometimes powerful physical manifestations.

3. Somatization may be an attempt by patients to strive for psychologic homeostasis.

D. Nonorganic findings

1. Many patients with nonorganic findings are incorrectly assumed to be malingerers but really have somatization.

2. Patients with nonorganic findings may be adult survivors of childhood physical and/or sexual abuse.

E. Factitious disorder

1. Factitious disorder is another form of somatization that resembles malingering.

2. It is a psychologic disorder in which patients have an unconscious need to assume an ill role by producing their disease (for example, patients who self mutilate, including seeking multiple surgeries); the most well known factitious disorder is Munchausen syndrome.

F. Depression

1. Depression may affect assignment of disability because depressed patients often have a heightened perception of disability

2. Depression can be a vicious cycle, arising from a protracted injury and then creating at least the perception of more physical illness.

VI. Issues Relating to Return to Work

A. Statistics

1. About 10% of injured employees who are off work have substantial problems returning to their jobs within usual timeframes.

2. Some studies cite the percentage of workers who return to full duty at only 50% after having been out of work for 6 months.

B. Early return to work

1. Disability itself can be pathogenic and even fatal; early return to duty usually is the best approach for all concerned in the workers' compensation system, especially the injured employee.

2. Early return to work

    a. Minimizes the sense of illness

    b. Lessens the loss of camaraderie and teamwork with associates

    c. Improves the self-respect and positive feedback that comes from knowing one is valued by society

    d. Lessens the effect of deconditioning

3. Exceptions to early return to work are indicated when appropriate light duty is not available and

for patients with posttraumatic stress after severe injuries such as amputations and burns.

4. Job satisfaction and early return to work

   a. Job satisfaction is the leading factor in early return to work.

   b. Workers with high levels of discretion are twice as likely to be working as those with less autonomy.

   c. An unpleasant, stressful work environment greatly reduces the chances that an injured employee will return to work.

5. Employer factors and early return to work

   a. The employer should show support for injured workers.

   b. Employer hostility intensifies worker stress.

   c. Some employers use disability as a way to dismiss workers.

C. Worker factors and return to work

   1. Some workers use time off and benefits to resolve home and family problems.

   2. Workers on disability tend to recover more slowly and have poorer outcomes than those with the same injuries covered by group health and other forms of insurance.

D. Other factors and return to work

   1. Union rules sometimes do not allow injured workers to be assigned to lighter jobs because other workers have more seniority.

   2. Work conditioning can be helpful as an intermediate step in transitioning patients from physical therapy to full duty.

Top Testing Facts

1. Workers are entitled to compensation when their diseases or injuries are caused by work-related factors.

2. It is crucial that the history, review of medical records, and physical examination findings support both the diagnosis and its causation analysis.

3. Workplace safety programs and OSHA activities resulted in a sharp reduction in the incidence of distinct workplace injuries in the late 20th century.

4. CTDs and MSDs have become more obvious with the decline of major work injuries.

5. Knowing the precise meanings of terms often used in workers' compensation matters (for example, impairment, disease, illness, disability) is important.

6. Key factors in a workers' compensation case include medical decisions about causation, treatment, light work status, and residual impairments.

7. Calling someone a malingerer is an accusation, not a diagnosis.

8. Somatization is far more common than malingering.

9. Patients with depression often have a heightened sense of impairment.

10. Early return to work is key to a successful outcome after a work injury.

Bibliography

American Academy of Orthopaedic Surgeons: Position statement: Defining musculoskeletal disorders in the workplace. Doc. No. 1165. 2004. www.aaos.org/about/papers/position.asp. Retired June 2011.

Brady W, Bass J, Moser R Jr, Anstadt GW, Loeppke RR, Leopold R: Defining total corporate health and safety costs—significance and impact: Review and recommendations. *J Occup Environ Med* 1997;39(3):224-231.

Brinker MR, O'Connor DP, Woods GW, Pierce P, Peck B: The effect of payer type on orthopaedic practice expenses. *J Bone Joint Surg Am* 2002;84-A(10):1816-1822.

Gerdtham UG, Johannesson M: A note on the effect of unemployment on mortality. *J Health Econ* 2003;22(3):505-518.

Harris I, Mulford J, Solomon M, van Gelder JM, Young J: Association between compensation status and outcome after surgery: A meta-analysis. *JAMA* 2005;293(13):1644-1652.

Jin RL, Shah CP, Svoboda TJ: The impact of unemployment on health: A review of the evidence. *CMAJ* 1995;153(5):529-540.

Lea RD: Independent medical evaluation: An organization and analysis system, in Grace TG, ed: *Independent Medical Evaluations.* Rosemont, IL American Academy of Orthopaedic Surgeons, 2001, pp 35-57.

2: General Knowledge

Melhorn JM, Talmage JB: Work-related illness, cumulative trauma, and compensation, in Flynn JM, ed: *Orthopaedic Knowledge Update*, ed 10. Rosemont, IL, American Academy of Orthopaedic Surgeons, 2011, pp 147-155.

Stone DA: *The Disabled State*. Philadelphia, PA, Temple University Press, 1984.

Waddell G, McCulloch JA, Kummel E, Venner RM: Nonorganic physical signs in low-back pain. *Spine (Phila Pa 1976)* 1980;5(2):117-125.

Chapter 20
Anesthesiology

Steve Melton, MD   Richard E. Moon, MD

I. Preoperative Assessment and Optimization

A. American Society of Anesthesiologists (ASA) Physical Status Classification System (**Table 1**)

   1. Provides uniform classification of a patient's state of health before surgery

   2. Does NOT provide a means to predict perioperative risk

B. History and physical examination includes airway examination, with or without laboratory tests, electrocardiogram, chest radiograph, or other evaluations, including but not limited to pulmonary function tests or cardiac tests.

C. Risk identification is the foundation of preoperative evaluation.

D. Signs and symptoms of instability or insufficient management of identified medical conditions and risks require further investigation and optimization.

E. The anesthesiologist and the surgeon must communicate directly to coordinate and optimize preoperative planning and surgical treatment.

II. Anesthetic Plan

A. Plan for the type of anesthesia and anesthesia monitoring based on the preoperative assessment, intraoperative and postoperative needs, and risk/benefit evaluation

B. The plan should include postoperative nausea and vomiting prophylaxis, when appropriate, and postoperative analgesia.

C. The anesthesiologist, surgeon, and patient must agree with the anesthetic plan.

D. Components of anesthesia

1. Amnesia

2. Anxiolysis

3. Analgesia

4. Akinesia

5. Attenuation of autonomic responses to noxious stimulation

E. Types of anesthesia

   1. Local anesthesia

      a. Infiltration of local anesthetic by surgeon, with or without sedation

      b. The anesthesiologist is not involved in the monitoring or care of the patient.

   2. Monitored anesthesia care

      a. The anesthesiologist is involved in monitoring and care of the patient, ensuring comfort, care, and safety.

      b. Sedation levels may range from no sedation to conscious sedation.

   3. General anesthesia

      a. Pharmacologically induced, reversible loss of consciousness, irrespective of airway management

      b. Inhalational anesthesia—Involves inspired volatile anesthetic gas

      c. Total intravenous anesthesia—Intravenous agents without inspired volatile anesthetic gas

   4. Regional anesthesia

      a. Regional block performed, anesthesiologist monitors patient, with or without sedation

      b. Provides targeted, site-specific (dermatome, myotome, osteotome) anesthesia and analgesia

      c. Minimizes opioid requirements and associated side effects

      d. Types of regional anesthetic

         • Central neuraxial

            ○ Epidural anesthesia: (1) epidural space injection of local anesthetic; (2) Delayed

Table 1

American Society of Anesthesiologists Physical Status Classification System

Physical Status Category	Preoperative Health Status	Examples
I	Normal healthy patient	No organic, physiologic, or psychiatric disturbance; excludes the very young and very old; healthy with good exercise tolerance
II	Patient with mild systemic disease	No functional limitations; has a well-controlled disease of one body system; controlled hypertension or diabetes without systemic effects, cigarette smoking without COPD; mild obesity, pregnancy
III	Patient with severe systemic disease	Some functional limitation; has a controlled disease of more than one body system or one major system; no immediate danger of death; controlled CHF, stable angina, old heart attack, poorly controlled hypertension, morbid obesity, chronic renal failure
IV	Patient with severe systemic disease that is a constant threat to life	Has at least one severe disease that is poorly controlled or at end stage; possible risk of death; unstable angina, symptomatic COPD, symptomatic CHF, hepatorenal failure
V	Moribund patients who are not expected to survive without the surgery	Not expected to survive >24 hours without surgery; imminent risk of death; multiorgan failure, sepsis syndrome with hemodynamic instability, hypothermia, poorly controlled coagulopathy
VI	A patient declared brain-dead whose organs are being removed for donor purposes	

CHF = congestive heart failure, COPD = chronic obstructive pulmonary disease.

ASA-emergency addendum: life threatening or loss of limb.

Adapted with permission from the ASA Physical Status Classification System, American Society of Anesthesiologists, Park Ridge, IL.

onset; (3) potential for incomplete block; and (4) epidural catheter for intraoperative or postoperative anesthesia or analgesia is a common practice—catheter allows local anesthetic redosing or infusion providing extension of anesthesia or analgesia

○ Spinal anesthesia: (1) subarachnoid, intrathecal injection of local anesthetic; (2) rapid onset; (3) dense block, more reliable than epidural; and (4) spinal catheter for intraoperative or postoperative anesthesia or analgesia is an uncommon practice, thus the duration of action is limited to the injected local anesthetic duration of action.

• Peripheral nerve blockade (**Table 2**)

○ Single-injection

○ Continuous catheter—Single injection of local anesthetic (range, 0.25% to 0.5%) followed by continuous infusion of local anesthetic (lower concentration, 0.2%) through perineural catheter.

• Intravenous regional anesthesia (Bier block)

○ After Esmarch exsanguination and tourniquet inflation, plain lidocaine is injected through a small, distal (hand) intravenous catheter on the surgical side.

○ Tourniquet is deflated after a minimum of 30 minutes to avoid venous release of local anesthetic and potential local anesthetic systemic toxicity (LAST).

○ Does not provide postoperative pain relief

○ Used for hand or forearm surgery 60 minutes or less in duration

e. Nerve localization for regional anesthesia techniques

• Electrical nerve stimulation (appropriate elicited motor response at greater than 0.2 mA and less than 0.5 mA approximates the needle-to-nerve distance associated with a successful block)

• Ultrasonographic guidance (direct visualization)

Table 2			
Peripheral Nerve Blocks			

Upper Extremity Peripheral Nerve Blocks

Block type	Level of Block	Surgery	Comments
Interscalene block	Roots/trunks	Shoulder/upper arm/elbow	Not ideal for hand surgery (may spare inferior trunk)
Supraclavicular block	Divisions	Shoulder/upper arm/elbow/hand	Not ideal for shoulder surgery (may spare supraclavicular, suprascapular, and subscapular nerves)
Infraclavicular block	Chords	Elbow/hand	
Axillary block	Individual nerves (proximal)	Elbow/hand	With musculocutaneous nerve block, if needed
Individual nerves at wrist/forearm	Individual nerves (distal)	Hand	

Lower Extremity Peripheral Nerve Blocks

Block Type	Roots of Origin	Surgery	Comments
Lumbar plexus	L1-4 (variable T12, L5)	Hip/knee	Risk of retroperitoneal bleeding; neuraxial guidelines
Femoral	L2-4 posterior divisions	Knee	Does not consistently cover obturator, lateral femoral cutaneous distribution
Obturator	L2-4 anterior divisions	Knee	In combination with femoral nerve block
Saphenous	L2-4	Foot	In combination with sciatic nerve block
Sciatic	Cutaneous branch of femoral nerve (L2-4)	Foot	In combination with saphenous nerve block; gluteal, subgluteal, popliteal approaches
Ankle	Individual nerves	Midfoot/forefoot	

f. Anticoagulation—Current anticoagulation status and future plan must be evaluated; central neuraxial blocks should not be performed in the anticoagulated patient; peripheral nerve blockade may provide an alternative in these patients, excluding lumbar plexus block.

g. Complications—Failed block, infection, bleeding, nerve injury, pneumothorax, intrathecal injection, epidural injection/spread, intravascular injection/uptake, LAST.

h. LAST

- Central nervous system (CNS) toxicity typically presents first, occurring at a lower plasma concentration than cardiac toxicity; preseizure excitation, seizures, coma, respiratory arrest

- Cardiovascular toxicity typically occurs at a higher plasma concentration than CNS toxicity; however, it may occur with no warning signs or symptoms of CNS toxicity; re-

duces cardiac conductivity and contractility at myocardium; arteriolar dilation; pacemaker cells; ectopy; prolonged ventricular conduction with widening of QRS followed by arrhythmia (ventricular fibrillation)

º Bupivacaine/ropivacaine-related cardiotoxicity—Cardiac toxicity occurs at a lower plasma concentration than with lidocaine (greater potency).

º Bupivacaine is associated with more difficult resuscitation than is ropivacaine. Bupivacaine is less expensive than ropivacaine, so it is still commonly used in practice.

- Intravenous lipid emulsion 20%

º Critical part of the treatment strategy for LAST (**Figures 1** and **2**)

º Administer 1.5 mL/kg bolus followed by 0.25 mL/kg/min infusion, bolus up to

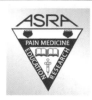

AMERICAN SOCIETY OF
REGIONAL ANESTHESIA AND PAIN MEDICINE

Checklist for Treatment
of Local Anesthetic Systemic Toxicity

The Pharmacologic Treatment of Local Anesthetic Systemic Toxicity (LAST) is Different from Other Cardiac Arrest Scenarios

☐ **Get Help**

☐ **Initial Focus**

    ☐ **Airway management:** ventilate with 100% oxygen

    ☐ **Seizure suppression:** benzodiazepines are preferred; **AVOID propofol** in patients having signs of cardiovascular instability

    ☐ **Alert** the nearest facility having **cardiopulmonary bypass** capability

☐ **Management of Cardiac Arrhythmias**

    ☐ **Basic and Advanced Cardiac Life Support (ACLS)** will require adjustment of medications and perhaps prolonged effort

    ☐ **AVOID vasopressin, calcium channel blockers, beta blockers, or local anesthetic**

    ☐ **REDUCE individual epinephrine doses to <1 mcg/kg**

☐ **Lipid Emulsion (20%) Therapy** (values in parenthesis are for 70-kg patient)

    ☐ **Bolus 1.5 mL/kg** (lean body mass) intravenously over 1 minute (~100mL)

    ☐ **Continuous infusion 0.25 mL/kg/min** (~18 mL/min; adjust by roller clamp)

    ☐ Repeat bolus once or twice for persistent cardiovascular collapse

    ☐ Double the infusion rate to 0.5 mL/kg/min if blood pressure remains low

    ☐ **Continue infusion** for at least 10 minutes after attaining circulatory stability

    ☐ Recommended upper limit: Approximately 10 mL/kg lipid emulsion over the first 30 minutes

☐ **Post LAST events** at www.lipidrescue.org and report use of lipid to www.lipidregistry.org

Figure 1   Chart shows the American Society of Regional Anesthesia and Pain Medicine checklist for treatment of local anesthetic systemic toxicity. (Reproduced with permission from the American Society of Regional Anesthesia and Pain Medicine, Pittsburgh, PA.)

3.0 mL/kg and infusion 0.5 mg/kg/min.

    ○ In patients unresponsive to resuscitation, cardiac bypass may provide the only life-saving measure.

  5. Combined general with regional anesthetic block

III. Monitors in Anesthesia

A. Standard ASA monitors

  1. Continuous electrocardiography

  2. Noninvasive arterial blood pressure (at least every 5 minutes)

  3. Continuous pulse oximetry

  4. Oxygen analyzer with a low oxygen concentra-

LipidRescue™

TREATMENT FOR LOCAL ANESTHETIC-INDUCED CARDIAC ARREST

PLEASE KEEP THIS PROTOCOL ATTACHED TO THE INTRALIPID BAG

In the event of local anesthetic-induced cardiac arrest that is <u>unresponsive to standard therapy,</u> in addition to standard cardio-pulmonary resuscitation, Intralipid 20% should be given i.v. in the following dose regime:

- Intralipid 20% 1.5 mL/kg over 1 minute

- Follow immediately with an infusion at a rate of 0.25 mL/kg/min,

- Continue chest compressions (lipid must circulate)

- Repeat bolus every 3-5 minutes up to 3 mL/kg total dose until circulation is restored

- Continue infusion until hemodynamic stability is restored. Increase the rate to 0.5 mL/kg/min if BP declines

- A maximum total dose of 8 mL/kg is recommended

In practice, in resuscitating an adult weighing 70kg:

- *Take a 500-ml bag of Intralipid 20% and a 50ml syringe.*

- *Draw up 50 ml and give stat i.v., X2*

- *Then attach the Intralipid bag to an iv administration set (macrodrip) and run it .i.v over the next 15 minutes*

- *Repeat the initial bolus up to twice more – if spontaneous circulation has not returned.*

If you use Intralipid to treat a case of local anaesthetic toxicity, please report it at <u>www.lipidrescue.org</u>. Remember to restock the lipid. Ver 7/06

Figure 2 Treatment of local anesthetic systemic toxity includes administration of 20% intralipid (LipidRescue). (Reproduced with permission from Guy Weinberg, MD, Lipid Rescue Resuscitation. http://lipidrescue.org.)

tion limit alarm

5. Capnography (end-tidal CO_2)

6. Temperature

B. Additional monitors

1. Invasive continuous arterial blood pressure

2. Central venous pressure—Surrogate of intravascular volume/preload in the absence of left ventricular dysfunction, pulmonary hypertension, or mitral valve disease

2: General Knowledge

3. Pulmonary arterial/capillary wedge pressure—Monitors cardiac filling pressures, cardiac output, derived hemodynamic parameters, mixed venous oxygen saturation

4. Peripheral nerve stimulators—Monitors neuromuscular function

5. Somatosensory evoked potentials, motor evoked potentials—Monitors neurologic injury

6. Electroencephalogram—Monitors cerebral ischemia

7. Cerebral oximetry—Monitors cerebral oxygenation; measures oxygenation of blood within the first few millimeters of the frontal cortex

8. Bispectral Index Scale—Uses electroencephalographic signals to measure depth of consciousness and sedation; 100, awake; 60 to 90, sedated; 40 to 60, general anesthesia; 0, coma

IV. Phases of Anesthetic Delivery

A. Stages of anesthesia

1. Stage 1, Induction—Time from awake state to unconscious state with amnesia and analgesia

2. Stage 2, Delirium/excitement—Begins with loss of consciousness, characterized by irregular and unpredictable respiratory and heart rate, breath holding, reflex activity including nonpurposeful muscle movements, vomiting, laryngospasm, arrhythmias

3. Stage 3, Surgical anesthesia—Characterized by achievement of minimum alveolar concentration, loss of reflex activity including laryngeal reflexes, muscle relaxation, shallow regular breathing

4. Stage 4, Overdose—Cardiorespiratory collapse

B. Induction of general anesthesia

1. Induces loss of consciousness (general anesthesia) through inhalational and/or intravenous administration of anesthetic agents

2. After loss of consciousness, prior to administration of paralytics in nonspontaneously breathing patient, ability to ventilate using a mask is evaluated.

3. If endotracheal intubation is used, paralytics are administered for vocal cord paralysis.

4. Airway placement

a. Natural airway—Patient spontaneously breathing without placement of artificial airway

b. Oral/nasal airway—First-line intervention for airway obstruction; potential for laryngo-

spasm in stage 2; advantage of nasal airway must be weighed against potential risk of epistaxis

c. Laryngeal mask airway—Supraglottic airway intervention; not a secure airway because it does not isolate lungs from potential aspiration; should be avoided in patients at risk for aspiration; important intervention in the difficult airway algorithm (**Figure 3**)

d. Endotracheal airway intubation

• Direct laryngoscopy

• Fiberoptic intubation—Fiberoptic scope can be utilized to assist with visualization for difficult airway; can be used in awake, lightly sedated patient or after induction of general anesthesia if the surgeon is confident the patient can be ventilated after potential loss of spontaneous respiration.

5. Rapid sequence induction—Intravenous induction agent followed immediately by succinylcholine, no mask ventilation, direct laryngoscopy. Pressure applied externally to the cricoid cartilage is intended to compress the esophagus and reduce the risk of gastric fluids refluxing into the pharynx and trachea. Used in setting of aspiration risk

C. Maintenance—Maintain components of anesthesia during intravenous or inhalation anesthesia.

D. Emergence

1. Evaluate depth of neuromuscular blockade, if used

2. Reverse neuromuscular blockade if needed

3. Remove or discontinue maintenance anesthetics

4. Ensure adequate ventilation and the ability to maintain and protect the airway

5. Ensure adequate postoperative analgesia

6. Extubate

V. Anesthetic Agents

A. Common anesthetic agents are described in **Table 3**.

VI. Postanesthesia Care

A. Postanesthesia care unit assessment and monitoring

1. Respiratory function—Respiratory rate, airway patency, oxygen saturation

2. Cardiovascular function—Blood pressure, pulse

3. Neuromuscular function

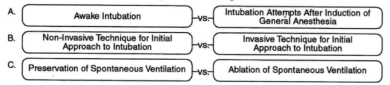

DIFFICULT AIRWAY ALGORITHM

1. Assess the likelihood and clinical impact of basic management problems:
   - A. Difficult Ventilation
   - B. Difficult Intubation
   - C. Difficulty with Patient Cooperation or Consent
   - D. Difficult Tracheostomy

2. Actively pursue opportunities to deliver supplemental oxygen throughout the process of difficult airway management

3. Consider the relative merits and feasibility of basic management choices:
   - A. Awake Intubation -vs- Intubation Attempts After Induction of General Anesthesia
   - B. Non-Invasive Technique for Initial Approach to Intubation -vs- Invasive Technique for Initial Approach to Intubation
   - C. Preservation of Spontaneous Ventilation -vs- Ablation of Spontaneous Ventilation

4. Develop primary and alternative strategies:

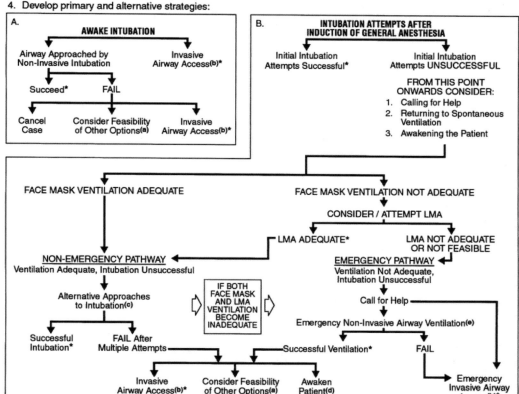

* Confirm ventilation, tracheal intubation, or LMA placement with exhaled CO_2

a. Other options include (but are not limited to): surgery utilizing face mask or LMA anesthesia, local anesthesia infiltration or regional nerve blockade. Pursuit of these options usually implies that mask ventilation will not be problematic. Therefore, these options may be of limited value if this step in the algorithm has been reached via the Emergency Pathway.

b. Invasive airway access includes surgical or percutaneous tracheostomy or cricothyrotomy.

c. Alternative non-invasive approaches to difficult intubation include (but are not limited to): use of different laryngoscope blades, LMA as an intubation conduit (with or without fiberoptic guidance), fiberoptic intubation, intubating stylet or tube changer, light wand, retrograde intubation, and blind oral or nasal intubation.

d. Consider re-preparation of the patient for awake intubation or canceling surgery.

e. Options for emergency non-invasive airway ventilation include (but are not limited to): rigid bronchoscope, esophageal-tracheal combitube ventilation, or transtracheal jet ventilation.

Figure 3 American Society of Anesthesiologists difficult airway algorithm. LMA = laryngeal mask airway. (Reproduced with permission from the American Society of Anesthesiologists, Park Ridge, IL.)

4. Mental status

5. Pain

6. Nausea, emesis

7. Drainage, bleeding

8. Fluids, voiding

9. Temperature

2: General Knowledge

Table 3

Anesthetic Agents

Inhalational Anesthetics

Isoflurane, sevoflurane, desflurane	Volatile liquids vaporized in a carrier gas Minimum alveolar concentration—Alveolar partial pressure of a gas at which 50% of humans will not respond to noxious stimuli Alveolar partial pressure is an indirect measure of brain partial pressure, the target of inhalational anesthetics

Intravenous Anesthetics

Nonopioids	Mechanism of Action	Other Effects
Propofol	GABA receptor agonist Sedative-hypnotic	Antiemetic
Etomidate	GABA receptor agonist Sedative-hypnotic	Emetogenic, adrenocortical suppression
Benzodiazepines	GABA receptor agonist Sedative-hypnotic	Amnestic and anxiolytic
Dexmedetomidine	Selective α-2 adrenoreceptor agonist Sedative-hypnotic	Analgesic, anxiolytic
Ketamine	Dissociative anesthetic—Inhibition of thalamocortical pathways and stimulation of limbic system Sedative-hypnotic	Analgesic, emergence delirium, increased secretions, bronchodilation

Other systemic effects of nonopioid intravenous anesthetics include reduced systemic blood pressure secondary to peripheral vasodilation and reduced systemic vascular resistance (ketamine increased); ventilatory depression (ketamine at induction doses); reduced cerebral blood flow and intracranial pressure (ketamine increased)

Opioids	Mechanism of Action	Other Effects
Fentanyl, alfentanil, sufentanil, remifentanil, morphine, hydromorphone	Interact with opioid receptors in brain and spinal cord	Analgesia, sedation

Neuromuscular Blocking Drugs

Depolarizing drugs bind to, depolarize, and transiently block acetylcholine receptor (agonist)	Short acting: succinylcholine	No long- or intermediate-acting agents
Nondepolarizing drugs bind to and transiently block acetylcholine receptor but do not depolarize (antagonists)	Intermediate acting: rocuronium, vecuronium, atracurium, cisatracurium Long acting: pancuronium	No short-acting agents

Local Anesthetics

Block sodium channels in the neuronal cell membrane	Short acting: chloroprocaine Intermediate-acting: lidocaine, mepivacaine Long acting: ropivacaine, bupivacaine	Intravenous lipid emulsion 20% is critical part of treatment strategy for local anesthetic–induced cardiotoxicity

(continued on next page)

VII. Positioning

A. Surgical positions include prone, Trendelenburg, reverse Trendelenburg, lithotomy, sitting (beach-chair), or lateral decubitus positions.

B. Positioning is the responsibility of both surgery and anesthesiology.

C. Priority must be directed toward the airway when planning for surgical positioning and during the process of active positioning.

D. All pressure points must be vigilantly identified, padded, and protected.

E. Potential changes in cardiorespiratory mechanics and function associated with positioning.

Table 3		

Anesthetic Agents (*continued*)

Reversal Agents (Neuromuscular Blockade Reversal)

Anticholinesterases	Mechanism of Action	Comments
Neostigmine: common Edrophonium: uncommon—longer neuromuscular blocking agents may outlast its short duration of action) Pyridostigmine: uncommon—can cross blood-brain barrier resulting in emergence delirium	Inhibit acetylcholinesterase (responsible for acetylcholine hydrolysis) resulting in increased acetylcholine to compete with nondepolarizing muscle blockers at neuromuscular junction (nicotinic receptors), increasing neuromuscular transmission	Side effects (muscarinic receptors): bradycardia resulting in potential sinoatrial arrest, increased salivation, bronchospasm, increased bladder tone, pupillary constriction, nausea/vomiting

Anticholinergics

Atropine, glycopyrrolate	Given in combination with anticholinesterases to minimize muscarinic effects	Glycopyrrolate typically is administered with neostigmine because onset of cardiac anticholinergic effect matches neostigmine onset of muscarinic effect.

Benzodiazepine Reversal

Flumazenil	Antagonizes benzodiazepine receptors	Caution with chronic benzodiazepine use; monitor for persistent or recurrent benzodiazepine effects

Opioid Reversal

Naloxone	Opioid antagonist	Monitor for persistent or recurrent opioid effects

Antiemetics

Ondansetron, granisetron, palonosetron	5-HT3 receptor agonists	Side effects: headache, elevated liver enzymes, constipation
Dexamethasone	Glucocorticoid	Side effects: transient elevation of blood glucose in patients with diabetes; no adverse effect on wound healing
Droperidol, haloperidol	Exact mechanism unknown; antagonizes dopamine and α-adrenergic receptors	Droperidol has an FDA black box warning secondary to QT prolongation
Scopolamine transdermal	Cholinergic antagonist Effective for 72 hours	Side effects: vision changes, dry mouth, confusion and delirium in elderly, other somnolence, central cholinergic system, urinary retention, skin irritation, headache
Aprepitant	Neurokinin-1 receptor agonist	Promising profiles, demonstrates improved antiemesis, outcomes are consistent with less expensive options
Promethazine	Nonselectively antagonizes central and peripheral histamine H1 receptors; anticholinergic properties	Side effects: sedation, confusion, delirium, particularly in elderly Skin necrosis when injected undiluted
Diphenhydramine	Antihistamine	Side effects: confusion, delirium
Metoclopramide	Dopamine antagonist	Side effects: confusion, delirium

GABA = gamma-aminobutyric acid.

1. Supine—Reduced functional residual capacity secondary to cephalad displacement of the diaphragm

2. Trendelenburg—Accentuated cephalad displace-

ment of the diaphragm; although sometimes used as an intervention to increase venous return to the heart in an effort to improve cardiac output, it may reduce cardiac output secondary to the abdominal viscera resting against the heart;

increased intracranial pressure

3. Prone—Cephalad displacement of the diaphragm with restricted caudad expansion, resulting in increased peak airway pressures; compression of inferior vena cava and aorta; turning patient's head may restrict vertebral artery flow and venous drainage

4. Lateral decubitus—Compression of the inferior vena cava; dependent lung is underventilated but has increased blood flow, whereas the independent lung is overventilated but has reduced blood flow, which may result in hypoxemia as a result of ventilation-to-perfusion mismatch; depends on axillary neurovascular compression

5. Sitting (beach chair)—Venous air embolism; may result in reduced cardiac output, perfusion pressure; hypotensive bradycardic events may be associated with shoulder arthroscopy in the beach chair position

6. Lithotomy—Cephalad displacement of the diaphragm; inferior vena cava obstruction with cephalad abdominal compression

F. Potential musculoskeletal, plexus/peripheral nerve injury associated with positioning

1. Supine/prone

a. Upper extremity—Brachial plexus, ulnar nerve

b. Median nerve injury from blood pressure cuff

c. Neutral neck positioning in prone position

2. Lateral decubitus neck positioning—Nondependent brachial plexus

3. Lithotomy

a. Lower extremity—Sciatic nerve, common peroneal nerve, femoral nerve, obturator nerve, saphenous nerve

b. Back pain exacerbation

VIII. Complications

A. Malignant hyperthermia

1. Rare, inherited, potentially lethal syndrome

2. Characterized by

a. Hypermetabolic activity

b. Marked CO_2 production

c. Altered skeletal muscle tone

d. Metabolic acidosis

e. Hyperkalemia

3. Triggers

a. Volatile inhalational anesthetics

b. Succinylcholine

4. Primary treatment—Dantrolene (Ca^{2+} blocker); active cooling may be required. Additional information can be obtained from the Malignant Hyperthermia Association of the United States at http://www.mhaus.org.

5. Diagnosis—Muscle biopsy. Specific malignant hyperthermia–related processing is available only at selected US sites.

B. Bone cement implantation syndrome

1. Associated with bone cement used during joint arthroplasty procedures

2. Characterized by hypotension, hypoxemia

3. Treatment—Hydration, vasopressors, 100% inspired oxygen

Top Testing Facts

1. Components of anesthesia include amnesia, anxiolysis, analgesia, akinesia, and attenuation of autonomic responses to noxious stimulation.

2. Alveolar partial pressure is an indirect measure of brain partial pressure, the target of inhalational anesthetics.

3. Minimum alveolar concentration is the alveolar partial pressure of a gas at which 50% of humans will not respond to noxious stimuli.

4. Peripheral nerve blockade provides targeted, site-specific (dermatome, myotome, osteotome) anesthesia and analgesia.

5. Intravenous lipid emulsion 20% is a critical part of the treatment strategy for LAST.

6. Hypotensive bradycardic events may be associated with shoulder arthroscopy in the beach chair position.

7. Malignant hyperthermia, triggered by volatile inhalational anesthetics and succinylcholine, is characterized by hypermetabolic activity and marked CO_2 production; the primary treatment is dantrolene.

8. Bone cement implantation syndrome, associated with bone cement used in joint arthroplasty procedures, is characterized by hypoxemia and hypotension.

Bibliography

Barash PG, Cullen BF, Stoetling RK, eds: *Clinical Anesthesia*, ed 4. Philadelphia, PA, Lippincot Williams & Wilkins, 1992.

Gan TJ, Meyer TA, Apfel CC, et al: Society for Ambulatory Anesthesia guidelines for the management of postoperative nausea and vomiting. *Anesth Analg* 2007;105(6):1615-1628.

Stoetling RK, Miller RD: *Basics of Anesthesia*, ed 4. Philadelphia, PA, Churchill Livingstone, 2000.

2: General Knowledge

Chapter 21
Electrophysiologic Assessment

Adam J. La Bore, MD

I. Principles of Neural Insult

A. Compression

  1. Compression of a peripheral nerve causes neural ischemia. This can produce relatively mild symptoms such as temporary regional numbness or weakness in an arm or leg resulting from pressure on it while in a sitting or sleeping posture.

  2. Sustained neural ischemia can result in necrosis of the nerve.

    a. Peripherally, the myelin sheath of the nerve is affected first, leading to localized demyelination. Axonal loss can eventually ensue.

    b. At the level of a spinal nerve root, a compression insult, such as from disk herniation, may produce this sequence of events.

    c. This sequence of events also occurs in advanced carpal tunnel syndrome, in which the tissue damage may result in neural deficits, even with maximum recovery after relief of the precipitating insult.

    d. Examples include permanent sensory and motor deficits after the release of chronic severe median nerve compression in carpal tunnel syndrome, and persistent footdrop due to L4 radiculopathy caused by disk herniation and resolved by diskectomy.

B. Neurapraxia

  1. Neurapraxia is an injury caused by the stretching of a peripheral nerve or nerve root that interrupts or completely disrupts the vascular supply of the nerve or root. It results in temporary neural impairment of varied degrees of severity, but with complete sensory and motor recovery.

  2. Neurapraxia can occur with any injurious event involving blunt injury and/or stretching of one or more nerves. An example is brachial plexopathy following traumatic shoulder dislocation.

C. Neurotmesis

  1. Neurotmesis occurs when axons, the myelin sheath, and supporting tissues are disrupted at a given site.

  2. With complete disruption, nerve function is not predictably recovered.

D. Axonotmesis

  1. Axons can also be disrupted within a nerve without disruption of the myelin sheath and its supporting tissue.

  2. Even with complete axonal disruption, some recovery can be expected if the nerve sheath is intact.

  3. The degree and rate of recovery vary with the severity of the insult.

E. Wallerian degeneration

  1. Wallerian degeneration is a sequence of cellular events that follow axonal injury, describing the degeneration of the involved axon.

  2. Complete neurotmesis most predictably results in complete wallerian degeneration.

II. Electrodiagnostic Testing

A. Principles of electrodiagnostic evaluation after neural insult

  1. Depending on the site of insult, acute nerve compression or demyelination can result in sudden conduction block of the nerve that is immediately identifiable on electrodiagnostic testing.

  2. Such testing can also reveal the sudden conduction loss across a nerve segment resulting from complete axonal disruption. In complete axonotmesis or neurotmesis, conduction distal to the insult is initially normal; however, with wallerian degeneration, the peripheral axons die and the distal response to a stimulus diminishes proportionately.

  3. Muscles change in a predictable fashion following partial or complete denervation. These changes are identifiable with needle electromyography (EMG).

2: General Knowledge

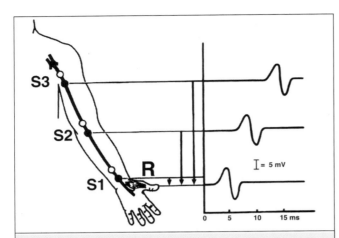

Figure 1 Motor nerve conduction velocity study of the median nerve. The recording electrodes are placed over the belly of the abductor pollicis brevis muscle (R). Stimulating electrodes are placed over the median nerve at the wrist (S1), elbow (S2), and axilla (S3). A reference electrode (black dot) is placed distal to the active stimulating electrode (white dot). The resultant compound muscle action potential is recorded on the right. (Reproduced with permission from Oh SJ: Nerve conduction study, in: *Principles of Clinical Electromyography: Case Studies*. Baltimore, MD: Williams & Wilkins, 1998, p 22.)

B. Motor nerve conduction studies

1. Motor nerves are most commonly tested by placing an electrode over the middle of a given muscle belly and proximally stimulating the nerve that innervates it.

2. A terminal nerve branch and the muscle fibers it innervates constitute a single motor unit.

3. The response of the muscle to nerve stimulation is the sum of all motor unit responses. This sum of motor unit responses is translated into the waveform known as the compound motor action potential (CMAP).

4. CMAPs are analyzed for the following:

   a. Onset latency: The time from nerve stimulation to the initial muscle response.

   b. Amplitude: The magnitude of the muscle response, indicating the number of motor units responding to the nerve stimulation. CMAP amplitudes are measured as the distance between the onset and the peak points of a waveform. Denervation of a muscle results in a loss of motor units; therefore, a decrease in CMAP amplitude may occur.

   c. Conduction velocity: The rapidity with which a motor nerve segment conducts an impulse.

      • Conduction velocity is calculated by stimulating the nerve distally and proximally, measuring both times to muscle response (onset latency), and dividing the difference between the two latency times by the distance between the distal and proximal nerve stimulation points.

   • This method is used to identify segmental insults to a nerve such as the compression of the ulnar nerve that produces cubital tunnel syndrome.

   • When calculating conduction velocity, conduction across the neuromuscular junction is not included because this occurs through a series of events entirely distinct from nerve conduction (**Figure 1**).

C. Sensory nerve conduction velocity studies

1. Sensory nerves are studied by placing electrodes over the distal nerve (for example, the digits) and stimulating the nerve at a proximal site (for example, the wrist).

2. Latency

   a. Sensory latency is the time from stimulation of a sensory nerve to depolarization of the nerve at a point distal to the point of stimulation.

   b. The waveform produced by this depolarization is referred to as the sensory nerve action potential (SNAP).

   c. The peak of the SNAP waveform is most commonly used to mark the sensory latency of a nerve.

   d. For example, the sensory latency of the median nerve is determined by stimulating it at the wrist and recording the response at a digit innervated by the nerve.

3. Amplitude

   a. The amplitude of a sensory nerve waveform indicates the magnitude of nerve response, reflecting the number of intact axons and thus the health of a studied nerve. It is measured by the distance between the peak and trough of a waveform.

   b. The amplitude represents the number of intact axons responding to stimulation (**Figure 2**).

4. Waveform quality

   a. The quality of the sensory nerve waveform is observed for temporal dispersion.

   b. With nerve compression at a site such as the carpal tunnel, the responding axons depolarize at the detecting electrode with varying delays, causing the translated waveform to degrade in sharpness and amplitude and spread over a longer period as axons depolarize in sequence. The more varied the delays, the greater the temporal dispersion (**Figure 2**).

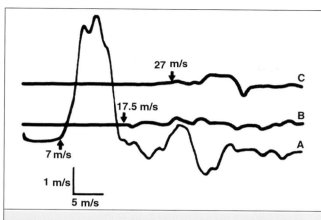

Figure 2 Conduction block in segmental demyelination. Median motor nerve conduction in a case of chronic demyelinating neuropathy. Tracing A: Normal amplitude of the compound muscle action potential (CMAP) with wrist stimulation. Tracing B: Dramatic reduction in the amplitude of the CMAP with elbow stimulation. Tracing C: CMAP with axillary stimulation. Conduction block is clearly seen between the wrist and elbow stimulation. The dispersion phenomenon is also observed. The motor nerve conduction velocity is 21.9 m/s over the wrist-elbow segment and 15.8 m/s over the elbow-axilla segment. The latency is prolonged at 7 m/s. (Reproduced with permission from Oh SJ: Nerve conduction study, in: *Principles of Clinical Electromyography: Case Studies.* Baltimore, MD: Williams & Wilkins, 1998, p 55.)

D. Needle EMG

1. Denervation of a muscle results in membrane destabilization, which produces spontaneous activity identifiable on needle EMG. Examples of spontaneous activity include fibrillations and positive sharp waves. Spontaneous activity occurs when there is no voluntary motor unit activity.

2. The activity follows denervation, evolves, and resolves in a predictable pattern and with a predictable chronology. Testing can therefore help identify the relative acuity and severity of the changes that follow denervation.

3. Motor unit recruitment refers to the pattern of voluntary motor unit activation that occurs with increased muscle effort against resistence. Clinical weakness after a denervating insult to a muscle is seen as decreased motor unit recruitment on needle EMG.

4. The morphology of waveform signals from voluntary motor units observed during needle EMG also changes with reinnervation.

III. Testing for Common Clinical Conditions

A. The goal of electrodiagnostic testing is to confirm the presence or absence of neuropathophysiology associated with clinical diagnoses such as carpal or cubital tunnel syndromes.

B. Carpal tunnel syndrome

1. Etiology

a. Carpal tunnel syndrome occurs with compressive ischemia of the median nerve as it crosses the wrist in the carpal tunnel.

b. Developmental anatomy, trauma, conditions that cause third-space fluid retention, and activities that demand specific sustained or repetitive wrist positions can contribute to the development of carpal tunnel syndrome.

2. Electrodiagnostic testing for carpal tunnel syndrome

a. Carpal tunnel syndrome is a clinical diagnosis. Electrophysiologic examination is performed to identify and grade any associated neuropathy.

b. Grading is based on the severity of neuropathy, which ranges from subtle prolongation of sensory latency (mild) to motor latency delays (moderate) to axonal loss with waveform degradations and possibly to denervation identified on needle EMG (severe).

- Prolonged sensory latency can be identified by internal comparison or by referencing normal average latencies. Examples of internal comparison:

  ○ Segments of the median nerve: transcarpal to the index or long finger compared with palm stimulation to the index or long finger.

  ○ Median versus ulnar nerve latencies to the ring finger

  ○ Median versus radial nerve latencies to the thumb

  ○ Median versus ulnar transcarpal segment latencies (palm to wrist for each nerve)

- Motor conduction velocity in the median nerve is calculated through the forearm.

C. Entrapment of the median nerve in the distal arm or proximal forearm

1. Depending on site of entrapment and axons affected, these conditions can produce symptoms resembling those of carpal tunnel syndrome. However, this insult results in a slowing of segmental motor conduction velocity in the forearm but not at the wrist.

2: General Knowledge

2. Studies in this situation may yield equivocal results because of the difficulty in assessing conduction in the proximal segment of the median nerve.

D. Entrapment of the anterior interosseous nerve (AIN)

1. The AIN can become entrapped distal to the pronator teres muscle after this nerve branches from the median nerve.

2. In this case, median nerve conduction study results should be normal, except for possible abnormalities on needle EMG of musculature innervated by the AIN.

E. Cubital tunnel syndrome

1. Ulnar neuropathy most commonly occurs at the level of the medial epicondyle in the ulnar groove and/or at the level of the humeroulnar aponeurosis (the cubital tunnel).

2. The below-elbow stimulation site for ulnar motor nerve examination should include the 3-cm segment distal to the medial epicondyle.

3. Because compression neuropathy most commonly occurs through this short segment, conduction through it should be carefully examined.

4. If conduction velocity is calculated over a long nerve segment, localized compression/slowing may be averaged out in the calculation, yielding an apparently normal result. Therefore, a report of normal conduction at the elbow may be a result of this averaging (**Figure 1**).

F. Ulnar neuropathy at the Guyon canal

1. Ulnar neuropathy can also occur at the Guyon canal, located at the wrist.

2. Neuropathy at this site spares the dorsal ulnar cutaneous nerve and palmar cutaneous branches of the ulnar nerve.

a. Electrodiagnostic abnormalities at the Guyon canal are limited to conduction through the ulnar nerve across the wrist.

b. Severe ulnar neuropathy at the wrist can result in denervation of the intrinsic muscles of the hand that are innervated by the ulnar nerve. If this occurs, needle EMG of the flexor digitorum profundus in the ring and little fingers will be normal, and the intrinsic muscles of the hand innervated by the ulnar nerve will demonstrate changes that indicate denervation. The first dorsal interosseous and/or the abductor digiti minimi are the muscles most commonly studied with EMG. Needle EMG of the flexor carpi ulnaris and the flexor digitorum profundus of the ring and little fingers should be normal.

G. Radial neuropathy

1. Principles of electrophysiologic assessment of the radial nerve

a. Motor function in radial neuropathy is investigated with an EMG electrode placed over the extensor indicis proprius (EIP) muscle.

b. Because of the small size of the EIP muscle and CMAP waveform, conduction velocities are often very fast, and segments are observed for relative decrements in velocity and changes in CMAP amplitude. These measurements can be compared with those in the contralateral nerve.

c. Any lesion proximal to the posterior interosseous branch of the radial nerve may cause sensory axonal loss in addition to motor deficits.

2. Neuropathy at the spiral groove

a. Lesions at the spiral groove can affect all radial nerve–innervated musculature distal to the supinator branch. Needle EMG of the triceps (routinely examined) should be normal.

b. The radial nerve must be stimulated in the arm above and below the spiral groove. Localized demyelination will result in normal test results distal to the spiral groove.

3. Neuropathy in the axilla

a. Neuropathic lesions at or proximal to the axilla affect the triceps muscle.

b. The deltoid muscle is not affected. Both the radial and axillary nerve branches arise from the posterior cord of the brachial plexus. Therefore, a lesion to the radial nerve branch does not affect the deltoid muscle.

4. Posterior interosseous neuropathy

a. Abnormalities are limited to muscles innervated by the posterior interosseous nerve.

b. Conduction abnormality, if identified, is limited to the forearm.

c. Radial nerve sensory function should be normal.

5. Superficial radial sensory neuropathy

a. The study should include comparison with the contralateral nerve.

b. Purely sensory lesions of the radial nerve should result in no clinical or electrodiagnostic motor deficits.

H. Peroneal neuropathy at the fibular head

1. If the neuropathy is the result of demyelinating compression, any abnormality in conduction should be limited to the segment that extends from the popliteal fossa to below the fibular head.

2. If partial denervation/axonal loss is present, abnormalities on needle EMG are typically limited to muscles distal to the lesion, sparing the short head of the biceps femoris.

3. If an axon is completely severed distally, proximal wallerian degeneration will occur, and denervation of musculature proximal to the site of injury may occur.

I. Tarsal tunnel syndrome

1. Abnormalities may be sensory, motor, or both.

2. Contralateral comparison and examination for lumbar radiculopathy and peripheral polyneuropathy are critical to diagnostic clarity.

J. Radiculopathy

1. Cervical and lumbar radiculopathy are always included in the differential diagnosis of any neuropathology in an extremity.

2. Conduction studies in the affected extremity or extremities are performed to rule out isolated or generalized peripheral neuropathy.

3. Needle EMG may be normal, may identify abnormalities in motor unit recruitment/activation, and may demonstrate denervation in a pattern most consistent with a single nerve root.

4. Because of overlapping and varying patterns of innervation, needle EMG alone has not been shown to consistently differentiate adjacent levels of radiculopathy. However, a well-administered test with careful differential testing helps narrow the diagnosis and identify pathophysiologic elements that correlate with the clinical presentation and anatomic studies.

K. Plexopathies

1. Plexopathies should be considered in every initial differential diagnosis.

2. These conditions produce findings that overlap with those of radiculopathy and peripheral neuropathy.

3. Brachial plexopathy is most common. Careful evaluation of conduction studies, with contralateral comparison of abnormalities and selection of muscles to examine on needle EMG, can often clearly localize the site of a lesion.

Top Testing Facts

1. Compression of a nerve results in nerve ischemia, resulting first in segmental conduction impairment and, if sustained, in demyelination and axonal loss.

2. Neurapraxia is an injury caused by the stretching of a peripheral nerve or nerve root that interrupts or completely disrupts the vascular supply of the nerve or root.

3. Neurotmesis occurs when axons, the myelin sheath, and supporting tissues are disrupted at a given site.

4. Axonotmesis results when axons are disrupted within a nerve without disruption of the myelin sheath and its supporting tissue.

5. Wallerian degeneration is a sequence of cellular events that follow axonal injury; it describes degeneration of the involved axon.

6. Latency refers to the time delay between nerve stimulation and the distal response waveform detected by electrodes. Sensory latency is most accurately measured at the peak of the waveform (peak latency) and motor latency at the onset of the waveform (onset latency).

7. Conduction velocity is calculated by stimulating the nerve distally and proximally, measuring both times to muscle response (onset latency), and dividing the difference between the two latency times by the distance between the distal and proximal nerve stimulation points. The conduction velocity calculation eliminates the time involved in neuromuscular junction events.

8. Denervation of a muscle results in membrane destabilization, which produces spontaneous activity identifiable on needle EMG. Examples of spontaneous activity include fibrillations and positive sharp waves. Spontaneous activity occurs when there is no voluntary motor unit activity.

9. Motor unit recruitment refers to the pattern of voluntary motor unit activation that occurs with increased muscle effort against resistance. Clinical weakness after a denervating insult to a muscle is seen as decreased motor unit recruitment on needle EMG.

10. Electrodiagnostic testing investigates the pathophysiology of nerves correlating with clinical syndromes.

Bibliography

Bromberg MB: An electrodiagnostic approach to the evaluation of peripheral neuropathies. *Phys Med Rehabil Clin N Am* 2013;24(1):153-168.

Brown WF, Bolton CF, Aminoff MJ: *Neuromuscular Function and Disease: Basic, Clinical, and Electrodiagnostic Aspects.* Philadelphia, PA, Saunders, 2002.

Brownell AA, Bromberg MB: Electrodiagnostic assessment of peripheral neuropathies. *Semin Neurol* 2010;30(4):416-424.

Buschbacher RM, Prahlow ND: *Manual of Nerve Conduction Studies,* ed 2. New York, NY, Demos Medical Publishing, 2005.

Craig AS, Richardson JK: Acquired peripheral neuropathy. *Phys Med Rehabil Clin N Am* 2003;14(2):365-386.

Dumitru D, Amato AA, Zwarts M: *Electrodiagnostic Medicine,* ed 2. Philadelphia, PA, Hanley & Belfus, 2001.

Gooch CL, Weimer LH: The electrodiagnosis of neuropathy: Basic principles and common pitfalls. *Neurol Clin* 2007; 25(1):1-28.

Kimura J: *Electrodiagnosis in Diseases of Nerve and Muscle: Principles and Practice,* ed 3. New York, NY, Oxford University Press, 2001.

Mallik A, Weir AI: Nerve conduction studies: Essentials and pitfalls in practice. *J Neurol Neurosurg Psychiatry* 2005; 76(Suppl 2):ii23-ii31.

Preston DC, Shapiro BE: *Electromyography and Neuromuscular Disorders: Clinical-Electrophysiologic Correlations,* ed 2. Newton, MA, Butterworth-Heinemann, 2005.

Ross MA: Electrodiagnosis of peripheral neuropathy. *Neurol Clin* 2012;30(2):529-549.

Chapter 22

Neuro-orthopaedics and Rehabilitation

Keith Baldwin, MD, MSPT, MPH   Mary Ann Keenan, MD

I. Spinal Cord Injuries

A. General principles

1. Approximately 400,000 people in the United States have spinal cord damage.

2. Leading causes of spinal cord injury are motor vehicle accidents, gunshot wounds, falls, and sports and water injuries.

3. Patients are generally categorized into two groups.

    a. Younger individuals who sustained the injury from substantial trauma

    b. Older individuals with cervical spinal stenosis caused by congenital narrowing or spondylosis; these patients often sustained the injury from minor trauma and commonly have no vertebral fracture causing spinal injury.

B. Definitions

1. Tetraplegia—Loss or impairment of motor or sensory function in the cervical segments of the spinal cord with resulting impairment of function in the arms, trunk, legs, and pelvic organs.

2. Paraplegia—Loss or impairment of motor or sensory function in the thoracic, lumbar, or sacral segments of the spinal cord; arm and hand function is intact, but, depending on the level of the cord injured, impairment in the trunk, legs, and pelvic organs may be present.

3. Complete injury—An injury with no spared motor or sensory function in the lowest sacral segments. Patients with complete spinal cord injury who have recovered from spinal shock have a negligible chance of any useful motor return (**Table 1**).

4. Incomplete injury—An injury with partial preservation of sensory or motor function below the neurologic level; includes the lowest sacral segments.

C. Neurologic impairment and recovery

1. Spinal shock

    a. Diagnosis of complete spinal cord injury cannot be made until spinal shock has resolved, as evidenced by the return of the bulbocavernosus reflex. To elicit this reflex, the clinician examines the patient's rectum digitally, feeling for contraction of the anal sphincter while squeezing the glans penis or clitoris.

Table 1		
ASIA Impairment Scale		
Level	**Injury**	**Description**
A	Complete injury	No motor or sensory function is preserved in sacral segments S4-S5.
B	Incomplete Injury	Sensory but not motor function is preserved below the neurologic level and includes sacral segments S4-S5.
C	Incomplete injury	Motor function is preserved below the neurologic level, and more than one half of key muscles below the neurologic level have a muscle grade <3.
D	Incomplete injury	Motor function is preserved below the neurologic level, and at least one half of key muscles below the neurologic level have a muscle grade ≥3.
E	Normal function	Motor and sensory functions are normal.

ASIA = American Spinal Injury Association.

b. If trauma to the spinal cord has caused complete injury, reflex activity at the site of injury will not return because the reflex arc is permanently interrupted.

c. When spinal shock has resolved, reflex activity returns in the segments below the level of injury.

2. Recovery

a. The booklet *International Standards for Neurologic and Functional Classification of Spinal Cord Injury*, published by the American Spinal Injury Association (ASIA) and the International Medical Society of Paraplegia, describes quantitative measurements of sensory and motor function. These standards represent the most reliable instrument for assessing neurologic status in the spinal cord.

b. Assessment

- The change in ASIA Motor Score (AMS) between successive neurologic examinations should be determined.

- The AMS is the sum of strength grades from 0 to 5 for each of the 10 key muscles, tested bilaterally, that represent neurologic segments C5 through T1 and L2 through S1, for a total possible AMS of 100 points.

D. Spinal cord syndromes

1. Anterior cord syndrome

a. Anterior cord syndrome results from direct contusion to the anterior cord by bone fragments or from damage to the anterior spinal artery.

b. Depending on the extent of cord involvement, only posterior column function (proprioception and light touch) may be present.

c. The ability to respond to pain and light touch signifies that the posterior half of the cord has some intact function.

2. Central cord syndrome

a. Central cord syndrome results from trauma to the central gray matter in the spinal cord. This gray matter contains nerve cell bodies and is surrounded by white matter consisting primarily of ascending and descending myelinated tracts. Central gray matter has a higher metabolic requirement and is therefore more susceptible to the effects of trauma and ischemia.

b. Central cord syndrome often results from a minor injury such as a fall in an older patient with cervical spinal canal stenosis and hyperextension of the cervical spine. It is the most common of the incomplete spinal cord injury patterns.

c. Most patients with central cord syndrome can walk despite severe paralysis of the upper limb. Their gait may be spastic and wide based, however.

3. Brown-Séquard syndrome

a. Brown-Séquard syndrome is caused by complete hemisection of the spinal cord. The classic mechanism is a stab wound. True Brown-Séquard syndrome is extremely rare.

b. Brown-Séquard syndrome results in a greater ipsilateral proprioceptive motor loss and greater contralateral loss of pain and temperature sensation (2 to 3 segments below).

c. Affected patients have an excellent prognosis and usually will be able to ambulate.

4. Mixed syndrome

a. Mixed syndrome is characterized by diffuse involvement of the entire spinal cord.

b. Affected patients have a good prognosis for recovery.

c. As with all incomplete spinal cord injury syndromes, early motor recovery is the best prognostic indicator.

E. General management strategies

1. Prevention of contractures and maintenance of range of motion should begin immediately following the injury.

2. Maintaining skin integrity is crucial to care of the patient with a spinal cord injury. Only 4 hours of continuous pressure on the sacrum is sufficient to cause full-thickness skin necrosis. Physical interventions such as a rotating bed or special mattresses allow for simpler nursing care.

3. Intermittent catheterization has been the factor most responsible for reducing urologic problems and increasing the life span of patients with spinal cord injuries.

F. Complications

1. Autonomic dysreflexia

a. Splanchnic outflow conveying sympathetic fibers to the lower body exits at the T8 region.

b. Patients with lesions above T8 are prone to autonomic dysreflexia.

c. Signs and symptoms include episodes of hypertension that may be heralded by dizziness, sweating, and headaches.

d. A classic cause is a kinked Foley catheter; relieving the kink can relieve the autonomic symptoms.

2. Heterotopic ossification (HO; see section V)

G. Management of tetraplegia

1. C4-level function

   a. The key muscles are the diaphragm and the trapezius and neck muscles.

   b. Head control is present.

   c. With a functioning diaphragm, long-term ventilatory support is generally not needed.

   d. Tracheostomy and mechanical ventilatory assistance may be required initially.

   e. Wheelchair mobility is possible using "sip-and-puff" controls.

   f. Newer assistive technology using voice controls for activities of daily living (ADLs) is becoming available.

   g. Most patients require around-the-clock care.

2. C5-level function

   a. Key muscles are the deltoid and biceps, which are used for shoulder abduction and elbow flexion.

   b. Surgical goals are to provide active elbow and wrist extension and to restore the ability to pinch the thumb against the index finger.

   c. Transferring the posterior deltoid to the triceps muscle provides active elbow extension.

   d. Transferring the brachioradialis to the extensor carpi radialis brevis provides active wrist extension.

   e. Attaching the flexor pollicis longus tendon to the distal radius and fusing the interphalangeal joint of the thumb provides key pinch by tenodesis when the wrist is extended.

   f. Patients with C5-level injuries may use a power wheelchair with hand controls. Some may even be able to use manual wheelchairs with grip enhancements, although this has tremendous energy requirements.

   g. These patients may assist with bed mobility and transfers, although they require attendant care for ADLs and instrumental activities of daily living (IADLs). Assistive devices are available for answering phones, using computers, and driving.

3. C6-level function

   a. Key muscles are the wrist extensors, which enable the patient to manually propel a wheelchair and transfer from one position to another. This is the highest level at which a patient conceivably can live without an attendant.

   b. Surgical goals are to restore lateral pinch and active grasp.

   c. Lateral pinch can be restored by tenodesis of the thumb flexor or transfer of the brachioradialis to the flexor pollicis longus.

   d. Active grasp can be restored by transfer of the pronator teres to the flexor digitorum profundus.

   e. These patients may use a manual wheelchair with grip enhancements, although most prefer a power wheelchair. Bed-to-chair transfers may be performed independently using a sliding board, although most patients prefer setup assistance. These patients can perform upper body dressing but need assistance with lower body dressing.

4. C7-level function

   a. The key muscle is the triceps.

   b. Patients with intact triceps function should be able to transfer and live independently if no other complications are present.

   c. Surgical goals are active thumb flexion for pinch, active finger flexion for grasp, and hand opening by extensor tenodesis.

   d. Transfer of the brachioradialis to the flexor pollicis longus provides active pinch.

   e. Transfer of the pronator teres to the flexor digitorum profundus allows active finger flexion and grasp.

   f. If the finger extensors are weak, tenodesis of these tendons to the radius provides hand opening with wrist flexion.

   g. Patients with C7-level function can perform most ADLs and IADLs independently or with very minimal assistance. A manual wheelchair can be used, although uneven surfaces can present challenges.

5. C8-level function

   a. Key muscles are the finger and thumb flexors, which enable a gross grasp.

   b. A functioning flexor pollicis longus enables lateral pinch between the thumb and the side of the index finger.

   c. Intrinsic muscle function is lacking, and clawing of the fingers usually is present.

   d. Capsulodesis of the metacarpophalangeal joints corrects clawing and improves hand function.

   e. Active intrinsic function can be achieved by splitting the superficial finger flexor tendon of the ring finger into four slips and transferring these tendons to the lumbrical insertions of each finger.

f. Patients with C8-level function and below generally are able to achieve total independence unless other significant medical comorbidities are present.

II. Stroke and Traumatic Brain Injury

A. Demographics

1. The annual incidence of stroke (cerebrovascular accident [CVA]) in the United States is 1 per 1,000.

   a. Cerebral thrombosis causes nearly 75% of cases.

   b. More than one half of stroke victims survive; of those, 50% have hemiplegia.

2. In the United States, 410,000 new cases of traumatic brain injury can be expected each year.

   a. Traumatic brain injury resulting from multiple traumatic injuries is twice as common in men as it is in women.

   b. Persons between the ages of 15 and 24 years are most commonly affected.

   c. One half of all traumatic brain injuries are caused by motor vehicle accidents.

B. Management during neurologic recovery

1. Spasticity must be managed aggressively to prevent permanent deformities and joint contractures.

2. Spasmolytic drugs such as baclofen can be administered orally or intrathecally.

3. Dantrolene is the drug of choice for treating clonus.

4. Casting and splinting have been shown to reduce muscle tone temporarily and are used to correct contractures. Dynamic splints must be monitored closely for skin effects.

5. Botulinum toxin injections into the spastic muscle provide a temporary focal decrease in muscle tone.

C. Definitive management

1. Most motor recovery occurs within 6 months of the event in patients with stroke or traumatic brain injury.

2. Surgery can be considered for correction of residual limb deformities after 6 months.

3. Surgical lengthening of musculotendinous units permanently decreases muscle tone and spasticity.

III. Lower Limb Deformities

A. Limb scissoring

1. Limb scissoring is a common problem caused by overactive hip adductor muscles.

2. It results in an extremely narrow base of support while standing and causes balance problems.

3. Surgical management options

   a. If no fixed contracture of the hip adductors is present, transection of the anterior branches of the obturator nerve is indicated to denervate the adductors, allowing the patient to stand with a broader base of support.

   b. If a fixed hip contracture is present, surgical release of the adductor muscles is indicated.

B. Stiff-knee gait

1. Characteristics—Inability to flex the knee during swing phase; unrestricted passive knee motion; a limb that appears to be functionally longer; no difficulty sitting.

2. Inappropriate activity in the rectus femoris from preswing through terminal swing blocks knee flexion.

3. Abnormal activity is also common in the vastus intermedius, vastus medialis, and vastus lateralis muscles.

4. Circumduction of the involved limb, hiking of the pelvis, or contralateral limb vaulting may occur as compensatory maneuvers.

5. Surgical management options

   a. Transfer of the rectus femoris to the gracilis tendon not only removes the rectus as a deforming muscle force but also converts it into a corrective flexion force.

   b. When any of the vasti muscles are involved, they can be selectively lengthened at their myotendinous junction.

C. Hip and knee flexion deformity

1. Hip and knee flexion occur in concert and result in a crouched posture, increasing the physical demand on the quadriceps and hip extensor muscles, which must continually fire to hold the patient upright.

2. Surgical management options

   a. Simultaneous surgical correction of the hip and knee flexion deformities is preferred.

   b. The hip is approached medially, and the adductor longus and pectineus muscles are released.

   c. The iliopsoas muscle is recessed from the lesser trochanter.

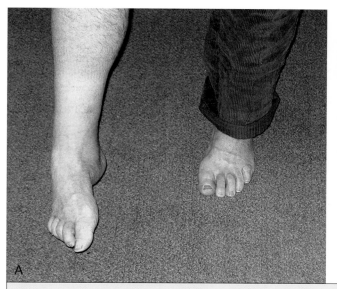 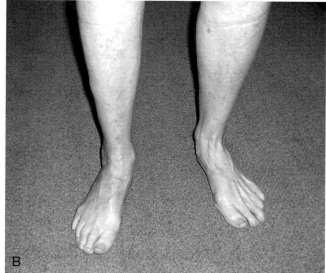

Figure 1 Photographs show a patient with equinovarus foot deformity that resulted from a stroke. The feet are shown before (**A**) and after (**B**) corrective surgery.

d. Hamstring tenotomy results in a 50% correction of the contracture at the time of surgery.

e. The residual joint contracture is corrected by physical therapy or serial casting.

D. Equinus, claw toe, and equinovarus foot deformity

1. Surgical correction of an equinus deformity is achieved with Achilles tendon lengthening or a Strayer procedure. At the time of surgery, the Silfverskiöld test may be performed. This test checks for contracture with the knee bent (soleus tightness) compared with tightness when the knee is straight (gastrocnemius tightness). If both are tight, Achilles tendon lengthening is performed. If only the gastrocnemius is tight, a Strayer procedure is performed.

2. Surgical correction of a claw toe deformity is achieved by releasing the flexor digitorum longus and brevis tendons at the base of each toe. Transfer of the flexor digitorum longus tendon to the calcaneus offers additional support to the weakened calf muscles.

3. Surgical correction of a hindfoot varus deformity

   a. Equinovarus is the most common musculoskeletal deformity seen following a stroke or traumatic brain injury.

   b. The tibialis anterior, tibialis posterior, and extensor hallucis longus are potentially responsible for the deformity.

   c. Tendon transfers are indicated to rebalance the foot (**Figure 1**).

      • A split anterior tibial tendon transfer diverts the inverting deforming force of the tibialis anterior to a corrective force. In this procedure, one half of the tendon is transferred laterally to the cuboid.

      • When the extensor hallucis longus muscle is overactive, it can be transferred to the dorsum of the foot.

      • Lengthening of the tibialis posterior is indicated when this muscle exhibits increased activity.

   d. After healing, 70% of patients can walk without an orthosis.

IV. Upper Limb Deformities

A. Shoulder deformities

1. Shoulder adduction and internal rotation deformities

   a. These deformities are caused by spasticity and myostatic contracture of four muscles: the pectoralis major, subscapularis, latissimus dorsi, and teres major.

   b. Muscle contractures in a nonfunctional arm are surgically released through an anterior deltopectoral incision.

   c. The subscapularis muscle can be released without violating the glenohumeral joint capsule.

2. Limited shoulder flexion

   a. Antagonistic activity of the latissimus dorsi, teres major, and long head of the triceps muscles can obscure the fact that volitional control of

2: General Knowledge

the agonist muscles (shoulder flexors) is present.

 b. Diminishing the increased muscle activity by fractional lengthening of the antagonist muscles can improve shoulder flexion.

3. Inferior subluxation of the glenohumeral joint

 a. This condition occurs in patients with flaccid upper extremity paralysis. Patients report pain when the limb is dependent.

 b. Physical examination reveals pain, which is exacerbated by dependency and relieved by support.

 c. These patients may undergo a biceps suspension procedure, in which the long head of the biceps is disconnected from its muscle belly distally and looped through a bone tunnel in the proximal humerus. The humeral head is then reduced, and the tendon is sewed to itself at the appropriate tension.

 d. Adduction and internal rotation contractures are often comorbid and can be treated by tendon lengthening at the time of suspension surgery.

B. Elbow flexion deformities—Treatment varies, depending on whether the patient has active movement.

1. Patients with active movement

 a. Myotendinous lengthening of the spastic elbow flexors is indicated to correct the flexion deformity and improve function.

 b. Surgical technique

  • The long and short biceps are lengthened proximally in the arm.

  • The brachialis is lengthened at the elbow.

  • The brachioradialis is lengthened in the forearm.

 c. The patient can begin active motion immediately after surgery.

2. Patients with no active movement and a fixed elbow flexion contracture

 a. The contracted muscles are released through a lateral incision.

 b. The brachioradialis muscle and biceps tendon are transected.

 c. The brachialis muscle is released.

C. Wrist and finger flexion deformities in a functional hand

1. In a hand with active movement, myotendinous lengthening of the spastic wrist and finger flexors in the forearm is indicated.

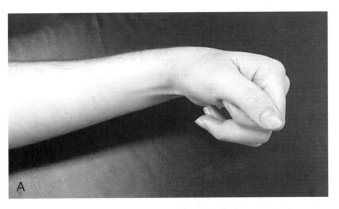

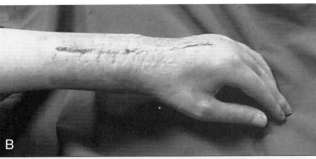

Figure 2 Photographs show a patient with a clenched-fist deformity in a nonfunctional hand before (**A**) and after (**B**) a superficialis-to-profundus transfer and wrist arthrodesis to correct the deformity.

2. The pronator teres and pronator quadratus muscles also can be lengthened.

D. Clenched-fist deformity in a nonfunctional hand (**Figure 2**)

1. Left untreated, this condition can cause palmar skin breakdown and hygiene problems, recurrent infections of the nail beds, and compression of the median nerve when combined with a wrist flexion contracture.

2. Adequate flexor tendon lengthening to correct the deformity cannot be attained by fractional or myotendinous lengthening without causing discontinuity at the musculotendinous junction.

3. The recommended surgical technique is a superficialis-to-profundus tendon transfer.

 a. This technique provides sufficient flexor tendon lengthening and preserves a passive tether to prevent a hyperextension deformity.

 b. The wrist deformity is corrected by release of the wrist flexors.

 c. Wrist arthrodesis maintains the hand in a neutral position and eliminates the need for a permanent splint.

d. Because intrinsic muscle spasticity occurs in conjunction with severe spasticity of the extrinsic flexors, a neurectomy of the motor branches of the ulnar nerve in the Guyon canal also is performed routinely to prevent the postoperative development of intrinsic deformities.

e. A neurectomy of the recurrent motor branch of the median nerve also is performed routinely to prevent a thumb-in-palm deformity.

V. Heterotopic Ossification

A. Characteristics

1. HO is characterized by the formation of bone in nonskeletal tissue, usually between the muscle and joint capsule (**Figure 3**).

2. HO usually develops within 2 months after a neurologic injury such as a traumatic brain injury or spinal cord injury.

   a. In patients with spinal cord injuries, the hip is the site most commonly involved, followed by the knee, elbow, and the shoulder (least common).

   b. In patients with traumatic brain injury, the hip is affected most often, followed by the elbow, shoulder, and knee.

3. HO is generally visible on plain radiographs.

4. The etiology of HO is unknown, but a genetic predisposition is suspected.

B. Risk factors

1. Trauma greatly increases the incidence of HO in patients with brain injuries.

2. Patients with massive HO usually have severe spasticity and a high recurrence rate following resection.

3. The completeness of a spinal cord lesion seems to be more predictive of HO than the level of injury, although cervical and thoracic lesions seem to produce HO more often than lumbar lesions.

4. Soft-tissue damage such as occurs with decubitus ulcers can be a predisposing factor.

5. Prolonged coma and young patient age (20 to 30 years) appear to increase the likelihood of HO formation.

C. Complications

1. Significant functional impairment, which can lead to a decline in a patient's ability to perform ADLs.

2. Decreased joint range of motion, which increases the likelihood of pathologic fractures of osteoporotic bone during transfers or patient positioning and can result in peripheral neuropathy by impinging adjacent nervous structures.

3. Soft-tissue contractures of the surrounding skin, muscles, ligaments, and neurovascular bundles, which can contribute to the formation of decubitus ulcers.

4. Skin maceration, often resulting in significant hygiene problems.

5. Complex regional pain syndrome, which is more prevalent in patients with HO.

6. Joint ankylosis, which frequently occurs as a result of HO.

D. Management

1. Early management and prophylaxis

   a. Although no proven prophylaxis is available, bisphosphonates and NSAIDs are the mainstays of early management.

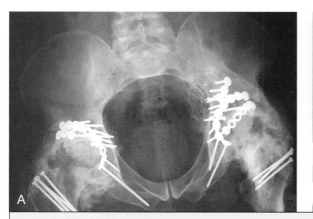
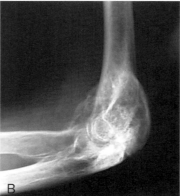
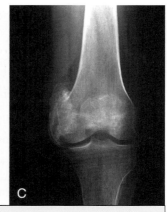

Figure 3 Radiographs of heterotopic ossification (HO) following traumatic brain injury. **A,** AP view of the pelvis shows HO of both hips. **B,** Lateral view of an elbow shows posterior HO. **C,** AP view demonstrates HO of the medial knee.

b. Radiation is thought to inhibit HO formation by disrupting the process whereby mesenchymal cells differentiate into osteoblasts; however, no data support this theory.

c. Maintaining joint motion is the goal of early management. This is achieved by treating spasticity and using gentle physical therapy.

2. Surgical management

a. Surgical excision is indicated when the HO interferes with function.

b. Preoperative assessment and planning are essential.

- Radiographs—The maturity of HO can be assessed by the appearance of a bony cortex on radiographs. Judet views of the pelvis are useful to assess hip HO. Limitations on mobility and the ability to position the patient make obtaining radiographic studies difficult.

- CT is used in planning the surgical approach, with three-dimensional reconstructions particularly helpful in complex cases.

3. Surgical techniques

a. Wide exposure and the identification of major vessels and nerves are important because HO often encases neurovascular tissues and can displace and/or compress adjacent tissues, distorting the normal anatomy.

b. Meticulous hemostasis and the elimination of dead space reduce the risk of infection; surgical drains can help with this.

4. Complications

a. Hematoma and infection

b. Fractures of osteoporotic bone, either during surgery or postoperatively, during physical therapy

c. Intraoperative bleeding requiring transfusion

d. Recurrence

e. Late development of osteonecrosis in patients who require extensive dissection

5. Postoperative management

a. Early gentle joint mobilization

b. Passive limb positioning for function

c. Prophylaxis to prevent recurrence, using bisphosphonates, NSAIDs, radiation, or a combination of these treatments. NSAIDs must be used with caution because of the risk of increased bleeding and hematoma formation.

VI. Physical Therapy and Occupational Therapy

A. Muscle weakness and physiologic deconditioning

1. Prolonged immobilization of the extremities, bed rest, and inactivity result in pronounced muscle wasting and physiologic deconditioning in a short time.

2. Disabled patients expend more energy than unaffected individuals when performing ADLs.

B. Aerobic metabolism

1. During sustained exercise, metabolism is mainly aerobic.

2. The principal fuels for aerobic metabolism are carbohydrates and fats.

3. In aerobic oxidation, substrates are oxidized through a series of enzymatic reactions that result in the production of adenosine triphosphate for muscular contraction.

4. A physical conditioning program can increase aerobic capacity by improving cardiac output, increasing hemoglobin levels, enhancing the capacity of cells to extract oxygen from the blood, and increasing the muscle mass by hypertrophy.

C. Areas of concern

1. Patient positioning

2. Mobility

3. Performance of ADLs

4. Enabling bedridden patients to sit can significantly improve quality of life and greatly enhance their opportunities to interact with other people.

5. For some patients, casts or orthotic devices may be required to maintain desired limb positions.

6. Aggressive joint motion exercises are necessary to prevent contractures.

D. Factors influencing a patient's ability to walk

1. Limb stability

2. Motor control

3. Good balance reactions

4. Adequate proprioception

E. Equipment and devices that aid in movement (for example, canes, walkers, wheelchairs)

1. These aids should always have the least complex design needed to accomplish the goal.

2. They should be selected based on the patient's cognitive and physical levels of function.

F. Developing appropriate exercises and activities

1. Considerations include joint range of motion, muscle tone, motor control, and cognitive function of the patient.

2. Cognitive function considerations

   a. Even confused and agitated patients may respond positively to simple, familiar functional activities such as face washing and teeth brushing.

   b. Patients with higher cognitive function should be encouraged to carry out hygiene, grooming, dressing, and feeding activities.

G. Physical therapy prescription

   1. Components include the diagnosis, functional deficits to be addressed, management goals, and any precautions or restrictions.

   2. The prescription also should specify whether modalities can be used, the need for orthoses, and the weight-bearing capacity of the arm or leg.

3. The frequency and duration of the therapy also should be specified.

H. Home exercise program

   1. A home exercise program may be initially appropriate for minor conditions or with motivated, intelligent patients.

   2. Home exercise has the advantage of convenience but the disadvantage that it lacks supervision and coaching.

   3. High-level home exercise programs may not be appropriate for patients with balance or other safety issues.

   4. Generally, a formal physical therapy program is followed up by a maintenance home exercise program.

Top Testing Facts

1. A diagnosis of a complete spinal cord injury cannot be made until spinal shock has resolved, as evidenced by the return of the bulbocavernosus reflex.

2. Neurologic recovery after spinal cord injury is assessed by determining the change in AMS (the sum of strength grades for each of the 10 key muscles, tested bilaterally, that represent neurologic segments C5 through T1 and L2 through S1) between successive neurologic examinations.

3. Treatment of the patient with spinal cord injury includes prevention of contractures, maintenance of range of motion and skin integrity, and intermittent catheterization.

4. The incidence of HO is approximately 20% in patients with spinal cord injury. Surgical excision is indicated when HO interferes with function.

5. C6 is the highest level of injury that conceivably allows independent living; patients with a level of injury at C7 and below are more likely to be functional when living alone.

6. A crouched posture increases the physical demand on the quadriceps and hip extensor muscles, which must continually fire to hold the patient upright. Simultaneous surgical correction of the hip and knee flexion deformities is the most desirable treatment.

7. Surgical correction of claw toe deformity requires release of the flexor digitorum longus and brevis tendons at the base of each toe.

8. Surgical correction of an equinovarus deformity is achieved with tendon transfers to rebalance the foot, including a split anterior tibial tendon transfer.

9. Wrist and finger flexion deformities in a functional hand are treated with myotendinous lengthenings.

10. The recommended surgical treatment of a clenched-fist deformity in a nonfunctional hand is a superficialis-to-profundus tendon transfer.

11. Factors that influence a patient's ability to walk include limb stability, motor control, balance reactions, and adequate proprioception.

Bibliography

American Spinal Injury Association: Reference Manual for the International Standards for the Neurological Classification of Spinal Cord Injury. Chicago, IL, American Spinal Injury Association, 2003.

Baldwin K, Hosalkar HS, Donegan DJ, Rendon N, Ramsey M, Keenan MA: Surgical resection of heterotopic bone about the elbow: An institutional experience with traumatic and neurologic etiologies. *J Hand Surg Am* 2011;36(5):798-803.

Ditunno JF Jr, Apple DF, Burns AS, et al: A view of the future Model Spinal Cord Injury System through the prism of past achievements and current challenges. *J Spinal Cord Med* 2003;26(2):110-115.

Garland DE: A clinical perspective on common forms of acquired heterotopic ossification. *Clin Orthop Relat Res* 1991; 263:13-29.

2: General Knowledge

Kaplan FS, Glaser DL, Hebela N, Shore EM: Heterotopic ossification. *J Am Acad Orthop Surg* 2004;12(2):116-125.

Keenan MA: The management of spastic equinovarus deformity following stroke and head injury. *Foot Ankle Clin* 2011; 16(3):499-514.

Keenan MA: Management of the spastic upper extremity in the neurologically impaired adult. *Clin Orthop Relat Res* 1988;233:116-125.

Keenan MA: Orthopaedic management of upper extremity dysfunction following stroke or brain injury, in Green DP, Hotchkiss RN, Pederson WC, eds: *Operative Hand Surgery*, ed 5. New York, NY, Churchill Livingstone, 2005, pp 287-324.

Keenan MA: Surgical decision making for residual limb deformities following traumatic brain injury. *Orthop Rev* 1988; 17(12):1185-1192.

Keenan MA, Korchek JI, Botte MJ, Smith CW, Garland DE: Results of transfer of the flexor digitorum superficialis tendons to the flexor digitorum profundus tendons in adults with acquired spasticity of the hand. *J Bone Joint Surg Am* 1987;69(8):1127-1132.

Keenan MA, Lee GA, Tuckman AS, Esquenazi A: Improving calf muscle strength in patients with spastic equinovarus deformity by transfer of the long toe flexors to the Os calcis. *J Head Trauma Rehabil* 1999;14(2):163-175.

Keenan MA, Mehta S: Neuro-orthopedic management of shoulder deformity and dysfunction in brain-injured patients: A novel approach. *J Head Trauma Rehabil* 2004;19(2): 143-154.

Keenan MA, Ure K, Smith CW, Jordan C: Hamstring release for knee flexion contracture in spastic adults. *Clin Orthop Relat Res* 1988;236:221-226.

Kirshblum SC, Priebe MM, Ho CH, Scelza WM, Chiodo AE, Wuermser LA: Spinal cord injury medicine: 3. Rehabilitation phase after acute spinal cord injury. *Arch Phys Med Rehabil* 2007;88(3, Suppl 1):S62-S70.

Mehta S, Keenan MA: Rehabilitation, in Skiner HB, ed: *Current Diagnosis and Treatment in Orthopedics*, ed 4. New York, NY, Lange Medical Books/McGraw-Hill, 2006, pp 671-727.

Namdari S, Alosh H, Baldwin K, Mehta S, Keenan MA: Outcomes of tendon fractional lengthenings to improve shoulder function in patients with spastic hemiparesis. *J Shoulder Elbow Surg* 2012;21(5):691-698.

Namdari S, Alosh H, Baldwin K, Mehta S, Keenan MA: Shoulder tenotomies to improve passive motion and relieve pain in patients with spastic hemiplegia after upper motor neuron injury. *J Shoulder Elbow Surg* 2011;20(5):802-806.

Namdari S, Horneff JG, Baldwin K, Keenan MA: Muscle releases to improve passive motion and relieve pain in patients with spastic hemiplegia and elbow flexion contractures. *J Shoulder Elbow Surg* 2012;21(10):1357-1362.

Namdari S, Keenan MA: Outcomes of the biceps suspension procedure for painful inferior glenohumeral subluxation in hemiplegic patients. *J Bone Joint Surg Am* 2010;92(15): 2589-2597.

Namdari S, Pill SG, Makani A, Keenan MA: Rectus femoris to gracilis muscle transfer with fractional lengthening of the vastus muscles: A treatment for adults with stiff knee gait. *Phys Ther* 2010;90(2):261-268.

Pappas N, Baldwin K, Keenan MA: Efficacy of median nerve recurrent branch neurectomy as an adjunct to ulnar motor nerve neurectomy and wrist arthrodesis at the time of superficialis to profundus transfer in prevention of intrinsic spastic thumb-in-palm deformity. *J Hand Surg Am* 2010;35(8): 1310-1316.

Chapter 23
Medicolegal Issues

David A. Halsey, MD

I. Patient Safety and Medical Errors

A. Institute of Medicine (IOM) effort—The IOM launched a concerted, ongoing effort focused on assessing and improving the nation's quality of care in 1996.

1. First phase (1996–1998)—Documented the serious and pervasive nature of the nation's overall quality problem, concluding that "the burden of harm conveyed by the collective impact of all of our healthcare quality problems is staggering."

2. Second phase (1999–2001)—The Committee on Quality of Health Care in America released two reports, establishing a vision for how the healthcare system and related policy environment must be radically transformed.

   a. *To Err Is Human: Building a Safer Health System* (1999) reported that tens of thousands of Americans die each year as a result of medical errors. It highlighted the importance of patient safety and quality issues for public and private policymakers.

   b. *Crossing the Quality Chasm: A New Health System for the 21st Century* (2001) stressed broader quality issues and described six aims of care: safe, effective, patient-centered, timely, efficient, and equitable.

3. Third phase (2002–present)—Operationalized the vision of a future health system described in the Quality Chasm report.

   a. Identifies stakeholders in creating a more patient-responsive health system: clinicians and healthcare organizations, employers and consumers, research foundations, government agencies, quality organizations.

   b. Focuses reform at three levels: environmental, the healthcare organization, the interface between clinicians and patients.

B. Collaborative efforts

1. Agency for Healthcare Research and Quality (AHRQ)

   a. Research arm of the US Department of Health and Human Services (HHS) and sister agency to the National Institutes of Health (NIH)

   b. Home to specialized research centers in major areas of healthcare research. These centers focus on:

   - Quality improvement in patient safety—Identifying factors that put patients at risk; using computer and other information technology to reduce and prevent errors; developing innovative approaches that reduce errors and produce safety in various healthcare settings and geographically diverse locations; disseminating research results; and improving patient safety education and training for clinicians and other providers.

   - Outcomes and effectiveness of care

   - Clinical practice and technology assessment

   - Healthcare organization and delivery systems

   - Primary care

   - Healthcare costs and sources of payment

   c. The AHRQ supports research on health disparities, drugs and other therapeutics, primary care practice, and integrated healthcare delivery systems.

   d. It focuses on evidence-based practice and the translation of research into clinical practice to improve patient care in diverse healthcare settings.

   e. It identifies strategies to improve healthcare access, foster appropriate use, and reduce unnecessary expenditures.

2. The Joint Commission

   a. The Joint Commission is the major accrediting agency for hospitals.

   b. It developed a sentinel reporting policy in 1996 that encourages accredited healthcare

Dr. Halsey or an immediate family member serves as a board member, owner, officer, or committee member of the American Academy of Orthopaedic Surgeons and the American Association of Hip and Knee Surgeons.

2: General Knowledge

organizations to voluntarily report "sentinel" events within 5 days and submit a root cause analysis within 45 days of discovery. A sentinel event is defined as "an unexpected occurrence involving death or serious physical or psychological injury, or the risk thereof." Serious injury specifically includes loss of limb or function. The phrase 'the risk thereof' includes any process variations the risk for which a recurrence would carry a significant chance of a serious adverse outcome."

c. Based on root cause analyses, The Joint Commission identified the need to establish national patient safety goals. The first National Patient Safety Goals were established in 2002. The Joint Commission reevaluates goals annually and identifies steps annually to accomplish goals. It allows alternatives to specific recommendations as long as the alternative is as effective as the original recommendation in achieving the specific patient safety goal.

d. The Joint Commission identified 15 National Patient Safety Goals; each year, specific steps are identified to accomplish the overarching goals. Examples of goals or steps specific to orthopaedics include:

- The Joint Commission 2013 National Patient Safety Goal #1: improve the accuracy of patient identification with the elimination of wrong-site surgery. Uses the American Academy of Orthopaedic Surgeons' (AAOS) Sign Your Site program. Requires a preprocedure "time-out" to confirm the correct patient, procedure, and site using active communication techniques.

- The Joint Commission 2013 National Patient Safety Goal #7: reduce the risk of healthcare-associated infections. Requires that healthcare organizations establish systems to ensure that the use of prophylactic antibiotic for total hip arthroplasty, total knee arthroplasty, and hip fracture management adheres to the best available evidence, including appropriate antibiotic selection, administration of the antibiotic within 60 minutes of the surgical incision, and discontinuation of prophylactic antibiotic therapy within 24 hours of wound closure.

3. National Patient Safety Foundation

a. Stakeholders include healthcare practitioners and institutions, manufacturers, educators, insurers, researchers, legal advisers, policymakers, and patients.

b. Mission

- Identify a core body of knowledge.

- Identify pathways to apply the knowledge.

- Develop and enhance the culture of receptivity to patient safety.

- Raise public awareness and foster communications about patient safety.

II. Compliance

A. Stark laws (**Table 1**)

1. Rationale for prohibitions

a. In some cases, excessive medical services were ordered for which the patient received unnecessary care, resulting in higher healthcare costs.

b. Costs for patients covered by government programs were ultimately passed on to taxpayers.

2. Stark I (1989)

a. Prohibits referral of Medicare patients who need clinical laboratory services to entities in which the physician has an ownership interest.

b. Prohibits referral of Medicare and certain Medicaid patients for "designated health services" to entities in which the physician or an immediate family member has a financial interest, unless an exemption applies.

c. Proscribes entities to which referrals are made from submitting payment claims to the government for specified services.

3. Stark II (1993)

a. Expands the list of referral services that are prohibited from physician ownership.

b. Expands the referral band to include patients covered by certain Medicaid managed care programs.

c. Identifies circumstances under which referrals are permitted activities, known as exceptions.

4. Final regulations for enactment of Stark II (1998)

a. Issued in 1995, but rolled out in two phases

Table 1

Chronology of Stark Laws

1989: Stark (I) enacted.

1993: Broadened version (Stark II) enacted.

1995: Final regulations for enactment of Stark I.

1998: Regulations proposed for two-phase enactment of Stark II.

2001: Phase I rolled out.

2004: Phase II rolled out.

b. Superseded the 1995 Stark I regulations

c. Consist of actual rules physicians must follow

5. Penalties for violating Stark II (phase I and II) regulations

   a. Denial of payment

   b. Mandatory refunding of payments that were made in error

   c. Civil monetary penalties of $15,000 per claim

   d. Prohibition from participation in Medicare and Medicaid programs

6. Phase II exceptions—Five are most important to orthopaedic surgeons.

   a. In-office ancillary service in a group practice or by a sole practitioner

   b. Bona fide employment

   c. Personal service arrangements

   d. Fair market value compensation

   e. Academic medical centers

B. Health Insurance Portability and Accountability Act (HIPAA; 1996)

1. Title I protects health insurance coverage for workers and their families when the workers change or lose their jobs.

2. Title II addresses "administrative simplification," as well as fraud, abuse, and medical liability reform.

3. Title III establishes medical savings accounts and health insurance deductions for the self-employed.

4. Title IV covers the enforcement of group health plan provisions.

5. Title V focuses on revenue offset provisions.

6. Privacy rules

   a. Create national standards to protect patient medical records and other personal health information

   b. Give patients more control over their health data

   c. Limit the way healthcare providers may use the information and release it to third parties

   d. Establish guidelines that must be followed to protect the privacy of the patient's "protected health information"

   e. Hold health plans, healthcare clearinghouses, and healthcare providers accountable for violations

C. Fraud

1. Centers for Medicare & Medicaid Services (CMS) definition—"Fraud is the intentional deception or misrepresentation that an individual knows to be false or does not believe to be true and makes, knowing that the deception could result in some unauthorized benefit to himself/herself or some other person. The most frequent kind of fraud arises from a false statement or misrepresentation made, or caused to be made, that is material to entitlement or payment under the Medicare program."

2. Most common types of fraud in Medicare

   a. Billing for services not rendered

   b. Misrepresenting a diagnosis to justify payment

   c. Soliciting, offering, or receiving a kickback

   d. Unbundling

   e. Falsifying treatment plans and medical records to justify payment

   f. Up-coding

III. Medical Malpractice Claims

A. Elements that the patient must prove

1. Duty—Physician's obligation to care for the patient in a manner that is consistent with the quality of care provided by other physicians in treating a patient's particular condition.

2. Breach of duty

   a. Facts show that the physician failed to meet the standard of care in treating the patient.

   b. Poor outcome, whether permanent or not, or a predictable complication does not necessarily mean that the physician has deviated from the standard of care.

3. Causation—Proof that the violation caused the patient's injury.

4. Damage—Proof that the physician's deviation from the standard of care resulted in physical, emotional, or financial injury to the patient.

B. Informed consent

1. Requires that a physician obtain consent before any treatment is rendered or operation is performed, and before many diagnostic procedures can be performed.

2. Requires a patient to give permission before being "touched" by another; without permission, contact may be considered an "assault," a "battery," or a "trespass" on the patient.

3. Without an informed consent, the orthopaedic physician may be held liable for violation of the pa-

tient's rights, regardless of whether the treatment was appropriate and rendered with due care.

4. Medical care cannot be provided without either expressed or implied permission for the physician to act.

IV. Patient Complaints

A. Factors that contribute to both the likelihood a patient will bring suit as well as the successful prosecution of medical malpractice claims

1. Miscommunication

2. Delay in response to patient/family concerns

3. Failure to diagnose

4. Failure to treat

5. Improper treatment

B. Factors that contribute to patient complaints

1. Inconsistency in communication

2. Promises that are not kept

3. Lack of sufficient details regarding the diagnosis and treatment plan

4. Perceived rudeness

5. Lack of understanding regarding known procedural/surgical complications

6. Perception that the physician and staff are too busy to be concerned with the patient's problem

7. Long wait times

8. Frustration with the inability to "fix" a painful condition

C. Patient-physician communication

1. Effective patient-physician communication will avert many patient complaints.

2. Tools to ensure high-quality patient-physician communication

a. Adequate time

b. Acknowledgment of emotional distress

c. Physician-obtained informed consent

d. Phone calls returned in a timely fashion

D. Skills to assist with addressing complaints when first expressed

1. Take all complaints seriously.

2. Acknowledge the patient's concern/complaint.

3. Provide accurate information to help clarify the situation.

4. Be frank and honest.

5. Avoid negative comments about other healthcare providers.

E. CMS requirements for complaints

1. All complaints must be addressed with a written response to the patient in a timely manner.

2. Situations requiring a written response to the patient

a. When a patient specifically asks for a written report

b. When there is a dispute about charges based on the patient's perception of quality of care

3. Components of the written response

a. Acknowledgment of the complaint

b. Addressing the issue to the extent possible

c. Reassurance that the patient's feedback will be used to avoid a similar problem for another patient in the future

V. Standard of Disclosure

A. Varies by state

B. Two standards for assessing adequacy of disclosure

1. Professional or reasonable physicians' standard—Based on what is customary practice in the medical community for physicians to divulge to patients (most common).

2. Patient viewpoint standard—Based on what a reasonable person in the patient's position would want to know in similar circumstances.

3. More information generally is revealed with patient viewpoint standard than in jurisdictions that adhere to the professional or reasonable physicians' standard.

C. Elements of informed consent

1. Stated diagnosis

2. Nature of the condition or illness requiring medical or surgical intervention

3. Nature and purpose of the treatment or procedure recommended

4. Risks and potential complications associated with the recommended treatment or procedure

5. All feasible alternative treatments or procedures noted, including the option of taking no action

6. Relative probability of success for treatment or procedure in terms the patient will understand

Top Ten Medicolegal Terms

1. *Abandonment*: Termination of the physician-patient relationship by the physician without reasonable notice to the patient at a time when the patient requires medical attention and without the opportunity to make arrangements for appropriate continuation and follow-up care.

2. *Burden of proof*: Typically, a plaintiff's responsibility to affirmatively prove a fact or facts in dispute on an issue raised between parties in a case.

3. *Causation*: The causal connection between the act or omission of the defendant and the injury suffered by the plaintiff. The plaintiff must show causation of an injury by the defendant to prove negligence.

4. *Damages*: Money receivable through judicial order by a plaintiff sustaining harm, impairment, or loss to his or her person or property as the result of the accidental, intentional, or negligent act of another. Damages can be grouped into two primary types: compensatory and punitive.
   * *Compensatory damages* are to compensate the injured party for the injury sustained and nothing more. Compensatory damages can be divided into economic, noneconomic, and special damages.
     ○ *Economic damages* include an estimate of lost wages, both past and future, of the plaintiff and affected family members, and all costs associated with residual disability of the patient.
     ○ *Noneconomic damages* include intangible damage resulting from the negligent act such as pain and suffering, disfigurement, and interference with the ordinary enjoyment of life.
     ○ *Special damages* are the actual out-of-pocket losses incurred by the plaintiff, such as medical expenses, rehabilitation expenses, and earnings lost during treatment and recovery.
   * *Punitive damages* are awarded to punish a defendant who has acted maliciously or in reckless disregard of the plaintiff's rights.

5. *Duty*: The obligation of the physician to care for the patient in a manner that is consistent with the quality of care provided by other physicians in treating a patient's particular condition.

6. *Fraud*: The intentional deception or misrepresentation that an individual knows to be false or does not believe to be true and makes, knowing that the deception could result in some unauthorized benefit to himself/herself or some other person.

7. *Informed consent*: Consent is "fully informed" only when the patient knows and understands the information necessary to make an informed decision about the treatment or procedure. There is no informed consent when the treatment or procedure extends beyond the scope of consent. For example, if the risk associated with the changed treatment or procedure is substantially different from that contemplated by the patient, the courts may find that the original informed consent was not sufficient. The certain circumstances for which special informed consent rules apply are medical emergencies, situations involving a minor, and those rare circumstances in which authorization for a treatment or procedure is obtained from a court.

8. *Malpractice*: In the case of a physician, failure to exercise the degree of care and skill that a physician or surgeon of the same specialty would use under similar circumstances (professional negligence); care below the "standard of care."

9. *Negligence*: In medical malpractice cases, a legal cause of action involving the failure of a defendant physician to exercise that degree of diligence and care that an average qualified physician practicing in the same specialty as that of the defendant physician would have exercised in a similar situation and that has resulted in the breach of a legal duty owed by the physician to the patient that proximately caused an injury that the law recognizes as deserving of compensation (damages).

10. *Res ipsa loquitur* ("The thing speaks for itself"): A doctrine that may be invoked in a negligence action when the plaintiff has no direct evidence of negligence but the injury itself results in the inference that it would not have occurred in the absence of a negligent act. It raises an inference of the defendant's negligence, thereby altering the burden of proof so that the defendant must produce evidence that he or she did not commit a negligent act.

Bibliography

American Academy of Orthopaedic Surgeons: Government relations. www.aaos.org/govern/govern.asp. Accessed Oct. 10, 2013.

American Academy of Orthopaedic Surgeons: Risk management continuing medical education. www5.aaos.org/oko/RiskManagement.cfm. Accessed Oct. 10, 2013.

Institute of Medicine of the National Academies. www.iom.edu. Accessed Oct. 10, 2013.

The Joint Commission: National patient safety goals. www.jointcommission.org/standards_information/npsgs.aspx. Accessed Oct. 10, 2013.

National Patient Safety Foundation: www.npsf.org. Accessed Oct. 10, 2013.

US Department of Health and Human Services: Agency for Healthcare Research and Quality. www.ahrq.gov. Accessed Oct. 10, 2013.

2: General Knowledge

Chapter 24
Medical Ethics

Ross E. McKinney Jr, MD

I. Professionalism and Code of Ethics

A. Medical professionalism is predicated on the Hippocratic Oath. Most physicians adhere to an updated version written by Louis Lasagna in 1964.

B. The best-known core principle in medical ethics is "Primum non nocere," or "First, do no harm." This aphorism, which probably was written in the 17th century by Thomas Sydenham, an English physician, does not appear in the Hippocratic Oath. It is intended to give a physician pause before automatically recommending surgery (which could have complications), prescribing a medicine (which could have side effects), or ordering a test (which could have false positive results, provoking anxiety or resulting in inappropriate management).

C. A fundamental tenet of professionalism is that the patient's interests should always be foremost. Maintaining this principle can be a challenge in a fee-for-service medical environment, in which volume- and price-related incentives can affect decision making.

D. Modern professional principles include an emphasis on privacy (which, in the United States, is codified in the Health Insurance Portability and Accountability Act of 1996 [HIPAA]) and on patient empowerment (informed consent).

E. Modern professionalism assumes good medical record keeping and accurate billing.

II. Informed Consent

A. Informed consent is predicated on the respect for persons and their right to make autonomous decisions.

B. Informed consent depends on providing adequate information so the patient can make a decision regarding which therapeutic option to follow or whether to enroll in a research study.

1. Alternative treatment options should be presented.

2. The risks and benefits of each option should be described.

3. The language should be clear and free of jargon.

C. Most of the clinical consent process is oral. The written document should highlight the most important points made during the oral discussion.

D. The physician obtaining consent should make a good faith effort to evaluate whether the patient understands the information that has been provided.

E. Patients have the right to decide their own course of treatment, even when their decisions are bad from the point of view of a physician.

F. Patients should be aware that their decision to proceed with treatment is voluntary.

G. In clinical care, deciding whether written consent or oral consent is required is usually based on risk. For most invasive procedures, written consent is expected. For minor procedures (phlebotomy, for example), consent is usually tacit (understood) or oral. Written informed consent underscores the point to the practitioner and the patient that a serious decision is being made.

H. True informed consent requires three key elements: the provision of adequate information, comprehension of the information by the person being asked to consent, and voluntariness.

III. Complications and the Peer Review Process

A. Complications

1. Complications are an inevitable but hopefully rare consequence of surgery.

2. Recent research suggests that directly admitting mistakes that have caused complications prevents malpractice suits more effectively than does evasion or avoiding discussion with the patient or the patient's family.

3. The possibility of complications should be addressed during the informed consent process. A balance should be struck between describing meaningful risks and providing an all-inclusive list of possible problems.

Dr. McKinney or an immediate family member serves as a paid consultant to or is an employee of Gilead Sciences.

B. Peer review

1. When a mistake is made, peer review is an important teaching and evaluative tool.

2. Peer review and other forms of quality improvement are legally protected in most states. Slanderous and inaccurate statements made during the review process are not protected, however. Transparently false accusations may result in peer-based condemnation of the accuser.

3. To be successful, peer review should focus on teaching, not retribution.

4. The best peer review looks forward, providing solutions that will prevent problems in the future.

5. Good peer review considers systems issues as well as individual physician performance.

IV. Industry Relationships

A. Medical research relationships with industry are not intrinsically bad.

B. Physician-industry relationships fall in several categories: employment, scientific collaborations, clinical, marketing.

1. Industry may sponsor research by a physician or group of physicians.

2. To minimize the potential for bias, physician researchers working with industry and charged with writing any study-related manuscripts should request access to the raw research data, although this is not the industry research norm.

3. Close relationships with industry may produce bias, particularly if personal compensation depends on a particular outcome. For example, if a physician invents and then licenses a product, resulting in a royalty stream, positive results from a study of that product could increase the inventor's personal income. This type of relationship can reduce the credibility of the research if the inventor takes a key role. Biased research results also may be harmful to future patients.

4. In academic medical centers, research contracts are generally agreements between the institution and the company, whereas for physicians in private practice, the contract is usually between the practice and the sponsor or contract research organization. Contracts with academic medical centers are more complicated because universities, as nonprofit entities, must work in the public benefit. In research, that usually means assurance that the work will be published. Also, many academic medical centers include language in their contracts that allows them to retain the rights to new intellectual property. Because private practices rarely pay attention to either of these issues, those practices have contractual advantages from the point of view of many sponsors.

5. For National Institutes of Health (NIH) grants, the US Public Health Service requires reporting of all major financial interests that could directly and substantially affect the design, conduct, or reporting of research. This responsibility falls on the institution that receives the grant, usually an academic institution or nonprofit organization. To help the institution identify which financial interests to report, investigators are required to fully disclose their financial relationships. After those relationships are disclosed to the institution, the conflict-of-interest program is expected to manage any conflicts.

   a. Typical management strategies include a requirement for disclosure of external financial relationships.

   b. Institutional review boards (IRBs) often require that informed consent documents provide information about external financial interests.

   c. The NIH expects the institution to describe how its management approach will mitigate the effects of conflict-of-interest–related bias in the research. The institution is required to file a formal report with the US Public Health Service.

C. As of 2013, the Physician Payments Sunshine Act (part of the Affordable Care Act of 2010) requires pharmaceutical companies, device manufacturers, and medical service providers to report all payments of $10 or more made to physicians and academic medical centers. These reports will be summarized in a publicly accessible, searchable website so that all physician-industry financial arrangements become public knowledge.

V. Institutional Review Boards

A. IRBs evaluate research protocols for scientific validity, ethical design, and proposed conduct.

B. Federally sponsored research is regulated by the Code of Federal Regulations (CFR). Regulation 45 CFR part 46, known as the Common Rule, is also applied to most other human investigation in the United States.

C. The Food and Drug Administration (FDA) has its own set of rules, set down in regulation 21 CFR parts 50 and 56, which are similar to the Common Rule but add requirements related to FDA jurisdiction.

D. The Common Rule is based largely on the Belmont Report, a 1979 document written by the National Commission for the Protection of Human Subjects of Biomedical and Behavioral Research (the National Commission).

1. The National Commission was created in response to several research scandals, including the Tuskegee syphilis study, in which investigators appeared to prioritize scientific objectives over the health and well-being of the persons who took part in the research. In some cases, the study participants were neither aware of nor even informed that they were involved in research.

2. The Belmont Report codifies three basic principles for the ethical conduct of clinical research.

   a. Respect for persons—Individuals have autonomous rights to participate (or not) in research, and their decisions should be made on the basis of an informed consent process.

   b. Beneficence—Research should benefit the participants in the research or people like them.

   c. Justice—The selection of research subjects should be fair.

E. Before human subjects are enrolled in a research study in the United States, the research proposal should be submitted to an IRB for review. Internationally, most institutions and countries have Ethics Review Boards that serve the same function as IRBs.

VI. Culturally Competent Care

A. Because many medical decisions involve issues surrounding values, physicians should be aware that different cultures may have different priorities.

B. Before a patient makes an important medical decision, the clinical team should help the patient achieve a full understanding of the important issues.

C. In some circumstances, when a physician does not agree with a decision made by the patient, the physician may decide not to continue to participate in providing care for that patient. A physician who so chooses still has a moral and legal obligation to make sure that another care provider is arranged for, or at least to give the patient sufficient time to find alternative care.

D. A patient who does not speak the same language as the physician will require a translator who is sufficiently skilled that medical information can be conveyed accurately. Privacy concerns should be considered when selecting a translator, particularly if the potential translator is a friend or family member of the patient, because many patients do not want their clinical status made public.

E. The physician should be aware that some patients may perceive a power imbalance between the patient and physician. They may believe they should accede to the physician's instructions solely because of the

physician's authority rather than because they agree with the physician's treatment plan. Although this behavior may be convenient for the physician, in medical care, the goal should be voluntary consent, not simple compliance.

VII. Elder Abuse and Child Abuse

A. A physician who encounters evidence of potential elder abuse or child abuse—for example, multiple poorly explained fractures in a single child—is required by law in almost all states to report their concerns to the local social service agency.

B. Deciding to report elder abuse or child abuse can be difficult because the act of reporting can rupture the therapeutic relationship between the patient, the family, and the medical provider. The highest priority is established by law, however: the person at risk should be protected.

C. Reporting suspected elder abuse or child abuse is protected by law. Only in cases of malicious reporting is the person filing the report legally liable. In contrast, failure to report is a potentially negligent act under the law.

VIII. End-of-Life Issues

A. Most states allow the use of advance care directives (also called a "living will"). These documents allow an individual to specify his or her expectations in the case of incapacitating medical illness, particularly situations in which the person is not able to express his or her wishes (for example, regarding feeding tubes, intubation, chest compressions).

B. Advance care directives are especially useful in diseases like cancer or progressive dementia. They also can facilitate conversation within a family regarding an individual's preferences about end-of-life decisions.

C. An advance care directive is not binding. Unanticipated circumstances may occur—for example, a need for short-term intubation for a surgical procedure—and family members may not agree with the patient. The physician should encourage the family to observe the spirit of the advance directive, but a living family member (who can sue) may make it difficult to follow the paper advance care directive.

D. Most advance care directives lack sufficient granularity to answer all questions that can arise. For example: Did the now-comatose patient intend to exclude feeding tubes, or only intubation? What is the realistic probability of recovery?

E. For patients who have dementia or who can anticipate periods in which they may not be able to make

2: General Knowledge

decisions (for example, postoperatively), assigning a medical power of attorney is important. The designee may be a family member, a friend, or an advocate. The person with medical power of attorney should pay close attention to the wishes of the patient as much as possible.

IX. Care of the Uninsured

A. Physicians are not required *by law* to provide care for the uninsured. Physicians also can require cash payments in their practice settings.

B. Under the Emergency Medical Treatment and Active Labor Act (EMTALA), hospitals must, in general, provide emergency care for people who need it, regardless of the patient's ability to pay.

C. Hospitals can require physicians to provide emergency care as part of their work contract with the hospital.

D. Patients who do not have the means to pay for care may require more careful discharge planning. For example, an elderly patient who has a fracture that suggests osteoporosis should be referred for the management of bone mineral density to prevent an avoidable second fracture. A patient who lacks financial resources may need to be referred to a publicly funded clinic.

E. Failure to pay bills is not sufficient reason to immediately terminate a patient in need of continued care, although it can prompt a notification advising the patient to seek other care providers. The physician or practice should give the patient enough time to arrange alternative care.

X. Sports Medicine Issues

A. Physicians engaged in sports medicine, particularly the care of professional athletes, are often caught in a conflict-of-interest situation in that their employer is the team and their patients are athletes who play for the team.

B. Rules surrounding privacy may not be clear in a team setting.

1. The team physician is part of the team.

2. Good medical care requires the confidence of the patient/player, including confidence in the privacy of information.

3. HIPAA generally does not cover physicians employed by a team in their communication with the team. Therefore, confidentiality decisions mainly reflect professional ethics and personal discretion, rather than legal principles.

C. Some decisions pit the player's best interests against those of the team. A decision to play despite the risk of long-term injury should be made by a fully informed player who has received independent advice. Players should be allowed to seek second opinions from independent physicians.

D. Return-to-play decisions should be made conservatively, particularly after a head injury.

1. A player who loses consciousness should not be returned to play without a full evaluation.

2. Confusion after a head injury should prompt a careful evaluation. Players often cannot judge their own medical condition after a head injury.

Top Testing Facts

1. "Primum non nocere" ("First, do no harm") means that a physician should consider whether a contemplated action or recommendation is more likely to do harm than good.

2. The three key elements of informed consent are adequate information, comprehension by the person providing consent (the patient or volunteer), and voluntariness.

3. Peer review generally is legally protected so that an honest discussion can occur with few worries about legal risks (for example, competitors suing each other).

4. The Physician Payments Sunshine Act increases the visibility of physician-industry financial relationships.

5. An IRB should review and approve all proposed research studies before any research subjects are enrolled.

6. When a physician disagrees with a patient's care decisions to the extent that the physician believes the patient-physician relationship should be severed, a legal obligation remains to arrange for substitute care in a timely fashion.

7. Physicians are legally required to report suspected child abuse and elder abuse to an appropriate social service agency.

8. Advance care directives are useful as guidance but are not binding documents.

9. In emergency situations, most hospitals are required to provide appropriate emergency care services under the EMTALA.

10. Sports medicine physicians employed by a team are exempt from HIPAA in their discussions with the team.

Bibliography

American Medical Association: Hot topics: Important and timely medical-legal issues. www.ama-assn.org/ama/pub/physician-resources/legal-topics/hot-topics.page. Accessed Nov. 13, 2013.

Beauchamp TL, Childress JF: *Principles of Biomedical Ethics*, ed 6. New York, NY, Oxford University Press, 2009.

Dunn WR, George MS, Churchill L, Spindler KP: Ethics in sports medicine. *Am J Sports Med* 2007;35(5):840-844.

Jonsen AR: *The Birth of Bioethics*. New York, NY, Oxford University Press, 1998.

Kachalia A, Kaufman SR, Boothman R, et al: Liability claims and costs before and after implementation of a medical error disclosure program. *Ann Intern Med* 2010;153(4):213-221.

Lawrence RE, Brauner DJ: Deciding for others: Limitations of advance directives, substituted judgment, and best interest. *Virtual Mentor* 2009;11(8):571-581.

National Academy of Sciences Committee on Science, Engineering, and Public Policy: *On Being a Scientist*. Washington, DC, The National Academies Press, 2009.

Smith CM: Origin and uses of primum non nocere—above all, do no harm! *J Clin Pharmacol* 2005;45(4):371-377.

Tyson P: The Hippocratic Oath today. www.pbs.org/wgbh/nova/body/hippocratic-oath-today.html. Accessed Nov. 13, 2013.

Weinfurt KP, Hall MA, King NM, Friedman JY, Schulman KA, Sugarman J: Disclosure of financial relationships to participants in clinical research. *N Engl J Med* 2009;361(9):916-921.

2: General Knowledge

Section 3

Trauma

Section Editors:
Kenneth A. Egol, MD
Michael J. Gardner, MD

Chapter 25

Evaluation of the Trauma Patient

Philip Wolinsky, MD   William Min, MD, MS, MBA

I. Definition and Epidemiology

A. Definition—A major trauma victim is an individual who has sustained potentially life-threatening and/or limb-threatening injuries and requires hospitalization.

B. Epidemiology

1. Trauma is the fourth leading overall cause of death in the United States, but is the leading cause of death in adults younger than 44 years. In 2004, 1 of 14 deaths were caused by traumatic injuries. Injury deaths accounted for more than one half of all deaths among those age 13 to 32 years, with 4 of 5 deaths caused by injury occurring among people age 18 and 19 years.

2. Worldwide, injuries cause 1 in 10 deaths.

3. Each year, 1.5 million individuals are admitted to hospitals and survive to discharge following injury, representing 8% of all hospital discharges. Of emergency department visits, 38% are for injury treatment.

4. The lifetime medical treatment costs for injuries are estimated to be $1.1 billion for fatal injuries, $33.7 billion for injury hospitalizations, $31.8 billion for injury emergency department visits, and $13.6 billion for other outpatient visits. Lifetime productivity costs are $142 billion for injury deaths, $58.7 billion for injury hospitalizations, and $125.3 billion for nonhospitalized injuries (adjusted for current dollars).

5. The elderly (65 years and older) have the highest risk for fatal or nonfatal injuries requiring hospitalization. The incidence of injuries that result in

death is 120 in 100,000 for patients age 65 years and older and 169 in 100,000 for patients age 75 years and older.

6. Fatal injuries

a. Major mechanisms of injury for traumatic injury and deaths in 2004 are listed in **Table 1**.

b. The leading causes of traumatic death are central nervous system injuries (40% to 50%) and hemorrhage (30% to 35%).

c. Nonaccidental deaths represent 31% of traumatic deaths; of these, 63% are suicides and 37% are homicides.

7. Nonfatal injuries

a. The leading cause of nonfatal injuries is falls (representing 39% of hospitalizations).

b. Injuries to the extremities is the most common reason for hospitalization (47%) and emergency department visits after nonfatal trauma. Approximately 33% of extremity injuries that require hospitalization have an Abbreviated Injury Scale (AIS) score of 3 or higher. They are moderately severe to severe injuries that may have a long recovery period and can result in permanent impairment.

Dr. Wolinsky or an immediate family member is a member of a speakers' bureau or has made paid presentations on behalf of Zimmer; serves as a paid consultant to or is an employee of Biomet and Zimmer; serves as a board member, owner, officer, or committee member of the Orthopaedic Trauma Association, the American Academy of Orthopaedic Surgeons, and the American Orthopaedic Association. Neither Dr. Min nor any immediate family member has received anything of value from or has stock or stock options held in a commercial company or institution related directly or indirectly to the subject of this chapter.

Table 1

Mechanisms of Injury in Accidental Deaths

Mechanism of Injury[a]	Percentage of Deaths
Motor vehicle accidents	34%
Gunshot wound poisonings	25%
All other	18%
Falls	18%
Suffocation	5%

[a]Data are from 2007.

3: Trauma

II. Mortality and the Golden Hour

A. Three peak times of death after trauma

1. About 50% occur within minutes, from a neurologic injury or massive hemorrhage.

2. Another 30% occur within the first few days after injury, most commonly from a neurologic injury.

3. The final 20% occur days to weeks after injury as a result of infection and/or multiple organ failure.

B. The Golden Hour

1. Defined as the period during which life-threatening and/or limb-threatening injuries should be treated so that the treatment results in a satisfactory outcome

2. Can range from minutes for a compromised airway to hours for an open fracture

3. Approximately 60% of preventable in-hospital deaths occur during the Golden Hour.

4. Sepsis is the major cause of mortality and morbidity in trauma patients following the Golden Hour.

III. Prehospital Care and Field Triage

A. General principles

1. Rapid assessment to identify life-threatening injuries

2. Proper field triage is critical to avoid wasting resources. Only 7% to 15% of trauma patients require the resources of a level I or II trauma center.

3. Appropriate intervention to address life-threatening conditions (airway, breathing, circulation, external hemorrhage control). The goal of prehospital care is to minimize preventable deaths.

4. Rapid transport

B. Goals of field triage

1. To match a patient's needs with the resources of a particular hospital

2. To transport all seriously injured patients to an appropriate hospital

3. To determine what resources will be needed at the time of patient arrival

4. To identify whether the patient is a major trauma victim

5. To monitor the rates of overtriage and undertriage

C. Components of field triage

1. Rapid decision making based on physiologic, anatomic, mechanism of injury (to assess the amount of energy absorbed at the time of injury), and comorbidity factors

a. Physiologic criteria include assessment of vital signs such as blood pressure, heart rate, respiration rate and effort, level of consciousness, and temperature. These changes or trends may take time to realize, particularly in younger patients.

b. Anatomic criteria include observations based on physical examination, such as penetrating injuries to the head, neck, or torso; obvious fractures; burns; and amputations. These assessments can be difficult in the field, however, particularly in a patient with an altered level of consciousness.

c. Mechanisms of injury that may result in major injuries include falls of more than 15 feet; motor vehicle accidents in which a fatality has occurred, a passenger has been ejected, extrication has taken longer than 20 minutes, or a pedestrian was struck; motorcycle accidents in which the vehicle was traveling faster than 20 mph; or an obvious penetrating injury. Using the mechanism of injury alone to assess injury severity may result in a high overtriage rate, but combining it with physiologic or anatomic data improves triage.

d. Comorbidity factors include increased patient age, the presence of chronic disease, and acute issues such as drug and alcohol intoxication.

2. Numerous field triage scoring systems have been developed that use all or parts of these data.

D. Components of field assessment

1. Goals

a. Should be quick and systematic

b. Patients with potentially life-threatening injuries must be transported quickly to the closest appropriate hospital. Definitive care for internal hemorrhage cannot be provided at the scene.

2. Primary survey (ABCDE—Airway, Breathing, Circulation, Disability, Exposure)

a. Performed just as in Advanced Trauma Life Support (ATLS) to establish priorities for management

b. Treatment is initiated as problems are identified (same as ATLS).

3. Indications for field intubation

a. Glasgow Coma Scale total score less than 8 (inability to maintain an airway)

b. Need for ventilation

c. Potentially threatened airway (for example, inhalation injuries or expanding neck hematoma)

d. Ventilation is required if respiration rate is less than 10 breaths per minute.

4. External bleeding is controlled with direct pressure.

5. Initiation of intravenous fluids in the field remains controversial. In general, transport should not be delayed just to start fluids.

6. Secondary survey

a. Performed after any acute issues have been addressed, perhaps during transport

b. AMPLE history (Allergies to medications, Medications the patient is taking, Pertinent medical history, Last time eaten, Events leading to the injury)

c. Head-to-toe examination; may need to be repeated in the obtunded or unconscious patient

7. Extremity trauma

a. Bleeding associated with fractures can be life-threatening.

b. External hemorrhage is controlled with direct pressure. Using an extremity tourniquet remains controversial. Blind clamping is not to be performed.

c. Immobilization of the extremity helps control internal bleeding. Gross correction of obvious deformities also helps improve tissue perfusion and lessens further soft-tissue compromise.

d. For critical injuries, immobilization with a backboard is sufficient. Otherwise, individual fractures should be splinted or placed in traction.

e. A traction splint should be used for suspected femur fractures because it stabilizes the fracture and controls pain. It is contraindicated in patients with obvious knee injuries or deformities.

8. Amputations

a. The amputated parts are cleaned by rinsing them with lactated Ringer solution.

b. The parts are covered with sterile gauze moistened with lactated Ringer solution and placed in a plastic bag.

c. The bag is labeled and placed in another container filled with ice.

d. The part must not be allowed to freeze or be immersed directly in an aqueous medium.

e. The part is transported with the patient.

IV. Trauma Scoring Systems

A. Components of present scoring systems include physiologic data, anatomic data, a combination of the two, and specialized data.

B. Although no single scoring system has been universally adapted, each has advantages and disadvantages.

C. Types of physiologic scores

1. Acute Physiology and Chronic Health Evaluation

a. Combines preexisting systemic diseases with current physiologic issues

b. Frequently used for the evaluation of medical and surgical patients in intensive care units, but not good for patients with acute trauma

c. One drawback for trauma care is that it requires data obtained after 24 hours of hospitalization.

2. Systemic Inflammatory Response Syndrome Score

a. Scores heart and respiratory rates, temperature, and white blood cell count

b. Predicts mortality and length of hospital stay for trauma patients

D. Types of anatomic scores

1. Glasgow Coma Scale

a. Attempts to score the function (level of consciousness) of the central nervous system

b. Components (**Table 2**)

2. Abbreviated Injury Scale

a. Developed to accurately rate and compare injuries sustained in motor vehicle accidents

b. Injuries are scored from 1 (minor injuries) to 6 (fatal within 24 hours).

c. A total of 73 different injuries can be scored, but it includes no mechanism to combine the individual injury scores into one score.

3. Injury Severity Score (ISS)

a. The sum of the squares of the three highest AIS scores of six regions provides an overall severity score (includes head and neck, face, thorax, abdomen, pelvis, extremities).

b. Each region is scored on a scale from 1 (minor injury) to 6 (almost always fatal).

c. Any region with an AIS score of 6 is automatically assigned an ISS value of 75, which represents a nonsurvivable injury.

3: Trauma

Table 2			

Glasgow Coma Scale

	Parameter		
Score	Eye Opening	Verbal Response	Motor Response
6			Obeys command
5		Oriented	Localized pain
4	Spontaneous	Confused	Withdraws from pain
3	To voice	Inappropriate	Flexion to pain
2	To pain	Incomprehensible	Extension to pain
1	None	None	None

d. A score of 15 or higher frequently is used as the definition of major trauma and correlates well with mortality.

e. Because ISS scores only one injury per body region, it does not reflect patient morbidity associated with multiple lower-extremity fractures.

4. New ISS

a. This modification of the ISS sums the squares of the AIS scores of the three most substantial injuries, even if they occur in the same anatomic area.

b. Better predictor of survival than the ISS

c. One study looking at orthopaedic blunt trauma patients found the New ISS to be superior to the ISS.

E. Combined systems

1. Trauma and Injury Severity Score

a. Predicts mortality based on postinjury anatomic and physiologic abnormalities

b. Uses age, the Revised Trauma Score (calculated in the emergency department), the ISS (calculated using discharge diagnosis), and whether the injury mechanism was blunt or penetrating.

c. The data from any institution can then be compared with the mortality data from the Major Trauma Outcomes Study conducted by the American College of Surgeons in 1990.

2. Harborview Assessment for Risk of Mortality— Consists of 80 variables, including ICD-9 codes, comorbidities, mechanism of injury, self-inflicted versus accidental injury, combined injuries, and age.

V. Initial Hospital Workup and Resuscitation

A. Goals

1. Diagnosis and treatment of life-threatening injuries takes priority over a sequential, detailed, definitive workup.

2. ATLS, which provides a systematic method to evaluate trauma patients, was developed to teach this concept and ultimately improve patient survival.

B. Components of ATLS

1. Primary survey

a. A systematic effort to identify life-threatening injuries immediately

b. Treatment and resuscitation are performed simultaneously as problems are identified.

c. Consists of evaluation of ABCDEs, which may need to be repeated because patient reevaluation constantly occurs during this step

2. Secondary survey

a. Performed later as part of a head-to-toe physical examination and detailed medical history

b. Intended to diagnose and treat injuries that are not an immediate threat to life when the patient's vital signs are normalizing

c. Additional radiography, CT, and laboratory tests are performed during this phase.

C. Shock

1. Hypovolemic shock is the most common type in trauma patients.

2. Signs and symptoms

a. Decreased peripheral or central pulses; peripheral vasoconstriction is an early compensatory mechanism for shock.

Table 3

Symptoms of Hypovolemic Shock by Hemorrhage Class

Hemorrhage Class	Blood Volume Loss (%)	Blood Loss	Symptoms
I	15	750 mL	Minimal
II	15–30	750–1,500 mL	Tachycardia, tachypnea, mild mental status changes, decreased pulse pressure
III	30–40	1,500–2,000 mL	Decreased systolic blood pressure
IV	> 40	> 2 L	

b. Pale and/or cool, clammy extremities; a tachycardic patient who has cool, clammy skin is in hypovolemic shock until proven otherwise.

c. Heart rate greater than 120 to 130 beats/min in adult trauma patients should be assumed to be caused by shock.

d. Altered level of consciousness may indicate a brain injury, hypovolemic shock, or both; the key to preventing secondary brain injury is to prevent (or treat, if present) hypoxia and hypotension.

e. Relying on systolic blood pressure measurements alone can be misleading. Because of compensatory mechanisms, up to 30% of blood volume can be lost before a patient becomes hypotensive (**Table 3**).

f. Pulse pressures may decrease with loss of as little as 15% of blood volume.

g. Urine output, although useful to judge resuscitation, is not used during the primary survey.

D. Shock resuscitation

1. Initial bolus of 2 L of crystalloid that can be repeated once if vital signs are not restored to normal

2. Patients who respond well to fluid resuscitation likely had a 10% to 20% blood volume deficit. Patients who do not respond have a higher volume deficit.

3. As the second bolus is given, blood should be obtained.

E. Initial radiographic evaluation

1. Views include a chest radiograph and an AP view of the pelvis. In patients who are not awake/alert or are suspected to have cervical spine injury (neurologic deficit, pain and/or tenderness, and/or presence of distracting injury), imaging of the cervical spine is required. The lateral view of the cervical spine offers no substantial information and has been supplanted by CT imaging.

2. The AP pelvis and chest radiographs can identify

potential bleeding sources.

3. Focused Assessment for the Sonographic Evaluation of the Trauma Patient (FAST) may be needed for patients with persistent hypotension. As with radiographic evaluation, FAST is obtained quickly and can be performed in the trauma bay.

4. FAST is accurate for the detection of free intraperitoneal fluid and visualizing blood in the pericardial sac and dependent regions of the abdomen, including the right and left upper quadrants and pelvis, but it cannot detect isolated bowel injuries and does not reliably detect retroperitoneal injuries.

5. CT scan: CT is recommended for the evaluation of patients with blunt abdominal trauma, associated neurologic injury, multiple extra-abdominal injuries, and equivocal findings on physical examination. Patients undergoing CT should be hemodynamically stable.

F. Patient may require diagnostic peritoneal lavage.

VI. Associated Injuries

A. Neck injuries

1. Any patient with an injury above the clavicle who is unconscious or has a neurologic deficit is assumed to have a cervical spine injury.

2. The neck is immobilized until it has been proven that no injury exists.

B. Pelvic (retroperitoneal) versus intra-abdominal bleeding

1. These two injuries may coexist.

2. If diagnostic peritoneal lavage is performed in the presence of a pelvis fracture, it should be supraumbilical and performed early, before the pelvic hematoma can track anteriorly. Alternatively, CT can be used (provided the patient is hemodynamically stable)

3. Diagnostic peritoneal lavage has a 15%

3: Trauma

false-positive rate in this setting. False-negative results are rare.

4. Unstable pelvic fractures should be stabilized early. Pelvic binders or bed sheets are a simple, quick, and effective means to accomplish this. The binders are not to be left for more than 24 hours, because they can lead to soft-tissue compromise.

5. Hemodynamically unstable patients with minimally displaced pelvic fractures or open-book pelvic fractures that do not respond to early stabilization should be considered for angiography.

C. Head injuries

1. Autoregulation of cerebral blood flow is altered after a head injury, and blood flow may become dependent on the mean arterial blood pressure.

2. Secondary brain injury may develop if hypoperfusion or hypoxia occurs after the initial insult.

3. Whether early definitive fracture surgery has an adverse effect on neurologic outcome remains subject to debate. At least one study that used neuropsychologic testing showed that this is not the case. Maintenance of cerebral perfusion and oxygenation remain the important goals during surgery.

4. Early surgery results in more blood and fluid requirements and may require invasive monitoring to ensure that adequate cerebral blood flow is maintained during surgery.

VII. Decision to Operate: Surgical Timing

A. Early considerations

1. Before the 1970s, definitive fracture surgery was performed on a delayed basis.

2. The philosophy of early total care became accepted as it became clear that early stabilization of long bone fractures in patients with multiple trauma (ISS ≥18) reduced pulmonary complications and perhaps mortality in the most severely injured patients.

B. Current considerations

1. It is unclear which subgroups of patients might be at risk from early surgery, particularly those with femoral shaft fractures stabilized with reamed intramedullary nails.

2. Previously, the initial focus was on patients with thoracic injuries, but the current consensus is that the extent of the pulmonary injury is related to the severity of the initial injury to the thorax.

3. Although the subject is still controversial, evidence exists that patients with "occult hypoten-

sion" have higher complication rates with early definitive surgery, as do those who clearly are underresuscitated.

C. Damage control orthopaedics

1. Long bones are stabilized temporarily with external fixation and converted to definitive fixation after the patient has been resuscitated. It has been recommended that, once patients are resuscitated adequately, conversion to definitive fixation be performed within 2 weeks to minimize the risks of surgical complications (infection).

2. Complication rates with this approach are lower than those of early definitive fixation.

D. Hypothermia

1. Must be detected and corrected before definitive fracture fixation

2. Leads to increased mortality in trauma patients

3. Defined as core body temperature <35°C.

4. Hypothermic patients with an International Normalized Ratio (INR) >1.5 are substantially coagulopathic, unless proven otherwise.

5. Patients with severe head injury are at risk for hypothermia.

VIII. Determination of the Extent of Resuscitation

A. Determining which patients are in compensated shock and which have been resuscitated fully often is difficult.

B. The distinction is critical, however, because inadequate resuscitation may allow local inflammation to progress to systemic inflammation, which can cause distant organ dysfunction, including adult respiratory distress syndrome and/or multiple organ failure.

C. Patients with abnormal perfusion also may be at risk for the "second hit" phenomenon, in which a primed immune system has a supranormal response to a second insult (surgical blood loss).

D. Vital signs, including blood pressure, heart rate, and urine output, are abnormal in patients with uncompensated shock but can normalize with compensated shock.

E. Level 1 evidence shows that the base deficit or lactate level on admission is predictive of complication rates and mortality, but standard hemodynamic parameters are not.

F. Level 2 evidence shows that following the base deficit and/or lactate (time to normalization) is predictive of survival and can be used to guide resuscitation.

G. Patients at risk for complications after early definitive treatment include those with:

1. Obvious shock: systolic blood pressure of greater than 90 mm Hg

2. An abnormal base deficit or lactate level

a. Depends on not only the absolute value but also the trend

b. Normalizing is a good sign, whereas worsening or failing to improve may indicate ongoing bleeding.

Top Testing Facts

1. A major trauma patient is an individual who has potentially life-threatening and/or limb-threatening injuries and requires hospitalization.

2. The goal of prehospital care is to minimize preventable deaths.

3. Field triage requires rapid decisions based on physiologic, anatomic, mechanism of injury, and comorbidity factors.

4. The rapid assessment and primary survey are systematic approaches to quickly identify life-threatening injuries.

5. During the initial treatment of a trauma patient, the diagnosis and treatment of critical injuries takes priority over a sequential, detailed, definitive workup.

6. The most common source of shock in a trauma patient is hypovolemic shock.

7. Resuscitation for shock begins with a bolus of 2 L of crystalloid that can be repeated once if the vital signs are not restored to normal.

8. Initial radiographic evaluation includes chest and AP pelvic views. In patients who are not awake/alert or are suspected to have cervical spine injury, imaging of the cervical spine is required. The lateral view of the cervical spine offers no substantial information and has been supplanted by CT.

9. It is difficult to determine which patients are in compensated shock and which patients have been resuscitated fully.

10. The base deficit or lactate level on admission is predictive of complication rates and mortality.

Bibliography

Balogh ZJ, Varga E, Tomka J, Süveges G, Tóth L, Simonka JA: The new injury severity score is a better predictor of extended hospitalization and intensive care unit admission than the injury severity score in patients with multiple orthopaedic injuries. *J Orthop Trauma* 2003;17(7):508-512.

Bergen G, Chen LH, Warner M, Fingerhut LA: *Injury in the United States: 2007 Chartbook.* Hyattsville, MD, National Center for Health Statistics, 2008.

Como JJ, Diaz JJ, Dunham CM, et al: Practice management guidelines for identification of cervical spine injuries following trauma: Update from the eastern association for the surgery of trauma practice management guidelines committee. *J Trauma* 2009;67(3):651-659.

Crowl AC, Young JS, Kahler DM, Claridge JA, Chrzanowski DS, Pomphrey M: Occult hypoperfusion is associated with increased morbidity in patients undergoing early femur fracture fixation. *J Trauma* 2000;48(2):260-267.

Englehart MS, Schreiber MA: Measurement of acid-base resuscitation endpoints: Lactate, base deficit, bicarbonate or what? *Curr Opin Crit Care* 2006;12(6):569-574.

Harwood PJ, Giannoudis PV, Probst C, Krettek C, Pape HC: The risk of local infective complications after damage control procedures for femoral shaft fracture. *J Orthop Trauma* 2006;20(3):181-189.

Harwood PJ, Giannoudis PV, van Griensven M, Krettek C, Pape HC: Alterations in the systemic inflammatory response after early total care and damage control procedures for femoral shaft fracture in severely injured patients. *J Trauma* 2005;58(3):446-454.

Lawson CM, Alexander AM, Daley BJ, Enderson BL: Evolution of a Level I Trauma System: Changes in injury mechanism and its impact in the delivery of care. *Int J Burns Trauma* 2011;1(1):56-61.

McKee MD, Schemitsch EH, Vincent LO, Sullivan I, Yoo D: The effect of a femoral fracture on concomitant closed head injury in patients with multiple injuries. *J Trauma* 1997; 42(6):1041-1045.

Moore E, Feliciano DV, Mattox KL, eds: *Trauma,* ed 5. New York, NY, McGraw-Hill, 2004.

3: Trauma

Moore FA, McKinley BA, Moore EE, et al: Inflammation and the Host Response to Injury, a large-scale collaborative project: Patient-oriented research core—standard operating procedures for clinical care. III: Guidelines for shock resuscitation. *J Trauma* 2006;61(1):82-89.

Nowotarski PJ, Turen CH, Brumback RJ, Scarboro JM: Conversion of external fixation to intramedullary nailing for fractures of the shaft of the femur in multiply injured patients. *J Bone Joint Surg Am* 2000;82(6):781-788.

Osler T, Baker SP, Long W: A modification of the injury severity score that both improves accuracy and simplifies scoring. *J Trauma* 1997;43(6):922-926.

Pape HC, Hildebrand F, Pertschy S, et al: Changes in the management of femoral shaft fractures in polytrauma patients: From early total care to damage control orthopedic surgery. *J Trauma* 2002;53(3):452-462.

Poole GV, Tinsley M, Tsao AK, Thomae KR, Martin RW, Hauser CJ: Abbreviated Injury Scale does not reflect the added morbidity of multiple lower extremity fractures. *J Trauma* 1996;40(6):951-955.

Schulman AM, Claridge JA, Carr G, Diesen DL, Young JS: Predictors of patients who will develop prolonged occult hypoperfusion following blunt trauma. *J Trauma* 2004;57(4):795-800.

Shafi S, Elliott AC, Gentilello L: Is hypothermia simply a marker of shock and injury severity or an independent risk factor for mortality in trauma patients? Analysis of a large national trauma registry. *J Trauma* 2005;59(5):1081-1085.

Tisherman SA, Barie P, Bokhari F, et al: Clinical practice guideline: Endpoints of resuscitation. *J Trauma* 2004;57(4):898-912.

Tuttle MS, Smith WR, Williams AE, et al: Safety and efficacy of damage control external fixation versus early definitive stabilization for femoral shaft fractures in the multiple-injured patient. *J Trauma* 2009;67(3):602-605.

Wafaisade A, Lefering R, Bouillon B, et al: Epidemiology and risk factors of sepsis after multiple trauma: An analysis of 29,829 patients from the Trauma Registry of the German Society for Trauma Surgery. *Crit Care Med* 2011;39(4):621-628.

Woodford MR, Mackenzie CF, DuBose J, et al: Continuously recorded oxygen saturation and heart rate during prehospital transport outperform initial measurement in prediction of mortality after trauma. *J Trauma Acute Care Surg* 2012;72(4):1006-1011.

Chapter 26
Gunshot Wounds and Open Fractures

John T. Riehl, MD   George J. Haidukewych, MD   Kenneth J. Koval, MD

I. Gunshot Wounds

A. Epidemiology

1. Firearm-related deaths in the United States totaled 31,224 in 2007.

2. Levy et al reported that 56% of patients with gunshot wounds (GSWs) had positive alcohol and/or drug screens; 24% tested positive for two or more drugs.

3. Hakanson et al found that 68% of these patients were substance abusers, 56% were unemployed, and 79% were uninsured.

4. The extremities are the most common location for a nonfatal GSW.

B. Ballistics

1. Velocity is only one of several factors that determine the extent of damage caused by a bullet. Other factors include the shape, weight, diameter, jacketing, and tumbling characteristics of the bullet, as well as characteristics of the target.

2. Low-velocity bullets are defined as those traveling <2,000 ft/s (for example, from handguns).

3. High-velocity bullets are defined as those traveling >2,000 ft/s (for example, from M16 military rifles, most hunting rifles).

4. Shotguns deliver ammunition at a low velocity (1,000 to 14,000 ft/s) but can cause a high degree of destruction at close range.

5. Shotgun blasts can inflict either high-energy injuries or low-energy injuries.

6. Damage caused by shotgun blasts is determined by three factors: distance from the target, load (mass of the individual pellets), and chote (shot pattern).

7. When a bullet strikes tissue, the following three things occur:

   a. Mechanical crushing of tissue, forming the permanent cavity

   b. Elastic stretching of the tissue at the periphery of the permanent cavity by the dissipation of imparted kinetic energy, causing a temporary cavity

   c. A shock wave, which may cause tissue damage at a distance from the immediate bullet contact area

8. With higher velocity injuries, the temporary cavity is larger and fills with water vapor at a low atmospheric pressure, causing a momentary vacuum to form, which may attract contaminating foreign material.

C. Energy

1. Energy imparted to human tissue by a bullet depends on three factors:

   a. The striking energy (the energy of the bullet on impact)

   b. The energy of the bullet on exiting the tissue (exit energy)

   c. The behavior of the bullet while within the target; eg, mushrooming, tumbling, fragmentation. Tumbling causes a greater amount of tissue displacement, than do other behaviors, and

Dr. Haidukewych or an immediate family member has received royalties from DePuy; serves as a paid consultant to or is an employee of Smith & Nephew and Synthes; has stock or stock options held in OrthoPediatrics and the Institute for Better Bone Health; and serves as a board member, owner, officer, or committee member of the American Academy of Orthopaedic Surgeons. Dr. Koval or an immediate family member has received royalties from Biomet; is a member of a speakers' bureau or has made paid presentations on behalf of Biomet and Stryker; serves as a paid consultant to or is an employee of Biomet; and serves as a board member, owner, officer, or committee member of the American Academy of Orthopaedic Surgeons and the Orthopaedic Trauma Society. Neither Dr. Riehl nor any immediate family member has received anything of value from or has stock or stock options held in a commercial company or institution related directly or indirectly to the subject of this chapter.

3:Trauma

more of the kinetic energy of the bullet is imparted to the tissue.

2. The kinetic energy (KE) of a bullet is proportional to its mass (m) and its velocity squared (v^2). This is represented by the equation $KE = \frac{1}{2}(mv^2)$. An M16 and a 0.22-caliber handgun fire a round of approximately the same size; however, the velocity of the M16 bullet is three times greater, thereby generating almost 10 times the kinetic energy.

D. Bullet entrance and exit

1. Secondary missiles can be created when a bullet contacts a dense object, such as a belt buckle or button, or tissue, such as bone or teeth. Secondary missiles may cause significant damage and additional permanent cavities.

2. An abrasion ring is produced at the entrance wound when the skin is damaged by clothing scraping the skin as the bullet penetrates it. The ring is stellate in the palm and sole.

3. Four categories of entrance wounds exist:

   a. Contact—The muzzle of the gun is against the target at the time the gun is fired, causing blackened, seared margins.

   b. Near-contact—The muzzle is a short distance away, causing powder soot deposit.

   c. Intermediate—Gunpowder tattooing is present.

   d. Distant—The muzzle is distant from the target.

4. Exit wounds are typically larger than entrance wounds, with a more irregular shape. When no exit wound is present, all of the kinetic energy of the bullet has been dissipated into the tissue.

E. Tissue parameters

1. The specific gravity of the tissue traversed by a bullet will have an effect on the degree of injury created. The higher the specific gravity, the greater the tissue damage.

2. The extent of injury to the tissue is related to the dissipation of kinetic energy for the crush or stretch of tissue, the production of secondary missiles, and cavitation.

3. Retained intra-articular bullet fragments can result in lead toxicity secondary to synovial fluid breakdown of the lead component of the bullet and absorption into the bloodstream.

4. Bullets are not sterilized by firing, and they introduce additional contaminants from clothing, the skin, and the bowel as they pass into sterile tissues.

F. Clinical evaluation

1. Initial assessment begins with Advanced Trauma Life Support (ATLS) protocols.

2. A thorough history should be obtained, including the type of firearm, its distance from the target, and the direction.

3. All clothing should be removed, and the skin should be examined for entrance and exit wounds.

4. Extremities should be evaluated for swelling, deformity, ecchymosis, and crepitus.

5. A thorough neurovascular examination should be performed on the injured extremity. Nerve injury can occur at a site remote from the immediate path of the bullet.

6. Biplanar radiographs of the injured limb should be obtained, including the joints above and below the injury.

7. A gunshot wound near a major joint should raise strong suspicion of penetration into that joint.

G. Treatment

1. Treatment depends on wound size, contamination, and the amount of devitalized tissue.

2. Tetanus immunization status should be updated if necessary. Antibiotics are administered in the emergency department.

3. Low-velocity wounds

   a. Outpatient treatment can be considered for stable fractures that exhibit minimal soft-tissue injury and are without neurovascular compromise. Superficial wound cleansing and skin-edge débridement can be performed in the emergency department. Upon discharge, patients are placed on oral antibiotics (for example, first-generation cephalosporin) for 7 to 10 days.

   b. Indications for surgical treatment include retained bullet fragments in the subarachnoid or joint space; vascular injury; gross contamination; a prominent missile in the palm or sole; and severe tissue damage, including compartment syndrome and an unstable fracture requiring fixation.

4. High-velocity wounds

   a. Surgical débridement—Evaluate muscle tissue for color, consistency, contractility, and capacity to bleed.

   b. Stabilization of fracture (**Figure 1**)

   c. Delayed wound closure, graft/flap planning as necessary

5. A GSW that passes through the abdomen requires débridement of the intra-abdominal and extra-

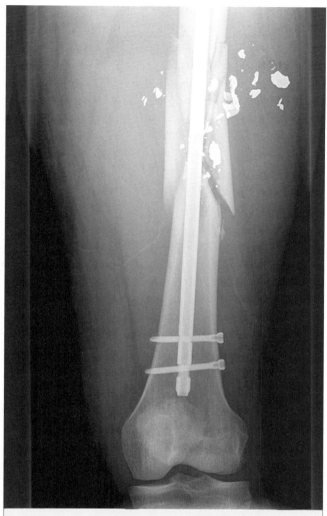

Figure 1 AP radiograph shows intramedullary nailing of a gunshot femoral shaft fracture. (Reproduced from Dougherty PJ, Najibi S: Gunshot fractures of the femoral shaft, in Dougherty PF, ed: *Gunshot Wounds*. Rosemont, IL, American Academy of Orthopaedic Surgeons, 2011, p 109.)

abdominal missile paths. Broad-spectrum antibiotics with coverage of gram-negative and anaerobic pathogens should be administered.

H. Complications

1. Infection—Occurs in 1.5% to 5% of patients; severity of injury is a contributing factor, and antibiotics help prevent infection after GSW.

2. Foreign bodies

   a. Historically, retained missile fragments have been presumed to be well tolerated.

   b. If symptoms develop late or with superficial or intra-articular location, surgical intervention is indicated.

c. Clothing may be drawn into the wound at the time of injury and should be removed if present.

d. In close-range shotgun injuries (< 4 ft), shotgun wadding may be present within the wound.

3. Neurovascular damage

   a. Greater in high-velocity injuries

   b. Temporary cavitation may result in traction or avulsion injuries to neurovascular structures outside the immediate path of the missile.

4. Lead toxicity

   a. Synovial or cerebrospinal fluid is caustic to lead components of bullet missiles, resulting in lead breakdown products that may produce severe synovitis and low-grade lead poisoning.

   b. Lead also may be introduced into the bloodstream through phagocytosis by macrophages. Rarely, this mechanism leads to lead toxicity.

II. Open Fractures

A. Definition—An open fracture is a soft-tissue injury that includes a fracture. Communication is present between the fracture site and an overlying break in the skin (**Figure 2**).

B. Clinical evaluation

1. Initial assessment begins with an evaluation of airway, breathing, circulation, disability, and exposure (ABCDE).

   a. Roughly one third of patients with open fractures have associated injuries; therefore, life-threatening injuries must be assessed, and treatment must begin immediately. The treating physician must take care not to allow the presence of an open fracture to distract from associated injuries to the head, chest, abdomen, pelvis, and spine.

   b. All four extremities must be assessed for injury and, when possible, a detailed neurovascular examination must be undertaken. A complete soft-tissue assessment, palpation for tenderness, and observation of any deformity also are included in the initial evaluation.

2. Emergency department care

   a. Tetanus prophylaxis should be given when appropriate (**Table 1**), and antibiotic treatment should begin immediately.

   b. Bleeding should be controlled by direct pressure rather than by limb tourniquets or blind clamping.

3: Trauma

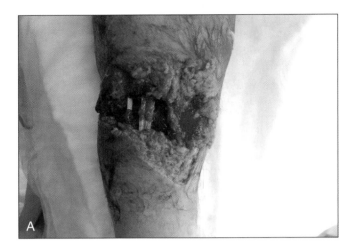

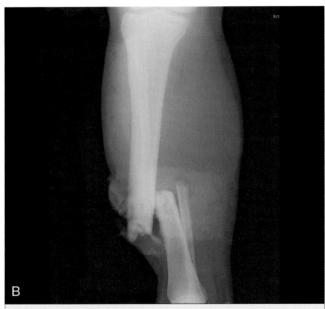

Figure 2 Clinical photograph (**A**) and AP radiograph (**B**) of a Gustilo grade IIIB open tibial shaft fracture.

Table 1

Requirements for Tetanus Prophylaxis

Immunization History	For clean, minor wound		For all other wounds	
	dT	TIG	dT	TIG
Incomplete (< 3 doses) or not known	+	-	+	+
Complete but > 10 years since last dose	+	-	+	-
Complete and < 10 years since last dose	-	-	-*	-

dT = diphtheria and tetanus toxoids; TIG = tetanus immune globulin; + = prophylaxis required; – = prophylaxis not required

* = required if > 5 years since last dose

the joints above and below. These radiographs should be obtained as soon as possible to allow preoperative planning to begin.

2. CT is ordered as clinically indicated. In cases of periarticular fractures when temporary spanning external fixation is planned, CT often is best delayed until after the joint has been spanned so as to provide the most information possible.

3. Angiography is obtained based on the clinical suspicion of vascular injury, the type of injury, and the following indications:

   a. Knee dislocation (or equivalent; for example, medial tibial plateau fracture) with asymmetric pulses

   b. A cool, pale foot with poor distal capillary refill

   c. High-energy injury in an area of compromise (eg, trifurcation of the popliteal artery)

   d. Any lower extremity injury with documented ankle brachial index < 0.9

D. Classification of open fractures—The Gustilo classification (**Table 2**) requires that surgical débridement be performed before assigning a grade. All factors are considered in assigning the grade, but typically the highest possible grade should be assigned based on each factor.

E. Nonsurgical treatment

1. Tetanus prophylaxis (**Table 1**)

   a. The dose of toxoid is 0.5 mL.

   b. The dose for immune globulin is 75 U for patients younger than 5 years, 125 U for patients aged between 5 and 10 years, and 250 U for patients older than 10 years.

   c. Both shots are administered intramuscularly, into different sites and from different syringes.

c. Manual exploration of the wound in the emergency department is not indicated if formal surgical intervention is planned. Exploration in the emergency department risks further contamination and hemorrhage as well as neurovascular injury.

d. The open wound can be covered with saline-moistened gauze, and the extremity can be splinted.

3. Compartment syndrome must be considered a possibility in all extremity fractures.

C. Radiographic evaluation

1. In any case of suspected open fracture, AP and lateral radiographs of the affected area should be obtained, in addition to radiographs that include

Table 2

Gustilo Classification of Open Fractures

Grade	Description
I	Wound <1 cm in length. Minimal contamination and soft-tissue damage. Usually an inside-to-outside injury.
II	Wound, between 1 cm and 10 cm in length. Soft-tissue injury and crushing are moderate; comminution is minimal.
III	Severe soft-tissue injury, contamination, and crushing. High-energy injury with comminution. Wound size may be >10 cm.
IIIA	Grade III fracture with adequate soft-tissue coverage after débridement; rotational or free flap coverage not needed.
IIIB	Any open fracture requiring soft-tissue flap coverage.
IIIC	Any open fracture with a vascular injury requiring repair.

2. Antibiotic coverage

 a. A Cochrane systematic review showed that in cases of open fracture, the administration of antibiotics reduces the risk of infection by 59%.

 b. Antibiotics should be given as soon as possible, preferably within 3 hours of the injury.

 c. In open fractures, gram-negative rods and gram-positive staphylococci are the most common infecting organisms.

 d. Data are lacking to indicate the optimal antibiotic treatment and duration of treatment for open fracture.

 e. Antibiotic therapy should be directed against both gram-positive and gram-negative organisms. First-generation cephalosporin (gram-positive) and an aminoglycoside (gram-negative) will provide the desired coverage in most cases. Clindamycin is an effective alternative to a first-generation cephalosporin.

 f. Some authors have recommended monotherapy with a first-generation cephalosporin for grade I and II open fractures, adding an aminoglycoside only in grade III fractures.

 g. When anaerobic infection is a significant risk (eg, vascular injury, farm injury), ampicillin or penicillin should be added to the antibiotic regimen.

 h. Antibiotic therapy is recommended to continue for 24 to 72 hours following each débridement.

 i. Local antibiotic therapy (in the form of polymethyl methacrylate beads) is a useful adjunct to systemic antibiotic therapy in the treatment of open fracture.

F. Surgical timing—No clear evidence exists to support the optimal timing of surgical débridement of an open fracture. When severe contamination is not present, several recent clinical studies have shown no difference in infection rate when surgical débridement occurred within 6 hours of the injury compared with treatment administered after 6 hours.

G. Surgical techniques

 1. The wound should be extended proximally and distally to expose and facilitate exploration of the zone of injury.

 2. Some authors recommend the routine use of a tourniquet to identify and remove all foreign debris and damaged tissues; others recommend avoiding tourniquet use to prevent further ischemic damage.

 3. Intraoperative culture is not indicated acutely in the case of open fracture because the organisms isolated from an initial culture typically are not the bacteria that ultimately will cause infection.

 4. Volume and method of irrigation

 a. Little has been published showing an ideal volume that should be used for open fractures. One common recommendation is 3 L for grade I open fractures, 6 L for grade II, and 9 L for grade III.

 b. Although high-pressure pulsatile lavage has been shown to be effective in removing bacteria, it may cause bone damage and deeper bacterial penetration into wounds. Clinical evidence regarding the use of high-pressure pulsatile lavage is insufficient.

 5. Contents of irrigation

 a. No consensus exists regarding the optimal irrigant solution. Recommendations include sterile normal saline, with or without additives such as antiseptics, antibiotics, or soaps. These additives function as surfactants only.

 b. In a prospective, randomized study, no significant difference was found in bone healing or infection rates when a soap solution was used compared with a bacitracin solution. Wound healing problems were more common in the bacitracin group.

 6. Fracture stabilization (**Figure 3**)

 a. Stabilization allows better patient mobility, helps prevent further damage to the surrounding soft tissues, and makes overall care of the patient more manageable.

3: Trauma

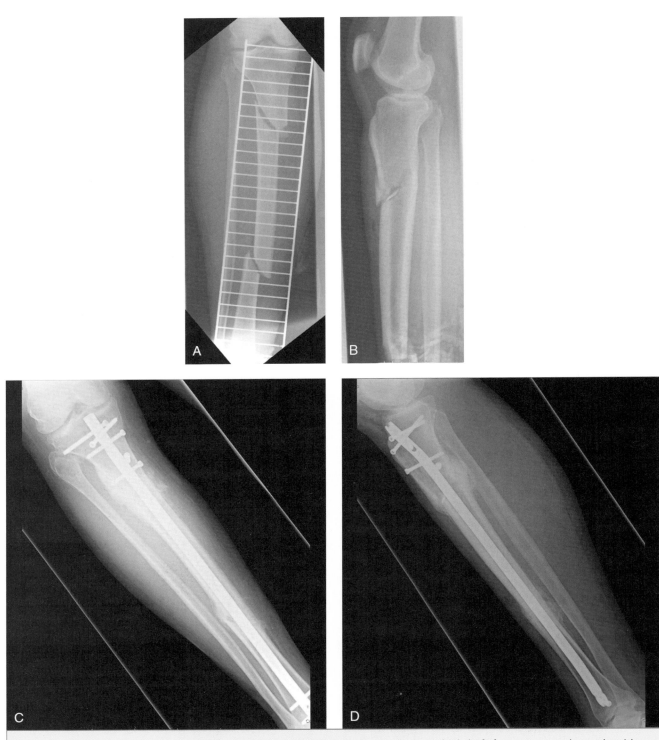

Figure 3   Preoperative AP (**A**) and lateral (**B**) radiographs show a segmental open tibial shaft fracture treated acutely with débridement and intramedullary nailing. Postoperative AP (**C**) and lateral (**D**) radiographs show the extremity at 3-month follow-up.

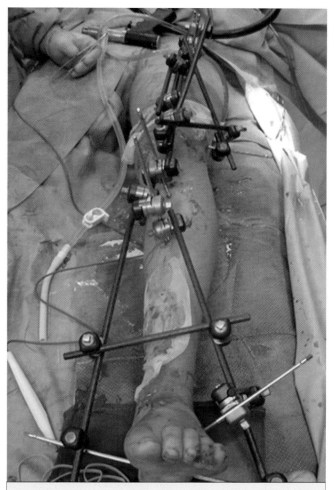

Figure 4 Clinical photograph shows external fixation of a lower extremity with multiple open fractures.

b. The type of fracture stabilization (ie, internal or external fixation) depends on fracture location and the degree of soft-tissue injury (**Figure 4**).

7. Soft-tissue coverage

a. Planning for soft-tissue closure should begin at the time of initial débridement.

b. Options for wound coverage before definitive closure include negative-pressure wound therapy, antibiotic bead pouches, and wet-to-dry dressings.

c. Immediate closure is permissible when the surgeon has determined that adequate débridement has been performed, a tension-free closure can be obtained, no farmyard or fecal contamination is present, and vascularity to the affected area is good.

d. When flap coverage is required, lower rates of infection have been reported when coverage is provided within 72 hours of injury (1.5%) versus between 72 hours and 3 months (17.5%).

8. Bone grafting/adjuncts

a. These procedures are performed when the wound is clean, closed, and dry.

b. In high-grade open tibia fractures, prophylactic bone grafting may decrease time to union.

c. Timing is controversial. Some authors advocate grafting at the time of definitive coverage; others advocate waiting a period (typically 6 weeks) after definitive closure.

d. The incidence of secondary intervention for open tibial fractures is diminished after recombinant human bone morphogenetic protein-2 (rhBMP-2) is used.

H. Limb salvage versus amputation

1. Indications for immediate or early amputation:

a. Nonviable limb, irreparable vascular injury, warm ischemia time > 8 hours, or a severe crush injury with minimal remaining viable tissue

b. Anticipated function following limb salvage will be less than that expected after amputation and prosthetic application.

c. The patient has medical comorbidities such that limb salvage will constitute a threat to the patient's life (for example, severe crush injury in a patient with chronic kidney disease).

d. The patient has sustained severe multiple trauma such that limb salvage may be life threatening. Attempted salvage of a marginal extremity may result in a high metabolic cost or a large necrotic/inflammatory load that could precipitate pulmonary or multiple organ failure.

e. Limb salvage is incompatible with the personal, sociologic, and economic consequences the patient is willing to withstand due to the demand of multiple surgical procedures and prolonged reconstruction time.

2. The indications for limb salvage versus amputation are controversial.

I. Outcomes

1. Infection risk following open fractures depends on the severity of the injury (**Table 2**).

2. The number of medical and immunocompromising comorbidities (for example, age older than 80 years, nicotine use, diabetes mellitus, malignant disease, pulmonary insufficiency, systemic immunodeficiency) has been shown to be a significant predictor of infection in open fractures of the long bones. Class A (no comorbidities) = 4%; class B (one or two comorbidities) = 15%; and class C (three or more comorbidities) = 31%.

3:Trauma

Top Testing Facts

Gunshot Wounds

1. Missile velocity is arbitrarily categorized into two groups: low-velocity (<2,000 ft/s) and high-velocity (>2,000 ft/s).

2. Shotgun blasts can inflict either high-energy injuries or low-energy injuries.

3. The permanent cavity is caused by mechanical crushing of soft tissues. The temporary cavity results from tissue that has been elastically stretched. The shock wave can cause tissue damage at a site distant from the path of the bullet.

4. Nerve injury can occur at a site remote from the immediate path of the bullet.

5. The energy imparted to human tissue by a bullet depends on the energy of the bullet on impact, the energy upon exit, and the behavior of the bullet while within the target.

6. Outpatient treatment may be appropriate in certain low-velocity GSWs.

7. A GSW that passes through the abdomen requires débridement of the entire missile path.

Open Fractures

1. One third of patients with open fractures will have associated injuries.

2. Antibiotics should be given as soon as possible in the treatment of open fractures.

3. Scientific evidence is lacking for the optimal timing of surgical débridement, antibiotic treatment and its duration, and irrigant solution for open fractures.

4. In open fractures, fracture stabilization provides protection from further soft-tissue injury.

5. For Gustilo grade III fractures, the indications for limb salvage versus amputation are controversial.

6. The number of medical comorbidities is a significant predictor of infection in patients with open fractures.

Bibliography

Anglen JO: Comparison of soap and antibiotic solutions for irrigation of lower-limb open fracture wounds: A prospective, randomized study. *J Bone Joint Surg Am* 2005;87(7): 1415-1422.

Artz CP, Sako Y, Scully RE: An evaluation of the surgeon's criteria for determining the viability of muscle during débridement. *AMA Arch Surg* 1956;73(6):1031-1035.

Bhandari M, Schemitsch EH, Adili A, Lachowski RJ, Shaughnessy SG: High and low pressure pulsatile lavage of contaminated tibial fractures: an in vitro study of bacterial adherence and bone damage. *J Orthop Trauma* 1999;13(8):526-533.

Blick SS, Brumback RJ, Lakatos R, Poka A, Burgess AR: Early prophylactic bone grafting of high-energy tibial fractures. *Clin Orthop Relat Res* 1989;240:21-41.

Bowen TR, Widmaier JC: Host classification predicts infection after open fracture. *Clin Orthop Relat Res* 2005;433: 205-211.

Boyd JI III, Wongworawat MD: High-pressure pulsatile lavage causes soft tissue damage. *Clin Orthop Relat Res* 2004; 427:13-17.

Dicpinigaitis PA, Fay R, Egol KA, Wolinsky P, Tejwani N, Koval KJ: Gunshot wounds to the lower extremities. *Am J Orthop (Belle Mead NJ)* 2002;31(5):282-293.

Dougherty PJ, Vaidya R, Silverton CD, Bartlett CS III, Najibi S: Joint and long-bone gunshot injuries. *Instr Course Lect* 2010;59:465-479.

Godina M: Early microsurgical reconstruction of complex trauma of the extremities. *Plast Reconstr Surg* 1986;78(3): 285-292.

Gosselin RA, Roberts I, Gillespie WJ: Antibiotics for preventing infection in open limb fractures. *Cochrane Database Syst Rev* 2004;1:CD003764.

Govender S, Csimma C, Genant HK, et al: Recombinant human bone morphogenetic protein-2 for treatment of open tibial fractures: A prospective, controlled, randomized study of four hundred and fifty patients. *J Bone Joint Surg Am* 2002; 84(12):2123-2134.

Gustilo RB, Anderson JT: Prevention of infection in the treatment of one thousand and twenty-five open fractures of long bones: Retrospective and prospective analyses. *J Bone Joint Surg Am* 1976;58(4):453-458.

Gustilo RB, Mendoza RM, Williams DN: Problems in the management of type III (severe) open fractures: A new classification of type III open fractures. *J Trauma* 1984;24(8): 742-746.

Hakanson R, Nussman D, Gorman RA, Kellam JF, Hanley EN Jr: Gunshot fractures: A medical, social, and economic analysis. *Orthopedics* 1994;17(6):519-523.

Leonard MH: The solution of lead by synovial fluid. *Clin Orthop Relat Res* 1969;64:255-261.

Levy RS, Hebert CK, Munn BG, Barrack RL: Drug and alcohol use in orthopedic trauma patients: A prospective study. *J Orthop Trauma* 1996;10(1):21-27.

National Center for Injury Prevention & Control: Centers for Disease Control & Prevention: Web-Based Injury Statistics Query & Reporting System (WISQARS) Injury Mortality Reports, 1999-2007. Available at: http://www.cdc.gov/injury/wisqars/index.html. Accessed October 5, 2013.

Oberli H, Frick T: The open femoral fracture in war—173 external fixators applied to the femur (Afghanistan war). *Helv Chir Acta* 1992;58(5):687-692.

Patzakis MJ, Harvey JP Jr, Ivler D: The role of antibiotics in the management of open fractures. *J Bone Joint Surg Am* 1974;56(3):532-541.

Patzakis MJ, Wilkins J: Factors influencing infection rate in open fracture wounds. *Clin Orthop Relat Res* 1989;243:36-40.

Rajasekaran S: Early versus delayed closure of open fractures. *Injury* 2007;38(8):890-895.

Swan KG, Swan RC: *Gunshot Wounds: Pathophysiology and Management*. Chicago, IL, Year Book Medical Publishers, 1989.

Trabulsy PP, Kerley SM, Hoffman WY: A prospective study of early soft tissue coverage of grade IIIB tibial fractures. *J Trauma* 1994;36(5):661-668.

Wang ZG, Feng JX, Liu YQ: Pathomorphological observations of gunshot wounds. *Acta Chir Scand Suppl* 1982;508:185-195.

Woloszyn JT, Uitvlugt GM, Castle ME: Management of civilian gunshot fractures of the extremities. *Clin Orthop Relat Res* 1988;226:247-251.

3: Trauma

Chapter 27

Nonunions, Malunions, and Osteomyelitis

David W. Lowenberg, MD

I. Nonunions

A. Definitions

1. Delayed union—Delayed union has been defined as a fracture that is showing slower progression toward healing than would normally be expected but in which pregression toward union remains possible.

2. Nonunion—Nonunion is an end result of a delayed union in which all reparative processes have ceased without bony union occurring. Once a fracture has lost the potential to progress with healing, it is a nonunion.

3. Fractures with large segmental defects—These fractures are functionally nonunions from the time of injury and should be treated as such.

B. Etiology

1. Common factors—Often, the cause of nonunions is multifactorial; however, a host of common denominators usually contribute to the development of a nonunion (**Table 1**). Of all potential causes, inadequate fracture stabilization and lack of adequate blood supply are the most common.

2. Infection—Infection alone does not preclude fracture healing; however, it can contribute to the failure of a fracture to progress to union. Even if the fracture does heal, the osteomyelitis must be treated. Hence, eradicating infection should be a concomitant goal with achieving bony union.

3. Fracture location—Location of the fracture can be an important contributing factor, because certain areas of the skeleton (eg, carpal, navicular, femoral neck, proximal diaphysis of the fifth metatarsal) are more prone to the development of nonunion.

4. Fracture pattern—Fracture pattern can influence the development of nonunion, especially when the fracture occurs in the diaphysis of a long bone. Segmental fractures and fractures with large butterfly fragments are more prone to nonunion, probably because of devascularization of the intermediary segment.

C. Evaluation

1. History

a. The mechanism of injury (**Table 2**), prior surgical and nonsurgical interventions, host quality (ie, underlying metabolic, nutritional, or immunologic disease), and NSAID or tobacco use are vital factors in determining the proper treatment of the patient.

b. Additional important factors are pain at the fracture site with axial loading of the involved

---

Table 1

Causes of Nonunion

Excess motion: Caused by inadequate immobilization

Gap between fragments
    Soft-tissue interposition
    Distraction by traction or hardware
    Malposition, overriding, or displacement of fragments
    Loss of bone substance

Loss of blood supply
    Damage to nutrient vessels
    Excessive stripping or injury to periosteum and muscle
    Free fragments, severe comminution
    Avascularity due to hardware

Possible infection
    Bone death (sequestrum)
    Osteolysis (gap)
    Loosening of implants (motion)

General: Age, nutrition, steroids, anticoagulants, radiation, burns, etc predispose to but do not cause nonunion.

Adapted with permission from Rosen H: Treatment of nonunions: General principles, in Chapman MW, ed: *Operative Orthopaedics*. Philadelphia, PA, JB Lippincott, 1988, p 491.

Dr. Lowenberg or an immediate family member is a member of a speakers' bureau or has made paid presentations on behalf of Stryker and serves as a paid consultant to or is an employee of Stryker and Ellipse Technologies.

3:Trauma

Table 2	
Forces Involved in Four Common Mechanisms of Injury[a]	
Fall off curb	100 ft-lb
Skiing (20 mph)	300-500 ft-lb
Gunshot wound	2,000 ft-lb
Bumper injury (20 mph)	100,000 ft-lb

[a]Based on the equation $E = 1/2mv^2$

Adapted with permission from Chapman M, Yaremchuk MJ, et al: Acute and definitive management of traumatic and osteocutaneous defects of the lower extremity. *Plast Reconstr Surg* 1987;80:1.

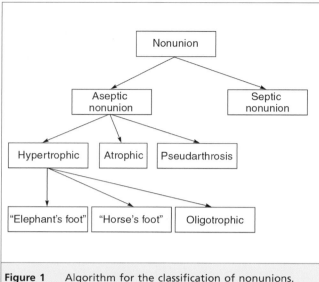

Figure 1   Algorithm for the classification of nonunions.

extremity and motion at the fracture site perceived by the patient.

2. Physical examination

   a. The examination should include a detailed evaluation of distal pulses and patency of vessels as well as motor and sensory function in the limb.

   b. Actual mobility of the nonunion, or lack thereof, is another important factor in determining treatment.

   c. The limb should be evaluated for deformity, including rotational deformity and any resultant limb-length discrepancy, because this might affect treatment decisions.

   d. All nonunions should be evaluated for signs of infection and the status of the soft-tissue envelope.

3. Imaging studies

   a. High-quality radiographs are the gold standard in evaluating fracture healing. To assess for a nonunion, four views of the affected limb segment are the first essential study.

   b. If these radiographs fail to clearly determine union, then CT with reformations and reconstruction can be quite helpful. The value of CT can be diminished, however, if significant hardware is present at the fracture site.

   c. If limb-length discrepancy or deformity of the lower extremity is a potential issue, a 51-in, full-length, weight-bearing view of both lower extremities is required.

   d. Bone scanning can be helpful; however, it is rarely used as a sole determinant of whether a nonunion exists.

4. Laboratory studies—If deep infection or chronic osteomyelitis is suspected, then screening laboratory studies (complete blood cell count [CBC],

erythrocyte sedimentation rate [ESR], and C-reactive protein [CRP] level) are warranted.

D. Classification—An algorithm for the basic classification of nonunions is provided in **Figure 1**. The subclassification of hypertrophic nonunions was originally described by Weber and Cech. The "elephant's foot" type of hypertrophic nonunion describes the radiographic appearance attributed to a vast widening of the bone ends on both sides of the nonunion as a result of hypertrophic callus. The "horse's foot" type describes slight widening of the bone ends at the nonunion site as a result of only modest callus formation at the nonunion site. The oligotrophic type has no callus present and often has the appearance of an atrophic nonunion, the primary difference being a paucity of motion at an oligotrophic nonunion (implying some healing has occurred) versus significant motion at the atrophic nonunion (indicating complete lack of a healing response).

E. General treatment issues—Nonsurgical treatment is a viable option in a small percentage of patients because some nonunions can be asymptomatic (eg, hypertrophic clavicular shaft nonunions). In some instances, however, surgical treatment can cause greater morbidity than leaving the nonunion untreated. This is occasionally true for an upper extremity nonunion in an elderly patient who has associated comorbidities and low functional demands.

F. Nonsurgical treatment

1. Fracture brace immobilization with axial loading of the limb is a viable treatment option for certain rigid/stable nonunions.

2. Bone growth stimulators (inductive or capacitive coupling devices) are an option in some patients. Published controlled clinical studies remain

scarce, however, and the use of these devices is limited to the United States. Clear contraindications to electrical stimulation include synovial pseudarthroses, mobile nonunions, and a fracture gap >1 cm.

G. Surgical treatment—The basic goal of surgery for nonunions is to create a favorable environment for fracture healing. This includes stable fixation with preservation of the blood supply to the bone and soft-tissue envelope, the minimization of shear forces, especially in nonunions with a high degree of fracture obliquity, and good bony apposition.

1. Hypertrophic nonunions

   a. The defining factor in hypertrophic nonunions is that they have viable bone ends, which are usually stiff in nature.

   b. Generally, these fractures "want to heal" and have the proper biology to heal, but they lack stable fixation.

   c. Treatment is therefore aimed at providing appropriate stabilization and is most easily achieved with internal fixation (for example, plates and screws, locked intramedullary rods).

   d. The nonunion itself usually does not need to be taken down unless this is required for proper fracture reduction to address accompanying deformity.

2. Oligotrophic nonunions

   a. Oligotrophic nonunions are generally lacking in callus. They often resemble atrophic nonunions radiographically but in fact have viable bone ends.

   b. Oligotrophic nonunions occasionally require further biologic stimulus and can behave like atrophic nonunions.

3. Atrophic nonunions

   a. The defining factor in atrophic nonunions is often the presence of avascular or hypovascular bone ends. They are usually mobile, so atrophic nonunions often are called mobile nonunions.

   b. Occasionally, oligotrophic fractures that go on to nonunion because of muscle interposition can look and behave like atrophic nonunions despite having viable bone ends.

   c. Treatment goals for atrophic nonunions

      • The apposition of well-vascularized bone ends

      • Stable fixation using hardware, be it internal or multiplanar external fixation if needed

      • Grafting to fill bony defects and provide osteoinductive agents to the local environment. Autologous iliac crest bone grafting is

the gold standard for osteoinductive agents. Recombinant bone morphogenetic proteins (rBMPs) initially appeared to represent a promising alternative, but they have not been found to be as effective as hoped, and complications from their use do exist. Other graft materials (for example, crushed cancellous allograft, demineralized allogenic bone matrix) are, for all practical purposes, osteoconductive only.

      • Preservation or creation of a healthy, well-vascularized local soft-tissue envelope. It is increasingly clear that the key to management of compromised bone and nonunions often involves a healthy soft-tissue envelope.

4. Pseudarthrosis

   a. A pseudarthrosis, which is in effect a "false joint," is often present if infection exists. The bone ends are atrophic with impaired vasculature.

   b. When a pseudarthrosis is exposed surgically, an actual joint capsule with enclosed synovial fluid is found.

   c. Complete surgical takedown with excision of the atrophic bone ends, followed by proper surgical stabilization with preservation of the remaining bone and soft-tissue vascularity, is required for an atrophic pseudarthrosis to heal.

5. Infected nonunions

   a. Although infection does not prevent a fracture from healing, if a fracture goes on to a nonunion and becomes infected, the chance of healing is low if the infection is not eradicated.

   b. Infected nonunions are often pseudarthroses and should be treated as such.

   c. Treatment goals for infected nonunions

      • Removal of all infected and devitalized bone and soft tissue

      • Sterilization of the local wound environment with the use of local wound management techniques (for example, antibiotic bead pouch, vacuum-assisted closure [VAC] sponge)

      • Creation of healthy, bleeding bone ends with a well-vascularized soft-tissue envelope

      • Stable fixation

   d. Achieving treatment goals most often requires a staged approach with multiple surgeries.

   e. Because the treatment often results in a substantial amount of bone loss, bone transport or later limb lengthening using the Ilizarov method often is beneficial.

f. Placement of a free muscle or fasciocutaneous flap can be crucial in managing the local soft-tissue environment if the soft-tissue envelope becomes deficient after treatment or the soft-tissue envelope is overly scarred and dysvascular.

H. Pearls and pitfalls

1. It is best to achieve as stable a fixation as possible to allow joint mobilization above and below the nonunion. The affected limb will have been through much trauma already, so the periarticular regions are prone to stiffness.

2. A healthy, well-vascularized soft-tissue envelope is necessary for the healing of tenuously vascularized diaphyseal bone ends. The generous use of free or rotational muscle transfers enhances the healing environment by providing more vascular access.

3. If union fails despite optimal treatment, metabolic or other endogenous problems that can inhibit fracture healing should be considered.

   a. NSAID use—One of the most common culprits is NSAID use. These medications can inhibit fracture healing by preventing calcification of the osteoid matrix.

   b. Tobacco use—Smoking and other tobacco use plays a role in inhibiting bone healing. An increased risk of nonunion is seen in patients who use tobacco-based products. Nicotine causes arteriolar vasoconstriction, thereby further inhibiting blood flow to bone and the already compromised area about an injury and acting as a secondary insult to the already compromised site of bone and soft-tissue injury.

4. BMPs—Currently, BMP-2 and BMP-7 are released for use. A recent review of the Cochrane Database demonstrating "the incremental effectiveness and costs of BMP on fracture healing in acute fractures and nonunions compared with standard care" was clouded by considerable industry involvement in the promotion of BMPs. Clear data supporting the efficacy of BMPs compared with conventional treatment are lacking.

II. Malunions

A. Definitions and overview

1. Malunions result from the incorrect healing and alignment of fractures.

2. Malunions can occur in fractures treated surgically or nonsurgically.

3. Malunions that occur following nonsurgical treatment (ie, cast immobilization) generally exhibit deformity in a random plane pattern, whereas fractures treated surgically more often exhibit malunion deformity in the true sagittal or coronal plane.

4. No inherent, predictable relationship exists between angulation and translation. The translation that occurs at a malunion can be either compensatory or contributory to the angulatory deformity as it relates to the mechanical axis of a limb.

5. The distinction between a malunion and mild deformity at a fracture site remains vague, and no absolute guidelines exist.

B. Upper extremity

1. Shortening is much better tolerated in the upper extremity, especially at the humeral level, than in the lower extremity.

2. Angulatory deformities of up to 30° are well tolerated by the humeral shaft.

3. Angulatory deformities at the supracondylar level are more poorly tolerated because of an altered carrying angle. These are limited to 10° of valgus and, occasionally, up to 15° of varus.

4. Forearm translation malunions are poorly tolerated because they interfere with rotation. Likewise, angulatory deformities greater than 5° often are poorly tolerated because they impede normal forearm pronation and supination. Isolated shortening of the radius or ulna of more than 3 to 5 mm also is poorly tolerated because of altered wrist mechanics.

C. Lower extremity

1. Shortening of more than 2 cm in the lower extremity clearly represents a malunion in the axial plane.

2. Angulatory malunions about the knee and ankle of 10° or more in the coronal plane are poorly tolerated and often require correction. In some patients, even less than 10° of malalignment can be poorly tolerated and necessitate correction.

3. Angulatory and translation deformities in the sagittal plane are tolerated much better because of the axis of motion of the knee and ankle in the sagittal plane. Because no clear criterion for acceptable deformity exists, it must be determined on an individual basis. The functional and aesthetic effects of the malalignment should be considered in terms of the functional demands of the patient.

III. Osteomyelitis

A. Etiology

1. Classically, osteomyelitis occurs via hematogenous seeding or direct inoculation, most typically secondary to trauma.

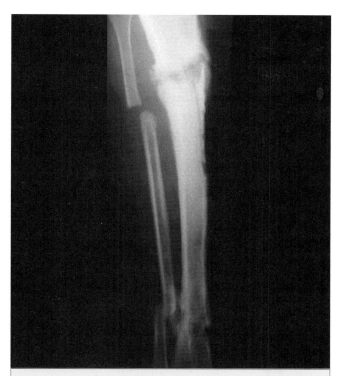

Figure 2   AP radiograph from a 24-year-old man 2 years after an open tibia fracture. The dense, necrotic cortical bone at the medial border of the tibia represents a sequestrum.

2. Hematogenous osteomyelitis, which occurs after seeding of the bacteria at metaphyseal end arterioles, is seen most commonly in the pediatric population.

3. Possible pathogens include not only bacteria but also fungi and yeasts, although most cases are caused by *Staphylococcus*, *Streptococcus*, *Enterococcus*, and *Pseudomonas*.

B. Types of osteomyelitis—Osteomyelitis can be acute or chronic.

1. Acute osteomyelitis

   a. Acute osteomyelitis, characterized by rapid presentation and a rapidly evident purulent infection, represents the first episode of bone infection.

   b. Acute osteomyelitis can become chronic over time.

2. Chronic osteomyelitis

   a. Chronic osteomyelitis can be present for decades.

   b. It can convert from a dormant to an active state without a known antecedent event or as a result of a local or systemic change in the host.

C. Biofilm-bacteria complex

1. The initial inoculum involves bacteria in a planktonic phase; they are mobile, float freely, and exhibit a high metabolic rate. Once the bacteria inhabit a biofilm, they assume a more dormant, slow metabolic rate. This altered metabolic rate can limit their antibiotic sensitivity.

2. The biofilm-bacteria complex is the entity comprising the bacteria in an extracellular matrix with a glycocalyx.

3. This matrix is avascular, making it difficult for antibiotics to penetrate.

4. Depending on the microbe, the biofilm layer usually forms between 8 and 14 days following planktonic colonization of the bone.

5. Biofilm represents the "first line response" of bacterial colonization, in which the initial colony invasion "falls on the sword" to create a bacteria-friendly environment for the rest of the colony to inhabit. It consists of a dead bacterial sludge milieu.

6. A mature biofilm complex represents the greatest barrier to treatment and effective eradication of musculoskeletal infections, especially if the infection involves bone or is implant related. This is due to the fact that the microbes enter into a sessile phase with markedly reduced metabolic rate, as well as the fact that the biofilm itself impairs efficacy because it represents a barrier to diffusion.

D. Evaluation

1. Clinical presentation

   a. A draining sinus tract with abscess formation is the classic presentation of osteomyelitis. Often, the sinus tracts are multifocal in nature.

   b. In acute osteomyelitis secondary to trauma, the clinical manifestation is exposed bone or a nonhealing, soupy, soft-tissue envelope over the bone.

   c. Indolent infections might present with only chronic swelling and induration, occasionally accompanied by recurrent bouts of cellulitis.

2. Imaging

   a. Radiographic evaluation of the affected limb segment is performed.

   b. Osteomyelitis can present radiographically as areas of osteolysis acutely, then chronically as areas of dense sclerotic bone because of the avascular, necrotic nature of osteomyelitic bone.

   c. When a necrotic segment of free, devascularized, infected bone is left in a limb over time, it becomes radiodense on radiographs and is called a sequestrum (**Figure 2**). Occasionally, it

Table 3

Cierny-Mader Staging System for Osteomyelitis

Stage	Anatomic Type	Typical Etiology	Treatment
1	Medullary	Infected intramedullary nail	Removal of the infected implant and isolated intramedullary débridement
2	Superficial; no full-thickness involvement of cortex	Chronic wound, leading to colonization and focal involvement of a superficial area of bone under the wound	Remove layers of infected bone until viable bone is identified
3	Full-thickness involvement of a cortical segment of bone; endosteum is involved, implying intramedullary spread	Direct trauma with resultant devascularization and seeding of the bone	Noninvolved bone is present at same axial level, so the osteomyelitic portion can be excised without compromising skeletal stability.
4	Infection is permeative, involving a segmental portion of the bone.	Major devascularization with colonization of the bone	Resection leads to a segmental or near-segmental defect, resulting in loss of limb stability.

will be engulfed and surrounded or walled off by healthy bone; it is then called an involucrum.

3. Laboratory studies

   a. Hematologic profiles can be useful in the workup for osteomyelitis. In chronic osteomyelitis, however, it is not uncommon for all laboratory indices to be normal.

   b. Blood tests that should be ordered include CBC with differential, ESR, and CRP.

   c. In acute osteomyelitis, elevated white blood cell count (WBC), platelet count, ESR, and CRP level may be present; a "left shift" of the differential often is present as well.

   d. In chronic osteomyelitis, the WBC and platelet count usually are normal. Often, the ESR is normal as well; occasionally the CRP level also is normal.

   e. Surgery or trauma also can elevate the platelet count, ESR, and CRP level. The platelet count generally returns to normal once the hemoglobin level has stabilized to a more normal range. The CRP value usually normalizes within 2 to 4 weeks, and the ESR returns to normal within 4 to 8 weeks.

4. Tissue culture

   a. The diagnosis of osteomyelitis depends on obtaining appropriate culture specimens.

   b. The gold standard for proper diagnosis is obtaining good tissue samples for culture. If an abscess cavity exists, this can sometimes be performed adequately with needle aspiration.

   c. Appropriate bacterial and fungal plating of the specimen is important.

   d. In chronic osteomyelitis, the culture specimens sometimes fail to grow. This does not mean that infection is absent, but rather that the offending organisms cannot be grown successfully. Often, patients with chronic osteomyelitis have received multiple courses of antibiotic therapy, making it hard to grow the organisms in a laboratory setting.

   e. Much new interest has focused on using polymerase chain reaction (PCR) analysis of specimens to determine whether microbial DNA is present as a way of diagnosing microbial infection. PCR analysis will no doubt become a cornerstone of diagnosis in the future.

E. Classification

1. The most widely accepted clinical staging system for osteomyelitis is the Cierny-Mader system (Table 3).

2. This system considers the anatomy of the bone involvement (Figure 3), then subclassifies the disease according to the physiologic status of the host (Table 4).

3. This staging method helps define the lesion and the ability of the host to deal with the process.

4. Prognosis has been well correlated with the physiologic host subclassification.

F. General treatment principles

1. Once the osteomyelitis has been staged and the condition of the host has been defined and optimized, a treatment plan individualized to the patient's condition and goals can be determined.

2. Ideally, the goal of treatment is complete eradication of the osteomyelitis with a preserved soft-

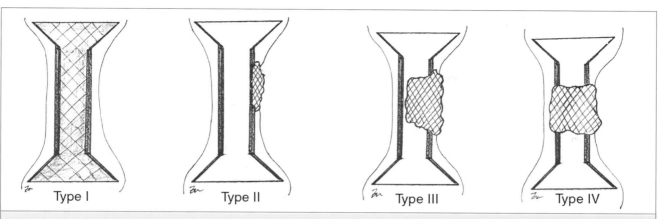

Figure 3 Illustrations show the Cierny-Mader anatomic classification of osteomyelitis. Type I is intramedullary osteomyelitis; type II is superficial osteomyelitis with no intramedullary involvement; type III is invasive localized osteomyelitis with intramedullary extension, but with a maintained, stable, uninvolved segment of bone at the same axial level; and type IV is invasive diffuse osteomyelitis, with involvement of an entire axial segment of bone such that excision of the involved segment leaves a segmental defect of the limb. (Reproduced from Ziran BH, Rao N: Infections, in Baumgaertener MR, Tornetta P III, eds: *Orthopaedic Knowledge Update: Trauma*, ed 3. Rosemont, IL, American Academy of Orthopaedic Surgeons, 2005, p 132.)

Table 4

Physiologic Host Classification Used With the Cierny-Mader Osteomyelitis Classification System

Type	Infection Status	Factors Perpetuating Osteomyelitis	Treatment
A	Normal physiologic responses to infection	Little or no systemic or local compromise; minor trauma or surgery to affected part	No contraindications to surgical treatment
B (local)	Locally active impairment of normal physiologic responses to infection	Cellulitis, prior trauma (such as open fracture, compartment syndrome, and free flap), or surgery to area; chronic sinus; free flap	Consider healing potential of soft tissues and bone, and anticipate the need for free-tissue transfer and hyperbaric oxygen.
B (systemic)	Systemically active impairment of normal physiologic responses to infection	Diabetes, immunosuppression, vascular disease, protein deficiency, or metabolic disease	Consider healing potential of soft tissues and treat correctable metabolic or nutritional abnormalities.
C	Severe infection	Severe systemic compromise and stressors	Because treatment of condition is worse than the condition itself, suppressive treatment or amputation is recommended.

Reproduced from Ziran BH, Rao N: Infections, in Baumgaertener MR, Tornetta P III, eds: *Orthopaedic Knowledge Update: Trauma*, ed 3. Rosemont, IL, American Academy of Orthopaedic Surgeons, 2005, p 133.

tissue envelope, a healed bone segment, and preserved limb length and function.

3. Because of the extreme variation in the way osteomyelitis presents and manifests itself in different people, there is a paucity of good evidence-based data to aid in making treatment guidelines.

G. Surgical treatment

1. Surgical débridement

   a. Surgical débridement is the cornerstone of osteomyelitis treatment.

   b. Aggressive débridement often is required to remove all infected and devitalized bone and tissue.

   c. The single most common mistake in treatment is inadequate débridement that leaves residual devitalized tissue in the wound bed.

   d. Débridement of any dense fibrotic scar is also necessary because it is often quite avascular and represents a poor soft-tissue bed for healing.

3: Trauma

e. Atrophic skin that has become adherent to the bone (eg, the medial border of the tibia) also requires débridement because of its impaired blood supply and compliance.

f. Although intermittent enthusiasm has been shown for using hyperbaric oxygen to treat osteomyelitis, only level IV data are available to suggest the efficacy of this treatment. Recent work in an animal model has shown hyperbaric oxygen to have no efficacy in the treatment of implant-associated osteomyelitis caused by methicillin-resistant *S aureus* and *Pseudomonas aeruginosa*.

2. Skeletal stabilization

a. Skeletal stabilization of the affected limb is necessary for all type IV lesions and some type III lesions where a large amount of bone has been removed.

b. Stabilization is accomplished most often with external fixation or a short course of external fixation followed by internal fixation. It also can be accomplished with antibiotic bone cement-impregnated nails.

c. If a segmental defect is created with the débridement, then proper planning in skeletal stabilization must occur from the start, with a clear and comprehensive plan established to gain bony stability of the limb.

d. For small defects (<2 cm), acute shortening remains a reasonable option for treatment; defects also can be stabilized with rods or plates once infection is eradicated, then the defect can be eliminated with bone grafting or osteomyocutaneous free-tissue transfer.

e. For some large osseous defects, the best option remains bone transport.

3. Dead-space management

a. Débridement creates a dead space; this space requires appropriate management while the infection is being eradicated.

b. The dead space can be filled by means of local muscle mobilization, a rotational muscle flap, a free muscle flap, a free fasciocutaneous flap, or a rotational perforator-based flap.

c. The VAC sponge is a useful short-term adjunct to assist in dead-space management until definitive soft-tissue coverage is achieved; however, the advisability of its long-term use is questionable, and if placed directly over cortical bone for an extended period, it can lead to desiccation and resultant death of the cortical bone in contact with it.

d. Antibiotic-impregnated polymethylmethacrylate (PMMA) beads are a time-honored method for managing dead space; they also provide an effective means of local, high-dose antibiotic delivery. Most surgeons make their own beads by mixing PMMA with tobramycin and vancomycin powder. Other antibiotics used include gentamycin, erythromycin, tetracycline, and colistin. Resorbable materials, including calcium sulfate, calcium phosphate, and hydroxyapatite ceramic beads with antibiotic impregnation, have recently been introduced, but their clinical efficacy has not yet been well established.

- Antibiotic-impregnated PMMA beads can be used effectively with or without a closed soft-tissue envelope.

- With an open soft-tissue envelope, the beads can be placed and then the limb and wound wrapped with an adhesive-coated plastic film laminate. This provides a biologic barrier with high-dose local antibiotic delivery and usually does well for 4 to 6 days before requiring changing because of leakage.

- With a closed soft-tissue envelope, the beads can be left in for an extended period to further ensure that infection has been controlled.

4. Soft-tissue coverage

a. A close working relationship with a microsurgeon experienced in soft-tissue mobilization and free-tissue transfer is imperative in managing combined type III or type IV osteomyelitis with soft-tissue void or an impaired soft-tissue envelope.

b. Microvascular free-tissue transfer is the gold standard for restoring a well-vascularized soft-tissue envelope after infection, trauma, or osteomyelitis.

c. Rotational flaps are a good adjuvant for certain soft-tissue defects or when a microsurgeon is not available. Rotational flaps are particularly useful about the pelvis, thigh, and shoulder girdle.

d. Flap coverage combined with bone transport to fill large bone and soft-tissue defects is safe and effective and has good long-term results.

5. Antibiotic coverage

a. Parenteral antibiotics are administered after débridement has been performed.

b. Treatment protocols frequently involve a 6-week intravenous antibiotic regimen; however, no empiric data have shown that this is necessary. Recent data suggest that, with proper and meticulous débridement, dead-space management, and soft-tissue management, a shorter duration of intravenous antibiotic delivery is as efficacious as a longer course of treatment.

c. With the sharp increase in organisms developing antibiotic resistance (such as methicillin-resistant *S aureus* and vancomycin-resistant *Enterococcus*) an appropriate antibiotic regimen may need to include daptomycin.

d. In certain instances (C hosts), long-term antibiotic suppression can be the treatment of choice.

6. Emerging treatments

a. Researchers now are focusing on therapeutic modalities to directly address the biofilm and its development and enable antibiotics to get to the microbes.

b. New ceramic scaffolds laden with time-release antibiotic cocktails have been developed and seem promising, but in vivo studies remain lacking.

c. It has become apparent that biofilm models of bacterial growth in vivo differ from planktonic models of growth. With this appreciation, research can be done to better understand quorum sensing among microbes and develop more effective treatments.

d. Interest has reemerged in vaccines that treat osteomyelitis against components of biofilm in an animal model. One study using a quadrivalent vaccine of antigenic components of biofilm combined with vancomycin showed significant eradication of infection in the chronic osteomyelitis model. This combined approach to infection eradication surely will be part of the orthopaedic armamentarium in the future.

Top Testing Facts

Nonunions

1. Stable fixation is of extreme importance in treating all nonunions. Particular attention should be paid to the elimination of shear in nonunions with a large degree of fracture obliquity.

2. It is best to achieve as stable a fixation as possible to allow joint mobilization above and below a nonunion.

3. A healthy, well-vascularized soft-tissue envelope is necessary for the healing of tenuously vascularized diaphyseal bone ends. Use of free or rotational muscle or skin flaps enhances the healing environment.

4. If union fails despite optimal treatment, the surgeon should look for metabolic or other endogenous problems that impede fracture healing.

5. If union still fails to occur following proper stabilization and a normal metabolic workup, then the vascularity and viability of the fracture ends should be evaluated and indolent infection should be considered.

Malunions

1. Translation of a fracture can be compensatory or contributory to the overall angulatory effect on mechanical axis deviation of a limb.

2. Angulation and translation are independent events that can both contribute to a malunion's deformity.

Osteomyelitis

1. All necrotic bone and soft tissue must be meticulously débrided.

2. Proper dead-space management and soft-tissue coverage are equally important.

3. The host and the bone involvement should be staged properly at the beginning of treatment so that an appropriate treatment plan can be established.

4. Biofilm currently represents the major limiting factor in eradicating microbes with antibiotics in the care of infection, especially implant-related and bone infections.

Bibliography

Bhandari M, Tornetta P III, Sprague S, et al: Predictors of reoperation following operative management of fractures of the tibial shaft. *J Orthop Trauma* 2003;17(5):353-361.

Bishop JA, Palanca AA, Bellino MJ, Lowenberg DW: Assessment of compromised fracture healing. *J Am Acad Orthop Surg* 2012;20(5):273-282.

Bosse MJ, McCarthy ML, Jones AL, et al: The insensate foot following severe lower extremity trauma: An indication for amputation? *J Bone Joint Surg Am* 2005;87(12):2601-2608.

Brady RA, O'May GA, Leid JG, Prior ML, Costerton JW, Shirtliff ME: Resolution of Staphylococcus aureus biofilm infection using vaccination and antibiotic treatment. *Infect Immun* 2011;79(4):1797-1803.

Garrison KR, Shemilt I, Donell S, et al: Bone morphogenetic protein (BMP) for fracture healing in adults. *Cochrane Database Syst Rev* 2010;6:CD006950.

Green SA, Gibbs P: The relationship of angulation to translation in fracture deformities. *J Bone Joint Surg Am* 1994; 76(3):390-397.

3: Trauma

Hak DJ, Lee SS, Goulet JA: Success of exchange reamed intramedullary nailing for femoral shaft nonunion or delayed union. *J Orthop Trauma* 2000;14(3):178-182.

Johansen LK, Iburg TM, Nielsen OL, et al: Local osteogenic expression of cyclooxygenase-2 and systemic response in porcine models of osteomyelitis. *Prostaglandins Other Lipid Mediat* 2012;97(3-4):103-108.

Lowenberg DW, Feibel RJ, Louie KW, Eshima I: Combined muscle flap and Ilizarov reconstruction for bone and soft tissue defects. *Clin Orthop Relat Res* 1996;332:37-51.

MacKenzie EJ, Bosse MJ, Kellam JF, et al: Early predictors of long-term work disability after major limb trauma. *J Trauma* 2006;61(3):688-694.

Mahaluxmivala J, Nadarajah R, Allen PW, Hill RA: Ilizarov external fixator: Acute shortening and lengthening versus bone transport in the management of tibial non-unions. *Injury* 2005;36(5):662-668.

Marsh JL, Prokuski L, Biermann JS: Chronic infected tibial nonunions with bone loss: Conventional techniques versus bone transport. *Clin Orthop Relat Res* 1994;301:139-146.

McKee MD, DiPasquale DJ, Wild LM, Stephen DJ, Kreder HJ, Schemitsch EH: The effect of smoking on clinical outcome and complication rates following Ilizarov reconstruction. *J Orthop Trauma* 2003;17(10):663-667.

Milner SA, Davis TR, Muir KR, Greenwood DC, Doherty M: Long-term outcome after tibial shaft fracture: Is malunion important? *J Bone Joint Surg Am* 2002;84(6):971-980.

Rao N, Santa E: Anti-infective therapy in orthopedics. *Oper Tech Orthop* 2002;12:247-252.

Rubel IF, Kloen P, Campbell D, et al: Open reduction and internal fixation of humeral nonunions: A biomechanical and clinical study. *J Bone Joint Surg Am* 2002;84(8):1315-1322.

Shandley S, Matthews KP, Cox J, Romano D, Abplanalp A, Kalns J: Hyperbaric oxygen therapy in a mouse model of implant-associated osteomyelitis. *J Orthop Res* 2012;30(2):203-208.

Watson JT: Distraction osteogenesis. *J Am Acad Orthop Surg* 2006;14(10 Spec No.):S168-S174.

Watson JT, Anders M, Moed BR: Management strategies for bone loss in tibial shaft fractures. *Clin Orthop Relat Res* 1995;315:138-152.

Weresh MJ, Hakanson R, Stover MD, Sims SH, Kellam JF, Bosse MJ: Failure of exchange reamed intramedullary nails for ununited femoral shaft fractures. *J Orthop Trauma* 2000;14(5):335-338.

Ziran B, Rao N: Treatment of orthopedic infections. *Oper Tech Orthop* 2003;12:225-314.

Chapter 28

Fractures of the Clavicle, Scapula, and Glenoid

Peter Cole, MD   Steven R. Gammon, MD

I. Clavicular Fractures

A. Anatomy and biomechanics

1. Clavicle osteology

   a. The clavicle is the only long bone to ossify by intramembranous ossification.

   b. It serves as the primary stabilizer between the axial skeleton (via the sternoclavicular [SC] joint) and the appendicular skeleton (via the acromioclavicular [AC] joint).

2. Coracoclavicular (CC) ligaments

   a. Conoid—medial; trapezoid—lateral

   b. The CC ligaments are the primary stabilizers to superior (vertical) translation of the distal clavicle.

3. Superior shoulder suspensory complex (SSSC)

   a. The SSSC is a bone–soft-tissue ring that provides a stable connection of the glenoid and scapula to the clavicle.

   b. The SSSC is composed of four bony landmarks—distal clavicle, acromion, coracoid process, and glenoid neck—and the supporting ligamentous complexes of the AC joint and the CC ligaments (**Figure 1**).

4. Blood supply

   a. The primary blood supply to the clavicle is periosteal; there is no nutrient blood supply.

   b. The clavicle is subcutaneous, with a poor muscle envelope and limited vascularity.

5. Radiographic appearance

Dr. Cole or an immediate family member serves as a paid consultant to or is an employee of Synthes and has received research or institutional support from Synthes. Neither Dr. Gammon nor any immediate family member has received anything of value from or has stock or stock options held in a commercial company or institution related directly or indirectly to the subject of this chapter.

   a. The clavicle forms a unique S-shaped curve on the axial view.

   b. The distal clavicle is flat in the anterior-posterior plane.

B. Overview and epidemiology

1. Clavicular fractures account for 3.8% of all fractures and 35.0% to 45.0% of all shoulder girdle injuries.

2. Approximately 15% of clavicular fractures are distal third, 80% are middle third, and 5% are medial third.

3. Medialization of a clavicular fracture more than 20 mm is associated with a measurable decrease in functional outcome.

C. Evaluation

1. History

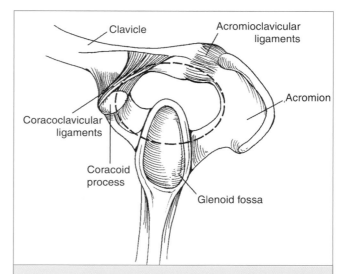

| **Figure 1** | Illustration shows a lateral view of the bone–soft-tissue ring of the superior shoulder suspensory complex. (Reproduced from Goss TP: Scapular fractures and dislocations: Diagnosis and treatment. *J Am Acad Orthop Surg* 1995; 3:22-23.) |

3:Trauma

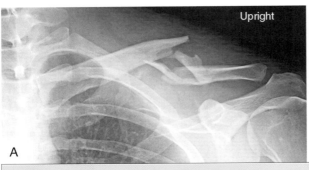

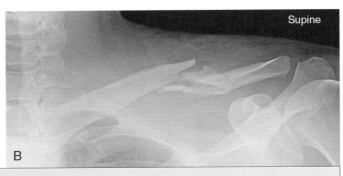

Figure 2 AP radiographs of a patient with a midshaft clavicle fracture show increased displacement when the patient is upright (**A**) compared with supine (**B**).

a. Injury—Most clavicular fractures are related to a lateral blow to the shoulder from a fall (most common) or a direct blow to the clavicle.

b. A small percentage of clavicular fractures are associated with more severe injuries, including scapulothoracic dissociation, scapular fractures, rib fractures, pneumothorax, and neurovascular compromise.

2. Physical examination

a. The typical deformity of middle third fractures is caused by a medial fragment pulled superiorly by the sternocleidomastoid muscle, with the weight of gravity pulling downward on the lateral fragment.

b. A distal neurovascular examination is critical because of the proximity of the brachial plexus and the vascular structures to the zone of injury.

c. Tenting of the skin should be evaluated carefully because it can be a sign of impending open fracture.

3. Imaging

a. Upright and supine radiographs, including an AP view of the clavicle and a 15° cephalad tilt view, should be obtained to define displacement when the patient is upright (**Figure 2**).

b. A bilateral panoramic view of both shoulders should be obtained to measure clavicular shortening.

D. Classification

1. The Allman classification defines fractures of the proximal (medial), middle (midshaft), and distal (lateral) thirds of the clavicle (**Figure 3**).

2. Neer classified lateral third fractures based on the integrity of the CC ligament complex and the involvement of the AC joint (**Figure 4**).

3. Medial third fractures are classified according to the displacement and involvement of the SC joint.

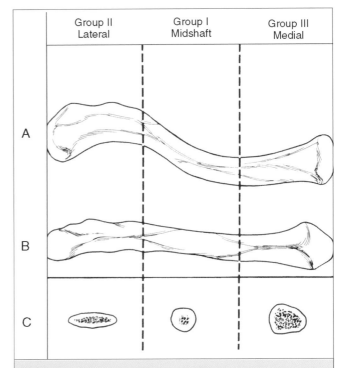

Figure 3 Diagram demonstrates the Allman classification system of clavicle fractures, which divides the clavicle into thirds. Group I (middle third) constitutes 69% to 85% of fractures, group II (distal [lateral] third) makes up 12% to 28%, and group III (medial third) represents 3% to 6%.

E. Treatment

1. Lateral third clavicular fractures

a. Nonsurgical treatment is reserved for all nondisplaced or minimally displaced fractures. Type II and type V fractures (especially type IIB) have a higher incidence of nonunion because of deforming forces.

b. Surgical treatment is considered for type II fractures because of the high incidence of nonunion.

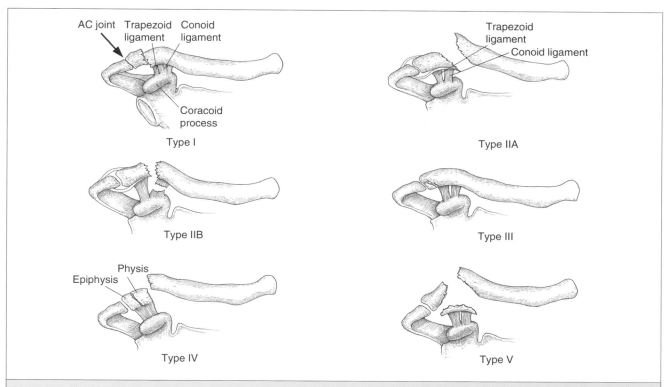

Figure 4 Illustration shows the Neer classification of distal clavicular fractures. Type I fractures occur lateral to the coraco-clavicular (CC) ligaments but do not extend into the acromioclavicular (AC) joint. Type II fractures are subdivided into type IIA or type IIB, based on the fracture pattern relative to the CC ligaments. Type IIA fractures occur just medial to the CC ligaments, resulting in greater displacement, and type IIB fractures occur between the conoid and the trapezoid ligaments. Type III fractures involve intra-articular extension into the AC joint without ligamentous disruption. Type IV fractures occur in skeletally immature individuals and mimic an AC joint dislocation. Type V fractures represent an avulsion of the CC ligaments from the clavicle with an associated distal clavicular fracture. (Reproduced from Banerjee R: Management of distal clavicle fractures. *J Am Acad Orthop Surg* 2011;19:392-401.)

c. Complications include AC joint arthritis in intra-articular variants, nonunion, and loss of fixation.

2. Middle third clavicular fractures

a. Nonsurgical treatment is appropriate for non-displaced or minimally displaced middle third fractures.

b. Surgical indications include open fractures or fractures with concomitant injuries to subclavian neurovascular structures, 100% displacement, more than 15 mm of shortening, highly comminuted fractures, and multiple upper or lower extremity fractures (polytrauma).

c. Implant choices include intramedullary screw fixation, superior plate fixation, and anteroinferior plate fixation. Both plating techniques have advantages. Recent literature has reported that superior plating may be better for axial compression and anteroinferior plating better for cantilever bending.

d. Surgical complications include iatrogenic neurovascular injury, subclavian thrombosis, pneu-mothorax, injury to the supraclavicular nerves, hardware prominence, and infection and nonunion following plate fixation.

3. Medial third clavicular fractures

a. Nonsurgical treatment is appropriate for most medial third clavicular fractures that are non-displaced or minimally displaced.

b. Surgical intervention is reserved for fractures with significant displacement or posterior displacement into the mediastinum.

c. Surgical procedures—Open reduction and internal fixation (ORIF) with plate and screws is used, with SC joint augmentation or reconstruction if the fracture is very medial and has little or no fixation to the medial clavicle.

d. Complications are similar to those seen in posterior SC dislocation.

- Retrosternal and mediastinal injuries are seen, including vascular, pulmonary, esophageal, cardiac, and neurologic injuries. Thoracic surgeon backup is important.

3: Trauma

- Hardware migration into the mediastinum also is seen, causing late intrathoracic or vascular injury when Kirschner wires are used.

F. Rehabilitation

1. Nonsurgically treated clavicular fractures require a short period of immobilization (2 to 4 weeks), with simple Codman exercises followed by full active-assisted and passive range of motion. Strengthening generally begins by 6 to 10 weeks.

2. Surgically treated clavicular fracture rehabilitation typically begins immediately with full active-assisted and passive range of motion. Strengthening is begun 4 to 6 weeks postoperatively.

G. Pearls and pitfalls

1. Scapulothoracic dissociation should be considered in the presence of severe displacement when substantial distraction of the clavicle fragments or forequarter is evident on chest radiographs, or when neurovascular injury to the upper extremity has occurred.

2. Displaced lateral-third clavicular fractures are inherently unstable and are prone to nonunion.

3. Completely displaced middle-third clavicular fractures treated nonsurgically have a nonunion rate of 15%.

4. Additional risk factors for nonunion after clavicular fractures include advanced age, distal-fifth fractures, displaced transverse fractures, female sex, and comminuted displaced middle-third fractures.

5. Nonsurgical management of completely displaced clavicular fractures is associated with slower functional return, more muscle fatigability, patient perception of poorer cosmesis, more symptomatic malunions, and a greater percentage of nonunions than such fractures managed surgically.

II. Scapular and Glenoid Fractures

A. Anatomy and biomechanics

1. Glenoid

    a. The labrum deepens the pear-shaped glenoid fossa by up to 50%.

    b. Glenoid version is 2° of anteversion relative to the scapular body.

2. Body of the scapula

    a. Ossification begins at the eighth week of gestation.

    b. Two thirds of shoulder motion is glenohu-

meral, and one third is scapulothoracic.

    c. The scapula is the origin or insertion for 18 muscles.

3. Spine

    a. The spine of the scapula is an osseous bridge that separates the supraspinatus from the infraspinatus origin.

    b. The spinoglenoid notch is a potential site of suprascapular nerve tethering or compression.

4. Acromion—Has three ossification centers: the meta-acromion (base), the mesoacromion (mid), and the preacromion (tip).

5. Coracoid process

    a. Site of muscular attachments for the coracobrachialis, the short head of the biceps, and the pectoralis minor

    b. Site of ligament attachments for the CC ligaments

6. Superior shoulder suspensory complex

    a. The SSSC is a bone–soft-tissue ring that provides a stable connection of the glenoid and scapula to the axial skeleton.

    b. The SSSC is composed of four bony landmarks—the distal clavicle, the acromion, the coracoid process, and the glenoid—and the supporting ligamentous complexes of the AC joint and the CC ligaments (**Figure 1**).

B. Overview and epidemiology

1. Scapula fractures account for only 3% to 5% of shoulder girdle injuries and less than 1% of all fractures.

2. Scapular fractures result from high-energy events such as motor vehicle or motorcycle accidents, which account for approximately 90% of all fractures.

3. Scapular fractures are associated with hemothorax or pneumothorax in 80% of cases, with ipsilateral extremity injury in 50%, head injury in 15%, cervical injury in 15%, and neurovascular injury in 10%.

4. Scapular fractures are missed or the diagnosis is delayed in 12.5% of multiply injured patients.

C. Pathoanatomy

1. Mechanism of injury

    a. Direct blunt force trauma causes scapular body, neck, and glenoid fractures.

    b. An axial load on an outstretched extremity can cause scapular neck and glenoid fractures.

    c. Glenohumeral dislocation can cause anterior

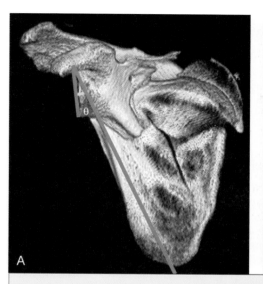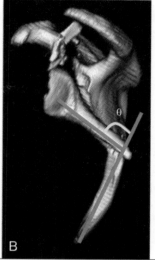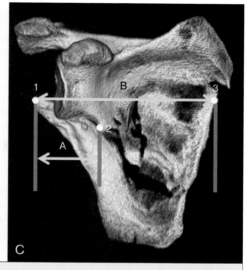

Figure 5   Three-dimensional CT reconstructions of the scapula demonstrate the accurate measurements of displacement and deformity for surgical decision making. **A,** Measurement of the glenopolar angle (GPA) represents the relationship of the glenoid surface on the AP view relative to the inferior wing. Normal GPA is 40° to 45°. **B,** Scapular Y view demonstrates the angulation of the scapular body. Translation can also be well visualized on this view. **C,** Measurement of the medialization of the glenoid relative to the scapular body on the AP view. 1 = lateral-most point of the distal fragment, 2 = lateral-most point of the proximal fragment, 3 = medial-most point on the scapula at the level of the fracture, line A = medial/lateral displacement, line B = width of the scapula at the level of the fracture. (Reproduced from Cole PA, Gauger EM, Schroder LK: Management of scapular fractures. *J Am Acad Orthop Surg* 2012;20[3]:130-141.)

(bony Bankart) or posterior (reverse bony Bankart) glenoid fractures.

2. Scapulothoracic dissociation is a lateral displacement of the scapula associated with severe soft-tissue injury and brachial and vascular injury of the extremity.

D. Evaluation

1. History—Patients typically present with a history of high-energy blunt trauma to the shoulder. Glenohumeral dislocations and penetrating trauma are less common. A history that includes baseline level of function and the patient's occupation, recreation, and handedness should be obtained.

2. Physical examination

   a. The incidence of injuries associated with scapular and glenoid fractures is high (90%). Identifying the mechanism of injury is helpful in determining other injuries.

   b. A thorough neurovascular examination of the affected extremity should be performed.

   c. The skin should be examined for abrasions or open wounds that should delay surgical intervention.

3. Imaging

   a. A true AP (Grashey), transscapular (Y), and axillary view should be obtained.

- Obtaining quality radiographs is often difficult secondary to patient discomfort and a lack of radiographic protocols.

- Radiographic parameters include intra-articular step-off, lateral border offset (medialization), glenopolar angle (angle on the true AP view of the glenoid surface relative to the inferior wing), and angulation seen on the transscapular view.

   b. CT scan with three-dimensional reconstruction is the gold standard for measuring radiographic parameters and visualizing the full picture of the scapula. If the scapular fracture is displaced more than 1 cm, CT should be obtained for accurate measurements (**Figure 5**).

E. Classification—Classification is based on the fracture's location on the scapula.

1. The Ogawa classification of coracoid fractures is shown in **Table 1**.

2. The Kuhn classification of acromial fractures is shown in **Table 2**. It is important not to mistake an os acromiale for an acute fracture.

3. The Ada and Miller classification of scapular body fractures is based on involvement of the acromion, the spine, the coracoid, the neck, the glenoid, and the body (**Figure 6**).

4. The Ideberg classification of glenoid fractures has been modified by Mayo to make a more practical

3: Trauma

Table 1

Ogawa Classification of Coracoid Fractures

Type of Fracture	Characteristics
1	Fracture occurs proximal to the coracoclavicular ligaments and is associated with other injuries to the superior shoulder suspensory complex, which results in double disruptions.
2	Fracture occurs toward the tip of the coracoid.

Table 2

Kuhn Classification of Acromial Fractures

Type of Fracture	Characteristics
I	Nondisplaced or minimally displaced
II	Displaced but does not compromise the subacromial space
III	Displaced and compromises the subacromial space

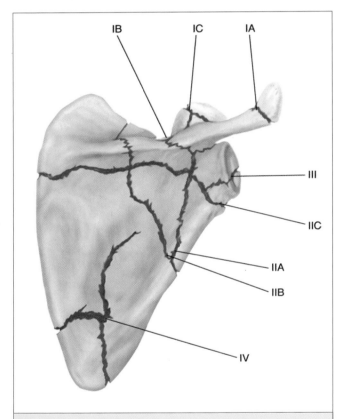

Figure 6 Illustration shows the Ada and Miller classification of scapular body fractures. Type IA: acromial fracture; type IB: scapular spine fracture; type IC: coracoid fracture; types IIA, IIB, and IIC: glenoid neck fractures; type III: glenoid fractures; type IV: scapular body fractures.

classification by adding fracture patterns that also involve the body, acromion, and/or coracoid process (**Figure 7**).

5. Disruption of the SSSC can be classified as a single, double, triple, or quadruple lesion.

6. Scapulothoracic dissociation can be classified by the presence or absence of a brachial plexus injury.

F. Nonsurgical indications—Most scapular fractures are minimally to moderately displaced and can be treated nonsurgically.

G. Surgical indications

1. Coracoid and acromion fractures—Surgical indications include painful nonunion, at least 1 cm of displacement, multiple disruption of the SSSC, or a concomitant ipsilateral scapular fracture requiring surgical intervention.

2. Glenoid fractures—Surgery is indicated when an intra-articular gap or step-off of 4 to 10 mm or glenohumeral instability is present after dislocation.

3. Scapular body fractures

a. Surgery is indicated when any of the following is present.

- Lateral border offset (medialization) of at least 20 mm

- Glenopolar angle of 20° or less

- Angulation as seen on the transscapular view of at least 45°

- Completely displaced double disruptions of the SSSC

b. If the fracture does not meet surgical criteria, weekly follow-up radiographs should be obtained for the first 2 to 3 weeks to ensure that no progressive displacement of an unstable fracture is present.

4. Double disruptions ("floating shoulder") as well as triple and quadruple disruptions of the SSSC can lead to discontinuity or malposition of the glenohumeral joint relative to the scapular body.

H. Surgical approach

1. The deltopectoral approach is used for anterior and superior glenoid fractures as well as coracoid fractures.

2. The transaxillary approach is sometimes beneficial for anteroinferior glenoid fractures that extend into the scapular neck.

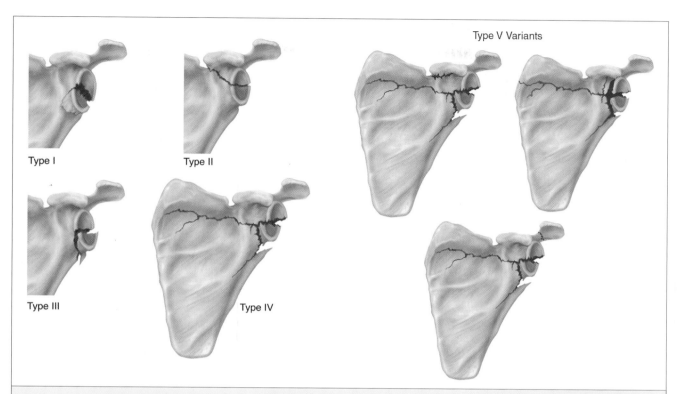

Figure 7   Illustrations depict the Mayo modification of the Ideberg classification of glenoid fractures. Type I injuries represent isolated involvement of the anteroinferior joint surface (bony Bankart) and may be associated with shoulder dislocation. Type II injuries consist of a displaced articular segment involving the superior third to one half of the articular surface in continuity with the coracoid. Type III fractures encompass the inferior or inferoposterior portion of the fossa in continuity with a variable portion of the lateral border. Type IV patterns involve the inferior articular surface, with extension into the body, frequently with a stellate pattern that at times can involve the spine. The displaced articular segment may be free or contiguous with the lateral border of the body. Type V fractures represent a type IV pattern plus an additional coracoid, acromial, or free superior articular component.

3. Posterior approaches

  a. A straight posterior approach is used for fractures isolated to the posterior glenoid, scapular neck, and/or the lateral border of scapula.

  b. The Judet approach is the most commonly used approach for scapular fractures. The incision begins at the acromion, courses along the spine of the scapula, and angles down along the vertebral border of the scapula. The surgeon can work in the interval between the infraspinatus and the teres minor or elevate the entire teres minor, infraspinatus, and posterior deltoid off the lateral border of the scapula.

I. Complications

  1. Complications of scapular fractures are related primarily to the severity of the traumatic injury and associated injuries.

  2. Axillary nerve injury is associated with fractures related to shoulder dislocation.

J. Pearls and pitfalls

  1. Suprascapular nerve injury is associated with scapular neck fractures that involve the spinoglenoid and suprascapular notches. Preoperative electromyography (EMG) is recommended if the fracture involves the spinoglenoid notch and more than 3 weeks have elapsed since injury.

  2. Deformity and dysfunction are related.

  3. Length, alignment, rotation, and articular congruity are treatment principles, as for any bone.

K. Rehabilitation

  1. Nonsurgically treated scapular and glenoid fractures typically are immobilized in a sling or shoulder immobilizer with gentle Codman exercises for 2 weeks and then advanced to full active and passive range of motion.

  2. For surgically treated scapular and glenoid fractures, full active and passive range of motion typically is prescribed for the first 4 weeks; then, a gradual strengthening program is initiated.

  3. Anterior approaches that involve subscapularis takedown require limitations in passive shoulder external rotation for 6 weeks.

3:Trauma

Top Testing Facts

1. The nonunion rate for displaced clavicular fractures treated nonsurgically approaches 15%.

2. Risk factors for nonunion after clavicular fractures include advanced age, clavicular fractures of the distal fifth, displaced transverse fractures, female sex, and comminuted displaced middle third fractures.

3. Nonsurgical management of completely displaced clavicular fractures is associated with slower functional return, more muscle fatigability, patient perception of poorer cosmesis, more symptomatic malunions, and a greater percentage of nonunions than such fractures managed surgically.

4. Scapular fractures are associated with hemothorax or pneumothorax in 80% of cases, ipsilateral extremity injury in 50%, head injury in 15%, cervical injury in 15%, and neurovascular injury in 10%.

5. The gold standard diagnostic test to measure angular deformities and displacement in scapular fractures with the greatest accuracy and reproducibility is the three-dimensional CT scan.

6. Surgical indications for scapular fractures include displaced intra-articular glenoid fractures, displaced double lesions of the SSSC, angulated scapular neck and body fractures greater than 45°, glenopolar angle of 20° or less, and lateral border offset (medialization) greater than 20 mm in active patients who demand optimal shoulder function.

Bibliography

Ada JR, Miller ME: Scapular fractures: Analysis of 113 cases. *Clin Orthop Relat Res* 1991;269:174-180.

Anavian J, Wijdicks CA, Schroder LK, Vang S, Cole PA: Surgery for scapula process fractures: Good outcome in 26 patients. *Acta Orthop* 2009;80(3):344-350.

Banerjee R, Waterman B, Padalecki J, Robertson W: Management of distal clavicle fractures. *J Am Acad Orthop Surg* 2011;19(7):392-401.

Canadian Orthopaedic Trauma Society: Nonoperative treatment compared with plate fixation of displaced midshaft clavicular fractures: A multicenter, randomized clinical trial. *J Bone Joint Surg Am* 2007;89(1):1-10.

Cole PA, Gauger EM, Schroder LK: Management of scapular fractures. *J Am Acad Orthop Surg* 2012;20(3):130-141.

DeFranco MJ, Patterson BM: The floating shoulder. *J Am Acad Orthop Surg* 2006;14(8):499-509.

Favre P, Kloen P, Helfet DL, Werner CM: Superior versus anteroinferior plating of the clavicle: A finite element study. *J Orthop Trauma* 2011;25(11):661-665.

Goss TP: Scapular fractures and dislocation: Diagnosis and treatment. *J Am Acad Orthop Surg* 1995;3(1):22-33.

Ideberg R, Grevsten S, Larsson S: Epidemiology of scapular fractures: Incidence and classification of 338 fractures. *Acta Orthop Scand* 1995;66(5):395-397.

Mayo KA, Benirschke SK, Mast JW: Displaced fractures of the glenoid fossa: Results of open reduction and internal fixation. *Clin Orthop Relat Res* 1998;347:122-130.

Nowak J, Holgersson M, Larsson S: Can we predict long-term sequelae after fractures of the clavicle based on initial findings? A prospective study with nine to ten years of follow-up. *J Shoulder Elbow Surg* 2004;13(5):479-486.

Zlowodzki M, Bhandari M, Zelle BA, Kregor PJ, Cole PA: Treatment of scapula fractures: Systematic review of 520 fractures in 22 case series. *J Orthop Trauma* 2006;20(3):230-233.

Zlowodzki M, Zelle BA, Cole PA, Jeray K, McKee MD; Evidence-Based Orthopaedic Trauma Working Group: Treatment of acute midshaft clavicle fractures: Systematic review of 2144 fractures. On behalf of the Evidence-Based Orthopaedic Trauma Working Group. *J Orthop Trauma* 2005;19(7):504-507.

Chapter 29

Proximal Humeral Fractures
Clifford B. Jones, MD, FACS

I. Epidemiology

A. Frequency—4% to 5% of all adult fractures (common)

B. Age and sex—bimodal distribution

 1. High-energy—younger men and boys

 2. Low-energy—older women

 3. Patterns can be similar based on the extent of the osteoporosis, however.

II. Pathoanatomy

A. Osseous

 1. The proximal humerus is composed of four parts: the head, greater tuberosity, lesser tuberosity, and diaphysis.

 2. The head is divided from the diaphysis via the surgical neck (distal to the tuberosities) and anatomic neck (proximal to the tuberosities).

 3. Fractures extending into the surgical neck versus the anatomic neck affect the surgical options based on the fixation techniques and the vascular supply (see II.B).

 4. The greater tuberosity has the supraspinatus, infraspinatus, and teres minor insertions. The lesser tuberosity has the subscapularis insertion. Fracture patterns with intact or detached tubercles affect muscle pull, deformity, and fracture reduction methods.

B. Vascular (**Figure 1**)

 1. The axillary artery courses medially to the humerus and supplies the proximal humerus via the anterior and posterior humeral circumflex arteries.

 2. The anterior humeral circumflex branches into the arcuate artery of Liang, which courses the bicipital groove and terminates as the major blood supply to the greater tuberosity and the humeral head.

 3. The posterior humeral circumflex artery traverses the posterior head via the capsule, terminating in the greater tuberosity and the posterior humeral head.

 4. Fracture patterns via the tuberosity and neck detachment disrupt the vascular supply to the humeral head and affect articular/head viability.

 5. The vascular viability of the humeral head is optimized with 8 mm or more of the intact medial calcar.

C. Neural

 1. The axillary nerve courses from anterior to posterior in close proximity to the humeral neck,

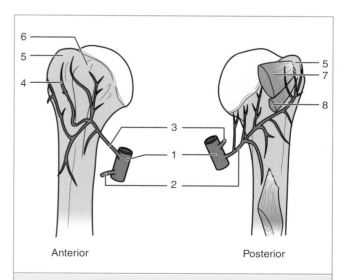

Figure 1 Illustration shows the proximal humeral vascular anatomy. 1. Axillary artery. 2. Proximal humeral circumflex artery. 3. Anterior humeral circumflex artery. 4. Lateral ascending branch of the anterior humeral circumflex artery. 5. Greater tuberosity. 6. Lesser tuberosity. 7. Infraspinatus tendon. 8. Teres minor tendon insertion.

3: Trauma

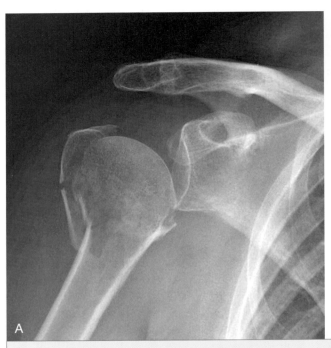
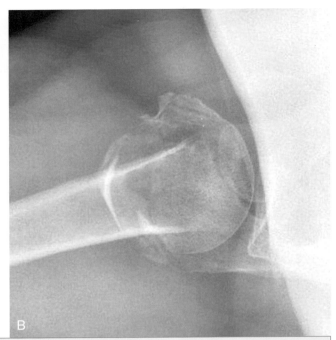

Figure 2 Radiographs depict the proximal humeral trauma series. **(A)** True AP view. No overlap of the humeral head on the glenoid is visualized. Translation, impaction, and angulation can be determined. **(B)** Axillary view. Angulation and dislocation can be determined. Unsupported arm positioning can exaggerate angulation.

inferior glenoid neck, and anterior-inferior capsular pouch; therefore, it is the site of the most common peripheral nerve injury.

2. Fracture-dislocations are associated with the highest risk of axillary nerve injury, which can occur in 20% to 50% of all fracture-dislocations (based on electromyographic analysis). This risk increases with glenohumeral dislocation and age.

III. Evaluation

A. History

1. The preinjury functioning and comorbidities as well as the level of patient compliance should be determined.

2. The mechanism of injury should be determined.

   a. Low-energy—The osseous quality should be confirmed.

   b. High-energy—Associated injuries, nerve function, and vascular integrity should be evaluated.

   c. Glenohumeral integrity (dislocation, labrum, rotator cuff) should be discerned.

B. Physical examination

1. The entire shoulder, neck, and thorax (pulmonary) are examined for associated injuries.

2. Neural examination is confirmed to best of ability (pain limits motor function)

C. Imaging (**Figure 2**)

1. Injury radiographs (shoulder trauma series), including true AP (Grashey), axillary (to ensure head reduction), and scapular Y views, are indicated in all fractures.

2. CT with reconstruction with three-dimensional averaging facilitates imaging of head-split fractures (marginal impaction, percentage of head involvement), fracture-dislocations, associated glenoid lesions (determine approaches), and extensive comminution with difficulty evaluating fracture patterns on plain radiography.

3. MRI has limited indications, including associated dislocation (labrum, anterior capsule, superior labrum anterior to posterior lesion, rotator cuff integrity).

IV. Classification

A. Based on fracture pattern and, therefore, vascular viability, healing, and outcomes

B. Codman classification—Fracture lines along physeal scars; therefore, four segments (head, greater tubercle, lesser tubercle, diaphysis)

C. Neer classification—Displaced with 1 cm or greater

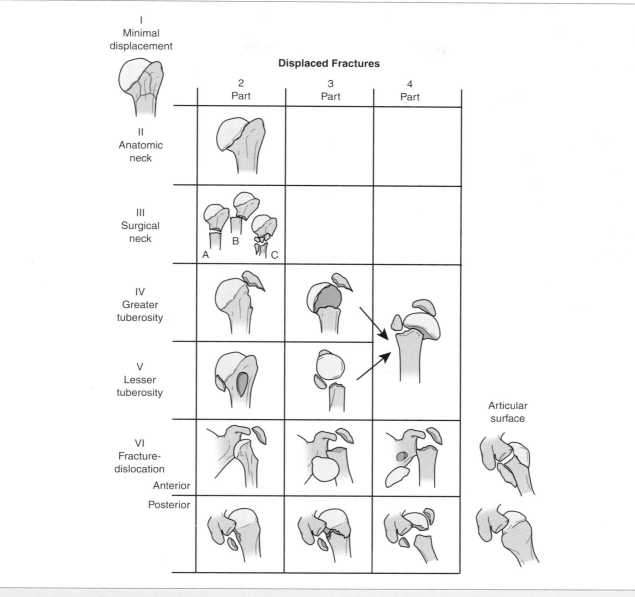

Figure 3   Chart shows the Neer classification of proximal humeral fractures.

and 45° (**Figure 3**); has poor interobserver reliability

D. Orthopaedic Trauma Association/AO Foundation classification—Comprehensive long-bone classification based on location, stability, comminution, and dislocation (**Figure 4**)

V. Treatment

A. Nonsurgical

1. Nonsurgical treatment is not simply "benign neglect." Frequent follow-up examination and imaging is required. Fracture realignment is facilitated with frequent sitting erect, which allows the weight of the arm to offset muscle forces about the shoulder. After the pain is diminished, callus formation is present, and the arm moves as a functional unit, self-directed or therapy-assisted exercises can begin. Starting therapy too early or too late may be detrimental. Nonsurgical intervention is successful most of the time.

2. Indications—Minimal displacement, medical comorbidities, osteoporosis

3. Includes a sling and rest until pain diminishes; then a rotator cuff program, range-of-motion (ROM) activities, and activities of daily living (ADLs) are initiated until the patient becomes skilled at a daily home program.

3: Trauma

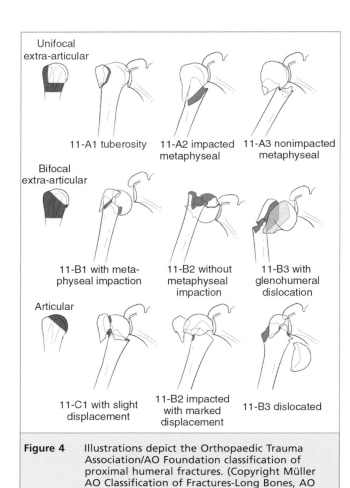

Unifocal
extra-articular

11-A1 tuberosity   11-A2 impacted   11-A3 nonimpacted
metaphyseal   metaphyseal

Bifocal
extra-articular

11-B1 with meta-   11-B2 without   11-B3 with
physeal impaction   metaphyseal   glenohumeral
impaction   dislocation

Articular

11-C1 with slight   11-B2 impacted   11-B3 dislocated
displacement   with marked
displacement

Figure 4   Illustrations depict the Orthopaedic Trauma Association/AO Foundation classification of proximal humeral fractures. (Copyright Müller AO Classification of Fractures-Long Bones, AO Trauma North America, Paoli, PA.)

B. Surgical

1. Indications—Cooperative patients, displaced fractures, dislocations, adequate bone quality

2. Closed reduction and percutaneous pinning (**Figure 5**)

   a. Limited indications are based on simple fracture pattern, patient compliance, and surgeon experience.

   b. Contraindications—Should not be used in dislocations (need for early ROM), metaphyseal comminution/diaphyseal extension (problems achieving a stable anchor point), severe osteoporosis (relative), or head-split fracture (unable to achieve early ROM and stable fixation).

   c. Pins are inserted initially under power and then advanced by hand terminally to avoid head penetration; two to four lateral-to-proximal and two greater tubercle pins (90-90 fixation) are inserted divergently and cut under the skin to avoid infection.

   d. Pins are removed at 6 weeks in the office or

surgical suite; then unlimited ROM and strengthening are initiated.

3. Open reduction and internal fixation (ORIF) (**Figure 6**)

   a. Indications—All types of fractures, including head split, diaphyseal extension, and comminution

   b. Contraindications—Unreconstructable fracture patterns

   c. Implants

   • Limited fixation—Combination of pin, cannulated screw, suture, and tension band wiring; best reserved for isolated tuberosity fractures and impacted (not comminuted) fractures.

   • Standard plate/screw implants—Reserved for very good quality bone

   • Locked plating implants—Used in compromised bone, comminution, and short-segment fixation. This has become the most common implant of choice for proximal humerus fixation based on the poor track record of other fixation methods. Despite this, failures are all too common based on many factors.

   d. Approaches

   • Deltopectoral—Workhorse, most common; can fix or replace through this approach

   • Extended anterolateral acromial, deltoid splitting—Increased risk to axillary nerve (6 cm distal to the lateral acromion); enhanced greater tuberosity reduction access, if displaced posteriorly; unknown risks of revision surgery (plate removal and/or arthroplasty conversion)

   e. Reduction techniques

   • Soft-tissue integrity should be maintained, especially medially along the calcar.

   • Rotator cuff attachments are used for tuberosity mobilization and stabilization with sutures.

   • With comminution and limited calcar stability, medially inserted fibular strut graft insertion and mechanics (endosteal substitution) may be considered.

   f. Plate application

   • Lateral to the bicipital groove to enhance screw insertion and diminish head penetration

   • Distal to the rotator cuff insertion to avoid subacromial impingement and enhance cal-

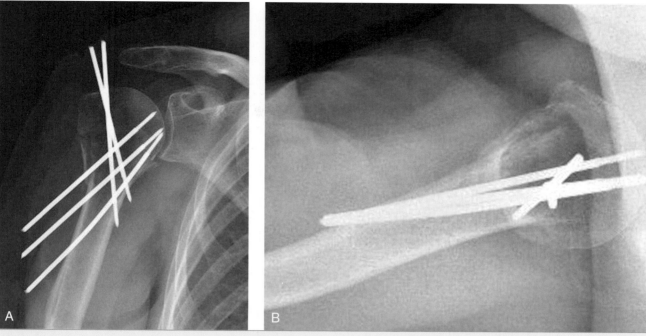

Figure 5 Radiographs show proximal humeral closed reduction and percutaneous pinning. Reduction AP (**A**) and axillary (**B**) radiographs demonstrate the restoration of anatomic relationships, three lateral terminally threaded 2.5-mm Schanz pins inserted manually in a divergent pattern deep into but not through the subchondral bone, and two pins inserted under power into the greater tuberosity, ending in the medial proximal diaphysis.

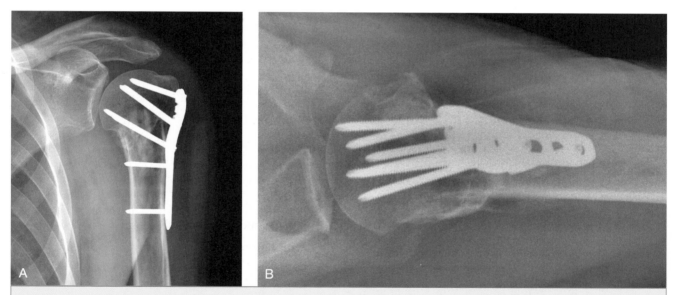

Figure 6 Radiographs demonstrate proximal humeral locked reduction plating. **A,** AP view shows medial reduction of the head to the diaphysis, inferior "kickstand" screws along the calcar, and appropriate plate positioning avoiding the subacromial prominence. **B,** Axillary view demonstrates the head to be centered on the diaphysis, divergent screws spread within the head, and no intra-articular screws.

car screw ("kickstand" screw) insertion

- Usually involves elevation of the deltoid insertion

- Care should be taken to avoid dissection or

plate application distal and/or posterior to the deltoid (radial nerve).

4. Intramedullary nailing

a. Indications—All fracture types, especially

3: Trauma

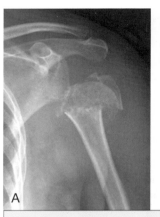
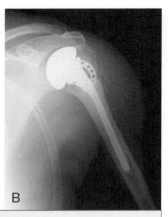

Figure 7 Grashey images show a complex head-splitting proximal humeral fracture (**A**) in an elderly woman with osteoporosis after a low-energy fall treated with proximal humeral arthroplasty (**B**).

diaphyseal extension, segmental, and comminution

b. Contraindications—Head-split fractures, osteoporosis (relative)

c. Rotator cuff approach

d. Intra-articular insertion (through the articular surface and medial to the greater tuberosity)

e. Joysticks should be used for reduction of the proximal segment in relation to the diaphysis.

5. Arthroplasty (**Figure 7**)

a. Indications—Unstable four-part fractures, fracture-dislocations, older population, osteoporosis, patterns that cannot be reconstructed

b. Acute head replacement with improved patient function compared with delayed or internal fixation revision techniques

c. Hemiarthroplasty

- Indications—Older physiologic age, severe osteoporosis

- Expected pain control with variable function

d. Total shoulder arthroplasty—Hemiarthroplasty indications (rare) with younger patient, preexisting glenohumeral arthrosis, skilled surgeon

e. Reverse shoulder arthroplasty—Hemiarthroplasty indications (controversial but becoming more popular) with tuberosity that cannot be reconstructed, preexisting cuff dysfunction/tear, surgeon experienced in the technique.

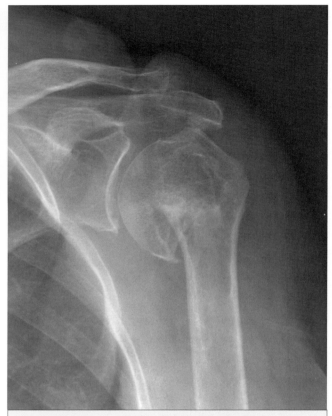

Figure 8 AP radiograph demonstrates the final pull of an intact rotator cuff into a varus alignment and malunion.

VI. Complications

A. Malunion (**Figure 8**)

1. Variable association with function and outcome

2. Posterior/cephalad greater tuberosity common and complex to revise

3. Usual varus and apex anterior

a. More common with nonsurgical techniques

b. Diminished with full intraoperative imaging

c. Results in increased implant failure

4. Options—Nonsurgical, osteotomy, arthroplasty

B. Nonunion (**Figure 9**)

1. Usually accompanies neck fractures

2. Usually atrophic and unstable

3. Difficult to reconstruct secondary to blood supply, osteoporosis (existing and disuse), scarring, and rotator cuff contracture

4. Options—ORIF with grafting and compression, arthroplasty (difficult with shortened and osteo-

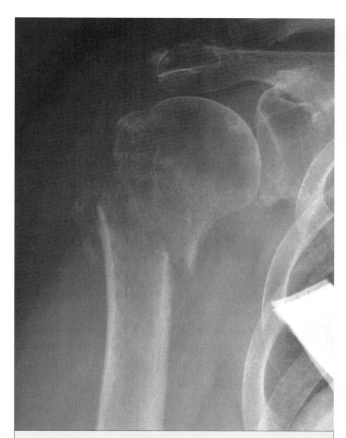

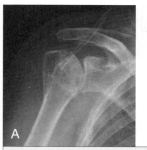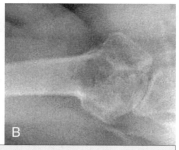

Figure 10   Radiographs show a posttraumatic osteonecrosis/avascular necrosis in the proximal humerus. AP (**A**) and axillary (**B**) radiographs obtained 18 months following closed reduction percutaneous pinning of a four-part valgus impacted fracture show symptomatic subsegmental collapse of the humeral head with chondrolysis.

Figure 9   AP radiograph demonstrates atrophic nonunion of the proximal humerus, resulting in pain and limited function.

porotic tubercles), and reverse shoulder arthroplasty (complex procedure, skilled/experienced surgeon, and possibly better for cuff dysfunction and tuberosity nonunion/resorption)

C. Posttraumatic osteonecrosis (**Figure 10**)

  1. Increased incidence with four-part fractures, small calcar (<8 mm), and dislocations

  2. Rates are lower than historic reports.

  3. Can be limited or extensive

D. Infection

  1. Open fracture increases incidence

  2. Complex problem to eradicate

  3. Usually results in chondrolysis and head resorption

E. Prominent and migrating implants (**Figure 11**)

  1. Proximal plate insertion can result in subacromial impingement.

  2. Intra-articular screw penetration more common with locked screws, diminished with calcium phosphate cement as bone void filler

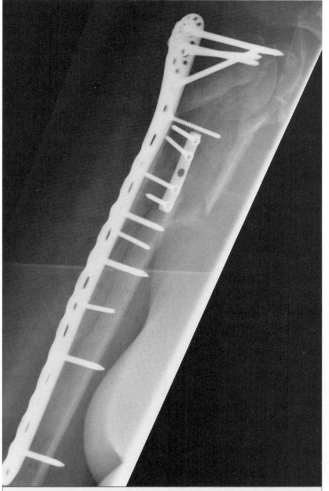

Figure 11   AP radiograph demonstrates fixation failure and intra-articular screws of proximal humeral fracture with diaphyseal extension.

  3. Screw loosening occurs with comminution and/or osteoporosis.

4. Avascular head collapse with locked screws can result in glenoid erosion.

5. Pin migration can occur when these implants are used in poor-quality bone.

F. Shoulder dyskinesia

1. Variable association based on ADLs

2. Occurs with or without malunions

3. Difficult problem to reverse

4. Many elderly or low-demand patients tolerate or accommodate for limitations

VII. Rehabilitation

A. Nonsurgical treatment

1. Sling and rest until pain dissipates; passive motion should be started within 2 weeks.

2. Gradual return to ADLs and rotator cuff program

3. Caution should be used with greater tuberosity fractures; to avoid further displacement, active motion should not begin for 6 weeks after frac-ture consolidation

B. Surgical treatment

1. Fixation should be stable enough to begin immediate passive ROM (forward flexion, abduction) but with limited external rotation to neutral.

2. When fracture consolidated is attained (usually 6 weeks), unlimited ROM, rotator cuff rehabilitation, and strengthening with an emphasis on ADLs should be initiated.

3. Transition to daily home program at 10 to 12 weeks

VIII. Outcomes

A. Variable, based on preexisting function, rotator cuff integrity, the extent of injury, reduction quality, patient expectations, and ADLs

B. Continued improvement can be expected for up to 1 year.

C. Optimal results usually require a compliant patient and extensive rehabilitation.

Top Testing Facts

1. The main or dominant arterial blood supply to the humeral head is the anterior humeral circumflex artery.

2. Head-split fractures have a high rate of osteonecrosis.

3. Minimally displaced fractures are best treated nonsurgically.

4. The axillary nerve is affected most commonly at the time of injury.

5. An axillary radiograph is key to ensure glenohumeral reduction.

6. Proximal humeral fractures are classified based on the number of parts and pattern.

7. Locking plate fixation has become the implant of choice for most proximal humerus fractures.

8. The deltopectoral approach is the approach most often utilized for fractures about the proximal humerus.

9. Arthroplasty is reserved for fractures in poor bone that cannot be reconstructed.

10. Screw penetration is the most common complication following ORIF with locked plates and screws.

Acknowledgments

The author wishes to recognize the work of Andrew Green, MD, for his contribution to *AAOS Comprehensive Orthopaedic Review* and this chapter.

Bibliography

Agel J, Jones CB, Sanzone AG, Camuso M, Henley MB: Treatment of proximal humeral fractures with Polarus nail fixation. *J Shoulder Elbow Surg* 2004;13(2):191-195.

Athwal GS, Sperling JW, Rispoli DM, Cofield RH: Acute deep infection after surgical fixation of proximal humeral fractures. *J Shoulder Elbow Surg* 2007;16(4):408-412.

Bengard MJ, Gardner MJ: Screw depth sounding in proximal humerus fractures to avoid iatrogenic intra-articular penetration. *J Orthop Trauma* 2011;25(10):630-633.

Court-Brown CM, Garg A, McQueen MM: The epidemiology of proximal humeral fractures. *Acta Orthop Scand* 2001; 72(4):365-371.

Duparc F, Muller JM, Fréger P: Arterial blood supply of the proximal humeral epiphysis. *Surg Radiol Anat* 2001;23(3): 185-190.

Egol KA, Ong CC, Walsh M, Jazrawi LM, Tejwani NC, Zuckerman JD: Early complications in proximal humerus fractures (OTA Types 11) treated with locked plates. *J Orthop Trauma* 2008;22(3):159-164.

Egol KA, Sugi MT, Ong CC, Montero N, Davidovitch R, Zuckerman JD: Fracture site augmentation with calcium phosphate cement reduces screw penetration after open reduction-internal fixation of proximal humeral fractures. *J Shoulder Elbow Surg* 2012;21(6):741-748.

Gardner MJ, Boraiah S, Helfet DL, Lorich DG: The anterolateral acromial approach for fractures of the proximal humerus. *J Orthop Trauma* 2008;22(2):132-137.

Gardner MJ, Voos JE, Wanich T, Helfet DL, Lorich DG: Vascular implications of minimally invasive plating of proximal humerus fractures. *J Orthop Trauma* 2006;20(9):602-607.

Gardner MJ, Weil Y, Barker JU, Kelly BT, Helfet DL, Lorich DG: The importance of medial support in locked plating of proximal humerus fractures. *J Orthop Trauma* 2007;21(3): 185-191.

Georgousis M, Kontogeorgakos V, Kourkouvelas S, Badras S, Georgaklis V, Badras L: Internal fixation of proximal humerus fractures with the polarus intramedullary nail. *Acta Orthop Belg* 2010;76(4):462-467.

Gerber C, Schneeberger AG, Vinh TS: The arterial vascularization of the humeral head: An anatomical study. *J Bone Joint Surg Am* 1990;72(10):1486-1494.

Harrison AK, Gruson KI, Zmistowski B, et al: Intermediate outcomes following percutaneous fixation of proximal humeral fractures. *J Bone Joint Surg Am* 2012;94(13): 1223-1228.

Hertel R, Hempfing A, Stiehler M, Leunig M: Predictors of humeral head ischemia after intracapsular fracture of the proximal humerus. *J Shoulder Elbow Surg* 2004;13(4): 427-433.

Jones CB, Sietsema DL, Williams DK: Locked plating of proximal humeral fractures: Is function affected by age, time, and fracture patterns? *Clin Orthop Relat Res* 2011;469(12): 3307-3316.

Keener JD, Parsons BO, Flatow EL, Rogers K, Williams GR, Galatz LM: Outcomes after percutaneous reduction and fixation of proximal humeral fractures. *J Shoulder Elbow Surg* 2007;16(3):330-338.

Levy JC, Badman B: Reverse shoulder prosthesis for acute four-part fracture: Tuberosity fixation using a horseshoe graft. *J Orthop Trauma* 2011;25(5):318-324.

Marsh JL, Slongo TF, Agel J, et al: Fracture and dislocation classification compendium - 2007: Orthopaedic Trauma Association classification, database and outcomes committee. *J Orthop Trauma* 2007;21(10, suppl):S1-S133.

Martinez AA, Bejarano C, Carbonel I, Iglesias D, Gil-Albarova J, Herrera A: The treatment of proximal humerus nonunions in older patients with reverse shoulder arthroplasty. *Injury* 2012;43(suppl 2):S3-S6.

Neer CS II: Displaced proximal humeral fractures: I. Classification and evaluation. *J Bone Joint Surg Am* 1970;52(6): 1077-1089.

Prasarn ML, Achor T, Paul O, Lorich DG, Helfet DL: Management of nonunions of the proximal humeral diaphysis. *Injury* 2010;41(12):1244-1248.

Solberg BD, Moon CN, Franco DP, Paiement GD: Surgical treatment of three and four-part proximal humeral fractures. *J Bone Joint Surg Am* 2009;91(7):1689-1697.

Südkamp NP, Audigé L, Lambert S, Hertel R, Konrad G: Path analysis of factors for functional outcome at one year in 463 proximal humeral fractures. *J Shoulder Elbow Surg* 2011;20(8):1207-1216.

Tejwani NC, Liporace F, Walsh M, France MA, Zuckerman JD, Egol KA: Functional outcome following one-part proximal humeral fractures: A prospective study. *J Shoulder Elbow Surg* 2008;17(2):216-219.

Voos JE, Dines JS, Dines DM: Arthroplasty for fractures of the proximal part of the humerus. *Instr Course Lect* 2011;60: 105-112.

Voos JE, Dines JS, Dines DM: Arthroplasty for fractures of the proximal part of the humerus. *J Bone Joint Surg Am* 2010;92(6):1560-1567.

Willis M, Min W, Brooks JP, et al: Proximal humeral malunion treated with reverse shoulder arthroplasty. *J Shoulder Elbow Surg* 2012;21(4):507-513.

3: Trauma

Chapter 30
Fractures of the Humeral Shaft and the Distal Humerus

Frank A. Liporace, MD

I. Fractures of the Humeral Shaft

A. Epidemiology

1. Humerus fractures account for 3% of all fractures and most commonly occur in the middle third of the bone.

2. They exhibit a bimodal age distribution, with peak incidence in the third decade of life for males and the seventh decade for females.

3. In the younger age group, high-energy trauma is more frequently the cause. Lower energy mechanisms are more common in older patients.

B. Anatomy

1. The anatomy of the humerus varies throughout its length (**Figure 1**).

   a. The shaft is generally cylindrical and provides origin and insertion points for the pectoralis, deltoid, biceps, coracobrachialis, brachialis, and triceps muscles.

   b. These origins and insertions determine the displacement of the major fracture fragments.

   c. Distally, the humerus becomes triangular, and its intramedullary (IM) canal terminates approximately 2 to 3 cm proximal to the olecranon fossa.

   d. Medial and lateral septae delineate the posterior and anterior compartments of the arm.

2. The main neurovascular structures of the arm and forearm traverse the soft tissues overlying the humerus. Posteriorly, the spiral groove houses the

radial nerve. Its location is approximately 14 cm proximal to the lateral-distal articular surface and 20 cm proximal to the medial-distal articular surface. It lies directly posterior to the deltoid tuberosity.

C. Surgical approaches

1. Anterolateral approach—May be extensile but usually is considered for proximal third to middle third humeral shaft fractures.

   a. The radial nerve can be identified between the

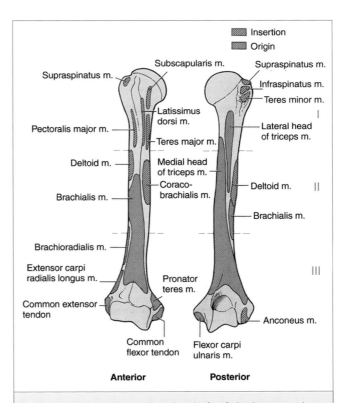

Figure 1   Illustrations show the shaft of the humerus, including the division into three surfaces (I, II, and III). m = muscle. (Adapted with permission from Browner BD, Jupiter JB, Levine AM, Trafton PG, eds: *Skeletal Trauma*, ed 2. Philadelphia, PA, WB Saunders, 2002, p 1524.)

Dr. Liporace or an immediate family member has received royalties from DePuy; is a member of a speakers' bureau or has made paid presentations on behalf of DePuy, Synthes, Smith & Nephew, Stryker, and Medtronic; serves as a paid consultant to or is an employee of DePuy, Medtronic, Synthes, Smith & Nephew, and Stryker; serves as an unpaid consultant to AO; and has received research or institutional support from Synthes, Smith & Nephew, and Acumed.

3: Trauma

brachialis and brachioradialis muscles and traced proximally as it pierces the intermuscular septum.

   b. The brachialis (innervated by the radial and musculocutaneous nerves) is split to spare its dual innervation and protect the radial nerve during retraction.

2. Posterior approach—Most effective for the distal two-thirds of the shaft from the deltoid insertion and distally. The deltoid muscle prevents extension of this approach proximally to the shoulder.

   a. The radial nerve can be identified in the spiral groove in this approach. The interval between the lateral and long heads of the triceps is used, with elevation of the medial (deep) head off the posterior aspect of the shaft.

   b. The ulnar nerve emerges medially from deep to the medial head of the triceps. It courses distally through the cubital tunnel. It can be palpated along the medial aspect of the triceps along the distal third of the humerus.

   c. The radial nerve can be identified approximately 4 cm proximal to the point of confluence through the posterior approach and can be used as a landmark for conducting a triceps splitting.

   d. Alternatively, from the posterior approach, a branch of the radial nerve (lower lateral brachial cutaneous nerve) can be identified off the posterior aspect of the intermuscular septum and can be used as a landmark to elevate the triceps musculature from lateral to medial, allowing 94% exposure of the humerus from the posterior approach.

3. Other approaches—The percutaneous, anterior, anteromedial, and direct lateral approaches have been described and may be used based on wound considerations, other injuries (for example, need for associated vascular repair), or the need for other approaches based on concomitant injuries.

D. Mechanism of injury and associated injuries

1. Distal humerus fractures may be caused by high-energy or low-energy trauma. In patients with osteoporosis or osteopenia, bone mineral density is decreased, so less force is required for injury (for example, a fall from a standing position).

2. Torsional, bending, axial, or a combination of these forces can result in humeral fractures. Direct impact or blast injury (for example, gunshot wounds) also can cause these fractures.

3. With any long bone injury, associated proximal or distal articular fractures or dislocations may be present, necessitating a complete radiographic examination of the bone, including the joints above and joint below.

4. In high-energy injuries, forearm and wrist radiographs are warranted to rule out associated forearm fractures (such as floating elbow).

E. Clinical evaluation

1. Patients typically present with pain, swelling, and deformity about the arm (most frequently shortening and varus).

2. The fracture pattern is related to the mechanism of injury and bone quality. Therefore, a careful history is important to rule out pathologic processes that would require further workup.

3. Careful neurovascular examination is important because radial nerve (distal shaft) and ulnar nerve (articular) injuries are not uncommon associated findings.

F. Radiographic studies

1. A standard radiographic series of AP and lateral views should be acquired.

2. When obtaining the transthoracic lateral view, rotating the patient prevents rotation of the distal fragment and avoids the risk of further soft-tissue or nerve injury.

3. Radiographic series should include the shoulder and elbow ("joint above and joint below") to rule out associated injuries.

4. Traction views for intra-articular fractures may aid in preoperative planning for severely comminuted fractures that meet surgical indications.

5. Advanced imaging studies need to be considered only when a concomitant intra-articular injury is present or a pathologic process is suspected based on the history and initial radiographic evaluation.

G. Classification—Several different systems have been used to classify humeral shaft fractures.

1. The Orthopaedic Trauma Association (OTA) classification system uses a combination of numbers and letters to describe the fracture: bone number (humerus = 1); location (diaphysis = 2); fracture pattern (simple = A, wedge = B, complex = C); and severity (1 through 3) (**Figure 2**).

2. The descriptive classification system is based on the location relative to the pectoralis and the deltoid. It provides information about the relative direction and displacement of the main fracture fragments.

3. A classification system based on fracture characteristics (transverse, oblique, spiral, segmental, comminuted) can aid in determining treatment (**Figure 3**).

H. Nonsurgical treatment

1. This is the treatment of choice for most humeral shaft fractures. A review of 922 patients showed

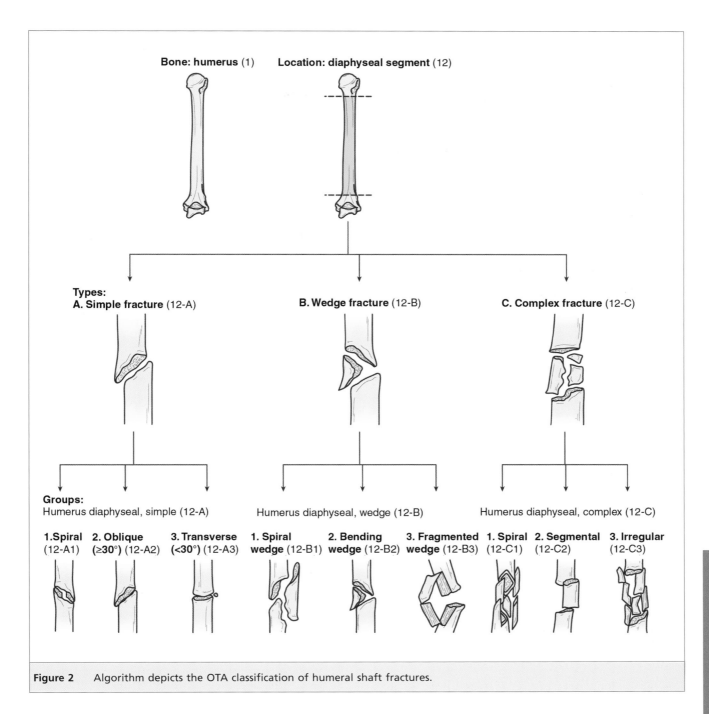

Figure 2   Algorithm depicts the OTA classification of humeral shaft fractures.

that closed treatment with a functional brace resulted in a fracture union rate greater than 98% in closed fractures and greater than 94% in open fractures; 98% exhibited less than 25° of angulation and had less than 25° of restricted shoulder motion at the time of brace removal.

2. Closed treatment may involve initial coaptation splinting followed by a functional brace or a hanging arm cast.

   a. The coaptation splint is used for 7 to 10 days, followed by application of a fracture brace in the office.

   b. Weekly radiographs are obtained for 3 weeks to ensure appropriate maintenance of the reduction; thereafter, they are obtained at 3- to 4-week intervals.

   c. Immediately on fracture brace application, the patient is encouraged to do pendulum exercises for shoulder mobility. Isometric biceps, triceps, and deltoid muscle exercises, as well as active wrist and hand exercises also are encouraged.

3: Trauma

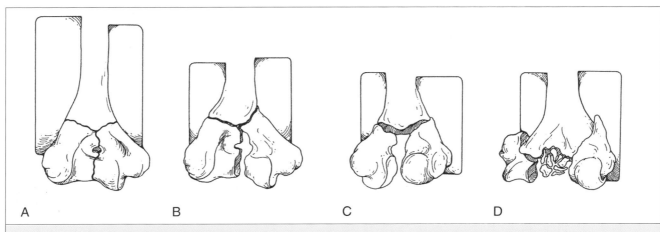

Figure 3 Illustrations depict the types of intercondylar fractures. **A,** Type I nondisplaced condylar fracture of the elbow. **B,** Type II displaced but not rotated T-condylar fracture. **C,** Type III displaced and rotated T-condylar fracture. **D,** Type IV displaced, rotated, and comminuted condylar fracture. (Reproduced with permission from the Mayo Foundation for Medical Education and Research, Rochester, MN.)

d. The patient is instructed to adjust the tension of the fracture brace twice per week and to sleep in a semierect position until 4 to 6 weeks after injury.

e. The fracture brace is worn for 10 to 12 weeks, until no pain is present with palpation at the fracture site, more than 90° of shoulder and elbow motion is painless, and bridging callus is seen radiographically on three of four cortices.

3. Hanging arm casts may be considered for shortened oblique, spiral, and transverse fractures. The cast should extend from 2 cm proximal to the fracture, across the 90° flexed elbow, and to the wrist; the forearm should be in neutral rotation. Suspension straps are attached to loops on the forearm aspect of the cast to aid in alignment.

4. No consensus exists on acceptable alignment, but it has been proposed that 20° apex anterior or posterior angulation and 30° varus/valgus angulation, 15° malrotation, and 3 cm of shortening are acceptable.

5. A recent meta-analysis review yielded no currently published studies that included randomized controlled trials to ascertain whether surgical intervention of humeral shaft fractures gives a better or worse outcome than nonsurgical management.

I. Surgical treatment

1. The absolute and relative indications for surgical treatment are listed in **Table 1**.

2. Outcomes—Open fractures have been shown to have a 12.0% infection rate without fixation and a 10.8% infection rate with fixation.

3. Surgical procedures

a. Open reduction and plate fixation

• This is the most common surgical treatment of humeral shaft fractures.

• Plate-and-screw constructs have union rates up to 94%, with low infection rates (0 to 6%) and low incidence of iatrogenic nerve injury (0 to 5%); they also allow the multiply injured patient to bear weight through the injured extremity.

• Conventional plating is usually performed with a broad 4.5-mm plate and three or four screws per side for axial and torsional stability.

• To improve resistance to bending when using a long plate, screw placement should include "near-near" and "far-far" relative to the site of the fracture.

• In osteoporotic bone, locked plating has been shown to improve stability and resistance to torsional stresses.

b. IM nailing

• Advocated by some as an alternative to plate fixation

• Originally, nonlocking flexible nails were used and inserted in an antegrade or retrograde fashion, but newer interlocking nails have become more common and allow better rotational control.

• IM nails can be useful in the medically unstable patient to avoid a large exposure, in segmental fractures, in the multiply injured patient to limit positioning changes, and in pathologic fractures.

Table 1

Indications for Surgical Treatment of Humeral Shaft Fractures

Absolute Indications	Relative Indications
Concomitant vascular injury	Multiply injured patient
Severe soft-tissue injury	Concomitant head injury
Open fractures	Inability to maintain an
Floating elbow	acceptable reduction
Concomitant displaced	closed
humeral articular injuries	Segmental fractures
Pathologic fractures	Transverse or short oblique
	fractures in a young
	athlete

- IM nails have been shown to withstand higher axial and bending loads than plates, although plated humerus fractures have been shown clinically to allow full weight bearing and have not shown a higher incidence of malunion or nonunion.

- IM nailing of humerus fractures has been shown to result in a higher incidence of shoulder pain and a potential risk to neurovascular structures when locking long nails distally.

- A recent meta-analysis comparing plating of humeral shaft fractures with nailing has shown that plating results in less need for revision, a lower nonunion rate, and fewer shoulder problems.

- A recent retrospective review of IM nails versus plating yielded no substantial difference in fracture union or nerve complications. Substantially more patients in the IM nailing group had restrictive pain and/or functional hindrance and postoperative complications.

- When using locked IM nails, a greater mismatch of nail diameter and shape occurred with retrograde nailing than antegrade nailing and necessitated substantially more reaming, which could increase bone weakness and the risk of a supracondylar fracture.

c. External fixation

- Indications—Staged external fixation is indicated for severe soft-tissue injury, bone defects, vascular injury with acute repair, the medically unstable patient, and infected nonunions.

- When applying external fixation, care must be taken to avoid neurovascular structures.

- Typically, the elbow joint is spanned with two lateral pins placed proximal to the frac-

ture in the humeral diaphysis and two pins in the ulna or radius, depending on whether a forearm injury is present.

- The ulna is the preferred location for pin placement, when possible, because of its subcutaneous location, the limited risk to neurovascular structures, and the ability to maintain pronation-supination mobility during the period of external fixation.

- An open approach is recommended for the humeral pins because of the variability of nerve courses in the region. An open approach also should be used if the distal pins are placed in the radius.

4. Surgical pearls

a. To minimize shoulder pain, an anterior starting point for antegrade IM nailing has been suggested.

- The interval between the anterior and middle thirds of the deltoid is split, and an inline-splitting incision of the rotator cuff is made. This allows a direct path to the IM canal and an easier side-to-side tendon closure.

- The surgeon must be aware that the humeral canal ends 2 to 3 cm proximal to the olecranon fossa and narrows distally, which can result in a risk for fracture distraction when impacting the nail.

b. When plating from a posterior approach, the radial nerve must be identified.

- The radial nerve can be located by bluntly dissecting deep to bone at a point approximately 4 cm superior to the proximal aspect of the triceps fascia.

- If necessary, the ulnar nerve can be located by finding the intermuscular septum that separates the posterior and anterior compartments approximately 2 to 3 cm proximal to the flare of the medial epicondyle.

J. Rehabilitation

1. Humeral shaft fractures treated nonsurgically should undergo rehabilitation as described previously.

2. Surgically treated fractures can be splinted for 3 to 7 days to rest the soft tissues. Subsequently, active and passive range of motion (ROM) of the shoulder, elbow, wrist, and hand can progress.

3. Resistance strengthening exercises may begin at 6 weeks postoperatively or, if nonsurgical treatment has been done, when callus with no motion or pain at the fracture sight is evident.

K. Complications

1. Radial nerve palsy

   a. Humerus fractures often are associated with radial nerve palsies, whether from the time of injury, from attempted closed reduction, or during surgical intervention.

   b. A recent meta-analysis of 4,517 fractures found an overall 11.8% incidence of concomitant radial nerve palsies in transverse and spiral fractures, with the middle and middistal third of the humeral shaft most frequently involved.

      • Overall, the recovery rate was 88.1%, whether the palsy was primary or secondary to iatrogenic intervention.

      • Substantially different rates of recovery were reported for complete (77.6%) versus incomplete (98.2%) palsies and closed (97.1%) versus open (85.7%) injuries.

      • The onset of spontaneous recovery was evident at a mean of 7.3 weeks, with full recovery at a mean of 6.1 months.

      • When nerve exploration was required, it was conducted at a mean of 4.3 months.

      • Barring open injury, vascular injury, a segmental fracture, or floating elbow, no difference in recovery between early and late exploration could be deduced.

   c. For a concomitant nerve injury in patients who do not require surgical treatment of the fracture, electromyography and/or nerve conduction velocity studies should be obtained 6 weeks postinjury. In patients who require surgical treatment, exploration is done at the time of surgery.

   d. For secondary palsies that occur during fracture reduction, it has not been clearly established that surgery improves the ultimate recovery rate when compared with the results of nonsurgical management. Delayed surgical exploration should be done after 3 to 4 months if no evidence of recovery is apparent using electromyography or nerve conduction velocity studies.

2. Vascular injury is rare and may be the result of a penetrating injury (for example, industrial accident, gunshot wound). Revascularization should be attempted within 6 hours.

3. Interlocking with humeral nails can place the axillary nerve at risk proximally and the lateral antebrachial cutaneous nerve, the median nerve, or the brachial artery at risk distally. These risks can be minimized by using a limited open approach, with careful blunt dissection to bone when applying interlocking screws.

4. When passing the reamer through an area of comminution, consider turning off the reamer and pushing it through the area manually to avoid damage to the radial nerve.

5. When radial nerve dysfunction is present preoperatively and IM nailing is chosen, a limited open approach should be considered to ensure that the fracture site is clear of neurovascular structures before nail placement.

6. Nonunions—Although union rates are relatively high with humeral shaft fractures, nonunions do occur.

   a. Motion, avascularity, gap, and infection are all potential causes of nonunion.

   b. In osteopenia and osteoporosis, stability can be difficult to achieve with standard compression plating.

7. Infected nonunions

   a. Eradication of the infection is important to help achieve union.

   b. In select cases of severe infection, temporary or definitive external fixation along with resection of affected tissue and antibiotic treatment may be required.

   c. Whether required by atrophic nonunion or infection, resection and shortening of up to 4 cm can be tolerated.

8. Nerve conduction velocity studies can be considered after 6 weeks to help determine a baseline for the prognosis and severity of the nerve injury.

9. Ultrasonography also has been suggested as a modality for nerve evaluation but depends on the quality of the technician, the radiologist, and the ultrasound machine.

10. A recent multicenter retrospective study showed no difference in time to union, infection, radial nerve palsy, or ultimate ROM between nonsurgically and surgically treated humeral shaft fractures, although the risks of nonunion (20.6% versus 8.7%) and malunion (12.7% versus 1.3%) were substantially greater in the nonsurgically treated group.

II. Distal Humerus Fractures

A. Epidemiology

   1. Intercondylar fractures are the most common distal humerus fracture pattern.

   2. Fractures of the capitellum constitute approximately 1% of all elbow injuries.

   3. Fractures of a single condyle (lateral is more com-

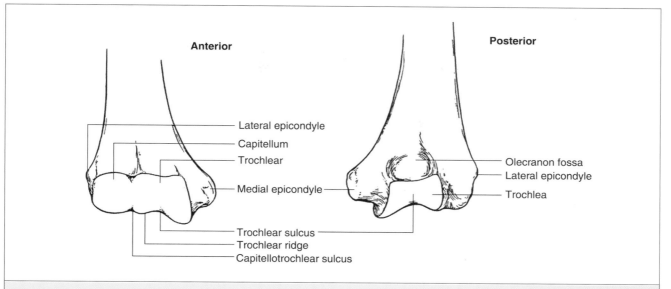

Figure 4   Illustrations show the anterior and posterior views of the anatomy of the distal articular surface of the humerus. The capitellotrochlear sulcus divides the capitellar and trochlear articular surfaces. The lateral trochlear ridge is the key to analyzing humeral condyle fractures. In type I fractures, the lateral trochlear ridge remains with the intact condyle, providing medial-to-lateral elbow stability. In type II fractures, the lateral trochlear ridge is a part of the fractured condyle, which may allow the radius and ulna to translocate in a medial-to-lateral direction in relation to the long axis of the humerus. (Reproduced with permission from Koval KJ, Zuckerman JD, eds: *Handbook of Fractures*, ed 2. Philadelphia, PA, Lippincott Williams and Wilkins, 2002, p 98.)

mon than medial) account for 5% of all distal humerus fractures.

B. Anatomy (**Figure 4**)

1. The elbow is a constrained, hinged joint. The ulna rotates around the axis of the trochlea, which is positioned in relative valgus and external rotation.

2. The capitellum articulates with the proximal radius and is involved with forearm rotation, not elbow flexion/extension. Posteriorly, the capitellum is nonarticular and allows for distal posterior hardware placement.

3. Medially, the medial collateral ligament originates on the distal surface of the medial epicondyle. The ulnar nerve resides in the cubital tunnel in a subcutaneous location.

4. Laterally, the lateral collateral ligament originates on the lateral epicondyle, deep to the common extensor tendon.

C. Classification

1. Classifications of fractures of the distal humerus traditionally were descriptive and based on the number of columns involved and the location of the fracture (supracondylar, transcondylar, condylar, and bicondylar; **Table 2**).

2. The OTA classification system divides these fractures into type A (extra-articular), type B (partial articular), and type C (complete articular).

   a. Each category is subclassified based on the degree and location of fracture comminution.

   b. It has been shown that the OTA classification has substantial stand-alone agreement for interobserver reliability in fracture type (A, B, and C) but is less reliable for subtype.

D. Surgical approaches

1. Extra-articular and partial articular fractures typically are approached through a posterior triceps-splitting or triceps-sparing approach.

   a. For a triceps-splitting approach, a posterior incision is made and carried deep to the triceps, which is subsequently split between the long and lateral heads and distally at its ulnar insertion.

   b. The triceps-sparing approach involves mobilization of the ulnar nerve and subsequent elevation of the entire extensor mechanism in continuity, progressing from medial to lateral.

   c. An alternative approach is the posterior triceps-preserving approach. It involves mobilization of the triceps off the posterior humerus from the medial and lateral aspects of the intermuscular septum. The ulnar nerve (medially) and the radial nerve (laterally and proximally) are identified and preserved.

   d. For the extensor mechanism approach, a recent study yielded mean elbow ROM arcs

3: Trauma

Table 2

Descriptive and Anatomic Classifications of Distal Humerus Fractures

Intra-articular Fractures	Extra-articular/Intracapsular Fractures	Extracapsular Fractures

Single-column fractures
  Medial (high/low)
  Lateral (high/low)
  Divergent
	High transcolumnar fractures
	  Extension
	  Flexion
	  Abduction
	  Adduction
		Medial epicondyle

Two-column fractures
  T pattern (high/low)
  Y pattern
  H pattern
  λ pattern (medial/lateral)
	Low transcolumnar fractures
	  Extension
	  Flexion
		Lateral epicondyle

Capitellar fractures		
Trochlear fractures		

exceeding 100° and reported 90% of triceps extension strength maintained.

2. Simple fractures often can be stabilized using one of these approaches with lag screws alone or screws and an antiglide plate.

3. For an isolated lateral column or capitellar fracture, a Kocher approach may be considered.

   a. A posterior skin incision or an incision going from the lateral epicondyle to a point 6 cm distal to the olecranon tip can be used. The incision can be extended proximally as needed.

   b. For capitellar exposure, the interval of the anconeus and extensor carpi ulnaris (Kocher interval) can be used.

4. Complete articular fractures can be repaired using one of the aforementioned approaches if adequate articular reduction and fixation can be achieved. Complex articular injury may require direct visualization through a transolecranon osteotomy.

   a. It is necessary to find and free the ulnar nerve before performing an olecranon osteotomy. A chevron-style osteotomy pointing distally is made at the level of the bare area of the olecranon.

   b. Some surgeons drill and tap the proximal ulna for larger screw insertion before osteotomizing the olecranon to facilitate later fixation.

   c. After the osteotomy is complete, the entire extensor mechanism can be reflected proximally to allow visualization of the entire distal humerus.

   d. Fixation of the osteotomy can be performed using Kirschner wires and a tension band, a long large-fragment IM screw fixation with a tension band, a plate, or two small-fragment lag screws.

   e. The olecranon osteotomy has potential complications, including nonunion and hardware discomfort.

5. Patients with open distal humerus injuries have been shown to have worse functional and ROM scores than those with closed fractures.

6. Regardless of the fixation approach used, the goals of fixation are anatomic articular reduction, stable internal fixation, and early range of elbow motion.

   a. In patients with irreconstructible or missing segments of the articular surface, care must be taken to avoid decreasing the dimensions of the trochlea and limiting the ability for flexion and extension.

   b. After articular reduction is accomplished, stable fixation of the distal end to the metadiaphyseal component with restoration of the mechanical axis is performed.

E. Mechanism of injury

1. Distal humerus fractures can result from low-energy falls (common in the elderly) or high-energy trauma with extensive comminution and intra-articular involvement (for example, gunshot wounds, motor vehicle accidents, falls from a height).

2. The amount of elbow flexion at the time of impact can affect the fracture pattern.

   a. A transcolumnar fracture results from an axial load directed through the forearm with the elbow flexed 90°.

   b. With the elbow in a similar position but with

direct impact on the olecranon, an olecranon fracture with or without a distal humerus fracture may result.

   c. With the elbow in more than 90° of flexion, an intercondylar fracture may result.

   d. Clinically may have similar presentation to a terrible triad injury (which involves fractures of the medial collateral ligament, the coronoid, and the radial head/neck).

F. Clinical evaluation

  1. Patients typically present with elbow pain and swelling. Crepitus or gross instability with attempted elbow ROM is often observed.

  2. Excessive motion testing should not be performed because of the risk of further neurovascular injury.

  3. A careful neurovascular examination should be performed because all neurovascular structures to the forearm and hand cross the area of injury, and sharp bone fragments can cause damage, especially to the radial nerve, the ulnar nerve, and the brachial artery.

  4. Serial compartment examinations may be required because of extreme cubital fossa swelling or in the obtunded patient to avoid missing a volar forearm compartment syndrome with resultant Volkmann contracture.

G. Radiographic evaluation

  1. AP and lateral views of the humerus and elbow are required.

  2. When concomitant elbow injuries are present, forearm and wrist radiographs may be needed.

  3. To aid in preoperative planning, traction radiographs, oblique radiographs, and CT scans may be of value.

  4. Recently, a blinded study comparing the evaluation of distal humerus fractures based on two-dimensional CT scans and plain radiographs versus three-dimensional CT scans showed that three-dimensional CT scans improved the intraobserver and interobserver reliability of two commonly used classification systems.

H. Supracondylar fractures are OTA type A fractures that are distal metaphyseal and extra-articular.

  1. Nonsurgical treatment is reserved for nondisplaced or minimally displaced fractures or for comminuted fractures in older, low-demand patients.

   a. A splint is applied for 1 to 2 weeks before initiating ROM exercises.

   b. At 6 weeks, with progressive evidence of heal-

ing, immobilization may be discontinued completely.

   c. Up to 20° of loss of condylar shaft angle may be acceptable.

  2. Surgical treatment is indicated for most displaced fractures and for those associated with an open injury or a vascular injury.

   a. Open reduction and internal fixation (ORIF) typically is performed, with plates placed on the medial and lateral columns.

   b. Biomechanical analysis demonstrates that 90-90 plating (medial and posterolateral), bicolumnar plating (medial and lateral), and locked plating constructs are effective in supplying adequate stability.

  3. ROM exercises may be initiated when the soft tissues allow.

I. Transcondylar fractures

  1. Epidemiology—Transcondylar fractures traverse both columns, reside within the joint capsule, and typically are seen in elderly patients.

  2. Mechanism of injury—These fractures occur with a flexed elbow or a fall on an outstretched hand with the arm in abduction or adduction.

  3. Clinical evaluation—The examiner must be wary of a Posadas fracture, which is a transcondylar fracture with anterior displacement of the distal fragment and concomitant dislocation of the radial head and proximal ulna from the fragment.

  4. Treatment

   a. Nonsurgical and surgical management follow recommendations and principles similar to those for supracondylar fractures.

   b. Total elbow arthroplasty may be considered in elderly patients with very distal fractures and poor bone quality.

J. Intercondylar fractures (**Figure 3**)

  1. Epidemiology—Intercondylar fractures are the most common distal humerus fracture; frequently they are comminuted.

  2. Classification

   a. According to the OTA classification, they are type C fractures.

   b. **Table 3** lists the descriptive types.

  3. Pathoanatomy—The medial flexor mass and lateral extensor mass are responsible for rotation and proximal migration of the articular surface.

  4. Treatment

   a. Treatment is primarily surgical, using medial and lateral plate fixation according to the

Table 3

Two-Column Intercondylar Distal Humerus Fractures

Type	Description
High T fracture	A transverse fracture line divides both columns at or proximal to the olecranon fossa
Low T fracture	Similar to the high T fracture except the transverse component is through the olecranon fossa, making treatment and fixation more difficult
Y fracture	Oblique fracture lines cross each column and join in the olecranon fossa, extending vertically to the joint surface
H fracture	The trochlea is a free fragment and at risk for osteonecrosis. The medial column is fractured above and below the medial epicondyle, whereas the lateral column is fractured in a T or Y configuration.
Medial λ fracture	The most proximal fracture line exits medially. Laterally, the fracture line is distal to the lateral epicondyle, rendering a very small fragment left for fixation on the lateral side.
Lateral λ fracture	The most proximal fracture line exits laterally. Medially, the fracture line is distal to the medial epicondyle, rendering a very small fragment left for fixation on the medial side.
Multiplane fracture	This represents a T fracture with concomitant coronal fracture lines

principles and fixation types described previously.

b. In some bicondylar fractures with simple fracture lines and adequate bone quality, lag screw or columnar screw fixation may be used alone or in concert with plate constructs if fracture morphology or osteopenia dictates.

c. The goal is stable fixation to allow early range of elbow motion.

d. In younger patients with extremely comminuted, distal, intra-articular fractures, minifragment fixation can help stabilize smaller fragments.

e. In patients who are older, medically unfit, or have dementia, the "bag of bones" nonsurgical treatment has been described. This involves approximately 2 weeks of immobilization in 90° of elbow flexion followed by gentle ROM to ultimately achieve a minimally painful, functional pseudarthrosis.

f. Total elbow arthroplasty may be selected in elderly patients with unreconstructible fractures. In a recent review of 49 elderly patients with distal humerus fractures treated with total elbow arthroplasty, the mean reported flexion arc was 24° to 131°, and the mean Mayo Elbow Performance Score was 93 out of a possible 100.

K. Condylar fractures

1. Classification

a. These represent OTA type B (partial articular) fractures of the distal humerus.

b. They can be divided into low or high medial/lateral column fractures.

- The following characteristics make a condylar fracture high: the involved column includes most of the trochlea, and the forearm follows the displacement of the fractured column.

- Because of the larger size of high column fractures, internal fixation is more straightforward and frequently can be achieved using lag screws with or without unilateral plating.

- Lateral column fractures are more common.

- The Milch classification system determines fracture stability based on pattern (**Figure 5**). It was suggested that type I fractures (in which the lateral wall of the trochlea is attached to the main mass of the humerus) were stable relative to type II fractures (in which the lateral wall of the trochlea is attached to the displaced fracture fragment).

2. Treatment

a. Surgical treatment is recommended for all but nondisplaced fractures.

b. Nonsurgical—The elbow is positioned in 90° of flexion with the forearm in supination or pronation for lateral or medial column fractures, respectively.

L. Capitellum fractures

1. Classification—Capitellum fractures can be classified into four types (**Figure 6**).

a. Type I (Hahn-Steinhal fragment)—These fractures involve a large osseous component of the capitellum that can include some involvement

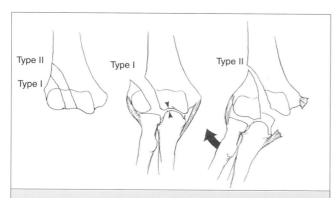

Figure 5 Illustrations show the types of Milch lateral column fractures. Type I: The lateral trochlear ridge remains attached, preventing dislocation of the radius and ulna; Type II: The lateral trochlear ridge is part of the fractured lateral condyle, resulting in dislocation of the radius and ulna. (Reproduced with permission from Koval KJ, Zuckerman JD, eds: *Handbook of Fractures*, ed 2. Philadelphia, PA, Lippincott Williams and Wilkins, 2002, p 98.)

of the trochlea.

   b. Type II (Kocher-Lorenz fragment)—These fractures are separations of articular cartilage with minimal attached subchondral bone.

   c. Type III—These are severely comminuted multifragmentary fractures.

   d. Type IV (added by McKee)—These fractures extend medially into the trochlea.

  2. Treatment

   a. Type I fractures usually require ORIF. Minifragment screw fixation from posterior to anterior or countersunk minifragment screws from anterior to posterior can be used. Alternatively, headless screws may be used.

   b. Typically, type II fractures and irreconstructible parts of type III fractures are excised.

  3. Complications—If instability is present or creeping substitution of devascularized fragments is unsuccessful, arthritis, osteonecrosis, decreased motion, cubital valgus, and tardy ulnar nerve palsy can result.

M. Trochlear fractures

  1. Epidemiology—These fractures are extremely rare in isolation. When they occur, a high index of suspicion is warrented for an associated elbow dislocation that caused a shearing of the articular surface.

  2. Treatment

   a. Nondisplaced fractures may be treated with 3 weeks of immobilization followed by ROM exercises.

   b. Displaced fractures require ORIF or excision if not reconstructible.

N. Epicondylar fractures

  1. Epicondylar fractures may occur on the medial or lateral aspect of the elbow.

  2. Treatment

   a. Epicondylar fractures that are nondisplaced and have a stable elbow joint during ROM may be treated nonsurgically.

   b. In children, medial epicondyle fractures with up to 5 mm of displacement may be treated nonsurgically if no concomitant instability or nerve deficits exist. No specific treatment is recommended for adults.

   c. If the fracture is displaced substantially or has concomitant elbow instability or ulnar nerve symptoms, ORIF with screws or Kirschner wires is recommended.

   d. Consider excision in patients who present late with a painful nonunion or a fragment that cannot be reconstructed.

O. Fracture of the supracondylar process

  1. Anatomy

   a. The supracondylar process is a bony protrusion on the anteromedial surface of the distal humerus and represents a congenital variant.

   b. The ligament of Struthers courses a path from the supracondylar process to the medial epicondyle.

   c. Fibers of the pronator teres or the coracobrachialis muscles may arise from this ligament.

  2. Treatment

   a. A fracture of the supracondylar process most frequently is treated nonsurgically.

   b. Excision is required only if an associated brachial artery injury or median nerve compression is present.

P. Surgical pearls

  1. When approaching the distal humerus from a posterior location, the ulnar nerve should be identified. Approximately 3 to 4 cm proximal to the superior aspect of the medial epicondyle, the nerve can be palpated as it emerges in the area of the intermuscular septum beneath the Osbourne ligament. Subsequently, it can be dissected to the first motor branch of the flexor carpi ulnaris.

  2. If surgical dissection must be carried proximally or laterally, the radial nerve can be found in one of two ways.

   a. Blunt deep dissection approximately 4 cm

3: Trauma

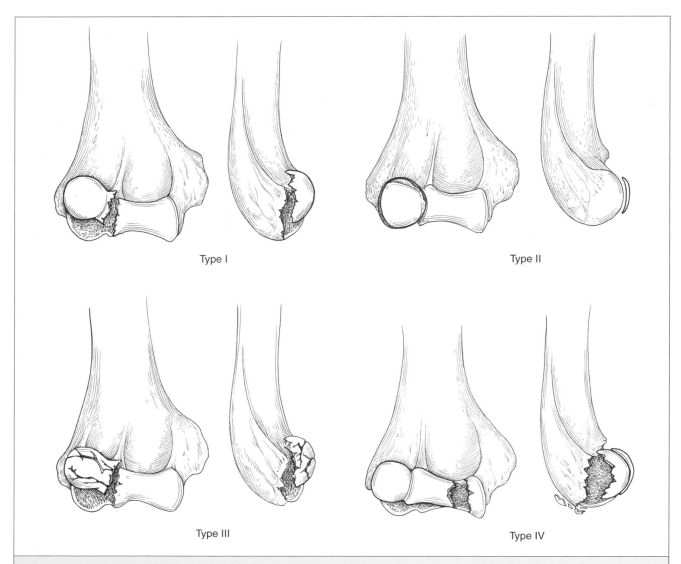

Figure 6   Illustrations depict the Bryan and Morrey classification of a capitellar fracture. Type I (Hahn-Steinthal), complete capitellar fracture with little or no extension into the lateral trochlea. Type II (Kocher-Lorenz), anterior osteochondral fracture with minimal subchondral bone. Type III (Broberg-Morrey variant), comminuted/compression fracture of the capitellum. Type IV extends medially to include most of the trochlea. (Reproduced from Ruchelsman DE, Tejwani NC, Kwon, YW, Egol KA: Coronal plane partial articular fractures of the distal humerus: Current concepts in management. *J Am Acad Orthop Surg* 2008;16[12]:716-728.)

proximal to the fascia of the confluence of the triceps mechanism allows the radial nerve to be palpated in the spiral groove.

  b. Posterolaterally, the radial nerve can be found by retracting the triceps medially to expose the lower lateral brachial cutaneous nerve that branches off the radial nerve on the posterior aspect of the lateral intermuscular septum. This can be traced proximally to identify the radial nerve proper. It is located directly posteriorly at the level of the deltoid tuberosity.

3. When performing an olecranon osteotomy, the apex of the chevron should point distally to en-

sure a larger proximal fragment. This minimizes the risk of fracture with later osteotomy repair.

4. The olecranon osteotomy can be initiated with an oscillating saw but should be completed with an osteotome to avoid making a curve that would decrease the olecranon chondral arc with fixation of the osteotomy.

5. Transient sensory ulnar nerve symptoms may occur. Patients should be warned of this preoperatively.

6. Although the ulnar nerve may be transposed, some surgeons return it to its native location, provided no tethering or abrasive hardware lies in

its path. Regardless, symptoms are seen postoperatively with or without transposition and likely are related to the devascularization following dissection.

7. When operating on a severely comminuted distal humerus fracture in an elderly individual, given the possibility of poor bone quality or a very distal fracture, surgeons should be prepared to perform a total elbow arthroplasty. If attempting internal fixation, a surgical exposure should be selected that will not affect arthroplasty placement negatively if the fracture cannot be reconstructed.

Q. Rehabilitation

1. Postoperatively, the elbow should be immobilized at 90° of flexion, with a wound check after 2 to 3 days.

2. Active and passive ROM of the shoulder, elbow, wrist, and hand usually are initiated within a few days of surgery. If the soft tissue is tenuous, elbow motion is deferred until 7 to 10 days postoperatively, but other therapy is initiated.

3. Typically, with a posterior approach, resistance exercises, especially extension, are delayed for 6 weeks.

R. Outcomes—Closed injuries treated with ORIF ultimately can expect results of approximately 105° arc of motion and the return of approximately 75% of flexion and extension strength. Loss of elbow extension typically is greater than loss of flexion.

S. Complications

1. Fixation failure and malunion are more common with inadequate fixation.

2. Nonunion can occur at the distal humerus fracture or the olecranon osteotomy. When appropriate principles are followed, the incidence is relatively low. In higher-energy trauma and greater soft-tissue injury, the risk is higher.

3. Infection is a relatively uncommon complication (0 to 6%) and has been described most commonly with grade 3 open fractures.

4. Ulnar nerve palsy can be very debilitating. Causes may include iatrogenic injury, inadequate release, impingement resulting from bony causes or hardware, and postoperative fibrosis.

5. Posttraumatic arthritis can result from inappropriate articular reduction or a devastating initial injury. Revision surgery, allograft, or total elbow arthroplasty may be considered in such instances.

Top Testing Facts

1. Most humeral shaft fractures can be treated nonsurgically.

2. Indications for surgical management of humeral shaft fractures include vascular injury, severe soft-tissue injury, open fracture, floating elbow, concomitant intraarticular elbow injury, and pathologic fractures.

3. Extension-type supracondylar fractures are encountered most frequently.

4. IM nailing of humeral shaft fractures is associated with a higher rate of shoulder pain.

5. The terrible triad of elbow injuries involves fractures of the medial collateral ligament, the coronoid, and the radial head/neck.

6. For patients with a concomitant radial nerve injury who do not require surgical treatment, electromyography and/or nerve conduction velocity studies should be performed 6 weeks postinjury. For those who require

surgical treatment, exploration is done at the time of surgery.

7. Total elbow arthroplasty should be considered in low-demand elderly individuals who sustain a complex distal humerus fracture.

8. The radial nerve can be found crossing the mid aspect of the posterior humeral shaft, traversing from proximal medial to distal lateral at the point of confluence, approximately 4 cm proximal to the most proximal aspect of the triceps aponeurosis.

9. In general, distal intercondylar fractures are managed surgically with medial and lateral plate fixation.

10. If a distally pointed chevron osteotomy is made for intraoperative access, the method of stable fixation (tension band, IM screw, plate) has no substantial difference on functional outcome or the need for secondary procedures.

3: Trauma

Bibliography

Ali A, Douglas H, Stanley D: Revision surgery for nonunion after early failure of fixation of fractures of the distal humerus. *J Bone Joint Surg Br* 2005;87(8):1107-1110.

Anglen J: Distal humerus fractures. *J Am Acad Orthop Surg* 2005;13(5):291-297.

Bhandari M, Devereaux PJ, McKee MD, Schemitsch EH: Compression plating versus intramedullary nailing of humeral shaft fractures—a meta-analysis. *Acta Orthop* 2006; 77(2):279-284.

Chalidis B, Dimitriou C, Papadopoulos P, Petsatodis G, Giannoudis PV: Total elbow arthroplasty for the treatment of insufficient distal humeral fractures: A retrospective clinical study and review of the literature. *Injury* 2009;40(6): 582-590.

Coles CP, Barei DP, Nork SE, Taitsman LA, Hanel DP, Bradford Henley M: The olecranon osteotomy: A six-year experience in the treatment of intraarticular fractures of the distal humerus. *J Orthop Trauma* 2006;20(3):164-171.

Denard A Jr, Richards JE, Obremskey WT, Tucker MC, Floyd M, Herzog GA: Outcome of nonoperative vs operative treatment of humeral shaft fractures: A retrospective study of 213 patients. *Orthopedics* 2010;33(8).

Denies E, Nijs S, Sermon A, Broos P: Operative treatment of humeral shaft fractures: Comparison of plating and intramedullary nailing. *Acta Orthop Belg* 2010;76(6):735-742.

Doornberg J, Lindenhovius A, Kloen P, van Dijk CN, Zurakowski D, Ring D: Two and three-dimensional computed tomography for the classification and management of distal humeral fractures: Evaluation of reliability and diagnostic accuracy. *J Bone Joint Surg Am* 2006;88(8):1795-1801.

Egol KA, Tsai P, Vazques O, Tejwani NC: Comparison of functional outcomes of total elbow arthroplasty vs plate fixation for distal humerus fractures in osteoporotic elbows. *Am J Orthop (Belle Mead NJ)* 2011;40(2):67-71.

Erpelding JM, Mailander A, High R, Mormino MA, Fehringer EV: Outcomes following distal humeral fracture fixation with an extensor mechanism-on approach. *J Bone Joint Surg Am* 2012;94(6):548-553.

Frankle MA, Herscovici D Jr, DiPasquale TG, Vasey MB, Sanders RW: A comparison of open reduction and internal fixation and primary total elbow arthroplasty in the treatment of intraarticular distal humerus fractures in women older than age 65. *J Orthop Trauma* 2003;17(7):473-480.

Gardner MJ, Griffith MH, Demetrakopoulos D, et al: Hybrid locked plating of osteoporotic fractures of the humerus. *J Bone Joint Surg Am* 2006;88(9):1962-1967.

Gerwin M, Hotchkiss RN, Weiland AJ: Alternative operative exposures of the posterior aspect of the humeral diaphysis with reference to the radial nerve. *J Bone Joint Surg Am* 1996;78(11):1690-1695.

Gosler MW, Testroote M, Morrenhof JW, Janzing HM: Surgical versus non-surgical interventions for treating humeral shaft fractures in adults. *Cochrane Database Syst Rev* 2012; 1:CD008832.

Hierholzer C, Sama D, Toro JB, Peterson M, Helfet DL: Plate fixation of ununited humeral shaft fractures: Effect of type of bone graft on healing. *J Bone Joint Surg Am* 2006;88(7): 1442-1447.

Mahaisavariya B, Jiamwatthanachai P, Aroonjarattham P, Aroonjarattham K, Wongcumchang M, Sitthiseripratip K: Mismatch analysis of humeral nailing: Antegrade versus retrograde insertion. *J Orthop Sci* 2011;16(5):644-651.

McKee MD, Jupiter JB, Bosse G, Goodman L: Outcome of ulnar neurolysis during post-traumatic reconstruction of the elbow. *J Bone Joint Surg Br* 1998;80(1):100-105.

Min W, Ding BC, Tejwani NC: Comparative functional outcome of AO/OTA type C distal humerus fractures: Open injuries do worse than closed fractures. *J Trauma Acute Care Surg* 2012;72(2):E27-E32.

Ruan HJ, Liu JJ, Fan CY, Jiang J, Zeng BF: Incidence, management, and prognosis of early ulnar nerve dysfunction in type C fractures of distal humerus. *J Trauma* 2009;67(6): 1397-1401.

Sarmiento A, Zagorski JB, Zych GA, Latta LL, Capps CA: Functional bracing for the treatment of fractures of the humeral diaphysis. *J Bone Joint Surg Am* 2000;82(4):478-486.

Schmidt-Horlohé K, Wilde P, Bonk A, Becker L, Hoffmann R: One-third tubular-hook-plate osteosynthesis for olecranon osteotomies in distal humerus type-C fractures: A preliminary report of results and complications. *Injury* 2012;43(3): 295-300.

Seigerman DA, Choung EW, Yoon RS, et al: Identification of the radial nerve during the posterior approach to the humerus: A cadaveric study. *J Orthop Trauma* 2012;26(4): 226-228.

Shao YC, Harwood P, Grotz MR, Limb D, Giannoudis PV: Radial nerve palsy associated with fractures of the shaft of the humerus: A systematic review. *J Bone Joint Surg Br* 2005; 87(12):1647-1652.

Tingstad EM, Wolinsky PR, Shyr Y, Johnson KD: Effect of immediate weightbearing on plated fractures of the humeral shaft. *J Trauma* 2000;49(2):278-280.

Ziran BH, Kinney RC, Smith WR, Peacher G: Sub-muscular plating of the humerus: An emerging technique. *Injury* 2010; 41(10):1047-1052.

Chapter 31

Fractures of the Elbow

Niloofar Dehghan, BSc, MD   Michael D. McKee, MD, FRCSC

I. Radial Head Fractures

A. Epidemiology and overview

  1. Approximately 20% of all elbow fractures involve the radial head.

  2. Radial head fractures can occur in isolation; however, they often are associated with more complex injuries, such as associated elbow fractures, dislocations, and soft-tissue injuries.

  3. The radial head plays an important role as a secondary valgus stabilizer of the elbow.

B. Pathoanatomy

  1. Radial head fractures typically result from a fall on an outstretched hand with the forearm in pronation, which results in an axial load on the elbow.

  2. Of patients with radial head fractures, 30% have other soft-tissue and skeletal injuries, including carpal fractures, distal radioulnar joint (DRUJ) and interosseous membrane disruption, coronoid fractures, Monteggia fracture-dislocations, capitellar fractures, and medial and lateral collateral ligament injuries.

C. Classification—The Mason classification of radial head fractures is shown in **Table 1**.

D. Evaluation

  1. History

    a. Fractures of the radial head typically occur following a fall on an outstretched hand.

    b. The patient should be questioned carefully about concomitant wrist, forearm, or shoulder pain.

  2. Physical examination

    a. Pain with palpation over the radial head

    b. The surgeon should examine elbow range of motion (ROM) and assess for a block to pronation/supination or flexion/extension.

    c. The surgeon should examine the forearm, wrist, and elbow for tenderness along the course of the interosseous membrane (Essex-Lopresti lesion), instability of the DRUJ, pain at the medial side of the elbow (medial collateral ligament [MCL]), and pain at the lateral side of the elbow (lateral collateral ligament [LCL]).

    d. Lateral elbow pain and tenderness or limitation in elbow or forearm motion should alert the examiner to the possibility of a radial head fracture.

  3. Imaging

    a. AP and lateral radiographs of the elbow are routinely obtained.

    b. Nondisplaced fractures of the radial head may not be visible; however, they may be diagnosed by elevation of the anterior and posterior fat pads (the sail sign) by an intra-articular hemarthrosis.

    c. The radiocapitellar view is accomplished by positioning the patient as for a lateral view but angling the tube 45° toward the shoulder.

    d. For comminuted fractures, CT can delineate the location, number, and size of the fragments and is rapidly emerging as a standard imaging method for more complicated radial head fractures.

  4. Joint aspiration—Aspiration of the intra-articular hematoma and injection of a local anesthetic can be helpful when assessing mechanical blocks to motion.

E. Treatment

  1. Nonsurgical—Most minimally displaced (< 3 mm) radial head fractures can be treated nonsur-

Dr. McKee or an immediate family member has received royalties from Stryker; is a member of a speakers' bureau or has made paid presentations on behalf of Synthes and Zimmer; serves as a paid consultant to or is an employee of Synthes and Zimmer; has received research or institutional support from Wright Medical Technology and Zimmer; and serves as a board member, owner, officer, or committee member of the American Shoulder and Elbow Surgeons, the Orthopaedic Trauma Association, and the Canadian Orthopaedic Association. Neither Dr. Dehghan nor any immediate family member has received anything of value from or has stock or stock options held in a commercial company or institution related directly or indirectly to the subject of this chapter.

3: Trauma

gically if no block to ROM is present, with a brief period of immobilization (7 to 10 days maximum) in a sling or posterior splint for pain relief followed by early ROM exercises.

Table 1

Mason Classification of Radial Head Fractures

Fracture Type	Characteristic(s)
I	Fracture is minimally displaced
II	Fracture is displaced
III	Fracture is comminuted and displaced
IV*	Fracture of the radial head with dislocation of the ulnohumeral joint

*Type IV added by Johnston.

2. Surgical—Radial head fractures that are significantly displaced, block motion (especially rotation), or are part of more complicated injury patterns are candidates for surgical repair.

3. Surgical procedures

a. Open reduction and internal fixation (ORIF) options

- Screws—Mini fragment screws (2.7 or 2.0 mm) or headless screws with differential pitch (for example, Herbert screw, headless compression screw) should be countersunk to prevent screw prominence.

- Plates and screws—Plates should be placed in the "safe zone," the part of the radial head that does not articulate with the proximal ulna, which is the arc between the lines drawn through the radial styloid and the Lister tubercle (**Figure 1**).

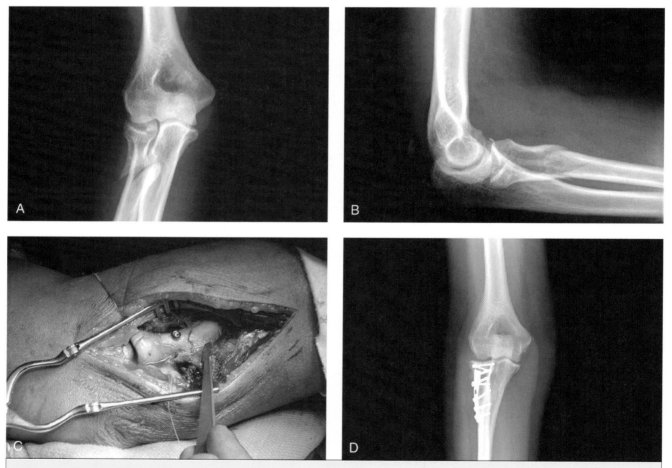

Figure 1   An active 32-year-old woman sustained a comminuted, displaced, intra-articular radial head and neck fracture. The patient had minimal, painful forearm rotation preoperatively. Preoperative AP (**A**) and lateral (**B**) radiographs demonstrate the fracture. **C,** Intraoperative photograph shows countersunk screw fixation of the head fracture and initial lag screw fixation of the neck fracture. The fixation was placed in the "safe zone," the nonarticular portion of the neck, in an arc subtended by lines through the radial styloid and the Lister tubercle. A mini-fragment plate was subsequently applied. **D,** Postoperative AP radiograph shows the completed procedure.

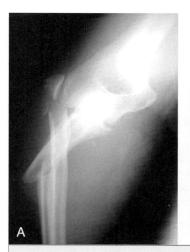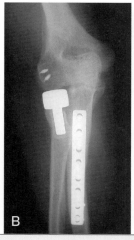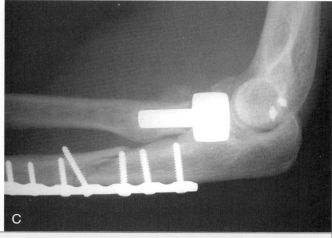

Figure 2 A 37-year-old patient sustained a Monteggia variant injury in a fall. **A,** Preoperative AP radiograph shows an angulated fracture of the proximal ulna with a comminuted posterolateral fracture-dislocation of the radial head. AP **(B)** and lateral **(C)** radiographs show the elbow following open reduction and internal fixation of the ulnar shaft; radial head replacement with a modular, metallic prosthesis; and repair of the lateral collateral ligament with suture anchors in the lateral column.

b. Radial head replacement for comminuted fractures

- This is a good treatment option in cases with more than three fracture fragments, which have a higher rate of failure with surgical fixation (**Figure 2**).

- The most commonly used radial head replacement prosthesis is a modular, metallic, uncemented prosthesis.

c. Radial head excision—The radial head is an important secondary stabilizer of the elbow; therefore, radial head excision alone is contraindicated in clinical settings in which extensive damage to the primary stabilizers (MCL: valgus instability; coronoid: posterior instability; interosseous membrane: longitudinal instability; LCL: posterolateral rotatory instability) is present.

F. Pearls and pitfalls

1. Isolated fractures heal best with early mobilization after 7 to 10 days.

2. Hardware should be applied to the safe zone.

3. Radial head fractures with three or more fragments have a higher incidence of unsatisfactory results with fixation. The surgeon should consider replacement, rather than fixation, for such fractures.

4. Radial head excision alone is contraindicated in the presence of other destabilizing injuries.

G. Rehabilitation

1. For nondisplaced radial head fractures: immobilization in a sling for 7 to 10 days followed by early ROM exercises

2. For other nonsurgically treated stable fractures and for surgically treated fractures: immobilization in a posterior splint for 7 to 10 days, followed by early ROM exercises

H. Complications of radial head fractures

1. Stiffness (especially forearm rotation)

2. Replacement of the radial head with a prosthesis that is too large (overstuffing the joint)

3. Fracture displacement (occurs in < 5% of cases)

4. Radiocapitellar arthritis

5. Infection

6. Loss of fixation

II. Olecranon Fractures

A. Epidemiology and overview

1. Olecranon fractures can result from several different mechanisms, including a direct blow, a fall on an outstretched hand with the elbow in flexion, or high-energy trauma that is associated with radial head fractures or elbow dislocation.

2. Sudden and violent triceps muscle contraction can produce an avulsion fracture of varying size of the olecranon tip.

3. A bimodal distribution of olecranon fractures is seen: young patients with high-energy trauma, and elderly patients with low-energy trauma such as a fall from standing.

3:Trauma

Table 2

Colton Classification of Olecranon Fractures

Fracture Type	Characteristics
I	Fracture is nondisplaced and stable, with < 2 mm of separation; the extensor mechanism is intact and the patient is able to extend the elbow against gravity with flexion to 90°.
II	Fracture is displaced. Type IIA—Avulsion Type IIB—Oblique and transverse Type IIC—Comminuted Type IID—Fracture-dislocation

B. Pathoanatomy

1. The olecranon and the coronoid process form the greater sigmoid notch, which articulates with the trochlea of the distal humerus. The intrinsic anatomy of this articulation allows flexion/extension movement of the elbow joint and provides stability for the elbow.

2. The olecranon also serves as the insertion for the triceps tendon, which blends with the periosteum of the proximal ulna.

3. The exposed position of the olecranon renders it vulnerable to direct trauma and violent muscular contractions (from the triceps).

C. Classification—The Colton classification of olecranon fractures is shown in **Table 2**.

D. Evaluation

1. History

   a. The history may help distinguish a triceps avulsion from an actual direct blow to the elbow.

   b. Pain usually is localized to the posterior part of the elbow.

2. Physical examination

   a. Given the subcutaneous location of the olecranon, the fracture itself may be palpable.

   b. Extensive posterior swelling is typical.

   c. A careful examination of the integrity of the extensor mechanism (with gravity eliminated) can aid surgical decision making.

   d. If present, open wounds are typically posterior and result from the direct impact of the posterior surface of the elbow against an unyielding structure.

3. Imaging

   a. Plain radiographs are usually sufficient for isolated fractures of the olecranon.

   b. A true lateral radiograph is necessary to accurately identify the plane of the fracture and the number of fracture fragments. The examiner also should assess for fracture comminution and impaction.

   c. In more complex cases, CT may help delineate the comminution or impaction better; however, this is not routinely required.

E. Treatment

1. Goals—The goals of olecranon fracture management include articular restoration, preservation of the extensor mechanism, elbow stability, avoidance of stiffness, and minimization of complications.

2. Nonsurgical—Nondisplaced fractures (Colton type I), although uncommon, can be treated effectively by immobilizing the limb in a long arm splint or cast with the elbow flexed at 60° to 90° for 4 weeks.

3. Surgical

   a. Displaced fractures (Colton type II and its subtypes) require surgical fixation in healthy, active patients to preserve the strength of the extensor mechanism and maintain intra-articular congruity.

   b. Contraindications include active infection and severe medical comorbidities.

4. Surgical procedures

   a. Tension band wiring technique over two Kirschner wires (K-wires)

   - Indications—Isolated, transverse fractures that are proximal to the coronoid, without significant comminution, and not associated with ligamentous instability

   - This technique does not resist angular forces or stabilize complex fracture patterns.

   - Contraindications—Significantly comminuted fractures of the proximal ulna (**Figure 3**), especially those with associated elbow instability

   - Insertion of K-wires into the anterior cortex of the ulna distal to the fracture line enhances fixation strength and may help prevent backing out. The surgeon must be aware of overpenetration of the anterior cortex, however, which may result in a decrease in ROM and risk injury to the anterior interosseous nerve.

b. Dorsal plate application to the posterior aspect of the proximal ulna (**Figure 4**)

- Dorsal plate application is the preferred fixation method if comminution or associated ligamentous injury with instability is present. (Question A-50)

- The terminal aspect of the triceps insertion can be elevated and then repaired following plate application to minimize prominence.

c. Fragment excision and triceps reattachment for osteoporotic, comminuted fragments composing less than 50% of the olecranon.

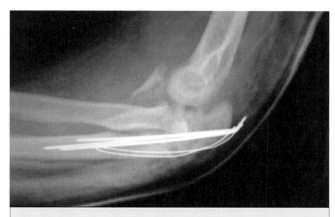

Figure 3   Lateral radiograph of the elbow of a 42-year-old man who sustained an early, recurrent posterior subluxation of the elbow following attempted fixation of a proximal ulnar fracture using a tension band technique demonstrates that the coronoid fragment has not been stabilized and the associated fracture of the radial head has not been addressed.

- May be beneficial for elderly (> 70 years), low-demand patients whose bones are osteoporotic enough to compromise fixation

- This procedure cannot be performed if associated ligamentous instability is present.

- Some evidence has shown that elderly, low-demand patients may function reasonably well with nonsurgical care of displaced fractures.

5. Pearls and pitfalls

a. The tension band technique should be used only for fractures that are proximal to the base of the coracoid and that occur secondary to eccentric loads.

b. Dorsal contoured plate application is the preferred fixation method in fractures secondary to bending mechanisms (including those distal to the coronoid), fractures with comminution, or associated ligamentous injury with instability.

6. Rehabilitation

a. Nonsurgically managed fractures that are minimally displaced with an intact extensor mechanism can be immobilized in a long arm splint with radiographic monitoring and mobilized at 4 weeks.

b. Surgically managed fractures are splinted for up to 1 week for pain control and to allow swelling to subside.

- Active and gentle passive motion is then initiated, but resisted extension is specifically restricted until clinical and radiographic evidence of fracture healing is apparent, usually at 6 weeks postoperatively.

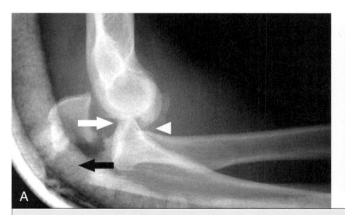
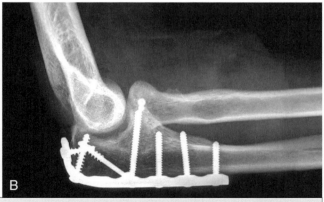

Figure 4   Lateral radiographs from a 17-year-old boy who sustained an elbow dislocation. **A,** Preoperative radiograph demonstrates the dislocation and associated olecranon (black arrow), coronoid (white arrowhead), and radial head (white arrow) fractures. **B,** Postoperative lateral radiograph shows the elbow following open reduction and internal fixation of the radial head fragment with a single countersunk Herbert screw, plate fixation of the ulna, and repair of the lateral collateral ligament through drill holes in the lateral column. A concentric reduction of the radiocapitellar and ulnohumeral joints was achieved, with sufficient stability to initiate immediate motion, enhancing the functional result.

• Older patients who typically use forceful elbow extension to rise from a chair or a toilet should be advised to avoid this activity until fracture union occurs.

7. Complications

a. Stiffness (typically with terminal extension)

b. Loss of reduction is rare if the proper principles of fixation are followed. As described previously, tension band wiring of fractures associated with comminution or elbow instability can lead to failure of the construct and loss of reduction and should be treated with plate fixation instead.

c. Nonunion is rare, but malunion (especially of unreduced, impacted articular fragments) may result in posttraumatic arthritic change and stiffness.

d. Hardware prominence and the need for hardware removal after fracture healing are common because of the subcutaneous nature of the olecranon.

e. Overpenetration of the anterior cortex with K-wires can result in a decrease in pronation/supination and puts the anterior interosseous nerve at risk for injury.

III. Proximal Ulnar Fractures

A. Epidemiology and overview

1. Although they may seem complex, proximal ulnar fractures tend to fall into one of three basic injury patterns.

   a. Simple olecranon fractures

   b. Olecranon fracture-dislocations

   c. Monteggia fractures and variants—Fracture of the proximal ulna with associated radial head dislocation or fracture

2. Most of these injuries require surgical intervention.

3. Posterior fracture-dislocations of the proximal ulna are associated with a high incidence of radial head fractures and LCL injuries.

B. Pathoanatomy

1. A fall directly on the elbow can produce a transolecranon fracture-dislocation because the distal humerus acts as a pile driver and drives through the trochlear notch of the ulna.

2. A fall on an outstretched hand results in a posteriorly directed force vector to the elbow and can produce a posterior fracture-dislocation or a (posterior) Monteggia fracture.

C. Classification—The Bado classification defines four types of Monteggia fractures according to the direction of displacement of the radial head and other characteristics (**Table 3**). A Bado type II injury, which is associated with a posterior radial head dislocation, is the most common type of injury pattern in adults. This subtype is associated with the highest complication rate.

D. Evaluation

1. History

   a. The history should include a clarification of the exact mechanism of injury, any sensation of dislocation with spontaneous reduction, and any associated upper extremity pain or discomfort.

   b. Any reports of wrist and/or forearm pain should alert the treating surgeon to the possibility of a more complex injury pattern.

2. Physical examination

   a. The elbow is typically swollen, especially posteriorly.

   b. If present, open wounds are usually posterior or posterolateral.

   c. Neurologic examination, especially of the posterior interosseous nerve, should be performed.

   d. The wrist should be examined for any evidence of a distal radioulnar injury (a bipolar forearm injury).

3. Imaging

   a. Radiographs

   • Plain radiographs are the mainstay of imaging; they usually show the general injury pattern.

   • On normal AP and lateral radiographs, a line drawn through the center of the proximal radial shaft and the center of the radial head should bisect the capitellum. If the radial head does not line up with the capitellum, concern should arise about subluxation or dislocation of the radial head (**Figure 5**).

   • Repeat radiographs obtained after a gentle reduction and splinting can provide more detailed information. It is important to look for associated bony injuries in this situation; radial head fractures, coronoid fragments, and collateral ligament avulsions are common.

   b. CT may help define the size and location of fracture fragments and in confirming associated injuries.

Table 3

Bado Classification of Monteggia Fractures

Fracture Type	Description		Direction of Displacement of the Radial Head	Characteristic(s)
I	Fracture of the middle or proximal third of the ulna		Anterior	More common in children and young adults
II	Fracture of the middle or proximal third of the ulna		Posterior	Comprise most (70% to 80%) Monteggia fractures in adults
III	Fracture of the ulna distal to the coronoid process		Lateral	More common in children
IV	Fracture of the middle or proximal third of the ulna and fracture of the proximal third of the radius		Any direction	Least common

Adapted from Turner RG, King GJW: Proximal ulnar fractures and fracture dislocations, in Galatz LM, ed: *Orthopaedic Knowledge Update: Shoulder and Elbow*, ed 3. Rosemont, IL, American Academy of Orthopaedic Surgeons, 2008, pp 517-529.

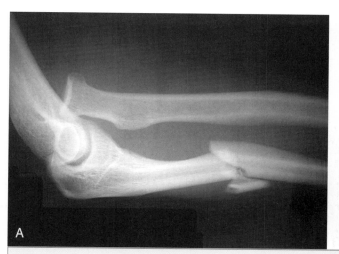 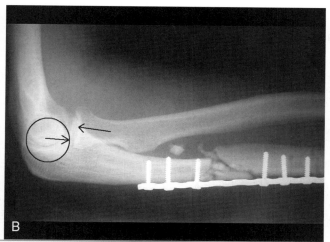

Figure 5   **A,** Preoperative lateral radiograph of the elbow shows a Monteggia fracture, with fracture of the proximal ulnar shaft and an associated anterior radial head displacement. **B,** Postoperative lateral radiograph obtained after attempted fixation that resulted in malreduction of the proximal ulnar shaft. This malreduction has caused anterior subluxation of the radial head. The circle represents the capitellum; the arrows bisect the radial head and the capitellum. In a reduced elbow, these arrows should line up; note that the arrow bisecting the radial head is more anterior than the arrow bisecting the capitellum.

3: Trauma

E. Treatment

1. Nonsurgical—Stable, noncomminuted fractures of the proximal ulna that are not associated with other injuries about the elbow can be treated nonsurgically. This injury pattern is relatively rare, however; most require surgical intervention.

2. Surgical

a. Complex proximal ulnar fractures often contain a substantial coronoid fragment, which is typically triangular and involves 50% to 100% of the coronoid process. This fragment is important for re-creating the anterior buttress of the greater sigmoid notch of the proximal ulna.

b. Coronoid reduction and fixation is a critical component of elbow stability.

c. Once the main proximal-distal fragment fracture line of the ulna is reduced, visualization and repair of the coronoid become difficult. Thus, it is important to fix the coronoid fragment (usually with lag screws) to the distal ulnar fragment before reducing the primary ulnar fracture line.

d. Fixation of the proximal ulnar fracture should be performed with a small fragment compression plate contoured to project proximally around the tip of the olecranon.

e. A similar approach is used for Monteggia fracture patterns: ORIF of the ulna with a 3.5-mm compression plate through a posterior approach.

f. Ulnar fracture malreduction is the usual cause of any residual subluxation or dislocation of the radiocapitellar joint (**Figure 5**).

F. Pearls and pitfalls

1. Failure to recognize associated radial head and LCL injuries can lead to recurrent instability.

2. Loss of fixation from inadequate plate selection, length, or placement is exacerbated by the osteoporotic bone of older individuals.

3. Extensive soft-tissue damage, the use of surgical approaches that expose radial and ulnar fracture sites together (often necessary), prolonged immobilization, or concomitant radial head injury can lead to radioulnar stiffness or even synostosis.

4. Ulnar fracture malreduction is the most common cause of residual radial head malalignment in a Monteggia fracture-dislocation.

G. Rehabilitation

1. Postsurgical rehabilitation depends largely on the fracture/ligament fixation obtained intraoperatively and on the results of stability testing at the conclusion of the procedure.

2. Typically, a well-padded posterior splint is applied with the elbow at 90° and the forearm in pronation to protect a lateral-side ligament repair.

3. If adequate stability has been achieved, early motion with active and gentle passive exercises is instituted within 1 week after surgery, and the patient is weaned from the splint.

4. Strengthening is instituted at 6 to 8 weeks. Even in marginally repaired fractures, active muscle contraction of the dynamic stabilizers, such as the flexor-pronator mass and the common extensor origin, may improve the concentric stability of the ulnohumeral joint, analogous to active deltoid exercises in a shoulder with inferior subluxation after trauma.

H. Complications

1. The reported complication rate for fractures of the proximal ulna is high.

2. Simple fractures tend to heal well, but management of complex fractures has been hampered by a poor understanding of injury patterns and deforming forces, inadequate fixation, and prolonged immobilization of tenuously repaired fractures (**Figure 3**).

3. The risk of proximal radioulnar synostosis is increased by multiple surgeries, extensive soft-tissue damage or dissection, exposure of the radius and ulna together, and concomitant radial head injuries.

IV. Coronoid Fractures

A. Epidemiology and overview

1. The coronoid acts as the anterior buttress of the greater sigmoid notch of the olecranon, and it is the primary resistor of posterior elbow subluxation or dislocation.

2. A coronoid fracture, identified in as many as 10% to 15% of elbow injuries, is pathognomonic of an episode of elbow instability.

3. Fractures at the base of the coronoid can exacerbate elbow instability because the sublime tubercle is the attachment site for the anterior bundle of the MCL, and the tip of the coronoid is the attachment site for the middle part of the anterior capsule.

4. Associated injuries are common, including fracture of the radial head or olecranon, injury to the LCL or MCL, or associated elbow dislocation.

B. Pathoanatomy

1. An intact coronoid resists posterior elbow displacement.

Table 4

Regan and Morrey Classification of Coronoid Fractures

Fracture Type	Characteristics
I	Fracture of the tip of the coronoid process
II	Fracture involves ≤ 50% of the coronoid process
III	Fracture involves > 50% of the coronoid process

2. The coronoid typically is fractured as the distal humerus is driven against it during an episode of posterior subluxation or severe varus stress.

3. Previously, type I and even some type II coronoid fractures (see Classification below) were considered avulsion fractures produced by the anterior capsule; however, this does not describe the mechanism of injury, which is primarily a shearing force.

4. The medial facet is important for varus stability, and the sublime tubercle just distal to it provides insertion for the MCL.

5. Anteromedial facet fractures occur from a primarily varus force, are often associated with an LCL injury, and represent a distinct subtype of injury.

6. Posteromedial rotatory instability results from anteromedial coronoid fracture and disruption of the LCL.

7. Posterolateral rotatory instability is associated with injury to the LCL; it is often associated with radial head fracture and coronoid tip fracture.

C. Classification

1. The Regan and Morrey classification is shown in **Table 4**.

2. O'Driscoll classification—O'Driscoll has proposed a more comprehensive classification scheme that subdivides the coronoid injury based on the location and the number of coronoid fragments. This scheme is important because it recognizes fractures of the anteromedial facet caused by a varus posteromedial rotatory force (**Figure 6**).

3. Anteromedial facet fractures are a different entity from the usual coronoid fractures. They may involve the rim, the tip, or the sublime tubercle and result in varus and posteromedial rotatory instability. These fractures result from a varus injury mechanism, commonly require surgical fixation with a buttress plate used medially, and usually are associated with LCL avulsions.

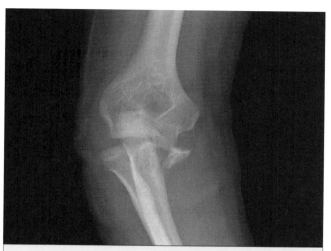

Figure 6 AP radiograph of the elbow of a young man demonstrates a posteromedial rotatory elbow injury from a varus deforming force. The varus position of the joint, with an avulsion of the lateral collateral ligament and a compression fracture of the anteromedial facet of the coronoid, is seen clearly. This injury pattern requires buttress plate fixation of the coronoid fracture and lateral ligament repair for an optimal outcome.

D. Evaluation

1. History

a. A history of dislocation with spontaneous reduction may be elicited.

b. Pain in the forearm or wrist may be a sign of associated injuries that require further evaluation and imaging.

2. Physical examination

a. Examination for instability is difficult but important for an accurate diagnosis.

b. A varus attitude of the elbow and pain on varus stress indicate a posteromedial rotatory injury (**Figure 6**).

3. Imaging

a. Standard AP and lateral radiographs should be obtained; however, the amorphous structure of the coronoid and the overlap of adjacent structures can make interpretation difficult.

b. CT can be useful in this setting, especially for higher grades of comminuted coronoid fractures.

E. Treatment

1. Nonsurgical

a. The decision to treat a coronoid fracture surgically or nonsurgically is based on the associated injuries (radial head fracture, collateral

3: Trauma

ligament tears) and the evaluation of elbow joint stability.

   b. A minimally displaced type I or II fracture with no associated injuries and a stable elbow on examination is rare but may be treated with a brief period of immobilization for pain control followed by early ROM exercises. Most elbow dislocations are more stable with the forearm in pronation.

2. Surgical

   a. Most coronoid fractures require surgical fixation because of elbow instability and are associated with other fractures or ligamentous injuries.

   b. Concurrent injuries (radial head fracture, ligament tears) also must be addressed.

   c. Surgical approach

- Lateral—This is ideal in cases associated with fracture of the radial head when the radial head will be replaced. The Kocher, Kaplan, or Hotchkiss approach may be used, depending on the presence of other injuries requiring fixation. After the radial head is removed, the coronoid can be visualized easily and repaired. The LCL complex also can be repaired at the end of the case.

- Medial—This is ideal for coronoid fractures that cannot be accessed from the lateral side because of the presence of the radial head or in situations with anteromedial facet fractures, which are visualized better from the medial side. Intervals include working between the two heads of the flexor carpi ulnaris or splitting the flexor pronator mass more anteriorly as described by Hotchkiss. The MCL may be repaired at the end of the case.

   d. Types of fixation

- Small type I or II coronoid fractures can be repaired with suture fixation by passing sutures through drill holes in the proximal aspect of the ulna and capturing the coronoid fragment and anterior elbow capsule for fixation.

- Larger type II or III coronoid fractures may require retrograde screws or plate insertion.

- Fractures involving the medial facet can be repaired with a buttress plate for rigid fixation.

- Hinged external fixation may be used to help maintain stability in difficult or revision cases.

F. Pearls and pitfalls

1. In the setting of a complex proximal ulnar fracture, the coronoid fragment is an important bulwark against recurrent posterior subluxation.

2. Larger coronoid fragments frequently include the insertion of the MCL.

3. In the setting of a complex proximal ulnar fracture, the coronoid fragment should be repaired before the main ulnar fracture is reduced.

4. Fixation of the coronoid fragment can be performed with cannulated screws from the posterior surface of the ulna.

5. Anteromedial facet fractures are best treated with a buttress plate via a medial approach.

G. Rehabilitation

1. Rehabilitation depends on an intraoperative examination at the conclusion of the procedure.

2. A thermoplastic resting splint is applied with the elbow at 90° and the forearm in the neutral position.

3. The terminal 30° of extension is restricted for the first 2 to 4 weeks.

4. Shoulder abduction, which places a varus moment on the arm, is avoided for the first 4 to 6 weeks in fractures/fracture-dislocations with varus instability.

5. Increasing evidence shows that some residual ulnohumeral "sagging" or gapping after the surgical repair of elbow injuries may rapidly improve under the influence of the dynamic muscle contraction that early active motion provides.

H. Complications

1. Complication and repeat surgery rates are high.

2. Complications include stiffness of the elbow, recurrent instability of the elbow, posttraumatic arthritic degeneration, and heterotopic ossification.

3. Failure to appreciate—and surgically repair—the underlying associated elbow instability results in early failure of fixation (**Figures 3 and 6**).

Top Testing Facts

Radial Head Fractures

1. The forearm and wrist should be examined carefully in all cases of radial head fracture.

2. Most radial head fractures can be treated nonsurgically.

3. Isolated radial head fractures do best with early mobilization, not prolonged casting. The patient should not be immobilized for more than 7 to 10 days.

4. Radial head fractures that block motion or are significantly displaced can be treated with ORIF.

5. If a plate is used for radial head fixation, it should be placed in the "safe zone," away from articulation with the proximal ulna, between the radial styloid and Lister's tubercle.

6. Comminuted fractures with more than three fragments benefit from radial head replacement using a metal, modular prosthesis.

7. Radial head excision alone is contraindicated in the presence of other destabilizing injuries.

Olecranon Fractures

1. The integrity of the extensor mechanism should be examined carefully.

2. The tension band technique is indicated for isolated, noncomminuted olecranon fractures proximal to the coronoid, without ligamentous instability. Failure to adhere to this principle may lead to failure of fixation.

3. Insertion of K-wires into the anterior cortex of the ulna distal to the fracture line enhances fixation strength and may help prevent backing out.

4. Plate fixation is preferred for comminuted fractures, fractures with coronoid extension, or fractures associated with elbow instability.

5. Fragment excision and triceps reattachment may be beneficial for elderly, low-demand patients whose bones are osteoporotic enough to compromise fixation.

Proximal Ulnar Fractures

1. Posterior fracture-dislocations of the proximal ulna are associated with a high incidence of radial head fractures and LCL injuries.

2. Type II (posterior radial head displacement) Monteggia fractures compose 70% to 80% of Monteggia fractures in adults.

3. Complex proximal ulnar fractures often contain a significant coronoid fragment, which is typically triangular and involves 50% to 100% of the coronoid process. This fragment is important for re-creating the anterior buttress of the greater sigmoid notch of the proximal ulna.

4. Coronoid reduction and fixation are critical components of elbow stability.

5. The risk of proximal radioulnar synostosis is increased by multiple surgeries, extensive soft-tissue damage or dissection, and concomitant radial head injuries.

6. Ulnar fracture malreduction is the most common cause of residual radial head malalignment in a Monteggia fracture-dislocation.

Coronoid Fractures

1. The presence of a coronoid fracture is pathognomonic of an episode of elbow instability, and associated injuries are common.

2. A coronoid fracture is not typically an avulsion fracture but is caused by a shearing mechanism.

3. Anteromedial facet fractures occur from a primarily varus force, are often associated with an LCL injury, and represent a distinct subtype of injury.

4. Hinged external fixation may be used to help maintain stability in difficult or revision cases.

5. In the setting of a complex proximal ulnar fracture, the coronoid fragment is an important restraint against recurrent posterior subluxation. In these situations, the coronoid fragment should be repaired before the main ulnar fracture is reduced.

6. Larger coronoid fragments are important because they frequently include the insertion of the MCL.

7. Fixation of the coronoid fragment can be performed with cannulated screws from the posterior surface of the ulna or with suture fixation if the fragment is small.

8. Fractures involving the anteromedial facet can be repaired with a buttress plate for rigid fixation via a medial approach.

Bibliography

Bryan RS, Morrey BF: Extensive posterior exposure of the elbow: A triceps-sparing approach. *Clin Orthop Relat Res* 1982;166:188-192.

Doornberg JN, Ring DC: Fracture of the anteromedial facet of the coronoid process. *J Bone Joint Surg Am* 2006;88(10): 2216-2224.

Flinkkilä T, Kaisto T, Sirniö K, Hyvönen P, Leppilahti J: Short- to mid-term results of metallic press-fit radial head arthroplasty in unstable injuries of the elbow. *J Bone Joint Surg Br* 2012;94(6):805-810.

Frankle MA, Koval KJ, Sanders RW, Zuckerman JD: Radial head fractures associated with elbow dislocations treated by immediate stabilization and early motion. *J Shoulder Elbow Surg* 1999;8(4):355-360.

Johnston GW: A follow-up of one hundred cases of fracture of the head of the radius with a review of the literature. *Ulster Med J* 1962;31:51-56.

Macko D, Szabo RM: Complications of tension-band wiring of olecranon fractures. *J Bone Joint Surg Am* 1985;67(9): 1396-1401.

Mathew PK, Athwal GS, King GJ: Terrible triad injury of the elbow: Current concepts. *J Am Acad Orthop Surg* 2009; 17(3):137-151.

McKee MD, Jupiter JB: Trauma to the adult elbow and fractures of the distal humerus, in Browner B, Jupiter J, Levine A, Trafton P: *Skeletal Trauma*, ed 3. Philadelphia, PA, WB Saunders, 2003, pp 1404-1480.

McKee MD, Pugh DM, Wild LM, Schemitsch EH, King GJ: Standard surgical protocol to treat elbow dislocations with radial head and coronoid fractures: Surgical technique. *J Bone Joint Surg Am* 2005;87(pt 1, suppl 1):22-32.

Moro JK, Werier J, MacDermid JC, Patterson SD, King GJ: Arthroplasty with a metal radial head for unreconstructible fractures of the radial head. *J Bone Joint Surg Am* 2001; 83(8):1201-1211.

O'Driscoll SW, Jupiter JB, Cohen MS, Ring D, McKee MD: Difficult elbow fractures: Pearls and pitfalls. *Instr Course Lect* 2003;52:113-134.

Pollock JW, Brownhill J, Ferreira L, McDonald CP, Johnson J, King G: The effect of anteromedial facet fractures of the coronoid and lateral collateral ligament injury on elbow stability and kinematics. *J Bone Joint Surg Am* 2009;91(6): 1448-1458.

Ring D: Fractures and dislocations of the elbow, in Bucholz RW, Heckman JD, Court-Brown CM, eds: *Rockwood and Green's Fractures in Adults*, ed 46. Philadelphia, PA, Lippincott Williams & Wilkins, 2001, pp 989-1049.

Ring D, Quintero J, Jupiter JB: Open reduction and internal fixation of fractures of the radial head. *J Bone Joint Surg Am* 2002;84(10):1811-1815.

Sanchez-Sotelo J, O'Driscoll SW, Morrey BF: Medial oblique compression fracture of the coronoid process of the ulna. *J Shoulder Elbow Surg* 2005;14(1):60-64.

Turner RG, King JWG: Proximal ulnar fractures and fracture-dislocations, in Galatz LM, ed: *Orthopaedic Knowledge Update: Shoulder and Elbow*, ed 3. Rosemont, IL, American Academy of Orthopaedic Surgeons, 2008, pp 517-529.

Chapter 32

Terrible Triad Injuries of the Elbow

Robert Z. Tashjian, MD

I. Overview

A. Elbow dislocations are categorized as simple (no associated fracture) and complex (associated fracture).

B. Terrible triad injuries refer to complex elbow dislocations that include posterolateral elbow dislocation, a radial head or neck fracture, and a coronoid process fracture. They are characterized by historically poor outcomes, secondary to persistent instability, stiffness, and arthrosis.

C. Generally, nonsurgical management has a limited role in the management of terrible triad injuries.

D. Surgical treatment using a standard protocol of coronoid fracture fixation, if possible, radial head fracture fixation or replacement, and lateral ligamentous repair can result in predictable results.

1. A standardized surgical protocol results in an average flexion arc of 112° and 77% good or excellent results.

2. Complications include stiffness, heterotopic bone formation, infection, ulnar neuropathy, persistent instability, nonunion, and malunion. Revision surgery is necessary in 20% to 25% of cases.

II. Pathoanatomy and Biomechanics

A. The primary stabilizing components of the elbow involved with terrible triad injuries include the radial head, the coronoid, the ligamentous structures (the lateral and medial collateral ligaments), and the common extensor mechanism.

1. Coronoid process—An important anterior and varus stabilizer to the ulnohumeral joint

a. Anatomic components of the coronoid process include the tip, body, anterolateral facet, and anteromedial facet. The O'Driscoll fracture classification is based on the fracture location

of these subregions.

b. Biomechanically, the coronoid process provides resistance to posterior subluxation beyond 30° of flexion. Small (<10% of height) fractures have been shown to have little effect on elbow stability.

c. In radial excision with intact ligaments, coronoid resection of 30% fully destabilizes the ulnohumeral joint, although stability is restored with radial replacement. In larger coronoid defects (50% to 70% resection), stability cannot be restored by radial head replacement alone.

d. The coronoid process fracture in this type of injury is typically simple, transverse, and small (O'Driscoll type 1; <30% of height); average height is 35% of total coronoid height. Based on biomechanical data on the restoration of joint stability, most should be repaired.

e. The coronoid fragment always has some anterior capsule attached, which can be useful for soft-tissue repair of the fracture.

2. Radial head

a. The radial head is an important secondary valgus stabilizer. It provides approximately 30% of valgus stability with intact medial ligaments.

b. The radial head also is a primary restraint to posterolateral rotatory instability.

c. In biomechanical studies with intact ligaments, isolated radial head excision leads to increased rotatory laxity. Radial head excision and a fracture of 30% of the coronoid with intact ligaments results in subluxation even with intact ligaments. Clinically, it has been shown that radial head excision in terrible triad injuries without ligament repair results in 50% redislocation at 2 months.

d. Complete restoration of the radial head articular surface, with repair or replacement, is required to restore elbow stability in terrible triad injuries.

3. Lateral ligamentous complex (**Figure 1**)

a. The lateral collateral ligament (LCL) is always

3: Trauma

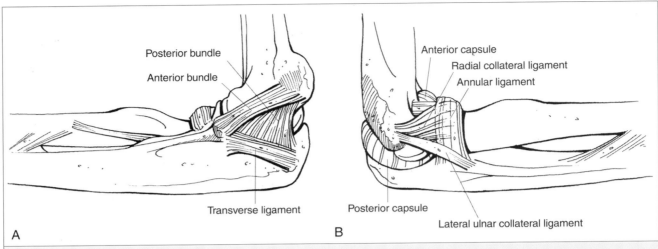

Figure 1 Illustration depicts the anatomy of the medial (**A**) and lateral (**B**) collateral ligaments of the elbow. (Reproduced from Tashjian RZ, Katarincic JA: Complex elbow instability. *J Am Acad Orthop Surg* 2006;14[5]:278-286.)

injured in a terrible triad injury and usually is avulsed off the lateral epicondyle with a portion of the extensor muscles.

   b. The LCL complex is the primary restraint to posterolateral rotatory instability of the elbow; it prevents external rotation of the radius and ulna relative to the humerus.

   c. The components of the LCL complex include the lateral ulnar collateral ligament (LUCL), the radial collateral ligament, and the annular ligament.

  4. Medial collateral ligament (MCL, **Figure 1**)

   a. The anterior bundle of the MCL is the most important stabilizer of valgus stress to the elbow.

   b. In an incompetent MCL, the radial head becomes a very important secondary stabilizer to valgus instability.

   c. In terrible triad injuries, excellent outcomes can be obtained without MCL repair if all articular fractures and the LCL are repaired or reconstructed. MCL repair may be performed in rare cases in which stability cannot be achieved.

B. Mechanism of injury

  1. Typically, a fall on an outstretched arm with an axial force and valgus moment on a forearm in supination; the injury begins with disruption of the LCL, followed by anterior capsule disruption and possibly MCL disruption, with fractures of the radial head and coronoid.

  2. Terrible triad injuries differ from anteromedial facet fractures of the coronoid, which also occur with a dislocation of the elbow. A varus defor-

mity, posteromedially directed, creates LCL injury and fracture of the anteromedial facet of the coronoid. The radial head is preserved.

III. Evaluation

A. History—Typically, the history reveals a fall on an outstretched arm; the dislocation can result from both high-energy and low-energy injuries.

B. Physical examination

  1. Skin: Medial ecchymosis may suggest a medial-side injury.

  2. Distal radioulnar joint: An Essex-Lopresti lesion must be ruled out.

C. Imaging

  1. AP and lateral radiographs of the elbow prereduction and postreduction; radiographs should be scrutinized for associated fractures of the capitellum and trochlea.

  2. PA and lateral wrist and forearm radiographs when indicated

  3. Advanced imaging is obtained routinely, specifically CT with three-dimensional reconstruction to further classify the proximal radius and coronoid fractures.

IV. Classification

A. Classification systems have been developed for individual parts of the terrible triad, specifically the radial head and coronoid process fractures (**Figures 2, 3, and 4**).

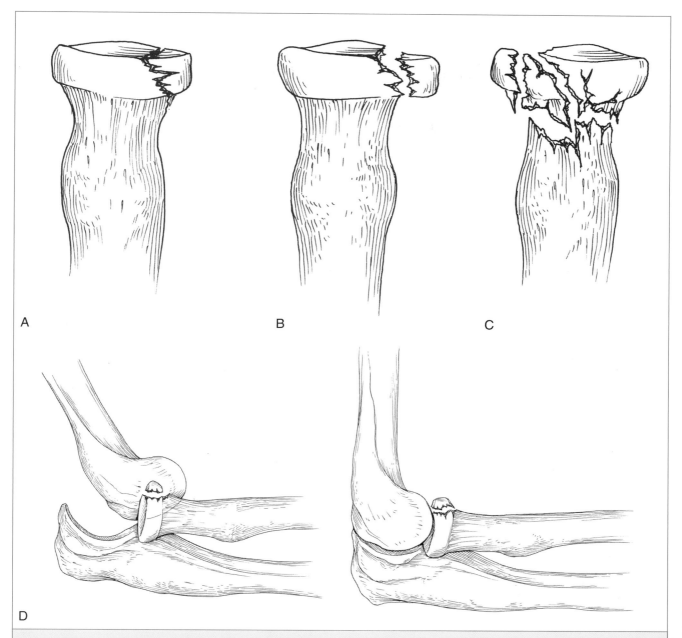

Figure 2   Illustrations demonstrate the Mason classification of radial head fractures. **A,** Type I, nondisplaced. **B,** Type II, displaced partial articular fracture. **C,** Type III, comminuted fracture. **D,** A type IV injury indicating an associated ipsilateral ulnohumeral dislocation. (Reproduced from Mathew PK, Athwal GS, King GJW: Terrible triad injury of the elbow: Current concepts. *J Am Acad Orthop Surg* 2009;17[3]:137-151.)

B. By definition, a terrible triad must include a posterolateral elbow dislocation, with fractures of the coronoid and the radial head.

V. Treatment

A. Nonsurgical management

1. Most patients require surgical treatment. Only those patients who, after reduction, have congruent ulnohumeral and radiohumeral articulations, have nondisplaced radial head or neck fractures, and whose elbow remains stable through a full range of elbow flexion/extension motion in neutral rotation can be managed nonsurgically.

2. Management includes 1 week of immobilization, followed by progressed range of motion. Serial radiographs should be performed at short intervals to confirm fracture healing and the maintenance of a stable reduction.

3: Trauma

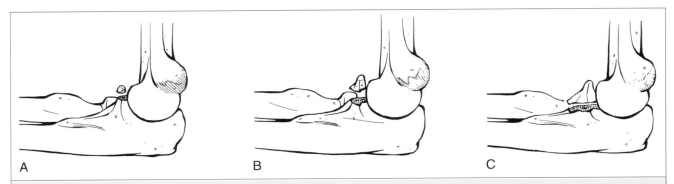

Figure 3   Illustrations show the Regan and Morrey classification of fractures of the coronoid process. **A,** Type I, simple avulsion. **B,** Type II, single or comminuted portion involving approximately 50% of the coronoid process. **C,** Type III, fracture involving more than 50% of the articulation. (Reproduced from Tashjian RZ, Katarincic JA: Complex elbow instability. *J Am Acad Orthop Surg* 2006;14[5]:278-286.)

O'Driscoll Coronoid Fracture Classification

Fracture	Subtype	Description
Tip	1	≤2 mm of coronoid height
	2	>2 mm of coronoid height
Anteromedial	1	Anteromedial rim
	2	Anteromedial rim and tip
	3	Anteromedial rim and sublime tubercle (± tip)
Basal	1	Coronoid body and base
	2	Transolecranon basal coronoid fracture

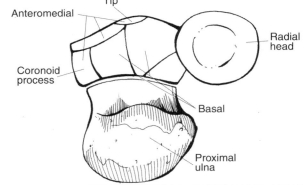

Figure 4   Table and illustration depict the O'Driscoll coronoid fracture classification system, including tip, anteromedial facet, and basal fractures. (Reproduced from Tashjian RZ, Katarincic JA: Complex elbow instability. *J Am Acad Orthop Surg* 2006;14[5]:278-286.)

B. Surgical management

1. Overview—A systematic approach should be applied, including repair or replacement of substantial radial head fractures, coronoid fracture fixation, and LCL repair, followed by additional procedures (MCL/flexor pronator repair, dynamic or static external fixation) only if stability is not obtained (**Figure 5**).

2. Surgical approach

a. Two primary incisions: lateral (with an additional medial approach if required) or posterior

b. The deep approach to the elbow is through the lateral extensor muscles, through the Kocher interval (between the extensor carpi ulnaris and the anconeus) or through an extensor digitorum communis (EDC) split. Distal extension of the EDC split may injure the posterior interosseous nerve, and the distal extension of the Kocher interval may injure the LCL. If the Kocher interval is used, the Kaplan interval (the extensor carpi radialis longus and the common extensor) also can be used to increase access to the anterior joint and the coronoid process (**Figure 6**).

3. Radial head fracture management—Surgical management of radial head fractures in terrible triad injuries includes fragment excision, open reduction and internal fixation, or radial head arthroplasty. Radial head fractures should be repaired or replaced unless they involve less than 25% of the articular surface and are not critical to elbow stability. The radial head should never be resected and left without replacement in a terrible triad repair.

a. Fragment excision is reasonable for small, unrepairable fragments (<25% to 30%) that do not articulate with the lesser sigmoid notch if stability of the elbow is achieved after coronoid and LCL repair. If stability is not restored, then arthroplasty should be performed.

b. Fixation of the proximal radius should be considered in radial neck fractures with limited neck comminution or in partial articular fractures with a single piece that is not comminuted (more than one piece increases the risk for failure).

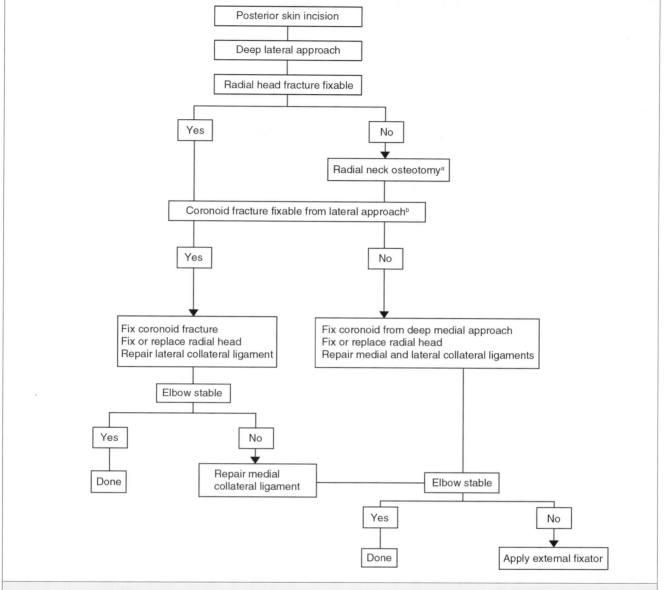

Figure 5   Algorithm depicts the surgical management of terrible triad injuries. [a]Neck osteotomy in preparation for radial head replacement; if the fragment size is less than 25% of the radial head, fragment excision may be considered. [b]Type I coronoid fractures may not require repair. (Reproduced from Mathew PK, Athwal GS, King GJW: Terrible triad injury of the elbow: Current concepts. *J Am Acad Orthop Surg* 2009;17[3]:137-151.)

c. Fixation of radial head fragments can be performed using countersunk headless screws.

d. Plate fixation is useful for neck fractures and should be placed in the "safe zone," where the radius does not articulate with the proximal radioulnar joint. The plate should be placed directly lateral with the arm in neutral rotation.

e. Radial head arthroplasty—Indicated in patients with comminuted Mason III fractures, surgical neck fractures with substantial neck comminution, or partial radial head fractures

with two or more pieces; if some neck comminution exists, two thirds of the shaft diameter may be used to support the prosthesis.

f. Overstuffing will substantially limit elbow range of motion, specifically flexion, and will result in pain and capitellar erosion.

g. The best radial head length permits the proximal surface of the radial head arthroplasty to line up with the proximal aspect of the lesser sigmoid notch.

h. Radial head excision is contraindicated in ter-

3: Trauma

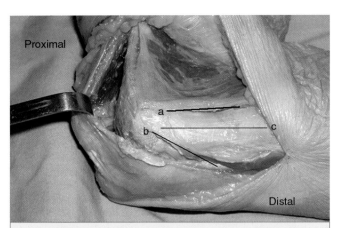

Figure 6 Intraoperative photograph shows a lateral view of the relative location of the Kaplan approach (line a), the Kocher approach (line b), and the EDC splitting approach (line c) in a right elbow. (Reproduced from Cheung EV, Steinmann SP: Surgical approaches to the elbow. *J Am Acad Orthop Surg* 2009;17[5]:325-333.)

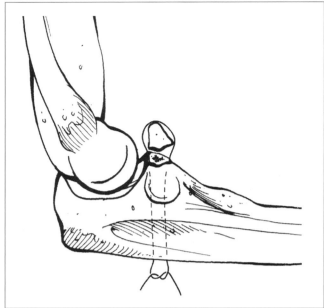

Figure 7 Coronoid fracture fixation using a Lasso repair, in which a suture is placed around a small coronoid piece and the anterior capsule and then passed through drill holes posteriorly in the ulna. (Reproduced from Tashjian RZ, Katarincic JA: Complex elbow instability. *J Am Acad Orthop Surg* 2006;14[5]:278-286.)

rible triad injuries with high rates of recurrent instability, progressive arthrosis, and pain.

4. Coronoid fracture management—Based on biomechanical data, most coronoid fractures should be fixed, with the possible exclusion of very small (<10% height) pieces.

   a. Most fractures can be repaired with a suture-grasping technique fixed through bone tunnels tied over the posterior aspect of the proximal ulna (**Figure 7**).

   b. Lasso suture repair has been shown to be more stable intraoperatively than suture anchor or screw fixation. Screw fixation is associated with a higher incidence of implant failure and anchor fixation with a higher incidence of nonunion.

   c. Basal or anteromedial facet fractures are associated much less commonly with a classic terrible triad injury (posterolateral dislocation).

   d. Larger coronoid fractures typically need fixation through a medial approach. Access to the medial coronoid is best performed between the two heads of the flexor carpi ulnaris. Fixation can be performed with a 2.0 or 2.4 T-shaped or L-shaped plate.

5. LCL complex

   a. The LCL complex must be repaired after fixation of the coronoid and radial head fixation or arthroplasty; repair can be accomplished using bone tunnels or suture anchors.

   b. The LCL complex often is avulsed with the common extensor from the epicondyle (midsubstance or distal ruptures are uncommon)

and should be repaired as a unit back to the origin of the LCL complex.

   c. The LUCL ligament needs to be repaired to its isometric point, which is at the center of the capitellum, approximately 2 mm anterior to the lateral epicondyle.

6. Additional procedures (MCL repair, external fixation)

   a. The elbow should be moved through a full range of flexion and extension in neutral rotation under fluoroscopy. If the ulnohumeral joint is persistently unstable (dislocating in extension), then further measures should be performed to restore stability.

   b. If instability persists, then the MCL, along with the flexor/pronators should be repaired. If instability still persists, then static or dynamic external fixation should be used. External fixation of the elbow can be used when repair of the bony injuries and the lateral and medial ligament complexes do not restore stability. This is usually an intraoperative decision based on stability during range of motion assessed fluoroscopically.

   c. Slight persistent ulnohumeral widening seen on the lateral radiograph can be monitored postoperatively; residual widening often results from incompetent forearm flexors, which should be treated with active flexor exercises and the avoidance of varus stress.

VI. Complications

A. Reoperation is relatively common (20% to 25%) after the fixation of terrible triad injuries.

B. Complications include severe stiffness, heterotopic bone formation, infection, posttraumatic arthritis, ulnar neuropathy, persistent instability, nonunion, and malunion.

1. Stiffness—About 10% of cases require release for pathologic stiffness; the procedure often includes excision of heterotopic ossification and hardware removal.

2. Heterotopic ossification—Occurs in approximately 10% of cases; can also result in synostosis, limiting forearm rotation, and restriction of the flexion arc

3. Infection—Relatively rare, except for pin site infections, which occur in about 40% to 50% of cases if an external fixator is used

4. Posttraumatic arthritis—Relatively common (60% to 70%), although it typically is not expressed clinically and usually does not affect outcomes or range of motion

5. Neurovascular injury—Ulnar neuritis is most common (about 10%).

6. Recurrent instability—Very uncommon (<5%) if the aforementioned contemporary standardized protocol was used, in contrast to relying on historical data, which show a high rate of persistent instability after surgical treatment.

VII. Rehabilitation

A. Postoperative rehabilitation is variable and surgeon dependent. Arms usually are splinted in 90° of flexion for the first week and then range-of-motion exercises are started. For an intact MCL, many authors place the arm in pronation to protect the LCL repair. For a compromised MCL with a repaired LCL, the elbow should be placed in neutral rotation.

B. Passive and active-assisted flexion/extension and supination/pronation are initiated at 1 week and continued from postoperative weeks 1 to 6.

C. Flexion/extension exercises are performed supine in the overhead position in full pronation to protect the LCL repair.

D. Terminal elbow extension is limited by 30°, and the limit is progressively decreased to full extension over the first 6 postoperative weeks. A hinged elbow brace limiting terminal extension but allowing flexion and extension may be used.

E. At 6 weeks, the hinged brace is removed, allowing limited lifting and continued stretching.

F. Strengthening is initiated at 8 to 12 weeks. Unrestricted use is allowed at 4.5 to 6 months postoperatively.

G. Static progressive stretching is initiated at 10 to 12 weeks, if concern for the development of stiffness exists, and continued for 8 to 12 weeks before consideration of contracture release.

3:Trauma

Top Testing Facts

1. Terrible triad injuries refer to complex elbow dislocations that include posterolateral elbow dislocation, a radial head or neck fracture, and a coronoid process fracture.

2. MCL repair is not required as part of a terrible triad injury repair unless persistent instability is present after coronoid fracture fixation, radial head repair or reconstruction, and LCL repair.

3. Anteromedial facet fractures of the coronoid typically are NOT associated with terrible triad injuries. The mechanism of elbow instability from an anteromedial facet injury results from a varus posteromedially directed force rather than the valgus posterolaterally directed force typically seen in a terrible triad injury.

4. Radial head fractures should be repaired or replaced unless they involve less than 25% of the articular surface and are not critical to elbow stability. The radial head should never be resected and left without replacement in a terrible triad repair.

5. Most coronoid process fractures should be repaired, with the possible exception of small tip fractures (<10% of height).

6. The LUCL ligament needs to be repaired to its isometric point, which is at the center of the capitellum, approximately 2 mm anterior to the lateral epicondyle.

7. Slight persistent ulnohumeral widening on the lateral radiograph can be monitored postoperatively.

8. Complications are very common, with 25% of patients requiring reoperation. The most common reasons are stiffness, heterotopic bone formation, and ulnar neuritis. Persistent instability, using contemporary fixation techniques and the surgical algorithm, is uncommon compared with that seen using historical procedures.

9. External fixation of the elbow can be used when repair of the bony injuries and the lateral and medial ligament complexes does not restore stability. This is usually an intraoperative decision based on stability during range of motion assessed fluoroscopically.

10. During rehabilitation with an intact MCL, many authors place the arm in pronation to protect the LCL repair. For a compromised MCL with a repaired LCL, the elbow should be placed in neutral rotation.

Bibliography

Cheung EV, Steinmann SP: Surgical approaches to the elbow. *J Am Acad Orthop Surg* 2009;17(5):325-333.

Cohen MS, Hastings H II: Rotatory instability of the elbow: The anatomy and role of the lateral stabilizers. *J Bone Joint Surg Am* 1997;79(2):225-233.

Doornberg JN, Linzel DS, Zurakowski D, Ring D: Reference points for radial head prosthesis size. *J Hand Surg Am* 2006; 31(1):53-57.

Doornberg JN, Parisien R, van Duijn PJ, Ring D: Radial head arthroplasty with a modular metal spacer to treat acute traumatic elbow instability. *J Bone Joint Surg Am* 2007;89(5): 1075-1080.

Doornberg JN, van Duijn J, Ring D: Coronoid fracture height in terrible-triad injuries. *J Hand Surg Am* 2006;31(5): 794-797.

Egol KA, Immerman I, Paksima N, Tejwani N, Koval KJ: Fracture-dislocation of the elbow functional outcome following treatment with a standardized protocol. *Bull NYU Hosp Jt Dis* 2007;65(4):263-270.

Forthman C, Henket M, Ring DC: Elbow dislocation with intra-articular fracture: The results of operative treatment without repair of the medial collateral ligament. *J Hand Surg Am* 2007;32(8):1200-1209.

Garrigues GE, Wray WH III, Lindenhovius AL, Ring DC, Ruch DS: Fixation of the coronoid process in elbow fracture-dislocations. *J Bone Joint Surg Am* 2011;93(20):1873-1881.

Lindenhovius AL, Jupiter JB, Ring D: Comparison of acute versus subacute treatment of terrible triad injuries of the elbow. *J Hand Surg Am* 2008;33(6):920-926.

Mathew PK, Athwal GS, King GJ: Terrible triad injury of the elbow: Current concepts. *J Am Acad Orthop Surg* 2009; 17(3):137-151.

McKee MD, Schemitsch EH, Sala MJ, O'driscoll SW: The pathoanatomy of lateral ligamentous disruption in complex elbow instability. *J Shoulder Elbow Surg* 2003;12(4): 391-396.

Pugh DM, Wild LM, Schemitsch EH, King GJ, McKee MD: Standard surgical protocol to treat elbow dislocations with radial head and coronoid fractures. *J Bone Joint Surg Am* 2004;86-A(6):1122-1130.

Ring D, Jupiter JB, Zilberfarb J: Posterior dislocation of the elbow with fractures of the radial head and coronoid. *J Bone Joint Surg Am* 2002;84-A(4):547-551.

Schneeberger AG, Sadowski MM, Jacob HA: Coronoid process and radial head as posterolateral rotatory stabilizers of the elbow. *J Bone Joint Surg Am* 2004;86-A(5):975-982.

Tashjian RZ, Katarincic JA: Complex elbow instability. *J Am Acad Orthop Surg* 2006;14(5):278-286.

Zeiders GJ, Patel MK: Management of unstable elbows following complex fracture-dislocations—the "terrible triad" injury. *J Bone Joint Surg Am* 2008;90(Suppl 4):75-84.

3: Trauma

Chapter 33

Forearm Trauma and Diaphyseal Fractures

Christopher McAndrew, MD

I. Epidemiology and Overview

A. Of hand, wrist, and forearm fractures, 44% involve the radius and/or ulna.

1. The most common age group affected is 5 to 14 years (34%).

2. Fractures of the distal radius and/or ulna are more common than diaphyseal fractures.

3. Common etiologies include falls at home (30%), highway accidents (14%), and sporting injuries (14%).

B. Nonsurgical and early surgical care of diaphyseal forearm fractures produce poor results.

1. The best report of closed treatment includes a loss of >50° of rotation for 30% of patients.

2. Early surgical treatment sometimes required supplemental above-arm casting and resulted in high nonunion rates and poor functional outcomes.

3. Anderson is credited with the first report of the compression plating technique advocated by the AO/Association for the Study of Internal Fixation (ASIF), resulting in reduced nonunion rates and better functional outcomes.

4. Treatment of adult diaphyseal fractures of the forearm with open reduction and plate fixation is considered the standard against which all other treatments are now compared.

5. Imaging of forearm trauma and fractures generally consists of plain radiographs of the forearm, wrist, and elbow. MRI may be considered in some patterns with associated ligamentous injury, such as Essex-Lopresti and Galeazzi fractures.

II. Anatomy and Biomechanics

A. Despite the diaphyseal nature of the central portions of the radius and ulna, the forearm is best considered a single articular unit composed of the proximal, middle, and distal radioulnar joints.

B. The axis of rotation for pronation/supination of the forearm extends from the center of the radial head through the ulnar styloid and is independent of elbow position.

C. The interosseous membrane (IOM) connects the ulna to the radius obliquely, 21° proximally to the transverse axis of the forearm (**Figure 1**).

1. Axial load is transmitted from the distal radius to the proximal ulna via the IOM.

2. The proportion of axial load is estimated to be 80% radius at the wrist, with an increasing amount of load borne proximally by the ulna, depending on elbow position.

3. The central fibers are on maximal tension in neutral rotation.

4. The distal fibers are on maximal tension in supination.

D. The radial bow accommodates pronation of the forearm.

1. The bow is not purely in the sagittal or coronal plane.

2. The mean maximal radial bow in the coronal plane is approximately 15 mm and is located 60% distally along the axis of the radius (**Figure 2**).

3. Failure to restore this anatomic relationship results in loss of rotation and grip strength.

4. Range of motion (ROM) of the forearm and wrist positively correlates with Disabilities of the Arm, Shoulder and Hand (DASH) scores following both-bone forearm fracture treatment.

3: Trauma

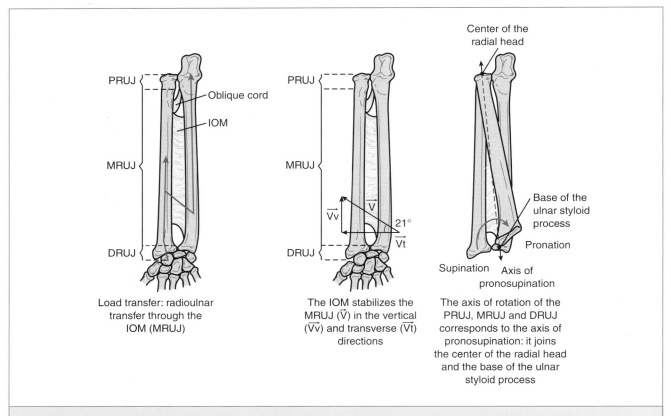

Figure 1 Illustrations show the relationship of the radius, ulna, and interosseous membrane (IOM). The orientation of the IOM transfers axial load from the distal radius to the proximal ulna. The axis of rotation of the forearm extends from the center of the radial head to the ulnar styloid. PRUJ = proximal radioulnar joint, MRUJ = middle radioulnar joint, DRUJ = distal radioulnar joint.

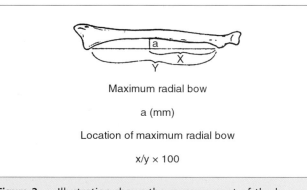

Maximum radial bow

a (mm)

Location of maximum radial bow

x/y × 100

Figure 2 Illustration shows the measurement of the location and magnitude of the maximal radial bow in the coronal plane. The maximal bow measures a mean 15 mm (a) and 60% distal along the length of the radius (x/y × 100). (Reproduced with permission from Schemitsch EH, Richards RR: The effect of malunion on functional outcome after plate fixation of fractures of both bones of the forearm in adults. *J Bone Joint Surg Am* 1992;74:1068-1078.)

III. Surgical Approaches for Fixation of Diaphyseal Fractures of the Radius and Ulna

A. The volar approach to the radius (Henry approach) is most commonly used.

1. The skin incision is longitudinal from lateral to the biceps tendon to the radial styloid, with the length dictated by the necessary exposure of the radius.

2. The lateral antebrachial cutaneous nerve lies in the subcutaneous fat, paralleling the cephalic vein and running along the border of the brachioradialis.

3. The internervous plane between the brachioradialis (radial nerve) and pronator teres/flexor carpi radialis (median nerve) is used.

4. The radial artery is located deep to the brachioradialis proximally, and its radial branches are ligated to allow ulnar retraction.

5. The superficial radial nerve is located deep to the brachioradialis proximally and is gently retracted radially with the muscle.

6. Proximally, the radius is exposed lateral/radial to the biceps insertion (the radial artery is medial/ulnar to the tendon).

   a. With the forearm in full supination, the insertion of the supinator muscle is identified and released.

   b. Subperiosteal dissection from ulnar to radial protects the posterior interosseous nerve (PIN) within the supinator muscle.

7. In the middle third of the forearm, slight pronation exposes the insertion of the pronator teres muscle. Subperiosteal release of the pronator teres and flexor digitorum superficialis from radial to ulnar exposes the radius shaft.

8. Distally, the pronator quadratus and flexor pollicis longus are released from their radial origins ulnarly, exposing the distal radius. Distally, the superficial radial nerve lies between the brachioradialis and extensor carpi radialis longus tendons, becoming superficial 9 cm proximal to the radial styloid.

B. The dorsal approach to the radius (Thompson approach) also can be used.

   1. The skin incision is longitudinal from the lateral epicondyle to the ulnar side of the Lister tubercle, with the length dictated by the necessary exposure of the radius.

   2. The internervous plane between the extensor carpi radialis brevis (radial nerve location) and the extensor digitorum communis/extensor pollicis longus (PIN location) is used.

   3. Proximally, the PIN must be identified and protected within the supinator.

      a. The PIN can be found distal to the radiocapitellar joint after it pierces the supinator at a distance of 3.2 cm in supination, 4.2 cm in neutral, and 5.6 cm in pronation (**Figure 3**).

      b. Fracture or osteotomy reduces the effect of forearm pronation, and the PIN is found closer to the radiocapitellar joint in these situations.

   4. The abductor pollicis longus and extensor pollicis brevis can be retracted distally (middle third) or proximally (distal third) to expose the radius.

C. Exposure of the ulna is performed along the subcutaneous border.

   1. The interval between the extensor carpi ulnaris (PIN) and the flexor carpi ulnaris (ulnar nerve) is used.

   2. The ulnar nerve and artery are volar to the flexor carpi ulnaris muscle and are placed at risk if this muscle is not carefully dissected directly off the ulna.

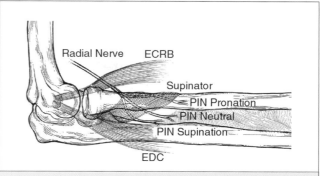

Figure 3 Illustration shows the relationship of the posterior interosseous nerve (PIN) to the radiocapitellar joint. With an intact radius, the distance from the radiocapitellar joint to the midaxial position of the PIN changes in supination (3.2 cm), neutral (4.2 cm), and pronation (5.6 cm). EDC = extensor digitorum communis tendon, ECRB = extensor carpi radialis brevis tendon. (Reproduced with permission from Calfee RP, Wilson JM, Wong AH: Variations in the anatomic relations of the posterior interosseous nerve associated with proximal forearm trauma. *J Bone Joint Surg Am* 2011;93[1]:81-90.)

3. The dorsal cutaneous branch of the ulnar nerve extends from the ulnar nerve 6.4 cm from the distal end of the ulna and becomes subcutaneous 5.0 cm from the proximal edge of the pisiform.

IV. Specific Forearm Fracture Types

A. Isolated radial shaft fracture

   1. Defined as a radius shaft fracture with less than 5 mm of ulnar positive variance on injury radiographs.

   2. Epidemiology—Approximately three fourths of radial shaft fractures without associated ulnar shaft fracture have less than 5 mm of ulnar positive variance on injury radiographs.

   3. Anatomy—Most fractures are in the middle third of the radius.

   4. Surgical approaches—The volar (Henry) or dorsal (Thompson) approach, as described in section III

   5. Mechanism of injury—Likely a direct blow to the radial side of the forearm without substantial rotational forces or axial load through the forearm

   6. Clinical evaluation—Includes examination of the distal neurovascular status and evaluation for compartment syndrome and associated joint injury of the elbow and wrist

   7. Radiographic evaluation—Includes radiographs of the wrist, forearm, and elbow. If no subluxation of the elbow exists and the ulnar variance

3: Trauma

on premanipulation radiographs is less than 5 mm, the diagnosis is isolated radial shaft fracture.

8. Treatment and rehabilitation—Open reduction and internal fixation (ORIF), restoring the anatomic relationship of the radius and ulna, should be followed by early (less than 2 weeks) active ROM and no weight bearing until the fracture heals.

9. Complications—All reported complications relate to iatrogenic nerve palsy (of the PIN) and missed diagnoses of associated elbow pathology.

B. Galeazzi fracture

1. A radial shaft fracture associated with a distal radioulnar joint (DRUJ) injury, which may or may not include an ulnar styloid fracture

2. Epidemiology—Approximately one fourth of radial shaft fractures, without ulnar shaft fracture, have an associated DRUJ injury.

3. Anatomy—More than one half of radial shaft fractures with associated DRUJ injury occur in the distal third and are associated with increased ulnar variance.

4. Surgical approaches

   a. Volar (Henry) or dorsal (Thompson) approach for internal fixation of the radius fracture, as described in section III.

   b. Longitudinal approach over the extensor carpi ulnaris tendon sheath, with protection of the superficial transverse ulnar nerve branches, is used for reduction and fixation of displaced ulnar styloid fractures.

5. Mechanism of injury—Axial loading, usually through the outstretched hand

6. Clinical evaluation—Includes examination of the distal neurovascular status and evaluation for compartment syndrome and associated joint injury of the elbow and wrist

7. Radiographic evaluation—Includes evaluation of the wrist, forearm, and elbow

8. Treatment

   a. ORIF of the radial shaft is the preferred method of treatment of this type of fracture. The DRUJ is stable in most cases after anatomic reconstruction of the radius.

   b. ORIF of the ulnar styloid through the extensor carpi ulnaris approach may be accomplished with fixation using headless screws or tension band wiring.

   c. If the DRUJ is not reduced after ORIF of the radius, the DRUJ should be explored to remove interposed soft tissues (most commonly the triangular fibrocartilage complex).

   d. Splinting of the unstable DRUJ in neutral or supinated rotation for 4 to 6 weeks is performed to treat DRUJ dislocation that is unstable in pronation after ORIF of the radius. If the DRUJ is still unstable, reduction and pinning with two Kirschner wires from the ulna to the radius in supination is performed and maintained for 4 to 6 weeks.

9. Rehabilitation—After ORIF of the radius (and the ulnar styloid), early (less than 2 weeks) active ROM and no weight bearing is recommended until fracture healing occurs. Immobilization in a splint/cast or with pin fixation for 4 to 6 weeks is reserved only for an unstable DRUJ, with active ROM initiated immediately after splint or pin removal.

10. Complications—Usually are related to undiagnosed associated injuries to the elbow or a missed diagnosis of DRUJ instability. Long-term follow-up demonstrates equivalent subjective and objective outcomes in patients with and without DRUJ instability at the time of injury, when treated appropriately.

C. Ulnar shaft fracture

1. Historically, good results have been obtained with bracing or compressive wraps and early ROM with proper patient selection (no associated injuries).

2. Anatomy—Most are in the middle third of the ulna, but particular attention should be given to those fractures in the proximal third that have higher associations with elbow pathology (for example, Monteggia fracture-dislocations) and nonunion.

3. Surgical approach—Direct approach to the subcutaneous border between the flexor carpi ulnaris and extensor carpi ulnaris, described in section III.C.

4. Mechanism of injury—Usually a direct blow to the ulnar forearm (defensive position); can occur with rotational stress, and these injuries (identified during the history) should alert the clinician to the possibility of associated elbow pathology.

5. Clinical evaluation—The distal neurovascular status, the soft-tissue envelope, and pain at the elbow and wrist should be evaluated. Exclusion of proximal radioulnar joint (PRUJ) injury is paramount.

6. Radiographic evaluation—Includes radiographs of the wrist, forearm, and elbow. Displacement of greater than 50% of the shaft width and angulation of greater than 10° have been associated with poor outcomes in function and nonunion and may warrant surgical treatment.

7. Treatment

a. Nonsurgical treatment with short-term (2 weeks) immobilization followed by active ROM is recommended for minimally displaced fractures that have no evidence of wrist, elbow, or interosseous instability.

b. Surgical treatment has been advocated for fractures with more than 10° of angulation and/or greater than 50% shaft-width displacement to maximize forearm function and decrease nonunion. Special attention also should be given to proximal and extreme distal ulnar shaft fractures, which have a higher nonunion rate.

8. Rehabilitation—Early (2 weeks) active ROM should be encouraged for stable fractures with minimal displacement. Following surgical treatment, early active ROM also is encouraged (described in section VI.)

9. Complications—When associated elbow injury is excluded, complication rates are low. Nonunion occurs in approximately 10% of cases treated nonsurgically, and appropriate patient/injury selection can reduce this rate.

D. Both-bone forearm fractures

1. The epidemiology has been described previously in section I, A.

2. The anatomy has been described previously in section II.

3. Surgical approaches have been described previously in section III.

4. Mechanism of injury—High-energy transfer is required to fracture the diaphyseal section of both bones of the forearm. This commonly results from motor vehicle accidents and falls from heights onto the upper extremities, with bending moments and direct blows causing the fractures. Low-energy injuries with resulting fractures should alert the clinician to possible associated elbow and wrist pathology.

5. Clinical evaluation—Should include distal neurovascular examination, soft-tissue envelope evaluation, and exclusion of compartment syndrome. A thorough history includes handedness and employment/hobby expectations.

6. Radiographic evaluation—Includes radiographs of the wrist, forearm, and elbow. Contralateral radiographs assist the treating surgeon by providing a template for reconstruction.

7. Treatment is described in section V. Surgical treatment is recommended for all both-bone forearm fractures, if the patient is able to tolerate surgery (**Figure 4**).

8. Rehabilitation is described in section VI.

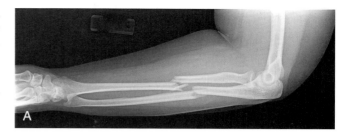

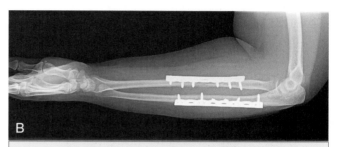

Figure 4 Preoperative (**A**) and postoperative (**B**) lateral forearm radiographs show a both-bone forearm fracture.

9. Outcomes

a. Mild losses in active ROM in pronation (7° less than normal), supination (9°), wrist flexion (11°), and wrist extension (5°) are expected after surgical fixation of both-bone forearm fractures with plate fixation with no complications.

b. Reduced strength in pronation (70% of normal), supination (68%), wrist flexion (84%), wrist extension (63%), and grip (75%) are expected after uncomplicated surgical care of both-bone forearm fractures with plate fixation.

c. Good subjective results (average DASH scores of 12 to 18) can be achieved overall, but worse outcomes are associated with decreased ROM, strength, and pain.

d. Currently, nonunion is less than 3% overall but increases with open fracture and bone loss.

e. Malunion of the radius with failure to restore the magnitude and location of the bow to within 5% of the normal opposite side results in a 20% loss of forearm rotation and loss of grip strength.

f. Infection rates of less than 3% are reported following both-bone forearm fractures, including those open fractures treated with débridement and immediate ORIF.

g. Radioulnar synostosis was reported historically, occurring in 2% of adult forearm fractures. Risk factors include a single approach to

3: Trauma

both bones for surgical fixation, errant placement of bone graft, fractures closer to or involving the elbow, delay to surgical repair of fractures, associated head trauma, and high-energy mechanisms.

h. Rates of refracture after plate removal have ranged from 4% to 25%. An increased risk for refracture is reported with early (<1 year) removal of plates, use of large fragment (4.5-mm) screws, and delayed union.

E. Longitudinal radioulnar dissociation (Essex-Lopresti lesion)

1. Most commonly associated with radial head fracture, which allows proximal migration to occur if excision or inadequate reconstruction is performed.

2. Proximal migration of the radius results in dorsal displacement of the ulna distally, limiting forearm supination and wrist extension.

3. Recognition of the acute injury and treatment are paramount for optimal function, because late reconstruction procedures result in limited success.

a. Restoration of radial length with anatomic reduction or reconstruction/arthroplasty is the first step to successful treatment.

b. Stabilization of the DRUJ in supination, possibly with pin fixation, is used if necessary.

V. Surgical Principles of Diaphyseal Fractures of the Radius and Ulna

A. ORIF with interfragmentary compression is the preferred method of treatment and the standard against which other approaches are compared.

1. Interfragmentary screw application with neutralization plating is appropriate for spiral and oblique fractures.

2. Compression plating with (oblique, **Figure 5**) or without (transverse) interfragmentary screw compression through the plate also can be used.

3. If the fracture is comminuted such that interfragmentary compression is not feasible, a bridge plating technique, with attention to reconstruction of the overall length, alignment, and rotation, is used (**Figure 6**). Contralateral radiographs of the uninjured elbow, forearm, and wrist are used as a template.

B. Intramedullary fixation has been studied in small case series and can produce comparable results in union rates and ROM.

1. The ulna is fixed antegrade, with an entry point in the olecranon process.

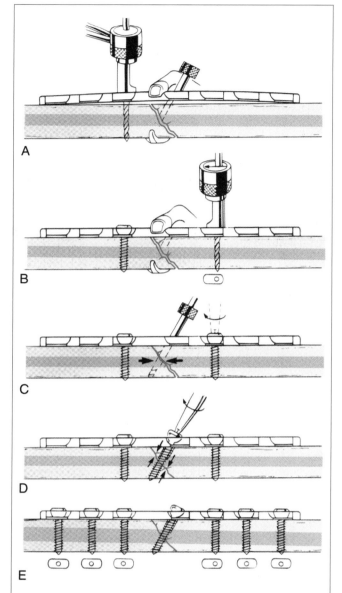

Figure 5 Illustrations demonstrate compression plate application using a dynamic compression plate. **A,** A plate with a slight concave bend is fixed to the fracture fragment to allow creation of an acute angle at the bone-plate interface (axilla). **B,** An eccentrically drilled (away from the fracture) hole is placed through the plate into the other fracture fragment, and compression at the fracture is achieved as the screw head articulates with the bevelled surface of the plate hole. **C,** An overdrilled pilot hole is created perpendicular to the fracture, and the core diameter drill bit is placed through a drill sleeve inserted into the pilot hole to drill the far cortex in the same orientation. **D,** The interfragmentary screw is applied. **E,** Plate fixation is completed in both fracture fragments.

2. The radius is fixed retrograde, with an entry point just ulnar to the Lister tubercle.

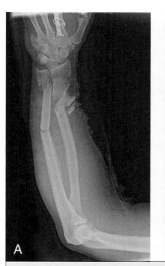 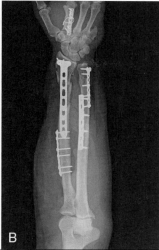

Figure 6 Preoperative (**A**) and postoperative (**B**) AP forearm radiographs show a both-bone forearm fracture treated using a bridge plating technique.

C. External fixation may be used temporarily in emergent situations or if soft-tissue compromise prevents safe ORIF. Safe half-pin fixation can be applied through the subcutaneous border of the ulna and the dorsal/radial border of the radius, with blunt dissection and retraction to protect soft-tissue structures.

D. Closed management is reserved for isolated single-bone fractures that are minimally displaced and not associated with proximal or distal joint compromise.

1. Isolated ulnar shaft fractures can be treated with and without immobilization with very high union rates and good functional outcomes.

   a. Indications for ORIF of unstable ulnar shaft fractures are aimed at prevention of nonunion and malunion causing ROM loss.

   b. Greater than 50% displacement and greater than 10° of angulation have been suggested as indications for ORIF.

2. Nonsurgical care of adult both-bone forearm fractures is reserved only for patients whose comorbid conditions prevent safe surgical and anesthetic care.

VI. Rehabilitation

A. Barring severe comminution, segmental bone loss, concomitant injuries to the extremity, or severe soft-tissue injury, the goal of surgical fixation should be to provide enough stability to allow immediate functional ROM of the elbow, forearm, and wrist.

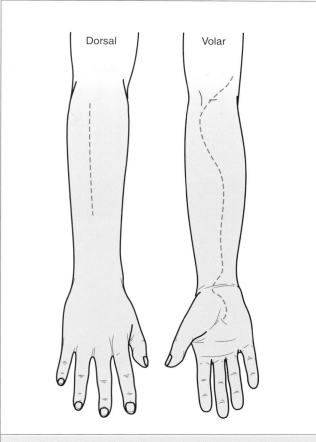

Figure 7 Illustration depicts the skin incisions for forearm fasciotomy. Adequate volar fasciotomy includes mobile wad fasciotomy, lacertus fibrosis release, volar extrinsic muscle fasciotomy, and carpal tunnel release. Dorsal compartment pressures often decrease with volar fasciotomy.

B. Weight bearing is limited until bone healing has progressed enough to tolerate loads (6 to 8 weeks).

C. DRUJ instability may require immobilization, with or without pin stabilization, for 4 to 6 weeks after ORIF, as described in section IV, B.

VII. Special Consideration—Compartment Syndrome of the Forearm

A. Causes include high-energy fracture, crush injury, spontaneous hematoma, constriction dressings, tight fascial closures, and revascularization.

B. Pain with passive stretch of the forearm muscles is the most commonly cited clinical finding, but concomitant traumatic injuries may make this symptom unreliable.

C. Loss of sensation (including subtle findings like decreased two-point discrimination) usually precedes motor dysfunction.

3: Trauma

D. Compartment pressures greater than 30 mm Hg for longer than 8 hours cause irreversible muscle and nerve damage.

E. A pressure gradient of less than 30 mm Hg (ΔP) between compartment pressure and diastolic blood pressure has been shown to be a reliable indication for fasciotomy of the leg.

F. The incidence of acute compartment syndrome associated with diaphyseal fractures of the forearm is approximately 3.1%.

G. Adequate volar fasciotomy includes release of the mobile wad fascia, lacertus fibrosis, volar compartment fascia, and carpal tunnel (**Figure 7**). Dorsal compartment pressures typically decrease with volar fasciotomy but should be remeasured intraoperatively to determine the need for a separate dorsal release.

H. The flexor digitorum profundus and flexor pollicis longus (deepest volar muscles) are typically affected most severely.

Top Testing Facts

1. Compression plating is the preferred method of fixation for both-bone forearm fractures in adults.

2. The axis of rotation of the forearm runs through the center of the radial head and the ulnar styloid.

3. Of the axial load, 80% is borne by the radius at the wrist and is nearly equivalent between the radius and ulna at the elbow (transferred via the intraosseous membrane).

4. The maximal coronal plane radial bow is 15 mm and is located 60% distally along the axis of the radius; it is critical to the restoration of rotational mechanics after fracture.

5. The Henry volar approach uses the internervous plane between the radial and median/anterior interosseous nerve myotomes.

6. The Thompson dorsal approach uses the internervous plane between the radial and PIN myotomes.

7. The PIN is located approximately 3 to 4 cm from the radiocapitellar joint dorsally; it is protected in volar approaches with supination and dorsal approaches with pronation.

8. Reduction in strength of 16% to 37% should be expected after ORIF of both-bone forearm fractures.

9. Refracture after plate removal has a reported occurrence of between 4% and 25%, and the risk is increased with early (<1 year) plate removal, large fragment implants, and delayed union.

10. Compartment syndrome occurs in 3.1% of forearm fractures, affects the flexor digitorum profundus and flexor pollicis longus most severely, and can be diagnosed with a gradient (ΔP) of less than 30 mm Hg between compartment pressure and diastolic blood pressure.

Bibliography

Anderson LD, Sisk D, Tooms RE, Park WI III: Compression-plate fixation in acute diaphyseal fractures of the radius and ulna. *J Bone Joint Surg Am* 1975;57(3):287-297.

Bot AG, Doornberg JN, Lindenhovius AL, Ring D, Goslings JC, van Dijk CN: Long-term outcomes of fractures of both bones of the forearm. *J Bone Joint Surg Am* 2011;93(6):527-532.

Calfee RP, Wilson JM, Wong AH: Variations in the anatomic relations of the posterior interosseous nerve associated with proximal forearm trauma. *J Bone Joint Surg Am* 2011;93(1):81-90.

Catalano LW III, Zlotolow DA, Hitchcock PB, Shah SN, Barron OA: Surgical exposures of the radius and ulna. *J Am Acad Orthop Surg* 2011;19(7):430-438.

Droll KP, Perna P, Potter J, Harniman E, Schemitsch EH, McKee MD: Outcomes following plate fixation of fractures of both bones of the forearm in adults. *J Bone Joint Surg Am* 2007;89(12):2619-2624.

Hollister AM, Gellman H, Waters RL: The relationship of the interosseous membrane to the axis of rotation of the forearm. *Clin Orthop Relat Res* 1994;298:272-276.

McQueen MM, Gaston P, Court-Brown CM: Acute compartment syndrome: Who is at risk? *J Bone Joint Surg Br* 2000;82(2):200-203.

Ring D, Allende C, Jafarnia K, Allende BT, Jupiter JB: Ununited diaphyseal forearm fractures with segmental defects: Plate fixation and autogenous cancellous bone-grafting. *J Bone Joint Surg Am* 2004;86-A(11):2440-2445.

Rozental TD, Beredjiklian PK, Bozentka DJ: Longitudinal radioulnar dissociation. *J Am Acad Orthop Surg* 2003;11(1):68-73.

van Duijvenbode DC, Guitton TG, Raaymakers EL, Kloen P, Ring D: Long-term outcome of isolated diaphyseal radius fractures with and without dislocation of the distal radioulnar joint. *J Hand Surg Am* 2012;37(3):523-527.

Chapter 34

Hand Trauma

David Ring, MD, PhD   Steven L. Moran, MD   Marco Rizzo, MD   Alexander Y. Shin, MD

I. Fractures of the Hand

A. General principles of fixation

1. Biomechanics

   a. Compression screws are stronger than Kirschner wires (K-wires).

   b. Plate and screw constructs are stronger than screws alone. Screws have resistance to bending only in the plane of the screw and little resistance to rotational or shear stress.

   c. Lag screws can be used without a plate when fracture length is at least twice the bone diameter.

2. Choice of fixation method

   a. Closed extra-articular fractures are treated with closed reduction and percutaneous pinning if possible to avoid the surgical dissection of the tendons, which creates scarring.

   b. Open reduction and internal fixation (ORIF) is generally reserved for fractures with associated soft-tissue injury or unstable articular fracture.

   c. Intramedullary fixation can be used for some fractures, such as small finger metacarpal shaft or neck fractures.

B. Fracture stability

1. Largely related to initial displacement

2. Fracture location, fracture type, bone quality/comminution, and soft-tissue injury are also important.

C. Treatment goals (all fractures)

1. Restoration of length, angular and rotational alignment, and optimization of articular congruity

2. Stabilization of the fracture

3. Repair of injured soft tissue and injury-specific exercises (for example, posttendon repair); ORIF allows a normal exercise regimen.

D. Incidence of hand fractures by location

1. Distal phalanx: 45% to 50%

2. Metacarpal: 30% to 35%

3. Proximal phalanx: 15% to 20%

4. Middle phalanx: 8%

E. Predictors of poorer outcome following fracture fixation

1. Open fractures

2. Intra-articular fractures

3. Associated nerve injury

4. Associated tendon injury

5. Crush injury

II. Fractures of the Metacarpals

A. Anatomy and biomechanics

1. Most metacarpal diaphyseal fractures are apex dorsal because of the pull of the interossei, which results in flexion of the distal fragment.

Dr. Ring or an immediate family member has received royalties from Wright Medical Technology, Inc.; serves as a paid consultant to or is an employee of Biomet, Skeletal Dynamics, and Wright Medical Technology, Inc.; has stock or stock options held in Illuminos; and serves as a board member, owner, officer, or committee member of the American Shoulder and Elbow Surgeons and the American Society for Surgery of the Hand. Dr. Moran or an immediate family member has received royalties from Integra; and is a member of a speakers' bureau or has made paid presentations on behalf of Integra. Dr. Rizzo or an immediate family member is a member of a speakers' bureau or has made paid presentations on behalf of Synthes; serves as a paid consultant to or is an employee of Synthes and Auxilium; serves as an unpaid consultant to Synthes; has received research or institutional support from SBI; and serves as a board member, owner, officer, or committee member of the American Academy of Orthopaedic Surgeons, the American Society for Surgery of the Hand, and the American Association for Hand Surgery. Dr. Shin or an immediate family member has received research or institutional support from the Musculoskeletal Transplant Foundation, Integra Life Sciences, and the American Association for Hand Surgery; and serves as a board member, owner, officer, or committee member of the American Society for Surgery of the Hand.

2. The hand can adjust dorsal angulation by compensating with metacarpophalangeal (MCP) hyperextension and carpometacarpal (CMC) motion. CMC motion is greatest at the little finger (30°), followed by the ring finger (20°). The long and index fingers have minimal CMC motion and thus can tolerate less angular deformity.

3. Rotational deformity of more than 5° can lead to finger scissoring.

4. Apex deformity at the metacarpal neck/metaphysis influences tendon balance less than at the diaphyseal level.

5. Cadaver experiments estimate 7° of extensor lag per 2 mm of metacarpal shortening, but compensation is variable. MCP hyperextension usually can compensate for up to 4 mm of shortening.

6. Metacarpal shortening or angulation >30° can result in shortening of the intrinsics, with the potential for extensor lag at the proximal interphalangeal joint.

7. Metacarpal shaft fractures are inherently stable because of the connections at the CMC joints and the intermetacarpal ligaments.

B. Fractures of the metacarpal neck

1. Metacarpal neck fractures are inherently unstable because of volar comminution.

2. The only way to prevent recurrence of deformity after closed reduction is surgical fixation with percutaneous K-wires, intramedullary fixation, or other methods.

3. For the little finger metacarpal neck, surgery is essentially cosmetic ("sunken knuckle") because deformity at the metacarpal neck level does not affect tendon balance, motion, or strength, although patients may have a "lump in palm" sensation with gripping because of the volar prominence of the metacarpal head.

C. Fractures of the metacarpal diaphysis

1. Radiographic evaluation

   a. PA and lateral views are indicated.

   b. The acceptable angulation is less than for metacarpal neck fractures because the deformity is felt to create more tendon imbalance.

      • 5° to 10° at the index and long fingers

      • 10° to 40° at the ring and little fingers

2. Treatment

   a. Most metacarpal diaphyseal fractures can be treated nonsurgically.

   b. Surgical treatment of these fractures is variable and may include percutaneous K-wire(s) placed transversely into the adjacent metacar-

pal, open plate or screw fixation, or intramedullary devices.

      • K-wire fixation minimizes soft-tissue injury.

      • Plate-and-screw fixation is usually performed dorsally.

   c. Treatment of metacarpal diaphysis bone loss

      • Distraction-fixation is used to restore length and alignment.

      • Soft-tissue coverage is crucial.

      • Secondary iliac crest bone graft can be used when contamination is present either immediately with limited contamination and good débridement or after the wound is clean following additional débridements, soft-tissue coverage as needed, and time.

   d. Malunion may be treated with opening or closing wedge osteotomies or derotational osteotomies in conjunction with internal fixation.

D. Fractures of the metacarpal base

1. Mechanism of injury and pathoanatomy

   a. Fractures of the metacarpal base can represent CMC fracture-dislocations.

   b. Fracture-dislocations are often associated with high-energy trauma, which may produce axial carpal injuries.

   c. Fracture-dislocations of the CMC joint of the little finger are sometimes called Stenneb (Bennett spelled backward), reverse Bennett, baby Bennett, or Busby fractures. The metacarpal diaphysis is displaced proximally and ulnarly as a result of the pull of the extensor carpi ulnaris tendon.

2. Evaluation

   a. Oblique radiographs must be obtained to assess displacement.

   b. Sagittal CT also is helpful.

3. Treatment

   a. Congruent joint reduction is important to maintain mobility of the fourth and fifth CMC joints.

   b. Treatment of these fractures may be accomplished through closed reduction using longitudinal traction and K-wire fixation.

   c. More comminuted fractures may require external fixation.

   d. In patients with posttraumatic arthritis, arthrodesis is considered.

E. Fractures of the metacarpal head

1. Evaluation—A Brewerton view (20° of MCP flex-

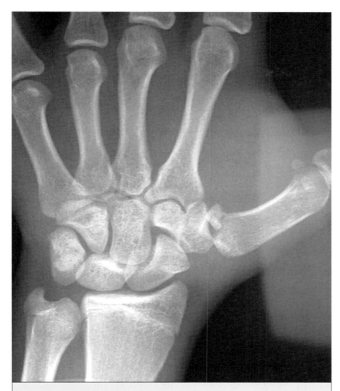

Figure 1   PA radiograph of the hand of an adolescent demonstrates a Bennett fracture.

ion) or CT scan may be needed for adequate visualization.

2. Surgical treatment—A dorsal approach is preferred.

F. Fractures of the thumb metacarpal

1. Extra-articular fractures

a. Up to 30° of angulation is acceptable because of the mobility of the saddle joint.

b. Fixation is usually accomplished with a percutaneous K-wire.

2. Bennett fracture—Base of the first metacarpal fracture (**Figure 1**)

a. Pathoanatomy—The volar oblique ligament is attached to the volar ulnar fragment of the base; the abductor pollicis longus displaces the distal metacarpal proximally, and the adductor pollicis displaces the metacarpal into adduction. The metacarpal base is displaced dorsally and rotated into supination.

b. Evaluation—The fracture is best visualized on the true lateral and hyperpronated AP (Robert) views.

c. Treatment

• Closed reduction can be obtained with lon-

gitudinal traction and extension/abduction/pronation of the metacarpal, as well as ulnarward pressure on the base of the metacarpal. The reduction is stabilized with a percutaneous K-wire fixation from the thumb metacarpal into the trapezium and another wire joining the thumb and index metacarpals.

• Open reduction is indicated if more than 2 to 3 mm of articular incongruity is present after closed reduction or severe central articular impaction.

3. Rolando fracture

a. Rolando fracture refers generally to more complex articular fractures of the base of the thumb metacarpal, although it is often described as specific to three-part Y or T intra-articular fractures.

b. Treatment

• ORIF with a plate and screws is possible for some simple fractures.

• Alternative treatment includes external fixator and K-wires or an external traction device.

• Bone graft may be helpful if realignment creates bone defects.

III. Metacarpophalangeal Dislocations

A. Dorsal MCP dislocations—The most frequently involved digit is the index finger.

B. Simple dislocation (subluxation)

1. Simple dislocations can be inadvertently converted to complete dislocation if improperly reduced.

2. Traction and hyperextension should not be used to reduce these dislocations.

a. To reduce these dislocations, the finger should be flexed to take tension off the flexor tendons, and the base of the proximal phalanx should be pushed volarly and distally to slide the displaced volar plate over the metacarpal head.

b. To reduce thumb MCP dorsal dislocations, the interphalangeal joint of the thumb and the wrist are flexed while the proximal phalanx is pushed volarly.

C. Complex/irreducible dislocation

1. Evaluation—The patient presents with the digit held in slight extension and a prominence in the palm.

2. Pathoanatomy—The key aspect is the interposed volar plate. The flexor tendon, lumbrical, and A1

pulley also wrap around the metacarpal head, but this rarely prevents reduction.

3. Treatment

   a. A volar approach puts the digital nerves at risk of injury because they are pushed into a subcutaneous position by the metacarpal head.

   b. Dorsal approach—A longitudinal incision is made and the proximal part of the sagittal band is divided on the ulnar side. The joint capsule is divided if needed for better joint exposure. The volar plate is attached to the proximal phalanx and covers the metacarpal head, blocking closed reduction. To reduce the joint, the volar plate is split longitudinally. A Freer elevator is then used to push the volar plate palmarly.

IV. Fractures of the Proximal and Middle Phalanx

A. Anatomy and biomechanics

1. Proximal phalanx

   a. Most transverse proximal phalanx fractures are apex palmar.

   b. The central extensor tendon pulls the distal fragment dorsal, and the interossei insertion flexes the proximal fragment.

   c. Proximal phalanx fractures have less stability than metacarpal fractures because they are not supported by adjacent bones as are the metacarpals. In addition, multiple tendon forces act on the fragments.

   d. Authors of cadaver studies estimate that shortening of the proximal phalanx produces an extensor lag at the proximal interphalangeal (PIP) joint, with each millimeter of bone loss equaling 12° of extensor lag, but the actual imbalance is more variable and multifactorial.

2. Fractures of the middle phalanx

   a. The angulation depends on the fracture position.

   b. Proximal middle phalanx fractures are apex dorsal because of the pull of the central slip.

   c. Distal middle phalanx fractures displace palmarly as a result of the pull of the superficialis insertion.

   d. Shortening of the middle phalanx following fracture may result in distal interphalangeal (DIP) joint extension lag.

B. Specific fractures

1. Fractures of the proximal phalanx base—Extra-articular base fracture

   a. Most proximal phalanx base fractures are unstable because of dorsal metaphyseal impaction.

   b. Closed reduction and cast immobilization can be attempted with stable fractures, and the MCP joint should be flexed >60°.

   c. Nonsurgical treatment of unstable fractures is an option. It leads to residual deformity with good hand function.

   d. Multiple options exist for better alignment with K-wire fixation; however, all risk tendon adhesions and stiffness.

   e. With complex trauma, including flexor tendon laceration, internal fixation with a mini condylar plate may enable early mobilization.

2. Fractures of the diaphysis of the proximal and middle phalanges

   a. The angulation is usually apex volar as a result of the pull of the central slip and lateral bands.

   b. Treatment—The type of fracture determines the treatment.

3. Fractures of the neck of the proximal and middle phalanges

   a. Epidemiology and pathoanatomy

     • These fractures are uncommon in adults.

     • In children, phalangeal neck fractures may displace and rotate 90° (apex dorsally).

     • With complete displacement, the volar plate may become entrapped in the fracture.

   b. Treatment—Closed reduction and a percutaneous K-wire

4. Condylar fractures of the proximal and middle phalanx

   a. Angulation and malrotation are evaluated.

   b. Treatment

     • Displaced condylar fractures require reduction and fixation, which is sometimes possible to achieve percutaneously.

     • If open reduction is necessary, screw fixation is attempted.

     • The PIP joint can be exposed by incising between the lateral band and the central tendon or through a midaxial incision opening the capsule above the collateral ligament.

V. PIP Joint Dislocations and Fracture-Dislocations

A. Epidemiology

1. Dorsal—These are the most common form of PIP joint dislocations. They are often associated with volar plate avulsion or fracture of the volar base of the middle phalanx.

2. Lateral—Sometimes associated with interposition of the collateral ligament.

3. Volar—Can be associated with injury to the central tendon.

B. Dorsal PIP joint dislocations and fracture-dislocations

1. Anatomy

   a. The accessory collateral ligaments insert onto the volar plate.

   b. The proper collateral ligaments insert onto the condyles.

   c. Fracture-dislocations involving >40% of the volar base of the joint surface are unstable.

   d. Boutonnière deformity involves compensatory hyperextension of the DIP joint (and an inability to flex the DIP joint actively) due to tightness in the lateral bands attempting to compensate for an inadequate central slip.

2. Treatment of PIP joint dislocations

   a. Most dorsal PIP joint dislocations are stable after closed reduction under digital block, even if a small volar plate avulsion fracture exists.

   b. The major risk is stiffness of the PIP joint. Treatment consists of immediate mobilization (with buddy straps for comfort as preferred) and stretching to maintain motion.

   c. Swelling improves for 1 year and is partially permanent. Stiffness and soreness can last for months and are particularly noticeable first thing in the morning.

   d. The unusual volar PIP dislocation should be evaluated for central slip injury and treated with extension splinting of the PIP joint for 4 to 6 weeks.

   e. Incomplete reduction and collateral ligament instability can be a result of interposition of the collateral ligament or other soft-tissue structures and are treated with open reduction.

3. Treatment of dorsal fracture-dislocations

   a. Stable—Dorsal extension block splint with the joint in 60° to 70° of flexion, decreasing flexion weekly over 2 to 3 weeks

   b. Unstable—The usual options include the following.

   - Extension block pinning

   - ORIF

   - Volar plate arthroplasty (currently out of favor)

   - Dynamic digital traction using force-couple splint fixation

   - Hemihamate arthroplasty

VI. Thumb MCP Ligament Injuries and Dislocations

A. Ulnar collateral ligament (UCL) disruption (gamekeeper's thumb)

1. Pathoanatomy

   a. The UCL ruptures off the base of the proximal phalanx.

   b. The avulsed ligament, with or without a bony fragment, can become displaced above the adductor aponeurosis, preventing healing (the so-called Stener lesion).

2. Treatment

   a. Tears of the UCL of the thumb MCP joint without a Stener lesion are believed to heal with 4 to 6 weeks of immobilization.

   b. Injuries that are unstable (difficult to define, but usually 30° more opening with radial stress than the opposite uninjured side) are believed to have Stener lesions and are treated surgically.

B. Radial collateral ligament (RCL) disruption

1. Pathoanatomy

   a. The RCL ruptures from its origin, from its insertion, or at the midsubstance.

   b. RCL ruptures are frequently associated with dorsal or dorsoradial capsular tears and with extensor pollicis brevis avulsions or tears.

   c. No equivalent of the Stener lesion exists, but RCL ruptures seem susceptible to chronic instability.

2. Treatment—The optimal treatment is unclear; percutaneous K-wire immobilization with or without open repair are options.

C. MCP Dislocation

1. Pathoanatomy—Both collateral ligaments and the volar plate are injured, but no Stener lesion is present, and healing of the ligaments is predictable.

3: Trauma

2. Treatment—Reduction and 3 to 4 weeks of immobilization

VII. Fractures of the Distal Phalanx

A. Types of fractures

1. Tuft

2. Diaphyseal

3. Volar (profundus tendon avulsion)

4. Dorsal (mallet finger)

5. Epiphyseal injury (Seymour fracture)

B. Tuft fractures

1. Closed tuft fractures are treated symptomatically. The roles of decompression of a subungual hematoma and nail bed repair are debated.

2. Open tuft fractures are usually treated with simple irrigation, débridement, and suturing in the emergency department.

C. Displaced unstable transverse distal phalanx fractures and flexor profundus avulsion fractures may best be treated with reduction and K-wire fixation.

D. Epiphyseal fractures (Seymour fracture)

1. Open epiphyseal fractures occur in children (typical mechanism: finger caught in car door).

2. The fracture results in nail matrix disruption. The plate may be avulsed lying dorsal to the proximal nail fold. The nail bed also may become interposed in fracture, resulting in nonunion or osteomyelitis.

E. Mallet fracture—Indications for ORIF of mallet fractures

1. Subluxation of the distal phalanx (volar subluxation seen with dorsal articular fracture fragment)

2. Indications with some debate

a. Articular fragment >40%

b. Gap in articular surface >2 mm

F. Profundus tendon avulsions are treated with ORIF when the fracture is large, and tendon advancement and reattachment when the fragment is small.

Top Testing Facts

1. Lag screws can be used without a plate when fracture length is at least twice the bone diameter.

2. Closed reduction and percutaneous pinning is favored for most closed, isolated fractures that can be adequately reduced. ORIF is generally reserved for fractures with associated soft-tissue injury or unstable articular fracture.

3. For metacarpal fractures, angular deformity is better tolerated at the neck than at the diaphyseal level and in the little and ring fingers compared with the index and long fingers.

4. The main deforming force for a little finger CMC fracture-dislocation is the extensor carpi ulnaris tendon.

5. Bennett fractures are best viewed on the Robert (hyperpronated) view.

6. The main deforming force in a thumb trapeziometacarpal fracture-dislocation (Bennett fracture) is provided by the abductor pollicis longus and the adductor pollicis.

7. In complex MCP dislocations, the volar plate remains attached to the proximal phalanx, becomes interposed between the metacarpal head and proximal phalanx, and prevents closed reduction.

8. The major risk of dorsal PIP joint dislocation is stiffness.

9. Dorsal PIP joint dislocations can usually be treated nonsurgically if the fracture of the volar base of the middle phalanx comprises less than 40% of the articular surface.

Bibliography

Beredjiklian PK: Small finger metacarpal neck fractures. *J Hand Surg Am* 2009;34(8):1524-1526.

Bloom JM, Khouri JS, Hammert WC: Current concepts in the evaluation and treatment of mallet finger injury. *Plast Reconstr Surg* 2013;132(4):560e-566e.

Huang JI, Fernandez DL: Fractures of the base of the thumb metacarpal. *Instr Course Lect* 2010;59:343-356.

Jupiter JB, Ring DC: *AO Manual of Fracture Management: Hand and Wrist.* Stuttgart, Germany, Thieme, 2005.

Kollitz KM, Hammert WC, Vedder NB, Huang JI: Metacarpal fractures: Treatment and complications. *Hand (N Y)* 2014;9(1):16-23.

McAuliffe JA: Dorsal fracture dislocation of the proximal interphalangeal joint. *J Hand Surg Am* 2008;33(10): 1885-1888.

Ugurlar M, Saka G, Saglam N, Milcan A, Kurtulmus T, Akp X0131 Nar F: Distal phalanx fracture in adults: Seymour-type fracture. *J Hand Surg Eur Vol* 2014;39(3):237-241.

3: Trauma

Chapter 35

Wrist Fractures and Dislocations, Carpal Instability, and Distal Radius Fractures

David Ring, MD, PhD   Steven L. Moran, MD   Marco Rizzo, MD   Alexander Y. Shin, MD

I. Carpal Fractures

A. Scaphoid fractures

1. Epidemiology—The scaphoid is the most frequently fractured carpal bone.

2. Anatomy

   a. More than one half of the bone is covered by articular cartilage.

   b. The blood supply to the scaphoid is limited. Proximal pole fracture fragments receive a limited blood supply from the scapholunate ligament and radioscapholunate ligament.

3. Evaluation

   a. Physical examination—The following findings are suggestive of a scaphoid fracture:

Dr. Ring or an immediate family member has received royalties from Wright Medical Technology, Inc.; serves as a paid consultant to or is an employee of Biomet, Skeletal Dynamics, and Wright Medical Technology, Inc.; has stock or stock options held in Illuminos; and serves as a board member, owner, officer, or committee member of the American Shoulder and Elbow Surgeons and the American Society for Surgery of the Hand. Dr. Moran or an immediate family member has received royalties from Integra; and is a member of a speakers' bureau or has made paid presentations on behalf of Integra. Dr. Rizzo or an immediate family member is a member of a speakers' bureau or has made paid presentations on behalf of Synthes; serves as a paid consultant to or is an employee of Synthes and Auxilium; serves as an unpaid consultant to Synthes; has received research or institutional support from SBI; and serves as a board member, owner, officer, or committee member of the American Academy of Orthopaedic Surgeons, the American Society for Surgery of the Hand, and the American Association for Hand Surgery. Dr. Shin or an immediate family member has received research or institutional support from the Musculoskeletal Transplant Foundation, Integra Life Sciences, and the American Association for Hand Surgery; and serves as a board member, owner, officer, or committee member of the American Society for Surgery of the Hand.

- Pain in the anatomic snuffbox

- Pain with axial compression of the first metacarpal

- Tenderness at the scaphoid tuberosity

   b. Imaging

- Radiographs may initially appear normal.

- Suspected scaphoid fracture. When there is tenderness of the scaphoid but the initial radiographs are normal (a suspected scaphoid fracture), the extremity can be splinted or casted, and one of the following options is then chosen. There is no consensus on the best management strategy for suspected scaphoid fractures.

  ∘ MRI, CT, or bone scan either immediately or within a few days. Bone scans must be delayed a few days to allow for increased metabolic activity.

  ∘ Repeat examination and radiographs 2 weeks later, with more sophisticated imaging used only for patients in whom scaphoid fracture is still suspected.

- Diagnosis of displacement

  ∘ On radiographs: More than 1 mm displacement or translation of the fracture; more than 15° of dorsal angulation of the lunate

  ∘ On CT scans: Any gap, translation, or angulation

4. Treatment

   a. Nonsurgical

- Nondisplaced scaphoid waist fractures—verification using CT should be considered, can be treated with cast immobilization.

- Inclusion of the thumb and the elbow in the cast are debated.

Table 1

Stages of Progressive Perilunate Instability and Reverse Perilunate Instability

Mayfield's Stages of Progressive Perilunate Instability

Stage	Characteristics
I	Scapholunate dissociation or scaphoid fracture
II	Capitolunate dislocation
III	Lunotriquetral dissociation or triquetral fracture
IV	Lunate dislocation

Stages of Reverse Perilunate Instability

Stage	Characteristics
I	Lunotriquetral dissociation
II	Capitolunate dislocation
III	Scapholunate dissociation

- The duration of cast immobilization is also debated—8 to 10 weeks is standard.

- Distal scaphoid tubercle fractures can be treated symptomatically (that is, splint, ice, medication)

  b. Surgical

- Displaced fractures merit surgery because the rate of nonunion is 50%. Scaphoid fractures associated with perilunate fracture-dislocations are repaired. Proximal pole fractures are increasingly considered for surgical treatment, even when they are nondisplaced.

- The surgical exposure can be dorsal, volar, or arthroscopic assisted.

- Internal fixation is usually performed with a single screw, typically one that has no head and generates compression via differential pitch in the screw threads.

B. Triquetral avulsion fractures

1. These injuries are considered wrist sprains and are treated symptomatically.

2. Stretching exercises help limit the potential for wrist stiffness.

C. Capitate fractures

1. Like the scaphoid bone, the capitate is covered mainly by cartilage. The blood supply is tenuous and can be compromised by transverse fractures.

2. Scaphocapitate syndrome refers to a greater arc injury pattern in which force passes from the scaphoid to the capitate neck, resulting in both scaphoid and capitate fractures. In this syndrome, the capitate head may be rotated 180°, requiring open reduction and internal fixation (ORIF) through a dorsal approach.

D. Hamate fractures

1. Fracture-dislocation of the ring and little metacarpal joints often result in fracture of the hamate.

  a. There is a shearing fracture of the dorsal part of the hamate with or without central articular impaction.

  b. Small fractures without articular impaction can be treated with closed reduction of the carpometacarpal joint and 4 weeks of Kirschner wire (K-wire) immobilization.

  c. Larger fractures and fractures with articular impaction are treated with open reduction and screw fixation.

2. Fracture of the hook of the hamate usually results from a direct blow from a golf club, baseball bat, or racket.

  a. Most hamate hook fractures are diagnosed months after injury as a nonunion causing tenderness with direct pressure.

  b. Surgery is elective and usually consists of excision of the hook of the hamate.

II. Carpal Ligament Injury and Perilunate Dislocation

A. Anatomy and biomechanics

1. The scapholunate interosseous ligament (SLIL) is the primary stabilizer of the scapholunate joint. It is composed of three distinct portions:

  a. The proximal or membranous portion, which has no significant strength

  b. The dorsal portion, which is the strongest portion and prevents translation

  c. The palmar portion, which acts as a rotational constraint

2. Distal scaphoid stabilizers include the scaphotrapezial interosseous ligaments (STIL).

3. The radioscapholunate ligament (ligament of Testut) is a volar intra-articular neurovascular structure and provides little mechanical stability.

4. The palmar stabilizers include the radioscaphocapitate ligament, long radiolunate ligament, and short radiolunate ligament. These ligaments are all

Table 2

Intercarpal Angles and Distances

Parameter	Mean Value	Abnormal Value/Significance
Scapholunate angle	46°	<30° or >60°
Radiolunate angle	0°	>15° dorsal suggests DISI deformity. >15° palmar suggests VISI deformity.
Capitolunate angle	0° (range, 30° dorsal to 30° palmar)	>30° in either volar or dorsal direction
Intercarpal distance		>2 mm between the scaphoid and lunate Increased distance, or diastasis, between the scaphoid and lunate or lunate and triquetrum may indicate an SLIL or LTIL injury.

DISI = dorsal intercalated segmental instability, LTIL = lunotriquetral interosseous ligament, SLIL = scapholunate interosseous ligament, VISI = volar intercalated segmental instability.

thought to be secondary stabilizers of the scaphoid.

5. The dorsal stabilizers are the dorsal radiocarpal ligament and the dorsal intercarpal ligament.

B. Pathomechanics (**Table 1**)

1. Mayfield described the four classic stages of progressive perilunate instability of the wrist, starting with scapholunate ligament disruption.

2. Reverse perilunate instability is a spectrum that might include isolated lunotriquetral (LT) ligament injury.

C. Evaluation

1. Imaging

a. Radiographic abnormalities (**Table 2**)

- Dorsal tilt of the lunate greater than 15° on a true lateral radiograph

- Volar tilt of the lunate on the lateral radiograph is highly variable and should be compared with the contralateral uninjured side.

- A gap of 4 mm or greater between the scaphoid and lunate on the PA view (sometimes with clenching of the hand or ulnar or radial deviation of the wrist) suggests scapholunate ligament injury.

- Ulnar translocation means the carpus is displaced ulnarward (>50% of the lunate lies ulnar to the lunate fossa).

- It can be very difficult to distinguish acute injuries from newly discovered old injuries. Radiographs with slight radioscaphoid arthritis (osteophyte or "beaking" of the radial styloid) represent old injuries. This is the earliest stage of the type of arthritis that occurs with the scapholunate ligament in-

jury known as scapholunate advanced collapse (SLAC). Later stages of SLAC are scaphocapitate and capitolunate arthritis.

- Carpal arcs of Gilula—Gilula described three parallel arcs observed on PA radiographs. The first arc corresponds to the proximal articular surface of the proximal row, the second arc corresponds to the distal articular surface of the proximal row, and the third arc represents the proximal articular surface of the distal carpal row. Disruption of one of these arcs suggests a carpal fracture or ligamentous injury (**Figure 1**).

- Carpal height ratio—This ratio is calculated by dividing the carpal height by the length of the third metacarpal. The normal ratio is 0.54 ± 0.03. In disease processes such as scapholunate dissociation, SLAC, and Kienböck disease, collapse of the midcarpal joint produces a reduction in this ratio.

b. MRI and arthroscopy

- The roles of MRI and MRI with gadolinium arthrography are debated.

- Arthroscopy is considered the reference standard for the diagnosis of intercarpal ligament injuries.

- The most common intercarpal ligament injury is disruption of the scapholunate interosseous ligament, which can be classified based on arthroscopic examination (**Table 3**).

D. Scapholunate (SL) ligament injuries

1. Epidemiology—SL ligament injuries are the most common form of interosseous carpal injury.

2. Pathomechanics

3:Trauma

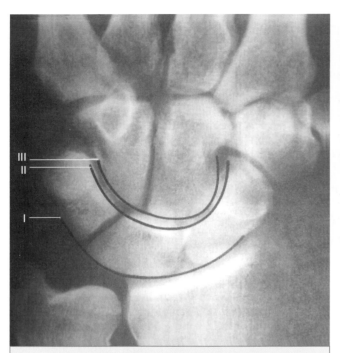

Figure 1 PA radiograph shows the carpal arcs of Gilula. I, smooth arc outlines the proximal surfaces of the scaphoid, lunate, and triquetrum. II, smooth arc outlines the distal surfaces of the scaphoid, lunate, and triquetrum. III, arc outlines the proximal surfaces of the capitate and hamate. (Reproduced from Blazar PE, Lawton JN: Diagnosis of acute carpal ligament injuries, in Trumble TE, ed: *Carpal Fracture-Dislocations*. Rosemont, IL, American Academy of Orthopaedic Surgeons, 2001, p 24.)

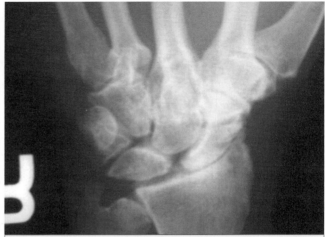

Figure 2 PA radiograph shows a patient with a scapholunate advanced collapse injury.

a. Unopposed extension forces on the lunate imparted by the triquetrum, leading to dorsal incalated segmental instability (DISI)

b. Abnormal scaphoid motion and dorsal subluxation of the scaphoid from the radial fossa during wrist flexion, leading to SLAC wrist arthritis (**Figure 2**)

3. Evaluation

   a. Physical examination

   • Positive scaphoid shift test—The wrist is moved from ulnar to radial deviation. With the examiner's thumb pressing against the scaphoid tubercle this maneuver will produce pain or a clunk, depending on the degree of instability.

   • This maneuver should be compared with the contralateral uninvolved wrist.

   b. Radiographs—PA and lateral views should be obtained.

   • Scapholunate angle—46° is normal; greater than 60° is considered abnormally elevated.

   • Diastasis between the scaphoid and lunate—greater than 4 mm is abnormal.

   • "Signet ring" sign—As the scaphoid flexes, the distal pole will appear as a ring on PA radiographs.

   • Radiolunate angle—greater than 15° dorsal indicates a DISI deformity on a true lateral radiograph.

   • Disruption of the Gilula lines suggests ligament injury.

4. Treatment

   a. Acute injuries—Treatment includes open repair with suture anchors or drill holes through bone, temporary stabilization of the carpus using K-wires or screws, and cast immobilization.

   b. Chronic injuries (dynamic or static)

   • Indications for open repair—Satisfactory ligament remains for repair; the scaphoid and lunate remain easily reducible; no degenerative changes within the carpus

   • Soft-tissue reconstruction (all with inconsistent and imperfect results)

     ○ Dorsal capsulodesis or tenodesis prevents dynamic or static scaphoid flexion.

     ○ Flexor carpi radialis tenodesis uses a strip of the muscle passed from volar to dorsal through a bone tunnel in the distal scaphoid and attached to the distal radius or lunate. Both link the scaphoid to the lunate and limit passive scaphoid flexion.

     ○ Ligament reconstruction—Attempts to reconstruct the SLIL with bone-ligament-

Table 3		

Stages of Scapholunate Instability

Stage	Pathoanatomy	Findings
Predynamic instability	Partial tear or attenuation of SLIL	Radiographs normal
Dynamic instability	Partial or complete tear of SLIL	Stress radiographs abnormal Arthroscopy abnormal (Geissler type II or III)
Static instability	Early: Complete SLIL tear with attenuation or attrition of supporting wrist ligaments Late: Lunate extends as a result of its sagittal plane shape and the unopposed extension force of the intact LT interosseous ligament and becomes fixed in dorsiflexion.	Early: Radiographs positive for scaphoid changes; scapholunate gap > 3 mm, scapholunate angle > 60° Arthroscopy abnormal (Geissler type IV) Late: Lateral radiograph shows DISI deformity (radiolunate angle > 15°)
SLAC wrist	With long-standing abnormal positioning of the carpal bones, arthritic changes occur. Arthritic changes are first seen at the styloscaphoid and radioscaphoid joints and move to the midcarpal joint in a standard progression.	1. Stage 1: arthritis noted at radial styloid 2. Stage 2: arthritis noted at radiocarpal joint 3. Stage 3: arthritis noted at capitolunate interface

DISI = dorsal intercalated segmental instability, LT = lunotriquetral; SLAC = scapholunate advanced collapse; SLIL = scapholunate interosseous ligament.

bone constructs from the carpus, foot, and extensor retinaculum

- ◦ Arthrodesis—Scaphotrapezial or scaphocapitate arthrodesis can be used to stabilize the scaphoid.

c. Chronic injuries with arthritis (SLAC changes)—See **Table 4.**

E. LT ligament injuries

1. LT injuries are much less common and difficult to diagnose.

2. Anatomy of the LT ligament

a. Like the SL ligament, the LT interosseous ligaments are C-shaped ligaments, spanning the dorsal, proximal, and palmar edges of the joint surfaces.

b. The palmar region of the LT is the thickest and strongest region.

c. The dorsal LT ligament region is most important in rotational constraint.

3. Most volar intercalated segmental instability on radiographs occurs in anatomically normal wrists. It is often associated with wrist laxity. It is important to compare radiographs of the symptomatic and asymptomatic sides.

4. Physical examination—The diagnostic performance characteristics of tests such as the LT ballottement, shear, and compression tests are uncertain.

5. Arthroscopy is the reference standard for LT injuries.

6. Treatment—Surgical treatment options include LT ligament repair, LT ligament reconstruction, and LT or capitate-hamate-lunate-triquetral arthrodesis.

F. Perilunate dislocations

1. Pathoanatomy

a. The lunate often remains bound to the carpus by stout radiolunate ligaments, and the carpus dislocates around it. The capitate may move dorsally to cause dorsal perilunate dislocation (common) or palmarly to cause palmar perilunate dislocation (rare).

b. Lunate dislocation occurs when the lunate dislocates from the radial fossa palmarly, resulting in palmar lunate dislocation (common), or dorsally, resulting in dorsal lunate dislocation (rare).

c. Fractures may pass through any bone found within the greater arc of the wrist, including the distal radius, scaphoid, trapezium, capitate, hamate, and triquetrum.

d. Lesser arc injuries pass only through ligamentous structures, with no corresponding fractures.

2. Evaluation

a. Diagnosis can be delayed because some radiographic findings may be subtle; 25% of these injuries are missed during the initial presentation.

b. The physical examination may reveal significant swelling, ecchymosis, and decreased range of motion.

3: Trauma

Table 4

Treatment of Scapholunate Advanced Collapse Changes

Stage	Characteristics	Treatment
I	Early arthritic changes, present only at radial styloid	STT fusion combined with radial styloidectomy for pain relief Scaphocapitate fusion with radial styloidectomy
II	Arthritis present at radioscaphoid joint	Four-corner fusion or proximal row carpectomy[a]
III	Arthritis present at the capitolunate joint	If the capitate is too arthritic to allow a proximal row carpectomy, options may be limited to the following: Four-corner fusion Total wrist fusion Total wrist arthroplasty

[a]Debate as to the benefits of four-corner fusion over proximal row carpectomy and vice versa is ongoing; however, no studies to date clearly show the superiority of one procedure over another.

STT = scaphotrapezial-trapezoid.

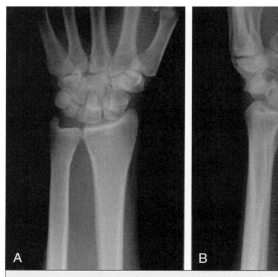

Figure 3   PA (**A**) and lateral (**B**) radiographs show a transscaphoid perilunate dislocation. Note the disruption of the carpal arcs of Gilula on the PA view.

c. The risk of acute carpal tunnel syndrome can be as high as 25% to 50%.

d. Radiographs

- PA views may show a disruption of the carpal arcs of Gilula and overlapping of the carpal bones (**Figure 3, A**).

- Lateral views will show dislocation of the capitate or lunate bones (**Figure 3, B**).

e. CT and MRI are usually not necessary or helpful.

3. Treatment

a. Acute presentation

- Closed reduction may be performed initially for pain relief, but surgery is the definitive treatment.

- Lunate dislocations may require an extended carpal tunnel approach initially for lunate reduction if the lunate cannot be reduced by closed means.

- Beware of acute carpal tunnel syndrome and forearm compartment syndrome. Both can develop over hours to days.

- If the injury can be reduced closed and no acute carpal tunnel syndrome or ulnar translocation is present, a dorsal approach may be adequate, and it can be performed many days later.

b. Surgical treatment

- After the SL ligament is repaired, the repair can be protected with a temporary screw or K-wires across the SL interval.

- Most surgeons place wires across the LT interval and midcarpal joint as well, but results using SL and LT screws leaving the midcarpal joint free to move are comparable, and some surgeons do not treat the LT ligament specifically. More data are needed to determine the best treatment approach.

III. Fractures of the Distal Radius

A. Overview

1. Fractures of the distal radius are among the most

common fractures seen in the emergency department.

2. Patients of advanced age with osteoporosis have an increased fracture risk during low-energy falls.

3. Fracture patterns vary depending on the mechanism of injury.

4. Principles of treatment—The goals of all treatment are to optimize the anatomy and restore function.

B. Management of distal radius fractures

1. Options include closed reduction and cast immobilization, closed reduction and percutaneous pinning with or without external fixation, and ORIF.

2. Surgical treatment indications relate to infirmity, functional demands, tolerance of deformity, and personal preferences. Injury and patient characteristics meriting a discussion of surgical treatment include the following:

   a. Loss of reduction, including ulnar variance 5 mm or more positive; dorsal articular tilt ≥15° (ie, volar apex angulation); and loss of radial inclination >10°

   b. Articular gap or step of 2 mm or more

   c. Unstable volar extra-articular fractures (Smith fracture)

   d. Intra-articular volar shear fracture (Barton fracture)

   e. Open fractures

   f. Fractures with associated neurovascular injuries

   g. Fractures with associated intercarpal ligament injuries

   h. Multiple trauma, such as bilateral distal radius fractures or the need to use crutches for a leg injury (relative indication)

3. Cast or splint immobilization

   a. The optimal reduction technique and immobilization are debated.

   b. Evidence shows that stability determines the final alignment, so wrist splints or short arm casts are usually used, and the elbow and forearm are usually left free.

   c. The total length of immobilization is approximately 6 weeks.

   d. It is important to encourage functional use of the limb to avoid stiffness of the fingers and forearm and to limit swelling.

4. Surgical treatment

   a. Closed reduction and percutaneous pinning

with or without external fixation—0.62-inch or 1.6-mm K-wires

   b. External fixator

   • Bridging external fixation can be used to protect pin fixation or to provide ligamentotaxis.

   • Beware of overdistraction or excessive flexion, which can lead to finger stiffness via tightening of the extrinsic digit flexors.

   • Full incisions over the radius and index metacarpal at the time of fixator pin placement minimize the risk of iatrogenic injury to the superficial branch of the radial nerve or tethering of the first dorsal interosseous muscle.

   • The fixator and pins typically remain in place for 6 weeks.

   • Bone graft or bone void fillers can be used to structurally support bone defects and perhaps allow earlier removal of the fixator.

   c. ORIF

   • Volar locking plates make it possible to stabilize dorsally displaced fractures from through the volar Henry approach (through the sheath of the flexor carpi radialis tendon).

   • Potential pitfalls include intra-articular screw placement and a prominent implant, leading to tendon rupture.

   • The most common tendon to rupture following application of a volar plate is the flexor pollicis longus.

   • Dorsal tendons such as the extensor pollicis longus can fray and rupture from screw tips that have been left prominent in the dorsal compartments following volar insertion.

   • Dorsal plates are now preferred for dorsal shearing fractures and complex articular fractures (in combination with volar plates). When used, the approach is between the third and the fourth dorsal compartments.

C. Volarly displaced extra-articular fractures (Smith fractures) can be treated with reduction and casting if no comminution is present and a good reduction is obtained, but these relatively uncommon injuries are usually treated surgically with a volar plate and screws.

D. Fractures of the radial styloid (chauffeur fractures)

1. These fractures may be associated with SL ligament injuries because the intra-articular fracture line extends into the joint at that level. Therefore, in the setting of isolated radial styloid fractures,

intercarpal ligament injuries must be suspected.

2. Treatment

   a. Nonsurgical—If the fracture is nondisplaced or minimally displaced, it may be treated nonsurgically.

   b. Surgical—Intra-articular displacement (or diastasis) greater than 2 mm is an indication for surgery. Compression screw fixation with partially threaded 3.5- or 4.0-mm cancellous screws can effectively compress the fragments and maintain the reduction. Alternative fixa-

tion options include K-wires and plate and screw fixation.

E. Distal radioulnar joint

1. The distal radioulnar joint must be assessed following stabilization of the radius. The presence of a displaced fracture at the base of the ulnar styloid is not in itself an indication for surgical fixation.

2. Preoperative physical examination of the distal radioulnar joint laxity of the unaffected side is helpful.

Top Testing Facts

1. Nondisplaced scaphoid waist fractures, as verified by CT, can be treated with cast immobilization.

2. A triquetral avulsion fracture is a simple wrist sprain and can be treated symptomatically.

3. Indications for surgical treatment of a scaphoid fracture include fracture displacement and perilunate ligamentous injuries.

4. The SLAC pattern of arthritis progresses from the radial styloid to the radioscaphoid joint, and to the capitolunate joint.

5. The potential for acute carpal tunnel syndrome with perilunate fracture-dislocations should always be considered.

6. Radiographic measures of alignment that prompt con-

sideration of surgical treatment for distal radius fractures include shortening ($\geq$5 mm), dorsal angulation ($\geq$15°), loss of radial inclination (>10°), or articular displacement ($\geq$2 mm).

7. Intra-articular volar shear fractures (Barton fractures) and unstable volar extra-articular fractures (Smith fractures) are treated with a volar plate and screws.

8. The tendon most at risk from a prominent volar plate is the flexor pollicis longus.

9. In the setting of isolated radial styloid fractures, scapholunate injury should be suspected.

10. The presence of a displaced fracture at the base of the ulnar styloid is not an indication for surgical fixation.

Bibliography

Cooney WP III, Linscheid RL, Dobyns JH: Carpal instability: Treatment of ligament injuries of the wrist. *Instr Course Lect* 1992;41:33-44.

Herzberg G, Comtet JJ, Linscheid RL, Amadio PC, Cooney WP, Stalder J: Perilunate dislocations and fracture-dislocations: A multicenter study. *J Hand Surg Am* 1993;18(5): 768-779.

Hildebrand KA, Ross DC, Patterson SD, Roth JH, MacDermid JC, King GJ: Dorsal perilunate dislocations and fracture-dislocations: Questionnaire, clinical, and radiographic evaluation. *J Hand Surg Am* 2000;25(6):1069-1079.

Kalainov DM, Cohen MS: Treatment of traumatic scapholunate dissociation. *J Hand Surg Am* 2009;34(7):1317-1319.

Lang PO, Bickel KD: Distal radius fractures: Percutaneous treatment versus open reduction with internal fixation. *J Hand Surg Am* 2014;39(3):546-548.

Mack GR, Bosse MJ, Gelberman RH, Yu E: The natural history of scaphoid non-union. *J Bone Joint Surg Am* 1984; 66(4):504-509.

Mayfield JK, Johnson RP, Kilcoyne RK: Carpal dislocations: Pathomechanics and progressive perilunar instability. *J Hand Surg Am* 1980;5(3):226-241.

Ring D, Lozano-Calderón S: Imaging for suspected scaphoid fracture. *J Hand Surg Am* 2008;33(6):954-957.

Souer JS, Rutgers M, Andermahr J, Jupiter JB, Ring D: Perilunate fracture-dislocations of the wrist: Comparison of temporary screw versus K-wire fixation. *J Hand Surg Am* 2007; 32(3):318-325.

Chapter 36
Pelvic, Acetabular, and Sacral Fractures

Raymond D. Wright Jr, MD

I. Pelvic Fractures

A. Epidemiology

   1. Most commonly occurs in men in their 40s

   2. Considerable diversity in associated visceral and soft-tissue injuries

   3. Morbidity and mortality rates range from 10% to 50%

B. Anatomy

   1. Osseous

      a. The pelvic ring is formed by two innominate bones joined posteriorly through the sacrum and anteriorly by the symphysis pubis (**Figures 1 and 2**).

      b. Each innominate bone is formed by the confluence of the ilium, ischium, and pubis.

      c. The pelvic ring has no inherent bony stability.

      • Anterior stability comes from the symphysis pubis, a fibrocartilaginous disk between the anterior portion of the innominate bones and the surrounding ligamentous attachments.

      • Posterior stability comes from the anterior and posterior sacroiliac ligaments (posterior are stronger than anterior).

      • The sacrospinous and sacrotuberous ligaments provide stability to the pelvic floor. The iliolumbar ligaments form a broad connection between the transverse processes of L4, L5, and the posterior ilium.

   2. Vascular

      a. The common iliac system begins near L4 at the bifurcation of the abdominal aorta.

      • The external iliac artery courses anteriorly along the pelvic brim to emerge as the common femoral artery distal to the inguinal ligament.

      • The internal iliac artery divides caudal and posterior near the sacroiliac joint. The posterior division gives rise to the superior gluteal artery and several other branches before exiting the posterior pelvis as the inferior gluteal and internal pudendal arteries. The anterior portion of the internal iliac artery becomes the obturator artery.

      b. The corona mortis is a connection between the obturator and iliac systems. One cadaver analysis demonstrated that the anastomosis is found a mean of 6.2 cm from the symphysis pubis in 84% of specimens and can be arterial, venous, or both. Traditionally, this structure is discussed in the context of retropubic dissection for acetabular fractures.

      c. A venous plexus in the posterior pelvis that results in the internal iliac system. Injury to this venous plexus and bony bleeding account for 90% of the hemorrhage associated with pelvic ring injuries.

   3. Neurologic

      a. The lumbosacral plexus is created from nerve roots L1-S4 (**Figure 3**).

      b. The lateral femoral cutaneous nerve (L2-3) runs deep to the inguinal ligament near the anterior superior iliac spine.

      c. The obturator nerve (L2-4) runs along the quadrilateral surface and exits peripherally and cranially in the obturator canal at the obturator sulcus.

      d. The femoral nerve (L2-4) travels with the iliopsoas tendon.

      e. The sciatic nerve (L4-S3) exits the greater sciatic notch.

3: Trauma

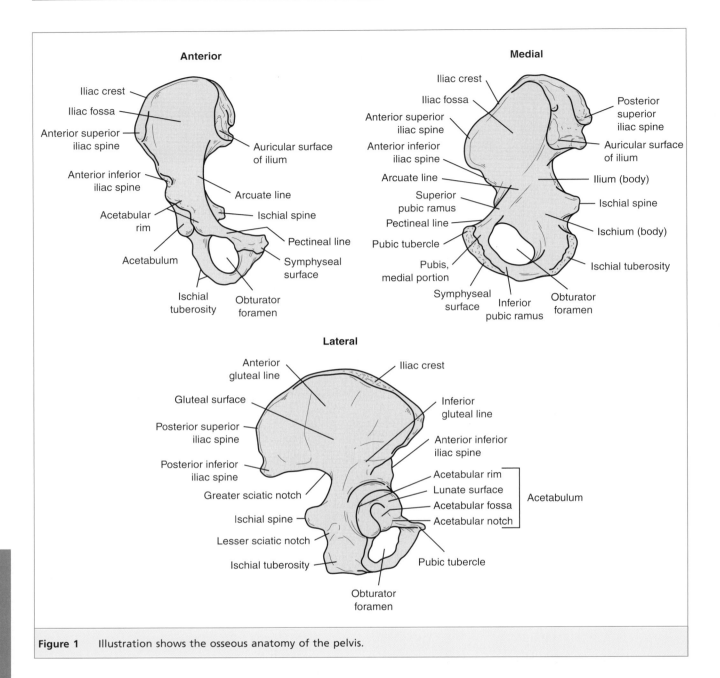

Figure 1   Illustration shows the osseous anatomy of the pelvis.

f. The L5 nerve root lies on the cranial anterior portion of the sacral ala 10 to 15 mm medial to the anterior portion of the sacroiliac joint.

C. Classification

1. AO Foundation/Orthopaedic Trauma Association (AO/OTA)

a. Classification based on the Tile and Pennal classification system with an additional numeric modifier (**Figure 4**)

b. The Tile classification system evaluated the potential instability of the pelvic ring injury.

- Type A, stable

- Type B, rotationally unstable, vertically stable

- Type C, rotationally and vertically unstable

2. Young-Burgess

a. Classification based on mechanism of injury (**Figure 5**)

b. Mechanisms divided into the following categories: lateral compression, anteroposterior compression, vertical shear, and combined mechanical injury (**Table 1**)

3. Letournel:

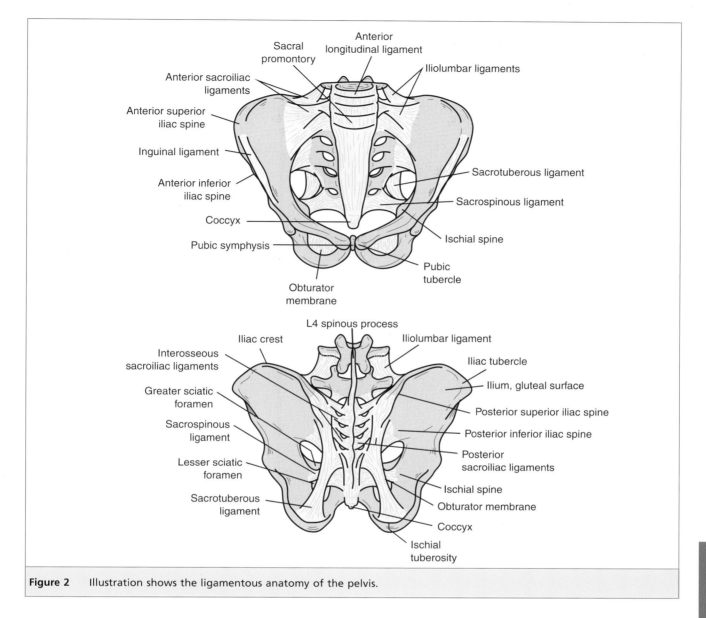

Figure 2   Illustration shows the ligamentous anatomy of the pelvis.

a. This system is based on anatomic site of injury.

b. The pelvis is divided into anterior and posterior portions.

c. This classification system is purely descriptive and provides no estimation of injury severity or pelvic stability (**Figure 6**).

D. Mechanism of injury

1. Most frequently high-energy trauma

2. Most common causes of injury (descending frequency):

   a. Motorcycle crashes

   b. Pedestrian-sustained automobile injuries

   c. Falls

   d. Motor vehicle crashes

   e. Crush injuries

3. Low-energy mechanisms may be possible in elderly patients with poor bone quality

E. Evaluation

1. Full Advanced Trauma Life Support (ATLS) workup because of high incidence of associated injuries

2. The skin and soft tissues should be inspected for evidence of open injury including the perineum and gluteal folds; a rectal and vaginal examination should be performed.

3. The skin is inspected for closed internal degloving lesions (Morel-Lavallee). The resulting necrotic fat and hematoma can contaminate the surgical exposure and may require débridement.

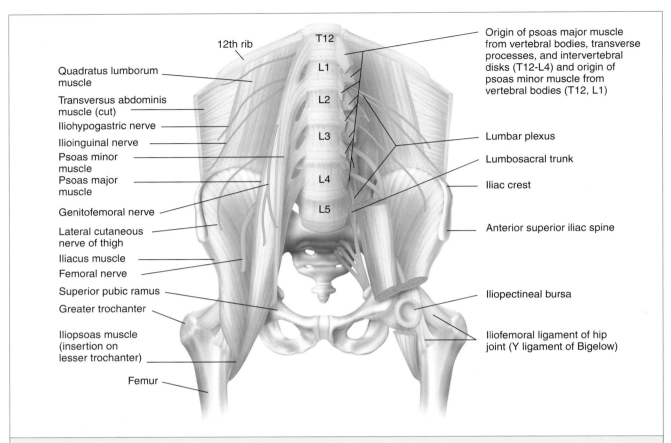

Figure 3   Illustration shows the anterior muscles of the lumbosacral plexus. (Reproduced from Della Valle CJ, Weber K: Hip and thigh: Anatomy of the hip and thigh, in Sarwark JF, ed: *Essentials of Musculoskeletal Care*, ed 4. Rosemont, IL, American Academy of Orthopaedic Surgeons, 2010, 530.)

4. Neurologic examination, including sacral nerve roots

5. Imaging

a. AP pelvic radiograph as a screening study in patients suspected of having a pelvic ring injury (routine screening study for trauma patients) (**Figure 7, A**)

b. Inlet pelvic view (**Figure 7, B**)

- Variable amount of caudal tilt, which depends on individual patient anatomy; ideally, the beam is perpendicular to the S1 end plate

- Demonstrates anteroposterior displacement of pelvic ring, horizontal rotation of injured hemipelvis

c. Outlet pelvic view (**Figure 7, C**):

- Variable amount of cranial tilt; ideally, the cranial portion of the symphysis pubis is centered at the level of the S2 body

- Demonstrates cranial-caudal displacement of the pelvic ring, sacral morphology

d. Computed tomography

- Improves detection and understanding of injury pattern; 30% of posterior injuries can be missed on plain radiographs

- May evaluate sacral nerve root tunnels for presence of bony debris or stenosis from fracture

- Soft tissue may be evaluated to detect hematoma formation, active arterial bleeding (in contrast-enhanced studies), and displacement of pelvic organs from hemorrhage

- CT confirms diagnosis and provides fine detail of the pelvic ring injury and enables the clinician to detect occult injuries that may not be visible on plain radiographs.

F. Treatment

1. Initial management

a. Consideration of the patient's hemodynamic status and injury pattern determines initial management.

b. ATLS protocol mandatory for all patients with osseous pelvic trauma

Groups:
Type A fracture: pelvis, ring, stable (61-A)

1. Fracture of innominate bone, avulsion (61-A1)

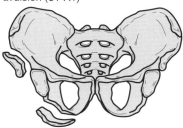

2. Fracture of innominate bone, direct blow (61-A2)

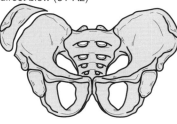

3. Transverse fracture of sacrum and coccyx (61-A3)

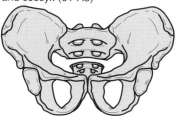

Type B fracture: pelvis, ring, partially stable (61-B)

1. Unilateral, partial disruption of posterior arch, external rotation ("open-book" injury) (61-B1)

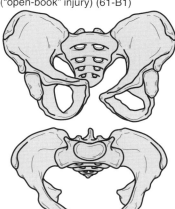

2. Unilateral, partial disruption of posterior arch, internal rotation (lateral compression injury) (61-B2)

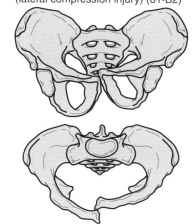

3. Bilateral, partial lesion of posterior arch (61-B3)

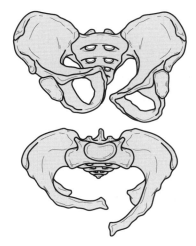

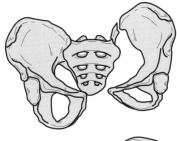
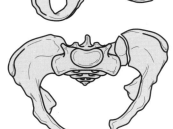
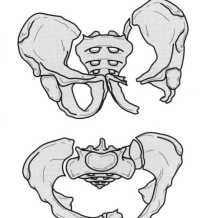

Type C fracture: pelvis, ring, complete disruption of posterior arch unstable (61-C)

1. Unilateral, complete disruption of posterior arch (61-C1)

2. Bilateral, ipsilateral complete, contralateral incomplete (61-C2)

3. Bilateral, complete disruption (61-C3)

Figure 4 The AO/Orthopaedic Trauma Association fracture compendium for pelvic fractures. Type A fractures are considered stable. Type B fractures are rotationally unstable and vertically stable. Type C fractures are rotationally and vertically unstable.

3: Trauma

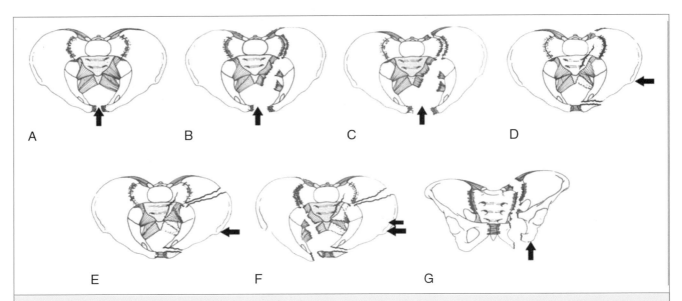

Figure 5   Diagram shows the Young-Burgess classification of pelvic fractures. **A,** Anteroposterior compression type I. **B,** Anteroposterior compression type II. **C,** Anteroposterior compression type III. **D,** Lateral compression type I. **E,** Lateral compression type II. **F,** Lateral compression type III. **G,** Vertical shear. (Reproduced from Hak DJ, Smith WR, Suzuki T: Management of hemorrhage in life-threatening pelvic fracture. *J Am Acad Orthop Surg* 2009;17[7]:451.)

Table 1

Comparison of the Young-Burgess Classification Fracture Types

Mechanism	I	II	III	Comments
LC	Horizontal fractures in rami with sacral impaction	Posterior ligamentous disruption of SI joint or equivalent bony disruption of posterior ilium	LC pattern on side ipsilateral to injury with contralateral external rotation deformity	Deaths with increasing LC grades because of increasing incidence of brain injury with only modest increases in complications related to ARDS, sepsis, and shock
APC	Anterior symphyseal widening ≤ 25 mm, incomplete anterior SI injury	Anterior symphyseal widening ≥ 25 mm, disruption of anterior SI, sacrospinous, and sacrotuberous ligaments	Anterior symphyseal injury with complete dissociation of SI joint	Circulatory shock, sepsis, and ARDS are substantial causes of death in increasing APC grades. APC III injuries have the highest fluid requirements, hemorrhage, and mortality
VS	Total disruption of posterior ligamentous structures resulting in craniocaudal as well as rotational instability			Associated systemic injury pattern similar to LC group
CMI	Fracture pattern does not fit any single classification			Associated systemic injury pattern similar to APC group

APC = anteroposterior compression, ARDS = acute respiratory distress syndrome, CMI = combined mechanical injury, LC = lateral compression, SI = sacroiliac, VS = vertical shear.

   c. Patients with unstable fracture patterns and hemodynamic instability may benefit from emergent skeletal stability to minimize intrapelvic hemorrhage.

   d. Emergent osseous pelvic stability may be achieved by various means.

• External fixation—Excellent anterior pelvic control; relatively little utility in pelvic fractures with complete posterior injury; may require fluoroscopy for safe placement; pins may contaminate definitive surgical incisions.

- C-clamp—Excellent posterior ring control; requires fluoroscopy for safe placement; may contaminate posterior approaches or insertion of iliosacral screws

- Pneumatic antishock garments—Application may diminish venous return, cause compartment syndrome, and cause injury to the skin and soft tissues.

- Pelvic binders—Can provide stability to the entire pelvic ring; may be applied in the field

- Sheets—Readily available; strategic application requires Kocher clamps, towel clips, and so forth for application; portions of sheet may be cut out for vascular access, angiography, external fixator placement, and percutaneous fixation; skin needs to be monitored regularly (**Figures 8** and **9**)

  - Traction—May be used for fractures with potential cranial-caudal instability

2. Nonsurgical treatment

   a. Indicated in patients with stable injuries or those in whom substantial medical comorbidities prohibit surgical intervention

   b. Patients are usually mobilized with toe-touch or flatfoot weight bearing on the side of the posterior ring injury.

   c. Radiographs may be obtained after mobilization to determine if occult instability is unmasked with mobilization.

3. Surgical treatment

   a. Generally reserved for unstable injuries

   b. Unstable symphyseal injuries generally are treated using open reduction and internal fixation (ORIF) with cranially applied plates and screws.

   c. Superior ramus fractures may be stabilized surgically, depending on the contribution of the fractures to the overall stability of the pelvic ring; surgical options include medullary ramus screws, plates, and external fixators

   d. Posterior ilium fractures may be treated with ORIF or percutaneous fixation, depending on the displacement and location of the iliac injury.

   e. Sacroiliac disruptions may be treated percutaneously if incomplete or complete with

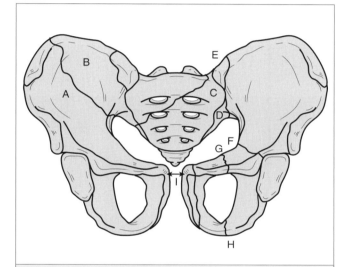

Figure 6 Illustration depicts the Letournel classification of pelvic fractures. This classification is descriptive and provides information about the location and types of injuries to the pelvic ring.

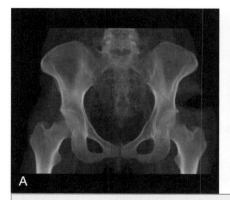
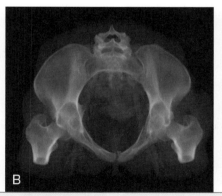
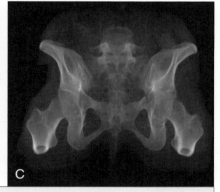

Figure 7 Images show the radiographic evaluation for pelvic fractures. **A,** The AP pelvic view is used to provisionally diagnose an injury and direct further workup. **B,** The inlet pelvic view is obtained so that the S1 and S2 bodies overlap and provides information regarding the anteroposterior translation of one hemipelvis relative to the contralateral side. Additionally, horizontal plane rotation can be demonstrated with this view. **C,** The outlet pelvic view demonstrates the upper and second sacral segment morphology and can demonstrate craniocaudal translation of an injured pelvic segment.

3: Trauma

displacement amenable to closed reduction; open reduction generally is required for complete injuries that do not reduce using closed or indirect means. Open reduction may be performed anteriorly through the lateral window of the ilioinguinal exposure or through posterior open exposure to the sacroiliac joint. Fixation methods include iliosacral screws, transsacral plates, transsacral bars, or a two-hole or three-hole plate applied across the anterior sacroiliac joint.

f. Sacral fractures that are part of a pelvic ring injury may be treated using percutaneous fixation techniques if acceptable reduction is present; these techniques include iliosacral screws and posterior transiliac bars. ORIF may be performed through a direct posterior exposure. After open reduction is achieved, fixation may be achieved with iliosacral screws, transiliac, transsacral screws, transiliac bars, or a transiliac plate.

g. Postoperative mobility is generally toe-touch or flatfoot weight bearing on the side of the posterior pelvic ring injury for approximately 6 weeks.

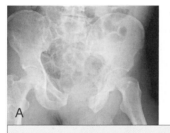
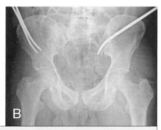

Figure 8 AP radiographs show an open pelvic fracture in a 52-year-old man. **A,** The symphysis pubis is widened with incomplete injury to the left anterior sacroiliac joint. **B,** The same pelvic ring injury after a sheet is applied to close the pelvic ring.

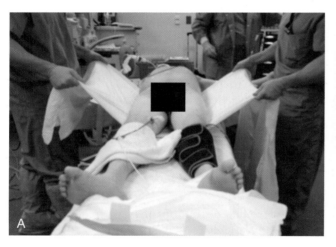
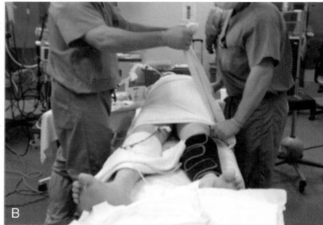
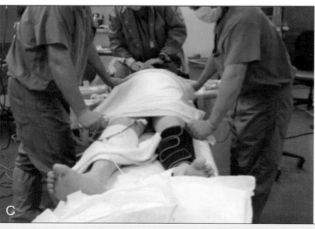
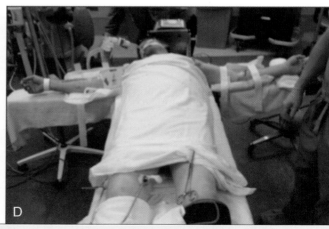

Figure 9 Photographs show the proper application of a draw sheet as a resuscitative aid. **A,** The draw sheet is pulled taut to minimize wrinkles in the sheet, preventing skin irritation and breakdown. **B,** One side of the sheet is moved to the contralateral side of the patient. **C,** Both sides of the sheet have been exchanged and are now pulled tightly across the patient. **D,** Large Kocher clamps hold the sheet in place.

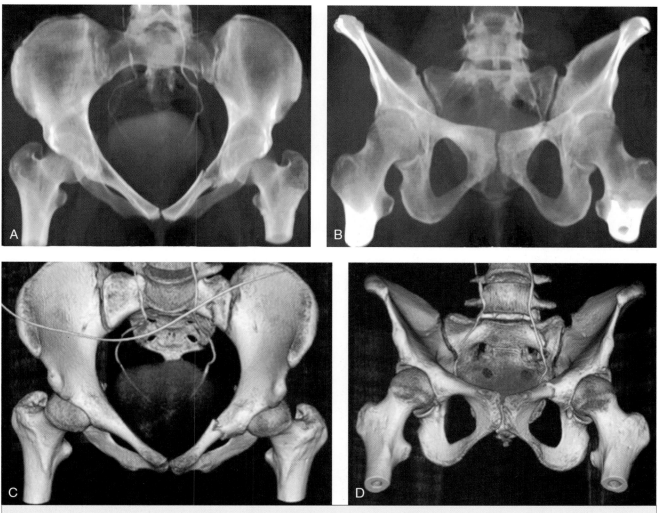

Figure 10 Comparison of normal (**A** through **D**) and dysmorphic (**E** through **H**) upper sacral segments using inlet (**A, E**) and outlet (**B, F**) radiographs with corresponding respective three-dimensional CT reconstructions (**C, D, G, H**). The dysmorphic upper sacral segment exhibits anterior and up-sloping sacral alar regions, irregular (not circular) appearing sacral nerve root tunnels, a residual S1 disk, and mammillary bodies. A "tongue-in-groove" appearance of the sacroiliac joint is a radiographic characteristic of sacral dysmorphism that can be best appreciated on an axial CT scan.

(continued on next page)

4. Specific surgical techniques

   a. External fixation

   • Pin placement options:

   ◦ Gluteus medius pillar directed toward the pelvic brim

   ◦ Anterior inferior iliac spine directed toward the sciatic buttress or posterior superior iliac spine

   ◦ Fluoroscopy is required for safe, durable pin placement.

   • Successful treatment of pelvic ring injury with an anterior frame can be accomplished only with some intact posterior structures; this allows the anterior frame to function as a tension band. One example is an anteroposterior compression type II pelvic ring injury with a disrupted and unstable pubic symphysis with intact posterior sacroiliac ligaments. Anterior external fixation cannot adequately stabilize a hemipelvis with a complete posterior injury.

   • Anterior external fixation is used more commonly as definitive fixation than for resuscitation. Definitive incisions to instrument the pelvic ring may be contaminated by external fixator pin tracts.

   b. Iliosacral screws

3: Trauma

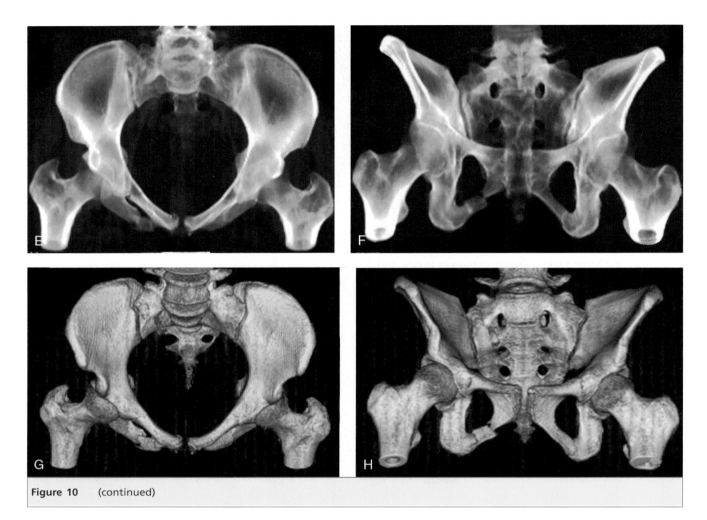

Figure 10 (continued)

- Indicated for sacroiliac disruptions, sacral fractures, and sacroiliac fracture-dislocations

- Sacral morphology may limit insertion options for safe screws. Identification of the dysmorphic upper sacral segment is important in planning for surgical treatment of the posterior pelvic ring. Sacral dysmorphism is present in approximately 30% to 40% of the population.

- Radiographic signs of sacral dysmorphism (**Figure 10**)

  - Anterior, up-sloping upper sacral ala

  - Irregular (not circular) sacral nerve-root tunnels

  - Residual S1 disk

  - Upper sacral body not recessed caudal to the peripheral ilium on the pelvic outlet

  - Mammillary bodies

  - Tongue-and-groove sacroiliac joint

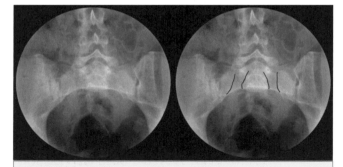

Figure 11 Inlet fluoroscopic views of the upper sacral segment. Lines indicate the course of the upper sacral segment nerve root tunnels.

- Intraoperative radiography of iliosacral screws

  - Inlet view—Demonstrates anteroposterior extents of osseous safety; sacral nerve root tunnel can be visualized as proceeding from posterior midline to anterior peripheral (**Figure 11**)

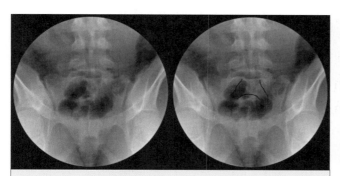

Figure 12 Outlet fluoroscopic views of the upper sacral segment. Lines indicate the course of the upper sacral segment nerve root tunnels.

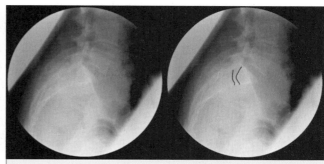

Figure 13 True lateral fluoroscopic views of the upper sacral segment. Lines indicate the course of the upper sacral segment nerve root tunnels.

- Outlet view—Demonstrates cranial-caudal extents of osseous safety; sacral nerve root tunnel can be visualized as proceeding from cranial midline to caudal peripheral (**Figure 12**)

- Sacral lateral view—This view is mandatory to ensure correct implant placement and avoid injury to the L5 and S1 nerve roots when placing instruments in the upper sacral segment. This view should be obtained when the drill is just peripheral to the upper sacral nerve root tunnel; the drill bit should be cranial and anterior to lateral projection of the upper sacral segment nerve root tunnel. If the patient has a nondysmorphic upper sacral segment, the drill should be caudal and posterior to the iliac cortical density because the iliac cortical density approximates the sacral alar slope in a nondysmorphic upper sacral segment (**Figure 13**).

5. Special circumstances and associated injuries

 a. Open pelvic fractures

 - An approximate 50% mortality rate exists for open pelvic fractures, not including direct fractures to the peripheral ilium.

 - Treatment includes thorough débridement and irrigation with skeletal stabilization.

 - Tetanus booster and broad-spectrum antibiotics at initial evaluation

 - Diversion colostomy for patients with wounds contaminated by the fecal stream

 - The importance of careful inspection of the perineum cannot be overemphasized. Occult open injuries may exist in the gluteal folds, scrotum, vagina, labia, and so forth (**Figure 14**).

 b. Neurologic injury

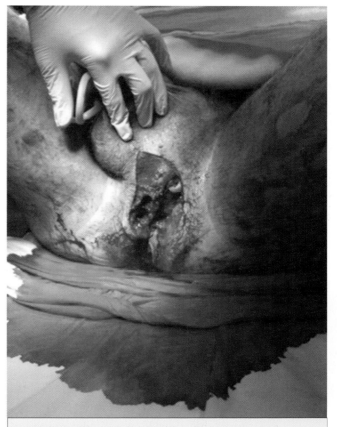

Figure 14 Photograph shows a patient with an open pelvic ring injury and a large wound in the perineum.

- Approximately 10% to 15% of patients will sustain neurologic injury. The most important predictor of outcome in these patients is the type and permanence of the neurologic injury.

- Focal neurologic deficits with corresponding bony entrapment (that is, sacral nerve root compressed in sacral fracture) should prompt decompression of the nerve roots in

3: Trauma

addition to fracture fixation.

c. Injury to genitourinary structures

- Injury to the urethra is more common in men than in women, secondary to urethral length.

- Bladder ruptures may be extraperitoneal, intraperitoneal, or both.

  ○ Extraperitoneal injuries may be treated closed by maintaining a urinary catheter for 10 to 14 days with broad-spectrum antibiotics.

  ○ Peritoneal injuries require surgical repair.

  ○ Pelvic instability causing continued bladder insult might require surgical stabilization.

d. Hypovolemic shock

- Treatment begins with multidisciplinary ATLS evaluation

  ○ Insertion of two large-bore peripheral intravenous needles

  ○ Infusion of 2 L of isotonic solution

- Pelvic stability should be part of resuscitation; this can be accomplished by wrapping the patient in a draw sheet.

- Resistance to fluid resuscitation should be augmented with administration of type O-negative blood.

- Other sources of bleeding (abdomen, chest, open wounds) should be considered in the patient refractory to aggressive fluid and blood resuscitation.

- Because 90% of hemorrhage associated with pelvic fractures is from bony bleeding or retroperitoneal venous bleeding, angiography should be used as an adjunct rather than the primary mode of hemorrhage control in most pelvic fracture patients.

- Retroperitoneal packing also may be used to control hemorrhage as an adjunctive measure.

6. Rehabilitation

a. Stable fractures treated nonsurgically

- Patients may mobilize immediately with protected weight bearing after a stable fracture pattern is confirmed.

- After radiographic healing occurs, patients may engage in quadriceps, hip, and core strengthening.

b. Unstable fractures treated surgically

- Patient mobility and weight bearing generally depend on the location of the posterior pelvic ring fracture.

- Mobility includes weight-of-limb weight bearing ipsilateral to the posterior pelvic injury with full weight bearing on the contralateral side.

- Patients with bilateral posterior injuries are mobilized with bed-to-chair transfers only, using the upper extremities to mobilize, if possible.

- When radiographic healing has occurred, weight bearing may be advanced gradually, as well as lower extremity strengthening.

7. Complications

a. Nonunion is rare in stable injuries but can occur in injuries that are treated closed with neglected instability.

b. Malunion is more common than nonunion, especially in patients with craniocaudal instability.

c. Sitting imbalance and limb-length discrepancy may result from cranial displacement of an unstable pelvic fracture.

d. Thromboembolic phenomena

- Incidence of deep vein thrombosis may be 35% to 50%

- Incidence of pulmonary embolism in up to 10% of cases

- Fatal pulmonary embolism in 2% of patients

e. Chemical prophylaxis is recommended for patients with pelvic fracture; the duration and type are debatable.

f. Patients with contraindications to deep vein thrombosis/pulmonary embolism prophylaxis may benefit from placement of an inferior vena cava filter.

g. Iatrogenic neurovascular injury is possible while instrumenting the pelvis. A thorough understanding of the osseous fixation pathways and their respective radiographic correlates is mandatory before attempting surgical fixation of pelvic ring injuries.

II. Acetabular Fractures

A. Epidemiology

1. Acetabular fractures frequently occur with associated injuries.

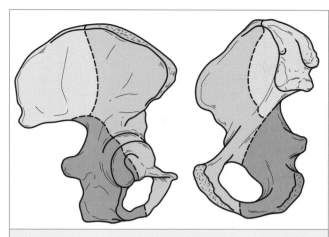

Figure 15 Illustrations show the columns of the acetabulum as described by Letournel. (Reproduced with permission from Letournel E: Acetabulum fractures: Classification and management. *Clin Orthop Relat Res* 1980;151:82.)

2. One of the largest series of acetabular fractures demonstrated the following associated injuries

   a. Extremity injury, 35%

   b. Head injury, 19%

   c. Chest injury, 18%

   d. Nerve palsy, 13%

   e. Abdominal injury, 8%

   f. Genitourinary injury, 6%

   g. Spine injury, 4%

B. Anatomy

   1. Letournel described the acetabulum as being contained within an arch forming an inverted Y (**Figure 15**).

      a. Anterior column—Extends from the anterior portion of the iliac crest to the symphysis pubis; includes the iliac fossa, medius pillar, anterior superior iliac spine (ASIS), anterior inferior iliac spine, and superior ramus.

      b. Posterior column—Cranial border is sciatic buttress; extends caudally to include ischial tuberosity, posterior wall, quadrilateral surface

   2. The column concept emphasizes the importance of osseous structures surrounding the articular surface for reduction, clamp application, and insertion of durable implants.

C. Classification

   1. AO/OTA classification—Pelvis (bone 6); acetabular location (region 2) (**Figure 16**)

   2. More commonly classified by Judet and Letournel as five elementary and five associated fracture patterns (**Figure 17**)

      a. Elementary patterns—Anterior wall, anterior column, posterior wall, posterior column, and transverse (**Table 2**)

      b. Associated patterns—Posterior column–posterior wall, transverse–posterior wall, T-shaped, anterior column–posterior hemitransverse, associated both-column (**Table 3; Figure 18**)

D. Surgical exposures

   1. Kocher-Langenbeck (**Figure 19**)

      a. Performed in the prone or lateral positions

      b. Exposure hazards

         • Sciatic nerve—Protected with visualization, knee flexion, and hip extension. Retractors should not be placed in the lesser sciatic notch.

         • Ascending branch of medial femoral circumflex artery—Protected by performing tenotomy of the piriformis and the obturator internus 1 cm midline to their respective femoral insertions

         • Superior gluteal neurovascular branches—Between medius and minimus

      c. Useful for the following fractures

         • Posterior wall

         • Posterior column

         • Posterior column–posterior wall

         • Transverse

         • Transverse posterior wall

         • Some T-shaped

   2. Ilioinguinal (**Figure 20**)

      a. Usually performed in the supine position; generally regarded as the most common exposure for associated both-column acetabulum fractures

      b. The skin incision classically is made along the iliac crest just posterior to the medius pillar and continued anterior to the ASIS. The incision is directed caudal and midline ending 2 cm cranial to the pubic symphysis in the midline. The lateral window is created by subperiosteal dissection of the iliacus muscle from the internal iliac fossa. The middle window is created by incising the external oblique aponeurosis and reflecting it distally, followed by splitting the inguinal ligament along its oblique course. The lateral femoral cutaneous nerve usually can be identified just deep to the inguinal ligament at the ASIS. The iliopectineal fascia divides the middle window into two

3: Trauma

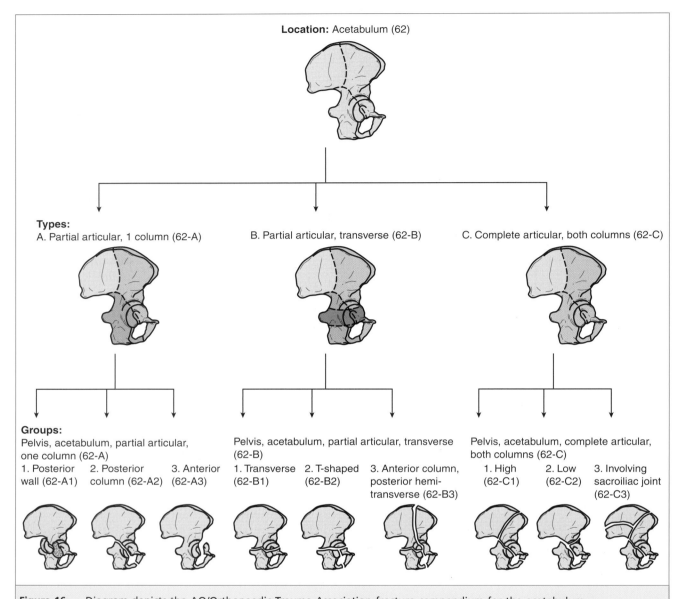

Figure 16   Diagram depicts the AO/Orthopaedic Trauma Association fracture compendium for the acetabulum.

portions: the lateral portion contains the ilio-psoas tendon and the femoral nerve, and the medial portion contains the inguinal artery, vein, and lymphatics. The iliopectineal fascia is divided sharply and under direct visualization. The classic description of the medial window includes lateral mobilization of the spermatic cord or round ligament with transection of the rectus abdominus tendon.

  c. Exposure hazards

- Iliac vessels—Protected with subperiosteal dissection in lateral window; keeping the patient's hip flexed while dissecting and working in the middle window removes tension from the vessels.

- Lateral femoral cutaneous nerve—This structure is identified deep to inguinal ligament, usually at the level of the ASIS, but its position may vary.

- Spermatic cord and ilioinguinal nerve—Careful dissection of external oblique aponeurosis

- Corona mortis—Communication between the obturator and iliac systems; this may be arterial, venous, or both

  d. Useful for the following fractures

- Anterior column

- Anterior column–posterior hemitransverse

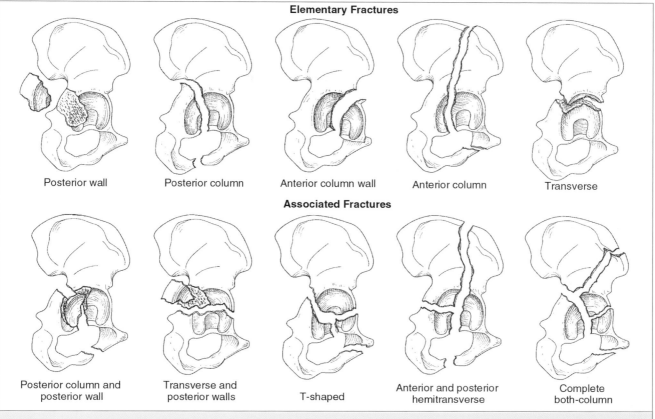

Elementary Fractures

Posterior wall   Posterior column   Anterior column wall   Anterior column   Transverse

Associated Fractures

Posterior column and posterior wall   Transverse and posterior walls   T-shaped   Anterior and posterior hemitransverse   Complete both-column

Figure 17   Diagram shows the acetabular subtypes as described by Letournel and Judet. (Reproduced from Webb LX: Open reduction and internal fixation of posterior wall acetabular fractures, in Flatow E, Colvin AC, eds: *Atlas of Essential Orthopaedic Procedures*. Rosemont, IL, American Academy of Orthopaedic Surgeons, 2013, p 385.)

- T-shaped

- Transverse

- Associated both-column

3. Extended iliofemoral

   a. Indicated by some authors for some complex acetabular fractures that contain a transtectal transverse component, comminution of the sciatic buttress, or associated both-column acetabulum fractures with comminution in the posterior column.

   b. This approach is classically indicated for surgical management of acetabular fractures that are at least 3 weeks old.

4. Stoppa

   a. This approach may substitute for the medial window in the ilioinguinal exposure or it can stand alone for certain acetabular fractures.

   b. Retropubic dissection is performed to expose the inner quadrilateral surface.

   c. This approach is useful for fracture visualization, reduction, clamp application, and in-

trapelvic plate placement.

   d. Used for associated both-column and anterior-column fractures

5. Smith-Petersen

   a. This exposure uses the internervous plane between the superior gluteal and femoral nerves.

   b. The interval may be useful for the surgical repair of select anterior wall fractures.

E. Mechanism of injury

   1. Frequently high-energy injuries: motor vehicle collisions, falls from a height, motorcycle crashes

   2. Low-energy mechanism possible in patients with poor bone quality

   3. Fracture pattern determined by force vector and position of hip at time of impact

   4. Energy mechanism may be direct to pelvis or indirect, with axial force through the femoral head

F. Evaluation

   1. Physical examination

      a. Full ATLS evaluation warranted because of

3: Trauma

Table 2

The Elementary Acetabular Fracture Types

Elementary Fracture	Description	Comments
Posterior wall	Separation of posterior articular surface	Frequently associated with posterior hip dislocation High incidence of posttraumatic DJD despite simple pattern Marginal impaction may complicate reduction tactics
Posterior column	Cranial fracture is frequently near the apex of the greater sciatic notch, divides the articular and quadrilateral surfaces; exits the inferior obturator ring	Superior gluteal neurovascular structures may be displaced or injured by fracture fragments
Anterior wall	Fracture line begins between the AIIS and iliopectineal eminence; involves varied amounts of anterior articular surface and the superior ramus	Fracture very infrequently encountered
Anterior column	Fracture through the innominate extends caudally to involve the articular surface and inferior obturator ring	Very low—cranial fracture limit at anterior horn articular surface Low—cranial fracture limit at psoas gutter Middle—cranial fracture limit at interspinous notch High—cranial fracture limit at iliac crest
Transverse	Divides the acetabulum into cranial and caudal segments	Only elementary fracture to include both columns Transtectal—traverses acetabular dome Juxtatectal—cranial portion of cotyloid fossa Infratectal—cotyloid fossa horizontally split

AIIS = Anterior inferior iliac spine, DJD = degenerative joint disease.

Table 3

The Associated Acetabular Fractures

Associated Fracture	Description	Comments
Posterior column–posterior wall	Association of posterior column and posterior wall fractures	Posterior column component is occasionally incomplete
Transverse-posterior wall	Extremely common fracture type	Often accompanied by a posterior hip dislocation
T-type	Transverse fracture associated with a vertical fracture that divides the ischiopubic segment	Also may be associated with a posterior wall fracture
Anteroposterior hemitransverse	May be fracture of anterior wall or anterior column combined with the posterior portion of a transverse fracture	Common fracture pattern of the elderly after a fall onto the hip
Associated both-column	Complete dissociation of acetabulum from axial skeleton	Radiographic "spur sign" (Figure 18) is diagnostic; represents the caudal portion of the intact ilium Secondary congruence results from medialization of anterior and posterior columns of acetabulum; may be indication for nonsurgical care in certain patients

high incidence of associated injuries

b. Ipsilateral lower extremity is evaluated for fracture, ligamentous knee injury, sciatic nerve palsy (especially in posterior wall fracture-

dislocation).

c. Skin and soft tissues are inspected for evidence of open injury, including the perineum, gluteal folds, rectum, and vagina.

d. Skin is inspected for closed internal degloving lesions (Morel-Lavallee); resulting necrotic fat and hematoma can contaminate surgical exposure and may require débridement.

2. Imaging

a. AP pelvic radiograph used as initial screening test

   • Six radiographic lines may be scrutinized to reach a provisional diagnosis of acetabular fracture as well as pattern (**Figure 21**, **Table 4**)

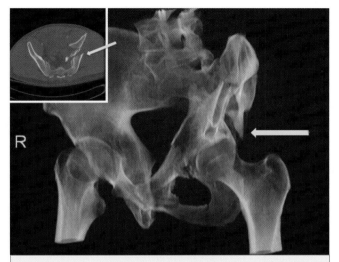

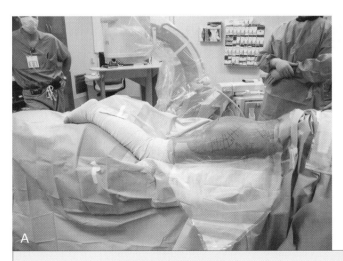

Figure 18 The obturator oblique view and corresponding axial CT scan cut (inset) of a left associated both-column acetabulum fracture. The spur sign (yellow arrows) is the radiographic representation of caudal portion of the intact ilium.

   • Lines are anatomy tangential to the radiographic beam and do not necessarily represent one particular anatomic structure.

b. Judet views (45° oblique)—Iliac oblique and obturator oblique views (**Figure 22**)

   • Iliac oblique view allows visualization of posterior column, anterior wall, sciatic notch, and iliac fossa.

   • Obturator oblique view demonstrates the anterior column, posterior wall, and obturator sulcus.

   • When obtained properly, the iliac oblique view of one side has the obturator oblique view of the contralateral side on the same radiograph.

c. CT scans confirm the articular pattern, highlight articular comminution, marginal impaction, and presence of occult ipsilateral femoral head fractures, and help detect loose bony fragments within the acetabulum. CT also can exclude the presence of associated pelvic ring injuries, which may be present in approximately 30% of acetabular fractures.

G. Treatment

1. Surgical treatment

a. ORIF is indicated for fractures resulting in hip instability, at least 2 mm articular displacement, marginal impaction, or loose intra-articular fractures trapped within the joint.

b. Recent support for percutaneous management of minimally displaced acetabular fractures to facilitate mobility in multiply injured patients

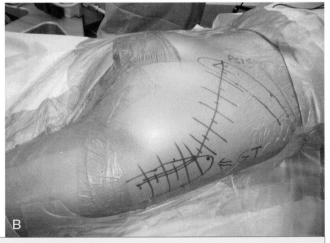

Figure 19 Photographs show the patient positioning and surgical marking of a patient undergoing open reduction and internal fixation for an acetabulum fracture via a prone Kocher-Langenbeck exposure. **A,** The patient is placed in the prone position with the ipsilateral limb prepared and draped circumferentially. **B,** The planned incision with pertinent landmarks.

3: Trauma

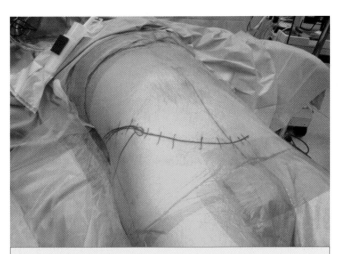

Figure 20 Photograph shows the surgical preparation and marking for open reduction and internal fixation of an acetabulum via an ilioinguinal exposure. The patient is in the supine position with the ipsilateral limb prepared and draped circumferentially.

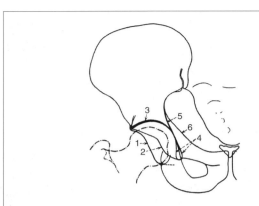

Figure 21 Illustration shows the radiographic lines described by Letournel to help evaluate acetabular fractures on plain pelvic radiographs. (Reproduced from Bellino MJ: Acetabular fractures: Acute evaluation, in Baumgaertner MR, Tornetta P III, eds: *Orthopaedic Knowledge Update: Trauma*, ed 3. Rosemont, IL, American Academy of Orthopaedic Surgeons, 2005, p 264.)

Table 4

Description of the Radiographic Lines Used for Evaluating Acetabular Fractures

Radiographic Line	Anatomic Structure	Comment
Posterior border of acetabulum	Posterior wall	Usually peripheral to the anterior wall Inferiorly overlies the outline of the upper ischial tuberosity
Anterior border of acetabulum	Anterior wall	Peripherally more transverse than the posterior border Medially confluent with the lower border of the teardrop
Roof	Acetabular dome	Represents only 2–3 mm of the cranial dome Does not indicate overall dome integrity
Teardrop (radiographic U)	None	External limb—outer cotyloid fossa Internal limb—outer wall of the obturator canal merging to the quadrilateral surface Lower border—located in the ischiopubic notch; forms the superior border of the obturator foramen
Ilioischial line	Posterior column	Results from beam tangent to a segment of the ischial quadrilateral surface Cranially confluent with the iliopectineal line
Iliopectineal line (pelvic brim)	Anterior column	Between the symphysis and ilioischial line (anterior three-fourths of the pelvis), this line corresponds exactly with the anatomic brim Posterior one-fourth corresponds with a surface 1–2 cm caudal to the anatomic brim

c. Total hip arthroplasty for select elderly patients

2. Nonsurgical treatment

   a. Indicated in minimally displaced (< 2 mm) fractures

   b. Roof-arc angles—Fractures that do not involve the acetabular dome, defined as the area within a 45° roof arc or the cranial 10 mm of the acetabulum defined on CT

   c. Posterior wall acetabulum fractures may be treated nonsurgically in the absence of marginal impaction and a negative stress examination performed under anesthesia with fluoroscopy.

   d. Associated both-column acetabulum fractures may exhibit secondary congruence; anterior and posterior columns medialize and conform to the femoral head, resulting in acceptable alignment.

H. Rehabilitation

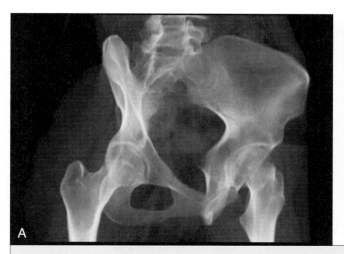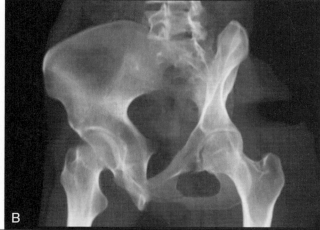

Figure 22 Judet views of the pelvis. **A,** Iliac oblique view demonstrates the anterior wall of the left acetabulum as well as the posterior column. **B,** Obturator oblique view demonstrates the anterior column of the left hip and a large displaced fracture of the left posterior wall. Notice that the iliac oblique of the injured hip also gives an obturator oblique of the contralateral hip, and vice versa.

1. Weight-of-limb weight bearing is used on the side of the injured acetabulum.

2. Patients with bilateral acetabulum fractures practice bed-to-chair transfers only, using the upper extremities to mobilize.

3. Early postoperative continuous passive motion may be used to prevent joint stiffness.

4. Active knee and ankle motion may be initiated immediately.

5. Patients who undergo posterior exposure via a Kocher-Langenbeck procedure should be placed on posterior hip precautions for patient comfort, to protect the posterior repair, and to prevent re-dislocation.

6. After 6 to 10 weeks, or after radiographic healing has occurred, the patient may advance gradually from weight-of-limb weight bearing to full weight bearing.

7. Quadriceps, hip, and core strengthening should be introduced gradually as weight bearing is advanced.

I. Complications

1. Thromboembolic phenomena, same as seen in pelvic fractures

2. Heterotopic bone formation

   a. Most commonly occurs when patients undergo surgical fixation via a Kocher-Langenbeck procedure (**Figure 23**) or extended iliofemoral exposures; heterotopic bone formation after ilioinguinal exposure is rare.

   b. Patients who undergo more than one exposure to the acetabulum are also at increased risk for

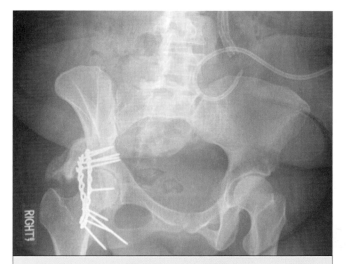

Figure 23 AP radiograph of a patient with heterotopic ossification following fixation for an acetabular fracture via a Kocher-Langenbeck exposure.

heterotopic bone formation.

   c. Prophylaxis options

   • Indomethacin 25 mg three times daily for 4 to 6 weeks

   • Radiation therapy (700 cGy); should be avoided in children or in women of child-bearing age

3. Femoral head aseptic necrosis

   a. Can occur most commonly when hip dislocation occurs in concert with acetabulum fracture.

3: Trauma

b. A dislocated femoral head should be reduced in an expedited fashion to minimize the thrombosis of vessels supplying the femoral head.

c. Intraoperative dissection should avoid injury to the ascending branch of the medial femoral circumflex artery.

4. Nerve or vessel injury

a. May be traumatic or iatrogenic

b. Careful handling of soft tissues is mandatory for preservation of nerve function (for example, keeping the hip extended and knee flexed during Kocher-Langenbeck exposure to protect the sciatic nerve).

c. Retractors should be placed carefully. The use of self-retaining retractors should be sparse.

III. Sacral Fractures

A. Epidemiology

1. Sacral fractures occur in 45% of injuries to the pelvic ring.

2. Some spare the pelvic ring and result from a direct blow (transverse sacral fracture, coccygeal fractures). These make up less than 5% of all sacral fractures.

B. Anatomy

1. The sacrum is roughly triangular in the coronal plane.

2. In the sagittal plane, the sacral anatomy varies but has some degree of lordosis, especially in the caudal segments.

3. Sacral nerve root tunnels arise from the sacral canal and proceed from midline, cranial, and posterior to lateral, caudal, and peripheral.

C. Fracture classification

1. Sacral fractures generally are organized into three categories.

a. Fractures associated with pelvic ring injuries

b. Fractures involving the lumbosacral junction

c. Fractures intrinsic to the sacrum

2. Sacral fractures associated with pelvic fractures are frequently vertical in nature. They are described by the AO/OTA, Young-Burgess, or Letournel classification systems (see I.C.).

3. Fractures involving the lumbosacral junction are best classified using the Isler system. This classification describes the fracture line in reference to the L5-S1 facet (**Figure 24**).

a. Type I fractures are lateral to the facet.

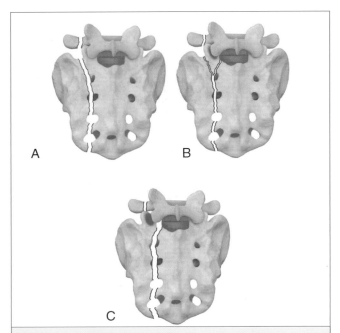

Figure 24 Illustrations depict the Isler classification system for sacral fractures. (Reproduced with permission from Vaccaro AR, Kim DH, Brodke DS, et al: Diagnosis and management of sacral spine fractures: Instructional course lecture. *J Bone Joint Surg Am* 2004;86[1]:165-175.)

- These are unlikely to affect lumbosacral stability.

- When combined with ramus fractures, they may affect pelvic ring stability.

b. Type II fractures traverse the L5-S1 facet.

- Extra-articular fractures of the lumbosacral junction

- Articular dislocation with facet displacement

c. Type III fractures are medial to the facet.

- This fracture type has increased potential to result in substantial instability.

- Bilateral fractures may result in lumbosacral dissociation.

4. Fractures intrinsic to the sacrum typically are classified according to the system of Denis. This system describes the fracture's relationship to the sacral nerve root tunnels (**Figure 25**).

a. Zone I fractures are lateral to the sacral nerve roots.

- This is the most common of the fracture locations (50% of the original series by Denis et al).

- Nerve root deficits occurred in 6% of cases

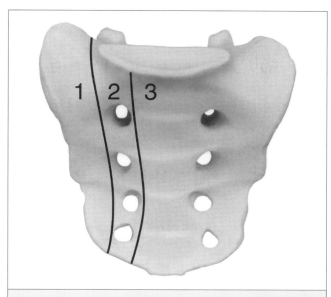

Figure 25 Illustration shows the sacral fracture classification system of Denis. (Reproduced with permission from Vaccaro AR, Kim DH, Brodke DS, et al: Diagnosis and management of sacral spine fractures: Instructional course lecture. *J Bone Joint Surg Am* 2004;86[1]:165-175.)

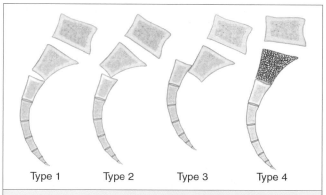

Figure 26 Illustrations show the subclassification of zone III injuries. (Reproduced with permission from Vaccaro AR, Kim DH, Brodke DS, et al: Diagnosis and management of sacral spine fractures: Instructional course lecture. *J Bone Joint Surg Am* 2004;86[1]:165-175.)

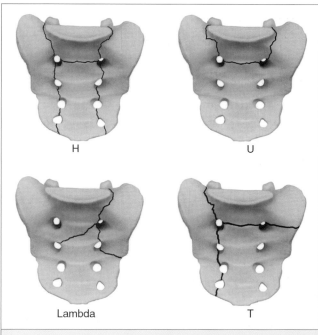

Figure 27 Illustrations show sacral fractures classified by the letter they most closely resemble. (Reproduced with permission from Vaccaro AR, Kim DH, Brodke DS, et al: Diagnosis and management of sacral spine fractures: Instructional course lecture. *J Bone Joint Surg Am* 2004; 86[1]:165-175.)

and involved the L5 root or sciatic nerve.

b. Zone II fractures pass through the neural foramina.

- Zone II fractures are the second most common fracture type (34% of fractures) in the series by Denis et al.

- Of these, 28% had unilateral L5, S1, or S2 injuries.

- Zone II fractures can be considerably unstable if a sheer component is present in the injury, or if comminution is present in the fracture.

c. Zone III fractures are medial to the sacral nerve root tunnels.

- These fractures have the highest rate of neurologic deficits.

- Dysfunction of the bowel, bladder, and sexual organs occurs in 76% of patients with zone III fractures.

- A transverse component can exist within zone III fractures. These are often misdiagnosed as bilateral zone I or zone II fractures (which are actually quite rare). Strange-Vognsen and Lebach, and Roy-Camille et al further classified the transverse portion of zone III injuries (**Figure 26**)

5. Fractures also can be classified by description of the letter they most closely resemble (**Figure 27**).

D. Mechanism of injury

1. Usually high energy: falls from a height, motor vehicle collisions, and motorcycle crashes. In patients with poor bone quality, sacral stress fractures may develop without supraphysiologic loading.

3: Trauma

2. A direct blow or fall onto the sacrum may result in transverse fractures.

3. Insufficiency fractures may occur in patients with poor bone quality.

E. Evaluation

1. Physical evaluation

   a. Identical to that of pelvic ring injuries; pelvic stability should be assessed by manual stress examination; patient should undergo a full ATLS workup because of the high energy required to fracture the sacrum

   b. Sacral fractures can be missed at initial presentation, and up to 30% are diagnosed late.

   c. Careful attention should be given to examination of the sacral nerve roots.

      • A careful lower-extremity examination, including motor function, sensory function, and reflexes, should be performed and documented.

      • Neurologic examination includes a digital rectal examination.

        ○ This should document voluntary and spontaneous rectal sphincter contraction.

        ○ The presence of sensation to light touch and pinprick to concentric dermatomes of S2 to S5 should be documented

      • Reflexes including the bulbocavernosus and cremasteric should be examined.

   d. Vascular examination of the bilateral lower extremities should be performed.

   e. Soft tissues in the pelvic region and perineum should be thoroughly examined for occult open injuries. Closed internal degloving (Morel-Lavallee) lesions also may be present.

2. Imaging

   a. AP, inlet, and outlet pelvic radiographs

   b. Sacral lateral view may be useful in transverse sacral body fractures or coccygeal fractures.

   c. CT with coronal and sagittal reconstructions for evaluation of sacral nerve root tunnels and preoperative planning

F. Treatment

1. When considering treatment options, sacral fractures may be categorized broadly into four subtypes.

   a. Fractures associated with a pelvic ring injury

   b. Fractures that also have a lumbosacral facet injury

   c. Sacral fractures with an associated dislocation of the lumbosacral junction

   d. Fractures with neurologic injury, persistent spinal cord injury, or cauda equina syndrome

2. For sacral fractures that are part of a pelvic ring injury, fracture treatment should coincide with treatment of the pelvic ring.

3. Fractures with lumbosacral facet injury

   a. Stable injuries or those with minimal displacement may be treated nonsurgically.

   b. Unstable injuries require surgical fixation to minimize the risk of residual facet incongruity.

4. Fractures with lumbosacral dislocation

   a. Patients without debris in the nerve root tunnels or central canal may be treated with percutaneous fixation in situ.

   b. Patients who have fractures with more displacement may require open treatment with decompression. Many techniques, including lumbopelvic fixation, have been described.

G. Rehabilitation

1. See section I.F.6 on pelvic fractures for sacral injuries that are part of a pelvic fracture

2. Additional spinal cord rehabilitation may be needed for patients with neurologic deficits

H. Complications

1. Infection occurs in 5% to 50% of surgical cases.

2. The incidence of sacral fracture nonunion is 10% to 15%.

3. Of patients sustaining a sacral fracture, 30% will have chronic pain.

Top Testing Facts

1. The radiographic workup of a patient with a pelvic fracture includes AP, inlet, and outlet pelvic views as well as CT, which should be a confirmatory study to evaluate the fine detail of the posterior ring and occult injuries.

2. The initial management of pelvic fractures includes measures to minimize hemorrhage, including pelvic binders, sheets, and skeletal traction.

3. Young-Burgess anteroposterior compression type III injuries have the highest fluid requirements as well as risk of hemorrhage and mortality.

4. Identification of the dysmorphic upper sacral segment is important in planning for the surgical treatment of the posterior pelvic ring.

5. The sacral lateral view is mandatory for placement of iliosacral screws in the upper sacral segment to avoid injury to the L5 and S1 nerve roots.

6. Acetabular fractures are most often classified according to the system of Judet and Letournel. The fractures are divided into elementary and associated patterns.

7. Judet views of the pelvis allow detailed understanding of the acetabular injury pattern. The obturator oblique view demonstrates the anterior column and posterior wall, whereas the iliac oblique view demonstrates the posterior column and anterior wall.

8. CT should be obtained as part of the radiographic workup and will demonstrate marginal impaction, articular comminution, bony fragments contained within the joint, and impaction lesions of the femoral head.

9. Small or peripheral posterior wall acetabular fractures may be treated nonsurgically in the absence of marginal impaction and with a negative, fluoroscopically assisted stress examination performed under anesthesia.

10. Lumbopelvic fixation may be required in addition to decompression for sacral fractures with nerve root or central canal deficit and anatomic compromise.

Bibliography

Bruce B, Reilly M, Sims S: OTA highlight paper predicting future displacement of nonoperatively managed lateral compression sacral fractures: Can it be done? *J Orthop Trauma* 2011;25(9):523-527.

Burgess AR, Eastridge BJ, Young JW, et al: Pelvic ring disruptions: Effective classification system and treatment protocols. *J Trauma* 1990;30(7):848-856.

Farrell ED, Gardner MJ, Krieg JC, Chip Routt ML Jr: The upper sacral nerve root tunnel: An anatomic and clinical study. *J Orthop Trauma* 2009;23(5):333-339.

Gardner MJ, Routt ML Jr: Transiliac-transsacral screws for posterior pelvic stabilization. *J Orthop Trauma* 2011;25(6):378-384.

Koo H, Leveridge M, Thompson C, et al: Interobserver reliability of the Young-Burgess and tile classification systems for fractures of the pelvic ring. *J Orthop Trauma* 2008;22(6):379-384.

Letournel E: Acetabulum fractures: Classification and management. *Clin Orthop Relat Res* 1980;151:81-106.

Marsh JL, Slongo TF, Agel J, et al: Fracture and dislocation classification compendium - 2007: Orthopaedic Trauma Association classification, database and outcomes committee. *J Orthop Trauma* 2007;21(10, Suppl)S1-S133.

Matta JM, Anderson LM, Epstein HC, Hendricks P: Fractures of the acetabulum: A retrospective analysis. *Clin Orthop Relat Res* 1986;205:230-240.

Mehta S, Auerbach JD, Born CT, Chin KR: Sacral fractures. *J Am Acad Orthop Surg* 2006;14(12):656-665.

Moed BR, Reilly MC: Acetabulum fractures, in Bucholz RW, Court-Brown CM, Heckman JD, Tornetta PT III, eds: *Rockwood and Green's Fractures in Adults*, ed 7. Philadelphia, PA, Lippincott, Williams, & Wilkins, 2010, pp 1463-1523.

Nork SE, Jones CB, Harding SP, Mirza SK, Routt ML Jr: Percutaneous stabilization of U-shaped sacral fractures using iliosacral screws: technique and early results. *J Orthop Trauma* 2001;15(4):238-246.

Pennal GF, Tile M, Waddell JP, Garside H: Pelvic disruption: Assessment and classification. *Clin Orthop Relat Res* 1980;151:12-21.

Routt ML Jr, Falicov A, Woodhouse E, Schildhauer TA: Circumferential pelvic antishock sheeting: A temporary resuscitation aid. *J Orthop Trauma* 2002;16(1):45-48.

Suzuki T, Smith WR, Hak DJ, et al: Combined injuries of the pelvis and acetabulum: Nature of a devastating dyad. *J Orthop Trauma* 2010;24(5):303-308.

Vaccaro AR, Kim DH, Brodke DS, et al: Diagnosis and management of sacral spine fractures. *Instr Course Lect* 2004;53:375-385.

3: Trauma

Chapter 37
Hip Dislocations and Femoral Head Fractures

Robert F. Ostrum, MD

I. Hip Dislocations

A. Epidemiology

1. Posterior dislocations represent 90% of all hip dislocations; most are secondary to motor vehicle accidents (MVAs) and knee-to-dashboard trauma with a posterior-directed force.

2. In MVAs, the right hip is involved much more often than the left.

B. Anatomy and surgical approaches

1. Anatomy

a. Strong capsular ligaments—The anterior iliofemoral and posterior ischiofemoral ligaments

Dr. Ostrum or an immediate family member serves as a paid consultant to or is an employee of Smith & Nephew and Synthes and has received research or institutional support from AO North America and Synthes.

run from the acetabulum to the femoral neck (**Figure 1**).

b. The ligamentum teres runs from the acetabulum (cotyloid fossa) to the femoral head (fovea centralis).

c. The main arterial blood supply comes from the superior and posterior cervical arteries, which are primarily derived from the medial circumflex artery (posterior); the lesser blood supply (10% to 15%) comes through the artery of the ligamentum teres (**Figure 2**).

2. Surgical approaches—For irreducible dislocations, "go where the money is."

a. Posterior approach (Kocher-Langenbeck)—Allows access to posterior dislocations.

b. Anterior approach (Smith-Petersen)—Allows access to anterior dislocations and also better visualization of the anterior joint.

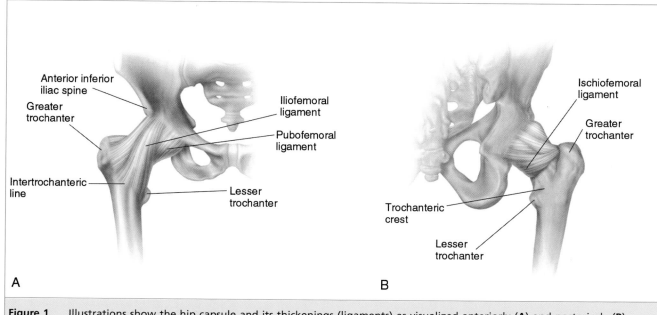

Figure 1   Illustrations show the hip capsule and its thickenings (ligaments) as visualized anteriorly (**A**) and posteriorly (**B**).

3: Trauma

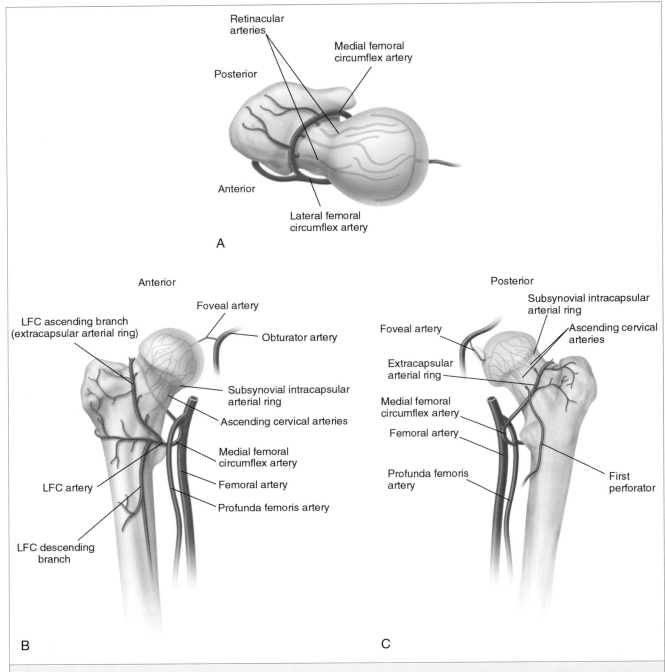

Figure 2   Axial (**A**), anterior (**B**), and posterior (**C**) illustrations depict the vascular supply to the femoral head, which arises from the medial and lateral circumflex vessels. These vessels create a ring, giving rise to the cervical vessels. A minor contribution comes from the obturator artery via the ligamentum teres. LFC = lateral femoral circumflex.

    c. Anterolateral approach (Watson-Jones)—Allows access to the posterior hip through the same incision.

C. Mechanism of injury

  1. Anterior dislocations

    a. These dislocations result from an abduction and external rotation force.

    b. A flexed hip leads to an inferior (obturator) dislocation; an extended hip results in a superior (pubic) dislocation.

    c. Femoral head impaction or osteochondral fractures are commonly seen.

  2. Posterior dislocations

    a. Posterior dislocations are most commonly seen

after dashboard injuries, in which the knee hits the dashboard, resulting in a posteriorly directed force through the femur.

    b. The presence of an associated fracture, as well as the location and extent of the fracture, is dictated by the flexion, abduction, and rotation of the hip joint at the time of the impact. Increased flexion and adduction favor a pure dislocation without fracture of the posterior wall.

D. Clinical evaluation

1. Associated injuries occur in up to 95% of patients with a hip dislocation secondary to an MVA.

2. Anterior hip dislocations present with the leg in a flexed (inferior) or extended (superior), abducted, and externally rotated attitude.

3. Posterior hip dislocations present with the limb in an adducted and internally rotated position.

4. Common associated injuries include those around the ipsilateral knee secondary to direct trauma.

    a. Patellar fractures

    b. Ligamentous tears and dislocations (posterior)

    c. Bone bruises

    d. Meniscal tears

5. Sciatic nerve injury may be seen in 8% to 20% of patients; a thorough neurologic examination should precede any attempts at reduction. Prereduction and postreduction neurologic examinations should be documented.

6. A high percentage of patients have ipsilateral knee pain and bruising; a good knee examination for effusion and stability is needed.

7. Some patients have associated femoral head impaction injuries visible on plain radiographs or CT scans.

E. Imaging evaluation

1. Standard AP radiographs show dislocation of the femoral head.

    a. The attitude of the limb and appearance of the femoral head can distinguish an anterior dislocation from a posterior one.

    b. In posterior dislocations, the femoral head appears small and is located superiorly; in anterior dislocations, the femoral head appears larger and overlaps the medial acetabulum or the obturator foramen.

2. Judet views (iliac and obturator oblique)

    a. These views can help diagnose the location of the dislocation and identify associated trans-

verse or posterior wall fractures.

    b. The obturator oblique view provides the best picture of the posterior dislocation and the posterior wall.

3. CT scans are necessary following all reductions of hip dislocations.

    a. They provide important information about concentric reduction, bony or cartilaginous fragments in the joint, associated fractures, marginal impaction of the posterior wall, avulsion fractures, and femoral head or neck fractures.

    b. The percentage of posterior wall fracture can be calculated. The need for internal fixation is assessed on the postreduction CT scan. The size of the posterior wall fragment and the dome involvement are identified. More than 25% involvement of the posterior wall is an indication for fixation.

4. Prereduction CT scans

    a. Prereduction scans are reserved for irreducible dislocations, to determine the block to reduction.

    b. In simple dislocations or fracture-dislocations, obtaining these CT scans before reduction provides little information and may result in prolonged dislocation and concomitant osteonecrosis or injury to the sciatic nerve or cartilage.

5. MRI of the hip can demonstrate labral injury and cartilage damage to the femoral head. This modality has been used to predict head survival.

6. In patients with hip dislocations who also report a painful knee or soft-tissue injury, the most common findings on MRI are effusions (37%), bone bruises (33%), and meniscal tears (30%).

F. Classification

1. Hip dislocations are classified as anterior or posterior.

2. Further clarification that also helps with prognosis is gained by using the Thompson-Epstein classification (**Table 1**).

G. Treatment

1. Preoperative—Abduction pillows are usually sufficient for postreduction stability while the patient awaits surgery. Skeletal traction is reserved for patients with instability or dome involvement.

2. Closed reduction

    a. Prompt closed reduction as an emergent procedure should be the initial treatment.

    b. Adequate pharmacologic muscle relaxation is

Table 1

Thompson-Epstein Classification of Hip Dislocations

Type	Characteristics
I	Dislocation with or without minor fracture
II	Dislocation with single large fracture of the rim with or without a large major fragment
III	Dislocation with comminuted fracture of the rim with or without a large major fragment
IV	Dislocation with fracture of the acetabular floor
V	Dislocation with fracture of the femoral head

necessary.

c. Reduction is performed by using traction in line with the thigh, with the extremity in an adducted attitude, and with countertraction exerted on the pelvis. Forceful reduction, which can lead to femoral head or neck fractures, should be avoided.

d. After successful reduction, abduction with external rotation and extension should maintain the reduction for posterior dislocations. For anterior dislocations, the limb is maintained in extension, abduction, and neutral or internal rotation. Traction is indicated for unstable injuries or for injuries with dome involvement.

e. Irreducible dislocations are seen in 2% to 15% of patients with these injuries. Irreducible anterior dislocations are due to buttonholing through the capsule or soft-tissue interposition. In posterior dislocations, reduction can be prevented by the piriformis, the gluteus maximus, the capsule, the labrum, or a bony fragment.

f. If one or two attempts at closed reduction with sedation are unsuccessful, then an emergent open reduction is necessary.

g. A CT scan should be obtained before open reduction to determine pathology.

h. Nonconcentric reductions can be missed even with careful scrutiny of postreduction radiographs of the hip. Postreduction CT is mandatory, to assess the hip joint following reduction.

3. Surgical treatment

   a. Indications include an irreducible dislocation, a nonconcentric reduction, an unstable hip joint, and an associated femoral or acetabular fracture.

   b. Assessing stability

- Stress testing under anesthesia to determine stability is controversial.

- Hip stability after reduction should not be assessed with range of motion. No real parameters have been established for stability, and further damage to cartilage or nerves may occur.

   c. Open reduction and internal fixation should be performed through an approach from the direction of the dislocation.

- For posterior dislocations, the Kocher-Langenbeck approach is used.

- For anterior dislocations, an anterior (Smith-Petersen) or anterolateral (Watson-Jones) approach is used.

H. Rehabilitation

1. Early mobilization

2. With posterior dislocations, hyperflexion is avoided for 4 to 6 weeks.

3. Immediate weight bearing is initiated for simple dislocations.

4. Delayed weight bearing is used with large posterior wall or dome fracture fixation.

I. Complications

1. Posttraumatic arthritis develops in 15% to 20% of patients because of cellular cartilage injury, nonconcentric reduction of the hip, articular displacement, or marginal impaction. Posttraumatic arthritis can develop years after the initial injury.

2. Osteonecrosis develops in approximately 2% to 10% of hips reduced within 6 hours.

   a. The rate of osteonecrosis increases with a delay in reduction.

   b. Osteonecrosis usually appears within 2 years after the injury but is evident at 1 year in most patients.

3. Sciatic nerve injury affects the peroneal division.

   a. The injury is seen in 8% to 19% of posterior dislocations.

   b. It is more common with fracture-dislocations than with simple dislocations.

4. Redislocation is reported in 1% of patients.

5. Myositis around the hip is uncommon after posterior dislocation.

II. Femoral Head Fractures

A. Epidemiology

1. Femoral head fractures occur in 6% to 16% of patients with posterior hip dislocations.

2. They may be the result of impaction, avulsions, or shear fractures.

3. Anterior dislocations are more commonly associated with impaction of the femoral head.

4. Femoral head fractures are produced by contact of the femoral head on the posterior rim of the acetabulum at the time of dislocation.

5. The location and size of the fracture and the degree of comminution are a result of the position of the hip at the time of the dislocation impact.

B. Anatomy and surgical approaches—Same as for hip dislocations, as described earlier.

C. Mechanism of injury and clinical evaluation—Same as for hip dislocations, as described earlier.

D. Imaging evaluation

1. Radiographs—AP and Judet views of the acetabulum are obtained both prereduction and postreduction.

2. CT—2-mm sections through the acetabulum are obtained. CT scans should be obtained postreduction only because a delay in reduction caused by waiting for a CT scan can result in further damage to the femoral head blood supply or to possible sciatic nerve injury.

E. Classification—The Pipkin classification system is used for femoral head fractures (**Figure 3**).

F. Treatment—Based on fragment location, size, displacement, and hip stability.

1. Excision of Pipkin I (infrafoveal) fractures after closed reduction and open reduction and internal fixation of Pipkin II (suprafoveal) fractures yield better clinical results than nonsurgical treatment (**Table 2**).

2. The Smith-Petersen approach is used most commonly for isolated femoral head fractures because the cartilaginous fragments are predominantly anterior and fixation or excision is easier from this exposure.

3. For femoral head fractures associated with a posterior wall of the acetabular fracture (Pipkin IV), a posterior Kocher-Langenbeck approach allows for fixation of the posterior wall with excision or fixation of the femoral head fracture.

G. Rehabilitation

1. Immediate early range of motion of the hip and weight bearing delayed for 6 to 8 weeks

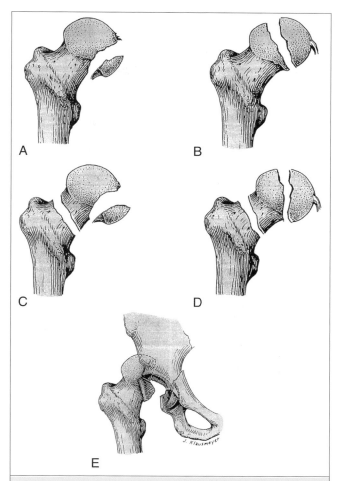

Figure 3 Illustration demonstrates the Pipkin classification of femoral head fractures. **A,** Intrafoveal fracture, Pipkin type I. **B,** Suprafoveal fracture, Pipkin type II. **C** and **D,** Intrafoveal fracture or suprafoveal fracture associated with femoral neck fracture, Pipkin type III. **E,** Any femoral head fracture configuration associated with an acetabular fracture, Pipkin type IV. (Reproduced with permission from Swionkowski MF: Intrascapular hip fractures, in Browner BD, Jupiter JB, Levine AM, Trafton PG, eds: *Skeletal Trauma: Basic Science, Management, and Reconstruction*, ed 2. Philadelphia, PA, WB Saunders, p 1756.)

2. Stress strengthening of the abductors and quadriceps

3. Radiographs after 6 months to evaluate for osteonecrosis and arthritis

3: Trauma

Table 2

Treatment of Femoral Head Fractures Based on the Pipkin Classification

Type	Characteristics	Treatment
I	Infrafoveal, disruption of the ligamentum teres from the head fragment	Nonsurgical treatment is most common because this is not a weight-bearing fragment Non–weight bearing, hip precautions, progressive weight bearing May need excision of small fragments, fixation of large fragments because they can heal as a malunion and limit hip motion
II	Suprafoveal, ligamentum teres attached to head fragment	Countersunk screws for open reduction and internal fixation Usually Smith-Petersen approach—Optimizes fracture visualization and fixation, minimizes complication rate Periacetabular capsulotomy to preserve femoral head blood supply
III	Associated femoral neck fracture	Simultaneous open reduction and internal fixation of femoral head and neck through a Watson-Jones or Smith-Petersen approach Consideration should be given to prosthetic replacement, especially in patients who are elderly, have osteoporosis, or have a comminuted fracture.
IV	Associated acetabular fracture	Posterior Kocher-Langenbeck approach for acetabular fixation, excision of small infrafoveal fragments through this approach Small posterior wall fragments may be treated nonsurgically and suprafoveal fractures can then be treated through an anterior approach. Use of anterior and posterior approaches together is controversial

H. Complications

1. The anterior approach is associated with reduced surgical time, better visualization, improved fracture reduction, and no osteonecrosis, but also with an increase in heterotopic ossification compared with the posterior approach. Heterotopic ossification is extra-articular and is rarely clinically significant.

2. Osteonecrosis is related to a delay in hip dislocation reduction.

   a. The effect of an anterior surgical incision on osteonecrosis is unknown.

   b. Osteonecrosis occurs in 0% to 23% of patients, depending on the injury, dislocation, and time to relocation and definitive treatment.

   c. Patients should be counseled about this complication preoperatively.

3. Fixation failure is associated with osteonecrosis or nonunion.

4. Posttraumatic arthritis is a result of joint incongruity or initial cartilage damage.

5. Decreased internal rotation is commonly seen after these femoral head fractures but may not be a clinical problem or cause disability.

Top Testing Facts

Hip Dislocations

1. Posterior dislocation is more common than anterior dislocation.

2. In posterior dislocations, the ipsilateral knee should be assessed for ligamentous or other injury.

3. The neurologic examination should be documented before and after reduction.

4. Hip stability, intra-articular fragments, and concentric reduction are assessed on the postreduction CT scan of the hip.

5. The postreduction CT scan is used to assess for marginal impaction of the posterior wall.

6. The need for internal fixation is assessed on the postreduction CT scan. The size of the posterior wall fragment and dome involvement should be identified. Any involvement of the posterior wall over 25% is an indication for fixation.

7. Good relaxation is required for an attempted closed reduction of posterior hip dislocations. Forceful reduction should be avoided because it can lead to femoral head or neck fractures.

8. In most patients, osteonecrosis is seen at 1 year following injury. Arthritis can develop later.

Femoral Head Fractures

1. High-quality Judet radiographic views should be assessed before and after reduction for femoral head fractures. A diagnosis can be made on the postreduction CT scan.

2. A prereduction CT scan is not needed; leaving the hip dislocated for a long period can lead to further damage to the femoral head blood supply or possible sciatic nerve injury.

3. It is important to identify whether the femoral head fracture is infrafoveal (below the weight-bearing dome) or suprafoveal (involves the weight-bearing surface) to determine appropriate treatment.

4. Usually, a Smith-Petersen approach to the hip is used for fixation, with a periacetabular capsulotomy to preserve blood supply.

5. A femoral head fracture is easier to see through an anterior approach and fix through an anterior approach with countersunk or headless screws.

6. With a large posterior wall fracture (Pipkin type IV), a Kocher-Langenbeck approach can be used with subluxation or dislocation of the femoral head. This allows access to the femoral head for fracture reduction and fixation.

7. Small fragments or foveal avulsion fractures can be excised through a posterior approach when associated with a posterior wall fracture.

8. Decreased internal rotation commonly is seen after femoral head fractures but may not be a clinical problem or cause disability.

Bibliography

Bastian JD, Turina M, Siebenrock KA, Keel MJ: Long-term outcome after traumatic anterior dislocation of the hip. *Arch Orthop Trauma Surg* 2011;131(9):1273-1278.

Bhandari M, Matta J, Ferguson T, Matthys G: Predictors of clinical and radiological outcome in patients with fractures of the acetabulum and concomitant posterior dislocation of the hip. *J Bone Joint Surg Br* 2006;88(12):1618-1624.

Brumback RJ, Holt ES, McBride MS, Poka A, Bathon GH, Burgess AR: Acetabular depression fracture accompanying posterior fracture dislocation of the hip. *J Orthop Trauma* 1990;4(1):42-48.

Chen ZW, Lin B, Zhai WL, et al: Conservative versus surgical management of Pipkin type I fractures associated with posterior dislocation of the hip: A randomised controlled trial. *Int Orthop* 2011;35(7):1077-1081.

Chen ZW, Zhai WL, Ding ZQ, et al: Operative versus nonoperative management of Pipkin type-II fractures associated with posterior hip dislocation. *Orthopedics* 2011;34(5):350.

Hak DJ, Goulet JA: Severity of injuries associated with traumatic hip dislocation as a result of motor vehicle collisions. *J Trauma* 1999;47(1):60-63.

Hougaard K, Thomsen PB: Traumatic posterior dislocation of the hip—prognostic factors influencing the incidence of avascular necrosis of the femoral head. *Arch Orthop Trauma Surg* 1986;106(1):32-35.

Keith JE Jr, Brashear HR Jr, Guilford WB: Stability of posterior fracture-dislocations of the hip: Quantitative assessment using computed tomography. *J Bone Joint Surg Am* 1988;70(5):711-714.

Moed BR, WillsonCarr SE, Watson JT: Results of operative treatment of fractures of the posterior wall of the acetabulum. *J Bone Joint Surg Am* 2002;84(5):752-758.

Sahin V, Karakaş ES, Aksu S, Atlihan D, Turk CY, Halici M: Traumatic dislocation and fracture-dislocation of the hip: A long-term follow-up study. *J Trauma* 2003;54(3):520-529.

Schmidt GL, Sciulli R, Altman GT: Knee injury in patients experiencing a high-energy traumatic ipsilateral hip dislocation. *J Bone Joint Surg Am* 2005;87(6):1200-1204.

3: Trauma

Stannard JP, Harris HW, Volgas DA, Alonso JE: Functional outcome of patients with femoral head fractures associated with hip dislocations. *Clin Orthop Relat Res* 2000;377: 44-56.

Swiontkowski MF, Thorpe M, Seiler JG, Hansen ST: Operative management of displaced femoral head fractures: Case-matched comparison of anterior versus posterior approaches for Pipkin I and Pipkin II fractures. *J Orthop Trauma* 1992; 6(4):437-442.

Tannast M, Pleus F, Bonel H, Galloway H, Siebenrock KA, Anderson SE: Magnetic resonance imaging in traumatic posterior hip dislocation. *J Orthop Trauma* 2010;24(12): 723-731.

Thompson VP, Epstein HC: Traumatic dislocation of the hip; a survey of two hundred and four cases covering a period of twenty-one years. *J Bone Joint Surg Am* 1951;33(3):746-778, passim.

Tonetti J, Ruatti S, Lafontan V, et al: Is femoral head fracture-dislocation management improvable: A retrospective study in 110 cases. *Orthop Traumatol Surg Res* 2010;96(6): 623-631.

Tornetta P III, Mostafavi HR: Hip dislocation: Current treatment regimens. *J Am Acad Orthop Surg* 1997;5(1):27-36.

Chapter 38

Fractures of the Hip

Steven J. Morgan, MD

I. General Considerations

A. Epidemiology

1. Hip fractures occur most commonly in patients 70 years or older.

2. The risk of hip fracture increases with decreasing bone mass.

3. Hip fractures are more common in women.

4. Intertrochanteric femur fractures account for approximately 50% of all proximal femur fractures.

5. Femoral neck fractures are slightly less common and account for approximately 40% of proximal femur fractures.

B. Anatomy

1. Fractures of the proximal femur are distinguished by their anatomic location in relationship to the joint capsule.

   a. Femoral neck fractures are considered intracapsular fractures, which are at higher risk of nonunion. Because of the absence of a periosteal or extraosseous blood supply, no callus forms during healing. Fracture healing occurs by intraosseous bone healing.

   b. Intertrochanteric fractures are considered extracapsular fractures. Callus formation is common in these fracture patterns, and nonunion is rare because of the absence of synovial fluid and the presence of an abundant blood supply.

2. Vascular anatomy (**Figure 1**)

   a. The medial femoral circumflex artery is the main blood supply to the femoral head. This artery terminates in the posterior aspect of the extracapsular arterial ring.

   b. The lateral femoral circumflex artery gives rise to the anterior aspect of the arterial ring.

   c. The superior and inferior gluteal arteries also contribute branches to the ring.

   d. The ascending cervical arteries originate from the extracapsular arterial ring and are divided into four distinct groups based on their anatomic relationship to the femoral neck: lateral, medial, posterior, and anterior. The lateral group of ascending branches is the main blood supply to the femoral head.

   e. The ascending branches give off multiple perforator vessels to the femoral neck and terminate in the subsynovial arterial ring located at the margin of the articular surface of the femoral head. The lateral epiphyseal artery then penetrates the femoral head and is believed to be the dominant blood supply to the femoral head from this system. Fractures that disrupt the ascending blood flow to the lateral epiphyseal vessel have an increased risk of osteonecrosis.

   f. The artery of the ligamentum teres arises from either the obturator or medial femoral circumflex artery. It does not provide sufficient blood supply to maintain the viability of the femoral head.

C. Surgical approaches

1. The anterior lateral (Watson-Jones) approach is used for the open reduction and internal fixation (ORIF) of femoral neck fractures or hemiarthroplasty.

   a. This approach is based on the interval between the gluteus medius and the tensor fascia lata. No internervous plane is present because both muscles are innervated by the superior gluteal nerve.

   b. The superior gluteal nerve can be damaged if the intermuscular plane is extended to the iliac crest.

2. The anterior (Smith-Petersen) approach can be used for ORIF of the femoral neck or hemiarthroplasty. If used for ORIF, a separate lateral approach to the proximal femur is required for fixation placement.

Dr. Morgan or an immediate family member has stock or stock options held in Johnson & Johnson and Emerge Medical; and or an immediate family member serves as a board member, owner, officer, or committee member of the Orthopaedic Trauma Association and the Western Orthopaedic Trauma Association.

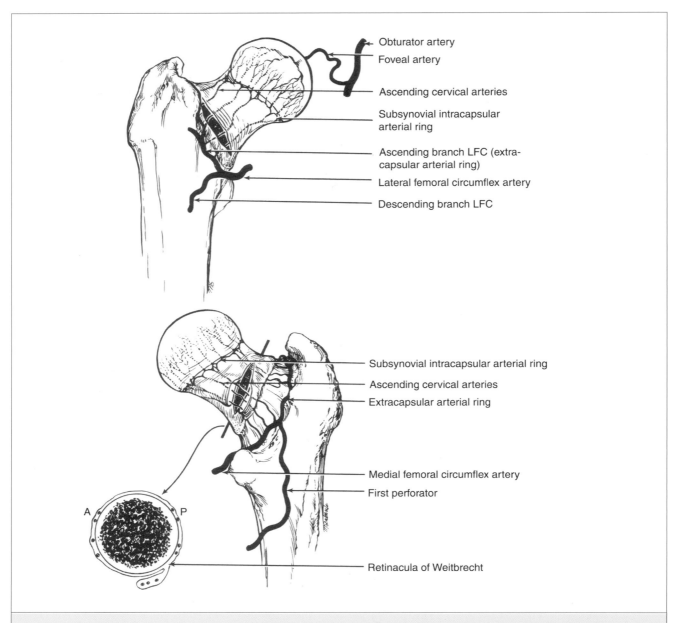

Obturator artery
Foveal artery
Ascending cervical arteries
Subsynovial intracapsular arterial ring
Ascending branch LFC (extra-capsular arterial ring)
Lateral femoral circumflex artery
Descending branch LFC

Subsynovial intracapsular arterial ring
Ascending cervical arteries
Extracapsular arterial ring

Medial femoral circumflex artery
First perforator

Retinacula of Weitbrecht

Figure 1   Illustrations depict the vascular anatomy of the femoral head and neck. LFC = lateral femoral circumflex artery. (Reproduced with permission from DeLee JC: Fractures and dislocations of the hip, in Rockwood CA Jr, Green DP, Bucholz RW, Heckman JD, eds: *Rockwood and Green's Fractures in Adults*, ed 4. Philadelphia, PA, Lippincott Williams & Wilkins, 2001, p 1662.)

a. The superficial dissection is between the tensor fascia lata (superior gluteal nerve) and the sartorius (femoral nerve).

b. The deep dissection is between the gluteus medius (superior gluteal nerve) and the rectus femoris (femoral nerve).

c. The lateral femoral cutaneous nerve is at risk with this approach.

d. The ascending branch of the lateral femoral circumflex artery is encountered between the tensor and the sartorius and must be sacrificed.

3. The lateral (Hardinge) approach is used primarily for hemiarthroplasty. This approach splits both the gluteus medius and the vastus lateralis, reflecting the anterior third of these structures medially. The superior gluteal nerve and artery are at risk in this approach.

4. The posterior (Southern) approach is used primarily for partial or total hip arthroplasty (THA).

a. The approach splits the gluteus maximus muscle (inferior gluteal nerve) and the fascia lata.

b. The tendons of the piriformis, obturator internus, and the superior and inferior gemelli are transected at their point of insertion and retracted posteriorly to protect the sciatic nerve.

c. The sciatic nerve is the main structure at risk with this exposure.

5. The lateral approach to the proximal femur is used for ORIF of intertrochanteric femur fractures.

a. This is a direct lateral approach that splits the fascia lata and either elevates the vastus lateralis from posterior to anterior or splits the muscle fibers.

b. No internervous plane is present; the vastus lateralis is innervated by the femoral nerve.

D. Hip biomechanics

1. The mean femoral neck-shaft angle in the adult is 130° ± 7°. The mean anteversion of the neck is 10° ± 7°.

2. Forces on the proximal aspect of the femur are complex. The osseous structure itself also is complex, consisting of both cortical and cancellous bone.

a. The two prime trabecular groups of the proximal femur are the principal tensile group and the principal compressive group. Secondary compressive and tensile trabecular groups (Figure 2) also exist. These trabecular bone patterns are the result of bone's response to stress, expressed as the Wolff law.

b. The weakest area in the femoral neck is located in the Ward triangle.

c. The calcar femorale is a medial area of dense trabecular bone that transfers stress from the femoral shaft to the inferior portion of the femoral neck.

d. Fractures of the proximal femur follow the path of least resistance.

e. The amount of energy absorbed by the bone determines the degree of comminution.

3. Standing position

a. The center of gravity is located at the midpoint between the two hips.

b. The weight of the body is supported equally by both hips.

c. The force vector acting on the hip is vertical.

d. The Y ligament of Bigelow resists hyperextension. Minimal muscle forces are required for balance in a symmetric stance, and the joint re-

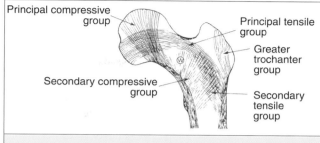

Figure 2 Illustration shows the trabecular groups of the proximal femur. W = the Ward triangle. (Adapted with permission from Singh M, Nagrath AR, Maini PS: Changes in trabecular pattern of the upper end of the femur as an index of osteoporosis. *J Bone Joint Surg Am* 1970;52:457-467.)

active force or compressive force across the hip is approximately one-half the body weight.

4. Single-leg stance

a. The center of gravity moves away from the hip. To counter the eccentric lever arm created by the weight of the body, the hip abductors function as stabilizers of the contralateral hemipelvis, contracting to maintain the pelvis in a level position. Because the lever arm created by the lateral offset of the greater trochanter is shorter than the lever arm created by the entire body opposite the hip, the magnitude of the muscle contracture is greater than the weight of the body. This results in a compressive load across the hip of approximately four times the body weight.

b. The resulting force vector in the standing phase is oriented parallel to the compressive trabeculae of the femoral neck.

c. In repetitive load situations, the tensile forces can cause microfractures in the superior femoral neck.

- Failure of these microfractures to heal in conditions of repetitive loading results in stress fracture.

- The frequency and degree of load influence the fatigue process.

5. Trendelenburg gait

a. Trendelenburg gait is noted when the hip abductors are no longer sufficient to counter the forces in single-leg stance. Without compensation, the pelvis cannot be maintained in a level position. Weakness of the abductors can be caused by disuse, paralysis, or by a diminished lever arm resulting from decreased femoral offset.

b. To compensate for the weakness of the abductors, the center of gravity can be shifted closer

3: Trauma

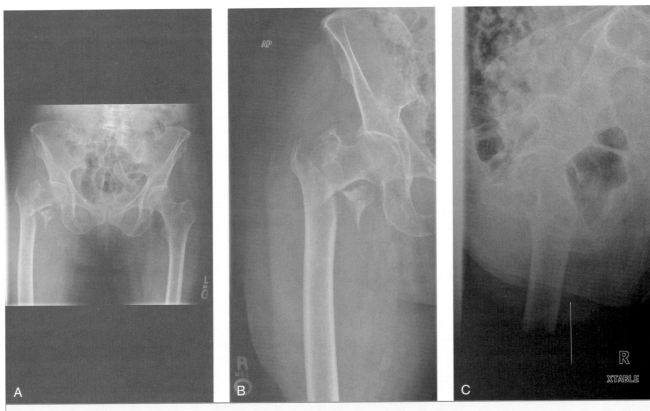

Figure 3   Radiographic evaluation should include an AP view of the pelvis (**A**), an AP view of the hip (**B**), and a cross-table lateral view (**C**). These radiographs demonstrate a displaced Evans type I intertrochanteric femur fracture with varus alignment, flexion of the proximal portion of the femur, and displacement of the lesser trochanter.

to the affected hip. This is done by shifting the upper body over the standing hip in single-leg stance, resulting in the characteristic gait. Alternatively, a cane used in the opposite hand can diminish the load on the hip in single-leg stance by nearly 40%.

E. Mechanism of injury

1. Hip fractures in the elderly are generally the result of low-energy trauma. Frequently, the patient sustains the fracture as a result of a fall from a standing height from either a direct blow or as a result of a rotational torsion of the femur.

    a. A fall to the side that impacts the greater trochanter is more likely to cause a fracture.

    b. External rotation of the distal extremity and the tethering of the anterior femoral capsule can result in posterior comminution of the femoral neck or anterior column fracture.

    c. One method of fracture prevention is training in fall prevention; protective padding has demonstrated efficacy but is often impractical.

2. Hip fractures in younger individuals are often the result of high-energy trauma that exerts an axial load on the femoral shaft, either through the distal femur or through the foot with the hip and knee extended.

F. Clinical evaluation

1. The injured extremity usually is shortened and externally rotated. A careful examination of the extremity should be performed, with particular attention given to skin condition and neurologic status.

2. In the geriatric population, a careful evaluation for medical comorbidities should be undertaken. The number of comorbidities is directly related to 1-year mortality figures: Patients with four or more comorbidities have been reported to have a higher 1-year mortality rate than patients with three or fewer.

3. In the high-energy trauma patient, a systematic search for other injuries should be undertaken, as well as a careful secondary assessment of the injured extremity for associated fractures.

G. Radiographic evaluation

1. An AP view of the pelvis, an AP view of the hip, and a cross-table or frog-lateral view are required for diagnosis and preoperative planning (**Figure 3**).

2. Normal radiographs do not exclude a hip fracture; of patients with hip pain, 8% have an occult fracture. MRI is recommended to evaluate for the presence of an occult fracture when it can be performed in the acute setting. Alternative imaging studies include CT and bone scanning. The sensitivity of bone scanning is increased by waiting 24 to 72 hours after injury.

H. Surgical indications

1. Most, if not all, fractures of the proximal femur should be stabilized surgically to prevent displacement and to allow early mobilization and weight bearing. For displaced fractures of the femoral neck in patients of advanced age or in those with preexisting arthritis, arthroplasty should be considered.

2. In the young patient with high-energy trauma, every effort should be made to obtain and maintain an anatomic reduction of the proximal femur fracture with internal fixation.

3. Nonsurgical management should be considered only in nonambulatory patients and in patients who are deemed too medically ill for surgical intervention.

I. Timing of surgery

1. In the elderly patient with substantial comorbidities, it is important to reverse easily correctible medical conditions before surgery, but surgery should be performed as soon as reasonably possible. Surgery should be performed when optimal medical support is available, preferably during normal surgical hours, because surgery performed in less optimal conditions is associated with an increased risk of malreduction and other technical errors.

2. In the younger trauma population, femoral neck fractures should be addressed as soon as possible after other life-threatening injuries have been stabilized. Performing surgery without delay helps to preserve and maintain the blood flow to the femoral head, preventing or limiting the development of osteonecrosis.

J. Anesthesia considerations

1. The goals of the anesthetic technique selected are to eliminate pain, allow appropriate intraoperative positioning, and achieve muscle relaxation to effect the reduction.

2. Spinal and general anesthetic techniques result in similar long-term outcomes, but spinal anesthesia may result in less postsurgical confusion, a reduced rate of deep vein thrombosis (DVT) and a diminished risk of early postsurgical death.

3. Spinal anesthetics are not successful in 20% of patients and must be converted to a general anesthetic.

K. Postoperative management

1. Postoperative management should focus on early mobilization of the patient and minimization of complications such as DVT, disorientation, bowel or bladder irregularities, and pressure sores.

2. Early hospital discharge with adequate outpatient medical and social assistance has been demonstrated to reduce the overall cost and improve recovery. Inpatient rehabilitation stays have not been associated with improved functional outcomes for community ambulators.

3. Elderly patients should be allowed to bear weight as tolerated. This population autoregulates its weight bearing based on the stability of the fracture pattern and fixation.

4. In younger individuals who sustain a high-energy femoral neck fracture, early weight bearing should be avoided because of the associated soft-tissue injury and the possible risk of fixation failure.

5. Antibiotic prophylaxis should be given within 1 hour of surgery and continued no longer than 24 hours following surgery to prevent postoperative wound infection.

6. DVT is reported to occur in up to 80% of patients who sustain a proximal femur fracture. Mechanical devices and chemical prophylaxis should be used as prophylactic measures against DVT. The risk of DVT is reduced substantially with prophylaxis, although the exact type of prophylaxis and the duration remain controversial.

II. Fractures of the Femoral Neck

A. Classification—Three main classification systems are used for fractures of the femoral neck.

1. Pauwels classification system

a. Not widely used, this system divides fractures into three groups based on the angle of the femoral neck fracture (**Figure 4**).

b. This system seems most applicable to high-energy femoral neck fractures.

c. Vertical fracture lines were believed to have the highest risk for nonunion and osteonecrosis; however, this system seems to have little predictive value.

2. Garden classification

a. This system divides fractures into four types based on the degree of displacement (**Figure 5**).

b. The interobserver agreement for this classification scheme as originally described is poor.

3: Trauma

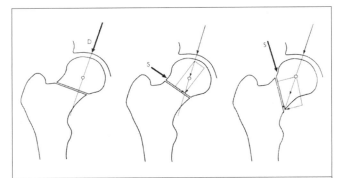

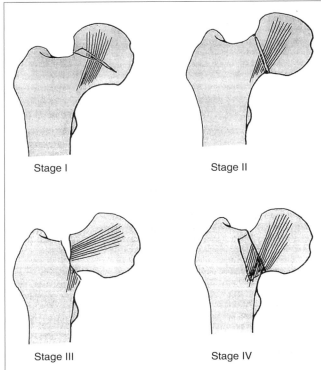

Figure 4 Illustrations depict the Pauwels classification of femoral neck fractures. **A,** In type I patterns, the fracture is relatively horizontal (< 30°), and compression forces caused by the hip joint reactive force predominate. **B,** In type II patterns, shear forces at the fracture are predicted. **C,** In type III patterns, when the fracture angle is 50° or higher, shear forces predominate. Arrows indicate the joint reactive force. (Adapted with permission from Bartonicek J: Pauwels' classification of femoral neck fractures. *J Orthop Trauma* 2001;15:359-360.)

Figure 5 Illustrations show the Garden classification of femoral neck fractures. Stage I is an incomplete, impacted fracture in valgus malalignment, which is generally stable. Stage II is a nondisplaced fracture. Stage III is an incompletely displaced fracture in varus malalignment. Stage IV is a completely displaced fracture with no engagement of the two fragments. The compression trabeculae in the femoral head line up with the trabeculae on the acetabular side. Displacement generally is more evident on the lateral view in stage IV. For prognostic purposes, these groupings can be lumped into nondisplaced/impacted (stages I and II) and displaced (stages III and IV), because the risks of nonunion and aseptic necrosis are similar within these grouped stages. (Reproduced with permission from Swiontkowski MF: Intracapsular hip fractures, in Browner BD, Jupiter JB, Levine AM, Trafton PG, eds: *Skeletal Trauma: Basic Science, Management, and Reconstruction*, ed 2. Philadelphia, PA, WB Saunders, 1998, p 1775.)

c. Interobserver agreement increases substantially, however, when type I and type II fractures are combined and considered nondisplaced and type III and type IV patterns are combined and considered displaced. The risk of nonunion and osteonecrosis is similar within the combined classification schemes.

3. AO/OTA classification

a. This classification system subdivides fractures based on the location in the femoral neck and the degree of displacement.

b. The femoral neck is divided into subcapital, transcervical, and basicervical regions.

c. This system is used mostly for research purposes.

B. Nonsurgical treatment

1. Nonsurgical treatment is reserved for the nonambulatory patient or the patient in the terminal stages of life. In general, acute pain can be controlled with narcotic medication and subsides in the first few days to 1 week, allowing transfers in the nonambulatory patient that are tolerable for the staff and patient.

2. Nonsurgical treatment can be considered for a nondisplaced femoral neck fracture, but the reported incidence of late displacement is between 15% and 30%.

3. Compression-related stress fractures also can be considered for nonsurgical treatment, but close follow-up and restricted weight bearing are required.

C. Surgical treatment

1. Nondisplaced fractures

a. The outcome is poor for displaced femoral neck fractures, so nondisplaced fractures should be stabilized to prevent late displacement. In surgically treated nondisplaced femoral neck fractures, the risk of late displacement is between 1% and 6%.

b. Transcervical and subcapital fractures are best treated with percutaneous placement of three partially threaded compression screws. The screws should be started at or above the level of the lesser trochanter on the lateral cortex to minimize the risk of subsequent subtrochanteric fracture. Screws should be placed in the periphery of the femoral neck to gain the support of the residual cortical bone to resist shear forces and within 5 mm of the articular surface to gain purchase in the subchondral bone. Care should be taken to avoid penetration of the articular surface, and multiplanar fluoroscopy should be used to confirm that no intra-articular penetration has occurred.

c. Basicervical fractures behave in a manner similar to intertrochanteric femur fractures and should be stabilized surgically with a sliding hip screw that allows controlled compression of the fracture. This fracture pattern has less inherent rotational stability than an intertrochanteric fracture, so an additional parallel screw should be placed to resist rotational forces.

2. Displaced fractures

a. Open reduction and internal fixation

- In the young patient with high-energy trauma or in the active elderly patient without preexisting arthritis, reduction and fixation of the displaced femoral neck fracture with the previously described techniques should be attempted.

- The key factor in preventing nonunion, loss of fixation, and osteonecrosis is the quality and maintenance of the reduction. Closed reduction can be attempted, but the reduction needs to be anatomic. If closed reduction is unsuccessful, open reduction with an anterolateral or anterior approach to the hip should be performed.

- When closed reduction techniques are used in high-energy fractures, a capsular release may help to diminish the risk of osteonecrosis by relieving the capsular pressure on the ascending branches.

- Femoral neck fractures that are the result of metastatic disease or pathologic process are contraindicated for ORIF.

b. Hemiarthroplasty

- Hemiarthroplasty should be considered in the low-demand individual of advanced physiologic age or in a patient who is chronologically older than 80 years.

- Short-term outcomes are similar for unipolar and bipolar prosthetic designs, but in patients followed for more than 7 years, those

with a bipolar prosthesis appeared to have better function.

- The use of cemented versus uncemented technique is controversial. Uncemented technique appears to be associated with a slightly higher short-term complication rate. Uncemented prostheses, which usually have been reserved for minimal ambulators in the past, can be considered for a broader spectrum of patients

c. Total hip arthroplasty

- The primary indication for THA has been an arthritic, symptomatic hip joint.

- Recent studies suggest that for displaced femoral neck fractures, functional outcomes are better with THA than with hemiarthroplasty, particularly in more active patients. This topic remains controversial.

- Pathologic fracture of the femoral neck is also an indication for THA.

- Dislocation rates for THA following femoral neck fracture may be greater than primary THA.

D. Surgical pearls

1. Pathologic fractures of the femoral neck should be treated with hemiarthroplasty or THA.

2. Screw fixation below the level of the lesser trochanter increases the risk of subtrochanteric femur fracture.

3. In patients between the ages of 65 and 80 years, surgical decision making should be based on physiologic, not chronologic, patient age.

4. Reversible medical comorbidities in geriatric patients should be minimized promptly. Surgical delay beyond 72 hours has been reported to increase the risk of 1-year mortality.

E. Complications

1. Osteonecrosis

a. In nondisplaced fractures, the incidence of osteonecrosis can be as high as 15%. In appropriately fixed displaced fractures, the rate of osteonecrosis has been reported to range between 20% and 30%.

b. Osteonecrosis alone is not necessarily of clinical importance unless late segmental collapse ensues. Segmental collapse can be seen as early as 6 to 9 months following injury, but it is most likely to be recognized in the second year following surgery. In most cases it can be excluded after the third year.

2. Nonunion

a. Nonunion rates are reported to be from 5% in

3: Trauma

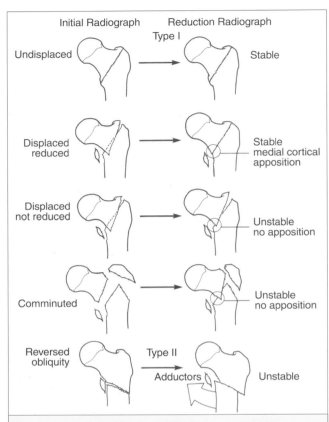

Initial Radiograph   Reduction Radiograph

Type I

Undisplaced → Stable

Displaced reduced → Stable medial cortical apposition

Displaced not reduced → Unstable no apposition

Comminuted → Unstable no apposition

Reversed obliquity — Type II

Adductors → Unstable

Figure 6 Illustrations show the Evans classification of intertrochanteric fracture. (Adapted with permission from DeLee JC: Fractures and dislocations of the hip, in Rockwood CA Jr, Green DP, Bucholz RW, Heckman JD, eds: *Rockwood and Green's Fractures in Adults*, ed 4. Philadelphia, PA, Lippincott Williams & Wilkins, 1996, p 1721.)

the elderly to 30% in the young, high-energy trauma population.

    b. Nonunion generally is associated with more vertically oriented fracture patterns and loss of reduction with varus collapse.

    c. Nonunion repair is based on the reorientation of the fracture line to a more horizontal position. A valgus osteotomy of the proximal femur is the treatment of choice in the physiologically young patient.

III. Intertrochanteric Fractures

A. Classification

    1. The Evans classification system divides intertrochanteric fractures into stable and unstable fracture patterns (**Figure 6**). The distinction between stable and unstable fractures is based on the integrity of the posterior medial cortex. The Evans

classification also recognizes the reverse obliquity fracture pattern, which is suseptible to medial displacement of the distal fragment.

    2. All other intertrochanteric fracture classification schemes, including the AO/OTA classification, are variations on the Evans classification.

    3. No classification of intertrochanteric fractures has gained wide acceptance, and all demonstrate suboptimal observer agreement.

    4. Intertrochanteric fractures may be classified best as stable or unstable based on the ability to resist compressive loads.

    5. In general, when the posterior medial cortex is comminuted, fractures are considered unstable, secondary to the likelihood the fracture will collapse into varus and retroversion.

B. Nonsurgical treatment

    1. Nonsurgical treatment should be reserved for patients who are nonambulatory or who are at substantial risk for perioperative mortality related to anesthesia or surgery.

    2. These patients should receive adequate analgesics and be mobilized to a chair.

    3. Nonsurgical treatment is associated with an increased mortality rate and an increased risk for decubiti, urinary tract infection, contracture, pneumonia, and DVT.

C. Surgical treatment

    1. General considerations

        a. Surgical fixation of intertrochanteric fractures is based on reestablishing a normal femoral neck-shaft alignment angle and allowing for the controlled collapse of both stable and unstable fracture types.

        b. Devices that allow controlled collapse have eliminated the need for restoring medial cortical contact by direct reduction techniques or medial displacement osteotomies. Regardless of the device, the main technical factors that eliminate the complications of treatment are the accurate restoration of alignment and placement of the lag screw in the femoral head. The lag screw should be placed in the center aspect of the head and in the subchondral bone. Measurement of the tip-apex distance (TAD) is predictive of fixation failure (**Figure 7**). A TAD greater than 25 mm has been associated with fixation failure.

    2. Internal fixation techniques—The two main devices used for internal fixation are the sliding hip screw/side plate and the intramedullary hip screw. Both devices have theoretical advantages, but no data indicate that one device is superior.

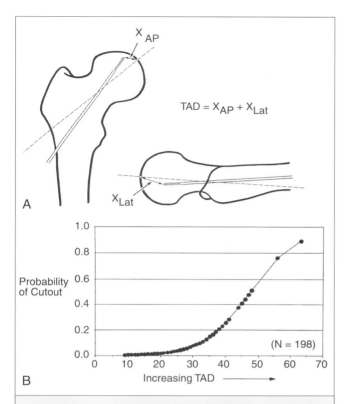

$$TAD = X_{AP} + X_{Lat}$$

Figure 7 Images show the measurement of the tip-apex distance (TAD). **A,** The TAD is estimated by combining the distance from the guide-pin tip to the tip of the apex of the femoral head (dashed line) on the AP and lateral (Lat) fluoroscopic views. **B,** The risk for cutout failure increases dramatically when the TAD exceeds 25 mm. (Reproduced from Baumgaertner MR, Brennan MJ: Intertrochanteric femur fractures, in Kellam JF, Fischer TJ, Tornetta P III, Bosse MJ, Harris MB, eds: *Orthopaedic Knowledge Update: Trauma*, ed 2. Rosemont, IL, American Academy of Orthopaedic Surgeons, 2000, pp 125-131.)

a. Sliding hip screw

- Advantages: ease of application, surgeon familiarity, availability, a high success rate, minimal complications, cost

- Disadvantages: open technique, increased blood loss, increased failure in reverse obliquity or subtrochanteric extension patterns, excessive collapse resulting in limb shortening and fracture deformity in unstable fracture patterns

b. Intramedullary hip screw

- Advantages: percutaneous application, limited blood loss, lateral buttress allowing limited collapse, increased resistance to varus forces

- Disadvantages: periprosthetic fracture, increased incidence of screw cutout, cost

3. Arthroplasty

a. Standard arthroplasty implants are not effective for most intertrochanteric fractures secondary to the presence of comminution in the proximal femur.

b. A calcar-replacing prosthesis or a proximal femoral replacement component frequently is required.

c. Secure fixation of the greater trochanter is problematic.

d. Because of the extensive nature of proximal femoral replacement and the associated increased surgical stress, arthroplasty is not warranted in most fractures.

e. Proximal femoral replacement should be reserved for the salvage of failed ORIF or pathologic fractures.

D. Unusual fractures

1. Reverse obliquity fracture

a. The reverse obliquity fracture is an unstable fracture pattern that does not have an intact lateral cortex to support controlled compaction with a sliding hip screw (**Figure 8**).

b. These fractures are best thought of as subtrochanteric femur fractures and therefore should be treated with either an intramedullary nail or a fixed-angle device such as a blade plate or dynamic condylar screw.

2. Fractures of the greater trochanter

a. Fractures of the greater trochanter are usually the result of a direct blow.

b. The primary deforming force is the external hip rotators, not the hip abductors.

c. Most of these fractures can be treated nonsurgically, regardless of the degree of displacement, but in the younger, more active patient, repair should be considered for fracture displacement greater than 1 cm.

3. Fractures of the lesser trochanter

a. Isolated fractures of the lesser trochanter are rare; they are seen in adolescents and generally represent an avulsion of the trochanter by the iliopsoas.

b. A more common etiology is a pathologic fracture resulting from tumor metastasis.

E. Complications

1. Loss of fixation

a. Usually occurs during the first 3 months following fracture treatment and is the most common complication

3: Trauma

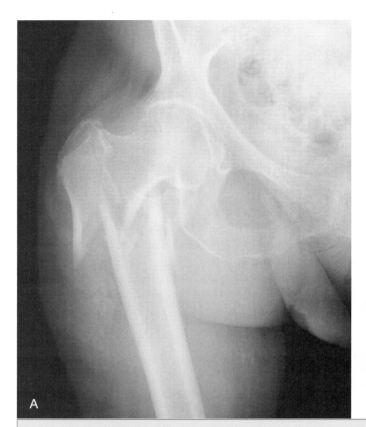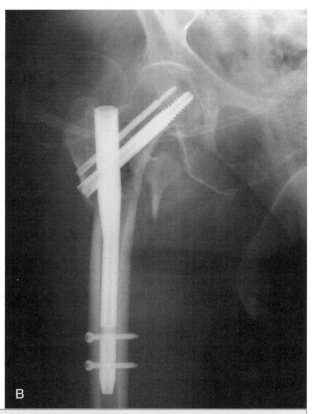

Figure 8   Radiographs depict a reverse obliquity fracture. **A,** AP view shows a four-part comminuted intertrochanteric fracture with reverse obliquity. **B,** AP view shows the same hip after treatment with an intramedullary hip screw. (Reproduced from Haidukewych GJ, Jacofsky DJ: Hip trauma, in Vaccaro AR, ed: *Orthopaedic Knowledge Update*, ed 8. Rosemont, IL, American Academy of Orthopaedic Surgeons, 2005, p 404.)

b. Varus malalignment at the time of fracture fixation, advanced age, and osteopenia are all contributory factors to screw cutout of the femoral head.

c. The most important predictor of cutout is the TAD. According to one study, a TAD less than 27 mm was not associated with screw cutout, but a TAD greater than 45 mm was associated with a failure rate of 60%.

2. Nonunion

a. Occurs in less than 2% of patients and is most commonly associated with unstable fracture patterns

b. Nonunion can be associated with fixation failure and varus collapse.

c. Failure of controlled impaction at the fracture site is also contributory.

d. The treatment options for this complication are revision internal fixation and valgus osteotomy versus proximal femoral replacement.

3. Malunion is common, in the form of a varus deformity or a rotational deformity.

a. Comminuted unstable fracture patterns have the greatest risk for an internal rotation deformity.

b. Corrective osteotomy is the best salvage procedure for this condition.

IV. Subtrochanteric Femur Fractures

A. Classification

1. Seinsheimer

a. The Seinsheimer classification system is a comprehensive scheme that subdivides the fracture patterns into eight groups (**Figure 9**).

b. Interobserver agreement is relatively low, and the system is not in widespread use.

2. Russell-Taylor

a. The Russell-Taylor classification system divides subtrochanteric fractures into four types, based on the involvement of the lesser trochanter and the piriformis fossa (**Figure 10**).

b. This system provides guidance on whether to

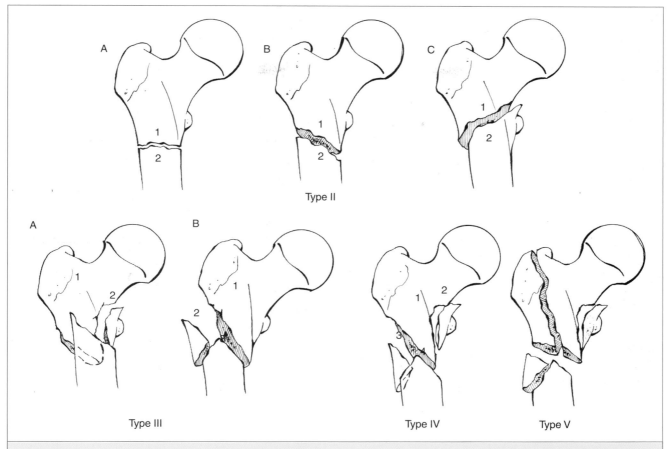

Figure 9   Illustrations show the Seinsheimer classification of subtrochanteric femur fractures. Type I fractures (not shown) are nondisplaced. (Reproduced with permission from Leung K: Subtrochanteric fractures, in Bucholz RW, Heckman JD, Court-Brown C, eds: *Rockwood and Green's Fractures in Adults*, ed 6. Philadelphia, PA, Lippincott Williams & Wilkins, 2006, p 1831.)

treat the fracture with a nail, the type of nail to use, and when nailing should be avoided.

  c. The Russell-Taylor classification has not been subjected to reliability tests.

B. Nonsurgical treatment—Nonsurgical treatment is appropriate only for the nonambulatory patient.

C. Surgical treatment

  1. General considerations

    a. Evaluation of the anatomic location and orientation of the fracture pattern guides the selection of the most appropriate device and its application for these fractures.

    b. The goals of internal fixation should be the anatomic restoration of femoral alignment, the maintenance of alignment, and the minimization of the surgical insult.

  2. Intramedullary nailing

    a. Intramedullary nailing can be used for all subtrochanteric femur fractures that do not ex-

tend to the piriformis fossa or greater trochanter.

    b. A standard nail with locking screws that do not enter the femoral head can be used in fractures below the level of the lesser trochanter as long as the device offers an oblique proximal locking option.

    c. For fractures that extend to or involve the lesser trochanter, a cephalomedullary nail is required for adequate fixation.

    d. Nailing can be performed in fractures that extend into the nail starting point, but it is not the preferred technique for most surgeons.

    e. The main pitfall of intramedullary nailing is varus deformity with the proximal fragment also assuming a flexed position. Alignment must be restored before reaming and placement of the intramedullary nail.

    f. Fracture reduction and intramedullary nailing can be facilitated with the patient in a lateral position on the fracture table. This allows the

3: Trauma

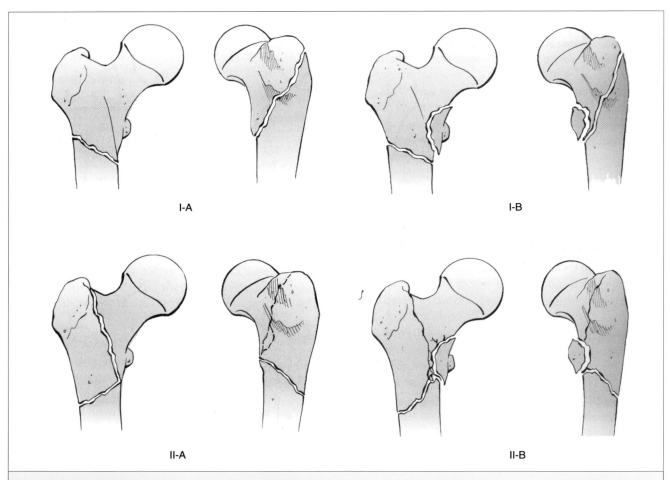

Figure 10   Illustrations depict the Russell-Taylor classification of subtrochanteric fractures. (Reproduced with permission from Leung K: Subtrochanteric fractures, in Bucholz RW, Heckman JD, Court-Brown C, eds: *Rockwood and Green's Fractures in Adults*, ed 6. Philadelphia, PA, Lippincott Williams & Wilkins, 2006, p 1832.)

femur to be flexed in relation to the hip, matching the unopposed flexion of the proximal fragment.

   g. Intramedullary nails are load-sharing devices, and early weight bearing frequently can be initiated.

3. Plate fixation

   a. Plate fixation with a fixed-angle device such as a blade plate or a dynamic condylar screw can be used on all subtrochanteric femur fractures regardless of location, but the open nature of the technique and the associated blood loss make its practical use limited to the most proximal fractures. Locking plate designs also can be used in this area and may be technically easier to apply than the older fixed-angle designs. Failure rates of locking-plate implants are reportedly higher.

   b. The surgical approach is a direct lateral approach to the proximal femur.

   c. Dissection of the medial fragments during fracture reduction should be avoided because of the relatively high rate of nonunion (30%) with excessive periosteal dissection.

   d. Fixed-angle plates are load-bearing devices, and early weight bearing should be avoided.

D. Complications

1. The deforming forces involved in subtrochanteric fractures of the femur are substantial; obtaining and maintaining an adequate reduction in subtrochanteric fractures while performing internal fixation can be difficult. Malunion in the form of varus and proximal fragment flexion is not uncommon.

2. Nonunion is associated with fracture comminution and excessive dissection in the area of the medial femur. Supplemental bone grafting is recommended when medial dissection is performed.

Top Testing Facts

Fractures of the Femoral Neck

1. Fractures of the femoral neck can result from direct force or indirect force (a fall onto the proximal thigh or a rotational force).

2. The main blood supply to the femoral head comes from the medial femoral circumflex artery.

3. The structure at risk during the anterior approach to the hip is the lateral femoral cutaneous nerve.

4. The Y ligament of Bigelow resists hip hyperextension.

5. Screw fixation below the level of the lesser trochanter increases the risk of subtrochanteric femur fracture.

6. Pathologic fractures of the femoral neck should be treated with hemiarthroplasty or THA.

Intertrochanteric Fractures

1. A TAD less than 25 mm should be maintained when placing the lag screw of a plate or nail device to minimize the risk of fixation failure.

2. Reverse obliquity fractures should be treated with an intramedullary nail or a fixed-angle plate.

3. Lesser trochanteric fractures often are associated with tumor metastasis.

Subtrochanteric Fractures

1. When using an open technique, medial dissection should be avoided.

Bibliography

Adams CI, Robinson CM, Court-Brown CM, McQueen MM: Prospective randomized controlled trial of an intramedullary nail versus dynamic screw and plate for intertrochanteric fractures of the femur. *J Orthop Trauma* 2001;15(6): 394-400.

Ahrengart L, Törnkvist H, Fornander P, et al: A randomized study of the compression hip screw and Gamma nail in 426 fractures. *Clin Orthop Relat Res* 2002;401:209-222.

Baumgaertner MR, Curtin SL, Lindskog DM, Keggi JM: The value of the tip-apex distance in predicting failure of fixation of peritrochanteric fractures of the hip. *J Bone Joint Surg Am* 1995;77(7):1058-1064.

Bhandari M, Devereaux PJ, Swiontkowski MF, et al: Internal fixation compared with arthroplasty for displaced fractures of the femoral neck: A meta-analysis. *J Bone Joint Surg Am* 2003;85-A(9):1673-1681.

Callaghan JJ, Liu SS, Haidukewych GJ: Subcapital fractures: A changing paradigm. *J Bone Joint Surg Br* 2012;94(11, suppl A):19-21.

Deangelis JP, Ademi A, Staff I, Lewis CG: Cemented versus uncemented hemiarthroplasty for displaced femoral neck fractures: A prospective randomized trial with early follow-up. *J Orthop Trauma* 2012;26(3):135-140.

Haidukewych GJ, Berry DJ: Hip arthroplasty for salvage of failed treatment of intertrochanteric hip fractures. *J Bone Joint Surg Am* 2003;85-A(5):899-904.

Haidukewych GJ, Israel TA, Berry DJ: Reverse obliquity fractures of the intertrochanteric region of the femur. *J Bone Joint Surg Am* 2001;83-A(5):643-650.

Koval KJ, Sala DA, Kummer FJ, Zuckerman JD: Postoperative weight-bearing after a fracture of the femoral neck or an intertrochanteric fracture. *J Bone Joint Surg Am* 1998;80(3): 352-356.

Marti RK, Schüller HM, Raaymakers EL: Intertrochanteric osteotomy for non-union of the femoral neck. *J Bone Joint Surg Br* 1989;71(5):782-787.

Oakes DA, Jackson KR, Davies MR, et al: The impact of the garden classification on proposed operative treatment. *Clin Orthop Relat Res* 2003;409:232-240.

Ong BC, Maurer SG, Aharonoff GB, Zuckerman JD, Koval KJ: Unipolar versus bipolar hemiarthroplasty: Functional outcome after femoral neck fracture at a minimum of thirty-six months of follow-up. *J Orthop Trauma* 2002;16(5):317-322.

Parker MJ, Handoll HH: Gamma and other cephalocondylic intramedullary nails versus extramedullary implants for extracapsular hip fractures in adults. *Cochrane Database Syst Rev* 2010;9:CD000093.

Rizzo PF, Gould ES, Lyden JP, Asnis SE: Diagnosis of occult fractures about the hip: Magnetic resonance imaging compared with bone-scanning. *J Bone Joint Surg Am* 1993;75(3): 395-401.

Szita J, Cserháti P, Bosch U, Manninger J, Bodzay T, Fekete K: Intracapsular femoral neck fractures: The importance of early reduction and stable osteosynthesis. *Injury* 2002; 33(suppl 3):C41-C46.

Tanaka J, Seki N, Tokimura F, Hayashi Y: Conservative treatment of Garden stage I femoral neck fracture in elderly patients. *Arch Orthop Trauma Surg* 2002;122(1):24-28.

3: Trauma

Taylor F, Wright M, Zhu M: Hemiarthroplasty of the hip with and without cement: A randomized clinical trial. *J Bone Joint Surg Am* 2012;94(7):577-583.

Trueta J, Harrison MH: The normal vascular anatomy of the femoral head in adult man. *J Bone Joint Surg Br* 1953; 35-B(3):442-461.

Vaidya SV, Dholakia DB, Chatterjee A: The use of a dynamic condylar screw and biological reduction techniques for sub-trochanteric femur fracture. *Injury* 2003;34(2):123-128.

Zuckerman JD, Skovron ML, Koval KJ, Aharonoff G, Frankel VH: Postoperative complications and mortality associated with operative delay in older patients who have a fracture of the hip. *J Bone Joint Surg Am* 1995;77(10):1551-1556.

Chapter 39

Fractures of the Femoral Shaft and Distal Femur

Lisa K. Cannada, MD

I. Fractures of the Femoral Shaft

A. Anatomy

1. The femur is the largest, strongest bone in the body and is enveloped by a thick mass of muscle (**Figure 1**).

2. The femoral shaft is defined as the diaphyseal portion of the bone, which extends from below the lesser trochanter to above the metaphyseal portion of the distal femur.

3. The bony anatomy of the femoral shaft includes an anterior bow.

4. Compartments of the thigh

   a. Anterior compartment with the quadriceps muscles

   b. Posterior compartment with the hamstrings

   c. Adductor compartment

5. Deforming forces after a fracture

   a. The abductors (gluteus medius and minimus) insert on the greater trochanter and abduct the proximal segment.

   b. The iliopsoas inserts on the lesser trochanter and flexes the proximal fragment.

   c. The adductor longus, adductor brevis, gracilis, and adductor magnus have a broad area of insertion on the distal femur and contribute to a varus force on the distal segment.

B. Mechanisms of injury

1. Femoral shaft fractures often are high-energy injuries, such as from a motor vehicle or motorcycle accident. The most common mechanism in motor vehicle accidents is impact of the knee against the car's dashboard. Associated injuries include pelvis/acetabulum fractures, hip fractures and/or dislocations, and fractures of the femoral head, distal femur, patella, tibial plateau, and knee ligaments.

2. A small percentage of fractures occurs as a result of repeated stress, such as that experienced by a young military recruit or runner following an increase in the intensity of physical training.

3. Pathologic fractures may be the first presentation of metastatic cancer. Radiographs should be evaluated for the possibility of bony lesions, especially when the injury is not consistent with the mechanism (for example, stepping off a curb or standing from a chair).

4. A fall from a standing height is a common mechanism in the elderly, underscoring the need for emphasis of osteoporotic fracture prevention.

5. Fractures may occur in the proximal femur from relatively low mechanisms of injury in patients who have a history of prolonged bisphosphonate use.

6. Bilateral femur fractures historically had a mortality rate of up to 25%. Recent studies demonstrate lower death rates, of less than 7%.

C. Clinical evaluation

1. Advanced Trauma Life Support principles should be initiated in patients with femoral shaft fractures.

2. Physical examination

   a. Obvious thigh deformity, with the limb shortened, rotated, and swollen compared with the contralateral extremity is a common presentation.

   b. The limb should be palpated for tenderness and deformity.

Dr. Cannada or an immediate family member is a member of a speakers' bureau or has made paid presentations on behalf of Smith & Nephew; serves as a paid consultant to or is an employee of Zimmer; has received research or institutional support from Zimmer, Synthes, the Department of Defense, and the Southeast Fracture Consortium; and serves as a board member, owner, officer, or committee member of the American Academy of Orthopaedic Surgeons, the Orthopaedic Trauma Association, and the Ruth Jackson Orthopaedic Society.

3: Trauma

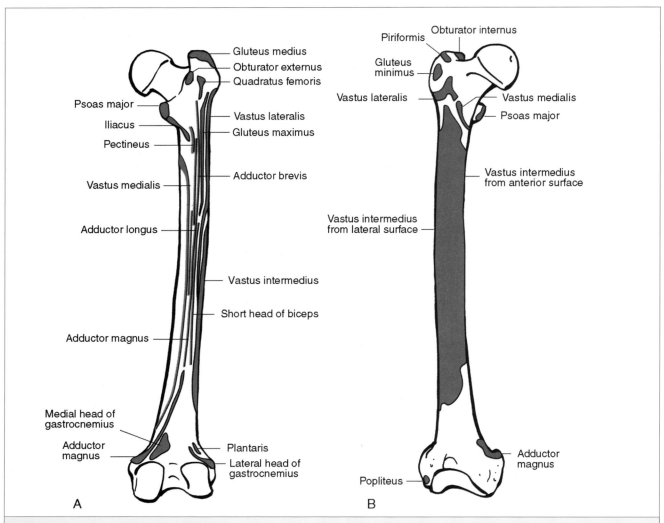

Figure 1 Illustrations depict the primary muscular attachments on the anterior (**A**) and posterior (**B**) aspects of the femur. (Adapted with permission from Nork SE: Fractures of the shaft of the femur, in Bucholz RW, Heckman JD, Court-Brown C, eds: *Rockwood and Green's Fractures in Adults*, ed 6. Philadelphia, PA, Lippincott Williams and Wilkins, 2001, p 1852.)

c. The distal extremity should be evaluated for pulses, sensation, and motor function.

d. The presence of pain to palpation, ecchymosis, crepitus, and deformity indicates that the patient should be examined for further injuries.

3. Additional injuries to the spine, pelvis, and ipsilateral lower extremity can occur, as can soft-tissue injuries, specifically ligamentous and/or meniscal injuries of the knee; therefore, patients with femur fractures always should be evaluated closely for associated injuries.

4. Ipsilateral femoral neck fracture also can occur, but is still missed routinely (in up to 50% of patients).

a. Initially, these fractures are nondisplaced or minimally displaced in up to 60% of patients.

b. The femoral neck fracture often is vertically oriented.

D. Radiographic evaluation

1. An AP view of the pelvis and AP and lateral views of the femur, including the knee joint, are indicated.

2. CT evaluation of the hip to detect associated nondisplaced femoral neck fracture is recommended in trauma patients who have sustained a femoral shaft fracture.

E. Fracture classification

1. The Winquist and Hansen classification system is based on the amount of comminution and has implications for weight-bearing status and the use of interlocking screws (**Figure 2**).

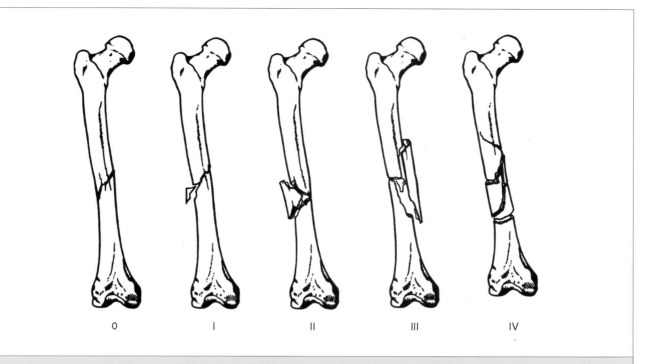

Figure 2 Illustrations show the Winquist and Hansen classification system of femoral shaft fractures. Type 0—no comminution; type I—minimal or no comminution; type II—at least 50% of the cortices intact; type III—comminution of at least 50% to 100% of the circumference of the bone; type IV—no cortical contact at the fracture site with circumferential comminution. (Reproduced from Poss R, ed: *Orthopaedic Knowledge Update*, ed 3. Park Ridge, IL, American Academy of Orthopaedic Surgeons, 1990, pp 513-527.)

2. The AO Foundation and Orthopaedic Trauma Association (AO/OTA) Classification of Fractures and Dislocations is used more commonly for research purposes and is not very useful in guiding treatment (**Figure 3**).

F. Nonsurgical treatment

1. Early stabilization (within the first 24 hours) of femur fractures minimizes the complication rates and can reduce the hospital length of stay.

2. Skeletal traction may be a reasonable treatment in patients who are too physiologically unstable for surgical treatment.

3. A long period of bed rest may be detrimental, however, and patients should be monitored closely.

   a. Patients should be evaluated closely for pin tract infection and decubiti secondary to prolonged immobilization.

   b. Serial radiographs should be obtained to monitor for distraction at the fracture site during treatment.

   c. Mechanical and chemical deep vein thrombosis (DVT) prophylaxis is important in these patients.

G. Surgical treatment

1. A statically locked, reamed intramedullary (IM) nail is the standard of care for femoral shaft fractures.

   a. An IM nail can be a load-sharing device, as opposed to a compression plate, which is a load-bearing device.

   b. Central placement of an IM nail within the femoral canal results in lower tensile and shear stresses on the implant.

   c. IM nailing has several benefits over plates and screws, including less extensive exposure and dissection, a lower infection rate, less quadriceps scarring, early functional use of the extremity, immediate full weight bearing, improved restoration of length and alignment with comminuted fractures, rapid fracture healing, and a low refracture rate.

   d. The starting point should be based on surgeon preference.

   e. At least two interlocking screws, one proximal and one distal, should be used for all fractures.

   f. For femur fractures with segmental comminution, multiple interlocking screws proximally and distally should be considered.

3: Trauma

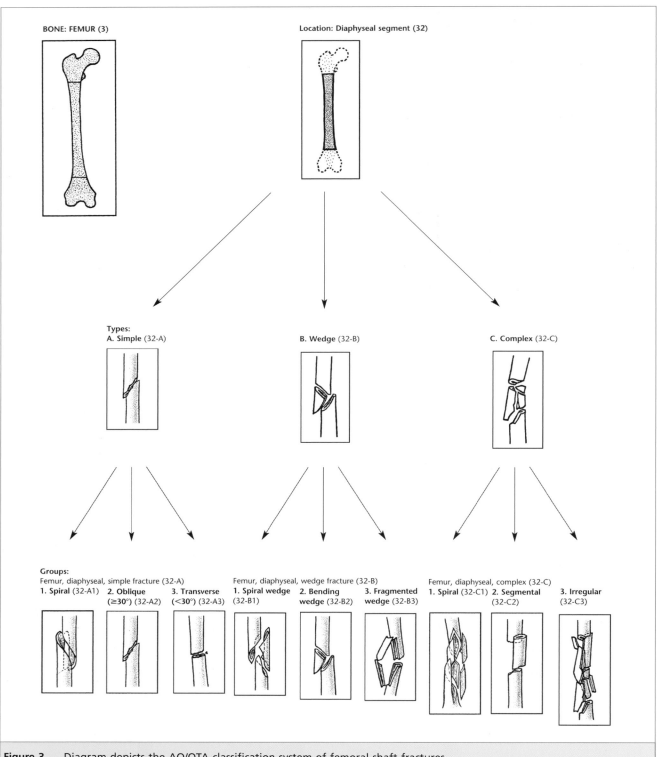

Figure 3 Diagram depicts the AO/OTA classification system of femoral shaft fractures.

2. Retrograde approach

    a. Indications for this approach include multiple-system trauma; trauma to the ipsilateral extremity, pelvis/acetabulum, and/or spine; bilat-

eral femur fractures; and morbid obesity.

    b. The overall union rate of retrograde nailing is comparable with that of antegrade nailing.

    c. The approach has several advantages, includ-

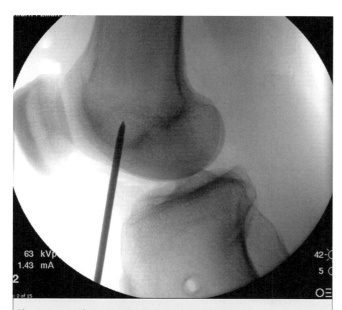

Figure 4 Fluoroscopic image demonstrates the lateral starting point for a retrograde intramedullary nail.

ing ease of entry point, the potential for shorter surgical times, and the avoidance of using a fracture table.

d. The recommended starting point for retrograde nailing is 10 mm anterior to the posterior cruciate ligament in the intercondylar notch and in line with the femoral canal.

e. The optimum starting point in the lateral plane is just anterior to the Blumensaat line (**Figure 4**). The Blumensaat line can be visualized on the lateral view. The line represents the intercondylar notch roof.

f. A true lateral radiograph should be obtained preoperatively, with both femoral condyles overlapping and appearing as a single condyle. The radiograph should be reviewed preoperatively to assess for patella baja, which may interfere with a percutaneous incision and require an arthrotomy (rare).

g. Surgical pearls: A radiolucent triangle or bump should be strategically placed to assist with reduction; The prepatellar skin and patella should be protected during reaming by seating the reamer in bone before starting; Before the patient wakes up, an AP pelvic radiograph should be obtained to rule out a femoral neck fracture, limb rotation and length should be evaluated, and the knee should be checked for ligamentous injuries.

h. Complications include malrotation and knee pain.

3. Piriformis entry point

a. This entry point is in line with the mechanical axis of the femur.

b. An excessively anterior entry point increases the risk for femoral neck fracture secondary to hoop stresses.

c. The piriformis entry point may result in more muscle and tendon damage and damage to the blood supply of the femoral head than the trochanteric entry point.

d. Using a piriformis entry point minimizes the risk of deformity, specifically varus, in proximal femoral fractures.

4. Trochanteric entry point

a. This entry point has several advantages over a piriformis entry point, including a more lateral location, less resultant abductor muscle damage, and shorter fluoroscopic and surgical times.

b. Complications include iatrogenic fracture if a straight piriformis-type nail is used, iatrogenic comminution with malreduction, anterior penetration distally with nail/curvature mismatch, and varus malreduction if the nail does not match the patient's anatomy.

H. Reamed versus nonreamed IM nailing

1. Reamed IM nailing is recommended over nonreamed nailing because it allows placement of a larger diameter nail with better cortical fit.

2. Previous concerns with reaming included an increased incidence of acute respiratory distress syndrome (ARDS) and lung complications in patients who had associated pulmonary injury. A study comparing open reduction and internal fixation with reamed IM nailing in this patient population showed no increased incidence, however.

I. Flat table versus fracture table

1. Whether to use a fracture table or a fluoroscopic flat table is a decision to be made with all antegrade nailings. Studies support either choice.

2. Considerations include the fracture pattern, the patient's body habitus, the number of assistants available, associated injuries, and surgeon preference.

3. Multiple complications have been reported with the use of a fracture table, including pudendal nerve neurapraxia and compartment syndrome of the unaffected leg. Additionally, positioning a patient with multiple injuries on a fracture table can be difficult.

J. Plate and screw fixation

1. Plate fixation of femur fractures is not used commonly and has few indications.

3: Trauma

2. Indications for compression plating include a fracture involving the distal metaphyseal-diaphyseal junction of the femur, periprosthetic fracture, preexisting deformity, or a small or obliterated intramedullary canal.

3. Complications of compression plating

   a. Failure of fixation

   b. Infection

   c. Nonunion

   d. Devitalization of fracture fragments with excessive periosteal stripping

   e. Stress shielding with possible refracture

K. External fixation

1. External fixation of femur fractures often is used temporarily as a form of orthopaedic damage control.

2. External fixation is useful for the unstable trauma patient and for patients whose skin does not permit initial definitive fracture fixation.

3. Concerns regarding external fixation include

   a. Pin tract infection

   b. The timing of external fixation removal and conversion to IM nailing. The literature supports safe conversion to IM nailing within the first 2 weeks to minimize the risk for infection.

L. Ipsilateral femoral neck and shaft fractures

1. Radiographic evaluation

   a. Most femoral neck fractures that are associated with an ipsilateral shaft fracture are vertically oriented and nondisplaced or minimally displaced, making radiographic detection difficult.

   b. Fine-cut CT may help detect femoral neck fractures before surgery.

2. Treatment

   a. The timing of discovery of the femoral neck fracture has implications for its treatment.

   b. No matter when the fracture is discovered, it is essential to obtain an anatomic reduction and optimize femoral neck fracture stabilization.

   c. One device or two devices may be used. With one device, a cephalomedullary nail or a centromedullary nail with cannulated screws strategically placed using the miss-a-nail technique may be used. With two devices, a retrograde nail with cannulated screws or a retrograde nail with a sliding hip screw may be used.

M. Open femoral shaft fractures

1. Open femoral shaft fractures should be treated with irrigation and débridement and primary IM nailing. This requires an incision that is adequate to allow visualization and débridement of the bone ends and the entire zone of injury.

2. No increased rate of infection is seen with retrograde nailing of open femur fractures.

3. The infection rate of open fractures of the femur is substantially lower than that of open tibia fractures.

N. Rehabilitation

1. With stable fracture fixation, early mobilization and weight bearing are permitted. Most patients are allowed to bear weight to varying degrees, but associated injuries, the fracture pattern, implant selection, and surgeon preference dictate the exact postoperative rehabilitation orders.

2. Early active motion of the hip and knee joint is encouraged.

O. Complications

1. Fat embolism syndrome

   a. This usually occurs 24 to 72 hours after initial trauma in a small percentage of patients with long bone fractures.

   b. It can be fatal in up to 15% of patients.

   c. Classic symptoms include tachypnea, tachycardia, hypoxemia, mental status changes, and petechiae.

   d. Treatment includes mechanical ventilation with high positive end-expiratory pressure levels.

   e. Prevention involves early (within 24 hours) stabilization of long bone fractures.

2. Thromboembolism

   a. DVT is a concern in trauma patients, especially those with long bone trauma, pelvic and acetabular fractures, and spine trauma. It may lead to a fatal pulmonary embolism (PE).

   b. Duplex ultrasonography may be used to diagnose DVT.

   c. In patients with suspected PE, a spiral CT scan, ventilation-perfusion scan, or pulmonary angiogram (the gold standard) may be used for diagnosis.

   d. The symptoms of a PE include acute onset tachypnea, tachycardia, low-grade fevers, hypoxia, mental status changes, and chest pain.

   e. Preventive measures include chemical prophylaxis (warfarin, subcutaneous heparin, low-molecular-weight heparin), sequential compression devices or foot pumps, and early surgical stabilization and subsequent mobilization, which are important, controllable measures.

3. Acute respiratory distress syndrome

   a. ARDS is acute respiratory failure with pulmonary edema.

   b. It can result from multiple etiologies and is known to occur after trauma and shock.

   c. The patient may be difficult to ventilate secondary to decreased lung compliance.

   d. Other signs and symptoms include tachypnea, tachycardia, and hypoxemia.

   e. Treatment consists of high positive end-expiratory pressure.

   f. The mortality rate can be as high as 50%.

   g. Early stabilization of long bone fractures minimizes ongoing soft-tissue injury and helps reduce the incidence of ARDS.

4. Compartment syndrome

   a. Compartment syndrome is rare after femur fractures. It is important to consider the mechanism of injury; a crush injury or an injury involving a prolonged extrication, in which the dashboard console was crushing the leg compartments, should be followed closely.

   b. Compartment syndrome has been reported after IM nailing on the fracture table.

5. Nerve palsy

   a. In femur fractures stabilized on the fracture table, pudendal nerve palsy may occur as a result of excessive traction and/or improper positioning with the perineal post.

   b. A peroneal nerve neurapraxia may occur secondary to excessive traction.

   c. These injuries may be missed unless the clinician asks about them.

6. Nonunion, delayed union, malunion

   a. The rate of nonunion after treatment of femoral shaft fractures with a locked IM nail is low.

   b. Treatment often includes reamed exchange nailing with a larger IM nail.

   c. For an infected nonunion (a rare complication), chronic suppressive antibiotic use until healing occurs is recommended, followed by implant removal.

   d. Delayed unions may occur because of technical concerns. Removal of the interlocking screw may allow compression across the fracture and allow union to occur.

   e. Up to 20% of patients may have limb rota-

tional deformities.

   f. Previously, it was thought that internal rotational deformities were not well tolerated, but in most patients, rotational deformities of less than 20° are well tolerated.

7. Hardware failure and recurrent fracture

   a. With reamed, statically locked IM nailing of femur fractures, the occurrence of hardware failure is low.

   b. The closer a fracture is to the interlocking screw placement, the higher the stresses on the hardware.

8. Heterotopic ossification

   a. The insertion site for an antegrade nail involves soft-tissue disruption of the abductors. Thus, heterotopic ossification about the hip may develop in some patients.

   b. Heterotopic ossification of minimal clinical significance has been reported to occur in up to 26% of patients with fractures stabilized using a piriformis starting point. The occurrence rate associated with a trochanteric starting point has not yet been reported.

P. New femoral fracture topics

1. Atypical femur fractures

   a. With prolonged use of bisphosphonates, bone turnover rate decreases considerably. It has been hypothesized that these are insufficiency fractures that resulted from severely suppressed bone turnover and accumulation of skeletal microdamage.

   b. Patients sustain these fractures from very low-energy mechanisms (for example, giving way at standing height).

   c. These fractures have a characteristic pattern.

      • They tend to be simple transverse or oblique fractures.

      • Cortical thickening occurs around the fracture site.

      • Lateral or medial beaking occurs.

   d. Treatment

      • IM nailing (but watchfulness for compromised bone quality and healing capacity should be maintained)

      • Plate fixation with compression applied across the fracture

      • Discontinuation of bisphosphonates

2. Interprosthetic fractures of the femoral shaft

   a. Interprosthetic fracture is a fracture between a

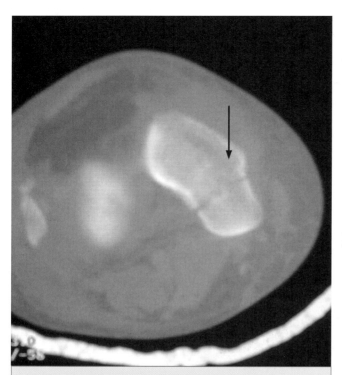

Figure 5   CT scan shows a Hoffa fracture (arrow).

hip prosthesis and a knee prosthesis.

b. The incidence is increasing.

c. Most often, affected patients already have compromised bone quality, and this must be considered in formulating treatment plans.

d. Plate fixation is the treatment of choice. It is important that the plate extend above the hip implant to provide overlap and below the knee implant to avoid stress risers.

II. Fractures of the Distal Femur

A. Epidemiology

1. Distal femur fractures are bimodally distributed.

2. Incidence is higher in young, healthy males (often from high-energy trauma) and elderly females with osteopenia (from low-energy mechanisms).

B. Anatomy

1. The geometric cross-section of the femoral shaft transitions from cylindrical to trapezoidal, with the medial condyle extending farther distally.

2. The distal femur is trapezoidal and is composed of cancellous bone.

3. The distal femur is in physiologic valgus of approximately 9°.

4. The posterior half of both femoral condyles lies posterior to the femoral shaft.

5. Deforming forces of the distal femur after a fracture

a. The origin of the gastrocnemius characteristically pulls the distal fragment into extension, resulting in an apex posterior angulation.

b. The patient must be closely evaluated preoperatively for a coronal plane Hoffa fracture (**Figure 5**). Hoffa fractures are intra-articular fractures characterized by a fracture line in the coronal plane. Most often, they are unicondylar and are best detected using CT.

C. Surgical approach

1. Depends on the choice of reduction type (indirect or direct) and plate

2. Minimally invasive surgical approaches include minimally invasive plate osteosynthesis.

a. This approach is ideal for extra-articular fractures, which can be reduced indirectly.

b. A lateral incision is made to facilitate plate placement, with stab incisions proximally for diaphyseal screw placement.

3. Lateral parapatellar approach

a. Affords excellent exposure of the femoral shaft and permits eversion of the patella

b. One disadvantage is that a different incision is needed for future total knee arthroplasties (TKAs).

c. The advantage of the approach is that it affords good visualization of the joint surface.

d. The lateral parapatellar approach should be used for the reduction of lateral Hoffa fracture fragments.

D. Mechanism of injury

1. Fractures involving the supracondylar femur often result from the same high-energy mechanisms seen in fractures of the femoral shaft.

2. Low-energy mechanisms, such as minor falls, are common in the older population.

E. Clinical evaluation

1. Consider the mechanism of injury: in high-energy mechanisms, a full trauma evaluation should be completed.

2. The patient usually presents with pain, swelling, and deformity in the distal femur region.

3. Neurovascular structures lie close to these fractures, so the neurovascular status should be assessed thoroughly.

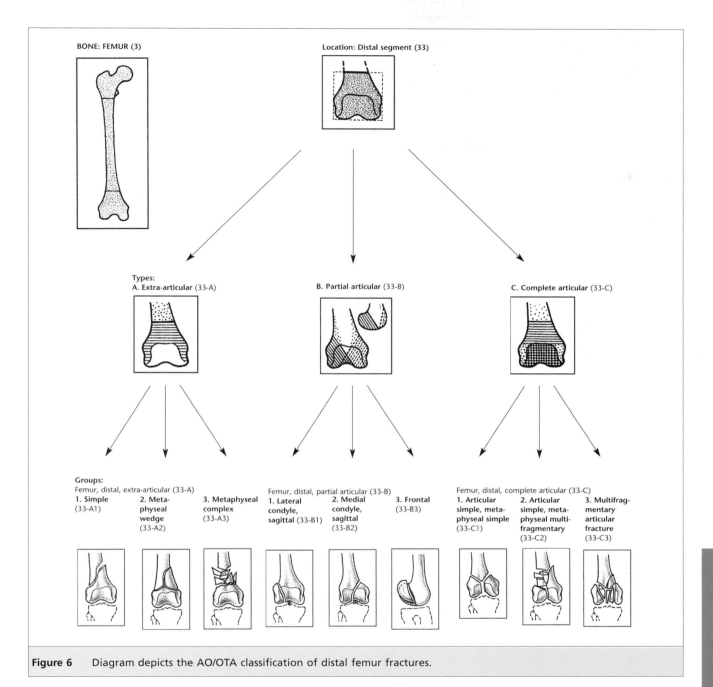

Figure 6 Diagram depicts the AO/OTA classification of distal femur fractures.

4. The skin should be examined closely for open wounds.

5. In the elderly patient, preexisting medical conditions and degenerative knee joint disease should be considered.

F. Radiographic evaluation

1. AP and lateral radiographs of the distal femur are standard.

2. Radiographic evaluation of the ipsilateral lower extremity should be considered because of the risk of associated injuries.

3. Oblique views may help provide further details regarding the intercondylar anatomy; however, CT scanning often eliminates the need for these additional radiographs.

4. Traction radiographs are helpful but may be too uncomfortable for the patient.

5. Contralateral views may help with preoperative planning and templating.

6. CT provides details about intra-articular involvement and can identify coronal plane deformities with reconstruction views.

3:Trauma

G. Classification—The AO/OTA classification is the universally accepted system for characterizing injuries of the distal femur (**Figure 6**).

1. Type A fractures are extra-articular injuries.

2. Type B fractures are partially articular and involve a single condyle.

3. Type C fractures are intercondylar or bicondylar intra-articular injuries with varying degrees of comminution.

H. Nonsurgical treatment—Nonsurgical treatment is indicated for nondisplaced distal femur fractures only. Nonsurgical treatment of displaced supracondylar and intercondylar femur fractures generally is associated with poor results and should be reserved for patients who represent an unacceptable surgical risk.

I. Surgical treatment

1. The goal of surgical treatment should be stable fixation to permit early mobility.

2. The trend in periarticular fracture treatment has changed recently from large, extensile approaches, subperiosteal dissection, circumferential clamps, absolute stability with compression by lag screws and using short plates with multiple screws to the concept of biologic reduction techniques that emphasize limited lateral exposures and the preservation of the soft-tissue attachments.

3. The locking plate has become quite popular. Multiple manufacturers offer locking plate systems.

   a. The main advantages of the newer plating systems are the ability to place the implant percutaneously, less periosteal stripping, and the application of a plate laterally without the need for additional medial plate stabilization.

   b. The locked nature of the screws in the femoral condyles allows the placement of multiple "internal external fixators" that have been shown to be axially superior to earlier fixation techniques. The improved axial strength of the newer implants should not instill a false sense of security, however.

   c. Another advantage of the newer design plates is the submuscular advancement of the plate to the bone, which minimizes periosteal stripping and preserves the blood supply. The implants do not rely on direct contact of the plate to the bone for stability. This concept is called relative stability, and longer plates and fewer screws are used.

   d. If using a long percutaneous plate, proximal visualization of plate placement may be difficult. The surgeon should consider making an incision to ensure proper placement proxi-

Table 1

Possible Implants for Distal Femur Fractures as Determined by the AO/OTA Classification System

Type A or C1/C2 Fractures
Dynamic condylar screw
95° blade plate
Antegrade femoral nail
Retrograde femoral nail
Locked internal fixator (lateral plate with locked distal screws)
Type B Fractures
Screw and/or plate fixation
Type C3 Fractures
Standard condylar buttress plate
Locked internal fixator (lateral plate with locked distal screws)

Reproduced from Kregor PJ, Morgan SJ: Fractures of the distal femur, in Baumgaertner MR, Tornetta P III, eds: *Orthopaedic Knowledge Update: Trauma*, ed 3. Rosemont, IL, American Academy of Orthopaedic Surgeons, 2005, pp 397-408.

mally on the femur.

   e. A concern with locking plates is that the construct is too stiff to allow healing. Recent studies discuss multiple screw options to decrease plate stiffness, with mostly nonlocking screws in the shaft position. Another screw option discussed is the far cortical locking screw. More research is needed on this topic.

J. Surgical technique

1. The patient should be positioned supine on a radiolucent table.

2. Open fractures should be treated in accordance with open fracture treatment principles. Temporizing knee-spanning external fixators should be used until the soft tissue permits the placement of internal fixators.

3. Once the soft tissues have been stabilized, the surgical approach and fixation tactic are dictated by the degree of articular comminution (**Table 1**).

   a. Type A fractures

   • Plate fixation is a viable option and is associated with good results.

   • Traditional plating options include a dynamic condylar screw, a 95° blade plate, or a locking plate. A dynamic condylar screw or blade plating requires using a more invasive incision for direct reduction techniques.

- Locked plating can be performed via a minimally invasive lateral approach to the distal femur, exposing only the portion of the distal lateral condyle necessary to facilitate placement of the implant.

b. Type B fractures

- Lag screw fixation

- Plate fixation

c. Type C fractures

- Open reduction and internal fixation with plates

- An anatomic articular reduction is critical for a good result.

K. IM nails

1. Retrograde IM nailing is a viable option for distal femur fractures not involving the articular surface.

2. When retrograde IM nailing of a distal femur fracture with extension into the articular surface is attempted, the articular surface should be stabilized with Kirschner wires and/or screws before nail placement.

3. Few indications exist for a short retrograde nail; any retrograde nails should be inserted proximally at least to the level of the lesser trochanter.

L. External fixation—Bridging external fixation may be advantageous as a temporizing measure in open fractures or in fractures with substantial comminution or soft-tissue compromise. When using bridging external fixation, the external fixator pins should be placed away from the planned plate.

M. Associated vascular injury

1. The neurovascular status should be evaluated carefully because of the proximity of vascular structures to these fractures.

2. If the fracture is associated with a knee dislocation, angiography may be considered because the risk of vascular injury is substantially greater with associated dislocation.

N. Supracondylar fracture after TKA

1. It is important to evaluate the stability of the prosthesis. If it is stable, then fixation strategy can be planned.

2. Locking plate

a. The locking plate is the fixation device of choice for very distal fractures in osteopenic bone.

b. The literature supports good results for locking plate fixation of periprosthetic fractures proximal to a TKA.

3. Retrograde nailing represents an alternative treatment option. Before proceeding with this treatment, it is important to learn the details of the TKA to assess if it will permit retrograde nail placement through the femoral prosthesis.

O. Rehabilitation

1. Postoperative treatment should include the administration of intravenous antibiotics for 24 hours following closure of all wounds and the routine use of mechanical and chemical prophylaxis for DVT.

2. Patients are assisted out of bed on the first postoperative day and should not bear weight on the affected limb when using ambulatory assistive devices.

3. Active-assisted range-of-motion exercises should be initiated in the early postoperative period. Early range-of-motion exercises are critical because functionally poor results most often are attributed to knee stiffness, and little improvement is gained after 1 year.

P. Complications

1. The metaphyseal location and preponderance of cancellous bone in these fractures can lead to significant comminution, even with low-energy injury mechanisms. Therefore, it is of paramount importance to pay meticulous attention to preoperative planning, with full consideration of all patient factors, including the condition of the soft tissues, concomitant injuries, comorbidities, and the functional level before injury.

2. Nonunions

a. The rate of nonunion has decreased with the use of more biologically friendly techniques such as minimally invasive plate application.

b. Nonunions should be treated with bone grafting and/or implant revision with plate compression or lag screw placement when possible.

3. Infection

a. Infection rates have decreased with the use of soft-tissue–friendly techniques.

b. Infection should be managed with thorough débridement, cultures, and appropriate antibiotics; removing the hardware should be considered if the fracture permits.

Top Testing Facts

Femoral Shaft Fractures

1. Fractures may occur in the proximal femur from relatively low mechanisms of injury in patients who have been on bisphosphonates for extended periods.

2. Bilateral femur fractures have a mortality rate of less than 7% with modern techniques.

3. The patient with a femur fracture should always be closely evaluated for associated injuries.

4. Early stabilization (within the first 24 hours) of femur fractures minimizes the complication rates and can reduce the hospital length of stay.

5. The type of nail used (antegrade, trochanteric, retrograde) should be based on surgeon preference and the fracture pattern.

6. A statically locked, reamed IM nail is the standard of care for femoral shaft fractures.

7. A bump or radiographic triangle strategically placed under the deformity may assist with reduction.

8. Before the patient wakes up, AP pelvic radiographic imaging should be performed to rule out a femoral neck fracture. Limb rotation and length should be evaluated, and the knee should be checked for ligamentous injuries.

9. No increased rate of infection is seen with retrograde nailing of open femur fractures.

10. The infection rate for open femur fractures is significantly lower than that of open tibia fractures.

11. Atypical femur fractures from bisphosphonate use tend to be simple transverse or oblique fractures with cortical thickening around the fracture site and cortical beaking.

Distal Femur Fractures

1. The origin of the gastrocnemius characteristically pulls the distal fragment into extension.

2. The patient must be closely evaluated preoperatively for a coronal plane Hoffa fracture.

3. The goal of surgical treatment should be stable fixation to permit early mobility.

4. A concern with locking plates is the construct being too stiff to allow healing. Recent studies discuss multiple screw options to decrease the plate stiffness, with mostly nonlocking screws in the shaft portion.

5. If using a long percutaneous plate, proximal visualization of the plate placement on the femur may be difficult. An incision should be made to ensure proper placement proximally on the femur.

6. When using a bridging external fixator, the external fixator pins should be placed away from the planned plate location.

7. Plate fixation provides good results for distal periprosthetic supracondylar femur fractures.

Bibliography

Black DM, Kelly MP, Genant HK, et al: Bisphosphonates and fractures of the subtrochanteric or diaphyseal femur. *N Engl J Med* 2010;362(19):1761-1771.

Bottlang M, Lesser M, Koerber J, et al: Far cortical locking can improve healing of fractures stabilized with locking plates. *J Bone Joint Surg Am* 2010;92(7):1652-1660.

Brumback RJ, Uwagie-Ero S, Lakatos RP, Poka A, Bathon GH, Burgess AR: Intramedullary nailing of femoral shaft fractures: Part II. Fracture-healing with static interlocking fixation. *J Bone Joint Surg Am* 1988;70(10):1453-1462.

Cannada LK, Taghizadeh S, Murali J, Obremskey WT, De-Cook C, Bosse MJ: Retrograde intramedullary nailing in treatment of bilateral femur fractures. *J Orthop Trauma* 2008;22(8):530-534.

Cannada LK, Viehe T, Cates CA, et al: A retrospective review of high-energy femoral neck-shaft fractures. *J Orthop Trauma* 2009;23(4):254-260.

Harwood PJ, Giannoudis PV, van Griensven M, Krettek C, Pape HC: Alterations in the systemic inflammatory response after early total care and damage control procedures for femoral shaft fracture in severely injured patients. *J Trauma* 2005;58(3):446-454.

Jaarsma RL, Pakvis DF, Verdonschot N, Biert J, van Kampen A: Rotational malalignment after intramedullary nailing of femoral fractures. *J Orthop Trauma* 2004;18(7):403-409.

Mamczak CN, Gardner MJ, Bolhofner B, Borrelli J Jr, Streubel PN, Ricci WM: Interprosthetic femoral fractures. *J Orthop Trauma* 2010;24(12):740-744.

Nork SE, Agel J, Russell GV, Mills WJ, Holt S, Routt ML Jr: Mortality after reamed intramedullary nailing of bilateral femur fractures. *Clin Orthop Relat Res* 2003;415:272-278.

Ostrum RF, Agarwal A, Lakatos R, Poka A: Prospective comparison of retrograde and antegrade femoral intramedullary nailing. *J Orthop Trauma* 2000;14(7):496-501.

O'Toole RV, Riche K, Cannada LK, et al: Analysis of postoperative knee sepsis after retrograde nail insertion of open femoral shaft fractures. *J Orthop Trauma* 2010;24(11):677-682.

Ricci WM, Bellabarba C, Evanoff B, Herscovici D, Di-Pasquale T, Sanders R: Retrograde versus antegrade nailing of femoral shaft fractures. *J Orthop Trauma* 2001;15(3): 161-169.

Tornetta P III, Kain MS, Creevy WR: Diagnosis of femoral neck fractures in patients with a femoral shaft fracture: Improvement with a standard protocol. *J Bone Joint Surg Am* 2007;89(1):39-43.

Watson JT, Moed BR: Ipsilateral femoral neck and shaft fractures: Complications and their treatment. *Clin Orthop Relat Res* 2002;399:78-86.

Weil YA, Rivkin G, Safran O, Liebergall M, Foldes AJ: The outcome of surgically treated femur fractures associated with long-term bisphosphonate use. *J Trauma* 2011;71(1): 186-190.

3: Trauma

Chapter 40

Knee Dislocations and Patellar Fractures

John T. Riehl, MD   Joshua Langford, MD   Kenneth J. Koval, MD

I. Knee Dislocations

A. Epidemiology

1. Knee dislocations represent less than 0.2% of all orthopaedic injuries.

2. The incidence reported in the literature is likely underrepresentative of the true incidence because 20% to 50% of knee dislocations spontaneously reduce in the field.

B. Anatomy

1. The stability of the knee joint is provided by bony articulations as well as dynamic and static soft-tissue stabilizers (**Table 1**).

2. The four major ligamentous stabilizers of the knee are the anterior cruciate ligament (ACL), the posterior cruciate ligament (PCL), the medial collateral ligament (MCL), and the lateral collateral ligament (LCL).

3. The posterolateral corner (PLC) and posteromedial corner (PMC) as well as the medial and lateral menisci confer additional stability to the knee.

4. The PLC is made up of the LCL, the iliotibial band, the popliteofibular ligament, and the popliteus tendon.

5. The relatively high incidence of neurovascular compromise in knee dislocation is explained by the anatomy of the knee (**Figure 1**).

   a. The popliteal artery travels through the adductor hiatus, where it is relatively immobile, and distally through the fibrous arch deep to the soleus muscle.

   b. The common peroneal nerve travels along the inferior edge of the biceps femoris and continues distally around the fibular head. The tibial nerve branches at a variable level but courses down the middle of the popliteal fossa. This makes the peroneal nerve more immobile and therefore more susceptible to injury.

C. Mechanism of injury

1. High-energy injuries include those from motor vehicle collisions, falls from a height, and industrial accidents.

Dr. Langford or an immediate family member serves as a paid consultant to or is an employee of Stryker and International Fixation Systems and has stock or stock options held in Internal Fixation Systems and the Institute for Better Bone Health. Dr. Koval or an immediate family member has received royalties from Biomet; is a member of a speakers' bureau or has made paid presentations on behalf of Biomet and Stryker; serves as a paid consultant to or is an employee of Biomet; and serves as a board member, owner, officer, or committee member of the American Academy of Orthopaedic Surgeons and the Orthopaedic Trauma Association. Neither Dr. Riehl nor any immediate family member has received anything of value from or owns stock in a commercial company or institution related directly or indirectly to the subject of this chapter.

Table 1

Soft-Tissue Stabilizers of the Knee

Structure	Function
ACL	Primary: Resists anterior translation of the tibia relative to the femur Secondary: Resists varus/valgus stresses in full extension
PCL	Primary: Resists posterior translation of the tibia relative to the femur Secondary: Resists tibial external rotation
MCL	Resists valgus stress
PMC	Resists valgus stress
LCL	Resists varus stress
PLC	Resists posterior translation, external rotation, and varus angulation of the tibia

ACL = anterior cruciate ligament, LCL = lateral collateral ligament, MCL = medial collateral ligament, PCL = posterior cruciate ligament, PLC = posterolateral corner, PMC = posteromedial corner.

3: Trauma

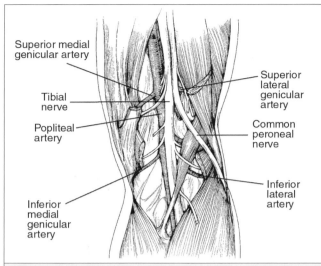

Figure 1 Illustration shows the posterior anatomy of the knee. Note the relationship between the popliteal artery and the tibial and common peroneal nerves. (Reproduced from Good L, Johnson RJ: The dislocated knee. *J Am Acad Orthop Surg* 1995;3:284-292.)

2. Low-energy injuries include sports-related injuries, often with a rotatory component.

3. Ultra-low–energy injuries include those from seemingly trivial trauma in morbidly obese patients.

D. Clinical evaluation

1. In high-energy mechanisms, other life-threatening injuries can be present. Evaluation should follow ATLS (Advanced Trauma Life Support) protocols.

2. Knee dislocation should be suspected in patients with uncontained hemarthrosis about the knee, contusions, and gross laxity. Additionally, any patient with two or more ligamentous injuries or with certain fractures about the knee should be evaluated for a suspected knee dislocation.

3. A thorough neurovascular examination is of the utmost importance. Pulses are assessed for symmetry and, when symmetric, should be accompanied by the ankle-brachial index (ABI) test. If these tests are normal, serial and frequent neurovascular examinations should follow. Neurovascular examination should be performed both prereduction and postreduction when possible.

4. Ligamentous examination should proceed in a systematic fashion to identify disrupted and intact structures. **Table 2** lists the soft-tissue stabilizers of the knee, their function, and the corresponding tests. The soft-tissue stabilizers of the knee and the test results that indicate disruption are listed below.

Table 2

Soft-Tissue Stabilizers of the Knee and Clinical Tests for Stability

Structure	Test
ACL	Lachman: With the knee flexed 20°, the examiner translates the tibia anteriorly.
PCL	Posterior drawer test: With the knee flexed 90°, the examiner translates the tibia posteriorly.
MCL	Valgus stress test: With the knee flexed 30°, the examiner applies valgus stress.
PMC	Posteromedial drawer test: With the knee at 0° and 30° of flexion, the examiner applies valgus stress.
LCL	Varus stress test: With the knee flexed 30°, the examiner applies varus stress.
PLC	Posterolateral drawer test: With the knee flexed 90° and in 15° of external rotation and with the foot flat on table, the examiner applies posterior force to knee. Varus stress at 0° and 30°: With the knee at 0° and 30°, the examiner applies varus stress at respective positions. Dial test: With the knees flexed 30°, the tibias are bilaterally externally rotated; increased rotation of 10° to 15° from affected side indicates PLC injury. Increased tibial external rotation at both 30° and 90° of flexion indicates combined PLC/PCL injury.

ACL = anterior cruciate ligament, LCL = lateral collateral ligament, MCL = medial collateral ligament, PCL = posterior cruciate ligament, PLC = posterolateral corner, PMC = posteromedial corner.

a. ACL: Positive Lachman test

b. PCL: Positive posterior drawer test

c. MCL: Valgus laxity at 30° of knee flexion

d. PMC: Positive posteromedial drawer test

e. LCL: Varus laxity at 30° of knee flexion

f. PLC: Positive posterolateral drawer test

g. Differentiating PLC injuries from combined PLC/PCL injuries: Positive dial test (increased tibial external rotation at 30° of flexion indicates PLC injury; increased tibial external rotation at 30° and 90° of flexion indicates combined PLC/PCL injury)

h. Collateral ligament, one or more cruciate ligaments, and capsular injury: Varus/valgus laxity at full knee extension

i. PCL, PMC, PLC, and posterior capsule: Positive supine heel-lift test

E. Associated injuries

1. Vascular injury

2. Neurologic injury

   a. Neurapraxia (stretch)

   b. Axonotmesis (axonal disruption, endoneurium intact)

   c. Neurotmesis (complete transection)

3. Chondral and meniscal injuries

4. Capsular injury

   a. Prevents immediate arthroscopic reconstruction

   b. May result in severe swelling

5. Compartment syndrome

6. Fracture

F. Vascular injury

1. Incidence in the literature ranges from 16% to 64%.

2. Hard signs of vascular injury (asymmetric pulses postreduction, active bleeding, expanding hematoma) warrant immediate vascular surgery consultation.

3. Injury range: transection, contusion, intimal tear, thrombus formation. Initial physical examination may be normal in the presence of an intimal flap tear, but such tears can progress to complete arterial occlusion.

4. Prolonged warm ischemia time is a major risk factor for amputation.

5. Vascular injury can present in a delayed fashion.

6. Angiography is unnecessary when physical examination and ABIs are normal (> 0.8).

7. In cases of obvious vascular injury and limb-threatening ischemia, immediate vascular surgical intervention is necessary. If angiography is to be performed, the operating room is the most appropriate setting.

8. The main indication for angiography is clinical signs of vascular injury without limb-threatening ischemia.

9. Vascular reconstruction often consists of a reverse saphenous vein graft.

10. With a warm ischemia time longer than 6 hours, prophylactic fasciotomies should be performed.

G. Neurologic injury

1. Incidence ranges from 10% to 42%.

2. Common peroneal nerve injury occurs more often than tibial nerve injury; it is commonly associated with posterolateral dislocations.

3. If the peroneal nerve recovers, improvement usually begins by 3 months from injury and is accompanied by a positive Tinel sign.

4. Observation is the treatment of choice for all incomplete peroneal nerve palsies.

5. If electromyographic (EMG) testing is to be performed, a baseline study can be obtained at approximately 4 to 6 weeks from injury; EMG testing can be repeated at 3 months.

6. Tibialis posterior transfer can be performed as a late reconstructive procedure to restore active dorsiflexion.

H. Imaging

1. AP and lateral radiographs should be obtained in all cases of suspected knee dislocation. If this can be accomplished without significant delay, the radiographs should be obtained both before and after any reduction attempt.

2. MRI is used to evaluate ligamentous, capsular, meniscal, cartilaginous, and other soft-tissue lesions, helping to guide surgical treatment. It should be obtained as soon as logistically and safely possible.

3. Magnetic resonance angiography has been suggested by some authors as an alternative to traditional angiography in the acute setting. Likewise, CT angiography, because of its speed and accuracy, has been adopted by many centers for use in the acute evaluation of knee dislocations.

I. Classification—Knee dislocation is most commonly classified by the direction of displacement of the tibia relative to the distal femur.

1. Anterior dislocation, the most common type, results from a hyperextension injury. It is commonly associated with intimal tears in the popliteal artery.

2. Posterior dislocation results from a posterior force on the proximal tibia (eg, dashboard injury). It can result in popliteal artery transection and extensor mechanism disruption.

3. Lateral, medial, and rotatory dislocations also can occur.

4. This classification system does not account for associated injuries or spontaneously reduced dislocations.

J. Closed reduction

1. Closed reduction is performed following neurovascular assessment and evaluation of plain radiographs.

2. The reduction maneuver is axial limb traction with translation of the tibia in the appropriate direction.

3: Trauma

3. For posterolateral dislocations where the medial femoral condyle has "buttonholed" through the medial capsule (the dimple sign), it is recommended to avoid attempts at closed reduction because it is associated with a high rate of skin necrosis. Emergent open reduction in the operating room is indicated in this circumstance.

4. Following reduction, a knee immobilizer or splint is placed. If the reduction cannot be maintained in a splint, external fixation is indicated, especially in obese patients.

K. Surgical treatment

1. Surgery is indicated in the acute setting in a physically active patient without medical comorbidities that prohibit surgery. In the chronic setting, surgical treatment is indicated for knee instability without significant arthrosis.

2. Treatment of associated PLC and PMC injuries is imperative to obtain good long-term results with ACL/PCL reconstructions.

3. Timing and materials for ligamentous reconstruction vary according to surgeon preference.

L. Nonsurgical treatment is indicated in patients unable to tolerate a surgical procedure and in less active patients.

M. Postoperative rehabilitation

1. The patient should be non–weight bearing for 6 weeks, with the knee braced in full extension.

2. Progressive range of motion in the brace and weight bearing begin at 6 weeks. Closed chain exercises also begin at this point.

3. At 10 weeks, the brace can be discontinued.

4. Return to unrestricted activity (sports, heavy labor) usually takes 9 months.

N. Complications

1. Stiffness

a. May be caused by heterotopic ossification about the capsule

b. The last few degrees of terminal extension and 10° to 15° of terminal flexion are commonly lost.

c. If the stiffness is severely limiting, manipulation under anesthesia or surgical lysis of the adhesions may be indicated. If stiffness is caused by heterotopic bone, resection may be performed.

2. Residual instability (often related to failure to recognize and treat all components of the initial injury)

3. Medial femoral condyle osteonecrosis

4. Sensory and motor disturbances

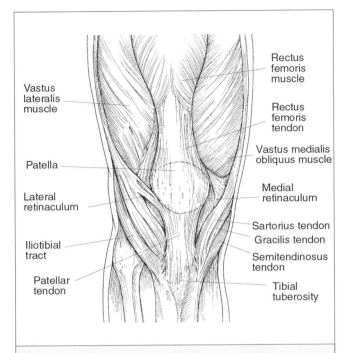

Figure 2   Illustration shows the anatomy of the extensor mechanism of the knee. (Reproduced from Matava MJ: Patellar tendon ruptures. *J Am Acad Orthop Surg* 1996;4:287-296.)

5. Iatrogenic neurovascular injury or tibial plateau fracture

II. Patellar Fractures

A. Epidemiology

1. Fractures of the patella most commonly occur in persons age 20 to 50 years.

2. The male-to-female ratio is 2:1.

3. Patellar fractures make up 1% of all skeletal injuries.

B. Anatomy (**Figure 2**)

1. The patella is the largest sesamoid bone in the body.

2. The subcutaneous location of the patella and the large joint reactive forces that it is subjected to make it prone to injury.

3. The patella has seven facets; the inferior pole is termed the apex.

4. The proximal portion of the patella is covered with the thickest articular cartilage in the body. The distal pole is devoid of articular cartilage.

5. Bipartite patella most commonly involves the superolateral portion.

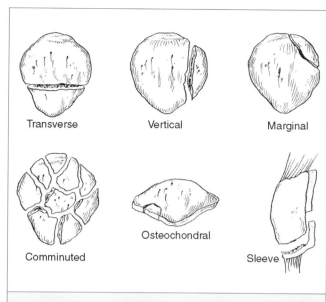

Transverse   Vertical   Marginal

Comminuted   Osteochondral   Sleeve

Figure 3   Illustrations demonstrate the classification of patellar fractures based on the configuration of fracture lines. (Reproduced from Cramer KE, Moed BR: Patellar fractures: Contemporary approach to treatment. *J Am Acad Orthop Surg* 1997;5:323-331.)

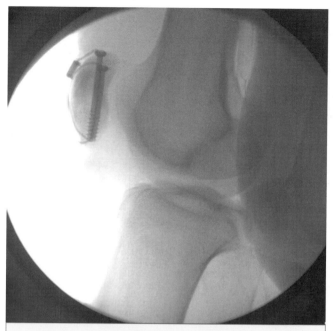

Figure 4   Lateral fluoroscopic image shows a displaced patellar fracture treated with cannulated screws and cable tension wire.

6. The patella increases the power of the extensor mechanism by 50% by anteriorly displacing the extensor mechanism away from the knee center of rotation (increased moment arm).

7. Its blood supply arises from the geniculate arteries.

C. Mechanism of injury

1. Direct blow (for example, from a fall)—Results in a simple or comminuted fracture pattern.

2. Indirect (more common)—Results from eccentric contraction; typically causes a transverse fracture pattern.

D. Clinical evaluation

1. The soft tissues should be inspected carefully for lacerations, abrasions, and ecchymosis.

2. Extensor lag and the ability to perform a straight leg raise should be evaluated.

3. The examiner should palpate for an extensor mechanism defect.

4. If pain limits the evaluation, intra-articular injection of local anesthetic can enable better assessment.

E. Radiographic evaluation

1. AP and lateral radiographs should be obtained. Oblique views also can be beneficial. A lateral view helps evaluate articular step-off; it should be obtained with the knee in 30° of flexion.

2. Bipartite patella can be differentiated from fracture by smooth, regular borders. Bipartite patella is often bilateral and involves the superolateral portion.

F. Fracture classification—Based on the fracture pattern, patellar fractures typically are classified as transverse, vertical, stellate (or comminuted), osteochondral, sleeve, or marginal (**Figure 3**).

G. Treatment

1. Anatomic reduction of the articular surface is paramount. Reduction may be assessed with palpation through retinacular defects, surgical arthrotomy, or fluoroscopy.

2. Indications for surgical treatment include open fractures, extensor mechanism dysfunction, articular step-off of 2 mm, and articular gap of 3 mm.

3. When nonsurgical treatment is chosen, the knee is kept in nearly full extension for 4 to 6 weeks. Isometric quadriceps exercises and straight leg raises are begun 1 week after injury.

4. Fixation construct options

a. Two longitudinal Kirschner wires with 18-gauge stainless steel wires in a figure-of-8 fashion; a second wire may be placed around the patella in a cerclage configuration.

b. Parallel cannulated screws with stainless steel wire in a figure-of-8 configuration. Screw tips must not extend beyond the edge of the patella.

3: Trauma

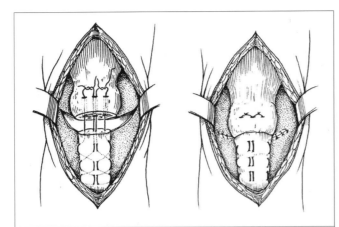

Figure 5   Illustrations demonstrate partial patellectomy. The ligament is sutured to the remaining patellar fragment. (Adapted from Cramer KE, Moed BR: Patellar fractures: Contemporary approach to treatment. *J Am Acad Orthop Surg* 1997; 5:323-331.)

   c. Wires or screws with braided cable tension wire in a figure-of-8 configuration (**Figure 4**)

   d. Minifragment screws/plates may be necessary in certain fracture types or in revision cases.

   e. Suture and biodegradable implants have been shown to be successful in some clinical series.

  5. In cases of severe comminution, fixation may not be possible. It is important to save as much of the patella as is reasonably possible. Partial patellectomy is performed, with reattachment of the patellar or quadriceps tendon to the remaining fragment, along with retinacular repair (**Figure 5**).

   a. Indication for partial patellectomy: A large, salvageable fragment in the presence of smaller comminuted polar fragments that are unreconstructible

   b. The tendon should be reattached close to the articular surface to prevent patellar tilt.

  6. In some cases, total patellectomy is necessary. In one clinical series of total patellectomies, advancement of the vastus medialis obliquus was shown to improve outcomes.

  7. Postoperative care includes splint immobilization in extension for 4 to 6 weeks. Weight bearing in full extension is allowed immediately.

H. Complications

  1. Painful implants (in some series, >50%) are the most likely reason for a return to the operating room.

  2. Decreased ROM (especially terminal knee flexion)

  3. Infection (3% to 10%)

  4. Loss of reduction (0% to 20%); more common in osteoporotic bone

  5. Posttraumatic osteoarthritis (50%)

  6. Osteonecrosis

  7. Nonunion (1% to 3%)

Acknowledgment

The authors would like to thank Dr. Stanley J. Kupiszewski for his contributions to this chapter.

Top Testing Facts

1. The popliteal artery travels through the adductor hiatus, where it is relatively immobile, and distally through the fibrous arch, deep to the soleus muscle.

2. The common peroneal nerve travels along the inferior edge of the biceps femoris and continues distally around the fibular head. The tibial nerve branches at a variable level but courses down the middle of the popliteal fossa. This makes the peroneal nerve more immobile and therefore more susceptible to injury.

3. Vascular status is of paramount importance in the setting of documented or suspected knee dislocation.

4. The incidence of vascular injury may be as high as 64%; it can present in a delayed fashion.

5. When warm ischemia time is longer than 6 hours, prophylactic fasciotomies should be performed.

6. Bipartite patella most commonly involves the superolateral portion and demonstrates smooth, regular borders on radiographs.

7. The patella increases the power of the extensor mechanism by 50%.

8. Indications for surgical treatment of patellar fractures include open fractures, extensor mechanism dysfunction, articular step-off of 2 mm, and articular gap of 3 mm.

9. In cases of severe comminution, fixation may not be possible. It is important to save as much of the patella as is reasonably possible. Partial patellectomy is performed, with reattachment of the patellar or quadriceps tendon to the remaining fragment, along with retinacular repair.

10. Painful implants are the most likely reason for a return to the operating room after surgical fixation of patellar fractures.

Bibliography

Brautigan B, Johnson DL: The epidemiology of knee dislocations. *Clin Sports Med* 2000;19(3):387-397.

Cramer KE, Moed BR: Patellar fractures: Contemporary approach to treatment. *J Am Acad Orthop Surg* 1997;5(6):323-331.

Fanelli GC, Harris JD, Tomaszewski DJ, Riehl JT, Edson CJ, Reinheimer KN: Multiple ligament knee injuries, in DeLee JC, Drez D Jr, Miller MD, eds: *DeLee & Drez's Orthopaedic Sports Medicine: Principles and Practice*, ed 3. Philadelphia, PA, Saunders, 2009, pp 1747-1765.

Günal I, Taymaz A, Köse N, Göktürk E, Seber S: Patellectomy with vastus medialis obliquus advancement for comminuted patellar fractures: A prospective randomised trial. *J Bone Joint Surg Br* 1997;79(1):13-16.

Hill JA, Rana NA: Complications of posterolateral dislocation of the knee: Case report and literature review. *Clin Orthop Relat Res* 1981;154:212-215.

LeBrun CT, Langford JR, Sagi HC: Functional outcomes after operatively treated patella fractures. *J Orthop Trauma* 2012;26(7):422-426.

Levy BA, Fanelli GC, Whelan DB, et al: Controversies in the treatment of knee dislocations and multiligament reconstruction. *J Am Acad Orthop Surg* 2009;17(4):197-206.

McDonough EB Jr, Wojtys EM: Multiligamentous injuries of the knee and associated vascular injuries. *Am J Sports Med* 2009;37(1):156-159.

Melvin JS, Mehta S: Patellar fractures in adults. *J Am Acad Orthop Surg* 2011;19(4):198-207.

Potter HG, Weinstein M, Allen AA, Wickiewicz TL, Helfet DL: Magnetic resonance imaging of the multiple-ligament injured knee. *J Orthop Trauma* 2002;16(5):330-339.

Scilaris TA, Grantham JL, Prayson MJ, Marshall MP, Hamilton JJ, Williams JL: Biomechanical comparison of fixation methods in transverse patella fractures. *J Orthop Trauma* 1998;12(5):356-359.

Seroyer ST, Musahl V, Harner CD: Management of the acute knee dislocation: The Pittsburgh experience. *Injury* 2008;39(7):710-718.

Smith ST, Cramer KE, Karges DE, Watson JT, Moed BR: Early complications in the operative treatment of patella fractures. *J Orthop Trauma* 1997;11(3):183-187.

Stannard JP, Sheils TM, Lopez-Ben RR, McGwin G Jr, Robinson JT, Volgas DA: Vascular injuries in knee dislocations: The role of physical examination in determining the need for arteriography. *J Bone Joint Surg Am* 2004;86(5):910-915.

Wascher DC, Dvirnak PC, DeCoster TA: Knee dislocation: Initial assessment and implications for treatment. *J Orthop Trauma* 1997;11(7):525-529.

3: Trauma

Chapter 41

Tibial Plateau and Tibial-Fibular Shaft Fractures

Erik N. Kubiak, MD   Kenneth A. Egol, MD

I. Tibial Plateau Fractures

A. Epidemiology

1. Historically, tibial plateau fractures were more common in young patients after high-energy trauma; now, a larger percentage results from a low-energy fall in older patients with osteoporotic bone (as a result of an aging active population).

2. Tibial plateau fractures account for approximately 2% of all fractures, with bimodal incidence in both men and women and a mean patient age of 48 years.

B. Anatomy (**Figure 1**)

1. Tibial plateau

a. The medial tibial plateau is larger than the lateral plateau and is concave in the sagittal and coronal planes. The lateral plateau is convex and extends higher than the medial plateau. Both articular surfaces are covered with hyaline cartilage.

b. Both plateaus are covered by a fibrocartilaginous meniscus. The coronary ligaments attach the menisci to the plateaus, and the intermeniscal ligament connects the menisci anteriorly.

2. Tibial spines are attachment points for the anterior cruciate ligament (ACL), the posterior cruciate ligament (PCL), and the menisci.

3. Tibial shaft

a. The tibial shaft is triangular in cross section.

b. Proximally, the tibial tubercle is located anterolaterally about 3 cm distal to the articular surface; it is the point of attachment for the patellar tendon.

c. Laterally on the proximal tibia is the Gerdy tubercle, which is the point of insertion for the iliotibial band. Medially is the pes anserinus, which is the point of insertion for the sartorius, gracilis, and semitendinosus muscles.

4. Soft-tissue structures

a. The medial (tibial) collateral ligament inserts into the medial proximal tibia.

b. The ACL and PCL provide anterior-posterior stability.

5. Neurovascular structures

a. The common peroneal nerve courses around the neck of the fibula distal to the proximal tibial-fibular joint before it divides into its superficial and deep branches.

b. The trifurcation of the popliteal artery into the anterior tibial, posterior tibial, and peroneal arteries occurs posteromedially at the level of the proximal tibia.

c. Vascular injuries to these structures are common following knee dislocation but also can occur in high-energy fractures of the proximal tibia.

6. Musculature

a. The anterior compartment musculature attaches to the proximal lateral tibia.

b. The proximal medial tibial surface is devoid of muscle coverage but serves as an attachment point for the pes tendons.

C. Mechanisms of injury

1. Tibial plateau fractures result from direct axial compression—usually with a valgus (more common) or varus (less common) moment—and indirect shear forces. Examples include the following:

Dr. Kubiak or an immediate family member serves as a paid consultant to or is an employee of Synthes, Tornier, Zimmer, DePuy, and Medtronic; and has received research or institutional support from Zimmer; and has received nonincome support (such as equipment or services), commercially derived honoraria, or other non–research-related funding (such as paid travel) from Biomet, Synthes, DePuy, and Zimmer. Dr. Egol or an immediate family member has received royalties from Exactech; has stock or stock options held in Johnson & Johnson; and has received research or institutional support from Stryker, Synthes, and the Orthopaedic Research and Education Foundation.

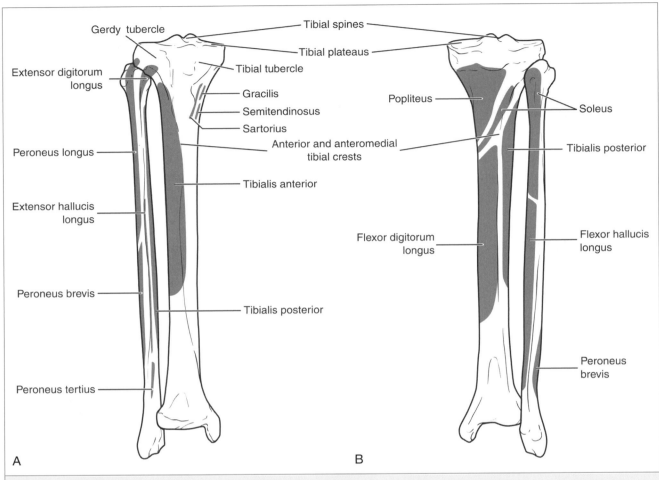

Gerdy tubercle
Tibial spines
Tibial plateaus
Extensor digitorum longus
Tibial tubercle
Gracilis
Popliteus
Semitendinosus
Soleus
Sartorius
Peroneus longus
Anterior and anteromedial tibial crests
Tibialis posterior
Tibialis anterior
Extensor hallucis longus
Flexor digitorum longus
Flexor hallucis longus
Peroneus brevis
Tibialis posterior
Peroneus tertius
Peroneus brevis

A

B

Figure 1   Illustrations show the anatomy of the tibia and fibula. Shaded areas indicate origins and insertions of the indicated muscles. **A,** Anterior view. **B,** Posterior view.

a. High-speed motor vehicle accidents

b. Falls from a height

c. Collisions between the bumper of a car and a pedestrian ("bumper injury")

2. The direction, magnitude, and location of the force as well as the position of the knee at impact determine the fracture pattern, location, and degree of displacement.

3. Associated injuries

a. Meniscal tears are associated with up to 50% of tibial plateau fractures.

b. Associated injury to the cruciate or collateral ligaments occurs in up to 30% of patients.

c. Skin compromise is frequently present in high-energy fracture patterns.

D. Clinical evaluation

1. Physical examination

a. The examiner should palpate over the site of potential fracture or ligamentous disruption to elicit tenderness.

b. Hemarthrosis typically is present; however, capsular disruption may result in extravasation into the surrounding soft-tissue envelope.

c. Any widening of the femoral-tibial articulation of more than 10° on stress examination, compared with the other leg, indicates instability.

2. Neurovascular examination

a. If pulses are not palpable, Doppler ultrasonographic studies should be performed.

b. The examiner should assess for signs and symptoms of an impending compartment syndrome (pain out of proportion to the injury, pain on passive stretch of the toes, pallor, pulselessness, or impaired neurologic status). Pallor, pulselessness, and/or impaired neurologic status are late signs of compartment syndrome; out-of-proportion pain is the most sensitive predictor.

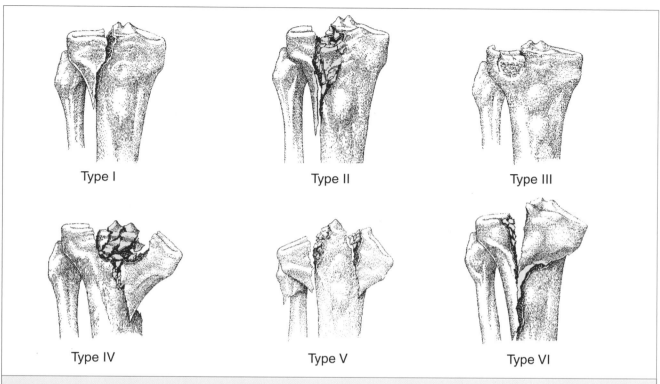

Type I   Type II   Type III

Type IV   Type V   Type VI

Figure 2   Illustrations depict the Schatzker classification of tibial plateau fractures. Type I: lateral plateau split; type II: lateral split-depression; type III: lateral depression; type IV: medial plateau fracture; type V: bicondylar injury; type VI: tibial plateau fracture with metaphyseal-diaphyseal dissociation. (Reproduced from Watson JT: Knee and leg: Bone trauma, in Beaty JH, ed: *Orthopaedic Knowledge Update*, ed 6. Rosemont, IL, American Academy of Orthopaedic Surgeons, 1999, p 523.)

c. Compartment pressures should be measured directly if the patient is unconscious and has a tense, swollen leg.

d. Ankle-brachial index (ABI) less than 0.9 requires consultation with a vascular surgeon.

3. Radiographic evaluation

a. Plain radiographs—Should include a trauma series (AP, lateral, and oblique views) and a plateau view (10° caudal tilt).

b. CT—Provides improved assessment of fracture pattern, aids in surgical planning, and improves the ability to classify fractures; CT should be ordered when better visualization of the bone fragments is required.

c. MRI—Used to evaluate ligamentous injury after fracture fixation when surgical intervention to repair or reconstruct the ligamentous injury is indicated.

E. Fracture classification

1. The Schatzker classification is used most commonly (**Figure 2**).

2. The Moore classification accounts for patterns

not described in the Schatzker classification (**Figure 3**).

3. The Orthopaedic Trauma Association (OTA) classification is the internationally accepted classification system (**Figure 4**).

F. Nonsurgical treatment

1. Nonsurgical treatment is indicated for nondisplaced and stable fractures

2. Patients are placed in a hinged fracture brace, and early range-of-motion exercises are initiated.

3. Partial weight bearing (30 to 50 lb) for 8 to 12 weeks is allowed, with progression to full weight bearing as tolerated thereafter.

G. Surgical treatment

1. Indications

a. If nonsurgical treatment fails to maintain the reduction, surgical treatment is indicated.

b. For closed fractures, the range of articular depression considered to be acceptable varies from 2 mm or less to 1 cm. Instability greater than 10° of the nearly extended knee compared with the contralateral side is an accepted

3: Trauma

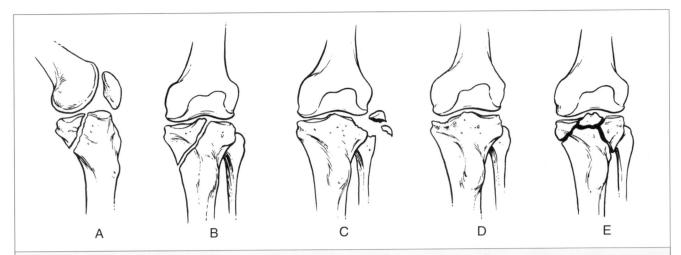

Figure 3 Illustrations show the Moore classification of tibial plateau fractures. **A,** Split fracture of the medial plateau in the coronal plane. **B,** Fracture of the entire condyle. **C,** Rim avulsion fracture. **D,** Pure compression fracture. **E,** Four-part fracture.

indication for surgical treatment of closed tibial plateau fractures.

   c. For open fractures, irrigation and débridement is required, with either temporary fixation or immediate open reduction and internal fixation. Regardless of approach, the knee joint should not be left open.

   d. If a delay in surgical intervention is expected, temporary spanning external fixation should be considered if the limb is shortened or the joint is subluxated.

2. Reduction techniques

   a. Indirect techniques have the advantage of minimal soft-tissue stripping and fragment devitalization. Centrally depressed articular fragments cannot be reduced indirectly by ligamentotaxis, however.

   b. With direct techniques, depressed articular fragments may be elevated through a cortical window placed inferiorly through a metaphyseal osteotomy.

   c. Arthroscopy can be used as a diagnostic tool to assess intra-articular structures in patients who sustain low-energy fractures; it also can be used as an adjunct to treatment by assessing the quality of fracture reduction.

3. Internal fixation techniques

   a. Most fracture patterns are treated with a lateral approach and buttress plating.

   b. A posteromedial approach is used to buttress posteromedial fragments. Splits in the medial plateau are reduced and secured. Consideration should also be given to repairing insertions of

the PCL and posterior horn of the lateral meniscus to the posterior tibia through the posterior medial approach by windowing the fracture open and working through the fracture.

   c. Screws alone can be used for simple split fractures that are anatomically reduced in young patients with healthy bone, for depression fractures that are elevated percutaneously, or for securing simple avulsion fractures.

   d. Plates may be placed percutaneously for fractures that extend to the metadiaphyseal region to secure the metaphysis to the diaphysis.

   e. The meniscus should be identified in all cases after a submeniscal arthrotomy is performed to visualize the articular surface and repair as indicated.

   f. Bone graft or calcium phosphate cement often is used to support metaphyseal defects; a lower incidence of articular subsidence is associated with the use of calcium phosphate cements than with autologous bone grafts.

4. External fixation techniques

   a. External fixation pins or wires should be placed 10 to 14 mm below the articular surface to avoid penetration of the synovial recess posteriorly.

   b. A circular frame is an alternative to a long percutaneous plate.

5. Bicondylar tibial plateau fractures

   a. Bicondylar fractures require dual-plate fixation or unilateral fixation with a locking plate. The use of a lateral locked plate is recommended only in the absence of medial comminution

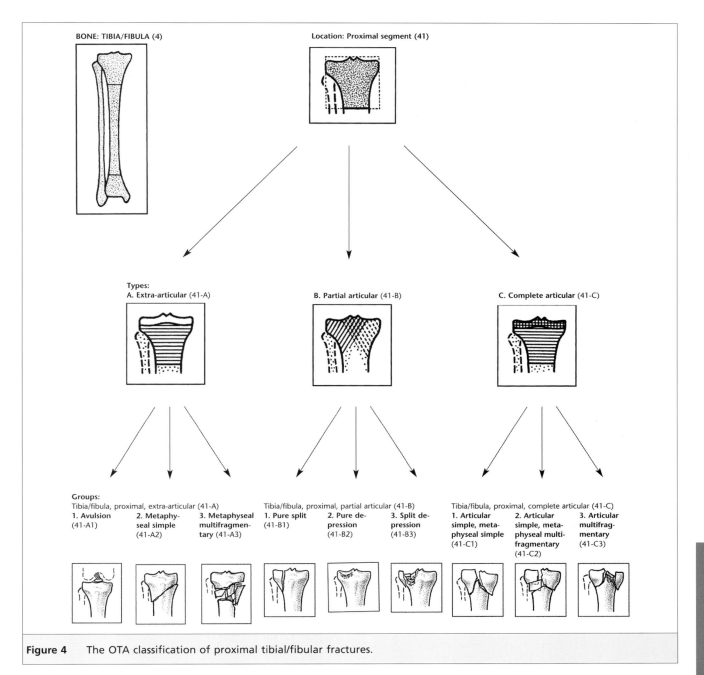

Figure 4   The OTA classification of proximal tibial/fibular fractures.

when the medial cortex is anatomically reduced.

b. An anterior midline incision should be avoided in bicondylar fractures because of the historically high rates of wound complications leading to the "dead bone sandwich" or high rates of wound complications.

H. Postoperative management

1. Continuous passive motion with a specific range of motion determined by the treating surgeon may be used. It can be initiated postoperatively and continued until the patient regains full range of knee motion.

2. Physical therapy should consist of active and active-assisted range-of-motion exercises, isometric quadriceps strengthening, and protected weight bearing.

3. Progressive weight bearing is generally initiated at 10 to 12 weeks postoperatively.

I. Complications

1. Early complications

a. Infection rates vary widely, from 1% to 38% of patients; superficial infections are more common (occurring in up to 38% of patients)

3: Trauma

than deep wound infections (occurring in up to 9.5%). Pin tract infections are common.

b. Deep vein thrombosis develops in up to 10% of patients; pulmonary embolism develops in 1% to 2%.

2. Late complications

a. Painful hardware is a late complication.

b. Posttraumatic arthrosis may be related to chondral damage that occurs at the time of the injury. At follow-up, articular incongruities appear to be well tolerated, whereas factors such as joint stability, coronal alignment, and retention of the meniscus may be more important in predicting arthrosis.

c. Nonunion is rare.

d. Loss of reduction, collapse, and/or malunion can occur if elevated fragments are not adequately buttressed.

II. Tibial-Fibular Shaft Fractures

A. Epidemiology

1. Most tibial shaft fractures result from low-energy mechanisms of injury. These fractures account for 4% of all fractures seen in the Medicare population. In younger patients, a high-energy injury such as a motor vehicle accident usually is the cause.

2. Isolated fibular shaft fractures are rare and usually are the result of a direct blow; they also can be associated with rotational ankle injuries (Maisonneuve fractures).

B. Anatomy

1. Bony structures

a. The anteromedial crest of the tibia is subcutaneous.

b. The proximal medullary canal is centered laterally.

c. The anterior tibial crest is composed of dense cortical bone.

d. The fibular shaft is palpable proximally and distally. The fibula is the site of the muscular attachment for the peroneal musculature and the flexor hallucis longus. It contributes little to load bearing (15%).

2. Musculature

a. The anterior compartment contains the tibialis anterior, extensor digitorum longus, the extensor hallucis longus, the anterior tibial artery, and the deep peroneal nerve.

b. The lateral compartment contains the peroneus longus and brevis and the superficial peroneal nerve.

c. The superficial posterior compartment contains the gastrocnemius-soleus complex, the soleus, the popliteus, and the plantaris muscles, as well as the sural nerve and saphenous vein.

d. The deep posterior compartment contains the tibialis posterior, the flexor digitorum longus, the flexor hallucis longus, the tibial artery, the peroneal artery, and the posterior tibial nerve.

C. Mechanism of injury

1. Tibial-fibular shaft fractures result from a torsional (indirect) or bending (direct) mechanism.

2. Indirect mechanisms result in spiral fractures.

3. Direct mechanisms result in wedge or short oblique fractures (low energy) or increased comminution (higher energy).

4. Associated injuries include open wounds, compartment syndrome, ipsilateral skeletal injury (that is, extension to the tibial plateau or plafond), and remote skeletal injury.

D. Clinical evaluation

1. Physical examination

a. The examiner should inspect the limb for gross deformity, angulation, and malrotation.

b. Palpation for tenderness and swelling is important as well. The fact that the anterior tibial crest is subcutaneous makes identification of the fracture site easier.

2. Neurovascular examination

a. The examiner should assess for signs and symptoms of impending compartment syndrome (tense compartment, pain out of proportion to the injury, or pain on passive stretch of the toes).

b. Compartment syndrome is more common in diaphyseal tibia fractures than in proximal or distal fractures.

c. Continuous intracompartmental monitoring is indicated in patients who are unable to communicate (for example, the intubated and sedated patient in the intensive care unit).

d. Compartment release by fasciotomy is indicated if the patient has one or more of the signs and symptoms listed above and the absolute pressure is greater than 40 mm Hg or there is less than 30 mm Hg difference between the compartmental pressure and the diastolic pressure.

Table 1

Oestern and Tscherne Classification of Closed-Fracture Soft-Tissue Injury

Grade	Description
0	Injuries from indirect forces with negligible soft-tissue damage
I	Superficial contusion/abrasion, simple fractures
II	Deep abrasions, muscle/skin contusion, direct trauma, impending compartment syndrome
III	Excessive skin contusion, crushed skin or destruction of muscle, subcutaneous degloving, acute compartment syndrome, and rupture of major blood vessel or nerve

Reproduced with permission from Oestern HJ, Tscherne H: Pathophysiology and classification of soft tissue injuries associated with fractures, in Tscherne H, Gotzen L, eds: *Fractures With Soft Tissue Injuries*. Berlin, Germany, Springer-Verlag, 1984, pp 1-9.

Table 2

Gustilo Anderson Classification of Open Fractures

Type	Description
I	Clean wound < 1 cm in length
II	Wound > 1 cm without extensive soft-tissue damage
III	Wound associated with extensive soft-tissue damage; usually > 5 cm Open segmental fracture Traumatic amputation Gunshot injuries Farmyard injuries Fractures associated with vascular repair Fractures > 8 hours old
IIIA	Adequate periosteal cover
IIIB	Presence of significant periosteal stripping
IIIC	Vascular repair required to revascularize leg

Adapted with permission from Bucholz RW, Heckman JD, Court-Brown C, eds: *Rockwood and Green's Fractures in Adults*, ed 6. Philadelphia, PA, Lippincott Williams & Wilkins, 2006, p 2084.

e. After the diagnosis of compartment syndrome is made, all four compartments must be released.

3. Radiographic evaluation

a. Plain radiographs should include a trauma series (AP, lateral, and oblique), with dedicated ankle or plateau views if the fracture extends to the surface of the joint. The entire tibia and fibula must be visualized, from knee to ankle.

b. After any fracture manipulation, postreduction views must also be obtained.

c. CT can be used to assess fracture healing or identify nonunion, but it plays no role in acute fracture management.

E. Fracture classification

1. Fractures are usually described based on the pattern, location, and amount of comminution.

2. The OTA classification includes types 42A (simple patterns—that is, spiral, transverse, or oblique), 42B (wedge), and 42C (complex, comminuted) (**Figure 5**).

3. Soft-tissue classification

a. The Oestern and Tscherne classification is used for closed fractures (**Table 1**).

b. The Gustilo-Anderson classification is used for open fractures (**Table 2**).

F. Nonsurgical treatment

1. Indications—Nonsurgical treatment is indicated for low-energy stable tibial fractures (such as axially stable fracture patterns) and virtually all isolated fibular shaft fractures.

2. Long leg casting is indicated, followed by functional bracing in a patellar tendon–bearing brace or cast, with weight bearing as tolerated after 2 to 3 weeks. Cast wedging may be used to correct deformity.

3. Following closed treatment, the mean shortening is 4 mm and mean angulation is less than 6°; nonunion occurs in 1.1% of patients.

G. Surgical treatment

1. Indications

a. When acceptable reduction parameters cannot be maintained, including less than 50% displacement, less than 10° of angulation, less than 1 cm of shortening, and less than 10° of rotational malalignment

b. In patients with open fractures, fractures with associated compartment syndrome, and inherently unstable patterns (segmental, comminuted, short, displaced), and in patients with multiple injuries (for example, floating knee)

2. Intramedullary (IM) nailing

a. Reamed IM nailing is the treatment of choice for unstable fracture patterns because it allows the use of a larger-diameter nail (with larger locking bolts) and paradoxically results in maintenance of periosteal perfusion. In addition, with tibial reaming, in contrast to femoral reaming, concern about embolization of the marrow contents is minimal.

3: Trauma

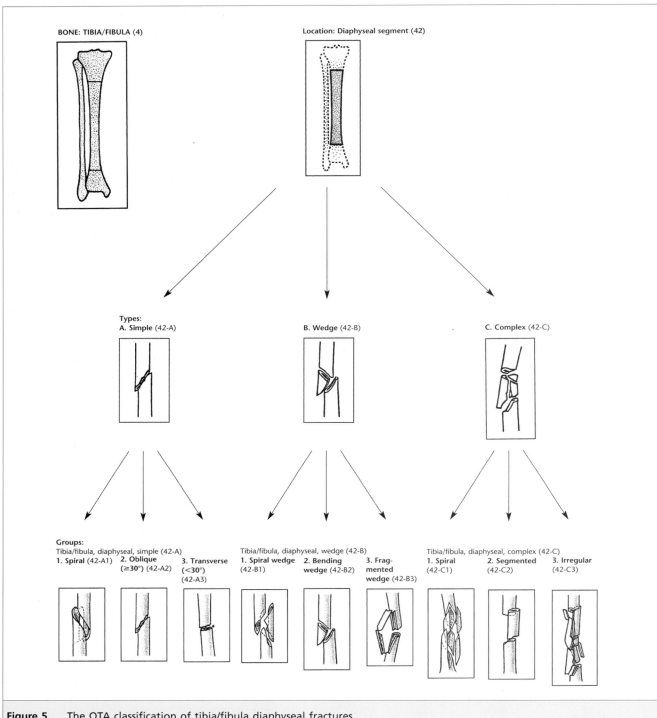

Figure 5   The OTA classification of tibia/fibula diaphyseal fractures.

b. A nonreamed IM nail is looser fitting than a reamed nail and is associated with less cortical necrosis. It is also associated with a higher rate of locking screw breakage than is reamed IM nailing.

c. Use of blocking screws, a unicortical plate, a lateral starting point, and IM nailing in a semi-extended position may help prevent displacement of proximal fractures into flexion and valgus.

d. Use of blocking screws and/or fibular plating may help prevent displacement of distal fractures into valgus (if at the same level as a fibular fracture) or varus (if the fibula is intact).

e. Contraindications to IM nailing include a pre-existing tibial shaft deformity that may preclude IM nail passage and a history of previous IM infection.

3. Plates and screws

   a. Open plating techniques typically have been associated with wound problems and nonunion.

   b. Newer plate designs and minimally invasive techniques have allowed these implants to play a role in the treatment of metadiaphyseal fractures or in tibial shaft fractures in which IM nailing is not possible; for example, following total knee arthroplasty or tibial plateau fixation.

   c. Lateral placement may be preferred to anteromedial placement when soft-tissue concerns exist.

4. External fixation

   a. External fixation has gained popularity in open tibial fractures with soft-tissue compromise because of dissatisfaction with outcomes following traditional techniques.

   b. Advantages of definitive external fixation are its low risk and its ability to provide access to wounds, provide a mechanically stable construct, and allow radiographic evaluation.

   c. Several types of frame constructs are available, including half-pin monolateral frames, which are considered safe and violate tissues on one side only; thin, circular wire frames that allow fixation in metaphyseal bone; and hybrid frames.

   d. Construct stiffness is increased with increased pin diameter, number of pins on either side of the fracture, rods closer to the bone, and a multiplane construct.

5. Treatment of open fractures

   a. Open fractures require urgent débridement and fracture stabilization

   b. Current evidence supports immediate closure of wounds if minimal contamination is present and closure can be performed without skin tension.

   c. If immediate closure is not possible, vacuum-assisted closure should be considered rather than early flap (rotational versus free).

   d. A first-generation cephalosporin should be given immediately in the emergency department. An aminoglycoside should be added for larger soft-tissue defects. Clostridial coverage should be considered in cases of soil contamination or farm injuries.

   e. Tetanus immunoglobin should be given if immune status is known and current; toxoid should be added if the status is unknown or if the patient has not received immunization for more than 10 years.

H. Rehabilitation

1. Following nonsurgical treatment of axially stable fractures, patients should be able to bear weight as tolerated after 1 to 2 weeks.

2. Following surgical treatment, weight-bearing status depends on the fracture pattern and implant type. For axially stable fracture patterns with bony contact, weight bearing as tolerated is allowed. For comminuted fractures, partial weight bearing is allowed until radiographic signs of healing are apparent.

3. Repeat radiographs should be obtained at 6 and 12 weeks.

4. External fixators should be dynamized before removal to ensure healing and prevent repeat fracture.

5. External bone stimulation has been shown to help in fracture healing.

I. Complications

1. Nonunion/delayed union

   a. Nonunion is defined as a fracture that has lost its capacity to unite.

   b. Delayed union is defined as a fracture that takes longer than expected to unite.

   c. Treatment can consist of dynamization, exchange nailing, or bone grafting.

2. Compartment syndrome—Failure to identify impending compartment syndrome is the most serious complication after tibial-fibular shaft fractures.

3. Knee pain occurs in up to 50% of patients following tibial nailing.

4. Infection

   a. Infection can be superficial or deep.

   b. Deep infection usually is associated with open fractures (fracture hematoma communication) and may lead to osteomyelitis.

5. Painful hardware can occur because locking bolts and plates are usually placed on the subcutaneous border of the tibia.

6. Nerve injury, usually affecting the peroneal (most common) or the saphenous nerve, may occur. The saphenous nerve can be injured during the placement of the locking bolts.

7. Malalignment often is associated with late loss of reduction such as may occur with casting or ex-

ternal fixation in proximal and distal metaphyseal fractures.

a. Immediate postoperative malalignment is preventable with careful surgical technique and awareness of this potential complication, particularly with nailing of proximal or distal tibia fractures.

b. Methods to prevent malalignment during tibial nailing include blocking screws, provisional plating, universal distractors, and fibular plating.

c. A more lateral proximal entry site should be considered to avoid valgus with a proximal one third fracture.

Top Testing Facts

Tibial Plateau Fractures

1. High-energy fracture patterns often are associated with compromised skin.

2. If surgical intervention will be delayed after tibial plateau fracture in which the limb is shortened or subluxated, temporary spanning external fixation should be considered.

3. All meniscal damage should be identified and repaired intraoperatively.

4. Calcium phosphate cement is associated with a lower rate of joint subsidence in depressed tibial plateau fractures than autologous bone graft.

5. Bicondylar tibial plateau fractures require dual-plate fixation or unilateral fixation with a locking plate, depending on the presence of comminution or a coronal plane medial plateau fracture.

6. An anterior midline incision should be avoided for bicondylar tibial plateau fractures because of the high rate of wound complications or "dead bone sandwich."

Tibial-Fibular Shaft Fractures

1. Failure to identify impending compartment syndrome is the most serious complication after tibial-fibular shaft fractures.

2. Immediate postoperative malalignment is preventable with careful surgical technique and awareness of this potential complication, particularly with nailing of proximal or distal tibial fractures.

3. Methods to prevent malalignment during tibial nailing include blocking screws, provisional plating, distractors, and fibular plating.

4. A more lateral proximal entry site should be considered to avoid valgus with a proximal one third fracture.

Bibliography

Baron JA, Karagas M, Barrett J, et al: Basic epidemiology of fractures of the upper and lower limb among Americans over 65 years of age. *Epidemiology* 1996;7(6):612-618.

Court-Brown CM, Gustilo T, Shaw AD: Knee pain after intramedullary tibial nailing: Its incidence, etiology, and outcome. *J Orthop Trauma* 1997;11(2):103-105.

Delamarter RB, Hohl M, Hopp E Jr: Ligament injuries associated with tibial plateau fractures. *Clin Orthop Relat Res* 1990;(250):226-233.

Egol KA, Weisz R, Hiebert R, Tejwani NC, Koval KJ, Sanders RW: Does fibular plating improve alignment after intramedullary nailing of distal metaphyseal tibia fractures? *J Orthop Trauma* 2006;20(2):94-103.

Gardner MJ, Yacoubian S, Geller D, et al: The incidence of soft tissue injury in operative tibial plateau fractures: A magnetic resonance imaging analysis of 103 patients. *J Orthop Trauma* 2005;19(2):79-84.

Giannoudis PV, Tzioupis C, Papathanassopoulos A, Obakponovwe O, Roberts C: Articular step-off and risk of posttraumatic osteoarthritis: Evidence today. *Injury* 2010;41(10):986-995.

Gopal S, Majumder S, Batchelor AG, Knight SL, De Boer P, Smith RM: Fix and flap: The radical orthopaedic and plastic treatment of severe open fractures of the tibia. *J Bone Joint Surg Br* 2000;82(7):959-966.

Krettek C, Stephan C, Schandelmaier P, Richter M, Pape HC, Miclau T: The use of Poller screws as blocking screws in stabilising tibial fractures treated with small diameter intramedullary nails. *J Bone Joint Surg Br* 1999;81(6):963-968.

Lansinger O, Bergman B, Körner L, Andersson GB: Tibial condylar fractures: A twenty-year follow-up. *J Bone Joint Surg Am* 1986;68(1):13-19.

Levy BA, Herrera DA, Macdonald P, Cole PA: The medial approach for arthroscopic-assisted fixation of lateral tibial plateau fractures: Patient selection and mid- to long-term results. *J Orthop Trauma* 2008;22(3):201-205.

Marsh JL, Smith ST, Do TT: External fixation and limited internal fixation for complex fractures of the tibial plateau. *J Bone Joint Surg Am* 1995;77(5):661-673.

McQueen MM, Court-Brown CM: Compartment monitoring in tibial fractures: The pressure threshold for decompression. *J Bone Joint Surg Br* 1996;78(1):99-104.

Muller M: The comprehensive classification of long bones, in Muller ME, Schneider R, Willenegger H, eds: *Manual of Internal Fixation*. Berlin, Germany, Springer-Verlag, 1995, pp 118-158.

Musahl V, Tarkin I, Kobbe P, Tzioupis C, Siska PA, Pape HC: New trends and techniques in open reduction and internal fixation of fractures of the tibial plateau. *J Bone Joint Surg Br* 2009;91(4):426-433.

Park SD, Ahn J, Gee AO, Kuntz AF, Esterhai JL: Compartment syndrome in tibial fractures. *J Orthop Trauma* 2009; 23(7):514-518.

Russell TA, Leighton RK; Alpha-BSM Tibial Plateau Fracture Study Group: Comparison of autogenous bone graft and endothermic calcium phosphate cement for defect augmentation in tibial plateau fractures: A multicenter, prospective, randomized study. *J Bone Joint Surg Am* 2008;90(10): 2057-2061.

3: Trauma

Chapter 42

Fractures of the Ankle and Tibial Plafond

David W. Sanders, MD, FRCSC   Kenneth A. Egol, MD

I. Rotational Fractures of the Ankle

A. Epidemiology

1. Rotational fractures of the ankle are among the most common injuries requiring orthopaedic care.

2. Ankle fractures vary from relatively simple injuries with minimal long-term effects to complex injuries with severe long-term sequelae.

3. Population-based studies have identified an increase in the incidence of ankle fractures. Data from Medicare enrollees suggest the rate of ankle fractures in the United States averages 4.2 fractures per 1,000 Medicare enrollees annually.

4. Rates of surgery vary depending on the type of fracture.

   a. For isolated lateral malleolar fractures, which account for two thirds of rotational ankle fractures, the surgical intervention rate is approximately 11%.

   b. For trimalleolar fractures, the surgical intervention rate is 74%.

5. Risk factors for ankle fracture include age, increased body mass, and a history of ankle fracture.

6. The highest incidence of ankle fractures occurs in elderly women.

B. Anatomy of the lower leg

1. Osseous anatomy and ligaments of the ankle joint (**Figure 1**)

Dr. Sanders or an immediate family member serves as a paid consultant to or is an employee of Smith & Nephew; has received research or institutional support from Smith & Nephew and Synthes; and serves as a board member, owner, officer, or committee member of the Orthopaedic Trauma Association (OTA). Dr. Egol or an immediate family member has received royalties from Exactech; serves as a paid consultant to or is an employee of Exactech; and has received research or institutional support from Synthes, the Orthopaedic Research and Education Foundation, OTA, and OMeGA.

a. The osseous anatomy of the ankle provides stability during weight bearing and mobility in plantar flexion.

b. The ankle joint behaves like a true mortise in dorsiflexion.

c. Stability is achieved by articular contact between the medial malleolus, the fibula, the tibial plafond, and the talus.

d. The talar dome is wider anteriorly than posteriorly so that, as the ankle dorsiflexes, the fibula rotates externally through the tibiofibular syndesmosis to accommodate the talus.

e. The lateral malleolus is surrounded by multiple strong ligaments.

   • These include the interosseous membrane and the tibiofibular ligamentous complex, consisting of the interosseous ligament and the syndesmotic ligaments (anterior inferior tibiofibular ligament [AITFL], posterior inferior tibiofibular ligament, inferior transverse tibiofibular ligament, inferior interosseous ligament).

   • These ligaments are responsible for the stability of the ankle in external rotation.

   • In addition, the lateral collateral ligaments of the ankle, including the anterior and posterior talofibular ligaments and calcaneofibular ligaments, provide support and resistance to inversion and anterior translation of the talus relative to the fibula.

2. Medial malleolus

   a. The medial malleolar surface of the distal tibia has a larger surface anteriorly than posteriorly.

   b. The posterior border of the medial malleolus includes the groove for the posterior tibial tendon.

   c. The medial malleolus includes the anterior colliculus, which is larger than and extends ap-

3: Trauma

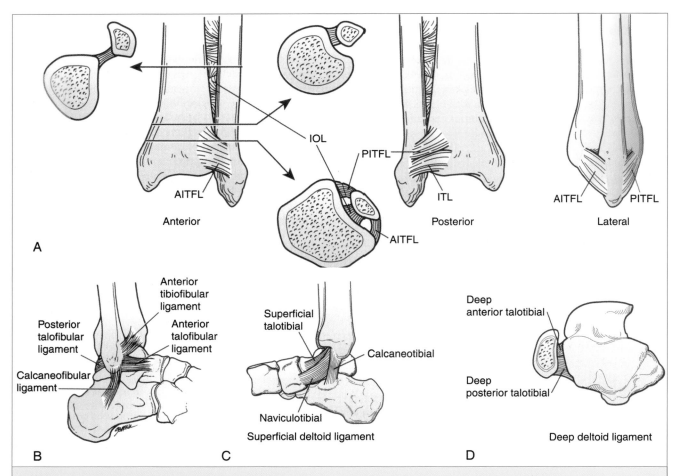

Figure 1   Illustrations show the osseous anatomy and ligaments of the ankle joint. **A,** Anterior, posterior, and lateral views of the tibiofibular syndesmotic ligaments. **B,** The lateral collateral ligaments of the ankle and the anterior syndesmotic ligament. Sagittal plane (**C**) and transverse plane (**D**) views of the medial collateral ligaments of the ankle. AITFL = anterior inferior tibiofibular ligament, PITFL = posterior inferior tibiofibular ligament, ITL = inferior transverse ligament, IOL = interosseous ligament. (Panels A, C, and D adapted with permission from Browner B, Jupiter J, Levine A, eds: *Skeletal Trauma: Fractures, Dislocations, and Ligamentous Injuries*, ed 2. Philadelphia, PA, WB Saunders, 1997. Panel B reproduced with permission from Marsh JL, Saltzman CL: Ankle fractures, in Bucholz RW, Heckman JD, Court-Brown CM, eds: *Rockwood and Green's Fractures in Adults*, ed 6. Philadelphia, PA, Lippincott Williams and Wilkins, 2006, pp 2147-2247.)

proximately 0.5 cm distal to the posterior colliculus.

  d. The deltoid ligament provides medial ligamentous support of the ankle.

- The important deep component of the deltoid ligament arises from the intercollicular groove and posterior colliculus.

- The deep layer of the deltoid ligament is a short, thick ligament inserting on the medial surface of the talus.

- The superficial deltoid ligament arises from the anterior colliculus of the medial malleolus.

3. Tendinous and neurovascular structures

  a. Posterior group

- The posterior group includes the Achilles and plantaris tendons.

- Immediately lateral to the Achilles tendon lies the sural nerve.

  b. Medial group

- On the medial side of the ankle, the flexor tendons—including the tibialis posterior, the flexor digitorum longus (FDL), and the flexor hallucis longus (FHL)—course posterior to the medial malleolus.

- The posterior tibial artery and tibial nerve lie between the FDL and FHL tendons.

- The saphenous vein and nerve course superior and anterior to the tip of the medial malleolus and are at risk during surgical repair of malleolar fractures.

c. Anterior group

- On the anterior aspect of the ankle, the extensor retinaculum contains the extensor tendons, including the tibialis anterior, extensor hallucis longus (EHL), extensor digitorum longus (EDL), and peroneus tertius.

- Between the EHL and EDL lie the deep peroneal nerve and the anterior tibial artery.

- The superficial peroneal nerve crosses the ankle anterior to the lateral malleolus, superficial to the extensor retinaculum.

- Because the superficial peroneal nerve may cross from the lateral compartment to the anterior compartment at varying levels, care must be exercised to avoid injury to this nerve in the treatment of fibular fractures.

d. Lateral group

- On the lateral side of the ankle, the peroneal tendons are contained by a stout retinacular structure posterior to the fibula.

- The peroneus longus is more external to the peroneus brevis.

- Lateral approaches to the ankle can injure the superficial nerve more proximally and the sural nerve more distally.

C. Classification—AO/Weber and Lauge-Hansen

1. AO/Weber classification (**Figure 2**)

a. Ankle fractures are classified based on the location of the fibular fracture.

b. The degree of instability depends on the location of the fibular fracture.

c. Weber A fracture

- Occurs when the fibular fracture is located distal to the tibiofibular syndesmosis

- Injury usually occurs according to an inversion mechanism.

- Because of the infrasyndesmotic location, Weber A fractures are less likely to result in instability.

- Indications for surgery are therefore dependent on the status of the medial ankle.

d. Weber B fracture

- Most common type of ankle fracture

- Includes a fibular fracture beginning at approximately the level of the ankle syndesmosis (the AITFL) and extending proximal and posterior

- May be associated with ankle instability, de-

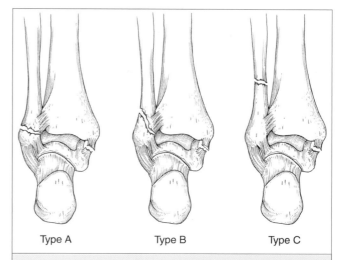

Figure 2 Illustrations show the AO/Weber classification of ankle fractures. The staging is determined solely by the level of fibular fracture. Type A occurs below the plafond; type C starts above the plafond. (Reproduced from Michelson JD: Ankle fractures resulting from rotational injuries. *J Am Acad Orthop Surg* 2003;11:403-412.)

Type A   Type B   Type C

pending on the status of the medial side of the ankle

e. Weber C fracture

- Associated with a fibular fracture above the level of the ankle syndesmosis

- Usually occurs with an external rotation mechanism

- Generally unstable because it usually is associated with medial injury

2. Lauge-Hansen classification (**Figures 3** and **4**)

a. Roughly corresponds to the Weber classification

b. Ankle fractures are classified according to the mechanism of injury.

- Two variables are described; the first is the position of the foot and the second relates to the deforming force applied to the ankle.

- In a cadaver study, most ankle fracture patterns were reproduced by placing the foot in supination or pronation and then applying deforming forces in abduction, adduction, or external rotation.

- When the foot is supinated, the medial deltoid ligament is relaxed and the initial injury is lateral.

- When the foot is pronated, the deltoid ligament is tense, and the initial injury occurs medially as a medial malleolar fracture or deltoid ligament disruption.

3:Trauma

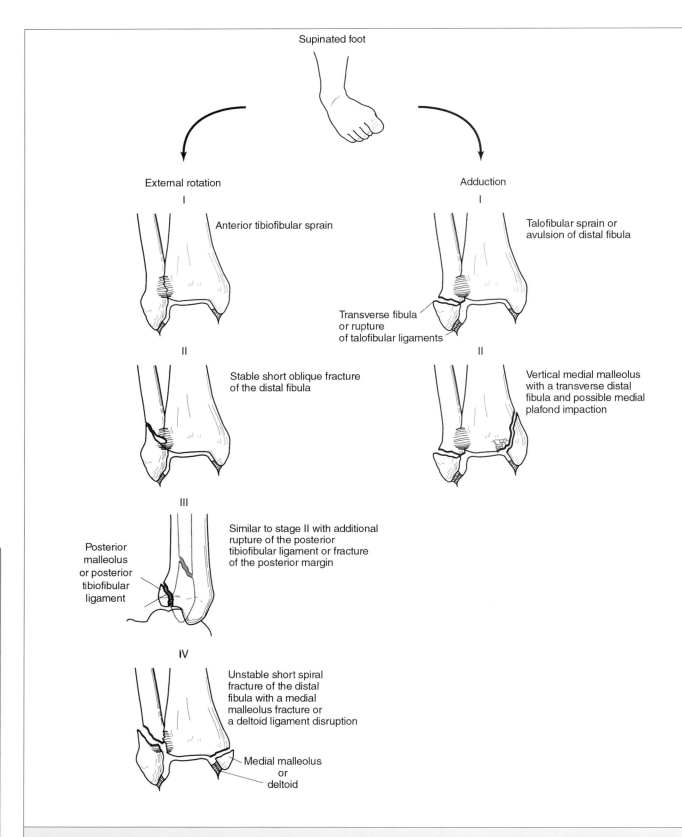

Figure 3   Illustrations show the Lauge-Hansen classification of ankle fractures, depicting the sequence of injury when the foot is supinated (supination–external rotation and supination-adduction injuries). (Adapted with permission from Marsh JL, Saltzman CL: Ankle fractures, in Bucholz RW, Heckman JD, eds: *Rockwood and Green's Fractures in Adults*, ed 5. Philadelphia, PA, Lippincott Williams and Wilkins, 2001, pp 2001-2090.

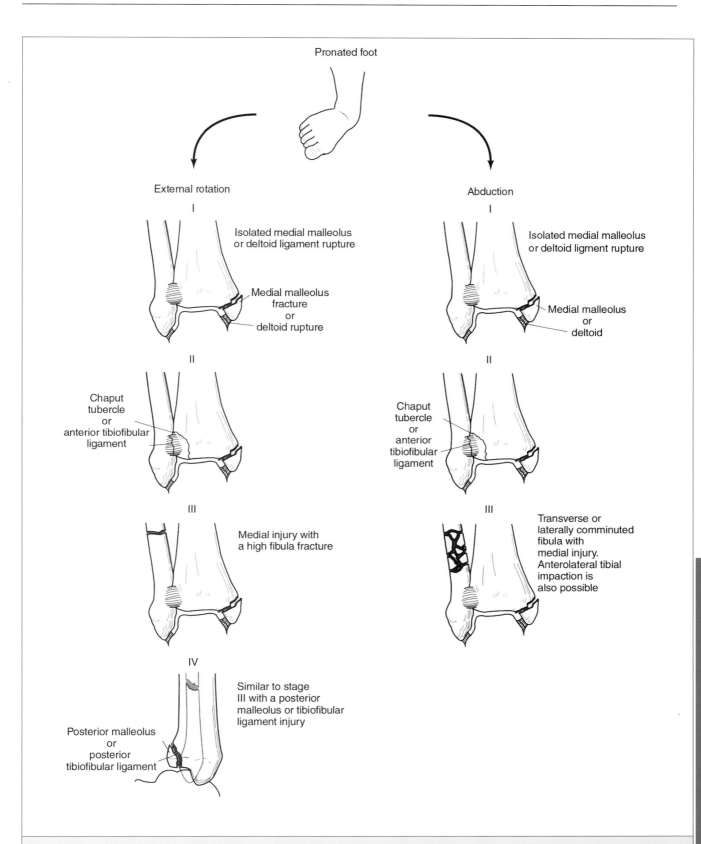

Pronated foot

External rotation

I

Isolated medial malleolus
or deltoid ligament rupture

Medial malleolus
fracture
or
deltoid rupture

II

Chaput
tubercle
or
anterior tibiofibular
ligament

III

Medial injury with
a high fibula fracture

IV

Posterior malleolus
or
posterior
tibiofibular ligament

Similar to stage
III with a posterior
malleolus or tibiofibular
ligament injury

Abduction

I

Isolated medial malleolus
or deltoid ligament rupture

Medial malleolus
or
deltoid

II

Chaput
tubercle
or
anterior
tibiofibular
ligament

III

Transverse or
laterally comminuted
fibula with
medial injury.
Anterolateral tibial
impaction is
also possible

Figure 4   Illustrations show the Lauge-Hansen classification of ankle fractures, depicting the sequence of injury when the foot is pronated (pronation–external rotation and pronation-abduction injuries). (Reproduced with permission from Marsh JL, Saltzman CL: Ankle fractures, in Bucholz RW, Heckman JD, eds: *Rockwood and Green's Fractures in Adults*, ed 5. Philadelphia, PA, Lippincott Williams and Wilkins, 2001, pp 2001-2090.)

3: Trauma

Table 1

Lauge-Hansen Classification of Ankle Fractures

Fracture Type	Sequence of Injury
SAD	Creates an infrasyndesmotic fibular fracture that may be associated with a vertical medial malleolar fracture and medial plafond impaction
SER	1. Disruption of the anterior inferior tibiofibular ligament 2. Short spiral fracture of the distal fibula analogous to a Weber B-type injury 3. Injury to the posterior malleolus or posterior tibiofibular ligament 4. Associated fracture of the medial malleolus or a deltoid ligament disruption
PER	1. Medial injury 2. Anterior tibiofibular ligament injury 3. High fibular fracture, analogous to a Weber C–type injury
PAB	1. Medial injury 2. Anterior tibiofibular ligament injury 3. Transverse or laterally comminuted fibular fracture 4. Anterolateral tibial impaction is also possible

SAD = supination-adduction, SER = supination–external rotation,
PER = pronation–external rotation, PAB = pronation-abduction.

c. The Lauge-Hansen classification describes four major fracture types—supination-adduction, supination–external rotation, pronation–external rotation, and pronation-abduction. In each type, the initial injury is followed by further injury to other structures around the ankle in a predictable sequence (**Table 1**).

d. As in the Weber classification, the Lauge-Hansen classification requires that particular attention be paid to the specific characteristics of the fibular fracture.

e. The Lauge-Hansen classification was first designed to assist in determining the forces required to obtain and maintain a closed reduction of an ankle fracture; however, it continues to assist in understanding the mechanism of injury of rotational ankle fractures.

D. Surgical approaches to ankle fractures

1. Direct lateral approach to the fibula

a. Commonly used to stabilize lateral malleolar fractures

b. The dissection is anterior to the peroneal tendons at the level of the ankle mortise.

c. Proximally, the peroneal tendons must be dissected to expose the fibula.

d. The dissection plane is between the peroneus tertius anteriorly and the peroneus longus and brevis posteriorly.

e. The superficial peroneal nerve should be considered when more proximal dissection is required for fibular fracture.

f. The posterior aspect of the lateral malleolus can be approached through this incision; this requires reflection of the peroneal tendons away from the posterior surface of the fibula to facilitate placement of internal fixation on the posterior surface of the fibula.

2. Posterolateral approach to the ankle joint

a. The posterolateral interval exists between the peroneal tendons and the Achilles tendon.

b. Direct exposure of the posterior aspect of the tibia is accomplished by elevating the FHL tendon off the fibula and away from the posterior aspect of the tibia in the deep portion of this incision.

c. This approach provides access to the posterior aspect of the distal tibia and fibula.

3. Anteromedial approaches to the medial malleolus

a. The medial malleolus can be approached through a longitudinal incision directly over the malleolus; the saphenous nerve and vein are frequently encountered.

b. A slightly more anterior incision facilitates direct inspection of the ankle joint and talar dome.

c. Using a more posteromedial incision, the posterior tibial tendon and neurovascular bundle can be elevated to access the posteromedial portion of the medial malleolus.

4. Percutaneous incisions

a. In addition to the lateral, posterolateral, and medial approaches, a variety of percutaneous incisions can be used to facilitate hardware placement.

b. An anterior percutaneous incision often is used to facilitate the indirect fixation of a posterior malleolar fracture.

c. Blunt dissection and placement of retractors and soft-tissue sleeves are required to avoid injury to the neurovascular structures surrounding the ankle.

E. Mechanism of injury

1. Most ankle fractures are low-energy, rotational injuries, in which the foot is planted and the body rotates around the fixed ankle.

2. Ankle fractures also occur commonly in sports, usually secondary to a rotational mechanism.

3. Fractures with a significant axial loading mechanism are more severe and often result in tibial plafond fractures.

4. Associated injuries

   a. Common with malleolar fractures

   b. Fractures of the talar dome occur in a substantial portion of ankle fractures and compromise long-term outcome.

   c. Associated osseoligamentous injuries such as avulsive injuries of the AITFL may occur.

   d. Avulsion fractures in which the AITFL avulses from the distal tibia (Chaput tubercle) or fibula (Wagstaffe tubercle) may occur and result in associated external rotation instability.

   e. With adduction-type ankle injuries, impaction injury to the medial distal tibia may occur.

      • To restore ankle joint congruency, this impaction injury may require treatment in addition to the malleolar fracture.

      • This injury pattern should be considered in particular when the medial malleolar fracture has a vertical orientation and is associated with a transverse distal fibular fracture.

   f. The lateral articular surface can be impacted in a pronation-abduction type of mechanism. Reduction and stabilization of the lateral articular impaction can be difficult and may also result in significant problems with long-term outcome.

F. Clinical evaluation

1. Clinical evaluation should include a description of the mechanism of injury.

2. An evaluation of medical comorbidities, with attention to peripheral vascular disease and diabetes mellitus, is important. Physical examination should include a thorough inspection for potentially communicating open wounds.

   a. An open ankle fracture is most commonly associated with an open medial wound with a punctate or transverse laceration in communication with the ankle joint.

   b. These fractures should be considered surgical emergencies.

3. An examination for deformity of the foot relative to the leg and the direction of displacement to the foot should be performed.

4. The complete circulatory and neurologic examination should be documented, including assessment of the superficial peroneal, deep peroneal, sural, and posterior tibial nerves, which can be examined using light touch and sharp/dull discrimination.

5. The condition of the skin must be considered.

6. Soft-tissue swelling should be assessed because it will affect surgical timing.

7. Fracture-dislocations should be reduced relatively quickly to avoid isolated skin and soft-tissue ischemia.

8. In patients without dislocation, the ankle should be palpated for areas of tenderness.

9. Ottawa ankle rules

   a. The Ottawa ankle rules assist physicians in deciding when it is appropriate to obtain radiographs in adults with ankle injuries.

   b. These guidelines are sensitive for ankle fracture, and they reduce the number of radiographs taken, along with associated costs.

   c. According to these rules, ankle radiographs are needed only if pain is present near the malleoli and one or more of the following conditions is present:

      • Age 55 years or older

      • Inability to bear weight

      • Bone tenderness at the posterior edge or tip of either malleolus

10. Physical examination and instability

   a. Although physical examination of acute ankle injuries is important, the ability to detect instability by physical examination alone has been questioned.

   b. This is particularly the case for isolated lateral malleolar fractures, in which it is often difficult to determine the degree of instability of the ankle.

   c. In patients with an isolated fibular fracture without talar shift, the ankle should be palpated directly over the deltoid ligament for swelling, ecchymosis, and tenderness as a clue to potential deltoid ligament injury; however, the value of this maneuver in predicting ankle instability is comparatively limited.

   d. Radiographic physician-assisted or gravity stress examination of isolated fibular fractures without talar shift has been advocated recently as a more sensitive examination of ankle instability.

G. Imaging

1. The standard trauma radiograph series of the ankle includes mortise, AP, and lateral views.

   a. The mortise view is obtained with the patient's leg in approximately 15° of internal rotation

3: Trauma

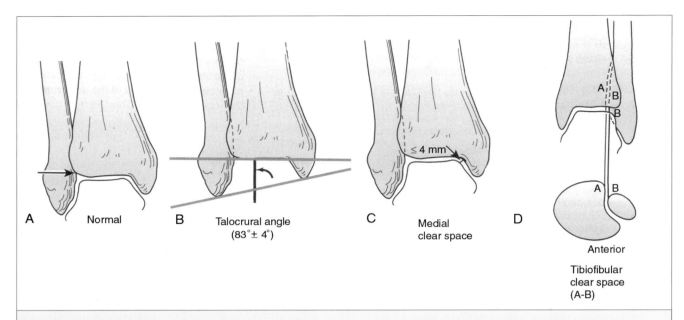

Figure 5 Illustrations depict the radiographic appearance of the normal ankle on the mortise view. **A,** The condensed subchondral bone should form a continuous line around the talus. **B,** The talocrural angle should be approximately 83°. **C,** The medial clear space should be equal to the superior clear space between the talus and the distal tibia and 4 mm or less on standard radiographs. **D,** The distance between the medial wall of the fibula and the incisural surface of the tibia, the tibiofibular clear space, should be 6 mm or less. (Panels A through C adapted with permission from Browner B, Jupiter J, Levine A, eds: *Skeletal Trauma: Fractures, Dislocations, and Ligamentous Injuries,* ed 2. Philadelphia, PA, WB Saunders, 1997. Panel D reproduced with permission from Marsh JL, Saltzman CL, Ankle fractures, in Bucholz RW, Heckman JD, Court-Brown CM, eds: *Rockwood and Green's Fractures in Adults,* ed 6. Philadelphia, PA, Lippincott Williams and Wilkins, 2006, pp 2147-2247.)

such that the x-ray beam is perpendicular to the transmalleolar axis.

    b. The AP radiograph is obtained with the x-ray beam in line with the second ray of the foot.

    c. If any suggestion of proximal tibial or fibular pain or tenderness or swelling and pain in the foot region is present, the radiographic evaluation should include full views of the tibia and fibula and foot.

2. Important considerations on standard radiographic views (**Figure 5**)

    a. The subchondral bone of the tibia and fibula should form a continuous line around the talus on all views.

    b. The talocrural angle (the angle between a line drawn perpendicular to the distal articular surface of the tibia and a line connecting the lateral and medial malleoli) should be 83° ± 4° or within 5° of the contralateral ankle on the mortise view.

    c. The medial clear space (the distance between the medial articular surface of the medial malleolus and the talar dome) should be 4-5 mm or less and should be equal to the superior clear space between the talus and the distal tibia on the mortise view.

    d. The tibiofibular clear space (the distance between the medial wall of the fibula and the tibial incisural surface) should be 6 mm or less on the mortise view.

3. In an ankle with an isolated fibular fracture and medial tenderness without evidence of initial talar displacement, a stress view has been recommended.

    a. This may be performed by simple gentle external rotation of the foot with the ankle in dorsiflexion and the leg stabilized, or by supporting the patient's leg with a pillow or cushion and allowing the ankle to rotate with the force of gravity.

    b. In these situations, a widening of the medial clear space of 5 mm or more may occur. This may indicate ankle instability secondary to medial ligamentous injury in conjunction with the fibular fracture.

H. Nonsurgical treatment

1. Nonsurgical treatment remains the standard of care for ankle fractures in many situations.

2. In stable fibular fractures without associated medial injury, closed treatment leads to excellent function in most cases.

    a. When the fracture is stable, a short leg cast or

functional brace can be applied for 4 to 6 weeks.

b. Weight bearing is permitted when symptoms allow.

c. Prolonged immobilization and casting is not necessary.

d. Some studies have reported good results using a simple supportive high-top shoe or elastic bandage.

3. Unstable fractures

a. With an unstable fracture, nonsurgical treatment requires frequent follow-up.

b. Radiographic confirmation that the talus has remained reduced in the mortise is required.

c. Casting and non–weight bearing for a minimum of 4 weeks is required to prevent the ankle from displacing; even so, maintaining the reduction is difficult and has several disadvantages.

- Prolonged casting presents challenges for elderly or infirm patients.

- As swelling diminishes, the reduction may be lost.

- Despite the disadvantages, casting is useful in selected cases such as neuropathic patients or patients too unwell to tolerate surgery.

I. Surgical treatment

1. General issues

a. Surgical treatment is indicated for unstable ankle fractures.

b. Distal tibiofibular diastasis also requires reduction and fixation.

c. The timing of surgery is important.

d. A closed reduction may assist in resolving swelling and help to avoid further articular damage.

e. Temporary immobilization and elevation allow swelling to resolve.

f. At the time of surgery, perioperative antibiotics are required.

2. Lateral malleolus

a. Fixation of the fibular fracture is usually performed before treatment of the medial or posterior malleolus or syndesmosis. Fixation of the fibula provides stability to the ankle and restores length. Exceptions to the fibula-first strategy.

- When the fibular fracture is extensively comminuted, stabilization of the medial side first may facilitate positioning the talus within the mortise, thus helping to achieve an anatomic reduction of the fibula.

- In many supination-adduction mechanisms, fixation of the fibula assists with stability but is not adequate to reduce the talus within the mortise.

b. Reduction of the fibula may be achieved directly, or indirectly with traction or a push/pull distraction technique.

c. Typically, simple patterns are stabilized with a lag screw to provide fracture compression and then with a one-third tubular plate, contoured to the lateral (neutralization) or posterolateral (buttress) fibula.

d. A posterior antiglide plate is useful for a very distal fibular fracture, a fracture associated with a posterior dislocation, or osteopenic bone.

- A posterior plate provides stable fixation in antiglide or buttress mode, even without the use of distal screws.

- The proximal portion of the plate is fixed with bicortical screws placed from posterior to anterior.

- When screws are needed in the distal fragment, they can be placed from posterior to anterior without penetrating the ankle joint.

- A lag screw can be placed from posterior to anterior through the plate or, alternatively, from anterior to posterior.

3. Medial malleolus

a. The medial malleolus can be stabilized using a variety of techniques, depending on the fracture pattern.

b. Most fractures are oblique and can be stabilized with two 4.0-mm partially threaded cancellous screws.

- Exceptions include the anterior colliculus fracture, which can occur with a deep deltoid ligament rupture.

- Stabilizing the anterior colliculus alone may not restore ankle stability.

c. Vertical shear fractures may be associated with articular impaction that requires reduction and bone void filling; antiglide or buttress plate fixation of the vertical shear fracture also may be necessary.

4. Posterior malleolus

a. Posterior malleolar fractures involving more than 25% to 33% of the articular surface or those associated with posterior subluxation following fixation of the fibula require reduction and fixation.

b. The posterior malleolus can be reduced using

3: Trauma

Table 2

Pearls for the Treatment of Ankle Fractures

Site of Fracture	Pearls
Lateral malleolus	Restore fibular length Avoid injury to the superficial peroneal nerve Fix fibula first unless comminuted PAB mechanism Check syndesmosis
Medial malleolus	2 × 4.0-mm partial threaded screws perpendicular to fracture Vertical shear: plate, reduce joint surface Tension band for small fragments
Posterior malleolus	Fix if > 25% of articular surface involved
Tibiofibular syndesmosis	Check after fibular fixation Ensure the fibula is reduced Leave screws in ≥ 3 months

PAB = pronation-abduction.

direct or indirect techniques.

c. The posterolateral approach described previously is useful for directly visualizing the extraarticular fracture line and facilitates placement of a posterior-to-anterior lag screw or buttress plate. A posteromedial approach is used for more complex patterns.

d. If indirect reduction is used, a reduction tenaculum is placed posteriorly through the fibular incision and anteriorly through a separate small anterior incision.

- Care should be taken to spread the soft tissues and avoid injuring the anterior neurovascular structures.

- A percutaneous anterior-to-posterior screw can then be inserted in lag mode, using fluoroscopic control.

e. Partially threaded screws require careful insertion, making sure the screw threads cross the fracture line for smaller posterior fragments.

5. Tibiofibular syndesmosis

a. Injuries to the tibiofibular syndesmosis are common with rotational ankle injuries.

b. Following fixation of both malleoli, all external rotation and eversion ankle fractures should be evaluated fluoroscopically because syndesmotic instability may be present.

c. Although more common in higher fibular fractures, approximately 33% to 50% of supination–external rotation–type ankle frac-

tures are associated with syndesmotic instability after fibular fixation.

d. The syndesmosis typically is stabilized with one or two 3.5- or 4.5-mm screws inserted from the fibula into the tibia. The most distal screw should be inserted at the superior margin of the syndesmosis.

e. An accurate anatomic reduction of the syndesmosis is required; overcompression and widening of the syndesmosis as well as anterior or posterior translation of the fibula can occur.

f. Achieving an accurate reduction is even more critical when only syndesmosis fixation is used, such as for a proximal fibular fracture associated with interosseous membrane disruption, ankle instability, and fibular shortening. In this instance, accurate restoration of fibular length and alignment is required before placement of the syndesmosis screw.

g. Screws can engage three or four cortices.

- Screws that engage all four cortices may be more likely to break.

- The indications for screw removal remain controversial; however, screws should be left in long enough (minimum, 12 weeks) to ensure that ligamentous healing has occurred to prevent redisplacement.

6. Pearls are listed in **Table 2**.

J. Rehabilitation

1. Following fracture fixation, the limb is immobilized in a splint.

2. Progression to weight bearing is based on the fracture pattern, the stability of fixation, patient compliance, and the philosophy of the surgeon.

K. Complications

1. Nonunion

a. Nonunion is rare, usually involves the medial malleolus when treated closed, and is associated with residual fracture displacement, interposed soft tissue, or associated lateral instability resulting in shear stresses across the deltoid ligament. Nonunion of the fibula also is described less commonly.

b. Symptomatic nonunions may be treated with open reduction and internal fixation (ORIF) and bone grafting.

c. Excision of the medial malleolus fragment may be necessary if not amenable to internal fixation and the patient is symptomatic.

2. Malunion

a. The lateral malleolus is usually shortened and malrotated. This is usually an iatrogenic problem.

b. A widened medial clear space and a large posterior malleolar fragment are most predictive of poor outcome.

c. The medial malleolus may heal in an elongated position, resulting in residual instability.

3. Wound problems

a. Skin edge necrosis occurs in 3% of patients.

b. Risk is reduced with minimal swelling, no tourniquet, and good soft-tissue technique.

c. If fracture surgery is performed in the presence of fracture blisters or abrasions, the complication rate more than doubles.

4. Infection

a. Occurs in less than 2% of closed fractures

b. Implants are left in situ if stable, even with deep infection. The implant may be removed after the fracture unites.

c. May require serial débridements with possible arthrodesis as a salvage procedure

5. Posttraumatic arthritis

a. Occurs secondary to damage at the time of injury, altered mechanics, or as a result of inadequate reduction

b. Rare in anatomically reduced fractures, but incidence increases with articular incongruity.

c. May be seen in asymptomatic patients at long-term follow-up

6. Complex regional pain syndrome (rare)—May be minimized by anatomic restoration of the ankle and early return to function

7. Compartment syndrome of foot (rare)

8. Loss of reduction—Found in 25% of unstable ankle injuries treated nonsurgically.

9. Loss of some ankle range of motion is the rule, not the exception.

II. Tibial Plafond (Pilon) Fractures

A. Epidemiology

1. A plafond fracture is a distal tibial fracture with articular surface involvement.

2. Tibial plafond fractures account for less than 10% of lower extremity injuries.

3. The mean patient age is 35 to 40 years.

4. More common in males than in females

5. The most common mechanisms of injury include motor vehicle collisions and falls from a height; injury generally is caused by an axial load of the talus upon the plafond.

6. Tibial plafond fractures appear to be increasing in incidence, similar to other severe lower extremity fractures

B. Anatomy

1. Relevant anatomy is the same as for rotational ankle fractures.

2. Fracture morphology

a. Fractures of the tibial plafond assume a varying course within the cartilage of the distal bone.

b. Fractures may include an impaction of the anterior articular surface, posterior articular surface, or both, as well as central impaction of the articular surface, depending on the exact direction of injury.

c. Careful evaluation of the direction and orientation of the fracture patterns is essential when determining the optimal surgical approach.

C. Classification

1. No universally accepted classification of tibial plafond fractures exists.

2. Important characteristics to consider include articular and metaphyseal comminution, shortening of the tibia resulting in proximal displacement of the talus, impaction of individual or multiple joint fragments, and associated soft-tissue injury.

3. A wide variation in fracture patterns can result, related to the position of the foot and the precise direction and magnitude of the force applied.

4. The Rüedi-Allgöwer classification, which is of historic value only, considers three variations of tibial plafond fractures (**Figure 6**). In this classification, comminution and displacement refer to involvement of the articular surface.

a. Type I: nondisplaced

b. Type II: displaced but minimally comminuted

c. Type III: highly comminuted and displaced

5. The Orthopaedic Trauma Association (OTA) classification system (**Figure 7**) is more precise than the Rüedi-Allgöwer system. In the OTA system:

a. Distal tibial fractures are divided into type A, or extra-articular fractures; type B, or partial articular fractures; and type C, or total articular fractures.

b. Each category is further subdivided into three groups based upon the amount and degree of

3: Trauma

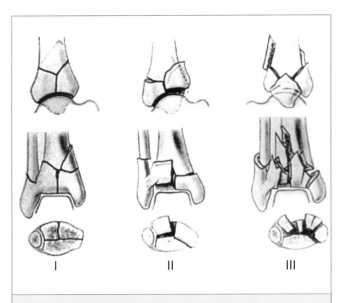

Figure 6 The Rüedi-Allgöwer classification of tibial plafond fractures is illustrated. (Reproduced with permission from Rüedi TP, Allgöwer M: Fractures of the lower end of the tibia into the ankle joint: Results 9 years after open reduction. *Injury* 1973;5:130.)

comminution.

c. Other characteristics of the fracture, such as the location and direction of fracture lines or the presence of metaphyseal impaction, also are included in further subdivisions.

d. Types B, C1, C2, and C3 are the fractures commonly considered to be tibial plafond fractures.

6. The Tscherne classification is used to grade the soft-tissue injury, which also is important.

a. Grade 0: closed fractures without appreciable soft-tissue injury

b. Grade 1: abrasions or contusions of skin and subcutaneous tissue

c. Grade 2: deep abrasion with some muscle involvement

d. Grade 3: extensive soft-tissue damage and severe muscle injury. Compartment syndrome and arterial rupture also are considered grade 3 injuries.

D. Surgical approaches

1. Rüedi and Allgöwer described the following surgical approaches to the distal tibia and fibula: ORIF of the fibula using a lateral approach, and ORIF of the tibia through a medial approach. Over time, this surgical technique has evolved to avoid some of the soft-tissue complications potentially associated with ORIF.

2. Some approaches to the distal tibia include skin incisions that do not pass directly over the thin subcutaneous skin of the medial subcutaneous border of the tibia.

3. The anterolateral approach may be useful, particularly when fractures are impacted in valgus and when the fibula is intact or is associated with a very proximal injury.

a. The anterolateral approach incision is just lateral to the anterior compartment tendons and neurovascular structures and crosses the ankle.

b. This incision may be long or short, as necessary to facilitate reduction.

c. The superficial peroneal nerve may be at risk with this incision and needs to be carefully avoided.

d. The skin incision for the anteromedial approach may be placed more anteriorly, just adjacent to the anterior tibial tendon, to avoid placing it directly over the subcutaneous border of the tibia.

e. The presence of a compromised soft-tissue envelope and blisters may preclude the use of an anteromedial approach.

f. When performed, the anteromedial approach should be done with great care to avoid unnecessarily risking further soft-tissue compromise.

4. The lateral incision to the fibula is placed slightly more posteriorly in the case of a tibial plafond fracture. This facilitates a larger skin bridge between the fibular incision and that used for placement of tibial fixation.

a. Placement of the incision posterior to the peroneal tendons may facilitate visualization, reduction, and fixation of the posterior articular surface of the tibia as well.

b. This incision courses between the peroneal tendons and the Achilles tendon; care must be taken to protect the sural nerve.

5. External fixation is also described for fractures of the ankle and distal tibia.

a. The medial subcutaneous border of the tibia is a safe position for wires, and transfibular wires may be safe.

b. If spanning temporary external fixation is used, the external fixation pins should be placed remote from the fracture site to avoid interference with definitive internal fixation.

c. Definitive articulating joint-spanning external fixation with limited internal fixation has been described and reported to produce similar outcomes to ORIF.

E. Mechanisms of injury

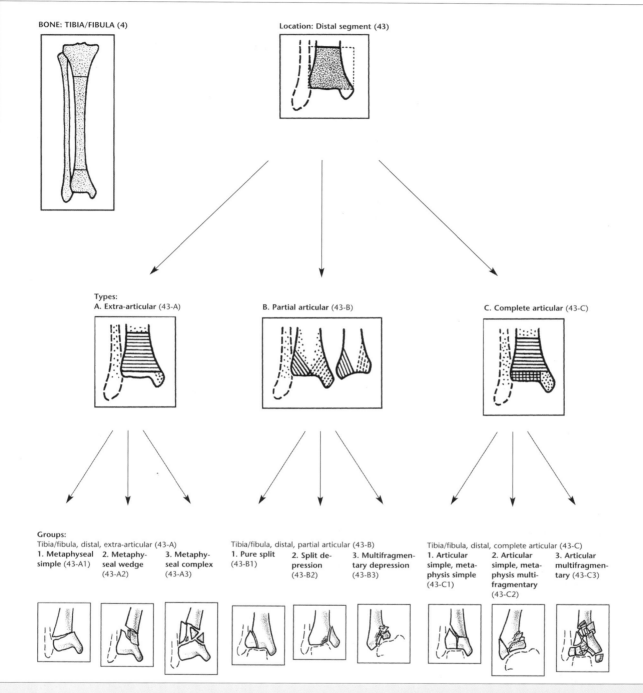

Figure 7   Diagram depicts the Orthopaedic Trauma Association classification of distal tibial fractures. Type A fractures are extra-articular, type B are partial articular, and type C are total articular. Types B3, C1, C2, and C3 are the fractures commonly considered tibial plafond fractures.

1. Axial compression (high energy; for example, fall from a height)

   a. The force is directed axially through the talus into the tibial plafond, causing impaction of the articular surface; may be associated with significant comminution.

   b. If the fibula remains intact, the ankle is forced into varus with impaction of the medial plafond.

   c. Plantar flexion or dorsiflexion of the ankle at the time of injury results in a primarily posterior or anterior plafond injury, respectively.

3: Trauma

2. Shear (low energy; for example, twisting injury)

  a. The mechanism is primarily torsion combined with a varus or valgus stress, producing two or more large fragments and minimal articular comminution.

  b. Usually, an associated fibular fracture is present, which is usually transverse or short oblique.

3. Combined compression and shear

  a. These fracture patterns demonstrate components of both compression and shear.

  b. The vector of the two forces determines the fracture pattern.

F. Clinical evaluation

1. Clinical evaluation of fractures of the tibial plafond includes an examination of the neurologic and vascular status of the entire limb.

2. An assessment of the stability and alignment of the ankle joint is useful. The orientation of the ankle is observed, including its length, alignment, and rotation.

3. The skin may be placed at risk by bone fragments that cause pressure on the skin and soft-tissue envelope; therefore, areas of blanching, abrasion, and contusion should be examined.

4. Large blood-filled fracture blisters should be noted, because they frequently preclude immediate ORIF.

G. Imaging

1. Plain radiographs

  a. The standard trauma series of the ankle includes AP, lateral, and mortise view radiographs centered on the joint.

  b. The AP view demonstrates the amount of articular impaction and shortening; the lateral view also demonstrates articular incongruity and is useful for determining the position of the posterior articular segment.

  c. Full-length views of the entire tibia and fibula rule out more proximal injury and assess the extent of metadiaphyseal involvement.

2. Computed tomography

  a. CT is essential for the proper evaluation of tibial plafond fractures.

  b. CT aids in identifying fracture fragments not seen on plain radiographs, assists in determining the extent of articular comminution, and is critical for planning surgery and guiding surgical approaches.

  c. CT may assist in determining whether a fracture can be reduced percutaneously or an open

approach is required.

  d. If temporary external fixation is planned, CT done following application of the external fixator and realignment of the limb provides the best information. If definitive external fixation is selected, the CT should be obtained preoperatively.

H. Nonsurgical treatment

1. Nonsurgical care is less common for tibial plafond fractures than for ankle fractures.

2. Indications

  a. Stable fracture patterns without displacement of the articular surface are treated nonsurgically; the nonsurgical treatment of fractures with articular displacement generally has yielded poor results.

  b. Nonambulatory patients or patients with significant neuropathy may be treated nonsurgically as well.

3. Nonsurgical treatment consists of casting for 6 weeks followed by a fracture brace and range-of-motion exercises, versus early range-of-motion exercises.

  a. Manipulation of displaced fractures is unlikely to result in the reduction of intra-articular fragments.

  b. Loss of reduction is common.

  c. The inability to monitor soft-tissue status and swelling is a major disadvantage.

I. Surgical treatment

1. Most treatment strategies for tibial plafond fractures currently are related to the safe management of the soft tissues.

2. External or internal fixation is used.

3. External fixation

  a. General issues

    • As definitive treatment, external fixation uses limited approaches to reduce the articular surface with minimal internal fixation of the joint surface.

    • It may bridge the ankle or may be localized to the distal tibia.

    • External fixation that spans the ankle may involve less disruption of the zone of injury, but it has the disadvantage of rigidly immobilizing the ankle.

    • Hybrid external fixation applied to a tibial side of the ankle joint allows greater motion at the ankle. The placement of pins and wires often disrupts the zone of injury.

- An additional alternative is articulated fixation, which allows some motion at the ankle but may be difficult to apply because the axis of the hinge of the fixator must correspond to the axis of the ankle joint.

  b. Techniques for application of definitive external fixation

    - In an ankle-bridging technique, pins are placed initially in the calcaneus and talar neck and proximal pins are placed in the medial subcutaneous border of the tibia.

    - A fixator is then placed, and the articular surface is reduced provisionally with ligamentotaxis.

    - Fracture reduction forceps or clamps can then be placed percutaneously directly over the fracture lines to reduce displaced fragments.

    - Articular fragments are stabilized using lag screws.

    - The external fixator is used to maintain length, alignment, and rotation of the extremity and to protect the joint as fracture healing occurs.

    - This technique preserves soft tissues and can be staged if necessary when the zone of injury is not thought to be safe enough to tolerate the limited approaches required for reduction.

4. Internal fixation

  a. General

    - Internal fixation using definitive plate fixation of high-energy tibial plafond fractures continues to evolve.

    - Initial successes using this technique, described by Rüedi and Allgöwer, were followed by many reports of failure, with the incidence of wound complications approaching 40% in large series of patients with high-energy tibial plafond fractures.

  b. Tips for minimizing complications

    - Various techniques have been recommended for minimizing the complications of plating, including delaying definitive surgical treatment using spanning external fixation until the soft tissues have settled; using lower-profile implants; minimizing anteromedial incisions; indirect reduction techniques that minimize soft-tissue stripping; and patient selection based on the injury pattern as necessary.

    - Recent literature has questioned the old guidelines regarding the distance between incisions about the ankle. It appears to be acceptable to place incisions closer to one another than previously believed.

    - With consideration of these principles, the rate of wound complications reported in more recent series ranges from 0% to 6%, down from the rates upward of 33% to 50% previously seen.

    - Using locked plates and percutaneously applied plates may further improve results.

  c. Definitive internal fixation is performed in two stages.

    - Stage 1—Fibular plating to regain lateral column length and application of a simple spanning external fixator.

      ○ Two proximal half-pins are placed on the anterior tibia.

      ○ Placing pins within or outside of the future zone of surgery is controversial and has not been definitively shown to affect complication rates.

      ○ A 5- or 6-mm centrally threaded pin can be placed across the calcaneus and attached to the proximal half-pins using a combination of struts. This technique is simple to perform and maintains stability and alignment. Extra care is necessary to avoid pressure from bony fragments on soft tissues, prevent shortening, and maintain forefoot positioning.

    - Typically, a delay of approximately 2 weeks is needed to allow the soft tissues to settle.

    - Stage 2—Formal articular reduction and internal fixation

      ○ Once ORIF is performed, incisions are made only as large as required to anatomically reduce the articular surface. Periosteal stripping is performed only at the edges of the fracture to achieve visualization of the reduction while preserving the blood supply.

      ○ Precontoured plates may be useful; both anteromedial and anterolateral plates facilitate percutaneous placement. Locking plates may be of benefit, particularly when articular surface comminution is present.

      ○ Void filling with bone graft or substitutes to fill metaphyseal voids was once described as a standard step in fixation of a tibial plafond fracture; however, with less extensive dissection in the metaphyseal region, the indications for grafting have become less routine.

5. Pearls are described in **Table 3**.

3: Trauma

Table 3

Pearls for the Treatment of Tibial Plafond Fractures

Treatment Step	Pearls
Soft-tissue management	Avoid surgery when swollen Use spanning fixator to control alignment and soft tissues
Spanning fixator	Simple construct Tibial pins should avoid future surgical site Reestablish length and alignment
Definitive open reduction and internal fixation	Approach guided by CT Limited incisions, avoid periosteal stripping Restore alignment and anatomically reduce joint Use distractor intraoperatively to facilitate reduction. Low-profile implants

J. Rehabilitation

1. Rehabilitation after tibial plafond fractures is prolonged. Patients should be counseled that weight bearing may be delayed for 3 months or more.

2. In patients treated by external fixation, the healing time is generally 12 to 16 weeks.

3. Tibial plafond fractures have a significant deleterious long-term effect on ankle function and quality of life. Worse outcomes are seen when complications occur.

4. When possible, motion of the ankle joint should be permitted and facilitated.

5. The use of a removable boot or brace may be of benefit as the patient transitions from immobilization and non–weight bearing to mobilization and protected weight-bearing status.

K. Complications

1. Malunion

   a. Malalignment of the tibia is relatively common.

   b. Articular malunion is probably even more common than recognized.

   c. Series using definitive external fixation have reported an increased incidence of fair or poor articular reduction compared with formal ORIF.

   d. Angular malalignment also may occur. Loss of alignment following treatment occurs in particular if union is delayed and implant failure occurs.

2. Nonunion and delayed union

   a. The rate of delayed union and nonunion for tibial plafond fractures is difficult to determine because surgical implants obscure radiographic visualization of the fracture.

   b. Some series report nonunion rates of approximately 5%.

   c. More comminuted fractures, open fractures, and fractures with greater devascularization of the fracture fragments are more likely to lead to nonunion; for this reason, soft-tissue dissection should be minimized.

3. Infection and wound breakdown

   a. Infection and wound breakdown is a devastating complication.

   b. Wound breakdown almost always is severe and frequently leads to unfavorable outcomes.

   c. The cost of treating this complication is extremely high because multiple surgical procedures are required, and amputation may be needed.

   d. Using modern techniques of soft-tissue preservation whenever possible appears to have substantially reduced the rate of infection and wound breakdown, but some risk of infection and wound breakdown remains. Patients should be counseled about this risk before surgical treatment of a tibial plafond fracture is undertaken.

4. Ankle arthritis

   a. Significant arthrosis of the ankle joint is common after tibial plafond fractures.

      • In one study, arthrosis was found in 74% of patients 5 to 11 years postinjury.

      • Arthrosis most commonly begins within 1 or 2 years postinjury.

   b. The presence of radiographic arthritis does not always correlate well with subjective clinical results, and, despite the devastating impact to the articular surface and the problems associated with fracture of the tibial plafond, arthrodesis is not commonly required until many years after the injury.

Top Testing Facts

1. The talar dome is wider anteriorly than posteriorly.

2. The superficial deltoid arises from the anterior colliculus, and the deep deltoid arises from the posterior colliculus of the medial malleolus.

3. According to the Ottawa ankle rules, ankle radiographs are indicated if the patient has an ankle injury and is older than 55 years, cannot bear weight, or has tenderness at the posterior edge or tip of either malleolus.

4. The best way to evaluate ankle stability associated with an isolated fibula fracture is a radiographic stress examination.

5. Fractures of the fibula are usually fixed first—before the medial malleolus, lateral malleolus, or syndesmosis—when treating ankle fractures surgically to obtain length.

6. A supination–external rotation type IV injury is associated with an unstable short spiral fracture at the distal fibula and a medial malleolus fracture or deltoid ligament disruption.

7. Posterior malleolar fractures involving more than 25% of the articular surface or posterior ankle instability should be reduced and stabilized.

8. The superficial peroneal nerve may be injured when using an anterolateral approach to treat a tibial plafond fracture.

9. Tibial plafond (pilon) fractures result from axial compression or shear.

10. Internal fixation of high-energy tibial plafond fractures should be delayed approximately 2 weeks after the injury, preceded by a period of temporary external fixation.

Bibliography

Amorosa LF, Brown GD, Greisberg J: A surgical approach to posterior pilon fractures. *J Orthop Trauma* 2010;24(3): 188-193.

Egol KA, Amirtharajah M, Tejwani NC, Capla EL, Koval KJ: Ankle stress test for predicting the need for surgical fixation of isolated fibular fractures. *J Bone Joint Surg Am* 2004; 86(11):2393-2398.

Egol KA, Pahk B, Walsh M, Tejwani NC, Davidovitch RI, Koval KJ: Outcome after unstable ankle fracture: Effect of syndesmotic stabilization. *J Orthop Trauma* 2010;24(1):7-11.

Graves ML, Kosko J, Barei DP, et al: Lateral ankle radiographs: Do we really understand what we are seeing? *J Orthop Trauma* 2011;25(2):106-109.

Honkanen R, Tuppurainen M, Kröger H, Alhava E, Saarikoski S: Relationships between risk factors and fractures differ by type of fracture: A population-based study of 12,192 perimenopausal women. *Osteoporos Int* 1998;8(1):25-31.

Jenkinson RJ, Sanders DW, Macleod MD, Domonkos A, Lydestadt J: Intraoperative diagnosis of syndesmosis injuries in external rotation ankle fractures. *J Orthop Trauma* 2005; 19(9):604-609.

Khurana S, Karia R, Egol KA: Operative treatment of nonunion following distal fibula and medial malleolar ankle fractures. *Foot Ankle Int* 2013;34(3):365-371.

Koval KJ, Lurie J, Zhou W, et al: Ankle fractures in the elderly: What you get depends on where you live and who you see. *J Orthop Trauma* 2005;19(9):635-639.

Lauge-Hansen N: Fractures of the ankle: II. Combined experimental-surgical and experimental-roentgenologic investigations. *Arch Surg* 1950;60(5):957-985.

Marsh JL, McKinley T, Dirschl D, et al: The sequential recovery of health status after tibial plafond fractures. *J Orthop Trauma* 2010;24(8):499-504.

McConnell T, Creevy W, Tornetta P III: Stress examination of supination external rotation-type fibular fractures. *J Bone Joint Surg Am* 2004;86(10):2171-2178.

Michelson JD, Varner KE, Checcone M: Diagnosing deltoid injury in ankle fractures: The gravity stress view. *Clin Orthop Relat Res* 2001;387:178-182.

Patterson MJ, Cole JD: Two-staged delayed open reduction and internal fixation of severe pilon fractures. *J Orthop Trauma* 1999;13(2):85-91.

Pollak AN, McCarthy ML, Bess RS, Agel J, Swiontkowski MF: Outcomes after treatment of high-energy tibial plafond fractures. *J Bone Joint Surg Am* 2003;85(10):1893-1900.

Sirkin M, Sanders R, DiPasquale T, Herscovici D Jr: A staged protocol for soft tissue management in the treatment of complex pilon fractures. *J Orthop Trauma* 1999;13(2):78-84.

Stiell IG, McKnight RD, Greenberg GH, et al: Implementation of the Ottawa ankle rules. *JAMA* 1994;271(11): 827-832.

Tochigi Y, Buckwalter JA, Martin JA, et al: Distribution and progression of chondrocyte damage in a whole-organ model of human ankle intra-articular fracture. *J Bone Joint Surg Am* 2011;93(6):533-539.

3: Trauma

Tornetta P III: Competence of the deltoid ligament in bimalleolar ankle fractures after medial malleolar fixation. *J Bone Joint Surg Am* 2000;82(6):843-848.

Tornetta P III, Weiner L, Bergman M, et al: Pilon fractures: Treatment with combined internal and external fixation. *J Orthop Trauma* 1993;7(6):489-496.

Chapter 43

Foot Trauma

Nirmal C. Tejwani, MD   Nelson Fong SooHoo, MD

I. Epidemiology

A. Calcaneal fractures are the most common fractures of the tarsal bones; many of these fractures involve the subtalar joint.

B. Fractures of the talus and fracture-dislocations of the midfoot are uncommon but can result in severe functional limitation.

C. Foot injuries are often missed in patients with polytrauma and are often a source of long-term disability.

II. Anatomy

A. Bones

1. The hindfoot includes the talus and calcaneus.

2. The midfoot includes the navicular, cuboid, and cuneiform bones and their articulations with the proximal metatarsal bones.

3. The forefoot includes the phalanges and distal metatarsal bones.

4. The heads of the first and fifth metatarsal bones and the calcaneus constitute a tripod necessary for foot stability.

B. Joints

1. The key joints in the foot for maintaining mobility are the hindfoot joints, including the tibiotalar, subtalar, and talonavicular articulations.

2. The lateral fourth and fifth tarsometatarsal joints

are important for normal foot function and are more mobile than other tarsometatarsal joints.

3. The remaining hindfoot and midfoot joints, including the calcaneocuboid and the first, second, and third tarsometatarsal joints, do not require a full range of motion (ROM) to maintain function of the foot.

4. The metatarsophalangeal (MTP) joints are important for gait and forefoot function. Motion of the interphalangeal joints is not critical for normal functioning of the foot.

III. Fractures of the Talus

A. Anatomy and blood supply of the talus

1. The talus consists of a head, neck, and body; it has five articulating surfaces, and 70% of its surface is covered by cartilage. The only muscle attached to the talus is the extensor digitorum brevis.

2. The limited blood supply to the talus puts the talar body at risk for osteonecrosis following fractures of the talar neck.

   a. Most of the blood supply to the body of the talus is from the artery of the tarsal canal, a branch of the posterior tibial artery.

   b. The deltoid artery in the deep portion of the deltoid ligament supplies blood to the medial portion of the body of the talus.

   c. Most of the blood supply to the head and neck of the talus is from the artery of the tarsal sinus, a branch of both the anterior tibial artery and peroneal artery.

B. Fractures of the talar neck

1. Mechanisms of injury

   a. Fractures of the talar neck occur with dorsiflexion of the talus against the tibia, usually as the result of a motor-vehicle accident or fall.

   b. Associated inversion with dorsiflexion can cause fracture of the medial malleolus, whereas eversion of the talus may be

Dr. Tejwani or an immediate family member has received royalties from Biomet; is a member of a speakers' bureau or has made paid presentations on behalf of Zimmer and Stryker; serves as a paid consultant to or is an employee of Zimmer and Stryker; and serves as a board member, owner, officer, or committee member of the American Academy of Orthopaedic Surgeons, the Orthopaedic Trauma Association, and the Foundation of Orthopaedic Trauma. Neither Dr. SooHoo nor any immediate family member has received anything of value from or has stock or stock options held in a commercial company or institution related directly or indirectly to the subject of this chapter.

3:Trauma

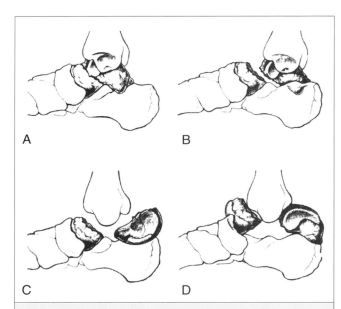

Figure 1 Hawkins classification of fractures of the talar neck. **A,** Type I: nondisplaced fracture of the talar neck. **B,** Type II: displaced fracture of the talar neck, with subluxation or dislocation of the subtalar joint. **C,** Type III: displaced fracture of the talar neck with associated dislocation of the body of the talus from both the subtalar and tibiotalar joints. **D,** Canale and Kelly type IV fracture: Displaced fracture of the talar neck with associated dislocation of the body of the talus from the subtalar and tibiotalar joints and dislocation of a fragment of the talar head/neck from the talonavicular joint. (Reproduced with permission from Sangeorzan BJ: Foot and ankle joint, in Hansen ST Jr, Swiontkowski MF, eds: *Orthopaedic Trauma Protocols.* New York, NY, Raven Press, 1993, p 350.)

associated with fracture of the lateral malleolus.

2. Radiographic evaluation

   a. Imaging studies in suspected or possible fractures of the talus should include three radiographic views (AP, lateral, and oblique) of the foot.

   b. CT is indicated if displacement cannot be ruled out on plain radiographs.

   c. MRI can be used to detect osteonecrosis or osteocartilaginous fragments of the talus.

3. Hawkins classification of fractures of the talar neck (**Figure 1**)

   a. Guides treatment decisions and helps predict the risk of osteonecrosis of the talus

   b. Types of Hawkins fracture are based on displacement of the fracture and the articulations of the talus

   c. Displaced type II, III, and IV fractures can in-

jure the arteries of the tarsal canal and tarsal sinus, creating the risk of osteonecrosis of the talar body.

4. Nonsurgical treatment

   a. Closed reduction of a talar fracture can be attempted by using plantar flexion with varus or valgus angulation of the heel, depending on the direction of displacement of the fracture fragments.

   b. Hawkins type I fractures are nondisplaced fractures of the talar neck and can be treated with casting and elimination of weight bearing on the affected foot, with follow-up radiographs to confirm maintenance of reduction.

5. Surgical treatment

   a. Urgent surgical treatment is required with open fractures of the talus or when subluxation or dislocation can result in soft-tissue compromise.

   b. Hawkins type I fractures may be treated with screws inserted percutaneously in a posterior-to-anterior direction.

   c. Open reduction and internal fixation (ORIF) (Hawkins types II, III, and IV fractures)

   - An anteromedial approach is combined with an anterolateral approach for adequate exposure of the fracture site. The anteromedial approach is between the posterior and anterior tibial tendons (**Figure 2**).

   - The sural nerve is encountered with a posterolateral approach through the interval of the peroneus brevis and flexor hallucis longus tendons.

   d. The talonavicular joint incongruity seen in type IV fractures should be reduced and pinned if unstable.

   e. Medial and/or lateral plating may be useful for comminuted talar fractures that may collapse with compression screws.

   f. Titanium screws are sometimes used for fixation, in allowing the use of MRI to evaluate for postoperative osteonecrosis.

6. Complications (**Table 1**)

   a. Posttraumatic arthritis is the most common complication of talar fractures and can affect the subtalar and/or tibiotalar joints.

   b. Osteonecrosis

   - The limited blood supply to the talus creates the risk of osteonecrosis with fractures of the talar neck.

   - The risk of osteonecrosis increases with each

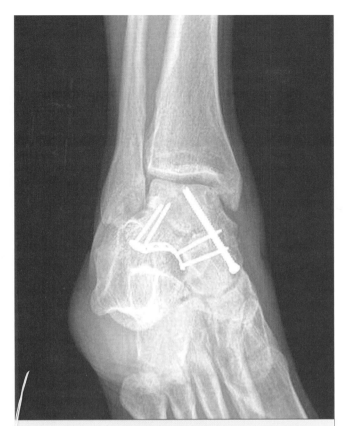

Figure 2   Postoperative radiograph of a fracture of the talus treated with medial screws and a lateral plate through two incisions.

Table 1

Complications of Talar Neck Fractures

Fracture Pattern	Osteonecrosis (%)	Posttraumatic Arthritis (%)	Malunion (%)
Type I	0–13	0–30	0–10
Type II	20–50	40–90	0–25
Type III/IV	80–100	70–100	18–27

Reproduced from Fortin PT, Balazsy JE: Talus fractures: Evaluation and treatment. *J Am Acad Orthop Surg* 2001;9:114-127.

successive Hawkins type of fracture. Restricting weight bearing beyond that needed for the healing of a fracture does not decrease the risk of osteonecrosis.

- The Hawkins sign, consisting of subchondral osteopenia seen at 6 to 8 weeks on plain radiographs, indicates revascularization of the talar body. It is 100% sensitive but only 58% specific for this and is therefore a reliable indicator of an intact blood supply when present, although its absence does not rule out an intact vascularity.

- Osteonecrosis of the talus may be seen as early as 3 to 6 months postoperatively on plain radiographs, accompanied by sclerosis. MRI is sensitive for detecting osteonecrosis, with decreased signal intensity on T1-weighted MRI, but rarely guides treatment.

- Osteonecrosis usually does not involve the entire talar body and often does not require further surgery. Tibiotalar fusion is an option for treating a talus damaged by osteonecrosis when nonsurgical treatment is unsuccessful.

- Extensive osteonecrosis may require excision of the talar body with tibiotalocalcaneal fusion or Blair fusion, which involves resection of the talar body with fusion of the talar head to the tibia and bone grafting for repair of the osteonecrotic defect to maintain overall limb length.

c. Varus malunion also can occur as a complication of a talar fracture and can limit eversion of the foot. It may be treated with a corrective osteotomy.

C. Fractures of the talar body

1. Fractures involving large portions of the talar body are usually the result of high-energy injuries.

2. CT provides the best visualization of fractures of the talar body and is used to identify fractures in the transverse, coronal, and sagittal planes.

3. ORIF with a dual lateral and medial approach is required when the articular surfaces of the talus are displaced by more than 2 mm. Medial and/or lateral malleolar osteotomy may be required for ORIF.

4. A posteromedial or posterolateral approach to fracture repair, with dorsiflexion and distraction, can expose most of the talar dome.

5. Complications of fractures of the talar body include posttraumatic arthritis (occurring in as many as 88% of cases) and osteonecrosis. Posttraumatic osteoarthritis is the most common complication.

D. Fractures of the lateral process of the talus

1. These fractures occur with dorsiflexion–external rotation injuries. A common mechanism is a snowboarding injury.

2. AP radiographs may show the fracture, but a CT scan may be needed to adequately visualize these injuries and for surgical planning.

3. Nondisplaced fractures of the lateral process of the talus can be treated with immobilization in a

3: Trauma

cast and no weight bearing.

4. ORIF is indicated for fractures displaced by more than 2 mm. Comminuted fractures not amenable to ORIF can be treated with casting. Excision of the fracture fragment is an option if symptoms persist.

5. The most common complication of fractures of the lateral process is posttraumatic subtalar arthritis.

E. Fractures of the posterior process of the talus

1. The posterior process of the talus includes a posteromedial and a posterolateral tubercle. Plain radiographs may not clearly show the area of fracture, whereas CT is useful for identifying these fractures.

2. Fractures of the posteromedial tubercle result from avulsion of the posterior talotibial ligament or posterior deltoid ligament.

   a. Small fragments of fractures of the posteromedial tubercle are treated with immobilization followed by late excision if symptoms persist.

   b. Large, displaced fragments are treated with ORIF.

3. Fractures of the posterolateral tubercle result from avulsion of the posterior talofibular ligament. Pain is aggravated by flexion and extension of the flexor hallucis longus tendon.

   a. Initial nonsurgical management with late excision for symptomatic lesions is indicated for fractures with no subtalar involvement.

   b. ORIF is indicated for fractures with subtalar involvement.

4. Nonunion in fractures of the posterior process of the talus is difficult to distinguish from symptomatic os trigonum. Both conditions can be treated with excision.

IV. Fractures of the Calcaneus

A. Intra-articular fractures

1. Mechanisms of injury

   a. The calcaneus is the most frequently fractured of the tarsal bones. Most (75%) of fractures of the calcaneus are intra-articular.

   b. Axial loading is the primary mechanism of fracture of the calcaneus, with falls from a height and motor vehicle accidents the most common causes of such loading.

   c. An oblique shear force causing fracture of the calcaneus results in a primary fracture line and two primary fragments:

   • The superomedial fragment includes the sustentaculum, which is stabilized by strong ligamentous and capsular attachments. This is called the constant fragment because it retains its anatomic position, making it a useful reference point for fracture reduction.

   • The superolateral fragment has an intraarticular component through the posterior facet and posterolateral tuberosity of the calcaneus.

   d. Secondary fracture lines signal whether there is joint depression or a tongue-type fracture. The two types of fracture are defined by whether or not the superolateral fragment and posterior facet of the calcaneus are separated from the posterolateral tuberosity. In tongue-type fractures, the superolateral fragment and posterior facet are attached posteriorly to the tuberosity.

2. Radiographic evaluation

   a. The lateral view of the foot and ankle can be used to determine the Böhler angle (normally 20° to 40°) and to assess loss of height. Double density of the posterior facet indicates subtalar incongruity.

   b. AP and oblique views can show the calcaneocuboid joint.

   c. The Broden view helps intraoperatively evaluate reduction of the posterior facet.

   d. The axial Harris view reveals widening, shortening, lateral translation, and varus positioning of the tuberosity fragment of a calcaneal fracture.

   e. An AP view of the ankle is useful for assessing extrusion of the lateral wall of the calcaneus with impingement against the fibula or peroneal tendons.

3. Sanders classification of calcaneal fractures (**Figure 3**)

   a. Used to guide treatment and to predict outcome of treatment of calcaneal fractures

   b. Based on CT visualization of the widest portion of the subtalar joint in the coronal oblique plane and the number of fracture fragments of the posterior facet of the calcaneus

   • Type I fractures: nondisplaced

   • Type II fractures: the posterior facet is in two fragments.

   • Type III fractures: the posterior facet is in three fragments.

   • Type IV fractures: comminuted, with more than three articular fragments

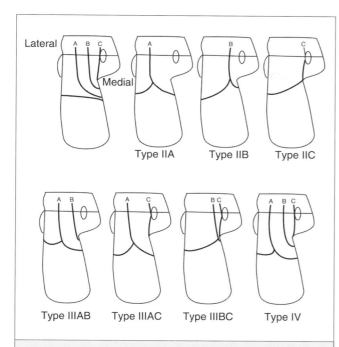

Figure 3   CT-based classification of displaced intra-articular calcaneal fractures. The first drawing shows the lateral (A), central (B), and medial (C) fracture lines. Type I (not shown) = nondisplaced calcaneal fracture. Type II = DIACF with a single displaced primary fracture line in the posterior facet. Type III = DIACF with two displaced fracture lines into the posterior facet. Type IV = comminuted DIACF with three or more displaced fracture lines in the posterior facet. This classification is prognostic (P = 0.06). (Reproduced from Buckley RE, Tough S: Displaced intra-articular calcaneal fractures. *J Am Acad Orthop Surg* 2004;12[3]:172-178.)

c. Other important characteristics of calcaneal features according to the Sanders classification include the degrees of shortening, widening, and lateral wall impingement, which may result in pathology of the peroneal tendon.

4. Nonsurgical treatment

a. Type I fractures are treated nonsurgically.

b. Patients do not bear weight for 6 to 8 weeks.

c. ROM exercises are initiated early, as soon as soft-tissue swelling allows.

5. Surgical treatment

a. Treatment of type II and III fractures remains controversial. Both ORIF and nonsurgical management have been advocated; nonsurgical management is the same as that for type I fractures. Improved outcomes are associated with age younger than 40 years, female sex, and simple fracture patterns. Negative factors include smoking, diabetes, workers' compensation, carrying heavy physical work loads, and comminution of fractures.

b. ORIF is generally delayed for 10 to 14 days to allow resolution of soft-tissue swelling (with the exception of fractures of the posterior tuberosity, which can cause skin tenting and may benefit from early surgery) (**Figure 4**).

- An extensile lateral L-shaped incision is the most common approach in the ORIF of calcaneal fractures.

- No-touch retraction techniques are used, a pin is placed in the tuberosity fragment to assist reduction, and a drain is inserted.

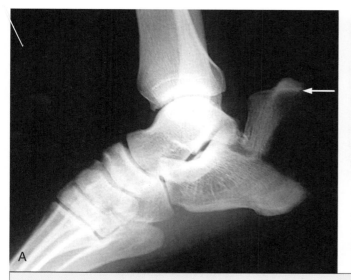
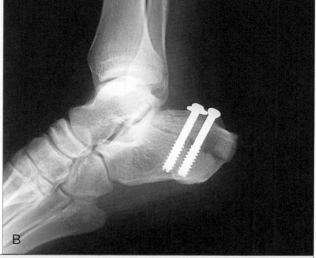

Figure 4   Lateral radiographs demonstrate avulsion of the calcaneal tuberosity requiring urgent reduction and fixation to prevent skin necrosis (arrow). Preoperative (**A**) and postoperative (**B**) views.

3: Trauma

- Bone grafting (autografting or allografting) has not been shown to be beneficial in treating calcaneal fractures. Injectable calcium phosphate cement has been shown to permit early weight bearing without loss of articular reduction.

    c. Type IV fractures can be treated through ORIF with possible primary fusion; ORIF alone (as well as nonsurgical treatment) is associated with poor results.

    d. Outcomes correlate with the accuracy of fracture reduction and the number of articular fragments. Type II fractures have better outcomes than type III fractures, whereas type IV fractures have the poorest outcomes.

6. Complications

    a. A complication rate of up to 40% has been reported in fractures of the calcaneus. Factors that increase the risk of complications include falls from a height, early surgery, and smoking. Approximately 10% of patients have associated injuries of the lumbar spine.

    b. Wound-related complications are the most common complications of calcaneal fractures. Other potential complications include malunion, subtalar arthritis, and lateral impingement with pathology of the peroneal tendon.

    c. Compartment syndrome develops in up to 10% of patients and may lead to a clawtoe deformity.

    d. Malunion can occur and result in loss of height and in widening of the heel and lateral impingement.

    - The talus may be dorsiflexed, with a decrease in the declination angle of the talus to less than 20°, which limits dorsiflexion of the ankle.

    - Impingement of the lateral wall associated with malunion may result in pathology of the peroneal tendon. Additionally, subtalar incongruity can result in subtalar arthritis. Difficulty with shoe wear also can occur, as a result of widening of the heel and loss of height. Malunions of the calcaneus are treated with lateral exostectomy. Fusion is also added to treat subtalar arthritis.

B. Extra-articular fractures (posterior tuberosity of the calcaneus)

    1. Mechanism of injury—Strong contraction of the gastrocnemius–soleus muscle complex and avulsion at its insertion on the posterior tuberosity of the calcaneus

    2. Treatment

    a. Early reduction is important because displaced fractures of the posterior tuberosity can cause pressure necrosis of the overlying skin.

    b. Full-thickness skin sloughing may require flap coverage.

    c. Small fracture fragments can be excised, but fractures with larger fragments require ORIF. Note, however, that screw fixation alone may fail in osteopenic bone but can be augmented with tension band fixation.

C. Fractures of the anterior process

    1. Mechanism of injury

    a. Inversion and plantar flexion

    b. Fractures result from avulsion of the bifurcate ligament.

    2. Treatment

    a. Small extra-articular fragments are treated with immobilization.

    b. Larger fragments (>1 cm) can involve the calcaneocuboid joint and require ORIF if joint displacement is present.

    c. Late excision is used for chronically painful nonunion.

V. Midfoot Fractures

A. Fractures of the navicular bone

    1. Anatomy

    a. The navicular bone articulates with the medial, intermediate, and lateral cuneiform bones, the cuboid bone, and the calcaneus and talus.

    b. The talonavicular articulation is critical to maintaining the ROM of inversion and eversion of the foot.

    c. The blood supply to the navicular bone is limited in its central watershed portion, making this area susceptible to fractures.

    2. Radiographic evaluation

    a. Plain radiographs including AP, lateral, internal oblique, and external oblique images of the foot are used for the initial evaluation of navicular fractures.

    b. CT is useful for characterizing the fracture pattern. MRI can be used for the detection of stress fractures.

    3. Avulsion fractures of the navicular bone

    a. Constitute one half of all navicular fractures; avulsion of the dorsal lip results from stress

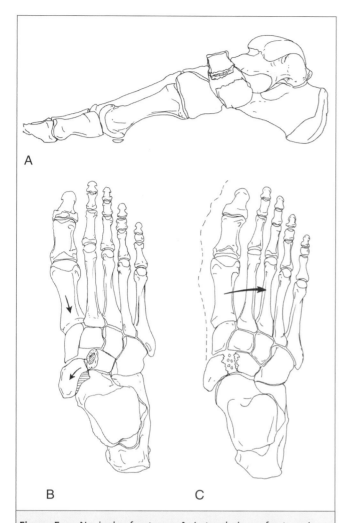

Figure 5 Navicular fractures. **A,** Lateral view of a type I navicular fracture (axial plane fracture line). **B,** AP view of a type II navicular fracture (sagittal plane fracture line). The arrows indicate the direction of applied force. Note the subluxation of the talonavicular joint and proximal migration of the first ray, a common component of type II fractures. **C,** AP view of a type III navicular fracture. Note the comminution, displacement, and incongruity of the talonavicular and naviculocuneiform joints. The arrow indicates the direction of applied force. (Reproduced from Stroud CC: Fractures of the midtarsals, metatarsals, and phalanges, in Richardson EG, ed: *Orthopaedic Knowledge Update: Foot and Ankle*, ed 3. Rosemont, IL, American Academy of Orthopaedic Surgeons, 2003, p 58.)

Table 2

Sangeorzan Classification of Navicular Fractures

Type	Features
I	Transverse Involves a dorsal fragment < 50% of the bone No associated deformity
II	Oblique Most commonly from dorsal-lateral to plantar-medial May be associated with forefoot adduction
III	Central or lateral comminution with abduction May be associated with cuboid or anterior process calcaneal fractures

involving more than 25% of the articular surface.

4. Fractures of the tuberosity of the navicular bone

   a. The principal mechanism of fracture is eversion and contraction of the posterior tibial tendon, which may result in the diastasis of a preexisting accessory navicular bone.

   b. Best visualized on an oblique radiograph and at 45° of internal rotation

   c. Most avulsion fractures of the tuberosity can be managed with immobilization.

   d. Acute ORIF is indicated with more than 5 mm of diastasis or with large intra-articular fracture fragments.

   e. Symptomatic nonunion is treated with late excision and reattachment of the tibialis posterior tendon.

5. Fractures of the navicular body (**Figure 5**)

   a. Mechanism of injury is axial loading.

   b. The Sangeorzan classification of fractures of the body of the navicular bone is based on the plane of the fracture and the degree of comminution (**Table 2**).

   c. Minimally displaced type I and II fractures are treated nonsurgically.

   d. ORIF through a medial incision is used for displaced type I and II fractures or with disruption of the talonavicular joint.

   e. Type III fractures require ORIF. A spanning external fixator or plate may be used to maintain the length of the medial column of the foot after fixation of the primary fracture fragments.

6. Stress fractures of the navicular bone

imposed by the deltoid ligament during eversion of the foot; medial avulsion results from stress imposed by the tibialis posterior muscle; plantar avulsion results from stress imposed by the spring ligament.

   b. Acute treatment consists of immobilization with delayed excision of painful fragments.

   c. ORIF is required for fractures with fragments

3: Trauma

a. Most common in runners and basketball players

b. When acute, these injuries can be treated either nonsurgically or surgically. Nonunion requires ORIF. Bone grafting may be used to encourage healing.

B. Tarsometatarsal (Lisfranc) fracture-dislocations

1. Anatomy

a. The bones of the midfoot include the navicular, cuboid, cuneiform bones, and bases of the metatarsal bones.

b. The midfoot has osseous stability through the recessed articulation of the base of the second metatarsal bone. The trapezoidal shape of the bases of the first three metatarsal bones contributes to stability of the foot, as do the plantar ligaments. The Lisfranc ligament runs from the base of the second metatarsal to the medial cuneiform bone.

c. The lateral tarsometatarsal joints (fourth and fifth metatarsal-cuboid joints) have 10° of motion in the sagittal plane. The medial three tarsometatarsal joints have limited motion.

d. Approximately 20% to 30% of tarsometatarsal fracture-dislocations may be missed in cases of multiple trauma.

2. Mechanisms of injury

a. Direct tarsometatarsal fracture-dislocations occur with dorsal force and may result in soft-tissue injuries and compartment syndromes. Involvement of both bony and soft-tissue components is common in direct injuries.

b. Indirect tarsometatarsal fracture-dislocations occur with axial loading and twisting on a loaded, plantarflexed foot. Patients commonly report a history of a fixed foot with rotation of the body around the midfoot.

3. Radiographic evaluation

a. Internal oblique, AP, and lateral views of the foot should be obtained.

b. Normal anatomic relationships should be maintained.

- The medial aspect of the second metatarsal should be aligned with the medial aspect of the middle cuneiform bone.

- The medial aspect of the fourth metatarsal should be aligned with the medial cuboid bone.

- Diastasis of greater than 2 mm between the base of the first and second metatarsal bones is pathologic.

- There should be no dorsal subluxation of the bases of the metatarsal bones on the lateral view.

c. The fleck sign is a small avulsed fragment of bone in the interval between the bases of the first and second metatarsal bones. This represents avulsion of the Lisfranc ligament from its insertion on the base of the second metatarsal.

d. Weight-bearing or stress radiographs can be obtained when the results of physical examination and plain radiography are equivocal.

4. Fracture classification—Tarsometatarsal injuries are divided into three categories (**Figure 6**).

a. Type A injuries: total incongruity of the midfoot joints. The most common direction of such incongruity is lateral, and homolateral injuries may be associated with compression fractures of the cuboid bone.

b. Type B injuries: partial incongruity of the midfoot joints. Common patterns include medial dislocation of the first metatarsal or lateral dislocation of some or all of the lateral rays.

c. Type C injuries: divergent incongruity of the midfoot joints in which the first metatarsal and some or all of the lateral rays displace in opposite directions.

5. Treatment

a. ORIF is indicated for displaced midfoot fractures and dislocations.

- One or two dorsal incisions can be used. The neurovascular bundle is lateral to the first metatarsal interspace. The medial three tarsometatarsal joints are stabilized with fully threaded screws or bridging plates after anatomic reduction.

- Percutaneous pins are commonly used in the fourth and fifth tarsometatarsal joints if there is no comminution or shortening (**Figure 7**).

b. Plate fixation or external fixation may be used for compression fractures of the cuboid bone (nutcracker injury) to maintain the length of the lateral column of the foot.

c. Reduction and screw fixation is indicated to stabilize intercuneiform instability.

d. Primary fusion has been advocated as an option in midfoot fractures, and recent studies show that it provides better results than fixation.

e. Late reconstruction of missed injuries (up to 30% of tarsometatarsal injuries) may include fusion of the first three tarsometatarsal joints.

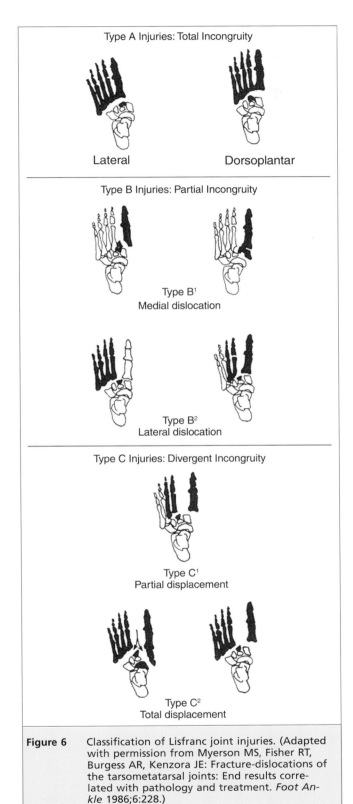

Type A Injuries: Total Incongruity

Lateral   Dorsoplantar

Type B Injuries: Partial Incongruity

Type B¹
Medial dislocation

Type B²
Lateral dislocation

Type C Injuries: Divergent Incongruity

Type C¹
Partial displacement

Type C²
Total displacement

Figure 6   Classification of Lisfranc joint injuries. (Adapted with permission from Myerson MS, Fisher RT, Burgess AR, Kenzora JE: Fracture-dislocations of the tarsometatarsal joints: End results correlated with pathology and treatment. *Foot Ankle* 1986;6:228.)

6. Complications

    a. Late posttraumatic osteoarthritis is common in tarsometatarsal injuries, occurring in up to

58% of patients. Anatomic reduction, open injury, and comminution predict outcomes.

    b. More than 2 mm or 15° of displacement is associated with a poorer prognosis.

    c. Purely ligamentous injuries also may have a poorer prognosis, leading some to advocate primary fusion as an alternative treatment for tarsometatarsal fracture-dislocations.

C. Fractures of the cuboid bone

1. Compression fractures of the cuboid bone resulting from a nutcracker mechanism can be part of a Lisfranc fracture-dislocation; isolated fractures of the cuboid bone are uncommon.

2. Oblique radiographs (oblique view with 30° internal rotation of the foot) and CT scans help identify and define the pattern of a fracture.

3. Fractures of the cuboid bone with substantial compression can result in collapse of the lateral column of the foot.

    a. External fixation can be used to restore length of the lateral column and disimpact fragments.

    b. Fixation and bone grafting may be required for impacted fractures of the cuboid bone.

    c. Avulsion fractures are treated symptomatically.

VI. Metatarsal and Phalangeal Fractures

A. Fractures of the first metatarsal bone

1. Mechanisms of injury include a direct blow, avulsion, twisting, or inversion.

2. The first metatarsal bone bears 40% of the weight of the foot (half on each sesamoid bone)

3. Indications for surgical treatment

    a. Displacement of more than 2 mm or intra-articular fracture. Proximal fractures are usually associated with Lisfranc injuries and require surgical repair.

    b. Malunion may result in dysfunction with plantar flexion of the foot, and shortening results in transfer metatarsalgia.

4. Options for fracture fixation include Kirschner wires (K-wires), screws, or plates. Fusion of the first tarsometatarsal joint may be needed for comminuted fractures or those in which diagnosis is late.

B. Fractures of the metatarsal neck and head (second to fourth metatarsal bones)

1. Most fractures of the metatarsal neck can be treated nonsurgically. Fractures of the metatarsal

3: Trauma

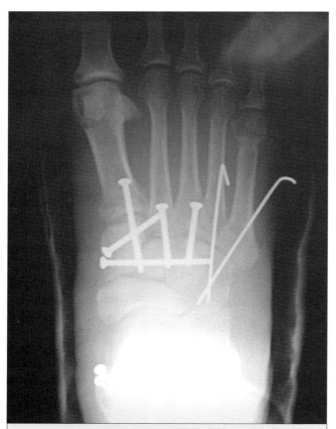

Figure 7 Radiograph demonstrating fixation of a Lisfranc injury with screws for the first, second, and third tarsometatarsal joints; Lisfranc joint and inter-cuneiform joints; and Kirschner wires for the fourth and fifth tarso-metatarsal joints.

neck in which there is severe angulation and plantar prominence may require reduction and fixation. Fractures in which there is dorsal angulation may require either closed or open reduction with fixation to prevent transfer metatarsalgia.

2. Fractures of the metatarsal head are rare and can generally be treated nonsurgically; however, severely displaced fractures may require closed or open reduction and fixation.

3. Stress fractures of the neck of the second metatarsal are commonly seen in athletes or military recruits and are treated nonsurgically, with posttreatment avoidance of impact exercises. Stress fractures of the proximal metatarsals may be seen in dancers.

4. Multiple displaced fractures of the metatarsals with shortening of more than 3 or 4 mm may result in loss of the normal "cascade" of the metatarsal heads and to pain. These fractures usually require restoration of metatarsal length and fixation.

C. Fractures of the fifth metatarsal

1. Type I fractures

   a. Avulsion of the long plantar ligament, the lateral band of the plantar fascia, or contraction of the peroneus brevis may result in type I fractures of the fifth metatarsal (pseudo-Jones fracture).

   b. Treatment consists of weight bearing as tolerated in a stiff-soled shoe.

   c. Surgery may be necessary, although rarely, for fractures with large displaced intra-articular fragments.

   d. Nonunion is uncommon, but can be treated by excision and repair of the peroneus brevis tendon, as needed.

2. Type II fractures

   a. The metadiaphyseal region of the fifth metatarsal is an area of circulatory watershed resulting in a limited blood supply to this region. Fractures at the metadiaphyseal junction, approximately 1.5 to 2.5 cm distal to the base of the fifth metatarsal, are commonly called Jones fractures (**Figure 8**).

   b. Because of the compromised blood supply in the metadiaphyseal region of the fifth metatarsal, fractures in this region are at risk of nonunion. Therefore, patients with such fractures should not bear weight for 6 to 8 weeks.

   c. Acute ORIF with screws, together with prolonged restriction of activity, is often used in athletes to minimize the possibility of nonunion of a type II fracture.

3. Type III fractures

   a. Type III fractures are stress fractures of the diaphysis of the fifth metatarsal. Cavovarus deformities of the foot increase the mobility of the first tarsometatarsal joint, increasing stress in the lateral column of the foot and predisposing to such fractures.

   b. Hereditary sensorimotor neuropathy and diabetic neuropathy may predispose to type III fractures by causing inability to sense overloading of the fifth metatarsal bone.

   c. Nonsurgical treatment, consisting of nonweight bearing, is used for proximal fractures in the vascular watershed area of the fourth and fifth metatarsals.

   d. Screw fixation is indicated for the repair of type III fractures in patients with established sclerosis and nonunion, and in athletes.

   e. Bone grafting and/or structural correction may be needed to achieve the healing of type III fractures and prevent their recurrence, particularly in cases of atrophic nonunion.

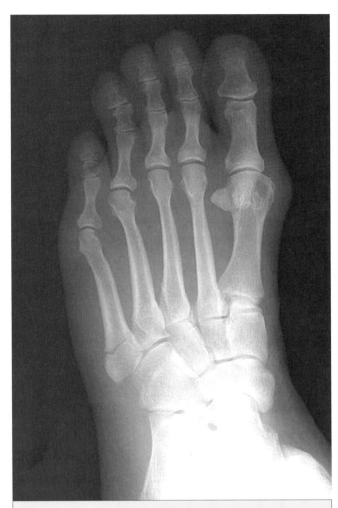

Figure 8   PA radiograph of a Jones fracture.

D. Phalangeal fractures

1. Mechanism of fracture is a crush injury or axial loading.

2. Painful subungual hematoma may be associated with distal phalangeal fracture and is usually treated nonsurgically; it can be evacuated through a hole in the nail.

3. Nonsurgical treatment consisting of closed reduction and buddy taping for 4 weeks generally is indicated for lesser injuries of the toes.

4. Surgical treatment is indicated for displaced articular injuries or angulated proximal phalangeal fractures of the hallux if closed reduction and percutaneous pinning fail. A failed closed reduction can be converted to an ORIF performed through an L-shaped incision dorsally.

E. Injuries to the sesamoid bone

1. Injuries can result from direct impact with compression, through hyperdorsiflexion with a transverse fracture, or with repetitive trauma.

2. Plain radiographs can include a sesamoid view to evaluate the articulation of the sesamoid bone with the plantar aspect of the metatarsal head. MRI is useful in determining the presence of a stress reaction or stress fracture.

3. Acute fractures or stress fractures of the sesamoid bone are treated with padding and immobilization in a hard-soled shoe for 4 to 8 weeks.

4. Excision of the sesamoid is used in cases of chronic symptomatic nonunion. The potential complication of medial sesamoidectomy is hallux valgus, whereas lateral sesamoidectomy may result in varus deformity of the hallux.

VII. Dislocations of the Foot

A. Subtalar dislocation

1. Mechanism of injury

a. Subtalar dislocations are high-energy injuries, but are closed in 75% of patients.

b. Most dislocations (65% to 80%) are medial, with the calcaneus translated medially. The remaining dislocations are generally lateral; anterior or posterior dislocation is rare.

2. Radiographic evaluation—CT is necessary after the reduction of a subtalar dislocation to rule out associated fractures and intra-articular fragments that may require surgery.

3. Treatment

a. Closed reduction of a subtalar dislocation is performed by flexing the patient's knee, recreating the deformity caused by the dislocation, plantarflexing the foot, and pushing on the head of the talus.

b. Medial dislocations that cannot be reduced are the result of buttonholing of the talus through the extensor digitorum brevis or talonavicular capsule and/or interposition of the peroneal tendons.

c. Lateral dislocations that cannot be reduced are the result of interposition of the posterior tibial tendon and buttonholing through the talonavicular capsule.

d. Open reduction with tendon relocation and stabilization with transarticular pins, as needed, is indicated for dislocations that cannot be reduced.

e. The most common long-term complication of subtalar dislocation is subtalar arthritis.

B. Midtarsal dislocation

1. Midtarsal dislocation involving the talonavicular and calcaneocuboid articulations (Chopart joint) can occur through axial loading (longitudinal) or crush injury.

2. Treatment involves prompt reduction to avoid skin necrosis. Displaced or subluxated joints should be reduced and pinned with K-wires if unstable.

C. Isolated tarsal dislocations

1. Isolated dislocations of the talonavicular joint, navicular bone, calcaneocuboid joint, cuboid bone, and cuneiform bones are uncommon.

2. Treatment involves prompt closed or open reduction to avoid skin necrosis. K-wires may be required to secure anatomic reduction.

D. Forefoot dislocations

1. First MTP joint

a. Dislocations of the first MTP joint are usually dorsal. Such dislocations are uncommon because of the thick plantar ligamentous complex.

b. Closed reduction is usually attempted first, but may not be possible if the first metatarsal bone buttonholes through the sesamoid–short flexor complex.

c. A dorsal approach is used for open reduction if necessary.

2. Lesser MTP joints

a. Dislocations are usually dorsal.

b. Closed reduction is usually attempted first, but may not be possible if the metatarsal head buttonholes through the plantar plate mechanism.

c. A dorsal incision is used for open reduction if needed.

3. Interphalangeal joints

a. Dislocations are uncommon and usually dorsal.

b. Closed reduction is usually attempted first, but may not be possible if the proximal phalanx buttonholes through the plantar plate.

c. A dorsal approach is used for open reduction if necessary.

VIII. Compartment Syndromes

A. Anatomy/pathophysiology

1. The foot has a total of nine compartments, which are divided into the following four main groups: medial (one compartment), lateral (one compart-

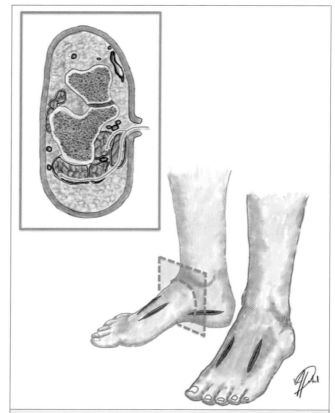

Figure 9   Illustration of the feet demonstrating incision sites for a three-incision fasciotomy. The blue panel indicates the level of the cross-section shown in the inset image. Inset, Cross-section of the medial, superficial central, deep central, and lateral compartments. The superior blue arrow indicates the entrance into the deep central compartment. The inferior blue arrow indicates the entrance into the medial, superficial, central, and lateral compartments (from medial to lateral). (Reproduced from Dodd A, Le I: Foot compartment syndrome: Diagnosis and management. *J Am Acad Orthop Surg* 2013;21[11]:657-664.)

ment), interosseous (four compartments), and central (three compartments, including the deep central, or calcaneal, which communicates with the deep posterior compartment of the leg).

2. Acute trauma to the foot, including fractures of the calcaneus, Lisfranc injuries, crush injuries, and injuries having other high-energy mechanisms can result in compartment syndromes.

B. Clinical evaluation

1. The primary method of diagnosis of compartment syndromes of the foot is clinical.

2. Loss of pulses and capillary refilling are unreliable signs of a compartment syndrome.

3. Loss of two-point discrimination and light touch sensation are more reliable than loss of pinprick

sensation as indicators of a compartment syndrome.

4. Pain with passive dorsiflexion of the foot results from stretching of the intrinsic muscles of the foot. This decreases compartment volume and increases pressure.

5. Pressure measurements can be helpful in clinically equivocal cases. Pressure thresholds exceeding 30 mm Hg or within 30 mm Hg of diastolic blood pressure have been advocated as indications for compartment release.

C. Treatment (**Figure 9**)

1. Fasciotomy is indicated when clinical symptoms are consistent with a compartment syndrome.

2. Medial and/or dorsal incisions can be used to release pressure in all nine compartments of the foot.

   a. Two dorsal incisions are commonly used.

3. Closure should be delayed because primary skin closure can increase intracompartmental pressure. A split-thickness skin graft may be required for closure.

4. Alternatively, "pie-crusting" dorsally may release hematoma and effectively decompress the dorsal compartments of the foot.

Top Testing Facts

Fractures of the Talus

1. The talus is 70% covered by cartilage and the extensor digitorum brevis is the only muscle attaching to it.

2. The blood supply to the talar body is mostly from the artery of the tarsal canal, a branch of the posterior tibial artery.

3. The blood supply to the talar neck is mainly from the artery of the tarsal sinus, a branch formed from the anterior tibial and peroneal arteries.

4. The deltoid artery supplies the medial body of the talus.

5. Posttraumatic osteoarthritis is the most common complication of talar fractures.

6. ORIF is required for all displaced talar neck fractures. ORIF is usually performed through combined anterolateral and anteromedial approaches.

7. Osteonecrosis occurs with increasing frequency as the Hawkins classification for a talar neck fracture increases in severity.

8. The Hawkins sign consists of subchondral osteopenia seen on plain radiographs at 6 to 8 weeks after fixation of a talar neck fracture and indicates revascularization of the talar body.

9. Varus malunion can occur as a complication of a talar fracture.

10. CT provides the best visualization of fractures of the talar body and is used to identify fractures in the transverse, coronal, and sagittal planes.

Fractures of the Calcaneus

1. The calcaneus is the most frequently fractured of the tarsal bones.

2. An oblique shear force causing fracture of the calcaneus results in a primary fracture line and two primary fragments.

3. The axial Harris view reveals widening, shortening, lateral translation, and varus positioning of the tuberosity fragment of a calcaneal fracture.

4. Negative prognostic factors for the surgical treatment of Sanders type II and III fractures include severity, advanced age, male sex, obesity, bilateral fractures, multiple trauma, and workers' compensation.

5. Malunion of calcaneal fractures can result in shortening, widening, and lateral impingement. The symptoms include difficulty with shoe wear and peroneal tendon symptoms.

6. Malunions that result in talar dorsiflexion with loss of the talar declination angle to less than 20° can limit ankle dorsiflexion.

7. Malunions of the calcaneus are treated with lateral exostectomy. Fusion is also added to treat subtalar arthritis.

8. Tension band fixation can be used to avoid failure of screw fixation in avulsion fractures of the calcaneal tuberosity.

9. Fractures of the anterior process of the talus occur with inversion and avulsion of the bifurcate ligament.

(continued on next page)

3: Trauma

Top Testing Facts (*continued*)

Midfoot Fractures

1. The central navicular has a limited blood supply and is susceptible to stress fractures.

2. The tarsometatarsal joints are constrained by the recessed articulation of the second metatarsal bone.

3. The Lisfranc ligament runs from the base of the second metatarsal to the medial cuneiform bone.

4. Lisfranc fracture-dislocations can occur with direct application of force or indirectly through axial loading and twisting on a fixed, plantar flexed foot.

5. Plain radiographs may show a fleck of bone in the proximal first metatarsal interspace. This fleck sign represents the avulsed Lisfranc ligament and is associated with poorer prognosis.

6. Homolateral dislocation of the tarsometatarsal joints may be associated with a compression injury to the cuboid.

7. Up to 30% of Lisfranc injuries are missed acutely. Weight-bearing or stress radiographs can be used to rule out injury.

8. Fusion of the fourth and fifth tarsometatarsal joints is poorly tolerated, and resection arthroplasty is used in conjunction with fusion of the medial tarsometatarsal joints for missed or late reconstruction of Lisfranc injuries.

Metatarsal and Phalangeal Fractures

1. Fractures of the metatarsal neck in which there is severe angulation and plantar prominence may require reduction and fixation.

2. Fractures of the metatarsal head are rare and can generally be treated nonsurgically.

3. Stress fractures of the proximal metatarsals may be seen in dancers.

4. Avulsion of the long plantar ligament, the lateral band of the plantar fascia, or contraction of the peroneus brevis may result in type I fractures of the fifth metatarsal (pseudo-Jones fracture).

5. Jones fractures occur where the proximal fifth metatarsal has poor blood supply; at the metadiaphyseal junction 1.5 to 2.5 cm distal to the base.

6. Acute ORIF with screws, together with a prolonged restriction of activity, is often used in athletes to minimize the possibility of nonunion of a type II fracture.

7. Diaphyseal stress fractures of the fifth metatarsal can be caused by cavovarus foot deformities or peripheral neuropathies. Second metatarsal neck stress fractures are seen in athletes and military recruits.

8. Bone grafting and/or structural correction may be needed to achieve the healing of type III fractures and prevent their recurrence, particularly in cases of atrophic nonunion.

9. Medial sesamoidectomy for nonunion may result in hallux valgus deformity.

10. Lateral sesamoidectomy for nonunion may result in hallux varus deformity.

Dislocations of the Foot

1. Medial subtalar dislocations may be irreducible if the talar head buttonholes through the extensor digitorum brevis, or with interposition of the peroneal tendons.

2. Lateral subtalar dislocations may be irreducible if buttonholed through the talonavicular capsule and the posterior tibial tendon is interposed.

3. Subtalar dislocations are reduced by flexing the knee to relax the gastrocnemius-soleus complex, recreating the deformity, plantarflexing the foot, and pushing on the talar head.

4. Dislocations of the first MTP joint are usually dorsal, and are uncommon because of the thick plantar ligamentous complex.

5. Midtarsal dislocation involving the talonavicular and calcaneocuboid articulations (Chopart joint) can occur through axial loading (longitudinal) or crush injury.

6. First MTP joint dislocations may be irreducible because of buttonholing through the sesamoid-short flexor complex. Irreducible first MTP joint dislocations are treated through a dorsal approach.

7. Lesser MTP joint dislocations may be irreducible because of buttonholing through the plantar plate.

Compartment Syndromes

1. The foot has a total of nine compartments divided into four main groups: the medial, lateral, four interosseous, and three central compartments.

2. Loss of pulses and capillary refilling are unreliable signs of a compartment syndrome.

3. Loss of two-point discrimination and light touch are more sensitive signs of compartment syndrome than loss of pinprick sensation.

4. Pain with passive dorsiflexion of the foot results from stretching of the intrinsic muscles of the foot. This decreases compartment volume and increases pressure.

5. Pressure measurements can be helpful in clinically equivocal cases. Pressure thresholds exceeding 30 mm Hg or within 30 mm Hg of diastolic blood pressure have been advocated as indications for compartment release.

6. Fasciotomy is indicated when clinical symptoms are consistent with a compartment syndrome.

7. Two dorsal incisions can be used to release pressure in all nine compartments of the foot.

8. Closure after incision to release pressure in the compartment of the foot should be delayed because primary skin closure can increase intracompartmental pressure. A split-thickness skin graft may be required for closure.

9. Dorsal pie-crusting may release hematoma and effectively decompress the dorsal compartments of the foot.

Bibliography

Buckley R, Tough S, McCormack R, et al: Operative compared with nonoperative treatment of displaced intra-articular calcaneal fractures: A prospective, randomized, controlled multicenter trial. *J Bone Joint Surg Am* 2002; 84-A(10):1733-1744.

Canale ST, Kelly FB Jr: Fractures of the neck of the talus: Long-term evaluation of seventy-one cases. *J Bone Joint Surg Am* 1978;60(2):143-156.

Kelly IP, Glisson RR, Fink C, Easley ME, Nunley JA: Intramedullary screw fixation of Jones fractures. *Foot Ankle Int* 2001;22(7):585-589.

Kuo RS, Tejwani NC, Digiovanni CW, et al: Outcome after open reduction and internal fixation of Lisfranc joint injuries. *J Bone Joint Surg Am* 2000;82-A(11):1609-1618.

Larson CM, Almekinders LC, Taft TN, Garrett WE: Intramedullary screw fixation of Jones fractures: Analysis of failure. *Am J Sports Med* 2002;30(1):55-60.

Ly TV, Coetzee JC: Treatment of primarily ligamentous Lisfranc joint injuries: Primary arthrodesis compared with open reduction and internal fixation. A prospective, randomized study. *J Bone Joint Surg Am* 2006;88(3):514-520.

Myerson MS: Experimental decompression of the fascial compartments of the foot—the basis for fasciotomy in acute compartment syndromes. *Foot Ankle* 1988;8(6):308-314.

Quill GE Jr: Fractures of the proximal fifth metatarsal. *Orthop Clin North Am* 1995;26(2):353-361.

Sanders R, Fortin P, DiPasquale T, Walling A: Operative treatment in 120 displaced intraarticular calcaneal fractures: Results using a prognostic computed tomography scan classification. *Clin Orthop Relat Res* 1993;290:87-95.

Schulze W, Richter J, Russe O, Ingelfinger P, Muhr G: Surgical treatment of talus fractures: A retrospective study of 80 cases followed for 1-15 years. *Acta Orthop Scand* 2002; 73(3):344-351.

Shah SN, Knoblich GO, Lindsey DP, Kreshak J, Yerby SA, Chou LB: Intramedullary screw fixation of proximal fifth metatarsal fractures: A biomechanical study. *Foot Ankle Int* 2001;22(7):581-584.

Teng AL, Pinzur MS, Lomasney L, Mahoney L, Havey R: Functional outcome following anatomic restoration of tarsal-metatarsal fracture dislocation. *Foot Ankle Int* 2002;23(10): 922-926.

Thordarson DB, Triffon MJ, Terk MR: Magnetic resonance imaging to detect avascular necrosis after open reduction and internal fixation of talar neck fractures. *Foot Ankle Int* 1996; 17(12):742-747.

Vallier HA, Nork SE, Barei DP, Benirschke SK, Sangeorzan BJ: Talar neck fractures: Results and outcomes. *J Bone Joint Surg Am* 2004;86-A(8):1616-1624.

Section 4

Orthopaedic Oncology/ Systemic Disease

Section Editor:
Kristy Weber, MD

Chapter 44

Overview of Orthopaedic Oncology and Systemic Disease

Frank J. Frassica, MD

I. General Information and Terminology

A. Overview

1. Approximately 2,900 new bone sarcomas and 11,300 new soft-tissue sarcomas are diagnosed annually in the United States.

2. Most of these sarcomas are high-grade malignancies with a high propensity to metastasize to the lungs.

B. Benign bone conditions

1. Developmental processes

2. Reactive processes (osteomyelitis, stress fractures, bone cysts)

3. Benign tumors (giant cell tumor, chondroblastoma)

C. Malignant bone conditions

1. Malignancies that arise from mesenchymal derivatives are called sarcomas.

2. Primary bone sarcomas include osteosarcoma and chondrosarcoma.

3. Bone malignancies that are not sarcomas include metastatic bone disease, multiple myeloma, and lymphoma.

D. Soft-tissue masses

1. Most common soft-tissue tumors

   a. Benign: lipoma

   b. Malignant: undifferentiated pleomorphic sarcoma (previously called malignant fibrous histiocytoma), liposarcoma, synovial sarcoma

2. Nonneoplastic reactive conditions include hematomas and heterotopic ossification.

Dr. Frassica or an immediate family member serves as a paid consultant to or is an employee of Synthes.

II. Bone Tumors

A. Classification/staging systems

1. Lichtenstein system—Modified by Dahlin to group conditions together based on the type of proliferating cell and whether the lesion is benign or malignant (**Table 1**).

2. Bone tumors can be classified according to whether the process involves the intramedullary area or the surface of the bone.

   a. Common intramedullary tumors

   • Enchondroma

   • Osteosarcoma

   • Chondrosarcoma

   • Undifferentiated pleomorphic sarcoma of bone

   b. Common surface tumors

   • Osteochondroma

   • Periosteal chondroma

   • Parosteal osteosarcoma

3. Bone sarcomas can also be characterized as primary or secondary.

   a. Common primary bone sarcomas

   • Osteosarcoma

   • Ewing sarcoma

   • Chondrosarcoma

   b. Common secondary bone sarcomas

   • Chondrosarcoma arising in an osteochondroma

   • Undifferentiated pleomorphic sarcoma arising in a bone infarct

   • Osteosarcoma occurring in a focus of Paget disease

4. Bone tumor grade (**Table 2**)

Table 1

Dahlin Modification of the Lichtenstein Classification System

Cell Type	Benign	Malignant
Bone	Osteoid osteoma Osteoblastoma	Osteosarcoma Parosteal osteosarcoma Periosteal osteosarcoma High-grade surface osteosarcoma
Cartilage	Enchondroma Periosteal chondroma Osteochondroma Chondroblastoma Chondromyxoid fibroma	Chondrosarcoma Dedifferentiated chondrosarcoma Periosteal chondrosarcoma Mesenchymal chondrosarcoma Clear cell chondrosarcoma
Fibrous	Nonossifying fibroma	Fibrosarcoma Undifferentiated pleomorphic sarcoma
Vascular	Hemangioma	Hemangioendothelioma Hemangiopericytoma
Hematopoietic		Myeloma Lymphoma
Nerve	Neurilemmoma	Malignant peripheral nerve sheath tumor
Lipogenic	Lipoma	Liposarcoma
Notochordal	Notochordal rest	Chordoma
Unknown	Giant cell tumor	Ewing sarcoma Adamantinoma

Table 2

Bone Tumor Grades

Grade	Characteristic	Examples
G1	Low grade (well differentiated)	Parosteal osteosarcoma Low-grade intramedullary osteosarcoma (rare) Adamatinoma Intramedullary grade 1 chondrosarcoma (represent two thirds of chondrosarcomas) Chordoma
G2	Intermediate grade (moderately differentiated)	Periosteal osteosarcoma Grade 2 chondrosarcoma of bone
G3, G4	High grade (poorly differentiated or undifferentiated)	Osteosarcoma Ewing sarcoma Undifferentiated pleomorphic sarcoma of bone

Table 3

Enneking Classification of Benign Bone Tumors

Stage	Description	Tumor Examples
1	Inactive (latent)	Nonossifying fibroma Enchondroma
2	Active	Giant cell tumor[a] Aneurysmal bone cyst[a] Chondroblastoma Chondromyxoid fibroma Unicameral bone cyst
3	Aggressive	Giant cell tumor[a] Aneurysmal bone cyst[a]

[a]Giant cell tumor and aneurysmal bone cyst can be either stage 2 (active) or stage 3 (aggressive) lesions, depending on the amount of bone destruction, soft-tissue masses, and joint involvement.

5. Enneking system—Staging system for benign and malignant bone tumors.

   a. Benign lesions—See **Table 3**.

   b. Malignant bone tumors—See **Table 4**.

6. American Joint Committee on Cancer (AJCC) classification system for bone tumors (**Table 5**)

   a. Based on the tumor grade, size, and presence or absence of discontinuous tumor or regional/systemic metastases.

   b. In this system, the order of importance of prognostic factors is:

   • Presence of metastasis (stage IV)

   • Discontinuous tumor (stage III)

   • Grade (I—low, II—high)

   • Size

      ○ T1 ≤ 8 cm

      ○ T2 > 8 cm

III. Soft-Tissue Tumors

A. Classification

1. Soft-tissue tumors are classified histologically, according to the predominant cell type.

2. Staging systems can include benign and malignant tumors and reactive conditions.

3. There are hundreds of different soft-tissue tumors; some of the most significant are listed in **Table 6**.

Table 4

Enneking Classification of Malignant Bone Tumors

Stage	Description
IA	Low grade, intracompartmental
IB	Low grade, extracompartmental
IIA	High grade, intracompartmental
IIB	High grade, extracompartmental
III	Metastatic disease

Suffix A = intracompartmental (confined to bone, no soft-tissue involvement); suffix B = extracompartmental (penetration of the cortex with a soft-tissue mass)

Table 5

Definitions of TNM Stage I through Stage IV

Stage	Tumor Grade	Tumor Size
IA	Low	<8 cm
IB	Low	>8 cm
IIA	High	<8 cm
IIB	High	>8 cm
III	Any tumor grade, skip metastases[a]	
IV	Any tumor grade, any tumor size, distant metastases	

[a]Skip metastases: discontinuous tumors in the primary bone site.

TNM = tumor, nodes, metastasis.

Reproduced with permission from Edge SB, Byrd DR, Compton CC, et al, eds: Bone, in *AJCC Cancer Staging Manual*, ed 7. New York, NY, Springer, 2010, pp 281-290.

Table 6

Histologic Classification of Soft-Tissue Tumors

Type	Benign	Malignant
Fibrous	Nodular fasciitis Proliferative fasciitis Elastofibroma Infantile fibromatosis Adult fibromatosis	Fibrosarcoma Infantile fibrosarcoma
Fibrohistiocytic	Fibrous histiocytoma	DFSP Undifferentiated pleomorphic sarcoma
Lipomatous	Lipoma Angiolipoma Hibernoma Atypical lipoma	Well-differentiated liposarcoma Myxoid round cell liposarcoma Pleomorphic liposarcoma Dedifferentiated liposarcoma
Smooth muscle	Leiomyoma	Leiomyosarcoma
Skeletal muscle	Rhabdomyoma	Rhabdomyosarcoma
Blood vessels	Hemangioma Lymphangioma	Angiosarcoma Kaposi sarcoma
Perivascular	Glomus tumor	Hemangiopericytoma
Synovial	Focal PVNS Diffuse PVNS	Malignant PVNS
Nerve sheath	Neuroma Neurofibroma Neurofibromatosis Schwannoma	MPNST
Neuroectodermal	Ganglioneuroma	Neuroblastoma Ewing sarcoma PNET
Cartilage	Chondroma Synovial chondromatosis	Extraskeletal chondrosarcoma
Bone	FOP	Extraskeletal osteosarcoma
Miscellaneous	Tumoral calcinosis Myxoma	Synovial sarcoma Alveolar soft-part sarcoma Epithelioid sarcoma

DFSP = dermatofibrosarcoma protuberans; PVNS = pigmented villonodular synovitis; MPNST = malignant peripheral nerve sheath tumor; PNET = primitive neuroectodermal tumor; FOP = fibrodyplasia ossificans progressiva

B. Staging—The most common system is the AJCC system (**Table 7**). The order of importance of prognostic factors is:

1. Presence of metastasis (stage IV)

2. Grade

   a. Low—stage I

   b. High—stage II

3. Size (>5 cm)

   a. T1 ≤5 cm

   b. T2 >5 cm

4. Location (superficial or deep)

Table 7

AJCC Version 7 Staging for Soft-Tissue Sarcomas

Primary Tumor (T)

TX	Primary tumor cannot be assessed
T0	No evidence of primary tumor
T1	Tumor 5 cm or less in greatest dimension
T1a	Superficial tumor
T1b	Deep tumor
T2	Tumor more than 5 cm in greatest dimension
T2a	Superficial tumor
T2b	Deep tumor

Note: Superficial tumor is located exclusively above the superficial fascia without invasion of the fascia; deep tumor is located either exclusively beneath the superficial fascia, superficial to the fascia with invasion of or through the fascia, or both superficial yet beneath the fascia.

Regional Lymph Nodes (N)

NX	Regional lymph nodes cannot be assessed
N0	No regional lymph node metastasis
N1	Regional lymph node metastasis

Note: Presence of positive nodes (N1) in M0 tumors is considered Stage III.

Distant Metastasis (M)

M0	No distant metastasis
M1	Distant metastasis

Anatomic Stage/Prognostic Groups

Stage IA	T1a	N0	M0	G1, GX
	T1b	N0	M0	G1, GX
Stage IB	T2a	N0	M0	G1, GX
	T2b	N0	M0	G1, GX
State IIA	T1a	N0	M0	G2, G3
	T1b	N0	M0	G2, G3
Stage IIB	T2a	N0	M0	G2
	T2b	N0	M0	G2
Stage III	T2a	N0	M0	G3
	T2b	N0	M0	G3
	Any T	N1	M0	Any G
Stage IV	Any T	Any N	M1	Any G

AJCC = American Joint Committee on Cancer.

Reproduced with permission from Edge SB, Byrd DR, Compton CC, et al, eds: *AJCC Cancer Staging Manual*, ed 7. New York, NY, Springer, 2010.

IV. Patient Evaluation

A. History

1. Current symptoms (pain, rate of growth, skin changes, presence of mass)

   a. Pain

   - Destructive bone tumors

     ○ Pain is intermittent and progresses to constant pain that does not respond to NSAIDs or weak narcotic medications.

     ○ A common presentation is severe pain that occurs at rest and with activity.

     ○ Night pain often present

   - Malignant soft-tissue tumors—Patients with these tumors often present without pain unless there is rapid growth or impingement on neural structures.

   b. Rate of growth—A rapidly growing soft-tissue mass may suggest malignancy. Some malignant soft-tissue tumors grow slowly (synovial sarcoma, epithelioid sarcoma).

   c. Presence of a mass—Assess when noticed in relation to other symptoms and rate of growth. A soft-tissue mass may also develop from a bone tumor.

2. Relevant history/family history

   a. History of cancer or family history of cancer/masses (neurofibromatosis)

   b. Exposure (for example, toxic chemicals, cats—cat scratch disease causes enlarged lymph nodes)

   c. History of infection or trauma (myositis ossificans)

B. Physical examination

1. Mass—With bone tumors, patients present with a hard, fixed mass adjacent to the bone lesion that is often tender on deep palpation. Soft-tissue masses can be compressible (lipoma) or firm (sarcoma, desmoid).

2. Range of motion—Range of motion of the joint adjacent to a bone or soft-tissue tumor is often diminished.

3. Muscle atrophy—Common, adjacent to painful lesion.

4. Lymphadenopathy—Lymph nodes can be enlarged as a result of infection or metastasis.

5. Pathologic fractures

   a. Fractures through a bone lesion occur in 5% to 10% of patients.

b. A history of antecedent pain is common.

c. Pathologic fractures generally occur with minor trauma or following activities of daily living.

C. Imaging

1. Plain radiographs

a. Primary bone lesion

- Plain radiographs alone (two planes) are often sufficient for benign bone lesions.

- Cortices should be inspected for bone destruction.

- Lesion should be assessed for mineralization.

  ○ Rings/stipples suggest a cartilage lesion.

  ○ Cloud-like lesions suggest bone formation.

- Periosteal reaction should be checked for.

b. Primary soft-tissue lesions

- Synovial sarcomas: Scattered calcifications are noted in 30%.

- Myositis ossificans: Peripheral mineralization is present.

- Hemangiomas: Phleboliths present in soft tissue.

- Lipomas: Radiolucent on plain radiographs.

2. Technetium Tc 99m bone scan

a. Technetium Tc 99m forms chemical adducts to sites of new bone formation.

b. Detects multiple sites of bone involvement or skip metastases

c. Very sensitive but not specific

d. High false-negative rate in multiple myeloma and occasionally in very osteolytic bone metastasis such as renal cell carcinoma

3. Computed tomography

a. Determines the mineral distribution in normal and abnormal bone

b. Helpful in evaluating pelvic and spine lesions

c. Thin-cut CT should be ordered if osteoid osteoma is suspected.

4. Magnetic resonance imaging

a. Sensitive and specific for detecting bone marrow involvement

b. Defines anatomic features (T1-weighted sequences)

c. Helpful in evaluating pelvic and spine bone lesions

d. Key study for evaluation of soft-tissue tumors

- Determinate masses—If nature of lesion can definitively be determined by analysis of MRI (lipoma, ganglion cyst, hemangioma, muscle injury). These can be definitively treated without a biopsy.

- Indeterminate masses—If nature of lesion cannot be determined by analysis of MRI. These require a biopsy before definitive treatment.

5. Pulmonary staging

a. CT is used as a baseline to detect pulmonary metastases and for future comparison.

b. Chest radiographs (or repeated CT scans) are used for future follow-up if initial CT of the chest is negative.

V. Biopsy

A. General

1. Biopsy is a key step in the evaluation and treatment of patients with bone or soft-tissue lesions.

2. Significant problems can occur when a biopsy is not done correctly.

a. Altered treatment

b. Major errors in diagnosis

c. Complications (for example, infection, nerve injury)

d. Nonrepresentative tissue

e. Adverse outcome (local recurrence)

f. Unnecessary amputation

B. Major types of biopsy

1. Needle biopsy—Most common method of establishing a diagnosis, but requires an experienced cytopathologist and surgical pathologist.

a. Fine needle aspiration—Needle aspiration of cells from the tumor.

b. Core needle biopsy—A larger bore needle is placed into the tumor and a core of tissue is extracted.

2. Open incisional biopsy—Surgical procedure to obtain tissue.

a. The biopsy tract should be designed to be excised at the time of the definitive resection if the tumor is malignant.

- The incision should be small and usually is oriented longitudinally.

Table 8

Tumor Suppressor Genes

Gene	Syndrome	Tumor Examples
RB	Hereditary neuroblastoma	Retinoblastoma, osteosarcoma
P53	Li-Fraumeni syndrome	Sarcomas, breast cancer
P16INK4a	Familial melanoma	Chondrosarcoma, osteosarcoma, melanoma
APC	Familial adenomatous polyposis	Colon adenomas, desmoids
NF1	Neurofibromatosis	Neurofibroma, sarcomas
EXT1/EXT2	Hereditary multiple exostosis	Osteochondromas, chondrosarcomas

Table 9

Chromosomal Alterations in Malignant Tumors

Tumor	Translocation	Genes
Ewing sarcoma, PNET	t(11;22)(q24;q12)	EWS, FLI1
Synovial sarcoma	t(X;18)(p11;q11)	SYT, SSX
Clear cell sarcoma	t(12;22)(q13;a12)	EWS, ATF1
Alveolar rhabdomyosarcoma	t(2;13)(q35;q14)	PAX3, FKHR
Myxoid liposarcoma	t(12;16)(q13;p11)	CHOP, TLS

PNET = primitive neuroectodermal tumor

- The following nonlongitudinal incisions are used occasionally:
  - A transverse incision for the clavicle
  - An oblique incision for the scapular body
  b. Soft-tissue flaps are not elevated; the biopsy is performed directly onto the tumor mass.
  c. Hemostasis is critical; usually, no indwelling drains are used.
  d. A frozen section analysis is often performed to ensure that diagnostic tissue has been obtained.

3. Excisional biopsy

  a. Indicated only when the surgeon is sure that the lesion is benign or when the tumor can be removed with a wide margin (for example, if the radiographic appearance suggests a superficial, small soft-tissue malignancy).

  b. Two low-grade malignancies for which an excisional biopsy is sometimes performed are parosteal osteosarcoma and low-grade chondrosarcoma.

VI. Molecular Markers/Genetic Considerations

A. Tumor suppressor genes and associated conditions are listed in **Table 8**.

B. Chromosomal alterations

  1. Chromosomal alterations in malignant tumors are generally translocations (**Table 9**).

  2. Alterations often produce unique gene products that may affect the prognosis.

Top Testing Facts

1. The most common site of metastases from bone and soft-tissue sarcomas is the lungs.

2. The most common low-grade bone sarcomas are chondrosarcoma, parosteal osteosarcoma, adamantinoma, and chordoma.

3. The most common high-grade sarcomas are osteosarcoma, Ewing sarcoma, and undifferentiated pleomorphic sarcoma.

4. The order of importance of prognostic factors in bone tumor staging is presence of metastases, discontinuous tumor, grade, and size.

5. A high rate of false-negative results occurs with technetium Tc 99m bone scanning in multiple myeloma.

6. The order of importance of prognostic factors in soft-tissue tumor staging is presence of metastases, grade, size, and depth.

7. The RB gene is the tumor suppressor gene associated with osteosarcoma.

8. EXT1/EXT2 are the tumor suppressor genes associated with hereditary multiple exostoses.

9. Ewing sarcoma and primitive neuroectodermal tumor have a characteristic chromosomal translocation t(11;22).

10. Synovial sarcoma has a characteristic chromosomal translocation t(X;18).

Bibliography

Edge SB, Byrd DR, Compton CC, et al, eds: Bone, in *AJCC Cancer Staging Manual*, ed 7. New York, NY, Springer, 2010, pp 281-290.

Enneking WF: A system of staging musculoskeletal neoplasms. *Clin Orthop Relat Res* 1986;204:9-24.

Enneking WF, Spanier SS, Goodman MA: A system for the surgical staging of musculoskeletal sarcoma. *Clin Orthop Relat Res* 1980;153:106-120.

General considerations, in Weiss SW, Goldblum JR, eds: *Enzinger and Weiss's Soft Tissue Tumors*, ed 5. St Louis, MO, Mosby, 2008, pp 1-20.

Hopyan S, Wunder JS, Randall RL: Molecular biology in musculoskeletal neoplasia, in Schwartz HSS, ed: *Orthopaedic Knowledge Update: Musculoskeletal Tumors*, ed 2. Rosemont, IL, American Academy of Orthopaedic Surgeons, 2007, pp 13-21.

Mankin HJ, Lange TA, Spanier SS: The classic: The hazards of biopsy in patients with malignant primary bone and soft-tissue tumors. The Journal of Bone and Joint Surgery, 1982; 64:1121-1127. *Clin Orthop Relat Res* 2006;450:4-10.

Mankin HJ, Mankin CJ, Simon MA; Members of the Musculoskeletal Tumor Society: The hazards of the biopsy, revisited. *J Bone Joint Surg Am* 1996;78(5):656-663.

Papp DF, Khanna AJ, McCarthy EF, Carrino JA, Farber AJ, Frassica FJ: Magnetic resonance imaging of soft-tissue tumors: Determinate and indeterminate lesions. *J Bone Joint Surg Am* 2007;89(Suppl 3):103-115.

Siegel R, Naishadham D, Jemal A: Cancer statistics, 2013. *CA Cancer J Clin* 2013;63(1):11-30.

Unni KK: Introduction and scope of study, in Unni KK, ed: *Dahlin's Bone Tumors: General Aspects and Data on 11,087 Cases*, ed 5. Philadelphia, PA, Lipppincott-Raven, 1996.

Chapter 45

Principles of Treatment of Musculoskeletal Tumors

Frank J. Frassica, MD

4: Orthopaedic Oncology/Systemic Disease

I. Overview

A. Biologic activity and potential morbidity

1. The treatment of musculoskeletal tumors is based on the biologic activity and potential morbidity of each lesion.

2. The important biologic aspects are the risk of local recurrence and metastasis.

B. Surgical margins are designed to reduce the risk of local recurrence.

1. Intralesional—The plane of dissection enters into the tumor.

2. Marginal—The plane of dissection is through the reactive zone at the edge of the tumor.

3. Wide—The entire tumor is removed with a cuff of normal tissue.

4. Radical—The entire compartment that the tumor occupies is removed.

C. Chemotherapy—Common mechanism is to induce programmed cell death (apoptosis). Chemotherapeutic agents achieve apoptosis in various ways.

1. Directly damage DNA: alkylating agents, platinum compounds, anthracyclines

2. Deplete cellular building blocks: antifolates, cytidine analogs, 5-fluoropyrimidines

3. Interfere with microtubule function: vinca alkaloids, taxanes

D. Radiation therapy—Causes DNA damage through production of free radicals or direct genetic damage.

II. Treatment of Bone Tumors

A. Benign processes/tumors

1. Observation—Used for asymptomatic inactive lesions.

2. Aspiration and injection

a. Unicameral bone cysts

   • Methylprednisolone acetate

   • Bone marrow

   • Synthetic bone grafts

b. Eosinophilic granuloma

   • Methylprednisolone acetate

3. Curettage

a. The margin is always intralesional.

b. For giant cell tumor, hand curettage is often extended with a high-speed burr.

c. Benign tumors commonly treated with curettage

   • Giant cell tumor

   • Chondroblastoma

   • Chondromyxoid fibroma

   • Osteoblastoma

   • Aneurysmal bone cyst

   • Unicameral bone cyst of the proximal femur

4. Surgical adjuvants for tumors prone to local recurrence (eg, giant cell tumor)

a. Phenol

   • Strong base that coagulates proteins

   • Potential soft-tissue injury with spillage

b. Liquid nitrogen

   • Freezes up to 1 cm of tissue

   • High stress-fracture rate (at least 25%)

c. Argon beam coagulation

d. Hydrogen peroxide

5. Materials used for reconstruction of the defect

a. Methylmethacrylate: often used for giant cell tumors

b. Bone graft (freeze-dried allograft, synthetic graft, autologous graft)

6. Excision/resection—Removal of the lesion and surrounding involved bone with the intent to definitively remove all tumor.

a. Benign, nonaggressive processes treated by excision/resection without reconstruction

- Osteochondroma

- Periosteal chondroma

b. Benign, aggressive lesions with major bone destruction, soft-tissue extension, cartilage loss, or fracture (often require reconstruction with prosthesis, allograft, or a combination)

- Giant cell tumor

- Osteoblastoma

B. Malignant bone tumors (sarcomas)

1. Overview

a. Malignant bone tumors must be removed with satisfactory margin to prevent local recurrence.

b. High risk of systemic metastases exists with high-grade tumors.

2. Surgery

a. Limb salvage versus amputation

- Limb salvage—Removal of the malignant tumor with a satisfactory margin and preservation of the limb.

- Amputation—Removal of the tumor with a wide or radical margin and removal of the limb.

b. Wide resection alone, with no current role for chemotherapy or radiation therapy

- Chondrosarcoma

- Adamantinoma

- Parosteal osteosarcoma

- Low-grade intramedullary osteosarcoma

c. Chemotherapy

- Used to kill micrometastases present in the pulmonary parenchyma and systemic circulation (neoadjuvant chemotherapy)

- An integral component of treatment, along with surgery, in the following malignancies:

  ○ Osteosarcoma

  ○ Ewing sarcoma/primitive neuroectodermal tumor

  ○ Undifferentiated pleomorphic sarcoma (malignant fibrous histiocytoma) of bone

d. Radiation therapy—External beam irradiation can be used for definitive or supplemental control of the tumor in the following primary malignant bone tumors:

- Ewing sarcoma/primitive neuroectodermal tumor

- Primary lymphoma of bone

- Hemangioendothelioma

- Solitary plasmacytoma of bone

- Chordoma (as a supplement to surgery with close margins)

III. Treatment of Soft-Tissue Tumors

A. Benign soft-tissue tumors

1. Observation—Inactive latent lesions (eg, subcutaneous/intramuscular lipomas)

2. Simple excision (intralesional or marginal margins)—Inactive/symptomatic or active lesions with minimal risk of local recurrence.

a. Intramuscular lipoma, intramuscular myxoma

b. Schwannoma—Careful dissection/separation of the tumor from normal nerve fibers.

3. Wide resection—Lesions prone to local recurrence (eg, extra-abdominal desmoid tumor)

B. Malignant soft-tissue tumors

1. Wide resection alone—Reserved for small, superficial low- or high-grade sarcomas that can be removed with a sufficient cuff of normal tissue.

2. Wide resection and external beam irradiation

a. Used to minimize the risk of local failure. (Local recurrence is 5% to 10% with wide resection and external beam irradiation.)

b. The modalities listed below have equivalent local control and survival rates but differing short- and long-term morbidities.

- Preoperative external beam irradiation followed by wide surgical resection

  ○ Higher risk of wound healing complications, lower risk of long-term fibrosis

  ○ Lower total dose (5,000 cGy) of irradiation

- Wide surgical resection with postoperative external beam irradiation

  ◦ Lower risk of wound healing complications

  ◦ Higher risk of long-term fibrosis

  ◦ Higher dose of irradiation (6,200 to 6,600 cGy)

IV. Indications for Amputation

A. Tumor that cannot be completely removed by a limb-salvage procedure (extremely large)

B. Locally recurrent tumors (relative indication)

C. The morbidity of the limb salvage procedure is too high.

D. Limb salvage will not result in a functional limb.

E. The tumor continues to grow after preoperative chemotherapy or radiation.

F. A major neurovascular bundle is involved (relative indication).

G. Lesions that are distal in the extremity (foot or hand) (relative indication)

H. Very young patients with malignant bone tumors with no reconstructive options available

Top Testing Facts

1. Chemotherapy drugs induce programmed cell death (apoptosis).

2. Radiation therapy induces DNA damage by the creation of free radicals.

3. Aspiration and injection is used for selected benign bone lesions: unicameral bone cyst (methylprednisolone, bone marrow, or synthetic graft) and eosinophilic granuloma (methylprednisolone).

4. Curettage—and bone graft or methylmethacrylate for reconstruction—is used for most active or aggressive benign bone tumors, including giant cell tumor, chondroblastoma, osteoblastoma, chondromyxoid fibroma, aneurysmal bone cyst, and unicameral bone cyst of the proximal femur.

5. Wide surgical margins alone are used for sarcomas without effective adjuvant therapy—chondrosarcoma, adamantinoma, parosteal osteosarcoma, and low-grade intramedullary osteosarcoma.

6. The major benefit of chemotherapy for osteosarcoma and Ewing sarcoma is to reduce the risk of pulmonary metastases.

7. Radiation can be used as the definitive method for local control of primary lymphoma of bone, solitary plasmacytoma, hemangioendothelioma of bone, and Ewing sarcoma.

8. Simple excision is chosen for most benign soft-tissue tumors, with the exception of extra-abdominal desmoid tumor, which requires wide margins.

9. Preoperative irradiation for soft-tissue sarcomas results in less fibrosis but a higher risk of early wound complications compared with postoperative irradiation.

10. Amputation surgery criteria: (1) an adequate surgical margin cannot be achieved, (2) locally recurrent tumors, (3) the morbidity is not acceptable, (4) the resulting limb will not be functional, (5) tumor growth continues after preoperative chemotherapy or irradiation, (6) the tumor involves major neurovascular bundles, (7) distal extremity lesions, (8) very young patients with malignant bone tumors and no reconstruction options.

Bibliography

Balach T, Stacy GS, Haydon RC: The clinical evaluation of soft tissue tumors. *Radiol Clin North Am* 2011;49(6): 1185-1196, vi.

Kirsch DG, Hornicek FJ: Radiation therapy for soft-tissue sarcomas, in Schwartz HSS, ed: *Orthopaedic Knowledge Update: Musculoskeletal Tumors*, ed 2. Rosemont, IL, American Academy of Orthopaedic Surgeons, 2007, pp 313-320.

Tuy BE: Adjuvant therapy for malignant bone tumors, in Schwartz HSS, ed: *Orthopaedic Knowledge Update: Musculoskeletal Tumors*, ed 2. Rosemont, IL, American Academy of Orthopaedic Surgeons, 2007, pp 205-218.

4: Orthopaedic Oncology/Systemic Disease

Chapter 46

Benign Bone Tumors and Reactive Lesions

Kristy Weber, MD

4: Orthopaedic Oncology/Systemic Disease

I. Bone

A. Osteoid osteoma—A distinctive, painful, benign osteoblastic bone tumor.

1. Demographics

   a. Male-to-female ratio = 2:1

   b. Most patients are between 5 and 30 years of age.

2. Genetics/etiology

   a. The etiology is unclear, but nerve fibers associated with blood vessels within the nidus likely play a role in producing pain.

   b. High prostaglandin and cyclooxygenase levels are present within the lesion.

3. Clinical presentation (Table 1)

   a. Classic symptom is night pain relieved by aspirin or NSAIDs.

   b. The pain is progressive in its severity, can be referred to an adjacent joint, and may be present for months to years before diagnosis.

   c. Most common locations include the femur, tibia, vertebral arch, humerus, and fingers. The proximal femur is the most common site; the hip is the most common intra-articular location.

   d. Osteoid osteomas usually occur in the diaphyseal or metaphyseal regions of long bones.

   e. When an osteoid osteoma is the cause of a painful scoliosis, the lesion is usually at the center of the concavity of the curve.

   f. Osteoid osteomas cause extensive inflammatory symptoms in the adjacent tissues (joint effusions, contractures, limp, muscle atrophy).

4. Imaging appearance (Figure 1)

   a. Round, well-circumscribed intracortical lesion with radiolucent nidus

   b. Lesions usually less than 1 cm in diameter

   c. Extensive periosteal reaction that may obscure the nidus (Figure 1, A)

   d. Lesions are occasionally intra-articular, subperiosteal, or medullary; these cause less surrounding periosteal reaction (Figure 1, C).

   e. Radiographic differential diagnosis includes osteomyelitis and Ewing sarcoma (because of the periosteal reaction).

   f. Intense and focal increased tracer uptake on technetium Tc-99m bone scans

   g. Thin-cut CT scan is often the key to diagnosis because it frequently identifies the small radiolucent nidus (Figure 1, B).

   h. MRI often shows extensive surrounding edema (Figure 1, D).

Table 1		
Factors Differentiating Osteoid Osteoma From Osteoblastoma		
Factor	**Osteoid Osteoma**	**Osteoblastoma**
Site	Diaphysis of long bone	Posterior elements of spine, metaphysis of long bone
Size	5–15 mm	>1.5 cm
Growth characteristic	Self-limited	Progressive
Symptoms	Exquisite pain, worse at night, relieved by aspirin	Dull ache

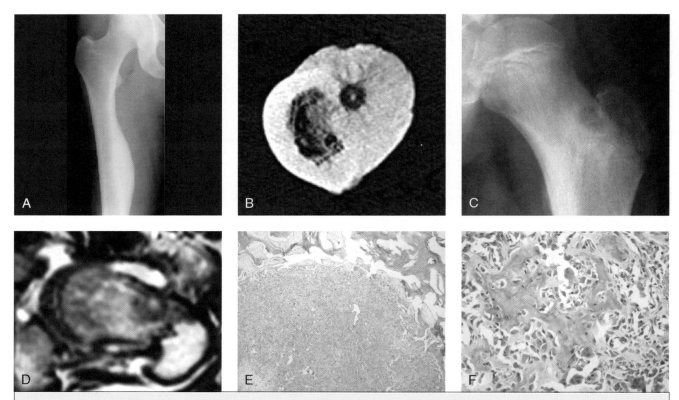

Figure 1   Osteoid osteomas. **A,** AP radiograph of a right femur shows extensive reactive bone formation and cortical thickening along the medial diaphysis. **B,** Axial thin-cut CT of the same patient shown in **A** reveals a clear radiolucent nidus with a central density that is classic for an osteoid osteoma. **C,** AP radiograph of a left femoral neck reveals a well-circumscribed subcortical lucency surrounded by sclerosis. **D,** MRI of the same patient shown in **C** reveals a nidus near the lateral cortex with surrounding edema. **E,** At low-power magnification, an osteoid osteoma has the histologic appearance of a sharply demarcated lesion (nidus) encased by dense cortical bone. **F,** High-power magnification shows osteoblastic rimming similar to that found in an osteoblastoma. The nuclei appear active but there is no pleomorphism. Marked vascularity is present within the stroma. (Parts E and F reproduced from Schwartz HS, ed: *Orthopaedic Knowledge Update: Musculoskeletal Tumors*, ed 2. Rosemont, IL, American Academy of Orthopaedic Surgeons, 2007, p 95.)

5. Pathology

   a. Microscopic appearance: uniform, thin osteoid seams and immature trabeculae (**Figure 1, E** and **F**)

   b. Trabeculae are lined with uniform, plump osteoblasts.

   c. A 1- to 2-mm fibrovascular rim surrounds the sharply demarcated nidus.

   d. No pleomorphic cells are present.

   e. The lesion does not infiltrate the surrounding bone.

   f. Similar in appearance to osteoblastoma but smaller in size (**Table 1**)

6. Treatment/outcome

   a. Standard of care is outpatient percutaneous radiofrequency ablation (RFA) of the lesion. A CT-guided probe is inserted into the lesion with the temperature raised to 90°C for 4 to 6 minutes to produce a 1-cm zone of necrosis.

      • Recurrence rates after RFA are less than 10%.

      • Contraindications include lesions close to the spinal cord or nerve roots.

   b. Other surgical treatments have included surgical resection or burring. The lesion must be localized preoperatively to identify its exact location.

   c. In lesions around the hip, patients often require internal fixation, sometimes with bone grafting, if a large portion of cortex is surgically removed with the lesion.

   d. Long-term medical management with aspirin or NSAIDs is useful to relieve symptoms because these lesions are self-limiting and burn out after an average of 3 years.

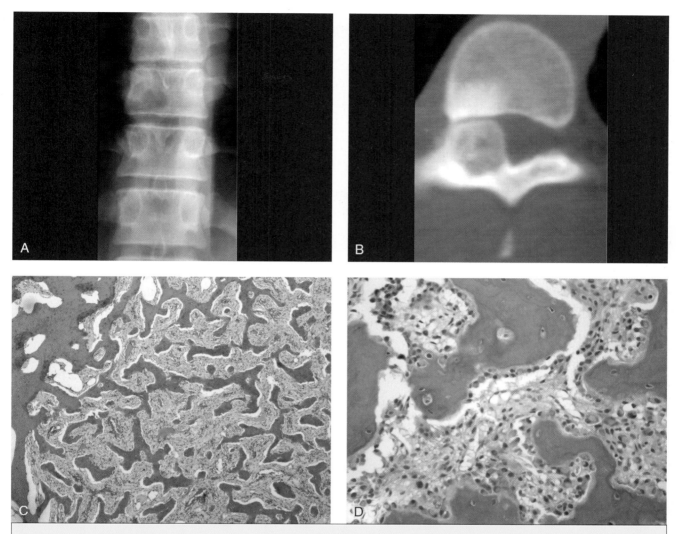

Figure 2   Osteoblastomas. **A,** AP radiograph of the lower portion of the thoracic spine of a 17-year-old boy shows a possible lesion on the right side of T10. **B,** A CT scan of the same patient shown in **A** better shows the location of the osteoblastoma in the pedicle of T10. **C,** The histologic appearance of an osteoblastoma shows interlacing trabeculae surrounded by fibrovascular connective tissue. The tumor merges into the normal bone at the periphery of the lesion. **D,** Higher power magnification shows osteoblastic rimming around the trabecular bone. The osteoblasts can appear plasmacytoid. (Reproduced from Weber KL, Heck RK Jr: Cystic and benign lesions, in Schwartz HS, ed: *Orthopaedic Knowledge Update: Musculoskeletal Tumors,* ed 2. Rosemont, IL, American Academy of Orthopaedic Surgeons, 2007, pp 87-102.)

e. Depending on the age of the child and duration of symptoms, removal of an osteoid osteoma associated with a painful scoliosis will allow resolution of the curve without further treatment.

B. Osteoblastoma—A rare, aggressive, benign osteoblastic tumor.

1. Demographics

   a. Male-to-female ratio = 2:1

   b. Osteoblastomas are much less common than osteoid osteomas.

   c. Most patients are between 10 and 30 years of age.

2. Genetics/etiology—Rare chromosomal rearrangements are reported.

3. Clinical presentation (**Table 1**)

   a. Slowly progressive, dull, aching pain of long duration; less severe than pain from an osteoid osteoma

   b. Night pain is not typical, and aspirin does not classically relieve the symptoms.

   c. Neurologic symptoms can occur because the spine (posterior elements) is the most common location for osteoblastoma (**Figure 2, A** and **B**).

   d. Other locations include the diaphysis or me-

4: Orthopaedic Oncology/Systemic Disease

taphysis of long bones (tibia and femur) and the mandible.

e. Related swelling, muscle atrophy, and a limp may occur because the lesions are large and present for a prolonged period.

4. Imaging appearance

a. Radiolucent lesion 2 to 10 cm in size with occasional intralesional densities

b. Two thirds of osteoblastomas are cortically based; one third are medullary.

c. Expansile with extension into the surrounding soft tissues and a rim of reactive bone around the lesion

d. 25% of osteoblastomas have an extremely aggressive appearance and are mistaken for malignancies.

e. Radiographic differential diagnosis includes osteosarcoma, aneurysmal bone cyst (ABC), osteomyelitis, and osteoid osteoma.

f. Three-dimensional imaging (CT, MRI) is necessary to fully evaluate the extent of the lesion before surgical treatment.

5. Pathology

a. Histology is similar to that of an osteoid osteoma, but more giant cells are present.

b. Irregular seams of osteoid separated by loose fibrovascular stroma are seen (**Figure 2, C**).

c. Osteoid is rimmed by prominent osteoblasts that are occasionally large and epithelioid (**Figure 2, D**).

d. Most commonly, a sharp demarcation from the surrounding bone is seen.

e. 10% to 40% are associated with secondary ABC formation.

f. Numerous mitotic figures may be present, but they are not atypical.

g. It is important to differentiate osteoblastoma from osteosarcoma; giant cell tumor and ABC are also similar in appearance.

6. Treatment/outcome

a. Osteoblastoma is not self-limiting, and it requires surgical treatment.

b. In most cases, curettage and bone grafting is adequate to achieve local control.

c. Nerve roots should be maintained when treating spinal lesions.

d. Occasionally, en bloc resection is required for lesions in the spine.

C. Parosteal osteoma—A rare, self-limiting deposition of reactive bone on the surface of the bone.

1. Demographics—Adults, most commonly in the fourth or fifth decade of life.

2. Females are affected more commonly than males.

3. Genetics/etiology—No known cause, but often a history of trauma is reported.

4. Clinical presentation

a. Long history of gradual swelling or dull pain

b. Occasionally, incidental radiographic findings are present.

c. Classically, osteomas are found in the craniofacial bones. Rarely, they present in other parts of the skeleton, including the long bones (tibia, femur), pelvis, and vertebrae.

d. Multiple osteomas are associated with Gardner syndrome (autosomal dominant), which also includes colonic polyps, fibromatosis, cutaneous lesions, and subcutaneous lesions.

5. Imaging appearance

a. Uniform radiodense lesion attached to the outer bone cortex with a broad base ranging from 1 to 8 cm in size (**Figure 3, A**)

b. Well-defined, with smooth, lobulated borders

c. No cortical or medullary invasion; this is best noted on CT scan (**Figure 3, B**).

d. Radiographic differential diagnosis includes parosteal osteosarcoma, healed stress fracture, and osteoid osteoma.

6. Pathology

a. Histologic appearance is of mature, hypocellular lamellar bone with intact haversian systems.

b. No atypical cells are present.

7. Treatment/outcome

a. Nonsurgical treatment is preferred for incidental or minimally symptomatic lesions.

b. Biopsy should be performed if the diagnosis is unclear.

c. Local recurrence of the lesion suggests it was initially not recognized as a parosteal osteosarcoma.

D. Bone island (enostosis)—A usually small (but occasionally large) deposit of dense, compact bone within the medullary cavity. Bone islands are nontumorous lesions.

1. Demographics—Bone islands occur frequently in adults, but their true incidence is unknown because they are usually found incidentally.

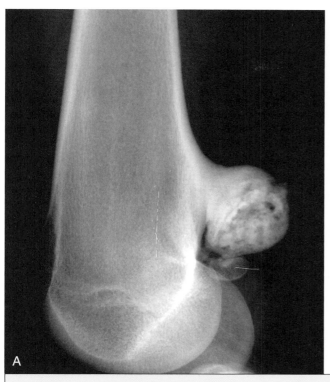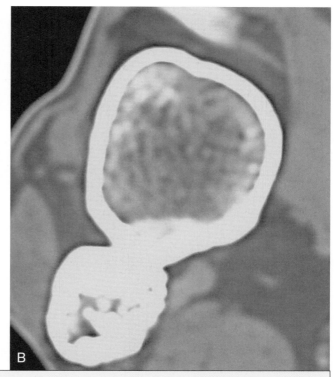

Figure 3 Parosteal osteoma. **A,** Lateral radiograph of the distal femur in a 37-year-old man reveals a heavily ossified surface lesion attached to the posterior femoral cortex. **B,** CT scan of the same patient reveals the relationship of the lesion to the cortex and differentiates it from myositis ossificans. An excisional biopsy revealed a parosteal osteoma.

2. Genetics/etiology—Possible arrested resorption of mature bone during endochondral ossification.

3. Clinical presentation

   a. Bone islands are asymptomatic and are found incidentally.

   b. Any bone can be involved, but the pelvis and femur are most common.

   c. Osteopoikilosis is a hereditary syndrome that manifests as hundreds of bone islands throughout the skeleton, usually centered about joints.

4. Radiographic appearance

   a. Well-defined, round focus of dense bone within the medullary cavity, usually 2 to 20 mm in diameter (**Figure 4**)

   b. Occasionally, radiating spicules of bone are present around the lesion that blend with the surrounding medullary cavity.

   c. Approximately one third of lesions show increased activity on bone scan.

   d. No surrounding bony reaction or edema on T2-weighted MRI.

   e. Low signal intensity on T1- and T2-weighted MRI

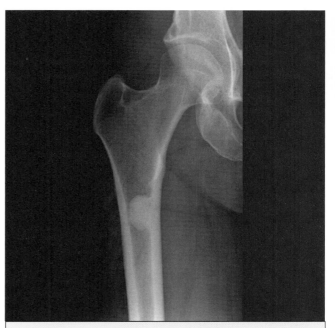

Figure 4 AP radiograph of the hip in an asymptomatic 45-year-old woman with a benign-appearing lesion in the proximal femur consistent with a bone island. (Reproduced from Weber KL, Heck RJ Jr: Cystic and benign bone lesions, in Schwartz HS, ed: *Orthopaedic Knowledge Update: Musculoskeletal Tumors*, ed 2. Rosemont, IL, American Academy of Orthopaedic Surgeons, 2007, p 98.)

4: Orthopaedic Oncology/Systemic Disease

f. Radiographic differential diagnosis includes well-differentiated osteosarcoma, osteoblastic metastasis, and bone infarct.

5. Pathology

   a. Bone islands appear histologically as cortical bone with a well-defined lamellar structure and haversian systems.

   b. The border between the lesion and surrounding medullary bone shows no endochondral ossification.

6. Treatment/outcome—No treatment is required, but follow-up radiographs should be taken if any question about the diagnosis exists.

II. Cartilage

A. Enchondroma—A benign tumor composed of mature hyaline cartilage and located in the medullary cavity.

1. Demographics

   a. Enchondromas can occur at any age, but they are most common in patients 20 to 50 years of age.

   b. The incidence is unclear because most lesions are found incidentally.

2. Genetics/etiology

   a. Thought to be related to incomplete endochondral ossification, in which fragments of epiphyseal cartilage displace into the metaphysis during skeletal growth.

   b. *IDH1* and *IDH2* mutations have been reported.

3. Clinical presentation

   a. Most enchondromas are asymptomatic and are noted incidentally on radiographs.

   b. Lesions in the small bones of the hands and feet can be painful, especially after pathologic fracture.

   c. In a patient with an enchondroma and pain in the adjacent joint, the pain often has a cause that is unrelated to the tumor.

   d. If a patient has pain and the radiographic appearance is suspicious, low-grade chondrosarcoma must be considered.

   e. One half of all enchondromas occur in the small tubular bones, with most in the hands. Enchondromas are the most common bone tumor in the hand.

   f. Other common locations include the metaphysis or diaphysis of long bones (proximal humerus, distal femur, proximal tibia); enchondromas are rare in the spine and pelvis.

   g. Enchondromas are classified by Enneking as inactive or latent bone lesions.

   h. The incidence of malignant transformation is less than 1%. Rarely, a dedifferentiated chondrosarcoma develops from an enchondroma.

4. Imaging appearance

   a. Enchondromas begin as well-defined, lucent, central medullary lesions that calcify over time; they appear more diaphyseal as the long bone grows.

   b. The classic radiographic appearance involves rings and stippled calcifications within the lesion (**Figure 5, A**).

   c. Lesions can be 1 to 10 cm in size.

   d. Small endosteal erosion (< 50% of the width of the cortex) or cortical expansion may be present.

   e. In hand enchondromas, the cortices may be thinned and expanded (**Figure 5, B**).

   f. Cortical thickening or frank destruction suggests a chondrosarcoma.

   g. The radiographic differential diagnosis includes a bone infarct and low-grade chondrosarcoma.

   h. The radiographic appearance is more important than the pathologic appearance in differentiating an enchondroma from a low-grade chondrosarcoma.

   i. Enchondromas frequently have increased uptake on bone scans due to continual remodeling of the endochondral bone within the lesion.

   j. MRI is not necessary for diagnosis, but it will show the lesion as lobular and bright on T2-weighted images with no bone marrow edema or periosteal reaction.

5. Pathology

   a. Gross: blue-gray, lobulated hyaline cartilage with a variable amount of calcifications throughout the tumor

   b. The low-power histologic appearance is of mature hyaline cartilage lobules separated by normal marrow, which is key to differentiating an enchondroma from a chondrosarcoma.

   c. Endochondral ossification encases the cartilage lobules with lamellar bone.

   d. Lesions in the small tubular bones and proximal fibula are more hypercellular than lesions in other locations.

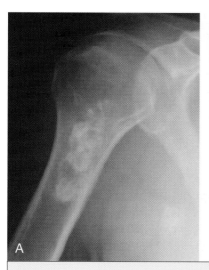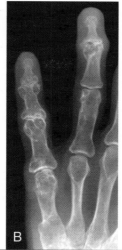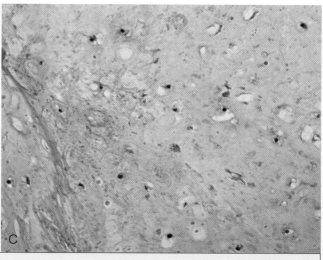

Figure 5 Enchondromas. **A,** AP radiograph of the right proximal humerus in a 49-year-old woman with shoulder pain reveals a calcified lesion in the metaphysis that is centrally located within the bone. The ring-like or stippled calcifications are consistent with an enchondroma. There is no endosteal erosion or cortical thickening. **B,** Radiograph demonstrates enchondromas in the hand of a patient with Ollier disease. Note the multiple expansile lytic lesions affecting the metacarpals and phalanges. Areas of calcified cartilage are evident within the lucent areas. **C,** Histologic appearance of an enchondroma. Note the normal chondrocytes in lacunar spaces with no mitotic figures. (Part C reproduced from Weber KL, O'Connor MI: Benign cartilage lesions, in Schwartz HS, ed: *Orthopaedic Knowledge Update: Musculoskeletal Tumors*, ed 2. Rosemont, IL, American Academy of Orthopaedic Surgeons, 2007, p 111.)

4: Orthopaedic Oncology/Systemic Disease

e. Enchondromas in long bones have abundant extracellular matrix but no myxoid component.

f. The cells are bland, with uniform, dark-stained nuclei; they have no pleomorphism, necrosis, mitoses, or multinucleate cells (**Figure 5, C**).

6. Treatment/outcome

a. Asymptomatic lesions require no treatment but can be followed with serial radiographs to ensure inactivity.

b. Rarely, when pain due to other causes is excluded, symptomatic enchondromas can be treated with curettage and bone grafting.

c. Pathologic fractures through enchondromas in small, tubular bones can be allowed to heal before curettage and bone grafting.

d. Surgery is necessary when radiographs are suspicious for a chondrosarcoma.

e. A needle biopsy is not reliable to differentiate enchondroma from low-grade chondrosarcoma and should be used only if confirmation of cartilage tissue type is needed.

7. Related conditions: Ollier disease; Maffucci syndrome

a. Ollier disease is characterized by multiple enchondromas with a tendency toward unilateral involvement of the skeleton (sporadic inheritance).

b. Multiple enchondromas are thought to indicate a skeletal dysplasia with failure of normal endochondral ossification throughout the metaphyses of the affected bones.

c. *IDH1* and, less commonly, *IDH2* mutations are present in patients with Ollier disease and Maffucci syndrome.

d. Patients with multiple enchondromas have growth abnormalities causing shortening and bowing deformities.

e. Maffucci syndrome involves multiple enchondromas and soft-tissue angiomas.

f. Radiographically, the enchondromas in Ollier disease and Maffucci syndrome have variable mineralization and often expand the bone markedly.

g. The angiomas in Maffucci syndrome can be identified on radiographs because of the presence of phleboliths (small, round, calcified bodies).

h. The histologic appearance of lesions in a patient with multiple enchondromas is similar to solitary lesions in small tubular bones (hypercellular with mild chondrocytic atypia).

i. Patients with multiple enchondromas may require surgical correction of skeletal deformities at a young age.

j. Patients with Ollier disease have an increased

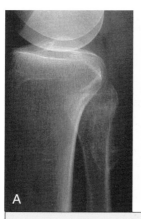
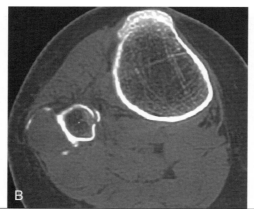
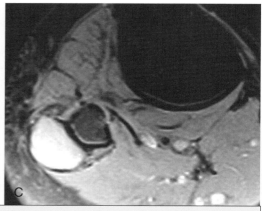

Figure 6   Periosteal chondroma. **A,** Lateral view of the right knee in a 28-year-old woman with lateral calf pain. Extraosseous calcification is seen around the proximal fibula. **B,** Axial CT reveals a surface lesion with a calcified rim and nondisplaced pathologic fracture in the fibula. **C,** T2-weighted MRI reveals bright signal intensity and defines this as a surface lesion without medullary involvement. A biopsy revealed a periosteal chondroma.

risk of malignant transformation of an enchondroma to a low-grade chondrosarcoma (25% to 30%).

   k. Patients with Maffucci syndrome have an increased risk of malignant transformation of an enchondroma to a low-grade chondrosarcoma (23% to 100%), as well as a high risk of developing a fatal visceral malignancy.

   l. Patients with Ollier disease or Maffucci syndrome should be followed long-term because of the increased chance of malignancy.

B. Periosteal chondroma—A benign hyaline cartilage tumor located on the surface of the bone.

   1. Demographics—Periosteal chondromas occur in patients from 10 to 30 years of age.

   2. Genetics/etiology—Periosteal chondromas are rare lesions thought to arise from pluripotential cells deep in the periosteum that differentiate into chondroblasts instead of osteoblasts.

   3. Clinical presentation

      a. Patients usually present with pain; sometimes the lesions are found incidentally in asymptomatic patients.

      b. Any bone can be involved, but the proximal humerus, the femur, and the small bones of the hand are the most common locations.

      c. The lesions can grow slowly after patients reach skeletal maturity, but they have no malignant potential.

   4. Imaging appearance

      a. The classic appearance is a well-defined surface lesion that creates a saucerized defect in the underlying cortex (**Figure 6**).

      b. The lesion ranges from 1 to 5 cm in size and is metaphyseal or diaphyseal.

      c. A rim of sclerosis is seen in the underlying bone.

      d. The edges of the lesion often have a mature buttress of bone.

      e. The amount of calcification is variable. Soft-tissue swelling may be present because of the surface location.

      f. The radiographic differential diagnosis includes periosteal chondrosarcoma and periosteal osteosarcoma.

   5. Pathology

      a. The low-power appearance is of well-circumscribed hyaline cartilage lobules.

      b. The histologic appearance is similar to that of an enchondroma, with mildly increased cellularity, binucleated cells, and occasional mild pleomorphism.

   6. Treatment/outcome

      a. No treatment is needed for asymptomatic patients.

      b. Symptomatic patients are treated with excision with an intralesional or marginal margin.

      c. Local recurrence is rare.

C. Osteochondroma—A benign osteocartilaginous tumor arising from the surface of the bone.

   1. Demographics

      a. Osteochondromas are the most common benign bone tumor.

b. The true incidence of osteochondromas is unknown because most lesions are asymptomatic.

c. Most lesions are identified in the first 2 decades of life.

2. Genetics/etiology

a. Osteochondromas are hamartomatous proliferations of both bone and cartilage.

b. They are thought to arise from trapped growth-plate cartilage that herniates through the cortex and grows via endochondral ossification beneath the periosteum.

c. A defect in the perichondrial node of Ranvier may allow the physeal growth to extend from the surface; as the cartilage ossifies, it forms cortical and cancellous bone that comprises the stalk of the lesion.

3. Clinical presentation

a. Most lesions are solitary and asymptomatic.

b. Most are less than 3 cm in size, but they can be as large as 15 cm.

c. Depending on size and location, patients can have pain from an inflamed overlying bursa, fracture of the stalk, or nerve compression.

d. When close to the skin surface, osteochondromas can be palpated as firm, immobile masses.

e. Osteochondromas continue to grow until the patient reaches skeletal maturity.

f. The lesions most commonly occur around the knee (distal femur, proximal tibia), proximal humerus, and pelvis; spinal lesions (posterior elements) are rare.

g. A subungual exostosis that arises from beneath the nail in the distal phalanx is a posttraumatic lesion and not a true osteochondroma.

h. When multiple lesions are present, the condition is called multiple hereditary exostoses (also called hereditary multiple exostoses).

i. The risk of malignant degeneration of a solitary osteochondroma to a chondrosarcoma is less than 1%.

j. Rarely, a dedifferentiated chondrosarcoma can develop from a solitary osteochondroma.

4. Imaging appearance

a. Osteochondromas can be sessile or pedunculated on the bone surface (**Figure 7, A**).

b. Sessile lesions are associated with a higher risk of malignant degeneration.

c. Lesions arise near the growth plate and appear to become more diaphyseal with time.

d. Pedunculated lesions grow away from the adjacent joint (**Figure 7, B** and **C**).

e. The medullary cavity of the bone is continuous with the stalk of the lesion.

f. The cortex of the underlying bone is continuous with the cortex of the stalk.

g. The affected bony metaphysis is often flared or widened.

h. The cartilage cap is usually radiolucent and involutes at skeletal maturity.

i. Metaplastic cartilage nodules can occur within a bursa over the cartilage cap.

j. The radiographic differential diagnosis includes parosteal osteosarcoma and myositis ossificans.

k. CT and MRI can evaluate the cartilage cap and surrounding soft tissues better than plain radiographs and are useful when malignant degeneration is a concern.

5. Pathology

a. The gross appearance of a pedunculated lesion is similar to that of a cauliflower, with cancellous bone beneath the cartilage cap.

b. Histologically, the cartilage cap consists of hyaline cartilage and is organized like a growth plate with maturation to bony trabeculae (**Figure 7, D**).

c. A well-defined perichondrium surrounds the cartilage cap.

d. The stalk consists of cortical and trabecular bone, with spaces between the bone filled with marrow.

e. The chondrocytes within the lesion are uniform, without pleomorphism or multiple nuclei.

f. A thick cartilage cap implies growth but is not a reliable indicator of malignant degeneration.

6. Treatment/outcome

a. Nonsurgical treatment is preferred in asymptomatic or minimally symptomatic patients who are still growing.

b. Relative indications for surgical excision of an osteochondroma (performed by excision at the base of the stalk)

- Symptoms secondary to inflammation of soft tissues (bursae, muscles, joint capsule, tendons) not controlled by NSAIDs or activity modification

- Symptoms secondary to frequent traumatic injury

- Significant aesthetic deformity

4: Orthopaedic Oncology/Systemic Disease

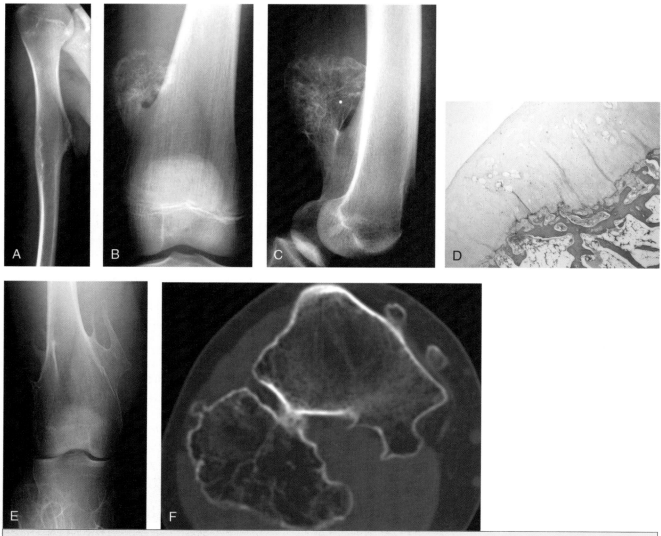

Figure 7   Osteochondromas. **A,** Sessile osteochondroma noted on an AP radiograph of the right humerus in a 14-year-old boy. AP (**B**) and lateral (**C**) radiographs of the distal femur in an 11-year-old boy reveal a pedunculated osteochondroma of the medial distal femur. The medullary portion of the lesional stalk is continuous with the medullary cavity of the distal femur. Note the cortical sharing. **D,** At low-power magnification, the histologic appearance of an osteochondroma shows the cartilage cap with the cartilage cells arranged in columns similar to a growth plate. **E,** AP radiograph of the right knee in an 18-year-old man with multiple hereditary exostosis. Note the multiple small lesions and the widened metaphysis. **F,** Axial CT scan of the same patient shown in **E** shows the posteromedial extension of a lesion in the proximal fibula. (Part F reproduced from Weber KL, O'Connor MI: Benign cartilage lesions, in Schwartz HS, ed: *Orthopaedic Knowledge Update: Musculoskeletal Tumors*, ed 2. Rosemont, IL, American Academy of Orthopaedic Surgeons, 2007, p 106.)

- Symptoms secondary to nerve or vascular irritation

- Concern for malignant transformation

c. The perichondrium over the cartilage cap must be removed to decrease the likelihood of local recurrence.

d. Delaying surgical excision until skeletal maturity increases the chance of local control.

e. The surgeon should be aware that patients with osteochondromas extending into the popliteal fossa can have pseudoaneurysms and are are at risk for vascular injury during excision.

7. Related condition: multiple hereditary exostoses

a. Multiple hereditary exostoses is a skeletal dysplasia that is inherited with an autosomal dominant pattern.

b. Patients may have up to 30 osteochondromas throughout the skeleton.

c. *EXT1* and *EXT2* are genetic loci associated with this disorder. Mutations in these genes are

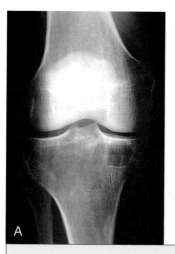
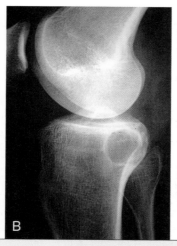
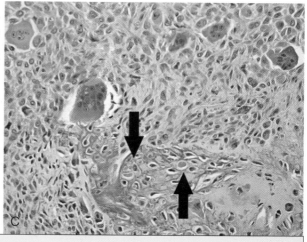

Figure 8   Chondroblastoma. AP (**A**) and lateral (**B**) views of the right knee in a 19-year-old man show a well-circumscribed round lesion in the proximal tibial epiphysis extending slightly into the metaphysis. Note the sclerotic rim. **C,** Histologic appearance of a chondroblastoma. Note the round or oval chondroblasts (arrows). On higher power magnification, areas of dystrophic calcification are visible around the individual cells in a "chicken-wire" pattern. (Part C reproduced from Weber KL, O'Connor MI: Benign cartilage lesions, in Schwartz HS, ed: *Orthopaedic Knowledge Update: Musculoskeletal Tumors,* ed 2. Rosemont, IL, American Academy of Orthopaedic Surgeons, 2007, p 116.)

found in most patients affected with the disorder; they are considered tumor-suppressor genes.

d. *EXT1* and *EXT2* proteins function in the biosynthesis of heparin sulfate proteoglycans, which are involved in growth factor signaling in normal growth plate. Decreased *EXT1* or *EXT2* expression results in defects in endochondral ossification, which is likely to be related to the formation of osteochondromas.

e. Clinically, patients with the disorder have skeletal deformities and short stature.

f. The lesions are similar radiographically and histologically to solitary osteochondromas.

g. Radiographs reveal primarily sessile lesions that may grow to be very large.

h. Metaphyseal widening is present in affected patients (**Figure 7, E** and **F**).

i. Deformities occur as a result of disorganized endochondral ossification in the growth plate and may require surgical correction, especially in the paired bones (radius/ulna, tibia/fibula).

j. The risk of malignant transformation is higher (~5% to 10%) in patients with this condition than in patients with solitary lesions.

k. The most common location of a secondary chondrosarcoma is the pelvis. The malignant tumors are usually low grade.

D. Chondroblastoma—A rare, benign bone tumor differentiated from giant cell tumor by its chondroid matrix.

1. Demographics

a. Male-to-female ratio = 2:1

b. 80% of patients are younger than 25 years.

2. Genetics/etiology

a. Chondroblastoma has been categorized as a cartilage tumor because of its areas of chondroid matrix, but type II collagen is not expressed by the tumor cells.

b. It is thought to arise from the cartilaginous epiphyseal plate.

3. Clinical presentation

a. Patients present with pain that is progressive at the site of the tumor.

b. Because these tumors often occur adjacent to a joint, decreased range of motion, a limp, muscle atrophy, and tenderness over the affected bone may be present.

c. Most chondroblastomas are found in the distal femur and proximal tibia, followed by proximal humerus, proximal femur, calcaneus, and flat bones.

d. Benign pulmonary metastasis develops from chondroblastoma in less than 1% of patients.

4. Imaging appearance

a. Chondroblastomas are small, round tumors that occur in the epiphysis or apophysis; they often extend into the metaphysis (**Figure 8, A** and **B**).

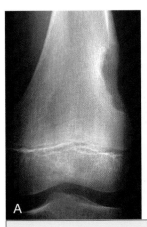 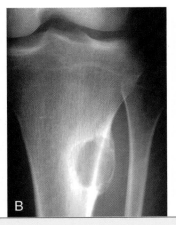 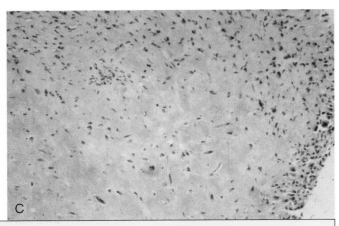

Figure 9 Chondromyxoid fibromas. **A,** AP radiograph of the right distal femur in a 12-year-old boy with knee pain shows an eccentric lytic lesion with a well-defined intramedullary border. A periosteal shell that is not easily seen is consistent with a chondromyxoid fibroma. **B,** AP radiograph of the proximal tibia in a 22-year-old woman with an eccentric lesion expanding the cortex with a visible rim. **C,** The histologic appearance of a chondromyxoid fibroma shows hypercellular regions at the periphery of the lobules. Note the spindled, stellate cells and myxoid stroma.

b. Most are 1 to 4 cm in size, have a sclerotic rim, and are centrally located in the epiphysis.

c. Cortical expansion of the bone may be present, but soft-tissue extension is rare.

d. A small subset have a more aggressive appearance due to secondary ABC formation.

e. Stippled calcifications are seen within the lesion in 25% to 40% of chondroblastomas.

f. The differential diagnosis includes giant cell tumor, osteomyelitis, and clear cell chondrosarcoma.

g. Three-dimensional imaging is not required, but a CT scan will define the bony extent of the lesion.

h. MRI shows extensive edema surrounding the lesion.

5. Pathology

a. The tumor consists of a background of mononuclear cells, scattered multinucleate giant cells, and focal areas of chondroid matrix.

b. The mononuclear stromal cells are distinct, round, S100+ cells with large, central nuclei that can appear similar to histiocytes; the nuclei have a longitudinal groove resembling a coffee bean (**Figure 8, C**).

c. Chicken-wire calcifications are present in a lace-like pattern throughout the tumor.

d. Mitotic figures are present but not atypical.

e. One third of chondroblastomas have areas of secondary ABC.

6. Treatment/outcome

a. Curettage and bone grafting is indicated for the treatment of chondroblastoma.

b. Surgical adjuvants such as phenol or liquid nitrogen can be used to decrease local recurrence.

c. The local recurrence rate is 10% to 15%.

d. Surgical resection is indicated for the rare cases of benign pulmonary metastasis.

E. Chondromyxoid fibroma (CMF)—A rare, benign cartilage tumor containing chondroid, fibrous, and myxoid tissue.

1. Demographics

a. Most CMFs occur in the second and third decades of life, but they may be seen in patients up to 75 years of age.

b. Slight male predominance

2. Genetics/etiology—CMF is thought to arise from remnants of the growth plate.

3. Clinical presentation

a. Most patients present with pain and mild swelling of the affected area.

b. Occasionally, the lesions are noted incidentally on radiographic examination.

c. The most common locations are the long bones of the lower extremities (proximal tibia) and pelvis. Small bones in the hands and feet are also affected.

4. Imaging appearance

a. CMF is a lucent, eccentric lesion found in the metaphysis of long bones (**Figure 9, A**).

b. It can cause thinning and expansion of the adjacent cortical bone (**Figure 9, B**).

c. It often has a sharp, scalloped sclerotic rim.

d. Radiographic calcifications within the lesion are rare.

e. CMFs range in size from 2 to 10 cm.

f. The radiographic differential diagnosis includes ABC, chondroblastoma, and nonossifying fibroma.

g. Increased tracer uptake is seen within the lesion on bone scan.

5. Pathology

a. On low-power magnification, the lesion is lobulated, with peripheral hypercellularity.

b. Within the lobules, the cells are spindled or stellate, with hyperchromatic nuclei.

c. Multinucleated giant cells and fibrovascular tissue are seen between the lobules.

d. Areas of myxoid stroma are present, but hyaline cartilage is rare (**Figure 9, C**).

e. The cellular areas may resemble chondroblastoma.

f. Areas with pleomorphic cells with bizarre nuclei are common.

g. The histologic differential diagnosis includes chondroblastoma, enchondroma, and chondrosarcoma.

6. Treatment/outcome

a. CMF is treated with curettage and bone grafting.

b. The local recurrence rate is 10% to 20%.

III. Fibrous/Histiocytic

A. Nonossifying fibroma (NOF)—A developmental abnormality related to faulty ossification; not a true neoplasm.

1. Demographics

a. Very common skeletal lesions

b. Occur in children and adolescents (age 5 to 15 years)

c. NOFs are found in 30% of children with open physes.

d. Also frequently called fibrous cortical defect or metaphyseal fibrous defect

2. Genetics/etiology—Possibly caused by abnormal subperiosteal osteoclastic resorption during remodeling of the metaphysis.

3. Clinical presentation

a. Usually an incidental finding

b. May be multifocal. Types include:

- Familial multifocal

- Neurofibromatosis

- Jaffe-Campanacci syndrome (congenital, with café-au-lait pigmentation, mental retardation, and nonskeletal abnormalities involving the heart, eyes, and gonads)

c. Most common in long bones of lower extremity (80%)

d. Patients occasionally present with a pathologic fracture.

4. Radiographic appearance

a. Eccentric, lytic, cortically based lesions with a sclerotic rim (**Figure 10, A and B**)

b. Occur in the metaphysis and appear to migrate to the diaphysis as bone grows

c. May thin the overlying cortex with expansion of the bone

d. Lesions enlarge (1 to 7 cm) as the patient grows.

e. As the patient reaches skeletal maturity, the lesions ossify and become sclerotic.

f. Occasionally associated with secondary ABC

g. Plain radiographs are diagnostic.

h. An avulsive cortical irregularity is the result of an avulsion injury at the insertion of the adductor magnus muscle on the posteromedial aspect of the distal femur and can be similar in appearance to an NOF.

5. Pathology

a. Prominent storiform pattern of fibrohistiocytic cells (**Figure 10, C and D**)

b. Variable numbers of giant cells

c. Areas of xanthomatous reaction with foamy histiocytes may be present.

d. Prominent hemosiderin

e. Occasional secondary ABC component

6. Treatment/outcome

a. Most are managed with observation; spontaneous regression usually occurs.

b. Large lesions should be monitored along with skeletal growth.

c. Curettage and bone grafting may be indicated for symptomatic and large lesions.

d. Pathologic fractures are often allowed to heal and then are observed or treated with curettage and grafting.

4: Orthopaedic Oncology/Systemic Disease

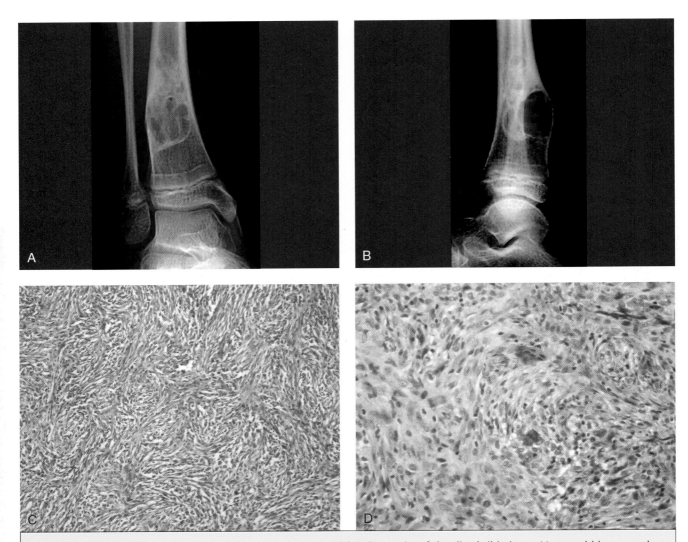

Figure 10 Nonossifying fibromas (NOFs). AP (**A**) and lateral (**B**) radiographs of the distal tibia in an 11-year-old boy reveal an NOF that has healed after a minimally displaced pathologic fracture. It is an eccentric, scalloped lesion with a sclerotic rim. Anteriorly, the lesion is filling in with bone. **C,** Histologic appearance of an NOF. Bands of collagen fibers and fibroblasts can be seen coursing throughout the lesion. **D,** High-power magnification of the same specimen shown in **C** reveals multinucleated giant cells and hemosiderin-laden histiocytes that are characteristic of an NOF. (Parts C and D reproduced from Pitcher JD Jr, Weber KL: Benign fibrous and histiocytic lesions, in Schwartz HS, ed: *Orthopaedic Knowledge Update: Musculoskeletal Tumors*, ed 2. Rosemont, IL, American Academy of Orthopaedic Surgeons, 2007, p 122.)

e. Internal fixation is rarely needed; depends on anatomic location.

B. Fibrous dysplasia—A common developmental abnormality characterized by hamartomatous proliferation of fibro-osseous tissue within the bone.

1. Demographics

   a. Can be seen in patients of any age, but approximately 75% are seen in patients younger than 30 years

   b. Females affected more commonly than males

2. Genetics/etiology

   a. Solitary focal or generalized multifocal inability to produce mature lamellar bone

b. Areas of the skeleton remain indefinitely as immature, poorly mineralized trabeculae.

c. Not inherited

d. Monostotic and polyostotic forms are associated with dominant activating mutations of GSα on chromosome 20q13, which produce a sustained adenylate cyclase–cyclic adenosine monophosphate activation.

e. Fibrous dysplasia tissue has high expression of fibroblast growth factor-23, thought to be the cause of hypophosphatemia in patients with McCune-Albright syndrome or oncogenic osteomalacia.

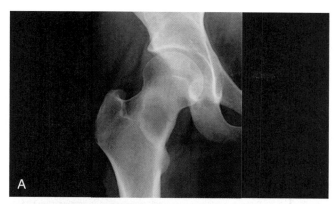

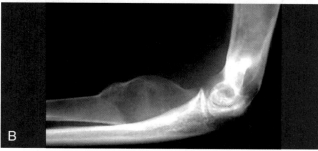

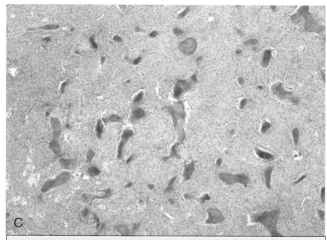

Figure 11 Fibrous dysplasia. **A,** AP radiograph of the right proximal femur in an 18-year-old woman with groin pain. A central, lytic bone lesion with a ground glass appearance fills the femoral neck, consistent with fibrous dysplasia. **B,** A lateral radiograph of an elbow reveals an expansile lesion in the proximal radius with a ground glass appearance. There is no evidence of cortical destruction. **C,** Histologic appearance on intermediate magnification. Metaplastic bone spicules can be seen scattered haphazardly; this pattern produces the characteristic radiographic ground glass appearance of fibrous dysplasia. (Part B reproduced from Prichard DJ, ed: *1999 Musculoskeletal Tumors and Diseases Self-Assessment Examination.* Rosemont, IL, American Academy of Orthopaedic Surgeons, 1999. Part C reproduced from Pitcher JD Jr, Weber KL: Benign fibrous and histiocytic lesions, in Schwartz HS, ed: *Orthopaedic Knowledge Update: Musculoskeletal Tumors,* ed 2. Rosemont, IL, American Academy of Orthopaedic Surgeons, 2007, p 125.)

3. Clinical presentation

   a. Usually asymptomatic and found incidentally

   b. Can be monostotic or polyostotic

   c. Can affect any bone but has a predilection for the proximal femur, rib, maxilla, tibia

   d. Fatigue fractures through the lesion can cause pain.

   e. Swelling may be present around the lesion.

   f. Severe cranial deformities and blindness with craniofacial involvement may be present.

   g. Patients occasionally present with pathologic fractures.

   h. McCune-Albright syndrome—Triad of polyostotic fibrous dysplasia, precocious puberty, and pigmented skin lesions (with irregular borders likened to the coast of Maine).

   • Unilateral bone lesions

   • Skin lesions usually on the same side as bone lesions

   • The syndrome is present in 3% of patients with polyostotic fibrous dysplasia.

   i. Myriad endocrine abnormalities are associated with polyostotic forms.

   j. Most common entity causing oncogenic osteomalacia (renal phosphate wasting due to fibroblast growth factor-23)

   k. Mazabraud syndrome—Fibrous dysplasia (usually polyostotic) associated with multiple intramuscular myxomas.

   • Females affected more commonly than males

   • Lower limbs more frequently affected

4. Radiographic appearance

   a. Central lytic lesions within the medullary canal, usually diaphysis/metaphysis

   b. Sclerotic rim

   c. May be expansile with cortical thinning

   d. Ground glass or shower-door glass appearance (**Figure 11, A**)

   e. Bowing deformity in proximal femur (shepherd's crook) or tibia

   f. Vertebral collapse and kyphoscoliosis may be seen.

   g. Long lesion in a long bone (**Figure 11, B**)

   h. Increased activity on bone scan; plain radiographs usually diagnostic

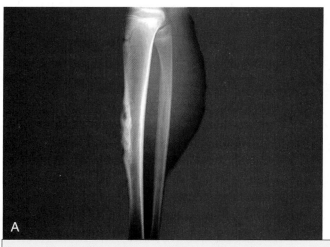
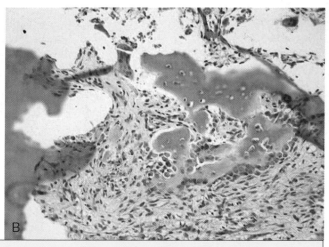

Figure 12   Osteofibrous dysplasia. **A,** Lateral radiograph of the tibia in a skeletally immature patient reveals a cortically based lytic lesion. There are multiple lucencies surrounded by dense sclerosis, consistent with osteofibrous dysplasia. There is no periosteal reaction. **B,** A high-power histologic section reveals woven bone arising from a fibrous stroma. The new bone is prominently rimmed by osteoblasts, thereby differentiating this from fibrous dysplasia. (Reproduced from Scarborough MT, ed: *2005 Musculoskeletal Tumors and Diseases Self-Assessment Examination.* Rosemont, IL, American Academy of Orthopaedic Surgeons, 2005.)

5. Bone scan—Increased activity is seen, but bone scan is not required because plain radiographs are usually diagnostic.

6. Pathology

   a. Gross: yellow-white gritty tissue

   b. Histology: poorly mineralized immature fibrous tissue surrounding islands of irregular, often poorly mineralized trabeculae of woven bone (**Figure 11, C**)

   c. "Chinese letters" or "alphabet soup" appearance

   d. Metaplastic bone arises from fibrous tissue without osteoblastic rimming.

   e. Common mitoses

   f. Metaplastic cartilage or areas of cystic degeneration may be present.

   g. Can be associated with secondary ABC

   h. Differential diagnosis includes low-grade intramedullary osteosarcoma

7. Treatment/outcome

   a. Asymptomatic patients may be observed.

   b. Surgical indications include painful lesions, impending/actual pathologic fracture, severe deformity, neurologic compromise (spine).

   c. Surgical treatment: curettage and bone grafting of the lesion. (It is important to use cortical allograft, not cancellous autograft, because cancellous autograft is replaced by dysplastic bone.)

   d. Internal fixation (intramedullary device more effective than plate) usually required to achieve pain control in the lower extremity

   e. Osteotomies for deformity

   f. Medical treatment with bisphosphonates provided pain relief in uncontrolled series.

   g. In approximately 1% of lesions, malignant transformation to osteosarcoma, fibrosarcoma, or undifferentiated pleomorphic sarcoma occurs, with extremely poor prognosis.

C. Osteofibrous dysplasia—A nonneoplastic fibro-osseous lesion affecting the long bones of young children.

   1. Demographics

      a. Affects males more commonly than females

      b. Usually noted in the first decade of life

   2. Genetics/etiology: Trisomies 7, 8, 12, and 22 have been reported.

   3. Clinical presentation

      a. Unique predilection for the tibia

      b. Anterior or anterolateral bowing deformity may be present.

      c. Pseudarthrosis develops in 10% to 30% of patients.

      d. Patients usually present with painless swelling over the anterior border of the tibia.

   4. Radiographic appearance

      a. Eccentric, well-defined anterior tibial lytic lesions (**Figure 12, A**)

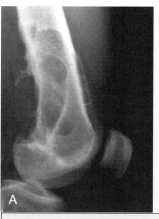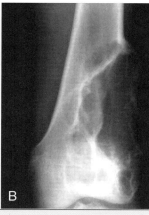

Figure 13 Desmoplastic fibroma. Lateral (**A**) and AP (**B**) radiographs of the distal femur reveal a lytic lesion expanding the posterolateral cortex and having an internal honeycomb appearance. This is consistent with the aggressive behavior of a desmoplastic fibroma.

b. Usually diaphyseal

c. Single or multiple lucent areas surrounded by dense sclerosis

d. Confined to the anterior cortex; may expand

e. No periosteal reaction

f. Differential diagnosis: adamantinoma (radiographic appearance can be identical)

5. Pathology

a. Moderately cellular fibroblastic stroma

b. Islands of woven bone with prominent osteoblastic rimming (**Figure 12, B**)

c. No cellular atypia

d. May have giant cells

e. Differential diagnosis: fibrous dysplasia

6. Treatment/outcome

a. Surgery should be avoided if possible; bracing may be used when necessary.

b. Lesions may spontaneously regress or stabilize at skeletal maturity.

c. Deformity correction may be required.

d. Controversy: whether a continuum exists from osteofibrous dysplasia to adamantinoma; the exact nature of this relationship is uncertain.

D. Desmoplastic fibroma—An extremely rare benign bone tumor composed of dense bundles of fibrous connective tissue.

1. Demographics—Most common in patients aged 10 to 30 years.

2. Genetics/etiology

a. Bone counterpart of the aggressive fibromatosis (desmoid) in soft tissue; may originate from myofibroblasts

b. Loss of 5q21-22 (gene location for familial adenomatous polyposis and Gardner syndrome) has been reported

c. Loss of 4p and rearrangement of 12q12-13; and trisomy 8 (0% to 33%), trisomy 20 (2% to 25%), or both (0% to 16%)

3. Clinical presentation

a. Can occur in any bone

b. Intermittent pain unrelated to activity

c. Palpable mass/swelling

4. Imaging appearance

a. Lytic lesion centrally located in metaphysis

b. Honeycomb/trabeculated appearance (**Figure 13**)

c. Usually no periosteal reaction unless a fracture is present (12%)

d. May appear aggressive with cortical destruction and soft-tissue extension

e. No calcification within lesion

f. Increased activity on bone scan

5. Pathology

a. Gross: dense, white, scarlike tissue

b. Histology: abundant collagen fibrils with intermixed spindle cells

c. Appearance is hypocellular and similar to scar tissue.

d. Monotonous, with uniform nuclei

e. Infiltrative growth pattern, trapping native trabeculae

f. Differential diagnosis includes low-grade fibrosarcoma.

6. Treatment/outcome

a. Surgical treatment is the standard of care.

b. Thorough curettage allows good results.

c. Wide resection is used for expendable bones or locally recurrent lesions.

d. Tumors do not metastasize but often recur locally.

E. Langerhans cell histiocytosis (LCH)—A clonal proliferation of Langerhans-type histiocytes; can have multiple clinical presentations.

4: Orthopaedic Oncology/Systemic Disease

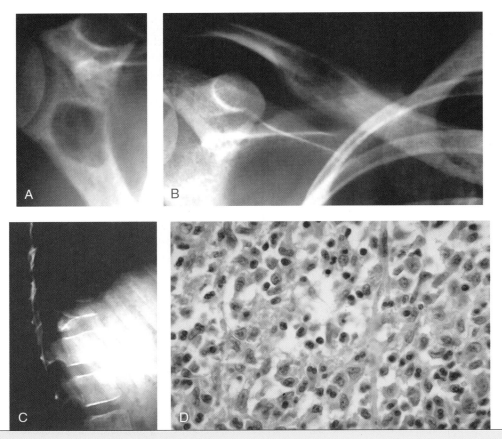

Figure 14   Eosinophilic granulomas/Langerhans cell histiocytosis. **A,** AP radiograph of a scapula with a well-defined lytic lesion having a classic "punched-out" appearance of an eosinophilic granuloma. **B,** AP radiograph of a lytic lesion in the right clavicle of a child demonstrates cortical expansion, periosteal reaction, and no sclerotic edges. This is an eosinophilic granuloma, but the radiographic appearance can also be consistent with osteomyelitis or Ewing sarcoma. **C,** A lateral radiograph of the thoracic spine shows the classic appearance of vertebra plana in a patient with eosinophilic granuloma. **D,** Histologic appearance of an eosinophilic granuloma shows a mixed inflammatory infiltrate with Langerhans histiocytes having large indented nuclei, lymphocytes, and eosinophils. (Part C reproduced from Prichard DJ, ed: *1999 Musculoskeletal Tumors and Diseases Self-Assessment Examination.* Rosemont, IL, American Academy of Orthopaedic Surgeons, 1999.)

1. Demographics

   a. Most common in children (80% younger than 20 years)

   b. Male-to-female ratio = 2:1

2. Genetics/etiology: An activating mutation of the *BRAF* gene is noted in LCH cells (more common in patients <10 years of age)

3. Clinical presentation

   a. Previously categorized as eosinophilic granuloma, Hand-Schüller-Christian disease (chronic, disseminated), and Letterer-Siwe disease (infantile, acute)

   b. Now believed to be three types

      • Solitary disease (eosinophilic granuloma)

      • Multiple bony sites

      • Multiple bony sites with visceral involvement (lungs, liver, spleen, skin, lymph nodes)

   c. Rarely, bone lesions are asymptomatic; usually, they cause localized pain/swelling/limp.

   d. Can occur in any bone; most commonly, the skull, ribs, clavicle, scapula, vertebrae (thoracic > lumbar > cervical), long bones, pelvis

4. Radiographic appearance

   a. Classic appearance: "punched-out" lytic lesion (**Figure 14, A**)

   b. May have thick periosteal reaction

   c. Can appear well-demarcated or permeative (**Figure 14, B**)

   d. Commonly causes vertebral collapse (vertebra plana) when affecting the spine (**Figure 14, C**)

Table 2

Unicameral Bone Cysts Versus Aneurysmal Bone Cysts

Factors	Unicameral Bone Cyst	Aneurysmal Bone Cyst
Presentation	Pathologic fracture	Pain, swelling
Common locations	Proximal humerus Proximal femur	Distal femur, proximal tibia Pelvis Posterior elements of spine
Radiographic characteristics	Central, lytic lesion Metaphyseal Symmetric expansion less than width of growth plate	Eccentric, lytic lesion Metaphyseal Can expand wider than growth plate Extends into soft tissues with a thin periosteal rim
Treatment	Intralesional steroid injection Curettage/grafting/internal fixation (proximal femur)	Curettage and bone grafting Embolization (spine, pelvis, and so forth)

e. Great mimicker of other lesions (osteomyelitis, Ewing sarcoma, leukemia)

5. Pathology

   a. The characteristic tumor cell is the Langerhans cell or histiocyte (**Figure 14, D**).

   b. Histiocytes have indented nuclei ("coffee bean" appearance), eosinophilic cytoplasm.

   c. Histiocytes stain with CD1a.

   d. Giant cells are present.

   e. Eosinophils are variable in number.

   f. Mixed inflammatory cell infiltrate

   g. Birbeck granules ("tennis racket" appearance) seen in Langerhans cells on electron microscopy

6. Treatment/outcome

   a. Solitary lesions can be treated effectively with an intralesional injection of methylprednisolone acetate.

   b. Curettage and bone grafting is done if open biopsy is being performed for diagnosis.

   c. In 90% of patients with vertebra plana caused by Langerhans cell histiocytosis, bracing alone will correct the deformity; 10% will need corrective surgery.

   d. Low-dose radiation is used in rare cases (spinal cord compression).

   e. Patients with disseminated disease and visceral involvement have a poor prognosis, with 50% survival at 5 years. The prognosis is improving with more effective chemotherapy but worsens with increasing number of extraosseous disease sites.

IV. Cystic

A. Unicameral bone cyst (UBC)—A common, serous fluid–filled bone lesion.

   1. Demographics—Most cases occur in patients younger than 20 years.

   2. Genetics/etiology

      a. Thought to result from a temporary failure of medullary bone formation near the epiphyseal plate during skeletal growth

      b. The cyst is active initially when adjacent to the growth plate. When medullary bone formation resumes, the cyst appears to move into the diaphysis.

      c. Possible causes and precursor lesions include lymphatic/venous obstruction, intraosseous hematoma, intraosseous synovial rest.

   3. Clinical presentation (**Table 2**)

      a. The most common presentation is a pathologic fracture after minor trauma.

      b. Painful symptoms resolve when the fracture heals.

      c. The most common locations include the proximal humerus and proximal femur, but UBCs can also occur in the ilium and calcaneus.

   4. Imaging appearance

      a. Purely lytic lesion located centrally in the medullary canal

      b. UBCs start metaphyseal, adjacent to the growth plate, and appear to progress toward the diaphysis with bone growth (**Figure 15, A**).

      c. Narrow zone of transition between cyst and normal bone

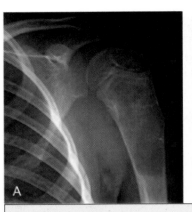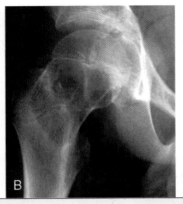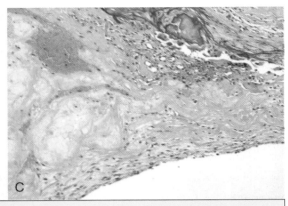

Figure 15 Unicameral bone cysts. **A,** AP radiograph of the proximal humerus in a 5-year-old girl shows a lytic lesion centrally located in the medullary canal of the metaphysis consistent with a unicameral bone cyst. The lesion does not expand the bone wider than the epiphyseal plate. The girl had had a prior pathologic fracture through the lesion. **B,** AP radiograph of a proximal femur demonstrates a lytic lesion in the metaphysis abutting the proximal femoral epiphyseal plate. The lesion is central in location and will likely require surgical treatment because of the high risk of fracture. **C,** Histologic appearance. A thin cyst lining consisting of fibroblasts is seen. Cementum is noted in the wall, and no cellular atypia is present. (Part C reproduced from Weber KL, Heck RK Jr: Cystic and benign bone lesions, in Schwartz HS, ed: *Orthopaedic Knowledge Update: Musculoskeletal Tumors*, ed 2. Rosemont, IL, American Academy of Orthopaedic Surgeons, 2007, p 91.)

  d. Cortical thinning but no soft-tissue extension (**Figure 15, B**)

  e. Bone expansion does not exceed the width of the physis.

  f. Trabeculations occur after multiple fractures.

  g. "Fallen leaf" sign is pathognomonic (cortical fragment that has fallen into base of empty lesion).

  h. Plain radiographs are usually diagnostic, but T2-weighted MRI shows a well-defined zone of bright, uniform signal intensity.

5. Pathology

  a. Lining of the cyst is a thin fibrous membrane; no true endothelial cells (**Figure 15, C**).

  b. Giant cells, inflammatory cells, hemosiderin within lining

  c. Clear or serous fluid within cavity (bloody after fracture)

  d. 10% of cysts contain cementum spherules (calcified eosinophilic fibrinous material) in the lining.

6. Treatment/outcome

  a. Natural history: fills in with bone as the patient reaches skeletal maturity.

  b. After acute fractures, lesions occasionally fill in with native bone (15%).

  c. Evidence-based treatment: intralesional injection of methylprednisolone acetate.

  d. Multiple injections may be required, especially in very young children.

  e. No evidence to suggest improved outcomes with injection of bone marrow or graft substitutes; however, they remain in use.

  f. Proximal femoral lesions with or without a pathologic fracture are often treated with curettage/bone grafting/internal fixation.

B. Aneurysmal bone cyst—A destructive, expansile reactive bone lesion filled with multiple blood-filled cavities.

1. Demographics: 75% of patients are younger than 20 years

2. Genetics/etiology

  a. Reactive, nonneoplastic process of unknown etiology

  b. Possibilities include a traumatic origin or a circulatory disturbance leading to increased venous pressure and hemorrhage.

  c. Can arise de novo or be associated with an underlying lesion that is identifiable in 30% of cases (most commonly chondroblastoma, giant cell tumor, chondromyxoid fibroma, nonossifying fibroma, osteoblastoma, or fibrous dysplasia).

  d. ABCs express a *TRE17/USP6* translocation.

3. Clinical presentation (**Table 2**)

  a. Pain and swelling are the most common symptoms.

  b. Pathologic fracture as a presenting symptom is rare.

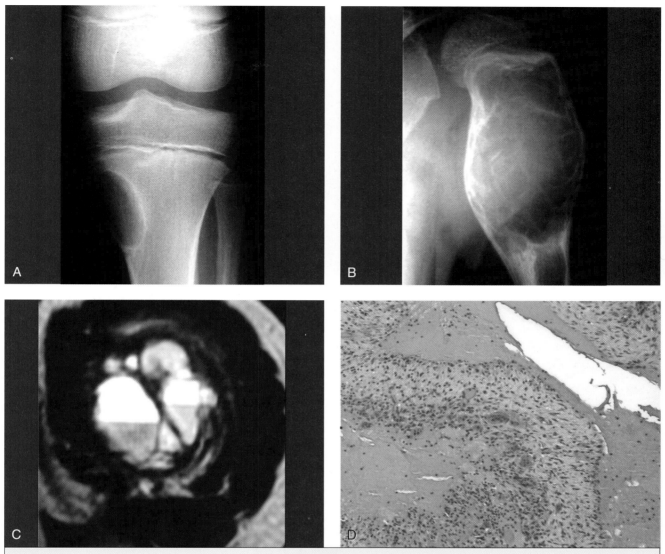

Figure 16   Aneurysmal bone cysts (ABCs). **A,** AP view of a proximal tibia shows an eccentric lytic lesion located in the metaphysis that expands into the soft tissues with a periosteal rim consistent with an ABC. **B,** AP view of a proximal humerus shows a septated expansile lesion wider than the epiphyseal plate in a very young child, consistent with an ABC. **C,** An axial MRI reveals the presence of fluid-fluid levels within the lesion. **D,** Higher power magnification of an ABC shows multinucleated giant cells within the fibrohistiocystic stroma. No cellular atypia is seen. (Part D reproduced from Weber KL, Heck RK Jr: Cystic and benign lesions, in Schwartz HS, ed: *Orthopaedic Knowledge Update: Musculoskeletal Tumors*, ed 2. Rosemont, IL, American Academy of Orthopaedic Surgeons, 2007, p 89.)

4: Orthopaedic Oncology/Systemic Disease

c. Neurologic symptoms are possible with lesions in the spine.

d. Most common locations are distal femur, proximal tibia, pelvis, spine (posterior elements).

4. Imaging appearance

a. Eccentric, lytic lesions located in the metaphysis (**Figure 16, A**)

b. Aggressive destruction of or expansion into the cortex and extension into the soft tissues may be seen.

c. Lesion can expand to greater than the width of the epiphyseal plate (**Figure 16, B**).

d. Usually maintains a periosteal rim around the lesion

e. Can grow contiguously across adjacent spinal segments or extend through the epiphyseal plate

f. No matrix mineralization

g. T2-weighted MRI shows fluid-fluid levels (separation of serum and blood products) (**Figure 16, C**).

h. Radiographic differential diagnosis includes UBC and telangiectatic osteosarcoma.

5. Pathology

   a. Blood-filled cyst without a true endothelial lining

   b. Lining contains giant cells, new (woven) bone, spindle cells (**Figure 16, D**).

   c. Solid areas are common.

   d. Histologic evidence of an underlying primary lesion may be seen.

   e. No cellular atypia, but mitoses are common

   f. Histologic differential diagnosis includes telangiectatic osteosarcoma and giant cell tumor.

6. Treatment/outcome

   a. Surgical treatment is curettage and bone grafting of the lesion.

   b. Local adjuvants (for example, phenol) can be used after curettage.

   c. Highest local recurrence is in young patients with an open physeal plate.

   d. For local recurrence, repeat curettage and grafting is indicated.

   e. Expendable bones (for example, proximal fibula) may be resected.

   f. Embolization or sclerotherapy can be useful for pelvic or spinal lesions alone or in combination with surgical treatment.

V. Giant Cell Tumor of Bone

A. Definition—Giant cell tumor of bone is a benign, aggressive bone tumor consisting of distinct undifferentiated mononuclear cells.

B. Demographics

   1. Most occur in patients 30 to 50 years of age (90% older than 20 years).

   2. Affects females more commonly than males

C. Genetics/etiology

   1. Etiology is unknown.

   2. Stromal cells have alterations in the *c-myc*, *c-Fos*, and *N-myc* oncogenes.

D. Clinical presentation

   1. Main symptoms: pain and swelling for 2 to 3 months

   2. Decreased range of motion around a joint

3. Some patients (10%) present with a pathologic fracture.

4. Located most commonly in the distal femur, proximal tibia, distal radius, proximal humerus, proximal femur, sacrum, and pelvis

5. 1% of cases are multicentric.

E. Imaging appearance

   1. Eccentric, lytic lesions located in the epiphysis/metaphysis of long bones

   2. May arise in an apophysis

   3. Lesions extend to the subchondral surface with no sclerotic rim (**Figure 17, A** and **B**).

   4. Can destroy the cortex and extend into the surrounding tissues (**Figure 17, C** and **D**)

   5. Located in the anterior vertebral body when the spine is involved

   6. Commonly have a secondary ABC component

   7. Associated soft-tissue calcifications may be present

   8. Bone scan shows increased uptake in the lesion.

   9. MRI is helpful only to define the extent of soft-tissue involvement; plain radiographs are usually diagnostic.

F. Pathology

   1. Gross: soft, red-brown, hemorrhagic, necrotic (**Figure 17, E**)

   2. Histology: uniformly scattered multinucleated giant cells within a background of mononuclear stromal cells (**Figure 17, F** and **G**)

   3. The stromal cell represents the neoplastic cell.

   4. Secondary changes of necrosis or fibrohistiocytic change may be seen.

   5. Mitoses are frequent, but no cellular atypia.

   6. No matrix production unless there is a pathologic fracture

   7. Frequent ABC component

   8. No histologic grading system exists for giant cell tumor; also no way to predict prognosis.

G. Treatment/outcome

   1. Most lesions can be treated with thorough curettage and a high-speed burr.

   2. Thorough intralesional treatment requires making a large cortical window.

   3. Local surgical adjuvants (phenol, cryotherapy, argon beam) are commonly used to decrease local recurrence.

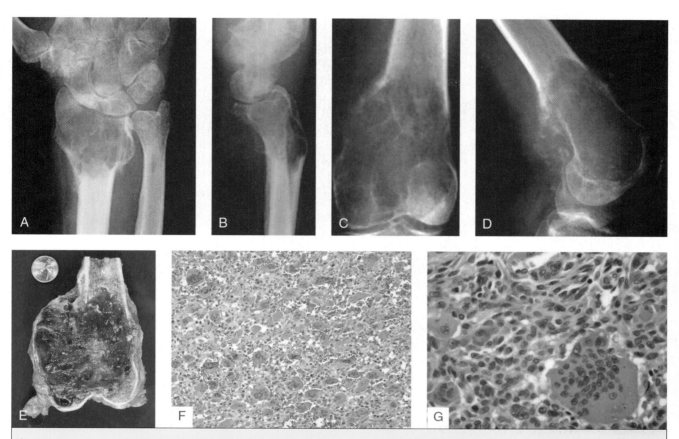

Figure 17 Giant cell tumors. AP (**A**) and lateral (**B**) radiographs of the wrist in a 54-year-old man reveal an expansile lesion located within the epiphysis of the distal radius. No matrix is produced, and there is no sclerotic rim. There has been a pathologic fracture through the lesion. AP (**C**) and lateral (**D**) radiographs of the distal femur in a 33-year-old woman demonstrate an aggressive lytic lesion expanding and destroying the medial and posterior cortices. The differential includes malignant bone tumors, but a biopsy revealed a giant cell tumor. **E,** Gross view of the resection specimen (an intralesional procedure was not deemed appropriate) from the same patient shown in **C** and **D**. **F,** Low-power photomicrograph shows abundant multinucleated giant cells amid a background of mononuclear stromal cells (hematoxylin and eosin, x100). **G,** A higher power photomicrograph shows the multinucleated giant cells with abundant nuclei (hematoxylin and eoxin, x400). The nuclei of the stromal cells resemble those of the giant cells. No cellular atypia or matrix production is noted. (Parts F and G reproduced from McDonald DJ, Weber KL: Giant cell tumor of bone, in Schwartz HS, ed: *Orthopaedic Knowledge Update: Musculoskeletal Tumors*, ed 2. Rosemont, IL, American Academy of Orthopaedic Surgeons, 2007, p 135.)

4. Defect can be filled with either bone graft or methylmethacrylate (equivalent recurrence rate), with or without internal fixation, depending on the defect size

5. Patient can bear weight as tolerated when methylmethacrylate is used; when bone graft is used, protection from weight bearing is required until consolidation.

6. Local recurrence with intralesional treatment is 10% to 15%.

7. Local recurrence can be in the adjacent bone or can manifest as soft-tissue masses.

8. Aggressive lesions may require resection and reconstruction.

9. Embolization should be used for large pelvic or spinal lesions alone or in combination with surgical treatment.

10. Denosumab is FDA-approved for the treatment of unresectable giant cell tumor of bone. Studies have shown disease and symptom control for advanced or refractory disease.

11. Radiation is occasionally used in multiply recurrent or surgically inaccessible lesions.

12. The tumor metastasizes to the lungs in 2% of patients (benign metastasizing giant cell tumor).

    a. Treatment includes thoracotomy, radiation, chemotherapy, or observation.

    b. 10% to 15% of patients with metastatic disease die of the disease.

13. Rarely, giant cell tumor is malignant (~1%).

Top Testing Facts

Bone

1. Osteoid osteoma has a radiolucent nidus with surrounding sclerosis.

2. The bone scan is always intensely positive in an osteoid osteoma.

3. Thin-cut CT scans most often identify the nidus and make the diagnosis of osteoid osteoma.

4. The proximal femur is the most common location for an osteoid osteoma.

5. Osteoid osteoma is the most common cause of a painful scoliosis in a young patient.

6. RFA is the current standard of care to treat osteoid osteoma.

7. An osteoid osteoma can be differentiated from an osteoblastoma by its smaller size and less aggressive behavior, although the histologic appearance is similar.

8. Osteoblastoma is a large radiolucent lesion that occurs most commonly in the posterior elements of the spine.

9. Parosteal osteoma must be differentiated from parosteal osteosarcoma.

10. A bone island is an inactive lesion most commonly found in the pelvis or proximal femur.

Cartilage

1. Enchondromas are usually asymptomatic; painful presentation is usually due to an unrelated condition.

2. The clinical presentation and radiographic appearance are more important than the histologic appearance in differentiating enchondroma from low-grade chondrosarcoma.

3. Patients with either Ollier disease or Maffucci syndrome have an increased risk of malignant transformation of an enchondroma to a low-grade chondrosarcoma.

4. A periosteal chondroma is a surface lesion that creates a saucerized defect in the underlying cortex.

5. The medullary cavity of the underlying bone is continuous with the stalk of an osteochondroma.

6. Secondary chondrosarcomas arising from osteochondromas are low grade and occur more often in patients with multiple lesions.

7. *EXT1* and *EXT2* are genetic loci commonly mutated in patients with multiple hereditary exostoses.

8. Chondroblastoma most commonly occurs in the epiphyses and apophyses of long bones.

9. Chondroblastoma rarely metastasizes to the lung.

10. Chondromyxoid fibroma is a lucent, eccentric lesion with a sclerotic, scalloped rim seen in long bones, pelvis, and hands/feet.

Fibrous/Histiocytic

1. Nonossifying fibromas are usually incidental findings that spontaneously regress and should be observed.

2. Nonossifying fibromas are developmental abnormalities that occur in 30% of children.

3. Nonossifying fibromas occur as scalloped lytic lesions with a sclerotic border within the metaphysis.

4. Fibrous dysplasia is a long lesion in a long bone with a ground glass appearance.

5. The histologic appearance of fibrous dysplasia is woven bone shaped like "Chinese letters" or "alphabet soup" in a cellular, fibrous stroma.

6. Polyostotic fibrous dysplasia occurs in McCune-Albright syndrome along with precocious puberty and café-au-lait spots.

7. Osteofibrous dysplasia affects children in the first decade of life; it has a predilection for the anterior cortex of the tibia.

8. The histologic appearance of osteofibrous dysplasia is a cellular, fibrous stroma with prominent osteoblastic rimming around the woven bone, which differentiates it from fibrous dysplasia.

9. Langerhans cell histiocytosis is the great mimicker; it should be considered with lytic lesions in children.

10. In Langerhans cell histiocytosis, the histiocyte (not the eosinophil) is the tumor cell and stains with CD1A.

Cystic/Miscellaneous

1. UBCs are centrally located in the metaphysis and appear to move to the diaphysis.

2. UBCs present with a pathologic fracture—rare fallen leaf sign on radiographs.

3. UBCs are treated with an intralesional steroid injection.

4. ABCs are destructive, expansile, blood-filled cysts.

5. ABCs occur around the knee, pelvis, and posterior elements of the spine.

6. At least 30% of ABCs are secondary to an underlying primary bone tumor.

7. Giant cell tumors of bone are epiphyseal or apophyseal and extend into the metaphysis and subchondral bone.

8. The mononuclear stromal cell is the neoplastic cell in giant cell tumor.

9. The treatment of giant cell tumor of bone is careful curettage with a large cortical window (low local recurrence rate of 10% to 15%).

10. Giant cell tumor metastasizes to the lung in 2% of patients.

Bibliography

Atesok KI, Alman BA, Schemitsch EH, Peyser A, Mankin H: Osteoid osteoma and osteoblastoma. *J Am Acad Orthop Surg* 2011;19(11):678-689.

Badalian-Very G, Vergilio JA, Fleming M, Rollins BJ: Pathogenesis of Langerhans cell histiocytosis. *Annu Rev Pathol* 2013;8:1-20.

Branstetter DG, Nelson SD, Manivel JC, et al: Denosumab induces tumor reduction and bone formation in patients with giant-cell tumor of bone. *Clin Cancer Res* 2012;18(16): 4415-4424.

De Mattos CB, Angsanuntsukh C, Arkader A, Dormans JP: Chondroblastoma and chondromyxoid fibroma. *J Am Acad Orthop Surg* 2013;21(4):225-233.

Donaldson S, Wright JG: Recent developments in treatment for simple bone cysts. *Curr Opin Pediatr* 2011;23(1):73-77.

Douis H, Saifuddin A: The imaging of cartilaginous bone tumours: I. Benign lesions. *Skeletal Radiol* 2012;41(10): 1195-1212.

Garcia RA, Inwards CY, Unni KK: Benign bone tumors—Recent developments. *Semin Diagn Pathol* 2011;28(1):73-85.

Guille JT, Kumar SJ, MacEwen GD: Fibrous dysplasia of the proximal part of the femur: Long-term results of curettage and bone-grafting and mechanical realignment. *J Bone Joint Surg Am* 1998;80(5):648-658.

Kitsoulis P, Galani V, Stefanaki K, et al: Osteochondromas: Review of the clinical, radiological and pathological features. *In Vivo* 2008;22(5):633-646.

Mankin HJ, Trahan CA, Fondren G, Mankin CJ: Non-ossifying fibroma, fibrous cortical defect and Jaffe-Campanacci syndrome: A biologic and clinical review. *Chir Organi Mov* 2009;93(1):1-7.

Most MJ, Sim FH, Inwards CY: Osteofibrous dysplasia and adamantinoma. *J Am Acad Orthop Surg* 2010;18(6): 358-366.

Motamedi K, Seeger LL: Benign bone tumors. *Radiol Clin North Am* 2011;49(6):1115-1134, v.

Ozaki T, Hamada M, Sugihara S, Kunisada T, Mitani S, Inoue H: Treatment outcome of osteofibrous dysplasia. *J Pediatr Orthop B* 1998;7(3):199-202.

Payne WT, Merrell G: Benign bony and soft tissue tumors of the hand. *J Hand Surg Am* 2010;35(11):1901-1910.

Rapp TB, Ward JP, Alaia MJ: Aneurysmal bone cyst. *J Am Acad Orthop Surg* 2012;20(4):233-241.

Raskin KA, Schwab JH, Mankin HJ, Springfield DS, Hornicek FJ: Giant cell tumor of bone. *J Am Acad Orthop Surg* 2013;21(2):118-126.

Riminucci M, Robey PG, Saggio I, Bianco P: Skeletal progenitors and the GNAS gene: Fibrous dysplasia of bone read through stem cells. *J Mol Endocrinol* 2010;45(6):355-364.

Romeo S, Hogendoorn PC, Dei Tos AP: Benign cartilaginous tumors of bone: From morphology to somatic and germ-line genetics. *Adv Anat Pathol* 2009;16(5):307-315.

Taconis WK, Schütte HE, van der Heul RO: Desmoplastic fibroma of bone: A report of 18 cases. *Skeletal Radiol* 1994; 23(4):283-288.

Thakur NA, Daniels AH, Schiller J, et al: Benign tumors of the spine. *J Am Acad Orthop Surg* 2012;20(11):715-724.

Turcotte RE, Wunder JS, Isler MH, et al: Giant cell tumor of long bone: A Canadian Sarcoma Group study. *Clin Orthop Relat Res* 2002;397:248-258.

Volkmer D, Sichlau M, Rapp TB: The use of radiofrequency ablation in the treatment of musculoskeletal tumors. *J Am Acad Orthop Surg* 2009;17(12):737-743.

Wuyts W, Van Hul W: Molecular basis of multiple exostoses: Mutations in the EXT1 and EXT2 genes. *Hum Mutat* 2000; 15(3):220-227.

Yasko AW, Fanning CV, Ayala AG, Carrasco CH, Murray JA: Percutaneous techniques for the diagnosis and treatment of localized Langerhans-cell histiocytosis (eosinophilic granuloma of bone). *J Bone Joint Surg Am* 1998;80(2):219-228.

4: Orthopaedic Oncology/Systemic Disease

Chapter 47

Malignant Bone Tumors
Kristy Weber, MD

I. Bone Tumors

A. Osteosarcoma

1. Definition and demographics

a. Classic intramedullary osteosarcoma is a malignant bone-forming tumor.

b. Male-to-female ratio = 1.5:1

c. Most common malignant bone tumor in children (1,000 new cases/year in United States)

d. Bimodal age distribution

- Most common in second decade of life

- Late peak in sixth decade of life

2. Genetics/etiology

a. Associated with retinoblastoma gene (RB1), a tumor-suppressor gene.

b. Increased incidence in patients with p53 mutations, Paget disease, prior radiation, Rothmund-Thomson syndrome, and retinoblastoma

c. MDM2, HER2/neu, c-myc, and c-fos are oncogenes overexpressed in osteosarcoma, although none are reproducible. Main characteristic is significant aneuploidy.

3. Clinical presentation

a. Commonly presents with intermittent pain progressing to constant (rest, night) pain unrelieved by medications

b. Swelling, decreased range of motion, limp, and weakness depending on location

c. Often present after injury or athletic activity (coincident with age group, no causality known to trauma)

d. Most commonly noted in metaphysis of distal femur, proximal tibia, proximal humerus, and pelvis

e. 10% of patients present with a pathologic fracture.

4. Imaging

a. Classically, osteosarcomas have a mixed appearance with bone destruction and bone formation (**Figures 1** and **2**).

b. In skeletally immature patients, most tumors do not extend past the epiphyseal plate.

c. Cortical destruction and soft-tissue mass with adjacent Codman triangle (normal reactive bone near tumor) are usually seen.

d. Classic osteosarcomas originate in the medullary canal.

e. Radiographic differential diagnosis includes osteomyelitis and Ewing sarcoma.

f. Technetium Tc-99m bone scan can identify skip lesions.

g. MRI delineates extent of marrow involvement, proximity of soft-tissue mass to adjacent neurovascular structures, and skip lesions (**Figure 1, C** and **Figure 2, C**).

h. Dynamic contrast-enhanced MRI correlates with histologic response to chemotherapy.

5. Pathology

a. The gross appearance varies from a soft, fleshy mass to a firm, fibrous, or sclerotic lesion (**Figure 1, D**).

b. The low-power histologic appearance is frankly sarcomatous stroma, which forms tumor osteoid that permeates existing trabeculae (**Figure 1, E**).

c. On high power, the osteoblastic cells are malignant and form the neoplastic new bone (**Figure 1, F**).

d. Osteosarcoma is defined by the presence of malignant osteoid.

e. Extensive pleomorphism and numerous mitotic figures are present.

f. Areas of necrosis, cartilage, or giant cells may be present within the lesion.

Dr. Weber or an immediate family member serves as a board member, owner, officer, or committee member of the Musculoskeletal Tumor Society and the Ruth Jackson Orthopaedic Society.

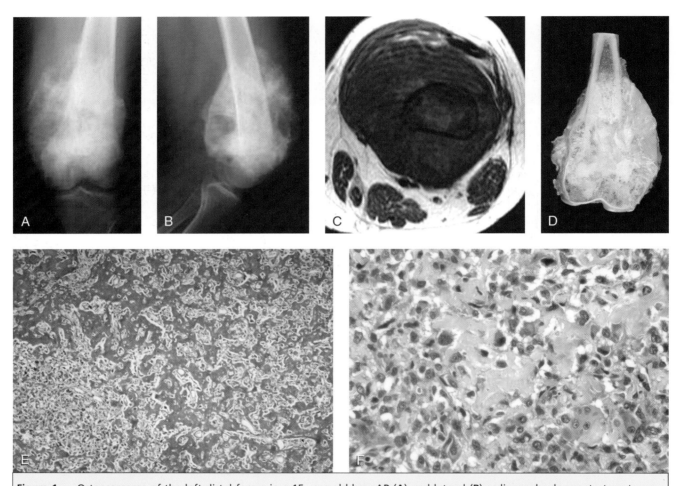

Figure 1 Osteosarcoma of the left distal femur in a 15-year-old boy. AP (**A**) and lateral (**B**) radiographs demonstrate extensive bone formation and an ossified soft-tissue mass after several cycles of chemotherapy. **C,** Axial T1-weighted MRI reveals an extensive circumferential soft-tissue mass abutting the neurovascular bundle posteriorly. **D,** Gross specimen after distal femoral resection shows a clear proximal margin and tumor extending into the epiphysis. **E,** Low-power histologic image shows the classic osteoid formed by malignant stromal cells. Note the lacelike pattern. **F,** High-power image reveals the pleomorphic cells producing the new bone. (Panel E reproduced from Scarborough MT, ed: *2005 Musculoskeletal Tumors and Diseases Self-Assessment Examination.* Rosemont, IL, American Academy of Orthopaedic Surgeons, 2005.)

g. The histologic differential diagnosis includes fibrous dysplasia.

6. Treatment/outcome

a. The standard treatment of osteosarcoma is neoadjuvant chemotherapy followed by surgical resection (limb-sparing or amputation), followed by additional adjuvant chemotherapy.

b. The most common chemotherapy agents include adriamycin (doxorubicin), cisplatinum, methotrexate, and ifosfamide (**Table 1**).

c. Radiation plays no role in the standard treatment of osteosarcoma, although it is used for palliative control in inoperable cases.

d. Limb-sparing surgery can be performed in 90% of cases.

e. Patients who present with a pathologic fracture can be treated with limb-salvage surgery but have a higher risk of local recurrence if the fracture is widely displaced.

f. Local recurrence after surgical resection is approximately 5%; these patients have a dismal prognosis.

g. Good histologic response and wide surgical margins are associated with a low risk of local recurrence.

h. The most common reconstructive options depend on patient age and tumor location and include metal prostheses, intercalary allografts, allograft-prosthetic composites, expandable prostheses, and vascularized fibular autografts.

i. Tumor stage is the most important prognostic indicator.

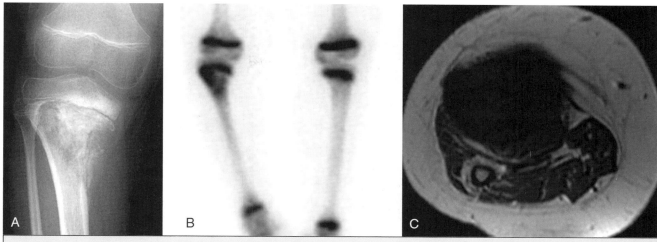

Figure 2   Osteosarcoma of the right proximal tibia in an 8-year-old boy. **A,** AP radiograph demonstrates collapse of the medial cortex with a minimally displaced fracture. Both bone destruction and formation are seen. **B,** Technetium Tc-99m bone scan reveals avid uptake in the area of the tumor. **C,** Axial T1-weighted MRI reveals a small, medial soft-tissue mass.

j. The percentage of necrosis within the tumor after neoadjuvant chemotherapy is related to overall survival (> 90% necrosis is associated with significantly increased survival).

k. Elevated lactate dehydrogenase (LDH) and alkaline phosphatase have been reported to be poor prognostic factors, as is overexpression of vascular endothelial growth factor (VEGF).

l. Survival

- The 5-year survival of patients with localized osteosarcoma in an extremity is 70%.

- The 5-year survival of patients with localized pelvic osteosarcoma is 25%.

- The 10-year overall survival of patients with metastatic disease is 25%.

- Intensifying treatment in response to poor prognostic variables allows no improvement in outcome.

- Outcomes have remained constant for several decades.

m. The most common site of metastasis is the lungs (61%), followed by the bones (16%).

- Aggressive treatment of late (> 1 year) pulmonary metastasis with thoracotomy allows 5-year survival of approximately 30%.

- Patients with bone metastasis usually die of the disease.

n. Skip lesions occur in 10% of patients; the prognosis in these patients is similar to that of patients with lung metastasis.

B. Osteosarcoma subtypes

Table 1

Chemotherapy Drugs Used in the Treatment of Osteosarcoma

Drug	Mechanism of Action	Major Toxicities
Adriamycin/ doxorubicin	Blocks DNA/RNA synthesis Inhibits topoisomerase II	Cardiotoxicity
Cisplatinum	DNA disruption by covalent binding	Hearing loss Neuropathy Renal failure
Methotrexate	Inhibits dehydrofolate reductase (inhibits DNA synthesis)	Mucositis
Ifosfamide	DNA alkylating agent	Renal failure Encephalopathy

1. Parosteal osteosarcoma

a. Definition and demographics

- Low-grade surface osteosarcoma composed of dense bone

- Female-to-male ratio = 2:1

- Accounts for 5% of all osteosarcomas

- Most patients are 20 to 45 years of age

b. Clinical presentation

- Classic presentation is swelling of long duration (often, years).

4: Orthopaedic Oncology/Systemic Disease

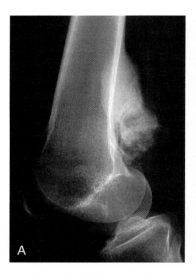
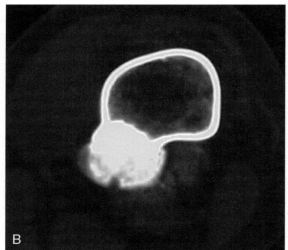
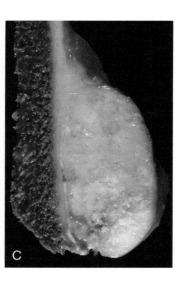
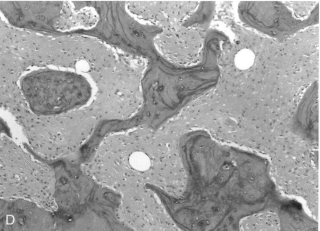
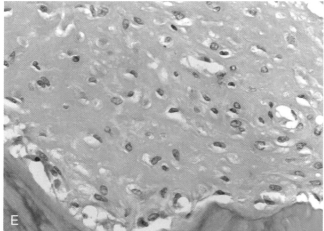

Figure 3   Parosteal osteosarcoma of the distal femur. **A,** Lateral radiograph of the knee reveals a densely ossified surface lesion on the posterior distal femur that is consistent with a parosteal osteosarcoma. **B,** CT scan demonstrates the relationship between the tumor and the femoral cortex. **C,** Gross specimen confirms that it is truly a surface osteosarcoma. **D,** Low-power histologic image reveals a bland appearance with regular, ordered, dense trabeculae and interspersed fibrous stroma. **E,** Higher power histologic image reveals minimal cellular atypia. (Panel A reproduced from Scarborough MT, ed: *2005 Musculoskeletal Tumors and Diseases Self-Assessment Examination.* Rosemont, IL, American Academy of Orthopaedic Surgeons, 2005.)

- Pain, limited joint range of motion, and limp all vary

- The most common location is the posterior aspect of the distal femur (75%), followed by the proximal tibia and the proximal humerus.

c. Imaging

- Dense, lobulated lesion on the surface of the bone (**Figure 3, A**)

- Underlying cortical thickening may be seen.

- Attachment to the cortex may be broad.

- Minor intramedullary involvement is occasionally seen.

- The tumor is most dense in the center and least ossified peripherally.

- Radiographic differential diagnosis includes myositis ossificans and osteochondroma.

- MRI or CT is helpful in defining the lesional extent before surgery (**Figure 3, B**).

- Dedifferentiated parosteal osteosarcoma has ill-defined areas on the surface of the lesion and hypervascularity on angiographic studies.

d. Pathology

- Regular, ordered osseous trabeculae (**Figure 3, D and E**)

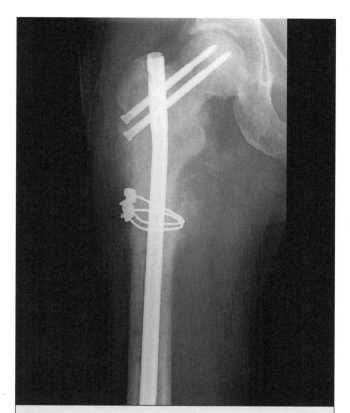

Figure 4 Radiograph shows the proximal femur of a 43-year-old man who was assumed to have metastatic disease; an intramedullary rod was placed in the right femur. Note the osteoblastic appearance of the proximal femur. A later biopsy obtained after continued pain revealed an osteosarcoma. The patient required a hindquarter amputation. This case highlights the importance of a preoperative biopsy.

- Bland, fibrous stroma with occasional slightly atypical cells (grade 1)

- Dedifferentiated parosteal osteosarcoma contains a high-grade sarcoma juxtaposed to the underlying low-grade lesion.

e. Treatment/outcome

- Wide surgical resection is the treatment of choice (**Figure 4**).

- High risk of local recurrence with inadequate resection

- Often, the knee joint can be maintained after resection of the lesion and posterior cortex of the femur.

- Survival is 95% if wide resection is achieved.

- Dedifferentiated variants occur in 25% of patients and are more common after multiple low-grade recurrences; survival is 50%.

2. Periosteal osteosarcoma

a. Definition and demographics

- Rare, intermediate-grade surface osteosarcoma

- Occurs in patients 15 to 25 years of age

- Extremely rare

b. Clinical presentation

- Pain is the most common presenting symptom.

- Most commonly occurs in the femoral or tibial diaphysis

c. Imaging

- Lesion has a sunburst periosteal elevation in the diaphysis of long bones (**Figure 5, A**).

- The underlying cortex may be saucerized.

- No involvement of the medullary canal

d. Pathology

- Gross appearance is lobular and cartilaginous (**Figure 5, B**)

- Histology reveals extensive areas of chondroblastic matrix, but the tumor produces osteoid (**Figure 5, C**).

- Without any osteoid production, the lesion would be a chondrosarcoma.

- Cellular appearance is grade 2 to 3.

e. Treatment/outcome

- Controversial whether to use chemotherapy; the current standard is neoadjuvant chemotherapy followed by wide surgical resection followed by additional chemotherapy.

- Recent study showed 10-year survival of 84% with surgical resection with or without chemotherapy.

- Metastasis develops in 25% of patients.

3. High-grade surface osteosarcoma

a. Definition—Rare, high-grade variant of osteosarcoma that occurs on the bone surface.

b. Demographics, genetics, etiology, clinical presentation, and pathology are the same as for classic osteosarcoma (see section I.A).

c. Radiographic appearance

- Similar to the appearance of a classic osteosarcoma except that high-grade surface osteosarcoma occurs solely on the cortical surface

- No intramedullary involvement

4: Orthopaedic Oncology/Systemic Disease

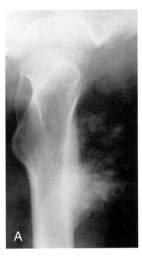
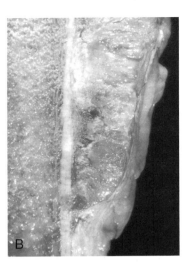
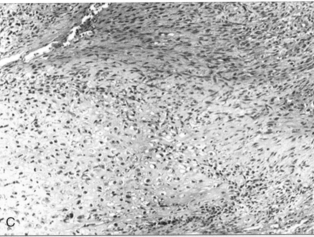

Figure 5 Periosteal osteosarcoma. **A,** Radiograph demonstrates a lesion in the proximal femur. **B,** Gross pathology. **C,** The histologic image reveals a lobular cartilaginous lesion with moderate cellularity. From this appearance, a malignant cartilage lesion would be suspected. One area reveals osteoid production confirming the diagnosis of periosteal osteosarcoma, which is typically chondroblastic in appearance. (Reproduced from Hornicek FJ: Osteosarcoma of bone, in Schwartz HS, ed: *Orthopaedic Knowledge Update: Musculoskeletal Tumors*, ed 2. Rosemont, IL, American Academy of Orthopaedic Surgeons, 2007, p 167.)

4. Telangiectatic osteosarcoma

    a. Definition—Rare histologic variant of osteosarcoma containing large, blood-filled spaces.

    b. Demographics, genetics/etiology, clinical presentation

        • Similar to classic osteosarcoma

        • Rare (only 4% of all osteosarcomas)

        • 25% of patients present with pathologic fracture.

    c. Imaging

        • Purely lytic lesion that occasionally obliterates entire cortex (**Figure 6**)

        • Differential diagnosis primarily includes aneurysmal bone cyst (ABC).

        • Osteosarcoma has more intense uptake than ABC on bone scan.

        • MRI may show fluid-fluid levels and extensive surrounding edema.

    d. Pathology

        • Grossly, the tumor is described as a "bag of blood."

        • Histology shows large blood-filled spaces (**Figure 6, C**).

        • Intervening septa contain areas of high-grade sarcoma with atypical mitoses (**Figure 6, D**).

        • May produce only minimal osteoid

        • Occasionally contains benign giant cells

        • Differential diagnosis: primarily ABC

    e. Treatment/outcome—Same as classic osteosarcoma (see section I.A.6).

II. Fibrous/Histiocytic Tumors

A. Undifferentiated pleomorphic sarcoma (previously called malignant fibrous histiocytoma)

    1. Definition and demographics

        a. Primary malignant bone tumor similar to osteosarcoma but with histiocytic differentiation and no osteoid (**Figures 7 and 8**)

        b. Occurs in patients 20 to 80 years of age (most older than 40 years)

        c. Slight male predominance

    2. Genetics/etiology—25% of cases occur as secondary lesions in the setting of a bone infarct, Paget disease, or prior radiation.

    3. Clinical presentation

        a. Pain is the primary symptom, followed by swelling, limp, decreased range of motion, and pathologic fracture.

        b. Undifferentiated pleomorphic sarcoma of bone most commonly occurs in the metaphyses of long bones, primarily the distal femur, proximal tibia, and proximal humerus.

    4. Imaging

        a. Lytic, destructive lesion with variable periosteal reaction (**Figure 7, A** and **B** and **Figure 8**)

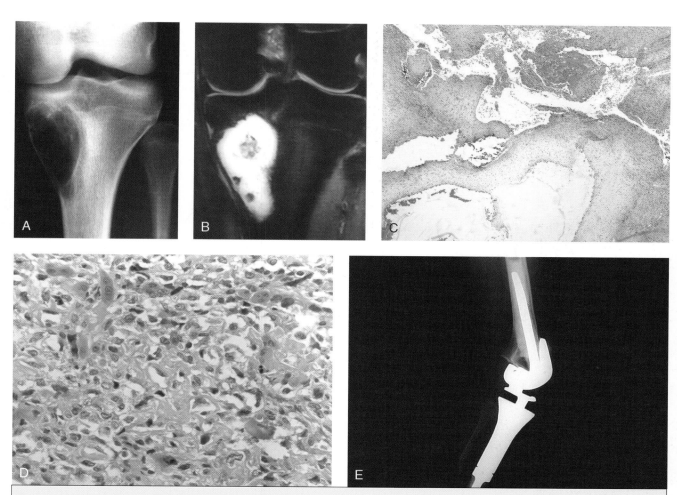

Figure 6   Telangiectatic osteosarcoma. **A,** AP radiograph of the knee of a 14-year-old girl reveals an osteolytic lesion in the medial aspect of the left proximal tibia. The differential diagnosis includes telangiectatic osteosarcoma and aneurysmal bone cyst. **B,** Coronal T2-weighted MRI reveals a lesion of high signal intensity, but no fluid levels are seen. **C,** Low-power histologic image reveals large blood-filled spaces with intervening fibrous septa. **D,** High-power histologic image is required to determine that this is a telangiectatic osteosarcoma with pleomorphic osteoblasts producing osteoid. **E,** Postoperative lateral radiograph obtained after wide resection of the proximal tibia and reconstruction with a modular proximal tibial endoprosthesis. (Panels A and B reproduced from Scarborough MT, ed: *2005 Musculoskeletal Tumors and Diseases Self-Assessment Examination.* Rosemont, IL, American Academy of Orthopaedic Surgeons, 2005.)

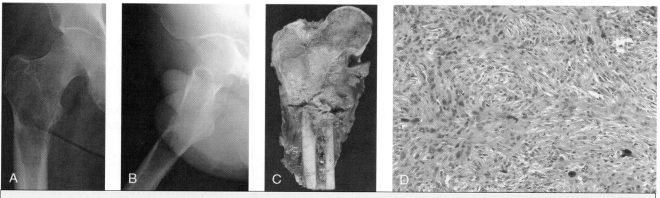

Figure 7   Undifferentiated pleomorphic sarcoma (UPS). AP (**A**) and lateral (**B**) radiographs of the hip of a 43-year-old man with a destructive lesion in the intertrochanteric region of the right femur. A needle biopsy revealed UPS of bone. The patient sustained a pathologic fracture during preoperative chemotherapy. **C,** Gross specimen after proximal femoral resection and reconstruction with a modular endoprosthesis. **D,** Histologic image reveals a storiform pattern with marked pleomorphism and a few multinucleated cells.

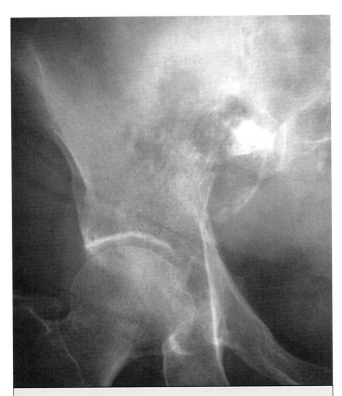

Figure 8   AP radiograph of the right hip and pelvis of a 54-year-old woman with a destructive lesion in the ilium. The lesion is poorly defined, and cortical disruption is seen along the medial wall. A biopsy was consistent with undifferentiated pleomorphic sarcoma of bone.

    b. No bone production

    c. Cortical destruction with a soft-tissue mass is often seen.

    d. Appearance is often nonspecific; the differential diagnosis includes any malignant bone tumor or metastasis.

  5. Pathology

    a. Storiform appearance with marked pleomorphism and mitotic figures (**Figure 7, D**)

    b. Fibrous fascicles radiate from focal hypocellular areas.

    c. Multinucleated tumor cells with histiocytic nuclei (grooved)

    d. Areas of chronic inflammatory cells

    e. Variable collagen production

  6. Treatment/outcome

    a. Undifferentiated pleomorphic sarcoma of bone is treated similarly to osteosarcoma, with neoadjuvant chemotherapy, wide surgical resection, and postoperative chemotherapy.

    b. As with osteosarcoma, reconstructive options depend on patient age and tumor location but include metal prostheses, intercalary allografts, allograft-prosthetic composites, expandable prostheses, and vascularized fibular autografts.

    c. Survival is slightly worse than for osteosarcoma, with metastasis primarily to the lung and bones.

    d. Secondary undifferentiated pleomorphic sarcoma in a preexisting lesion has a worse prognosis than primary undifferentiated pleomorphic sarcoma.

B. Fibrosarcoma of bone

  1. Definition and demographics

    a. Rare malignant bone tumor characterized by spindle cells

    b. Presents in patients 20 to 70 years of age (most older than 40 years).

  2. Clinical presentation

    a. Pain is the predominant symptom.

    b. Variable swelling, limp, decreased range of motion

    c. Occurs most commonly in the femur

    d. Twenty-five percent of patients present secondary to preexisting lesions such as Paget disease, prior radiation, or an infarct.

  3. Imaging

    a. Purely lytic lesion that occurs primarily in the metaphysis

    b. Focal periosteal reaction

    c. Poorly defined margins

    d. A soft-tissue mass best defined with MRI may be present.

    e. Appearance is often nonspecific; the differential diagnosis includes any malignant bone tumor or metastasis.

  4. Pathology

    a. Histology is spindle cells arranged in a herringbone pattern—fascicles at right angles (**Figure 9**).

    b. Low- to high-grade variants exist.

    c. Differential diagnosis includes desmoplastic fibroma.

    d. The number of mitotic figures correlates with the grade of the lesion.

  5. Treatment/outcome

    a. The standard treatment of high-grade fibrosarcoma is similar to that for osteosarcoma: neoadjuvant chemotherapy, wide surgical resection, and postoperative chemotherapy.

b. Overall survival is correlated with grade of the tumor (30% for high grade, 80% for low grade).

c. Overall survival is slightly worse than for osteosarcoma.

III. Cartilage Tumors

A. Chondrosarcoma

1. Definition and demographics

   a. Classic intramedullary chondrosarcoma is a malignant cartilage-producing bone tumor that arises de novo or secondary to other lesions.

   b. Occurs in adult patients (40 to 75 years)

   c. Slight male predominance

   d. Central and surface lesions occur with equal frequency.

   e. Incidence

   • Grade 1 = 60%

   • Grade 2 = 25%

   • Grade 3 = 5%

   • Dedifferentiated = 10%

2. Genetics/etiology—Correlation exists between high expression of telomerase reverse transcriptase and metastasis.

3. Clinical presentation

   a. Pain of prolonged duration (lesional pain can differentiate low-grade chondrosarcoma from benign enchondroma)

   b. Slow-growing firm mass (surface lesion)

   c. Bowel/bladder symptoms may develop with large pelvic lesions.

   d. Most common locations, in order of occurrence, include pelvis, proximal femur, scapula

   e. Location is important for diagnosis (scapula usually malignant, hand usually benign).

   f. Wide range of aggressiveness, depending on grade

   g. Secondary chondrosarcomas occur in the setting of a solitary osteochondroma (< 1%), multiple hereditary osteochondromas (5% to 10%), Ollier disease (25% to 30%), or Maffucci disease (23% to 100%).

4. Imaging

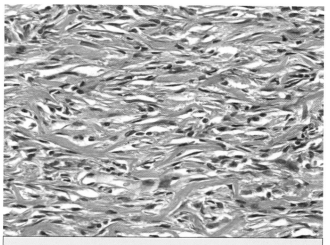

Figure 9   High-power histologic image of a bone fibrosarcoma reveals moderately atypical spindle cells arranged in a herringbone pattern along with collagen fibers.

   a. Radiographic appearance varies by grade of tumor.

   b. Low-grade intramedullary lesions are similar to enchondromas but they have cortical thickening/expansion, extensive endosteal erosion, and occasional soft-tissue extension (Figure 10).

   c. Low-grade lesions have rings, arcs, and stipples and are usually mineralized.

   d. Low-grade chondrosarcomas in the long bones are usually larger than 8 cm.

   e. Low-grade pelvic chondrosarcomas can grow to large size (> 10 cm) with extensive soft-tissue extension toward surrounding viscera.

   f. Intermediate- or high-grade chondrosarcoma is less well defined, involves frank cortical destruction, and often has an associated soft-tissue mass (Figures 11, 12, and 13).

   g. Dedifferentiated chondrosarcoma is a high-grade sarcoma juxtaposed to a benign or low-grade malignant cartilage lesion, noted radiographically by a calcified intramedullary lesion with an adjacent destructive lytic lesion (Figure 14).

   h. Secondary chondrosarcomas appear with ill-defined edges or rapid thickening of cartilage caps next to an enchondroma or osteochondroma, respectively (Figure 15).

   i. Bone scan shows increased uptake in all variants and grades of chondrosarcoma.

   j. CT or MRI is helpful in defining cortical destruction and marrow involvement, respectively.

4: Orthopaedic Oncology/Systemic Disease

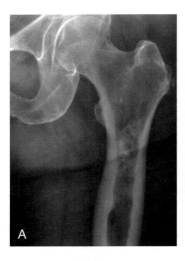
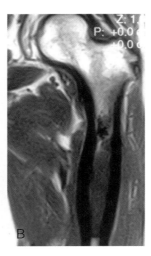
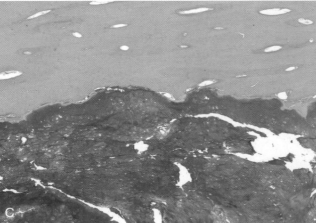
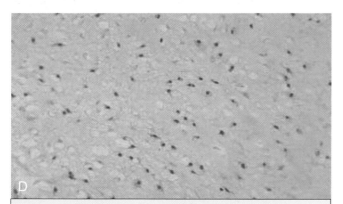

Figure 10   Low-grade chondrosarcoma in a 65-year-old woman who presented with constant thigh pain. **A,** AP radiograph of the left proximal femur shows thickened cortices and proximal intramedullary calcification within the lesion. These findings are consistent with a low-grade chondrosarcoma. **B,** Coronal T1-weighted MRI reveals the intramedullary extent of the lesion. No soft-tissue mass is evident. **C,** Low-power histologic image reveals the interface between the bone and a relatively hypocellular cartilage lesion. **D,** Higher power histologic image reveals a grade 1 chondrosarcoma with a bland cellular appearance, extensive basophilic cytoplasm, and no mitotic figures.

5. Pathology

   a. Low-grade tumors are grossly lobular; higher grade tumors may be myxoid.

   b. Needle biopsy is not helpful in determining the grade of a cartilage tumor.

   c. Low-grade chondrosarcomas have a bland histologic appearance, but permeation and entrapment of the existing trabeculae are present (**Figure 10, C** and **D**).

   d. Mitotic figures are rare.

   e. Higher-grade chondrosarcomas have a hypercellular pattern with binucleate forms and occasional myxoid change (**Figure 11, C**).

   f. Dedifferentiated chondrosarcomas reveal a high-grade sarcoma (undifferentiated pleomorphic sarcoma, fibrosarcoma, osteosarcoma) adjacent to a low-grade or benign cartilage tumor (**Figure 14, D**).

6. Treatment/outcome

   a. Grade 1 chondrosarcomas in the extremities can be treated with careful intralesional curettage or wide resection.

   b. All pelvic chondrosarcomas should be resected with an adequate margin (may require amputation).

   c. Local recurrence rate at 10 years is approximately 20%.

   d. Recurrent lesions have a 10% chance of increasing in grade.

   e. Grade 2 or 3 or dedifferentiated chondrosarcomas require wide surgical resection regardless of location.

   f. Metastasis to the lungs is treated with thoracotomy.

   g. Slow progression of disease requires long-term follow-up (approximately 20 years).

   h. Overall survival depends on the grade of the tumor.

   • Grade 1 > 90%

   • Grade 2 = 60% to 70%

   • Grade 3 = 30% to 50%

   • Dedifferentiated = 10%

   i. No current role for chemotherapy or radiation except in dedifferentiated chondrosarcoma (chemotherapy may be used for high-grade sarcomas, depending on patient age/condition)

B. Chondrosarcoma subtypes

   1. Clear cell chondrosarcoma

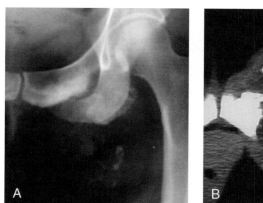
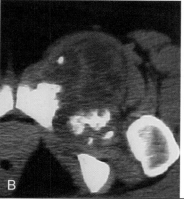
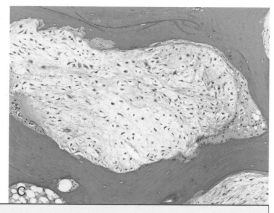

Figure 11   High-grade chondrosarcoma in a 42-year-old woman. **A,** AP radiograph of the left pelvis reveals a destructive lesion of the inferior pubic ramus with a soft-tissue mass. **B,** CT scan defines the mass. Evidence of intralesional calcium within the mass is seen. This radiographic appearance is consistent with a chondrosarcoma. **C,** Histologic image reveals a hypercellular lesion with atypical cells and permeation of the trabecular spaces consistent with a high-grade lesion. (Panels A and B reproduced from Scarborough MT, ed: *2005 Musculoskeletal Tumors and Diseases Self-Assessment Examination.* Rosemont, IL, American Academy of Orthopaedic Surgeons, 2005.)

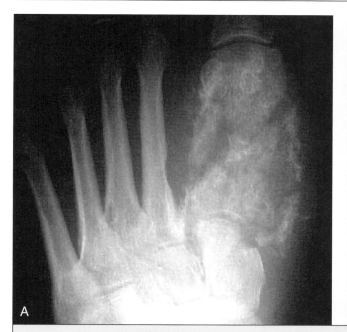
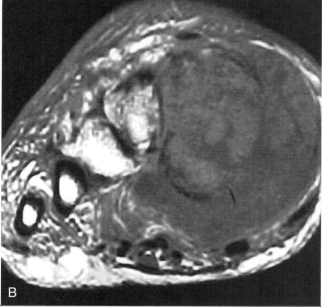

Figure 12   Grade 2 chondrosarcoma of the left foot in a 68-year-old man. **A,** AP radiograph reveals a destructive lesion in the metatarsal. **B,** Axial T1-weighted MRI reveals an extensive soft-tissue mass; the tissue diagnosis was a grade 2 chondrosarcoma. The patient required a transtibial amputation.

a. Definition—Rare malignant cartilage tumor with immature cartilaginous histiogenesis.

b. Demographics, genetics/etiology, and clinical presentation are the same as for classic chondrosarcoma (see section II.A.1-3).

c. Radiographic appearance

   • Clear cell chrondrosarcoma occurs in the epiphysis of long bones, most commonly in the proximal femur or proximal humerus.

   • Lytic, round, expansile well-defined lesion

   • No periosteal reaction

   • Mineralization may be evident within the lesion.

   • Most often confused with a benign chondroblastoma

d. Pathology

   • Intermediate- to high-grade lesion formed of immature cartilage cells (**Figure 16**)

   • Lobular growth pattern

- Benign giant cells throughout the tumor

- Extensive clear cytoplasm with minimal matrix

e. Treatment/outcome

- Wide surgical resection required for cure

- Chemotherapy and radiation not effective

- Metastasis to bones and lungs

- Good prognosis (5-year survival is 80%)

2. Mesenchymal chondrosarcoma

a. Definition and demographics

- Rare primary bone tumor composed of a biphasic pattern of cartilage and small round cell components (**Figure 17**)

- Occurs in younger individuals (10 to 40 years of age) than classic chondrosarcoma.

b. Clinical presentation

- Most common in the flat bones (ilium, ribs, skull), but can occur in the long bones

- Thirty percent of cases involve only soft tissue.

- May involve multiple skeletal sites at presentation

- Pain and swelling of long duration are the most common symptoms.

c. Radiographic appearance

- Lytic destructive tumors with stippled calcification within the lesion (**Figure 17, A**)

- Expansion of bone with cortical thickening and poor margination

- Nonspecific appearance can be included in a differential of any malignant or metastatic lesion.

d. Pathology—Biphasic histologic pattern of low-grade islands of cartilage alternating with sheets of small anaplastic round cells (**Figure 17, B and C**).

e. Treatment/outcome

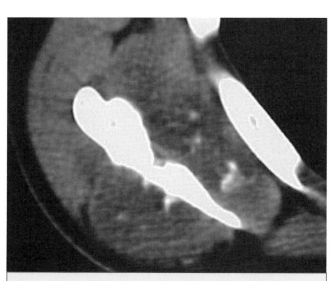

Figure 13 CT scan of the scapula reveals a large soft-tissue mass with tissue consistent with a grade 3 chondrosarcoma. Note the intralesional calcifications. The scapula is a common location for this tumor.

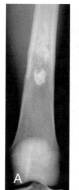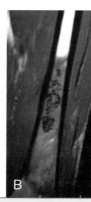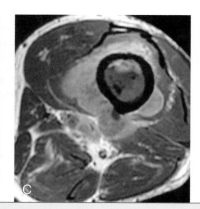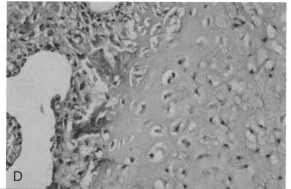

Figure 14 Dedifferentiated chondrosarcoma of the femur in a 73-year-old man. **A,** AP radiograph reveals a lesion similar to an enchondroma within the medullary canal but there is an ill-defined lucency distal to the lesion. **B,** Coronal T1-weighted MRI reveals the intramedullary extent of the lesion, which is much different from an enchondroma and raises the concern for a dedifferentiated chondrosarcoma. **C,** Axial T1-weighted MRI demonstrates a circumferential soft-tissue mass consistent with a high-grade lesion. **D,** A high-power histologic view shows low-grade cartilage juxtaposed to a high-grade sarcomatous lesion, indicating a dedifferentiated chondrosarcoma. (Panels A and B reproduced from Scarborough MT, ed: *2005 Musculoskeletal Tumors and Diseases Self-Assessment Examination*. Rosemont, IL, American Academy of Orthopaedic Surgeons, 2005.)

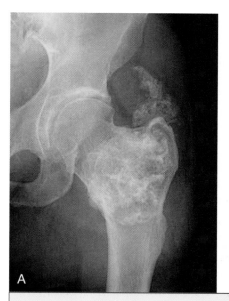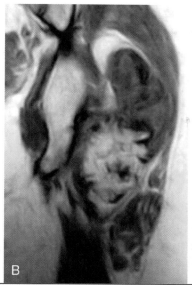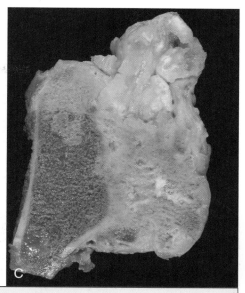

Figure 15 Chondrosarcoma in a 35-year-old woman with multiple hereditary osteochondromas who presented with new-onset hip pain that had become constant. **A,** AP radiograph of the proximal femoral osteochondroma with an ill-defined area proximal to the lesion. **B,** Coronal T1-weighted MRI reveals the osteochondroma to have the same appearance as the adjacent pelvic marrow, but the proximal aspect is composed of soft tissue consistent with malignant degeneration. **C,** Gross appearance of the lesion after resection of the proximal femur. The histology revealed a grade 1 chondrosarcoma.

- Treatment is chemotherapy and wide surgical resection.

- The 5-year survival is 30% to 60%.

- Few series in the literature

IV. Round Cell Lesions

A. Ewing sarcoma/primitive neuroectodermal tumor (PNET)

1. Definition and demographics

   a. Malignant bone tumor composed of small round blue cells

   b. Male-to-female ratio = 3:2

   c. Uncommon in African Americans and Chinese

   d. Second most common primary malignant bone tumor in children (3 cases/million persons/year; 80% younger than 20 years)

   e. Can also be a soft-tissue tumor

2. Genetics/etiology

   a. Cell of origin unknown

   b. Hypothesized to be of neuroectodermal differentiation. PNET is thought to be the differentiated neural tumor, and Ewing sarcoma the undifferentiated variant.

   c. Possible mesenchymal stem cell derivation

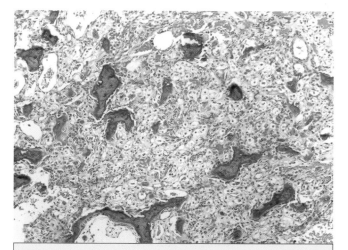

Figure 16 Low-power histologic image of a clear cell chondrosarcoma reveals a cellular lesion with minimal matrix. The cartilage cells have clear cytoplasm. Additional benign giant cells are within the lesion.

   d. Classic 11:22 chromosomal translocation (*EWS/FLI1* is the fusion gene) in 85% of cases

3. Clinical presentation

   a. Pain is the most common symptom.

   b. Swelling, limp, and decreased range of motion are variable.

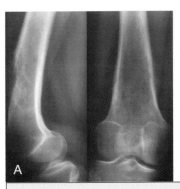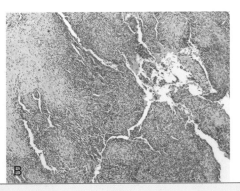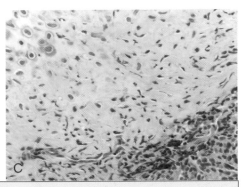

Figure 17 Chondrosarcoma of the distal femur in a 28-year-old woman. **A,** Composite lateral and AP radiographs reveal a poorly defined lytic lesion with destruction of the anterior cortex. **B,** Low-power histologic image reveals a biphasic appearance to the lesion with cartilage as well as small round cells consistent with a mesenchymal chondrosarcoma. **C,** Higher-power histologic image shows the junction between the low-grade cartilage and the sheets of small cells.

   c. Frequent fever, occasional erythema (mistaken for infection)

   d. Elevated erythrocyte sedimentation rate, LDH, white blood cell count

   e. The most common locations are the pelvis, diaphysis of long bones, and scapula.

   f. Twenty-five percent of patients present with metastatic disease.

   g. Staging workup includes a bone marrow biopsy in addition to the standard studies (CT chest, radiograph/MRI of primary lesion, bone scan).

4. Imaging

   a. Purely lytic bone destruction

   b. Periosteal reaction in multiple layers (the classic reaction, called "onion skin") or sunburst pattern (**Figure 18, A** and **B**).

   c. Poorly marginated and permeative

   d. Extensive soft-tissue mass often present despite more subtle bone destruction (**Figures 19** and **20**)

   e. MRI necessary to identify soft-tissue extension and marrow involvement (**Figure 18, C**)

   f. Radiographic differential diagnosis includes osteomyelitis, osteosarcoma, eosinophilic granuloma, osteoid osteoma, lymphoma.

5. Pathology

   a. Gross appearance may be a liquid consistency, mimicking pus.

   b. Small round blue cells with round/oval nuclei (**Figure 18, D** and **E**)

   c. Indistinct cell outlines

   d. Prominent nuclei and minimal cytoplasm

   e. Reactive osseous or fibroblastic tissue may be present.

   f. Can be broad sheets of necrosis and widely separated fibrous strands

   g. Differential diagnosis includes lymphoma, osteomyelitis, neuroblastoma, rhabdomyosarcoma, eosinophilic granuloma, leukemia.

   h. Immunohistochemical stains helpful; CD99+ (013 antibody)

   i. 11:22 chromosomal translocation produces *EWS/FLI1*, which can be identified by polymerase chain reaction in 85% of cases and differentiates Ewing sarcoma from other round cell lesions.

   j. Additional features seen only in PNET include a more lobular pattern and arrangement of the cells in poorly formed rosettes around an eosinophilic material (**Figure 21**).

6. Treatment/outcome

   a. Standard treatment of Ewing sarcoma is neoadjuvant chemotherapy.

   b. Most common chemotherapy drugs include vincristine, adriamycin (doxorubicin), ifosfamide, etoposide, cytoxan, and actinomycin D.

   c. Local control of the primary tumor can be achieved by either wide surgical resection or external beam radiation.

   d. Most isolated extremity lesions are treated with surgical resection rather than radiation because of short-term and long-term side effects of radiation and better potential local control with surgery.

   e. Radiation is often used for the primary lesion in patients who are inoperable or present with metastatic disease.

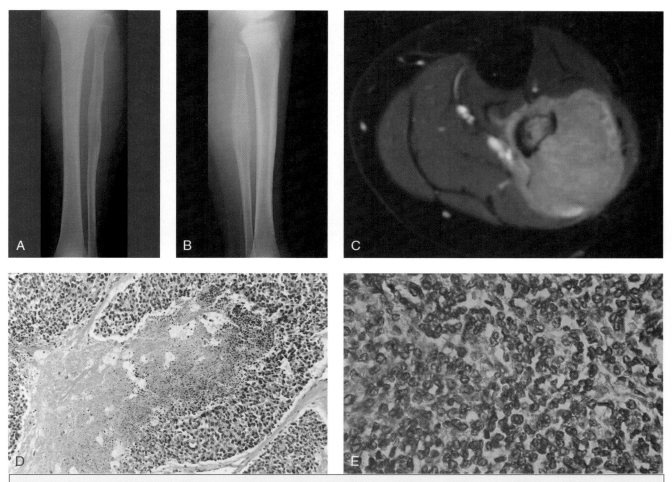

Figure 18 Ewing sarcoma/primitive neuroectodermal tumor (PNET) in an 11-year-old boy. AP (**A**) and lateral (**B**) radiographs of the left tibia/fibula reveal a lesion in the fibular diaphysis. Needle biopsy was consistent with Ewing sarcoma. The initial periosteal reaction ossified slightly after two cycles of neoadjuvant chemotherapy. **C,** Axial T2-weighted fat-saturated MRI obtained at diagnosis reveals an extensive soft-tissue mass at diagnosis consistent with a small round cell lesion. **D,** Low-power histologic image reveals a small round blue cell lesion with large sheets of necrosis. **E,** Higher power image reveals the monotonous small cells with prominent nuclei and scant cytoplasm characteristic of Ewing sarcoma/PNET.

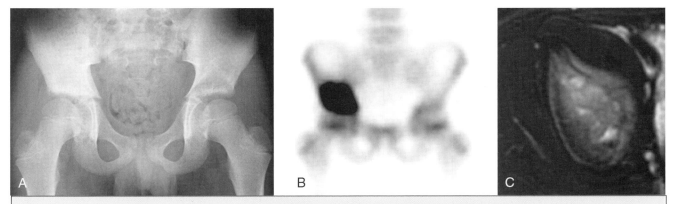

Figure 19 Ewing sarcoma of the pelvis. **A,** AP radiograph reveals an indistinct abnormality in the right supra-acetabular region. **B,** Technetium Tc-99m bone scan reveals avid uptake in this area. **C,** Axial MRI of the acetabular region reveals an elevated periosteum. A biopsy was consistent with Ewing sarcoma.

4: Orthopaedic Oncology/Systemic Disease

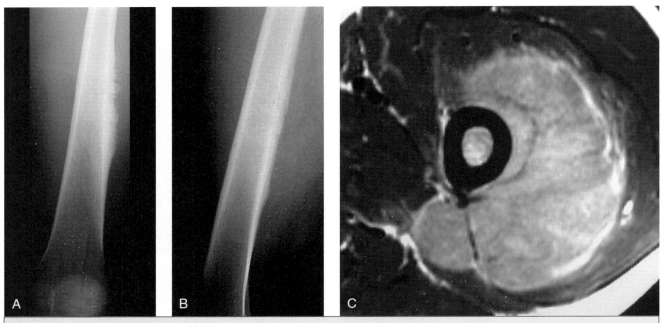

Figure 20   Ewing sarcoma in the femur of a 14-year-old boy. AP (**A**) and lateral (**B**) radiographs of the femur reveal a diaphyseal lesion with a sunburst pattern of periosteal reaction. **C,** Axial MRI reveals an extensive soft-tissue mass. A biopsy revealed Ewing sarcoma.

f. Local control is controversial for localized pelvic Ewing sarcoma: surgery or radiation or both are used.

g. Complications of radiation in skeletally immature patients include joint contractures, fibrosis, growth arrest, fracture, and secondary malignancy (usually 10 to 20 years later).

h. Response to chemotherapy (percent necrosis) is used as a prognostic indicator for overall survival.

i. Patients with localized extremity Ewing sarcoma have 5-year event-free survival of 73%.

j. Patients who present with metastatic disease have a poor prognosis (5-year survival < 20%).

k. Metastases occur primarily in the lungs (60%) but also in the bone (43%) and bone marrow (19%). With recurrent disease, the event-free survival is less than 10% at 3 years.

l. Adverse prognostic factors include nonpulmonary metastasis, less than 90% necrosis, large tumor volume, and pelvic lesions.

m. Different *EWS-FLI* fusion protein subtypes do not predict different outcomes.

n. PNET is thought to have a slightly worse prognosis than Ewing sarcoma.

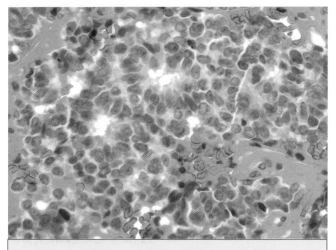

Figure 21   High-power histologic image of a primitive neuroectodermal tumor. Note that the cells are arranged in a rosette pattern around a central eosinophilic substance.

V. Notochordal and Miscellaneous Tumors

A. Chordoma

1. Definition and demographics

a. Slow-growing malignant bone tumor arising from notochordal rests and occurring in the spinal axis

b. Male-to-female ratio = 3:1 (most apparent in sacral lesions)

c. Occurs in adult patients (> 40 years)

d. Lesions at base of skull present earlier than sacral lesions

2. Genetics/etiology

a. Chordoma is thought to develop from residual notochordal cells that eventually undergo neoplastic change.

b. Brachyury gene duplication is a major susceptibility mutation in familial chordoma. No clear marker for sporadic forms is known.

3. Clinical presentation

a. Insidious onset of low back or sacral pain

b. Frequently misdiagnosed as osteoarthritis, nerve impingement, disk herniation

c. Infrequent distal motor/sensory loss because most lesions occur below S1

d. Bowel/bladder symptoms are common.

e. Fifty percent can be identified on a careful rectal examination. (Transrectal biopsy should not be performed.)

f. Fifty percent occur in the sacrococcygeal region, 35% in the spheno-occipital region, and 15% in the mobile spine.

4. Imaging

a. Chordomas occur in the midline, consistent with prior notochord location.

b. Findings on plain radiographs of sacrum are subtle because of overlying bowel gas.

c. Cross-sectional imaging with CT or MRI required (**Figure 22, A through C**)

d. CT reveals areas of calcification within the lesion.

e. MRI (low signal intensity on T1-weighted images, high signal intensity on T2-weighted images) defines the extent of the frequently anterior soft-tissue mass and the bony involvement (usually involves multiple sacral levels).

f. Radiographic differential diagnosis includes chondrosarcoma, multiple myeloma, metastatic disease, giant cell tumor, and lymphoma (**Table 2**).

5. Pathology

a. Grossly, chordoma appears lobulated and jelly-like, with tumor tracking along the nerve roots.

b. The signature cell is the physaliferous cell, which contains intracellular vacuoles and appears bubbly (cytoplasmic mucous droplets) (**Figure 22, D and E**).

c. Lobules of the tumor are separated by fibrous septa.

d. Physaliferous cells are keratin positive, which differentiates this tumor from chondrosarcoma.

e. Weakly S100 positive

f. Differential diagnosis includes chondrosarcoma and metastatic carcinoma.

6. Treatment/outcome

a. The main treatment is wide surgical resection.

b. Local recurrence is common (50%) and is directly related to the surgical margin achieved.

c. To achieve a satisfactory wide margin, the surgeon must be willing to sacrifice involved nerve roots, viscera, and so forth.

d. Radiation (protons or photons) can be used as an adjunct for locally recurrent disease, positive margins, or as primary treatment of inoperable tumors (protons or photons).

e. Radiation alone is generally not effective for long-term local control.

f. Chemotherapy is not effective and is currently not indicated.

g. Chordoma metastasizes late to the lungs and, occasionally, bone; requires long-term follow-up (20 years).

h. Long-term survival is 25% to 50%, due in part to local progression.

B. Adamantinoma

1. Definition and demographics

a. Unusual, rare, slow-growing malignant bone tumor with a predilection for the tibia (**Figure 23**)

b. No sex predilection

c. Patients are generally 20 to 40 years of age.

d. Fewer than 300 cases in the literature

2. Genetics/etiology—Controversial whether adamantinoma evolves from osteofibrous dysplasia; most believe it does not.

3. Clinical presentation

a. Pain of variable duration and intensity is the major symptom.

b. Occasional tibial deformity or a mass

c. Tenderness over the subcutaneous tibial border

d. History of preceding trauma is common.

e. Ninety percent of lesions occur in the tibial diaphysis.

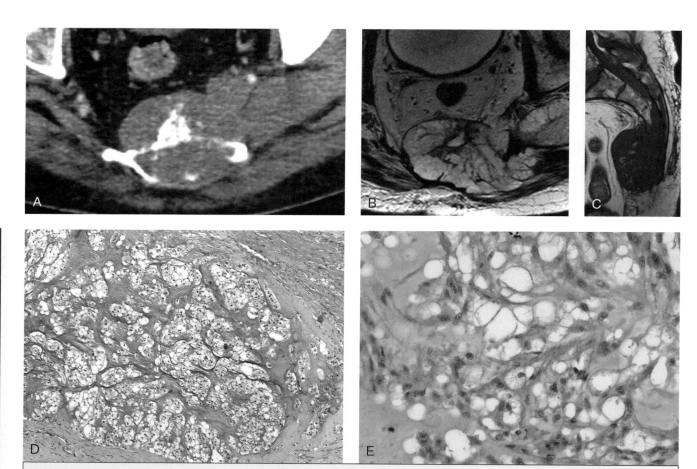

Figure 22 Chordoma of the sacrum in a 66-year-old man. **A,** CT scan reveals a destructive lesion with an anterior soft-tissue mass containing calcifications. **B,** Axial MRI further defines the soft-tissue extension anteriorly and toward the left pelvic sidewall. **C,** Sagittal T1-weighted MRI shows the lesion at S3 and below. Note that the anterior extension abuts the rectum. **D,** Low-power histologic image of this lesion reveals a tumor lobule surrounded by fibrous tissue. **E,** Higher power histologic image reveals the physaliferous cells of a chordoma with a bubbly appearance to the cytoplasm.

4. Imaging

   a. Classic radiographic appearance is multiple well-circumscribed lucent defects, usually with one dominant defect that may expand the bone locally (**Figure 23, A**).

   b. Sclerotic bone between defects

   c. "Soap bubble" appearance

   d. Lesions may be intracortical or intramedullary, with occasional (10%) soft-tissue mass.

   e. No periosteal reaction

5. Pathology

   a. Nests of epithelial cells in a benign fibrous stroma (**Figure 23, C**)

   b. Epithelial cells are columnar in appearance and keratin positive.

   c. Epithelial cells are bland without mitosis.

6. Treatment/outcome

Table 2

Tumors Occurring in the Vertebrae

Anterior (Vertebral Body)

Giant cell tumor
Metastatic disease
Multiple myeloma
Ependymoma
Chordoma
Lymphoma
Primary bone tumors (chondrosarcoma, osteosarcoma)

Posterior Elements

Osteoid osteoma
Osteoblastoma
Aneurysmal bone cyst

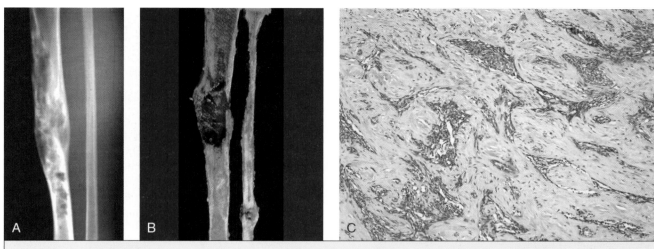

Figure 23 Adamantinoma of the tibia in a 38-year-old woman. **A,** AP radiograph reveals multiple diaphyseal lucent lesions separated by sclerotic bone. They have a bubbly appearance consistent with adamantinoma. **B,** A gross specimen from a different patient reveals lesions in both the tibia and fibula that expand the bone. **C,** The histologic appearance is nests of epithelial cells in a fibrous stroma.

a. Standard of care is wide surgical resection.

b. Chemotherapy and radiation are not indicated.

c. Local recurrence is more common when adequate margins are not achieved.

d. Given diaphyseal location, common reconstruction is intercalary allograft

e. Late metastasis to lungs, bones, lymph nodes in 15% to 20% of patients

f. Requires long-term follow-up

g. Case series from 2000 described 87% survival at 10 years.

VI. Systemic Disease

A. Multiple myeloma

1. Definition and demographics

   a. Neoplastic proliferation of plasma cells producing a monoclonal protein.

   b. Considered the most common primary malignant bone tumor (20,000 persons/year) in the United States

   c. Affects patients older than 40 years

   d. Twice as common in African Americans as in Caucasians

   e. Affects males more commonly than females

2. Genetics/etiology

   a. Immunoglobulins (Igs) are composed of two heavy chains and two light chains.

   • Heavy chains = IgG, IgA, IgM, IgD, and IgE (IgG and IgA are common in myeloma)

   • Light chains = κ and λ (Bence Jones proteins)

   b. In myeloma, both heavy and light chains are produced.

   c. Major mediators of osteoclastogenesis in myeloma include receptor activator of nuclear factor-κ B ligand (RANKL), interleukin-6, and macrophage inflammatory protein-1α.

   d. Osteoblastic bone formation is suppressed by tumor necrosis factor and Dickkopf-related protein 1 (Dkk-1).

3. Clinical presentation

   a. Common symptoms include bone pain, pathologic fractures, cord compression, and recurrent infections.

   b. Lesions occur throughout the skeleton but are common in bones that contain hematopoietic marrow, including the skull, spine, and long bones (**Figure 24**)

   c. Laboratory findings: normochromic, normocytic anemia; hypercalcemia; renal insufficiency; amyloidosis; elevated erythrocyte sedimentation rate

   d. Electrophoresis—99% of patients have a spike in serum or urine or both.

   • Serum: identifies types of proteins present

   • Urine: identifies Bence Jones proteins

   e. 24-hour urine collection quantifies protein in urine.

f. β₂-microglobulin and serum albumin—Tumor markers with prognostic ability (increased β_2-microglobulin and decreased serum albumin = poor prognosis).

g. Diagnosis—One major and one minor (or three minor) diagnostic criteria must be present.

- Major criteria

  ◦ Plasmacytoma: tissue diagnosis on biopsy

  ◦ More than 30% plasma cells in bone marrow

  ◦ Serum IgG greater than 3.5 g/dL, IgA greater than 2 g/dL or urine greater than 1 g/24 hours, or Bence Jones protein

- Minor criteria

  ◦ 10% to 30% plasma cells in bone marrow

  ◦ Serum/urine protein levels lower than listed for major criteria

  ◦ Lytic bone lesions

  ◦ Lower-than-normal IgG levels

4. Imaging

a. Classic appearance is multiple "punched-out" lytic lesions throughout the skeleton (**Figure 25, A** and **B**, and **Figure 26, A**)

b. No surrounding sclerosis

c. Skull lesions and vertebral compression fractures are common (**Figure 25, B** and **Figure 26, A**).

d. Diffuse osteopenia (**Figure 26, A**)

e. Bone scan is usually negative because there is minimal osteoblastic response in myeloma.

f. Skeletal survey has been the screening tool of choice. MRI and fludeoxyglucose–positron emission tomography (FDG-PET) currently identifying bone lesions earlier.

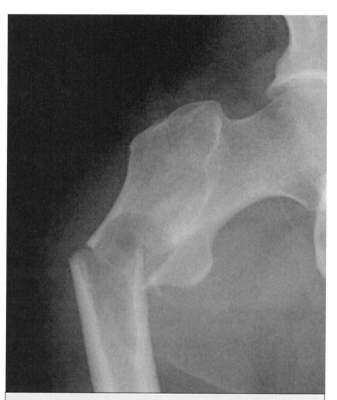

Figure 24 AP radiograph of the hip of a 47-year-old woman who presented with a pathologic fracture of the proximal femur through a lytic lesion. Open biopsy at the time of surgery showed a plasma cell lesion consistent with multiple myeloma.

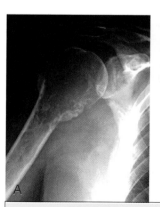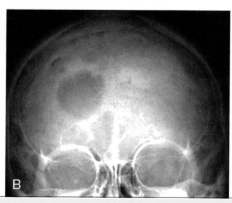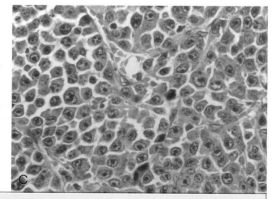

Figure 25 Multiple myeloma in a 67-year-old woman who presented with constant right shoulder pain. **A,** AP radiograph shows a lytic lesion in the humeral head. The workup included a skeletal survey after a positive result for serum protein electrophoresis. **B,** AP radiograph demonstrated a punched-out lytic lesion in the skull, consistent with multiple myeloma. **C,** A high-power histologic image reveals numerous plasma cells with eccentric nuclei and extensive vascularity.

g. MRI is also helpful in defining vertebral lesions (**Figure 26, B**).

5. Pathology

   a. The lesion consists of sheets of plasma cells with eccentric nuclei; little intercellular material is present (**Figure 25, C**).

   b. Nuclear chromatin arranged in a "clock face" pattern

   c. Abundant eosinophilic cytoplasm

   d. Rare mitotic figures

   e. Extremely vascular, with an extensive capillary system

   f. Immunohistochemistry stains: CD38+

6. Treatment/outcome

   a. Dramatic improvement in survival over the past 10 years

   b. Standard of care is high-dose chemotherapy with autologous stem cell support.

   c. Risk stratification of patients allows for individualized treatment

   d. Five sets of active agents in myeloma

     • Alkylating agents (melphalan, cyclophosphamide)

     • Anthracyclines (doxorubicin, liposomal doxorubicin)

     • Corticosteroids (dexamethasone, prednisone)

     • Immunomoduatory drugs (thalidomide, lenalidomide)

     • Proteosome inhibitors (bortezomib, carfilzomib)

   e. Bisphosphonates help decrease number of lesions, bone pain, and serum calcium.

   f. Delayed autologous stem cell transplant improves survival.

   g. Radiation effective to decrease pain, avoid surgery

   h. Surgical stabilization of pathologic fractures or impending fractures (principles similar to those used in metastatic disease)

   i. Kyphoplasty/vertebroplasty common to treat vertebral compression fractures

   j. Survival worse with renal failure

   k. Median survival is 8 years.

B. Plasmacytoma

1. Plasma cell tumor in a single skeletal site

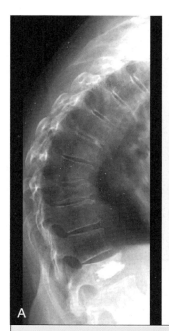
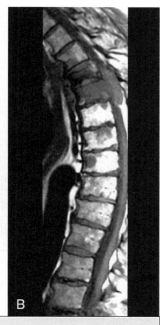

Figure 26   Multiple myeloma. **A,** A lateral radiograph of the thoracic spine demonstrates the severe osteopenia present in multiple myeloma contributing to compression fractures. Note the prior injection of cement to stabilize a vertebral body in the lower part of the figure. **B,** Sagittal MRI of the thoracic spine in a patient with long-standing multiple myeloma shows multiple vertebral lesions with an area of epidural extension.

2. Represents 5% of patients with plasma cell lesions

3. Negative serum/urine protein electrophoresis

4. Negative bone marrow biopsy/aspirate

5. Treated with radiation alone (4,500 to 5,000 cGy)

6. Progresses to myeloma in approximately 55% of patients

C. Osteosclerotic myeloma

1. Accounts for 3% of myeloma cases

2. POEMS syndrome = *p*olyneuropathy, *o*rganomegaly, *e*ndocrinopathy, *M*-spike, *s*kin changes

D. B cell lymphoma

1. Definition and demographics

   a. Clonal proliferation of B cells commonly presenting as nodal disease and occasionally affecting the skeleton

   b. Can occur at any age; most common in patients 35 to 55 years of age

   c. Affects males more commonly than females

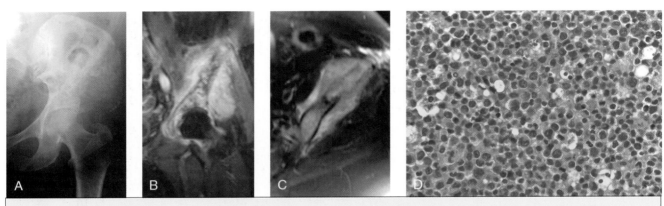

Figure 27 Lymphoma in a 72-year-old woman who presented with lateral hip pain. **A,** AP radiograph of the left pelvis reveals an extensive lytic lesion of the ilium and a resultant pathologic fracture. Coronal (**B**) and axial (**C**) MRIs reveal the extent of the surrounding soft-tissue mass. **D,** A high-power histologic image reveals a small round blue cell lesion (larger than lymphocytes). A CD20 stain was positive for a B cell lymphoma.

d. Non-Hodgkin lymphoma most commonly affects the bone (B cell much more common than T cell variants).

e. Ten percent to 35% of patients with non-Hodgkin lymphoma have extranodal disease.

f. Primary lymphoma of bone can occur but is quite rare.

2. Genetics/etiology—Risk factors for B cell lymphoma include immunodeficiency (HIV, hepatitis) and viral/bacterial infection.

3. Clinical presentation

a. Constant pain unrelieved by rest

b. A large soft-tissue mass that is tender or warm is common.

c. Lymphoma affects bones with persistent red marrow (femur, spine, pelvis).

d. Neurologic symptoms from spinal lesions

e. Twenty-five percent of patients present with pathologic fracture.

f. B-symptoms = fever, weight loss, night sweats

g. Primary lymphoma of bone is rare; occurs when there are no extraskeletal sites of disease (other than a single node) for 6 months after diagnosis.

4. Imaging appearance

a. Lytic, permeative lesions that can show subtle bone destruction (**Figure 27, A**)

b. Generally involves the diaphysis in long bones

c. Can involve multiple sites in the skeleton

d. Intensely positive on bone scan

e. Extensive marrow involvement noted on MRI

f. Large soft-tissue mass (**Figure 27, B and C**) is common.

g. PET helpful in staging and follow-up

h. Radiographic differential diagnosis includes metastatic disease, myeloma, and osteomyelitis.

5. Pathology

a. Difficult to diagnose on needle biopsy because the tissue is often crushed

b. Diffuse infiltrative rather than nodular pattern

c. Lesion comprised of small round blue cells (2× size of lymphocytes; can be variable) (**Figure 27, D**)

d. Immunohistochemistry stains

- B cell (CD20+, CD79a+)

- Atypical/large cells (CD15+, CD30+, CD45+)

e. Increased percentage of cleaved cells improves prognosis in primary lymphoma of bone.

6. Treatment/outcome

a. Bone marrow biopsy and CT of the chest, abdomen, and pelvis are required as part of staging/workup.

b. Chemotherapy is the primary treatment. Chemotherapeutic agents include cyclophosphamide, doxorubicin, prednisone, and vincristine.

c. Radiation of the primary site is used in some individuals for persistent disease.

d. Surgical treatment is necessary only for pathologic fractures because chemotherapy alone is effective for most lesions.

e. Reported 5-year survival is as high as 70% when chemotherapy and radiation are used for disseminated disease.

f. Secondary involvement of bone in lymphoma has a worse prognosis than primary lymphoma of bone.

VII. Secondary Lesions

A. Overview (**Table 3** and **Figures 28** and **29**)

1. Secondary lesions can be benign (secondary ABC), but most commonly they are malignant (postradiation sarcoma, Paget sarcoma, sarcomas emanating from infarct or fibrous dysplasia, secondary chondrosarcomas from benign cartilage tumors, squamous carcinomas from osteomyelitis/draining sinus).

2. Secondary chondrosarcomas are described in section III.A.

3. These lesions develop from a preexisting tumor, process, or treatment.

B. Postradiation sarcoma

1. Definition and demographics

a. A postradiation sarcoma develops with a latent period after radiation has been used to treat a benign or malignant bone, soft-tissue, or visceral tumor.

b. These lesions can occur at any age after radiation of a prior tumor (Ewing sarcoma, cervical/breast/prostate cancer, giant cell tumor, soft-tissue sarcoma, retinoblastoma).

c. More common in children exposed to radiation than in adults

d. Latent period is variable (range, 4 to 40 years; median, approximately 10 years)

Table 3

Secondary Lesions

Type	Histology
Benign	Aneurysmal bone cyst
Postradiation (for Ewing sarcoma, carcinoma, giant cell tumor)	Osteosarcoma Undifferentiated pleomorphic sarcoma Fibrosarcoma Chondrosarcoma
Paget sarcoma	Osteosarcoma Undifferentiated pleomorphic sarcoma Fibrosarcoma
Secondary to infarction	Undifferentiated pleomorphic sarcoma
Secondary to fibrous dysplasia	Osteosarcoma Undifferentiated pleomorphic sarcoma Fibrosarcoma
Secondary to benign cartilage lesion (enchondroma/osteochondroma)	Chondrosarcoma
Secondary to chronic osteomyelitis/draining sinus	Squamous cell carcinoma

4: Orthopaedic Oncology/Systemic Disease

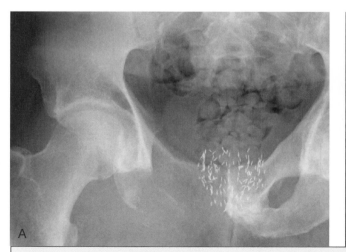
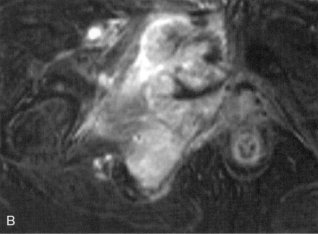

Figure 28 Secondary sarcoma in a 68-year-old man with a history of treatment for prostate cancer. **A,** AP radiograph of the right pelvis shows a destructive lesion in the right pubic rami. Note the radiation seeds. **B,** Axial MRI shows the extent of the surrounding soft-tissue mass. The biopsy revealed a high-grade sarcoma that was presumably radiation-induced.

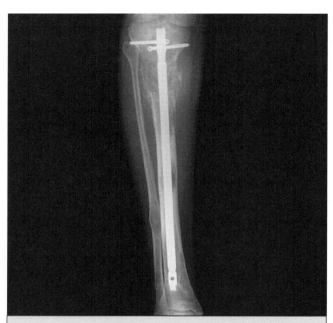

Figure 29 AP radiograph of the right lower extremity of a 64-year-old man with a diagnosis of polyostotic fibrous dysplasia. He sustained a pathologic fracture of the right proximal tibia through a lytic lesion, and an intramedullary device was placed without a preoperative biopsy. The eventual biopsy revealed a high-grade osteosarcoma developing from an area of fibrous dysplasia. The patient required a transfemoral amputation.

e. Literature suggests children with Ewing sarcoma treated with radiation have a 5% to 10% risk of postradiation malignancy at 20 years (7% for a postradiation sarcoma).

2. Genetics/etiology

a. Ionizing radiation causes DNA damage and creates free radicals.

b. Incidence depends on dose, type, and rate of radiation treatment. In survivors of atomic bombs, dose threshold is 0.85 Gy (lower than previously thought to be associated with secondary development of sarcoma)

c. May be affected by the use of chemotherapy (especially alkylating agents)

3. Clinical presentation

a. Gradual onset of intermittent, then constant, pain in a previously radiated site

b. Can affect any skeletal site

4. Imaging appearance

a. Lytic, aggressive, destructive bone lesion (**Figure 28, A**)

b. Possible soft-tissue mass (**Figure 28, B**)

c. MRI used to define the extent of the lesion

5. Pathology

a. Histology shows high-grade sarcoma (osteosarcoma, undifferentiated pleomorphic sarcoma, fibrosarcoma, chondrosarcoma).

b. May be histologic evidence of prior irradiation in the surrounding tissues

6. Treatment/outcome

a. Treatment is chemotherapy and surgical resection.

b. Poor prognosis, with 25% to 50% 5-year survival (worse in sites not amenable to surgical resection)

c. Metastasis primarily to the lung

C. Paget sarcoma

1. Definition and demographics

a. Sarcoma that arises from a skeletal area affected by Paget disease

b. Occurs in older patients (older than 50 years)

c. Occurs in approximately 1% of patients with Paget disease

2. Clinical presentation

a. New onset of pain in an area affected by Paget disease

b. Possible swelling or pathologic fracture

c. Commonly affects pelvis, proximal femur

3. Imaging appearance

a. Marked bone destruction and possible soft-tissue mass in a skeletal site affected by Paget disease

b. Helpful to have prior documentation of the radiographic appearance

c. MRI helpful to define the extent of the sarcoma within the abnormal bone

4. Pathology—Histology shows a high-grade sarcoma (osteosarcoma, undifferentiated pleomorphic sarcoma, fibrosarcoma, chondrosarcoma) within an area of pagetoid bone.

5. Treatment/outcome

a. Poor prognosis; survival is less than 10% at 5 years.

b. Treat as a primary bone sarcoma, with chemotherapy and surgical resection

c. Radiation is palliative only.

d. High rate of metastasis to the lung

Top Testing Facts

Osteosarcoma and Undifferentiated Pleomorphic Sarcoma

1. Osteosarcoma is the most common malignant bone tumor in children.

2. Osteosarcoma classically occurs in the metaphysis of long bones and presents with progressive pain.

3. Osteosarcoma has a radiographic appearance of bone destruction and bone formation starting in the medullary canal.

4. The osteoblastic stromal cells are malignant in osteosarcoma.

5. The 5-year survival of patients with localized osteosarcoma in an extremity is 70%.

6. Parosteal and periosteal osteosarcomas occur on the surface of the bone.

7. Parosteal osteosarcoma is a low-grade lesion that appears fibrous histologically and is treated with wide surgical resection alone.

8. Periosteal osteosarcoma is an intermediate-grade lesion that appears cartilaginous and is treated with chemotherapy and surgical resection.

9. Telangiectatic osteosarcoma can be confused with an ABC.

10. Undifferentiated pleomorphic sarcoma of bone (previously called malignanat fibrous histiocytoma) presents and is treated like osteosarcoma, but no osteoid is noted histologically.

Chondrosarcoma

1. Chondrosarcoma occurs de novo or secondary to an enchondroma or osteochondroma.

2. Chondrosarcoma occurs in adults, whereas osteosarcoma and Ewing sarcoma occur primarily in children.

3. The pelvis is the most common location for chondrosarcoma.

4. Secondary chondrosarcomas can occur in prior enchondromas or osteochondromas (more commonly in patients with Ollier disease, Maffucci syndrome, or multiple hereditary osteochondromas).

5. Pelvic chondrosarcomas require wide resection regardless of grade.

6. Chemotherapy is used only in the dedifferentiated and mesenchymal chondrosarcoma variants.

7. Tumor grade is a major prognostic factor for chondrosarcoma.

8. Grade 1 chondrosarcomas rarely metastasize and have a > 90% survival.

9. The survival for patients with dedifferentiated chondrosarcoma is the lowest of all bone sarcomas (10%).

10. Clear cell chondrosarcoma has a radiographic appearance similar to chondroblastoma.

11. Radiation is not used in the treatment of chondrosarcoma.

Ewing Sarcoma/PNET

1. Ewing sarcoma is one of a group of small round blue cell tumors not distinguishable based on histology alone.

2. Ewing sarcoma is the second most common primary malignant bone tumor in children.

3. Ewing sarcoma is found most commonly in the diaphysis of long bones as well as in the pelvis.

4. No matrix is produced by the tumor cells, so the radiographs are purely lytic.

5. There may be extensive periosteal reaction and a large soft-tissue mass.

6. Ewing sarcoma is CD99 positive and has the 11:22 chromosomal translocation.

7. Ewing sarcoma is radiation sensitive, but surgery is used more commonly for local control unless the patient has metastatic disease or cannot undergo surgery.

8. Ewing sarcoma requires multiagent chemotherapy.

9. Ewing sarcoma can metastasize to the lungs, bone, and bone marrow.

10. The 5-year survival rate of patients with isolated extremity Ewing sarcoma is 73%.

Chordoma and Adamantinoma

1. Chordoma occurs exclusively in the spinal axis, although many lesions should be considered in the differential of a destructive sacral lesion.

2. Chordoma occurs in adults and has a prolonged course; misdiagnosis is common.

3. Plain radiographs often do not identify sacral destruction from chordoma—cross-sectional imaging is required.

4. CT scan of a chordoma shows calcified areas within the tumor.

5. Chordoma consists of physaliferous cells on histologic examination.

6. Surgical cure of chordoma requires a wide resection, possibly removing nerve roots, bowel, bladder, and so forth.

7. Radiation can be used in an adjunct fashion for chordoma, but chemotherapy has no role.

8. Adamantinoma occurs primarily in the tibial diaphysis and has a soap bubble radiographic appearance.

9. Adamantinoma consists of nests of epithelial cells in a fibrous stroma and is keratin positive.

10. Adamantinoma requires a wide surgical resection for cure.

4: Orthopaedic Oncology/Systemic Disease

Top Testing Facts

Multiple Myeloma and Lymphoma

1. Multiple myeloma is the most common primary malignant bone tumor.

2. Myeloma often presents with normochromic, normocytic anemia.

3. Myeloma presents radiographically with multiple punched-out lytic lesions.

4. Bone scan is typically negative with myeloma.

5. Myeloma lesions are composed of sheets of plasma cells.

6. Myeloma is treated with chemotherapy, bisphosphonates, and possibly autologous stem cell transplant.

7. Lymphoma affecting bone is usually non-Hodgkin B cell subtype.

8. Subtle radiographic bone destruction with extensive marrow and soft-tissue involvement is typical.

9. Lymphoma B cells are CD20+ on immunohistochemistry staining.

10. B cell lymphoma is treated with chemotherapy and radiation; rarely requires surgery.

Secondary Lesions

1. Secondary lesions can be benign (secondary ABC) but are most commonly sarcomas.

2. Secondary sarcomas arise in areas of Paget disease, prior radiation, or previous lesions (bone infarcts, fibrous dysplasia).

3. New-onset pain in the site of a previous lesion or site of radiation is suspicious for a secondary lesion.

4. Radiographic appearance of a secondary sarcoma is an aggressive, destructive bone tumor.

5. Histologic appearance is of a high-grade sarcoma (osteosarcoma, undifferentiated pleomorphic sarcoma, fibrosarcoma, chondrosarcoma).

6. Secondary sarcomas have a uniformly poor prognosis; treatment is with chemotherapy and surgery.

7. Undifferentiated pleomorphic sarcoma of bone can arise in a prior infarct and has a poor prognosis.

8. Fewer than 1% of fibrous dysplasia lesions undergo malignant change to undifferentiated pleomorphic sarcoma or osteosarcoma.

9. Secondary squamous cell carcinoma can arise in long-standing osteomyelitis with a draining sinus tract.

Bibliography

Bacci G, Longhi A, Versari M, Mercuri M, Briccoli A, Picci P: Prognostic factors for osteosarcoma of the extremity treated with neoadjuvant chemotherapy: 15-year experience in 789 patients treated at a single institution. *Cancer* 2006;106(5): 1154-1161.

Cesari M, Alberghini M, Vanel D, et al: Periosteal osteosarcoma: A single-institution experience. *Cancer* 2011;117(8): 1731-1735.

Chou AJ, Malek F: Osteosarcoma of bone, in Biermann JS, ed: *Orthopaedic Knowledge Update: Musculoskeletal Tumors*, ed 3. Rosemont, IL, American Academy of Orthopaedic Surgeons, 2014, pp 159-170.

Douis H, Saifuddin A: The imaging of cartilaginous bone tumours: II. Chondrosarcoma. *Skeletal Radiol* 2013;42(5): 611-626.

Durie BG, Salmon SE: A clinical staging system for multiple myeloma: Correlation of measured myeloma cell mass with presenting clinical features, response to treatment, and survival. *Cancer* 1975;36(3):842-854.

Fuchs B, Dickey ID, Yaszemski MJ, Inwards CY, Sim FH: Operative management of sacral chordoma. *J Bone Joint Surg Am* 2005;87(10):2211-2216.

Gorlick R, Janeway K, Lessnick S, Randall RL, Marina N; COG Bone Tumor Committee: Children's Oncology Group's 2013 blueprint for research: Bone tumors. *Pediatr Blood Cancer* 2013;60(6):1009-1015.

Hickey M, Farrokhyar F, Deheshi B, Turcotte R, Ghert M: A systematic review and meta-analysis of intralesional versus wide resection for intramedullary grade I chondrosarcoma of the extremities. *Ann Surg Oncol* 2011;18(6):1705-1709.

Kim HJ, McLawhorn AS, Goldstein MJ, Boland PJ: Malignant osseous tumors of the pediatric spine. *J Am Acad Orthop Surg* 2012;20(10):646-656.

Kuttesch JF Jr, Wexler LH, Marcus RB, et al: Second malignancies after Ewing's sarcoma: Radiation dose-dependency of secondary sarcomas. *J Clin Oncol* 1996;14(10):2818-2825.

Lessnick SL, Ladanyi M: Molecular pathogenesis of Ewing sarcoma: New therapeutic and transcriptional targets. *Annu Rev Pathol* 2012;7:145-159.

Maheshwari AV, Cheng EY: Ewing sarcoma family of tumors. *J Am Acad Orthop Surg* 2010;18(2):94-107.

Mavrogenis AF, Ruggieri P, Mercuri M, Papagelopoulos PJ: Dedifferentiated chondrosarcoma revisited. *J Surg Orthop Adv* 2011;20(2):106-111.

McGough RL III: Chondrosarcoma of bone, in Biermann JS, ed: *Orthopaedic Knowledge Update: Musculoskeletal Tumors*, ed 3. Rosemont, IL, American Academy of Orthopaedic Surgeons, 2014, pp 1818-194.

Mikhael JR, Dingli D, Roy V, et al: Mayo Clinic: Management of newly diagnosed symptomatic multiple myeloma: Updated Mayo Stratification of Myeloma and Risk-Adapted Therapy (mSMART) consensus guidelines 2013. *Mayo Clin Proc* 2013;88(4):360-376.

Ostrowski ML, Unni KK, Banks PM, et al: Malignant lymphoma of bone. *Cancer* 1986;58(12):2646-2655.

Qureshi AA, Shott S, Mallin BA, Gitelis S: Current trends in the management of adamantinoma of long bones: An international study. *J Bone Joint Surg Am* 2000;82(8):1122-1131.

Schwab JH, Springfield DS, Raskin KA, Mankin HJ, Hornicek FJ: What's new in primary bone tumors. *J Bone Joint Surg Am* 2012;94(20):1913-1919.

Steensma M: Ewing sarcoma, in Biermann JS, ed: *Orthopaedic Knowledge Update: Musculoskeletal Tumors*, ed 3. Rosemont, IL, American Academy of Orthopaedic Surgeons, 2014, pp 171-180.

Unni KK: *Dahlin's Bone Tumors: General Aspects and Data on 11,087 Cases*, ed 5. Philadelphia, PA, Lippincott-Raven, 1996, pp 71-342.

Wold LE, Adler CP, Sim FH, Unni KK: *Atlas of Orthopedic Pathology*, ed 2. Philadelphia, PA, WB Saunders, 1990, pp 179-396.

4: Orthopaedic Oncology/Systemic Disease

Chapter 48

Benign Soft-Tissue Tumors and Reactive Lesions

Kristy Weber, MD

4: Orthopaedic Oncology/Systemic Disease

I. Lipoma

A. Definition and demographics

1. Lipoma—A benign tumor of adipose tissue.

2. Slightly more common in men than in women

3. Occurs primarily in patients 40 to 60 years of age

4. Superficial/subcutaneous lesions are common; deep lesions are uncommon.

5. Hibernomas are tumors of brown fat; they occur in slightly younger patients (20 to 40 years).

B. Genetics/etiology

1. Lipomas (white fat) are common.

2. Lipomas occur when white fat accumulates in inactive people.

3. Chromosomal abnormalities have been described.

4. Brown fat usually occurs in hibernating animals or human infants.

C. Clinical presentation

1. A soft, painless, mobile mass characterizes the common superficial variety.

2. Five percent to 8% of patients with superficial lipomas have multiple lesions.

3. Superficial lipomas are common in the upper back, the shoulders, the arms, the buttocks, and the proximal thighs.

4. Deep lipomas are usually intramuscular, fixed, and painless and can be large.

5. Deep lesions are found frequently in the thigh, shoulder, and calf.

6. Most are stable after an initial period of growth.

Dr. Weber or an immediate family member serves as a board member, owner, officer, or committee member of the Musculoskeletal Tumor Society and the Ruth Jackson Orthopaedic Society.

D. Imaging appearance

1. Plain radiographs—Not helpful for diagnosing lipomas; in deep lipomas, a radiolucency may be seen.

2. CT—Appearance of subcutaneous fat.

3. Magnetic resonance imaging

a. Bright on T1-weighted images, moderate on T2-weighted images (**Figure 1, A** and **B**)

b. Lipomas image exactly as fat on all sequences (suppress with fat-suppressed images); hibernomas have increased signal intensity on T1-weighted images but not always the same appearance as fat.

c. Homogeneous, although minor linear streaking may occur

d. Appearance is usually classic on MRI; biopsy not required.

4. Occasionally, lipomas contain calcific deposits or bone.

E. Pathology

1. Gross appearance

a. Lipoma: soft, lobular, white or yellow, with a capsule.

b. Hibernoma: red-brown in color because of profusion of mitochondria and more extensive vascularity than lipoma.

2. Histology

a. Mature fat cells with moderate vascularity (**Figure 1, C**)

b. Occasionally, focal calcium deposits, cartilage, or bone

c. Histologic variants include spindle cell lipoma, pleomorphic lipoma, angiolipoma. (All are benign but can be confused histologically with malignant lesions.)

F. Treatment/outcome

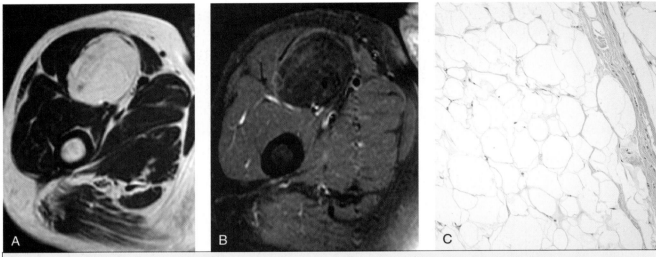

Figure 1   Intramuscular lipoma. Axial T1-weighted fat-suppressed (**A**) and T2-weighted fat-suppressed (**B**) MRIs of the right thigh reveal a well-circumscribed lesion with the same signal as the subcutaneous fat. Note that the lesion is suppressed on the fat-suppressed images, as is classic for an intramuscular lipoma. **C,** The histologic appearance is of mature fat cells without atypia (hematoxylin and eosin). A loose fibrous capsule is visible.

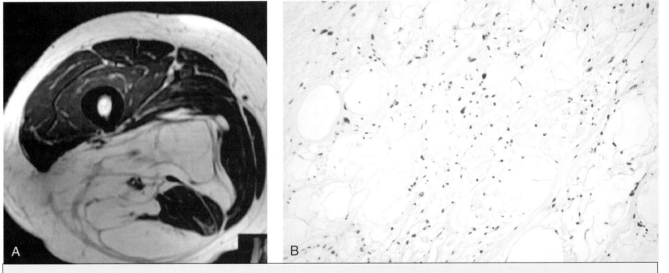

Figure 2   Atypical lipoma. **A,** Axial MRI reveals an extensive intramuscular lipomatous lesion infiltrating the posterior thigh musculature. Note the extensive stranding within the lesion. From this appearance, an intramuscular lipoma cannot be differentiated from an atypical lipoma. **B,** The histologic appearance of this atypical lipoma is more cellular than a classic lipoma (hematoxylin and eosin).

1. Treatment is observation or local excision (excisional biopsy with marginal margin can be performed if imaging studies clearly document a lipoma).

2. Local recurrence is less than 5% if removed.

3. Malignant transformation is not clinically relevant; few cases have been reported.

G. Atypical lipoma/well-differentiated liposarcoma

1. Often called atypical lipoma in the extremities and well-differentiated liposarcoma in the retroperitoneum

2. Usually very large, deep tumors

3. May look identical to classic lipomas or may have increased stranding on MRI (**Figure 2, A**)

4. Histology shows greater cellularity than classic lipoma (**Figure 2, B**).

5. Treatment is marginal excision; often not differentiated from classic lipoma until after excision (based on histology).

6. Higher chance of local recurrence (50% at 10 years) compared with lipoma, but does not metastasize

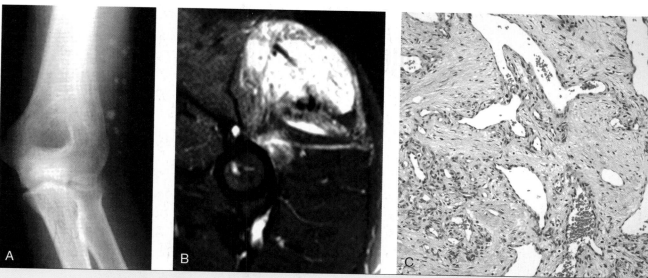

Figure 3 Intramuscular hemangiomas. **A,** Phleboliths seen in the lateral arm on this plain radiograph suggest a hemangioma. **B,** Axial T2-weighted MRI of the thigh reveals a poorly circumscribed soft-tissue lesion with both fatty and vascular features within the muscle, consistent with a hemangioma. **C,** Histologic image of this capillary hemangioma shows large blood-filled spaces but no cellular atypia (hematoxylin and eosin).

II. Intramuscular Hemangioma

A. Definition and demographics

1. Intramuscular hemangioma—A benign vascular neoplasm occurring in the deep tissues.

2. Accounts for less than 1% of all benign vascular tumors

3. Males and females affected equally

4. Usually seen in patients younger than 30 years

5. Hemangioma may be of several types (capillary, cavernous, infantile, pyogenic granuloma). Intramuscular hemangiomas are more commonly capillary than cavernous.

6. Often confused with vascular malformations (arteriovenous malformations, vascular ectasias), which are clusters of blood vessels that develop in arteries or veins and occur during fetal development

B. Genetics/etiology

1. Not well understood, as different types have different etiologies

2. Some hemangiomas are caused by errors in morphogenesis affecting any segment of the vascular system.

3. Hormonal modulation is a possible etiology; some hemangiomas develop and resolve in association with hormonal changes of pregnancy.

4. Twenty percent are associated with a history of trauma (but no known causal relationship).

C. Clinical presentation

1. Lesions are usually deep in the lower extremities, but they can involve any muscle.

2. Growth is variable and often fluctuates with activity.

3. Pain is variable and can increase with activity.

4. Usually, no overlying skin lesions or bruits are seen.

5. Lesions are usually isolated, but a rare form called diffuse hemangioma manifests in childhood and involves a limb extensively.

D. Imaging appearance

1. Plain radiographs

   a. May reveal phleboliths or calcifications within the lesion (**Figure 3, A**)

   b. Adjacent bone erosion may be seen.

2. Ultrasonography—Can help differentiate types of vascular lesions based on flow.

3. Magnetic resonance imaging

   a. Increased signal intensity on T1- and T2-weighted images (**Figure 3, B**)

   b. Focal areas of low signal intensity are due to blood flow or calcifications.

   c. Lesions are often ill-defined or described as a "bag of worms"; they can appear infiltrative within the muscle.

   d. Frequently mistaken for a malignant soft-tissue tumor

4. Magnetic resonance angiography—Differentiates high-flow from low-flow lesions.

E. Pathology

1. Gross appearance

   a. Varies, depending on whether the lesion is the capillary (more common) or cavernous type

   b. Color varies from red to tan to yellow.

2. Histology

   a. Capillary-sized vessels with large nuclei (**Figure 3, C**)

   b. Well-developed vascular lumens, infiltration of muscle fibers

   c. No significant cellular pleomorphism

   d. Cavernous type composed of large vessels with a large degree of adipose tissue

3. Differential diagnosis includes angiosarcoma.

F. Treatment/outcome

1. Most intramuscular hemangiomas should be treated with observation, anti-inflammatory medications, and compression sleeves.

2. Many are amenable to interventional radiology techniques of embolization or sclerotherapy to decrease the size of the lesion or relieve symptoms.

3. Surgical excision carries a high risk of local recurrence.

4. No incidence of malignant transformation

III. Neurilemoma (Schwannoma)

A. Definition and demographics

1. Neurilemoma (schwannoma)—An encapsulated benign soft-tissue tumor composed of Schwann cells.

2. Commonly discovered in patients 20 to 50 years of age (may also occur in older patients)

3. Affects males and females equally

4. Can affect any motor or sensory nerve

5. More common than neurofibroma

B. Genetics/etiology

1. *NF2* tumor suppressor gene encodes schwannomin

2. Inactivating *NF2* mutations are linked to neurofibromatosis type 2 (NF2; hallmark is schwannomas).

C. Clinical presentation

1. Usually asymptomatic; sometimes causes pain with stretch or activity

2. Occurs frequently on the flexor surfaces of the extremities as well as the head/neck

3. Pelvic lesions can become quite large.

4. May change in size given frequent occurrence of cystic degeneration

5. Multiple lesions occur rarely.

6. Positive Tinel sign may be seen.

D. Appearance on MRI

1. Low signal intensity on T1-weighted MRI, high signal intensity on T2-weighted MRI (**Figure 4, A** and **B**)

2. Diffusely enhanced signal with gadolinium administration

3. On sagittal or coronal images, the lesion may appear in continuity with the affected nerve (**Figure 5**).

4. Difficult to differentiate neurilemoma and neurofibroma

E. Pathology

1. Gross appearance

   a. Well-encapsulated lesion, gray-tan in color (**Figure 6**)

   b. Grows eccentrically from the nerve

2. Histology

   a. Alternating areas of compact spindle cells (Antoni A) (**Figure 4, C**) and loosely arranged cells with large vessels (Antoni B) (**Figure 4, D**)

   b. The appearance of Verocay bodies (two rows of aligned nuclei in a palisading formation) is pathognomonic.

   c. Strongly uniform positive staining for S100 antibody

F. Treatment/outcome

1. Treatment is observation or marginal/intralesional excision with nerve fiber preservation as symptoms dictate.

2. Small risk of sensory deficits or long-standing palsies after dissection

3. Extremely rare risk of malignant degeneration

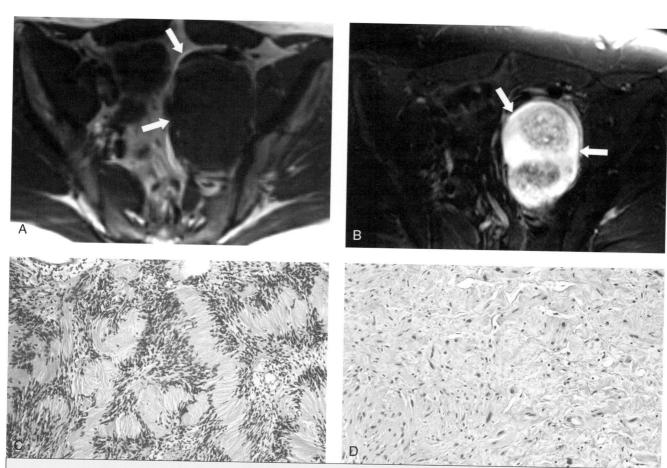

Figure 4   Neurilemoma of the pelvis. Axial T1-weighted (**A**) and T2-weighted (**B**) MRIs reveal a large soft-tissue mass (arrows) that has low signal intensity on T1 sequences and high signal intensity on T2 sequences. It would enhance after gadolinium administration. **C**, Low-power histologic image reveals the compact spindle cell areas (Antoni A) of a neurilemoma (hematoxylin and eosin). Note the palisading nuclei and Verocay bodies. **D**, Another histologic image from within the same tumor reveals areas of loosely arranged cells within a haphazard collagenous stroma (Antoni B; hematoxylin and eosin). Antoni B areas contain numerous blood vessels.

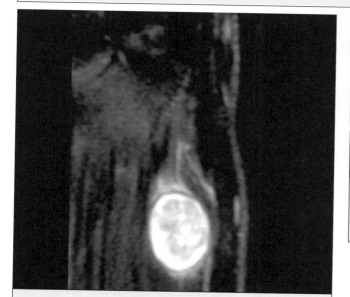

Figure 5   Coronal T2-weighted MRI of the wrist reveals a small, oval soft-tissue mass in continuity with a nerve, consistent with a neurilemoma.

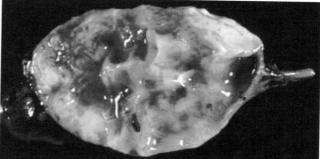

Figure 6   Photograph shows gross appearance of a bisected neurilemoma (schwannoma). Note the cystic degeneration of the well-encapsulated lesion.

4: Orthopaedic Oncology/Systemic Disease

IV. Neurofibroma

A. Definition and demographics

  1. Neurofibroma—A benign neural tumor involving multiple cell types.

  2. Occurs in patients 20 to 40 years of age (or younger when associated with neurofibromatosis)

  3. Affects males and females equally

B. Genetics/etiology

  1. Most neurofibromas arise sporadically.

  2. Neurofibromatosis type 1 (NF1) is an autosomal dominant syndrome characterized by multiple neurofibromas.

    a. NF1: abnormal chromosome 17 (1 in 3,000 births)

    b. NF2: abnormal chromosome 22 (1 in 33,000 births)

C. Clinical presentation

  1. Can affect any nerve; may be cutaneous or plexiform (infiltrative)

  2. Most are asymptomatic, but sometimes neurologic symptoms are present.

  3. Tumors are slow growing.

  4. Positive Tinel sign may be seen.

  5. National Institutes of Health criteria for NF1:

    a. Six or more café-au-lait spots

    b. Two or more Lisch nodules (melanocyte hamartoma affecting the iris)

    c. Axillary or inguinal freckling

    d. Two neurofibromas or one plexiform neurofibroma

    e. Optic glioma

    f. Bone scalloping

    g. First-degree relative with NF1 disease

  6. Rapid enlargement of a neurofibroma suggests malignant transformation.

D. Imaging appearance

  1. Varies in size; usually a fusiform expansion of the nerve

  2. Magnetic resonance imaging

    a. Low signal intensity on T1-weighted sequences, high on T2-weighted sequences (**Figure 7, A**).

    b. Dumbbell-shaped lesion that can expand a neural foramen

    c. More likely than neurilemoma to have "target sign" (peripheral high signal intensity and center of low signal intensity on T2-weighted sequences)

    d. Plexiform neurofibroma has extensive signal on MRI; infiltrative

  3. Radiographs—Orthopaedic manifestations include penciling of the ribs, sharp vertebral end plates, tibial congenital pseudarthrosis, nonossifying fibromas, osteopenia, and scoliosis.

E. Pathology

  1. Gross appearance

    a. Fusiform expansion of the nerve

    b. Usually unencapsulated

  2. Histology

    a. Interlacing bundles of elongated cells with wavy, dark nuclei (**Figure 7, B and C**)

    b. Cells are associated with wirelike collagen fibrils.

    c. Cells are sometimes arranged in fascicles or a storiform pattern.

    d. Mixed cell population of Schwann cells, mast cells, lymphocytes

    e. Stroma may have a myxoid appearance.

    f. S100 staining is variable.

F. Treatment/outcome

  1. If asymptomatic, treatment is observation.

  2. Surgical excision; can leave significant nerve deficit and may require grafting.

  3. In 5% of patients with neurofibromatosis, malignant transformation of a lesion develops (often a plexiform neurofibroma).

  4. Malignant transformation of a solitary lesion is rare.

V. Nodular Fasciitis

A. Definition and demographics

  1. Nodular fasciitis—A self-limited reactive process often mistaken for a fibrous neoplasm.

  2. Most common in adults 20 to 40 years of age

  3. Males and females affected equally

  4. Most common fibrous soft-tissue lesion

B. Genetics/etiology—Reactive rather than neoplastic process.

C. Clinical presentation

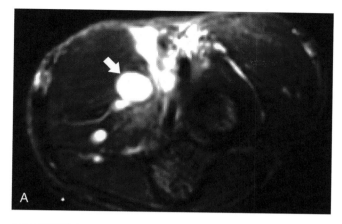

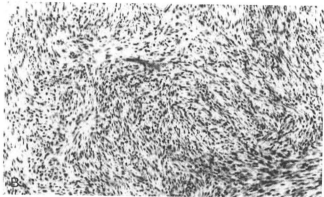

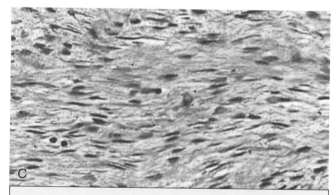

Figure 7 Neurofibroma of the elbow. **A,** Axial T2-weighted MRI of the elbow of a 26-year-old man with neurofibromatosis reveals an area of high signal intensity (arrow) consistent with a neurofibroma within the volar forearm muscles. The same lesion would be dark on T1-weighted sequences. **B,** Low-power histologic image reveals a cellular lesion with a wavy or storiform appearance (hematoxylin and eosin). **C,** Higher power histologic image reveals elongated cells with dark nuclei and no atypia (hematoxylin and eosin).

1. Rapid growth of a nodule over 1 to 2 weeks

2. Pain and/or tenderness in 50% of patients

3. Lesion usually 1 to 2 cm

4. Commonly occurs on volar forearm, back, chest wall, head/neck

5. Solitary lesion

D. Imaging appearance

1. MRI shows nodularity, extension along fascial planes, and avid enhancement with gadolinium.

2. Usually small

3. Occurs superficially (most common), intramuscularly, or along the superficial fascial planes

E. Pathology

1. Gross appearance—Nodular without a surrounding capsule.

2. Histology

   a. Cellular with numerous mitotic figures (**Figure 8, A**)

   b. Cells are plump, regular fibroblasts arranged in short bundles or fascicles (**Figure 8, B**).

   c. Additional cells include lymphoid cells, erythrocytes, giant cells, and lipid macrophages.

F. Treatment/outcome

1. Treatment is marginal or intralesional excision; has a low risk of local recurrence.

2. No risk of malignant transformation

3. Reports of resolution of lesion after needle biopsy

VI. Intramuscular Myxoma

A. Definition and demographics

1. Intramuscular myxoma—A benign, nonaggressive myxomatous soft-tissue tumor.

2. Occurs in adults 40 to 70 years of age

3. Male-to-female ratio = 1:2

B. Clinical presentation

1. Usually presents as a painless mass

2. Pain/tenderness in approximately 20% of patients

3. Possible numbness or paresthesias in patients with large lesions

4. Usually solitary

5. Most commonly located in the thigh, buttocks, shoulder, and upper arm

6. Often close to neurovascular structures

7. The presence of multiple intramuscular myxomas is associated with fibrous dysplasia (Mazabraud syndrome). In Mazabraud syndrome, fibrous dysplasia develops at a young age and the myxomas

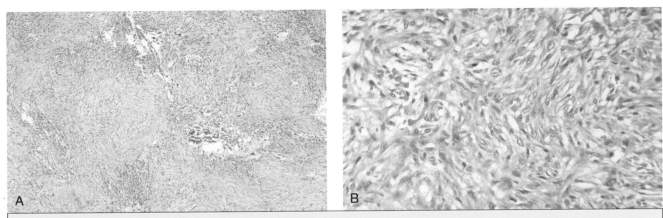

Figure 8 Nodular fasciitis. **A,** Low-power histologic image reveals a highly cellular lesion with a nodular pattern (hematoxylin and eosin). **B,** Higher power histologic image shows regular, plump fibroblasts with vessels, erythrocytes, and lipid macrophages consistent with nodular fasciitis (hematoxylin and eosin).

occur later in the same general anatomic area.

C. Imaging appearance

1. MRI appearance is homogeneous.

2. Low signal intensity (lower than muscle) on T1-weighted sequences, high on T2-weighted sequences (**Figure 9, A and B**)

3. Located within the muscle groups; usually 5 to 10 cm in size

D. Pathology

1. Gross appearance—Lobular and gelatinous with cyst-like spaces (**Figure 9, C**)

2. Histology

   a. Minimal cellularity with cells suspended in abundant mucoid material (**Figure 9, D**)

   b. Loose network of reticulin fibers

   c. No atypia, and only sparse vascularity

   d. "Cellular myxoma" has increased cellularity and can be mistaken for a malignant myxoid neoplasm.

E. Treatment/outcome

1. Marginal excision is the preferred treatment.

2. Very rarely recurs locally and does not metastasize

VII. Desmoid Tumor (Extra-abdominal Fibromatosis)

A. Definition and demographics

1. Desmoid tumor—A benign, locally aggressive fibrous neoplasm with a high risk of local recurrence.

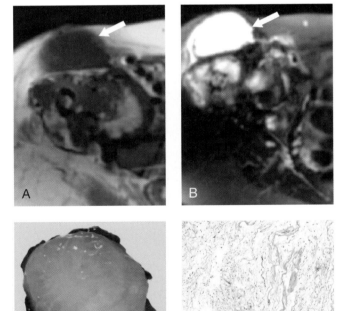

Figure 9 Intramuscular myxoma. Axial T1-weighted (**A**) and T2-weighted (**B**) MRIs in a 52-year-old woman with Mazabraud syndrome show a large soft-tissue lesion (arrows) along the anterior aspect of the right hip consistent with an intramuscular myxoma. It has lower signal intensity than muscle on the T1-weighted image and is bright on the T2-weighted image. **C,** Photograph shows the gross appearance of a bisected intramuscular myxoma; note the white, gelatinous surface. **D,** The histologic appearance reveals a paucicellular lesion with extensive reticulin fibers and a mucoid stroma (hematoxylin and eosin).

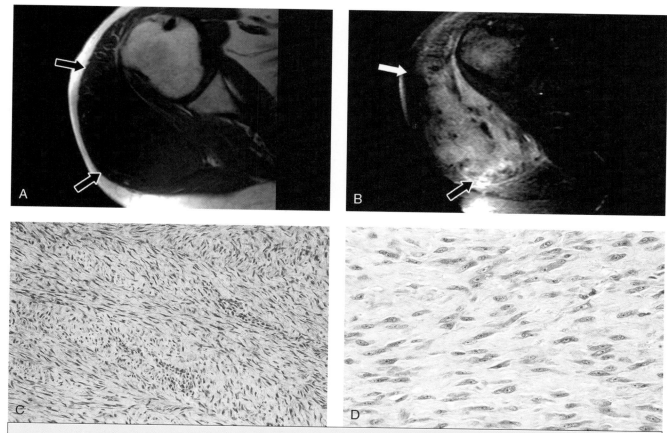

Figure 10   Desmoid tumors. Axial T1-weighted (**A**) and short tau inversion recovery (STIR) (**B**) MRIs of the right shoulder of a 58-year-old woman reveal a desmoid tumor (arrows). The STIR sequence is fluid-sensitive and reveals findings similar to those found on a fat-sensitive T2-weighted image. Low signal intensity is seen on both images. **C,** Low-power histologic image reveals sweeping bundles of collagen (hematoxylin and eosin). **D,** Higher power histologic image demonstrates bland, elongated, fibrous cells without atypia (hematoxylin and eosin).

4: Orthopaedic Oncology/Systemic Disease

2. Approximately 900 cases annually in the United States

3. Occurs in young persons (15 to 40 years)

4. Slight female predominance

5. Desmoid tumors occur within a family of fibromatoses that also includes superficial lesions in the palmar and plantar fascia (Dupuytren contracture, Ledderhose disease).

B. Genetics/etiology

1. Most spontaneous desmoid tumors are associated with mutations of the β-catenin gene (85% of cases), which results in decreased activation of Wnt/catenin signaling.

2. A minority of desmoid tumors are associated with Gardner syndrome and have mutations in the adenomatous polyposis coli (APC) gene.

3. Cytogenetic abnormalities include trisomy of chromosomes 8 or 20.

C. Clinical presentation

1. Usually a painless mass

2. Rock hard, fixed, and deep on examination

3. Most commonly occurs in the shoulder, chest wall/back, thigh

4. More than 50% are extra-abdominal; the rest are intra-abdominal (pelvis, mesentery).

5. Occasionally multicentric; usually a subsequent lesion occurs more proximal in the same limb.

D. Imaging appearance

1. Typical MRI appearance: low signal intensity on T1-weighted sequences, low to medium signal intensity on T2-weighted sequences (**Figure 10, A and B**)

2. Enhanced appearance with gadolinium administration

3. Infiltrative within the muscles; usually 5 to 10 cm in size

4. Adjacent osseous changes (erosion) may be seen.

E. Pathology

1. Gross appearance: gritty, white, poorly encapsulated

2. Histology

a. Bland fibroblasts with abundant collagen (**Figure 10, C** and **D**)

b. Uniform spindle cells with elongated nuclei and only occasional mitoses

c. Moderate vascularity

d. Sweeping bundles of collagen less defined than in fibrosarcoma

e. Often infiltrates into adjacent tissues and has no tumor capsule

f. Nuclear staining for β-catenin helps differentiate from other fibrous lesions

g. Positive staining for estrogen receptor β

3. Differential diagnosis includes fibrosarcoma nodular fasciitis, hypertrophic scar

F. Treatment/outcome

1. If surgery is possible, treatment is similar to that for sarcoma, with wide resection.

2. High risk of local recurrence given infiltrative pattern

3. Difficult to differentiate recurrent tumor from scar tissue

4. External beam radiation (up to 60 Gy) can be used for recurrent lesions.

5. Overall treatment should be determined by a multidisciplinary team.

a. Surgery if resectable

b. Radiation as an adjuvant (although risk exists for secondary sarcoma)

c. Medical treatment of large or inoperable tumors is becoming more common, including anti-hormonal drugs (tamoxifen), NSAIDs (cyclo-oxygenase [COX]-2 inhibitors), or classic chemotherapy.

d. Results are highly variable.

6. Unusual natural history: hard-to-predict behavior, occasional spontaneous regression

7. Treatment should not be worse than the disease; avoid amputation.

8. No risk of metastasis or malignant transformation except related to radiation

VIII. Elastofibroma

A. Definition and demographics

1. Elastofibroma—An unusual, tumorlike reactive process that frequently occurs between the scapula and chest wall.

2. Occurs in patients 60 to 80 years of age

3. More common in females than in males

B. Genetics/etiology

1. High familial incidence

2. Often occurs after repeated trauma

C. Clinical presentation

1. Usually asymptomatic; found in approximately 17% of elderly people at autopsy

2. Snapping scapula on examination

3. Firm, deep lesion

4. Occurs almost exclusively in the soft tissues between the tip of the scapula and the chest wall

5. Bilateral in 10% of cases (can be noted incidentally on chest CT scans)

D. Imaging appearance

1. CT—Ill-defined lesion with appearance of muscle.

2. MRI—Mixed low and high signal intensity on T1- and T2-weighted sequences (**Figure 11, A**).

E. Pathology

1. Gross appearance: gray with cystic degeneration, 5 to 10 cm in length.

2. Histology

a. Elastic fibers having a beaded appearance with characteristic staining for elastin (**Figure 11, B**)

b. Equal proportion of intertwined collagen fibers

F. Treatment/outcome

1. Treatment for asymptomatic lesions is observation.

2. Simple excision is curative.

3. No risk of malignant transformation

IX. Glomus Tumor

A. Definition and demographics

1. Glomus tumor—A benign tumor of the normal glomus body usually occurring in the subungual region.

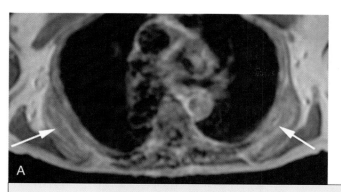
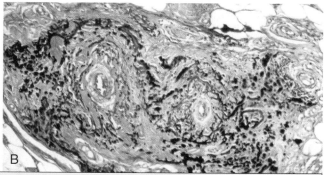

Figure 11   Elastofibroma. **A,** Axial MRI of the chest of a 73-year-old woman reveals bilateral soft-tissue masses (arrows) between the inferior tip of the scapula and the underlying chest wall consistent with elastofibromas. **B,** High-power histologic image reveals the beaded appearance of the elastic fibers admixed with the extensive collagen fibers. The elastin stain highlights the elastic fibers throughout the lesion (hematoxylin and eosin). Note the extensive vascularity.

2. Extremely rare

3. Occurs in patients 20 to 40 years of age

4. Males and females are affected equally (except subungual tumors, for which the male-to-female ratio = 1:3).

B. Clinical presentation

1. Small (<1 cm) red-blue nodule in the subungual region or other deep dermal layers in the extremities

2. More difficult to see color in subungual region; may have ridging of the nail or discoloration of the nail bed

3. Characteristic triad of symptoms: paroxysmal pain, cold insensitivity, localized tenderness

4. Frequent delay in diagnosis

5. Less common locations include the palm, wrist, forearm, and foot.

6. Multiple tumors in 10% of cases

C. Imaging appearance

1. Magnetic resonance imaging

   a. Best imaging modality to identify glomus tumors

   b. Sensitivity: 90% to 100%; specificity: 50%

   c. Low signal intensity on T1-weighted sequences, high on T2-weighted sequences

2. Plain radiographs

   a. Not very helpful in diagnosis

   b. Can show a scalloped osteolytic defect with a sclerotic border in the distal phalanx

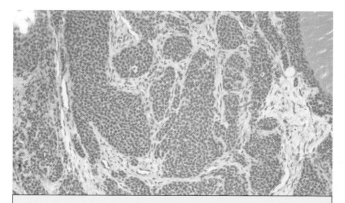

Figure 12   Low-power histologic image of a glomus tumor reveals small, rounded cells with dark nuclei in well-defined clumps. On higher power, the glomus cells and the admixed capillaries would be present within a myxoid stroma (hematoxylin and eosin).

D. Pathology

1. Gross appearance—Small, red-blue nodule.

2. Histology

   a. Well-defined lesion of small vessels surrounded by glomus cells in a hyaline or myxoid stroma (**Figure 12**)

   b. Uniform, round cell with a prominent nucleus and eosinophilic cytoplasm

   c. Periodic acid-Schiff stain gives a chicken-wire appearance to the matrix between cells.

E. Treatment/outcome

1. Marginal excision is curative.

2. Extremely rare reports of malignant glomus tumors

X. Synovial Chondromatosis

A. Definition and demographics

1. Synovial chondromatosis—A metaplastic proliferation of hyaline cartilage nodules in the synovial membrane.

2. Occurs in patients 30 to 50 years of age

3. Male-to-female ratio = 2:1

B. Genetics/etiology

1. Generally thought to be a metaplastic condition

2. Occasional chromosomal aberrations have been identified.

C. Clinical presentation

1. Joint pain, clicking, limited range of motion

2. Pain worse with activity

3. Warmth, erythema, or tenderness may be present, depending on location.

4. Slow progression of symptoms over years

5. Most common in the hip and knee, followed by shoulder and elbow

6. Occasionally occurs in the bursa overlying an osteochondroma

D. Imaging appearance

1. Plain radiographs show variable appearance, depending on early or late disease.

2. Cartilage nodules are not visible initially, except on MRI.

3. Nodules calcify over time, then undergo endochondral ossification (**Figure 13, A and B**).

4. Densities are smooth, well defined, and remain within the confines of the synovial membrane.

5. Erosion of cartilage and underlying bone may be seen.

6. CT scan can define intra-articular loose bodies.

7. MRI shows lobular appearance with signal dropout consistent with calcification.

E. Pathology

1. Gross appearance—There may be hundreds of osteocartilaginous loose bodies within an affected joint.

2. Histology

a. Discrete hyaline cartilage nodules in various phases of calcification or ossification (**Figure 13, C**). Ossification starts on the periphery of the nodules.

b. Cellular appearance of chondrocytes includes mild atypia, binucleate cells, and occasional

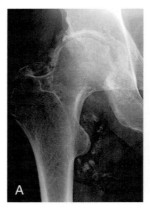
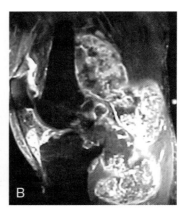
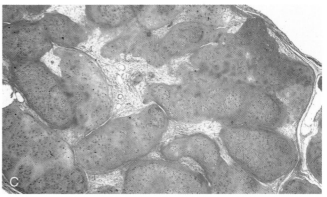
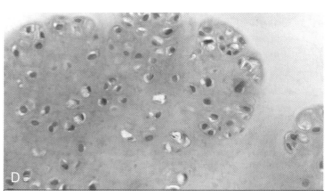

Figure 13   Synovial chondromatoses. **A,** AP radiograph of the right hip of a 46-year-old man with synovial chondromatosis demonstrates discrete calcifications superior and inferior to the femoral head, both within and external to the hip capsule. **B,** Sagittal T2-weighted MRI of the knee in a 33-year-old man with extensive synovial osteochondromatosis. Multiple ossified nodules within the joint required open synovectomies of the anterior and posterior compartments of the knee. **C,** Low-power histologic image of synovial osteochondromatosis reveals discrete hyaline cartilage nodules (hematoxylin and eosin). **D,** Higher power reveals increased cellularity with occasional binucleate cells (hematoxylin and eosin).

mitoses (more cellular atypia than allowed in an intramedullary benign cartilage tumor) (**Figure 13, D**).

F. Treatment/outcome

1. Treatment is open or arthroscopic synovectomy.

2. Less than adequate removal of nodules increases risk for local recurrence.

3. Natural history is self-limited, but the process can damage the joint.

XI. Pigmented Villonodular Synovitis

A. Definition and demographics

1. Pigmented villonodular synovitis (PVNS)—A benign, clonal neoplastic proliferation arising from synovium and characterized by mononuclear stromal cells, hemorrhage, histiocytes, and giant cells.

2. Most commonly affects patients 30 to 50 years of age; occasionally affects teenagers

3. Males and females affected equally

4. Occurs in focal or diffuse forms

5. Can be intra-articular or extra-articular (giant cell tumor of tendon sheath)

B. Genetics/etiology

1. An earlier traumatic incident is reported by 50% of patients.

2. Minor population of intratumoral cells harbor a recurrent translocation, and these cells overexpress colony-stimulating factor-1 (CSF1).

C. Clinical presentation

1. Pain, swelling, effusion, erythema, and decreased joint range of motion with diffuse joint involvement

2. Mechanical joint symptoms with focal involvement

3. Most commonly affects the knee (80%), followed by hip, shoulder, ankle

4. Extra-articular form (giant cell tumor of tendon sheath; not related in any way to giant cell tumor of bone) usually affects the hand/wrist with a small, painless, superficial soft-tissue nodule.

D. Imaging appearance

1. Plain radiographs—Well-defined erosions on both sides of a joint signify advanced, diffuse disease (**Figure 14, A**).

2. Magnetic resonance imaging

a. Either a focal low-intensity-signal nodule within a joint or a diffuse process with low signal intensity (due to hemosiderin deposits) on T1- and T2-weighted images (**Figure 14, B and C**)

b. Fat signal within the lesion

c. Extra-articular extension of the process may be seen.

3. Differential diagnosis includes reactive or inflammatory synovitis, hemophilia, synovial chondromatosis.

E. Pathology

1. Gross appearance—Reddish-brown stained synovium with extensive papillary projections (**Figure 14, D**).

2. Histology

a. Diagnostic mononuclear stromal cell infiltrate within the synovium (**Figure 14, E**)

b. Cells are round with a large nucleus and eosinophilic cytoplasm.

c. Hemosiderin-laden macrophages, multinucleated giant cells, and foam cells present; not required for diagnosis

d. Mitotic figures relatively common

F. Treatment/outcome

1. Treatment is arthroscopic or open removal of a focal PVNS lesion.

2. Diffuse form requires aggressive total synovectomy using arthroscopic, open, or combined arthroscopic and open techniques.

3. An anterior arthroscopic synovectomy can be combined with open posterior removal of any extra-articular disease.

4. High local recurrence rate suggests frequent incomplete synovectomy.

5. Total joint arthroplasty is indicated for advanced disease with secondary degenerative changes.

6. External beam radiation is used occasionally following multiple local recurrences.

7. Giant cell tumor of tendon sheath is treated with marginal excision.

8. Inhibition of CSF1 receptor (CSF1R) using small-molecule inhibitors can be tried for unresectable or multiply recurrent disease.

XII. Myositis Ossificans

A. Definition and demographics

1. Myositis ossificans—A reactive process characterized by a well-circumscribed proliferation of fibroblasts, cartilage, and bone within a muscle (or, rarely, within a nerve, tendon, or fat).

2. Occurs in young, active individuals (most com-

4: Orthopaedic Oncology/Systemic Disease

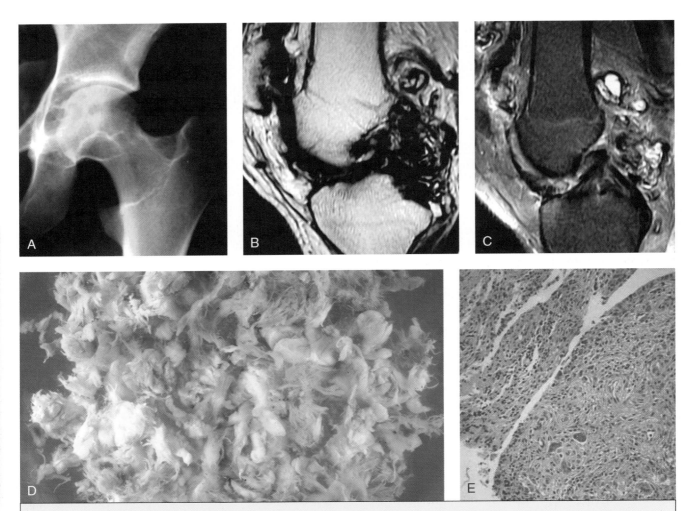

Figure 14 Examples of pigmented villonodular synovitis (PVNS). **A,** AP radiograph of the left hip of a patient with advanced PVNS reveals osteolytic lesions with sclerotic rims on both sides of the joint. Sagittal T1-weighted (**B**) and T2-weighted (**C**) MRIs of a knee show extensive disease in the posterior aspect of the knee. The lesion is both intra-articular and extra-articular. Dark signal is seen on both of the images as a result of the hemosiderin deposits within the synovium. **D,** Gross appearance of the reddish-brown synovial fronds seen in PVNS. **E,** Histologic image reveals a cellular infiltrate within the synovium with multinucleated giant cells and faint hemosiderin (hematoxylin and eosin). The round, mononuclear stromal cells are the key to the diagnosis.

mon in individuals 15 to 35 years of age)

   3. More common in males than in females

B. Genetics/etiology—Almost always a posttraumatic condition.

C. Clinical presentation

   1. Pain, tenderness, swelling, and decreased range of motion, usually within days of an injury

   2. Mass that increases in size over several months (usually 3 to 6 cm); then growth stops and mass becomes firm

   3. Commonly occurs in the quadriceps, brachialis, gluteal muscles

D. Imaging appearance

   1. Mineralization begins 3 weeks after injury.

   2. Initially, irregular, fluffy densities in the soft tissues are noted on plain radiographs (**Figure 15, A**).

   3. Adjacent periosteal reaction in the bone may be seen.

   4. Rim enhancement is seen on MRI with gadolinium within the first 3 weeks.

   5. With time and maturation, a zoning pattern occurs, with increased peripheral mineralization and a radiolucent center.

   6. CT defines the ossified lesion, which looks like an eggshell (**Figure 15, B**).

   7. Differential diagnosis includes extraskeletal and

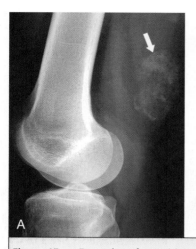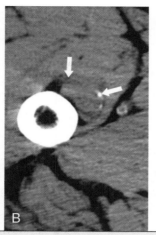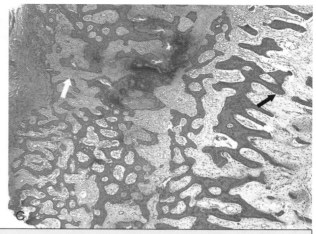

Figure 15 Examples of myositis ossificans. **A,** Lateral radiograph of a knee obtained 4 weeks after a football injury to the posterior thigh in a 19-year-old man reveals fluffy calcifications (arrow) in the posterior thigh musculature consistent with early myositis ossificans. **B,** CT scan of the thigh of a patient with traumatic myositis ossificans reveals the calcified outline of the lesion (arrows) with more mature tissue on the periphery. **C,** Histologic image of a myositis ossificans lesion reveals a zonal pattern (hematoxylin and eosin), with more mature bone toward the periphery (white arrow) and looser fibrous tissue toward the center (black arrow).

parosteal osteosarcoma (more ossified in the center with peripheral lucencies).

E. Pathology

1. Gross appearance—Immature tissue in center of lesion with mature bone around outer edge.

2. Histology

   a. Zonal pattern (**Figure 15, C**)

     • Periphery: mature lamellar bone

     • Intermediate: poorly defined trabeculae with osteoblasts, fibroblasts, and large ectatic blood vessels

     • Center: immature, loose, fibrous tissue with moderate pleomorphism and mitoses

   b. Skeletal muscle can be entrapped in the periphery of the lesion.

   c. No cytologic atypia

3. Differential diagnosis includes extraskeletal osteosarcoma (periphery is least ossified and cells show extreme pleomorphism).

F. Treatment/outcome

1. Myositis ossificans is a self-limited process, so observation and physical therapy to maintain motion are indicated.

2. Repeat radiographs should be obtained to confirm maturation and stability of the lesion.

3. Excision is indicated only when the lesion is mature (approximately 6 to 12 months) and if symptomatic; excision at initial stages predisposes to local recurrence.

4. The size of the mass often decreases after 1 year.

4: Orthopaedic Oncology/Systemic Disease

Top Testing Facts

1. Lipomas should image the same as fat on all MRI sequences.

2. Intramuscular hemangiomas or other vascular malformations are best treated nonsurgically.

3. Neurilemomas have Antoni A (cellular) and Antoni B (myxoid) areas on histology.

4. NF1 involves an abnormal chromosome 17; malignant transformation of a lesion will occur in 5% of patients.

5. Desmoid tumors are one of the few benign soft-tissue lesions that require a wide resection.

6. Treatment of desmoid tumors requires a multidisciplinary team with consideration of medical management for large or inoperable tumors.

7. Elastofibromas commonly occur between the scapula and chest wall; they stain positive for elastin.

8. Glomus tumors usually occur in a subungual location.

9. Synovial chondromatosis and diffuse forms of PVNS require a complete synovectomy to achieve local control.

10. The imaging and histologic appearance of myositis ossificans shows a zonal pattern with increased peripheral mineralization and immature tissue in the center.

Bibliography

Cassier PA, Gelderblom H, Stacchiotti S, et al: Efficacy of imatinib mesylate for the treatment of locally advanced and/or metastatic tenosynovial giant cell tumor/pigmented villonodular synovitis. *Cancer* 2012;118(6):1649-1655.

El-Merhi F, Garg D, Cura M, Ghaith O: Peripheral vascular tumors and vascular malformations: Imaging (magnetic resonance imaging and conventional angiography), pathologic correlation and treatment options. *Int J Cardiovasc Imaging* 2013;29(2):379-393.

Feldman DS, Jordan C, Fonseca L: Orthopaedic manifestations of neurofibromatosis type 1. *J Am Acad Orthop Surg* 2010;18(6):346-357.

Flors L, Leiva-Salinas C, Maged IM, et al: MR imaging of soft-tissue vascular malformations: Diagnosis, classification, and therapy follow-up. *Radiographics* 2011;31(5):1321-1341.

Furlong MA, Fanburg-Smith JC, Miettinen M: The morphologic spectrum of hibernoma: A clinicopathologic study of 170 cases. *Am J Surg Pathol* 2001;25(6):809-814.

General considerations, in Weiss SW, Goldblum JR, eds: *Enzinger and Weiss's Soft Tissue Tumors*, ed 5. St Louis, MO, Mosby, 2008, pp 1-14.

Jee WH, Oh SN, McCauley T, et al: Extraaxial neurofibromas versus neurilemmomas: Discrimination with MRI. *AJR Am J Roentgenol* 2004;183(3):629-633.

Kransdorf MJ, Meis JM, Jelinek JS: Myositis ossificans: MR appearance with radiologic-pathologic correlation. *AJR Am J Roentgenol* 1991;157(6):1243-1248.

Lim SJ, Chung HW, Choi YL, Moon YW, Seo JG, Park YS: Operative treatment of primary synovial osteochondromatosis of the hip. *J Bone Joint Surg Am* 2006;88(11):2456-2464.

Murphey MD, Vidal JA, Fanburg-Smith JC, Gajewski DA: Imaging of synovial chondromatosis with radiologic-pathologic correlation. *Radiographics* 2007;27(5):1465-1488.

Okuno S: The enigma of desmoid tumors. *Curr Treat Options Oncol* 2006;7(6):438-443.

Parratt MT, Donaldson JR, Flanagan AM, et al: Elastofibroma dorsi: Management, outcome and review of the literature. *J Bone Joint Surg Br* 2010;92(2):262-266.

Ravi V, Wang WL, Lewis VO: Treatment of tenosynovial giant cell tumor and pigmented villonodular synovitis. *Curr Opin Oncol* 2011;23(4):361-366.

Walker EA, Fenton ME, Salesky JS, Murphey MD: Magnetic resonance imaging of benign soft tissue neoplasms in adults. *Radiol Clin North Am* 2011;49(6):1197-1217, vi.

Wodajo FM: Benign vascular soft-tissue tumors, in Schwartz HS, ed: *Orthopaedic Knowledge Update: Musculoskeletal Tumors*, ed 2. Rosemont, IL, American Academy of Orthopaedic Surgeons, 2007, pp 225-231.

Wu JS, Hochman MG: Soft-tissue tumors and tumorlike lesions: A systematic imaging approach. *Radiology* 2009;253(2):297-316.

Chapter 49

Malignant Soft-Tissue Tumors

Kristy Weber, MD

4: Orthopaedic Oncology/Systemic Disease

I. Soft-Tissue Sarcomas

A. Overview

1. Ratio of benign to malignant soft-tissue masses is 100:1 (sarcomas rare).

2. Males are affected more commonly than females.

3. Sixty percent of sarcomas affect the extremities (upper and lower).

4. Eighty-five percent occur in individuals older than 15 years.

5. Diagnostic appearance of most sarcomas on MRI is indeterminate; a biopsy is required.

6. Staging—The most common staging system is the American Joint Committee on Cancer system, which relies on tumor size, tumor depth, nodal status, and whether distant metastases are present.

B. Surgery

1. The goal of surgery is to achieve an acceptable margin to minimize local recurrence and maintain reasonable function; limb salvage procedures are performed in approximately 90% of patients.

2. Sarcomas have a centripetal growth pattern.

3. A reactive zone around the tumor includes edema, fibrous tissue (capsule), inflammatory cells, and tumor cells.

4. "Shelling out" a sarcoma usually means excising it through the reactive zone, which leaves tumor cells behind in most cases.

5. Definition of surgical margins (Enneking)

   a. Intralesional: resection through the tumor mass for gross total resection

   b. Marginal: resection through the reactive zone

   c. Wide: resection with a cuff of normal tissue

   d. Radical: resection of the entire compartment (for example, quadriceps)

6. Indications for amputation

   a. When necessary to resect the entire tumor

   b. When major nerves cannot be saved

   c. In some locally recurrent sarcomas

   d. When the patient has significant comorbidities that preclude limb-sparing surgery

7. Standard oncologic techniques are used to resect soft-tissue sarcomas, including use of a tourniquet without exsanguination, excision of the biopsy tract, and use of drains distal, close, and in line with the incision.

8. Surgical resection alone of large, deep, high-grade tumors has an unacceptably high rate of local recurrence and requires adjuvant treatment (radiation with or without chemotherapy).

9. Soft-tissue reconstruction by free or rotational tissue transfer frequently is necessary; it minimizes wound complications after major resection, especially when preoperative radiation is used (**Figure 1**).

C. Radiation

1. Radiation is used routinely as an adjuvant to surgery in the treatment of soft-tissue sarcoma.

2. Noted exceptions to the use of radiation are when an amputation is performed or when the sarcoma is small, superficial, low grade, and amenable to a wide surgical resection.

3. Radiation can be administered by external beam techniques (photons or protons), brachytherapy (**Figure 2**), or intraoperatively.

4. Early radiation effects: desquamation, delayed wound healing, infection. Late effects: fibrosis, fractures, joint stiffness, secondary sarcoma (depending on treatment dose, volume, and length of follow-up).

5. Preoperative radiation requires a lower dose (~50 Gy) than postoperative radiation (~66 Gy), decreases the surrounding edema, and helps form a fibrous capsule around the tumor. Surgery is delayed 3 to 4 weeks after completion of radiation.

Dr. Weber or an immediate family member serves as a board member, owner, officer, or committee member of the Musculoskeletal Tumor Society and the Ruth Jackson Orthopaedic Society.

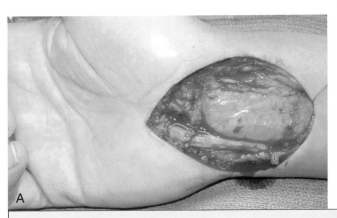

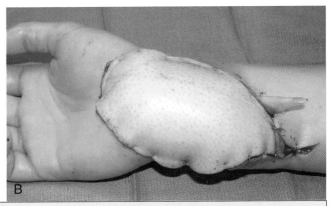

Figure 1   Clinical photographs show the wrist of a patient after soft-tissue sarcoma resection. **A,** Soft-tissue defect after wide resection of a clear cell sarcoma of the volar wrist. **B,** Soft-tissue reconstruction using free tissue transfer. This procedure is commonly performed to minimize wound breakdown and infection, especially when the patient has undergone preoperative radiation.

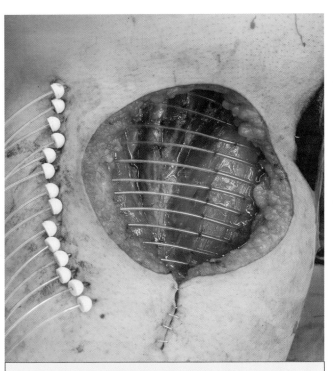

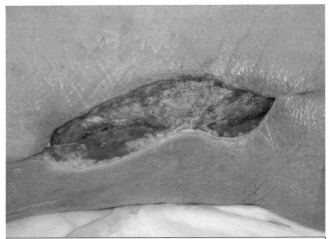

Figure 3   Clinical photograph shows wound breakdown in a patient who underwent preoperative radiation and surgical resection of a high-grade liposarcoma of the medial thigh.

Figure 2   Clinical photograph shows brachytherapy catheters overlying a tumor bed after resection. A free flap was used to cover the defect.

6. Preoperative radiation incurs a higher wound complication rate (35%) than postoperative radiation (17%) (**Figure 3**).

7. No difference in overall survival or functional outcomes related to timing of radiation has been reported.

8. External beam radiation combined with extensive periosteal stripping during tumor resection increases the risk of postradiation fracture. In these cases, immediate or delayed prophylactic intramedullary or plate stabilization should be considered.

9. Brachytherapy (percutaneous flexible catheters placed directly on tumor bed and loaded with radiation sources [beads or wires] over 48 to 96 hours) can be given as the sole radiation treatment dose or as a boost before or after external beam treatment. It is currently used infrequently and only at institutions with extensive experience.

D. Chemotherapy

1. Chemotherapy is a key component of treatment of rhabdomyosarcoma and soft-tissue Ewing sarcoma/primitive neuroectodermal tumor.

2. Objective evidence of benefit for many other types of localized soft-tissue sarcoma is lacking.

Studies show a substantial effect on local or systemic disease recurrence but no difference in survival with or without chemotherapy.

3. Given the high risk of metastasis in high-grade, large soft-tissue sarcomas, chemotherapy is frequently used, often in a clinical trial setting. Patients with metastatic disease often receive systemic therapy given that surgical options are often lacking.

4. Common agents include ifosfamide and doxorubicin, which have considerable toxicity in high doses. Taxanes can be used for angiosarcoma. Gemcitabine and docetaxel are used for leiomyosarcoma.

5. Patients with soft-tissue sarcoma who are older and have more comorbidities often cannot tolerate high-dose systemic treatment.

E. Outcomes

1. The use of radiation and surgery minimizes the risk of local recurrence to less than 10%.

2. Stage is the most important factor in determining overall prognosis/outcome.

3. Other prognostic factors include presence of metastasis, grade, size, and depth of tumor.

4. Tumor grade is related to risk of metastasis (low grade, < 10%; intermediate grade, 10% to 25%; high grade, > 50%).

5. The most common site of metastasis is the lungs.

6. Lymph node metastasis (normally <5%) occurs more frequently in rhabdomyosarcoma, synovial sarcoma, epithelioid sarcoma, and clear cell sarcoma.

7. The outcome of individual soft-tissue sarcoma subtypes is rarely reported; approximately 50% of patients with high-grade soft-tissue sarcomas die of the disease.

8. Resection of pulmonary metastasis can cure up to 25% of patients.

9. Patients require follow-up imaging of primary site of resection (MRI with contrast, or ultrasonography) and chest (radiography or CT) every 3 to 4 months for 2 years and then every 6 months for 3 years. Thereafter, annual chest studies are required.

II. Undifferentiated Pleomorphic Sarcoma

A. Definition and demographics

1. Undifferentiated pleomorphic sarcoma (previously called malignant fibrous histiocytoma) is pleomorphic in histologic appearance.

2. It is the most common soft-tissue sarcoma in adults 55 to 80 years of age.

3. Male-to-female ratio = 2:1

4. More common in Caucasian than in African American or Asian populations

B. Genetics/etiology—No data yet.

C. Clinical presentation

1. Usually a deep, slow-growing, painless mass

2. More common in the extremities (lower more common than upper) than retroperitoneum

3. Patients occasionally present with fever, elevated white blood cell count, and hypoglycemia.

D. Imaging appearance (indeterminate)—Low signal intensity on T1-weighted MRI; high signal intensity on T2-weighted MRI (**Figure 4, A and B**).

E. Pathology

1. Gross: a gray-white multinodular mass

2. Histologic subtypes include pleomorphic (80% to 85%), giant cell (10%), and inflammatory (< 10%).

3. Storiform or cartwheel growth pattern is seen on low-power histologic images (**Figure 4, C**).

4. Cells are plump, spindled, and arranged around narrow vessels.

5. Haphazard histiocytic cells

6. Multinucleate eosinophilic giant cells (**Figure 4, D**)

7. Marked atypia, mitotic activity, and pleomorphism

F. Treatment/outcome

1. Radiation and wide surgical resection

2. Chemotherapy in selected cases

3. Overall 5-year survival of 50% to 60% (depending on size, grade, depth, presence of metastasis)

III. Liposarcoma

A. Definition and demographics

1. Composed of a variety of histologic forms related to the developmental stages of lipoblasts

2. Second most common soft-tissue sarcoma in adults

3. Occurs most commonly in patients 50 to 80 years of age

4. Affects males more commonly than females

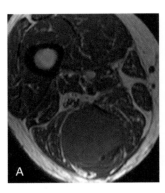
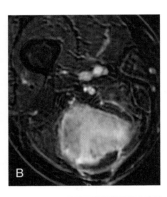
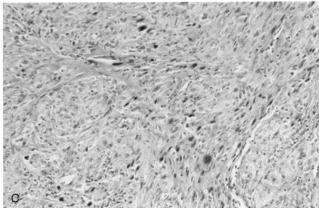
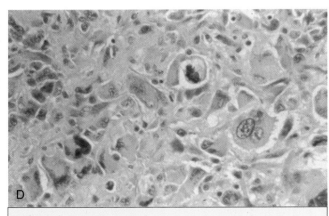

Figure 4 Undifferentiated pleomorphic sarcoma in a 68-year-old man who presented with a painless soft-tissue mass in the right posterior thigh. Axial T1-weighted MRI (**A**) and T2-weighted post-contrast MRI (**B**) show a mass indeterminate in appearance; a biopsy is required. **C,** Low-power histologic image reveals a storiform pattern with bizarre pleomorphic tumor cells and hyalinized collagen bundles consistent with undifferentiated pleomorphic sarcoma. **D,** Higher power histologic image reveals anaplastic tumor cells, multinucleated cells, and mitotic figures.

B. Genetics/etiology

   1. Liposarcoma originates from primitive mesenchymal cells; diagnosis does not require adipose cells.

   2. Simple lipomas do not predispose a patient to liposarcomas.

   3. Histologic types include well-differentiated, myxoid (most common, 50%), round cell, pleomorphic, and dedifferentiated.

   4. Well-differentiated variants have giant marker and ring chromosomes and overexpression of *MDM2*.

   5. Well-differentiated and dedifferentiated liposarcoma are both characterized by chromosome 12q13-15 amplification.

   6. Myxoid liposarcoma is associated with a translocation between chromosomes 12 and 16.

C. Clinical presentation

   1. Wide spectrum of disease, depending on histologic type

   2. Slow growing; may become extremely large (10 to 20 cm), painless masses

   3. Pain may occur in larger lesions.

   4. Occur in extremities (lower [thigh] more common than upper) and retroperitoneum (15% to 20%) (present at later age)

   5. Well-differentiated liposarcoma is essentially the same entity as atypical lipoma/atypical lipomatous tumor; some authors use the former term for retroperitoneal lesions and the latter term for extremity lesions.

   6. Well-differentiated liposarcomas rarely dedifferentiate. Rapid growth of a long-standing (usually > 5 years) painless mass should be watched for.

D. Imaging appearance

   1. Plain radiographs occasionally show foci of calcification or ossification in well-differentiated variants.

   2. MRI appearance of well-differentiated variant is the same as a lipoma. Rare areas of dedifferentiation should be watched for (**Figure 5, A and B**).

   3. MRI appearance of high-grade liposarcoma is indeterminate and similar to all sarcomas (low signal intensity on T1-weighted images; high signal intensity on T2-weighted images) (**Figure 6, A and B**).

   4. Myxoid liposarcomas can metastasize to sites other than the lungs (such as the abdomen), so staging for this tumor should include a CT scan of the abdomen and pelvis with contrast as well as a chest CT scan.

E. Pathology

   1. Gross: large, well-circumscribed, lobular

   2. Well-differentiated liposarcoma

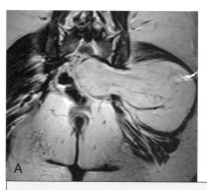
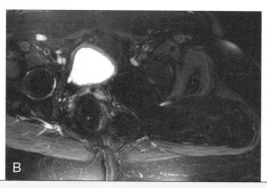
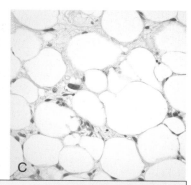

Figure 5   Well-differentiated liposarcoma. **A,** Coronal T1-weighted MRI reveals a large left retroperitoneal lipomatous lesion extending through the sciatic notch into the gluteal muscles. **B,** Axial T2-weighted fat-suppressed MRI reveals that the lesion completely suppresses with no concern for high-grade areas. **C,** Histologic image of the resected specimen reveals slight variation in the size and shape of the fat cells with hyperchromatic nuclei, consistent with a well-differentiated liposarcoma.

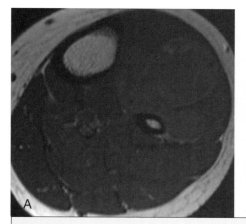
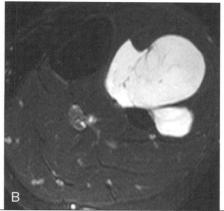
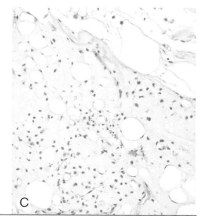

Figure 6   Myxoid liposarcoma in the left calf of a 27-year-old woman. Axial T1-weighted MRI (**A**) and T2-weighted short tau inversion recovery MRI (**B**) sequences reveal an indeterminate lesion that has low signal intensity on T1-weighted images and high signal intensity on T2-weighted images. No bony involvement is seen, but the mass is adjacent to the proximal fibula. **C,** Histologic image reveals lipoblasts (some with signet ring appearance), numerous capillaries, and a myxoid stroma between the tumor cells. No significant round cell component is noted.

4: Orthopaedic Oncology/Systemic Disease

a. Low-grade tumor

b. Lobulated appearance of mature adipose tissue (**Figure 5, C**)

3. Myxoid liposarcoma

   a. Low- to intermediate-grade tumor with lobulated appearance

   b. Composed of proliferating lipoblasts, a plexiform capillary network, and a myxoid matrix (**Figure 6, C**)

   c. Signet ring (univacuolar) lipoblasts occur at the edge of the tumor lobules.

   d. Few mitotic figures

4. Round cell liposarcoma

   a. Also considered a poorly differentiated myxoid liposarcoma

b. Characteristic small round blue cells

c. Rare intracellular lipid formation and minimal myxoid matrix

5. Pleomorphic liposarcoma

   a. High-grade tumor with marked pleomorphic appearance

   b. Giant lipoblasts with hyperchromatic bizarre nuclei

   c. Deeply eosinophilic giant cells

6. Dedifferentiated liposarcoma

   a. High-grade sarcoma (undifferentiated pleomorphic sarcoma, fibrosarcoma, leiomyosarcoma)

   b. Juxtaposed to well-differentiated lipomatous lesion

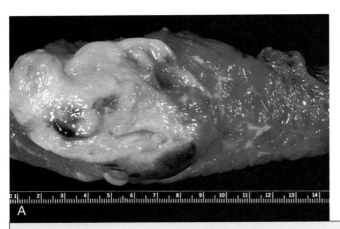
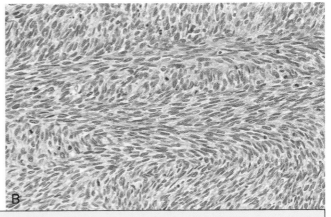

Figure 7 Fibrosarcomas. **A,** Gross appearance of a fibrosarcoma within the muscles of the anterior thigh. Areas of hemorrhage and cyst formation are present. **B,** High-power view of a fibrosarcoma reveals the distinct fascicular appearance of cells with little variation in size or shape. When the cells are cut in cross section, they appear round. The overall appearance is that of a herringbone pattern of spindle cells.

F. Treatment/outcome

1. Well-differentiated liposarcoma

   a. Marginal resection without radiation or chemotherapy

   b. Metastasis extremely rare

   c. Risk of local recurrence is 25% to 50% at 10 years.

   d. Dedifferentiation risk is 2% for extremity lesions and 20% for retroperitoneal lesions.

2. Intermediate- and high-grade variants

   a. Radiation and wide surgical resection

   b. Chemotherapy in selected patients

   c. Incidence of pulmonary metastasis increases with grade.

   d. Myxoid liposarcomas with more than 10% round cells have a higher likelihood of metastasis.

   e. Local recurrence is higher in retroperitoneal lesions.

   f. Agents that target chromosome 12 gene products (*MDM2* and *CDK4*) are in trials for well-differentiated and dedifferentiated liposarcoma.

IV. Fibrosarcoma

A. Definition and demographics

1. Fibrosarcoma is a rare soft-tissue sarcoma of fibroblastic origin that shows no tendency to other cellular differentiation.

2. Occurs in adults 30 to 55 years of age

3. Affects males more commonly than females

B. Genetics/etiology—No data yet.

C. Clinical presentation

1. Slow-growing, painless mass (4 to 8 cm) most commonly noted around the thigh or knee

2. Ulceration of the skin in superficial lesions

D. Imaging appearance (indeterminate)—Low signal intensity on T1-weighted MRI; high signal intensity on T2-weighted MRI.

E. Pathology

1. Gross: shown in **Figure 7, A**

2. Histology

   a. Uniform fasciculated growth pattern (herringbone) (**Figure 7, B**)

   b. Spindle cells with minimal cytoplasm

   c. Collagen fibers commonly aligned in parallel throughout tumor

   d. Mitotic activity varies

F. Treatment/outcome

1. Wide surgical resection and radiation

2. Chemotherapy for selected patients

3. Metastasis in approximately 50% of high-grade lesions

V. Dermatofibrosarcoma Protuberans

A. Definition

1. Rare, low-grade malignancy affecting dermal layers of skin

2. Occur in subcutaneous locations; 1 to 5 cm

3. Ninety percent have chromosomal translocation: t(17:22)(q22;q13).

4. Ten percent have fibrosarcomatous areas.

5. Two percent to 5% can metastasize to lungs

B. Treatment

1. Treatment is surgical resection with wide margins because of propensity for local recurrence.

2. Tyrosine kinase inhibitors (imatinib) can be used.

VI. Synovial Sarcoma

A. Definition and demographics

1. Distinct lesion occurring in para-articular regions

2. Most common soft-tissue sarcoma in young adults

3. Occurs most commonly in patients 15 to 40 years of age

4. Affects males more commonly than females

B. Genetics/etiology

1. Characteristic translocation (X;18)

2. Represents the fusion of *SYT* with either *SSX1* or *SSX2*

C. Clinical presentation

1. Slow-growing soft-tissue mass; 3 to 5 cm

2. In some patients, 2 to 4 years can elapse before a correct diagnosis.

3. Pain in 50% of patients; some have a history of trauma

4. Most commonly occur in para-articular regions around the knee, shoulder, arm, elbow, and foot (lower extremity in 60%)

5. Can arise from tendon sheath, bursa, fascia, and joint capsule, but only rarely involve a joint (**Figure 8, A and B**)

D. Imaging appearance

1. Calcification noted on plain radiographs in 15% to 20% of synovial sarcomas

2. MRI appearance indeterminate: low signal intensity on T1-weighted images; high signal intensity on T2-weighted images (**Figure 8, A and B**)

E. Pathology

1. Classically occurs as biphasic type, with epithelial cells forming glandlike structures alternating with elongated spindle cells (**Figure 8, C**)

2. Epithelial cells are large and round with distinct cell borders and pale cytoplasm.

3. Epithelial cells are arranged in nests or chords and stain positive with keratin.

4. Fibrous component involves plump, malignant spindle cells with minimal cytoplasm and dark nuclei; mast cells are common in fibrous sections.

5. Calcification more common at periphery

6. Variable vascularity

7. Less commonly, a purely monophasic histology is seen (either fibrous or epithelial) (**Figure 8, D**).

F. Treatment/outcome

1. Wide resection and radiation

2. Chemotherapy effectiveness is variable; younger patients tolerate it better.

3. Lymph node metastasis occurs in 10% to 12% of patients; sentinel node biopsy may be indicated.

4. Five-year survival = 50%, 10-year survival = 25%; better in heavily calcified lesions

VII. Epithelioid Sarcoma

A. Definition and demographics

1. Distinct soft-tissue sarcoma often mistaken for a benign granulomatous process

2. Occurs in adolescents and young adults (10 to 35 years)

3. Male-to-female ratio = 2:1

B. Genetics/etiology—*CA125* is highly expressed in the tumor.

C. Clinical presentation

1. Small, slow-growing soft-tissue tumor that can be superficial or deep

2. Frequently involves hand, forearm, fingers; 3 to 6 cm (**Figure 9, A**)

3. Most common soft-tissue sarcoma in the hand/wrist

4. Occurs as firm, painless nodule(s); may ulcerate when superficial

5. When deep, attached to tendons, tendon sheaths, or fascia

6. Confused with granuloma, rheumatoid nodule, or skin cancer, often resulting in delay in diagnosis or inappropriate treatment

D. Imaging appearance

1. Occasional calcification within lesion

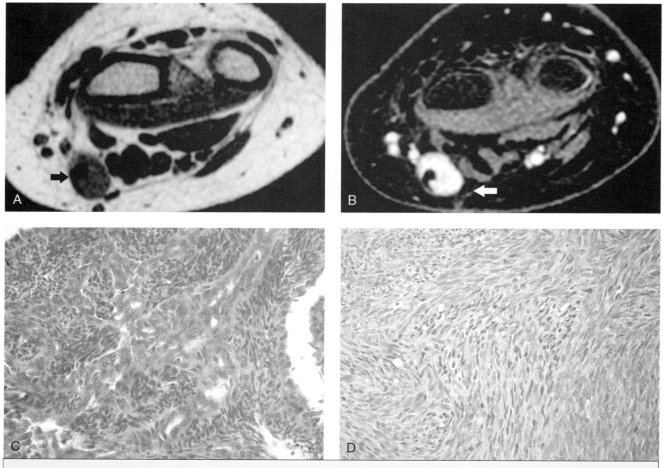

Figure 8   Synovial sarcomas. Axial T1-weighted (**A**) and T2-weighted (**B**) MRIs of the wrist reveal a small soft-tissue mass associated with the flexor carpi radialis tendon sheath (arrows). The mass is indeterminate in appearance; a biopsy revealed it to be a synovial sarcoma. **C,** Histologic image of a biphasic synovial sarcoma shows the typical pattern of epithelial cells and fibrosarcoma-like spindle cells. **D,** Monophasic synovial sarcoma variant shows only spindle cells (would be keratin positive).

2. Can erode adjacent bone

3. MRI reveals nodule along tendon sheaths of upper or lower extremity.

    a. Low signal intensity on T1-weighted images; high signal intensity on T2-weighted images

    b. Indeterminate in appearance; requires biopsy

E. Pathology

    1. A nodular pattern with central necrosis within granulomatous areas is seen on low-power histologic images (**Figure 9, B**).

    2. Higher power reveals an epithelial appearance with eosinophilic cytoplasm.

    3. Minimal cellular pleomorphism

    4. Intercellular deposition of dense hyalinized collagen

5. Calcification/ossification in 10% to 20% of patients

6. Cells are keratin positive

F. Treatment/outcome

    1. Wide surgical resection and radiation (if limb-sparing)

    2. Regional lymph node metastasis is common. Sentinel node biopsy may be indicated.

    3. Often mistaken for a benign lesion and inadequately excised, leading to a high rate of multiple recurrences

    4. Amputation is frequently necessary to halt spread of disease.

    5. Late regional or systemic metastasis to lungs is common.

    6. Overall, extremely poor prognosis

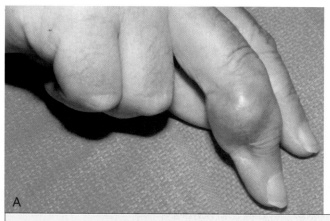
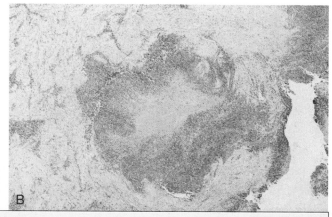

Figure 9 Epithelioid sarcoma. **A,** Clinical photograph shows an epithelioid sarcoma in the dorsal aspect of the distal long finger. Note the nodule in the superficial tissues. **B,** Low-power histologic image reveals a nodule with central necrosis consistent with an epithelioid sarcoma; these are often mistaken for a benign granulomatous process. (Reproduced from Scarborough MT, ed: *2008 Musculoskeletal Tumors and Diseases Self-Assessment Examination.* Rosemont, IL, American Academy of Orthopaedic Surgeons, 2008.)

VIII. Clear Cell Sarcoma

A. Definition and demographics

1. Rare soft-tissue sarcoma that has the ability to produce melanin

2. Occurs in young adults (age range, 20 to 40 years)

3. Affects females more commonly than males

4. Also called "malignant melanoma of soft parts"

B. Genetics/etiology

1. Frequent translocation of chromosomes 12 and 22 (not seen in malignant melanoma)

2. Etiology thought to be neuroectodermal

C. Clinical presentation

1. Occurs in deep tissues associated with tendons, aponeuroses

2. Most common soft-tissue sarcoma of the foot; also occurs in ankle, knee, and hand

3. 2 to 6 cm

4. Slow-growing mass; pain in 50% of patients; present for many years before diagnosis

5. Often mistaken for a benign lesion and inadequately excised

D. Imaging appearance

1. Nonspecific appearance; may be nodular in foot

2. MRI: indeterminate; requires a biopsy; low signal intensity on T1-weighted images; high signal intensity on T2-weighted images (**Figure 10, A**)

E. Pathology

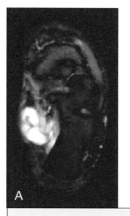
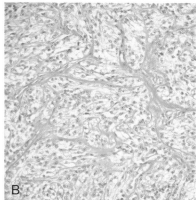

Figure 10 Clear cell sarcoma. **A,** Short tau inversion recovery MRI sequence of the left foot reveals a soft-tissue lesion abutting the medial calcaneus. Additional views revealed involvement of the neurovascular bundle. **B,** Histologic image shows fibrous septa separating the tumor into well-defined fascicles of cells with clear cytoplasm, consistent with a clear cell sarcoma.

1. Gross: no connection to overlying skin, but may be attached to tendons

2. Nests of round cells with clear cytoplasm are seen on histologic images (**Figure 10, B**).

3. Uniform pattern of cells with a defined fibrous border that might be continuous with surrounding tendons or aponeuroses

4. Occasional multinucleate giant cells but rare mitotic figures

5. With appropriate staining, intracellular melanin noted in 50% of patients

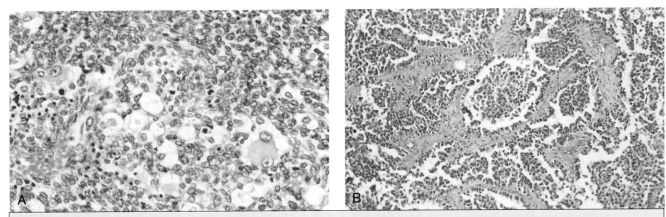

Figure 11   Rhabdomyosarcomas. **A**, Histologic image of embryonal rhabdomyosarcoma shows undifferentiated small round cells in addition to rhabdomyoblasts in various stages of differentiation. **B**, Histologic image of alveolar rhabdomyosarcoma shows aggregates of small round tumor cells separated by fibrous septa.

F. Treatment/outcome

1. Wide surgical resection and radiation

2. Local recurrence is common.

3. Frequent regional lymph node metastasis; sentinel node biopsy may be indicated

4. High rate of pulmonary metastasis with extremely poor prognosis

5. No effective chemotherapy

IX. Rhabdomyosarcoma

A. Definition, demographics, and genetics

1. Soft-tissue sarcoma of primitive mesenchyme, occurring primarily in children

2. Most common soft-tissue sarcoma in children/adolescents (embryonal and alveolar types); 4.5 per million children

3. Fifty percent occur in first decade of life.

4. Embryonal type occurs in infants/children, peaks at 0 to 4 years of age. Affects males more commonly than females.

5. Alveolar type occurs in adolescents/young adults, equal incidence from 0 to 19 years of age. No male predilection.

6. Histologic subtypes include embryonal (most common), alveolar, botryoid, and pleomorphic (affects adults 40 to 70 years of age).

7. Most cases are sporadic.

8. In alveolar rhabdomyosarcoma, translocation between chromosomes 2 and 13 is common and forms the *Pax3-FKHR* fusion protein.

B. Clinical presentation

1. Most lesions occur in head/neck, genitourinary, and retroperitoneal locations.

2. Fifteen percent occur in extremities—forearm, thigh, foot, hand—with incidence equal in upper and lower.

3. Often rapidly enlarging, deep, painless soft-tissue masses

4. Staging should include bone marrow biopsy.

C. Imaging appearance

1. Indeterminate: low signal intensity on T1-weighted MRI; high signal intensity on T2-weighted MRI

2. Positron emission tomography (PET) or bone scanning can identify other sites of disease

D. Pathology

1. Immunohistochemical markers for rhabdomyosarcoma: desmin, myoglobin, *MyoD1*

2. Embryonal—Composed of small round cells that resemble normal skeletal muscle in various stages of development, with cross striations visible in 50% of patients.

   a. Alternating dense hypercellular areas with loose myxoid areas (**Figure 11, A**)

   b. Mixture of undifferentiated, hyperchromatic cells and differentiated cells with eosinophilic cytoplasm

   c. Matrix with minimal collagen and more prominent myxoid material

3. Alveolar—Aggregates of poorly differentiated round tumor cells and irregular alveolar spaces.

   a. Cellular aggregates surrounded by dense, hyalinized fibrous septa arranged around dilated vascular spaces (**Figure 11, B**)

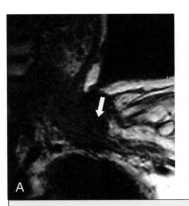 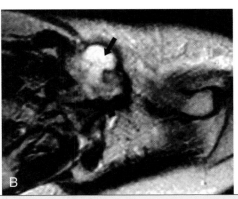 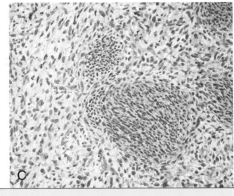

Figure 12 Malignant peripheral nerve sheath tumor (MPNST) arising from a solitary neurofibroma. Coronal T1-weighted (**A**) and axial T2-weighted (**B**) MRIs of the left neck area show that the tumor (arrows) is indeterminate in appearance; it involves the brachial plexus, causing decreased motor function of the left arm. **C,** Histologic image shows an appearance similar to a fibrosarcoma, with spindle cells arranged in long fascicles. The nuclei, however, are wavy or comma-shaped in appearance, which is unique to MPNSTs.

b. Multinucleated giant cells prominent

4. Pleomorphic—Loosely arranged polygonal tumor cells with eosinophilic cytoplasm.

   a. Difficult to differentiate from other pleomorphic sarcomas

   b. Requires either cells with cross striations or positive staining for desmin and myoglobin

E. Treatment/outcome

1. Treatment is mutimodal chemotherapy in conjuction with surgery, radiation, or both.

2. Surgical resection is preferred for local control. For unresectable lesions, incomplete resections, positive regional lymph nodes, or poor response to chemotherapy, radiation is indicated.

3. Common chemotherapy agents include vincristine, dactinomycin, cyclophosphamide, ifosfamide.

4. Regional lymph node metastasis is common. Sentinel lymph node biopsy may be considered.

5. Tendency to metastasize to the bone marrow

6. Poor prognostic factors

   a. Alveolar (versus embryonal) subtype

   b. Patient age younger than 1 year or older than 9 years

   c. Stage 2 or 3 disease

7. Five-year survival for localized disease of embryonal form is 82%; for alveolar, 65%.

8. For pleomorphic variant in adults, treatment is wide resection and radiation. Chemotherapy is not effective (5-year survival of 25%).

X. Malignant Peripheral Nerve Sheath Tumor

A. Definition and demographics

1. Malignant peripheral nerve sheath tumor (MPNST), or neurofibrosarcoma, is a sarcoma arising from a peripheral nerve or neurofibroma.

2. MPNSTs that arise from solitary neurofibromas occur in patients 30 to 55 years of age.

3. MPNSTs that arise in the setting of neurofibromatosis type 1 (NF1) occur in patients 20 to 40 years of age.

4. In NF1 setting, males more commonly affected than females; males and females affected equally in sporadic cases

B. Genetics/etiology

1. Most cases (50%) associated with NF1

2. Patients with NF1 have an approximate 5% risk of malignant transformation (latent period of 10 to 20 years).

C. Clinical presentation

1. Slow or rapid enlargement of a long-standing benign soft-tissue mass

2. Pain is variable but more common in patients with NF1.

3. Most arise from large nerves (sciatic, sacral roots, brachial plexus); 5 to 8 cm.

D. Imaging appearance

1. Indeterminate MRI appearance: low signal intensity on T1-weighted images; high signal intensity on T2-weighted images (**Figure 12, A and B**)

2. Fusiform appearance; eccentrically located within a major nerve

4: Orthopaedic Oncology/Systemic Disease

3. Serial MRIs that document enlargement of a previously documented benign nerve sheath tumor suggest malignant degeneration.

E. Pathology

1. Spindle cells closely resemble fibrosarcoma; pattern is sweeping fascicles (**Figure 12, C**).

2. Histology reflects Schwann cell differentiation; cells arranged asymmetrically

3. Spindle cells have wavy nuclei.

4. Dense cellular areas alternate with myxoid areas.

5. Mature islands of cartilage, bone, or muscle present in 10% to 15% of lesions.

6. Staining for S100 is positive in most tumors but usually focal.

7. Keratin staining is negative.

F. Treatment/outcome

1. Wide surgical resection (requires nerve resection) and radiation

2. Chemotherapy has not been effective.

3. Previous data showed 75% survival at 5 years in patients with a solitary lesion and 30% survival at 5 years in patients with NF1; however, survival for NF1 patients has improved in the past decade, and the difference is diminishing.

Top Testing Facts

1. Soft-tissue sarcomas are usually categorized as indeterminate lesions on MRI (low signal intensity on T1-weighted images and high signal intensity on T2-weighted images) and require a biopsy for definitive diagnosis.

2. Liposarcomas (other than low-grade well-differentiated subtypes) do not resemble fat on MRI studies.

3. Myxoid liposarcoma has a classic 12;16 chromosomal translocation.

4. Synovial sarcoma has a classic X;18 chromosomal translocation.

5. Epithelioid sarcoma is the most common soft-tissue sarcoma found in the hand/wrist.

6. Common sarcomas that metastasize to regional lymph nodes include rhabdomyosarcoma, synovial sarcoma, clear cell sarcoma, and epithelioid sarcoma.

7. Chemotherapy has not been shown to have a proven benefit in the treatment of most soft-tissue sarcomas (exceptions include rhabdomyosarcoma and soft-tissue Ewing sarcoma).

8. Patients with a history of NF1 have a 5% chance of malignant degeneration of a neurofibroma to an MPNST.

9. Most high-grade soft-tissue sarcomas are treated with radiation and wide surgical resection.

10. Compared with postoperative radiation, preoperative radiation allows a lower dose, but wound complications are increased.

Bibliography

Asano N, Susa M, Hosaka S, et al: Metastatic patterns of myxoid/round cell liposarcoma: A review of a 25-year experience. *Sarcoma* 2012;2012:345161.

Cohen RJ, Curtis RE, Inskip PD, Fraumeni JF Jr: The risk of developing second cancers among survivors of childhood soft tissue sarcoma. *Cancer* 2005;103(11):2391-2396.

Crago AM, Singer S: Clinical and molecular approaches to well differentiated and dedifferentiated liposarcoma. *Curr Opin Oncol* 2011;23(4):373-378.

Crew AJ, Clark J, Fisher C, et al: Fusion of SYT to two genes, SSX1 and SSX2, encoding proteins with homology to the Kruppel-associated box in human synovial sarcoma. *EMBO J* 1995;14(10):2333-2340.

Crozat A, Aman P, Mandahl N, Ron D: Fusion of CHOP to a novel RNA-binding protein in human myxoid liposarcoma. *Nature* 1993;363(6430):640-644.

Guillou L, Aurias A: Soft tissue sarcomas with complex genomic profiles. *Virchows Arch* 2010;456(2):201-217.

Gupta G, Mammis A, Maniker A: Malignant peripheral nerve sheath tumors. *Neurosurg Clin N Am* 2008;19(4):533-543, v.

Holt GE, Griffin AM, Pintilie M, et al: Fractures following radiotherapy and limb-salvage surgery for lower extremity soft-tissue sarcomas: A comparison of high-dose and low-dose radiotherapy. *J Bone Joint Surg Am* 2005;87(2):315-319.

Kolberg M, Høland M, Agesen TH, et al: Survival meta-analyses for >1800 malignant peripheral nerve sheath tumor patients with and without neurofibromatosis type 1. *Neuro Oncol* 2013;15(2):135-147.

Llombart B, Serra-Guillén C, Monteagudo C, López Guerrero JA, Sanmartín O: Dermatofibrosarcoma protuberans: A comprehensive review and update on diagnosis and management. *Semin Diagn Pathol* 2013;30(1):13-28.

Matushansky I, Charytonowicz E, Mills J, Siddiqi S, Hricik T, Cordon-Cardo C: MFH classification: Differentiating undifferentiated pleomorphic sarcoma in the 21st Century. *Expert Rev Anticancer Ther* 2009;9(8):1135-1144.

Meza JL, Anderson J, Pappo AS, Meyer WH; Children's Oncology Group: Analysis of prognostic factors in patients with nonmetastatic rhabdomyosarcoma treated on intergroup rhabdomyosarcoma studies III and IV: The Children's Oncology Group. *J Clin Oncol* 2006;24(24):3844-3851.

O'Sullivan B, Davis AM, Turcotte R, et al: Preoperative versus postoperative radiotherapy in soft-tissue sarcoma of the limbs: A randomised trial. *Lancet* 2002;359(9325): 2235-2241.

Patrikidou A, Domont J, Cioffi A, Le Cesne A: Treating soft tissue sarcomas with adjuvant chemotherapy. *Curr Treat Options Oncol* 2011;12(1):21-31.

Walker EA, Salesky JS, Fenton ME, Murphey MD: Magnetic resonance imaging of malignant soft tissue neoplasms in the adult. *Radiol Clin North Am* 2011;49(6):1219-1234, vi.

Weiss SW, Goldblum JR, eds: *Enzinger and Weiss's Soft Tissue Tumors*, ed 5. St Louis, MO, Mosby, 2008.

Wodajo FM: Benign vascular soft-tissue tumors, in Schwartz HS, ed: *Orthopaedic Knowledge Update: Musculoskeletal Tumors*, ed 2. Rosemont, IL, American Academy of Orthopaedic Surgeons, 2007, pp 225-231.

Zagars GK, Ballo MT, Pisters PW, Pollock RE, Patel SR, Benjamin RS: Surgical margins and reresection in the management of patients with soft tissue sarcoma using conservative surgery and radiation therapy. *Cancer* 2003;97(10): 2544-2553.

4: Orthopaedic Oncology/Systemic Disease

Miscellaneous Lesions

Frank J. Frassica, MD

I. Melorheostosis

A. Definition and demographics

1. Melorheostosis is a rare, painful disorder of the extremities characterized by large amounts of periosteal new bone formation.

2. Affects both sexes equally

3. Usually discovered by age 40 years

B. Genetics/etiology

1. Nonhereditary

2. Often follows a sclerotomal pattern

C. Clinical presentation

1. Pain, reduced range of motion, contractures

2. Soft tissues: tense, erythematous skin, induration and fibrosis of subcutaneous tissue

D. Radiographic appearance (**Figure 1**)

1. More common in the lower extremities; usually involves one extremity

2. Cortical hyperostosis (dripping candle wax appearance)

3. Wavy appearance that flows across and involves joints

E. Pathology

1. Enlarged bony trabeculae

2. Normal haversian systems

F. Treatment

1. Symptomatic treatment of pain

2. Occasionally, correction of contractures by excision of hyperostotic and fibrotic areas

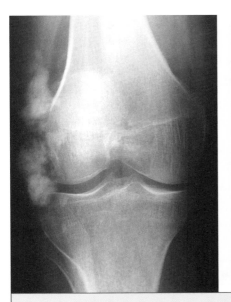 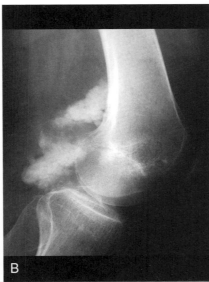 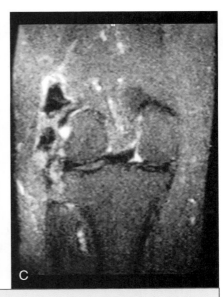

Figure 1   Melorheostosis. **A,** AP radiograph shows periosteal new bone formation on the lateral aspect of the knee. Note the nodular appearance of the heavily ossified bone formation. **B,** Lateral radiograph shows a large amount of nodular bone formation arising from the posterior aspect of the distal femur. **C,** T2-weighted coronal MRI of the knee shows nodular masses of very low signal intensity (corresponding to bone formation) and areas of high signal intensity (corresponding to edema) around the nodules.

II. Massive Osteolysis

A. Definition and demographics

1. Massive osteolysis, also called Gorham-Stout disease or vanishing bone disease, is a very rare condition that is characterized by massive resorption of entire segments of bone.

2. Affects both sexes equally

3. Most common in patients younger than 40 years

B. Etiology/clinical presentation

1. May be related to trauma

2. Abrupt or insidious onset

C. Radiographic appearance

1. Massive osteolysis

2. Progressive lytic bone loss

3. End of the remaining bone is often tapered

4. Often spreads to adjacent bones (crosses joints)

D. Pathology

1. Begins with numerous vascular channels

2. Ends with fibrosis

E. Treatment

1. No effective treatment

2. May resolve spontaneously

III. Gaucher Disease

A. Definition and demographics

1. Gaucher disease results from an enzyme deficiency that causes accumulation of glucocerebrosides in the marrow, leading to bone deformities and osteonecrosis.

2. Most common in Ashkenazi Jews

B. Genetics/etiology

1. Autosomal recessive

2. Caused by deficiency of glucocerebrosidase (acid β-glucosidase, lysosomal enzyme)

C. Clinical presentation

1. Types

a. Type I: adult nonneuropathic

b. Type II: acute neuropathic (infants); lethal form

c. Type III: juvenile subacute neuropathic (children); death occurs by second decade of life

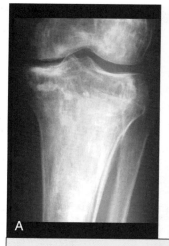
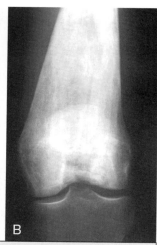

Figure 2 Gaucher disease. **A,** AP radiograph of the tibia shows sclerosis in the medullary cavity. **B,** AP radiograph of the distal femur shows the Erlenmeyer flask deformity, typical of Gaucher disease. Note the widened metaphyses.

2. Hematologic problems: pancytopenia, thrombocytopenia

3. Easy bruisability, fatigue

4. Bone problems

a. Osteonecrosis

b. Fractures

D. Radiographic appearance (**Figure 2**)

1. Abnormal bone remodeling: Erlenmeyer flask deformity

2. Lucent expansile lesions

3. Subchondral collapse

4. Vertebral collapse

E. Pathology

1. Macrophages are enlarged and filled with abnormal material (crumpled cytoplasm).

2. Periodic acid–Schiff–positive, acid phosphatase–positive

F. Treatment: enzyme replacement

IV. Stress Fractures

A. Definition and demographics

1. Stress fractures are overuse injuries in which normal bone is subjected to abnormal stresses, resulting in microfractures.

2. Stress fractures occur following repetitive stress in either normal or abnormal bone.

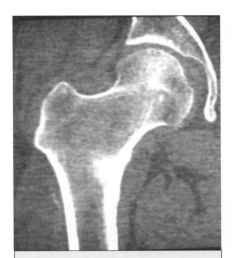

Figure 3 Coronal CT reconstruction shows a stress fracture of the proximal femur. Note the focal endosteal new bone formation and the periosteal new bone formation on the medial femoral cortex.

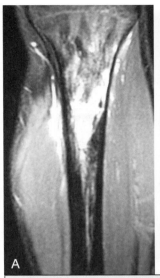
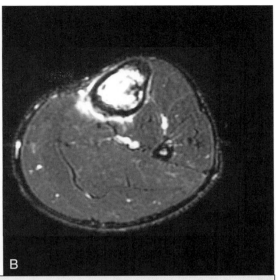

Figure 4 Stress fracture of the tibia. **A,** Coronal T2-weighted MRI shows high signal intensity in the medullary cavity and on the periosteal surface. **B,** Axial T2-weighted MRI shows high signal intensity in the medullary cavity and over the posteromedial cortical surface of the tibia.

a. Fatigue fracture—Occurs in normal bone, such as in military recruits following marching drills or in marathon runners.

b. Insufficiency fracture—Occurs in abnormal bone with femoral shaft bowing (Paget disease, polyostotic fibrous dysplasia).

3. Stress fractures in patients on bisphosphonates—Typically occur in the subtrochanteric region of the femur (lateral cortex).

B. Etiology/clinical presentation

1. Linear microfractures in trabecular bone from repetitive loading

2. Pain during activity located directly over the involved bone

3. Pain during activity following a prolonged course of bisphosphonates

C. Imaging appearance

1. Radiographs/CT

a. Diaphysis

• Linear cortical radiolucency

• Endosteal thickening

• Periosteal reaction and cortical thickening

• Beaking in the lateral cortex of the subtrochanteric region of the femur

b. Metaphysis: focal linear increased mineralization (condensation of the trabecular bone)

c. Endosteal and periosteal new bone formation (**Figure 3**)

2. Technetium Tc-99m bone scan—Area of focal uptake in the cortical and/or trabecular region.

3. MRI (**Figure 4**)

a. Periosteal high signal intensity on T2-weighted images (earliest finding)

b. Linear zone of low signal intensity on T1-weighted images

c. Broad area of increased signal intensity on T2-weighted images

d. When a stress fracture is advanced in clinical course, low signal intensity lines representing the fracture may be seen.

D. Pathology

1. Callus formation

2. Woven new bone

3. Enchondral bone formation

E. Treatment

1. Rest

2. Protected weight bearing until symptoms resolve and fracture heals

3. Prophylactic fixation in selected cases

a. Tension-side femoral neck fractures in athletes

b. Patients with low bone mass, especially pa-

4: Orthopaedic Oncology/Systemic Disease

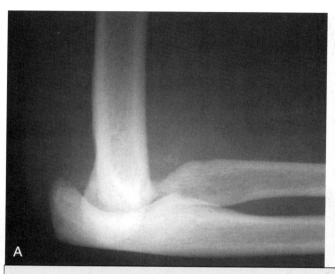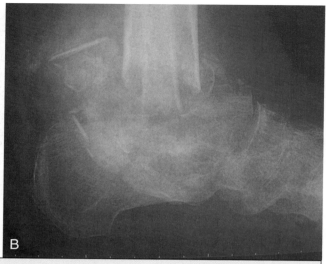

Figure 5 Neuropathic arthropathy. **A,** Lateral radiograph of the elbow of a patient with syringomyelia. Note the prominent neuropathic changes with complete destruction of the articular surfaces. **B,** Lateral radiograph of the ankle of a patient with diabetes mellitus. Note the complete destruction of the articular surfaces with dissolution and fragmentation.

tients older than 60 years and those with lesions on the tension side of the subtrochanteric region of the femur

V. Neuropathic Arthropathy

A. Definition and demographics

1. Neuropathic arthropathy is the destruction of a joint following loss of protective sensation.

2. Common locations include the foot, ankle, elbow, and shoulder.

B. Etiology—Disease processes that damage sensory nerves.

1. Diabetes mellitus: affects the foot and ankle

2. Syringomyelia: affects the shoulder and elbow

3. Syphilis: affects the knee

4. Spinal cord tumors: affect the lower extremity joints

5. Leprosy: can affect any joint

C. Clinical presentation

1. Swollen, warm, and erythematous joint with little or no pain

2. Often mimics infection, especially in patients with diabetes

D. Radiographic appearance (**Figure 5**)

1. Characteristic feature: destruction of the joint

2. Initial changes may simulate osteoarthritis

3. Late changes

a. Fragmentation of the joint

b. Subluxation/dislocation

c. Fracture

d. Collapse

E. Pathology

1. Productive/hypertrophic changes secondary to conditions involving the spinal cord (generally do not involve the sympathetic nervous system)

a. Spinal cord traumatic injury

b. Neoplasms

c. Spinal cord malformations

d. Syphilis

e. Syringomyelia

2. Destructive/atrophic changes usually secondary to peripheral nerve damage. Conditions that cause atrophic changes:

a. Diabetes

b. Alcoholism

3. Histologic changes

a. Synovial hypertrophy

b. Fragments of bone and cartilage in the synovium (detritic synovitis)

F. Treatment

1. Rest, elevation, protected weight bearing

2. Total contact casting when ulcers are present in the foot and ankle

VI. Hemophilic Arthropathy

A. Definition and demographics

1. Hemophilic arthropathy is the destruction of a joint secondary to repetitive bleeding into the synovial cavity.

2. Classic hemophilia, or hemophilia A (deficiency of factor VIII); Christmas disease, or hemophilia B (deficiency of factor IX)

3. Locations: knee, ankle, elbow

B. Genetics/etiology—X-linked recessive.

C. Clinical presentation

1. Hemarthrosis: often seen in young males, 3 to 15 years of age.

2. Temporal changes

a. Acute hemarthrosis: tense, painful effusion

b. Subacute hemarthrosis: occurs after two previous bleeds

c. Chronic hemarthrosis: arthritis, contractures

D. Radiographic appearance

1. Arnold/Hilgartner stages

a. Stage I: soft-tissue swelling

b. Stage II: osteoporosis

c. Stage III: bone changes (subchondral cysts) with intact joint

d. Stage IV: cartilage loss

e. Stage V: severe arthritic changes

2. Radiographic changes

a. Knee

• Overgrowth of distal femur and proximal tibia

• Distal condylar surface appears flattened.

• Squaring of the inferior portion of the patella

b. Ankle: arthritic changes of the tibiotalar joint

c. Elbow: arthritic changes and contractures

E. Pathology

1. Synovial hypertrophy and hyperplasia

2. Synovium covers and destroys the cartilage.

F. Treatment

1. Factor replacement

2. Prophylaxis against recurrent hemarthroses

Top Testing Facts

1. Melorheostosis is characterized by nodular, heavily mineralized bone on the surface of bones and in the soft tissues, which gives a dripping candle wax appearance on radiographs.

2. Massive osteolysis (Gorham-Stout disease) is purely lytic resorption of large segments of bone.

3. Radiographic findings for Gaucher disease include Erlenmeyer flask deformity (widened metaphyses).

4. Gaucher disease is caused by a deficiency of the enzyme glucocerebrosidase (acid β-glucosidase, lysosomal enzyme); treatment consists of enzyme replacement.

5. Imaging findings for stress fractures: radiographs show periosteal new bone formation; T1-weighted MRIs show normal marrow except for linear areas of low signal intensity; T2-weighted MRIs show high signal intensity in the medullary cavity and on the periosteal surface.

6. Stress fractures from prolonged bisphosphonate therapy often occur on the lateral diaphyseal area of the subtrochanteric region and have a beaked appearance on radiographs.

7. The area affected by neuropathic arthropathy varies with the condition: syringomyelia—shoulder and elbow; syphilis—knee; diabetes mellitus—foot and ankle; spinal cord tumors—lower extremity joints; leprosy—any joint.

8. Radiographic findings for neuropathic arthropathy include fragmentation, subluxation, and dissolution of the joint.

9. Hemophilic arthropathy is characterized by factor deficiencies, including factor VIII (hemophilia A) and factor IX (hemophilia B).

10. Key radiographic findings for hemophilic arthropathy include squaring of the inferior patellar pole and femoral condyles.

Bibliography

Chisholm KA, Gilchrist JM: The Charcot joint: A modern neurologic perspective. *J Clin Neuromuscul Dis* 2011;13(1): 1-13.

Ihde LL, Forrester DM, Gottsegen CJ, et al: Sclerosing bone dysplasias: Review and differentiation from other causes of osteosclerosis. *Radiographics* 2011;31(7):1865-1882.

Jain VK, Arya RK, Bharadwaj M, Kumar S: Melorheostosis: Clinicopathological features, diagnosis, and management. *Orthopedics* 2009;32(7):512.

Katz R, Booth T, Hargunani R, Wylie P, Holloway B: Radiological aspects of Gaucher disease. *Skeletal Radiol* 2011; 40(12):1505-1513.

McCarthy EF, Frassica FJ: Genetic diseases of bones and joints, in *Pathology of Bone and Joint Disorders With Clinical and Radiographic Correlation*. Philadelphia, PA, Saunders, 1998, pp 54-55.

Resnick D: Neuropathic osteoarthropathy, in Resnik D, ed: *Diagnosis of Bone and Joint Disorders With Clinical and Radiographic Correlation*, ed 3. Philadelphia, PA, Saunders, 1995, pp 3413-3442.

Ruggieri P, Montalti M, Angelini A, Alberghini M, Mercuri M: Gorham-Stout disease: The experience of the Rizzoli Institute and review of the literature. *Skeletal Radiol* 2011;40(11): 1391-1397.

Vigorita VJ: Osteonecrosis, Gaucher's disease, in *Orthopaedic Pathology*. Philadelphia, PA, Lippincott Williams & Wilkins, 1999, pp 503-505.

Chapter 51

Metastatic Bone Disease

Kristy Weber, MD

I. Evaluation/Diagnosis

A. Overview

1. Demographics

   a. Metastatic bone disease occurs in patients older than 40 years.

   b. Most common reason for destructive bone lesion in adults

   c. More than 1.6 million cases of cancer per year in the United States; bone metastasis develops in about 50% of patients

   d. Bone is the third most common site of metastasis (after lung and liver).

   e. Most common primary cancer sites that metastasize to bone are breast, prostate, lung, kidney, and thyroid.

2. Genetics/etiology

   a. Two main hypotheses

      • 1889: Paget's "seed and soil" hypothesis (ability of tumor cells to survive and grow in addition to the compatible end-organ environment)

      • 1928: Ewing's circulation theory

         ○ Tumors colonize particular organs because of the routes of blood flow from the primary site.

         ○ Organs are passive receptacles.

         ○ Batson plexus—Valveless plexus of veins around the spine allows tumor cells to travel to the vertebral bodies, pelvis, ribs, skull, and proximal limb girdle (eg, prostate metastases).

   b. Mediators of bone destruction include tumor necrosis factors; transforming growth factors (TGFs); 1,25 dihydroxyvitamin D3; and parathyroid hormone-related protein (PTHrP).

B. Clinical presentation (**Table 1**)

1. History

   a. Progressive pain that occurs at rest and with weight bearing

   b. Constitutional symptoms (weight loss, fatigue, loss of appetite)

   c. Personal or family history of cancer

   d. History of symptoms related to possible primary sites (hematuria, shortness of breath, hot/cold intolerance)

   e. Primary tumors may metastasize quickly or take 10 to 15 years or longer (breast, renal, prostate).

2. Physical examination findings

   a. Occasional swelling, limp, decreased joint range of motion, neurologic deficits (10% to 20%) at metastatic bone sites

   b. Possible breast, prostate, thyroid, or abdominal mass

Table 1

Workup of Patients Older Than 40 Years With a Destructive Bone Lesion[a]

Thorough history (history of cancer, weight loss, malaise, gastrointestinal bleeding, pain, etc)
Physical examination (focus on breast, lung, prostate, thyroid, lymph nodes)
Laboratory studies (electrolyte panel [calcium], alkaline phosphatase, complete blood cell count, tumor-specific markers as appropriate (eg, PSA, CA 125), serum protein electrophoresis/urine protein electrophoresis)
Plain radiographs of the bone lesion (two planes, include entire bone)
CT scan of chest, abdomen, pelvis
Total body bone scan

[a]Identifies primary site in 85% of patients.

CA 125 = cancer antigen 125, PSA = prostate-specific antigen.

Dr. Weber or an immediate family member serves as a board member, owner, officer, or committee member of the Musculoskeletal Tumor Society and the Ruth Jackson Orthopaedic Society.

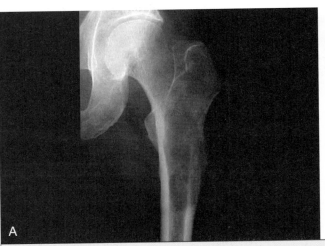
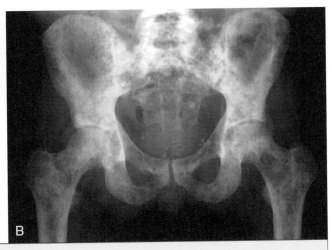

Figure 1   Osteolytic and osteoblastic metastases. **A,** Lung cancer metastases are generally purely osteolytic, as demonstrated in this AP radiograph of a left hip. Note the lesion in the left proximal femur that is destroying the lateral cortex. **B,** Prostate cancer metastases are osteoblastic, as noted throughout the pelvis, spine, and proximal femurs in this AP pelvic radiograph.

c. Stool guaiac

d. Regional adenopathy

3. Laboratory studies

    a. Complete blood cell count (anemia suggests myeloma)

    b. Serum protein electrophoresis/urine protein electrophoresis (abnormal in myeloma)

    c. Thyroid function tests (may be abnormal in thyroid cancer)

    d. Urinalysis (microscopic hematuria in renal cancer)

    e. Basic chemistry panel: calcium, phosphorus, alkaline phosphatase, lactate dehydrogenase (LDH)

    f. Specific tumor markers: prostate-specific antigen (PSA) (prostate); carcinoembryonic antigen (CEA) (colon, pancreas); cancer antigen 125 (CA 125) (ovarian)

4. Common scenarios

    a. Known cancer patient with multiple bone lesions—Does not usually require confirmatory biopsy.

    b. Known cancer patient with bone pain and normal radiographs—May be symptomatic from chemotherapy/bisphosphonates or may require bone scan or MRI to define an early destructive lesion.

    c. Patient without history of cancer with a destructive bone lesion—Must differentiate between metastatic disease and primary malignant bone tumor.

C. Radiographic appearance/workup

1. Appearance

    a. Osteolytic (most bone metastases): lung, thyroid, kidney, gastrointestinal (**Figure 1, A**)

    b. Osteoblastic: prostate, bladder (**Figure 1, B**)

    c. Mixed osteolytic/osteoblastic: breast

    d. Most common locations include spine (40%), pelvis, proximal long bones, and ribs.

    e. The thoracic spine is the most common vertebral location of metastasis.

    f. Metastatic carcinoma to the spine spares the intervertebral disk.

    g. Lesions distal to the elbow/knee are most commonly from the lung as a primary site.

    h. Pathologic fracture is a common presentation (25%) and occurs more commonly in osteolytic versus osteoblastic lesions.

    i. An avulsion of the lesser trochanter implies a pathologic process in the femoral neck with impending fracture.

2. Workup (**Table 1**)

    a. Plain radiographs—Images in two planes and of the entire bone should be obtained (consider referred pain).

    b. Differential diagnosis of lytic bone lesion in patient older than 40 years includes metastatic disease, multiple myeloma, lymphoma, and, less likely, primary bone tumors, Paget sarcoma, and hyperparathyroidism (**Table 2**).

    c. Bone scan

Table 2

Differential Diagnosis of Destructive Bone Lesion in Patients Older Than 40 Years

Metastatic bone disease

Multiple myeloma

Lymphoma

Primary bone tumors (chondrosarcoma, osteosarcoma, undifferentiated pleomorphic sarcoma, chordoma)

Pelvic/sacral insufficiency fractures

Postradiation/Paget sarcoma

Giant cell tumor

Hyperparathyroidism

Infection

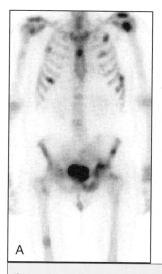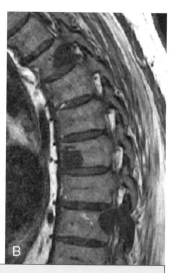

Figure 2 Metastases seen on a total body bone scan and MRI. **A,** Total body bone scan shows increased uptake in the sacroiliac region and metastases in the anterior pelvis, ribs, and shoulder girdle. **B,** Sagittal MRI of the thoracic spine shows vertebral lesions.

- Detects osteoblastic activity (may be negative in myeloma, metastatic renal cancer)
- Identifies multiple lesions, which are common in metastatic disease (**Figure 2, A**)

d. CT scan of chest, abdomen, pelvis to identify primary lesion

e. Staging evaluation of lytic bone lesion will identify primary site in 85% of patients (**Table 1**).

f. Bone marrow biopsy when considering myeloma as a diagnosis

g. MRI scan of the primary lesion is generally not necessary unless defining disease in the spine (**Figure 2, B**).

h. Difficult to differentiate osteoporosis from metastatic disease with a single vertebral compression fracture; tumor is suggested by soft-tissue mass and pedicle destruction.

D. Biopsy/pathology

1. A biopsy of a destructive bone lesion must be performed unless the diagnosis is certain.

2. Placing an intramedullary device in a 65-year-old patient with a lytic lesion in the femur without appropriate workup is risky (could be a primary malignant bone tumor).

3. An open incisional biopsy or closed needle biopsy (fine needle aspiration/core) can be performed.

4. Histologic appearance of metastatic carcinoma is islands of epithelial cells with glandular or squamous differentiation (**Figure 3, A** and **B**).

5. The carcinoma cells have tight junctions and reside within a fibrous stroma.

6. Thyroid (follicular): follicles filled with colloid material (**Figure 3, C**)

7. Renal cancer often has a clear appearance to the cytoplasm within the epithelial cells (**Figure 3, D**); in some cases, it may be poorly differentiated or have a sarcomatoid pattern.

8. Epithelial cells are keratin-positive.

9. Special immunohistochemistry stains can sometimes determine the primary site of disease.

a. Thyroid transcription factor-1: lung, thyroid

b. Estrogen and progesterone receptors: breast

c. PSA: prostate

II. Pathophysiology/Molecular Mechanisms

A. Metastatic cascade

1. Primary tumor cells proliferate and stimulate angiogenesis.

2. Tumor cells cross the basement membrane into capillaries and must avoid host defenses.

3. Tumor cells disseminate to distant sites.

4. Cells arrest in distant capillary bed, adhere to vascular endothelium, and extravasate into end-organ environment (integrins, cadherins, matrix metalloproteinases).

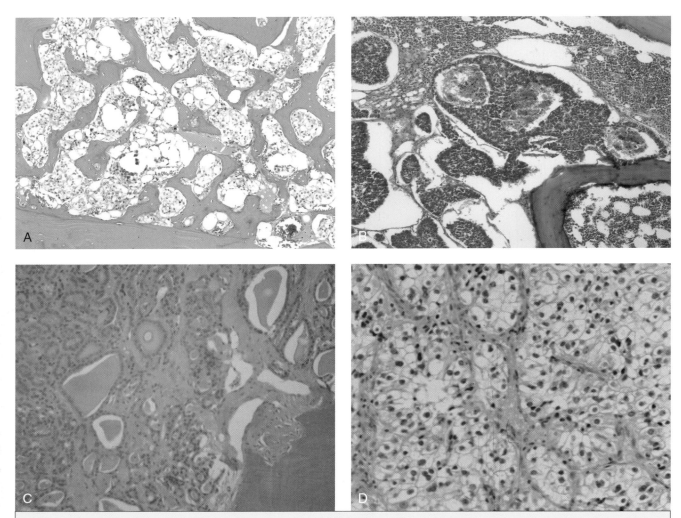

Figure 3   Histologic specimens show bone metastasis from the most common primary lesions. **A,** Prostate—note the new bone formation by the osteoblasts that are stimulated by factors secreted by the tumor cells. **B,** Lung—note the clumps of epithelial cells characterized by tight cell-cell junctions. **C,** Thyroid (follicular)—the epithelial cells are forming follicles surrounding a central colloid substance. **D,** Renal—the epithelial tumor cells are characterized by clear cytoplasm.

5. Tumor cells interact with local host cells and growth factors (TGF-β, insulin-like growth factor, fibroblast growth factor, bone morphogenetic protein).

6. Tumor cells proliferate to become a site of metastasis.

B. RANKL/osteoprotegerin

1. Tumor cells do not destroy bone; cytokines from the tumor stimulate osteoclasts or osteoblasts to destroy or generate new bone, respectively.

2. Osteoblasts/stromal cells secrete receptor activator of nuclear factor κ B ligand (RANKL).

3. Osteoclast precursors have receptors for RANKL (RANK).

4. Increased secretion of RANKL by osteoblasts causes an increase in osteoclast precursors, which eventually results in increased bone destruction.

5. Osteoprotegerin (OPG) is a decoy receptor that binds to RANKL and inhibits an increase in osteoclasts.

C. Vicious cycle in breast cancer

1. TGF-β is stored in the bone and released during normal bone turnover.

2. TGF-β stimulates metastatic breast cancer cells to secrete PTHrP.

3. PTHrP from cancer cells stimulates osteoblasts to secrete RANKL.

4. RANKL from osteoblasts stimulates osteoclast precursors and increases osteoclasts.

5. Osteoclasts destroy bone and release TGF-β, and the cycle of destruction repeats.

D. Other disease-specific factors

1. Breast cancer cells also secrete osteoclastic stimulants (interleukin [IL]-6, IL-8).

2. Prostate cancer—Endothelin-1 stimulates osteoblasts to produce bone.

3. Overexpression of growth factors and their receptors is common in renal cell carcinoma (epidermal growth factor receptor [EGFR], vascular endothelial growth factor receptor [VEGFR], platelet-derived growth factor receptor [PDGFR]).

E. Fracture healing in pathologic bone

1. Likelihood of pathologic fracture healing: multiple myeloma > renal carcinoma > breast carcinoma > lung carcinoma (ie, pathologic fracture healing is most likely in patients with myeloma and least likely in patients with metastatic lung cancer)

2. Most important factor in determining healing potential is the length of patient survival.

F. Other physiologic disruptions

1. Calcium metabolism—Hypercalcemia is present in 10% to 30% of cases.

   a. Common with lung, breast cancer metastasis

   b. Does not correlate with number of bone metastases or osteolytic nature

   c. Early symptoms: polyuria/polydipsia, anorexia, weakness, easy fatigability

   d. Late symptoms: irritability, depression, coma, profound weakness, nausea/vomiting, pruritus, vision abnormalities

   e. Treatment requires aggressive hydration and intravenous bisphosphonate therapy.

2. Hematopoiesis—Normocytic/normochromic anemia is common with breast, prostate, lung, and thyroid cancer metastasis.

3. Thromboembolic disease

   a. Patients with malignancy have increased thromboembolic risk.

   b. Requires prophylaxis, especially after lower extremity/pelvic surgery

4. Pain control/bowel abnormalities

   a. Use narcotics for pain control.

   b. Requires laxatives/stool softener to avoid severe constipation

Table 3			
Mirels Scoring System for Prediction of Pathologic Fracture in Patients With Metastatic Bone Lesions			
Factor	**Points**		
	1	2	3
Radiographic appearance	Blastic	Mixed	Lytic
Size (as a proportion of shaft diameter)	<1/3	1/3 to 2/3	>2/3
Site	UE	LE	Peritrochanteric
Pain	Mild	Moderate	Mechanical

UE = upper extremity, LE = lower extremity.

Adapted with permission from Mirels H: Metastatic disease in long bones: A proposed scoring system for diagnosing impending pathologic fractures. *Clin Orthop* 1989;249:256-265.

III. Biomechanics

A. Stress riser in bone occurs whenever there is cortical destruction.

B. Defects

1. Open section defect—When the length of a longitudinal defect in a bone exceeds 75% of diameter, there is a 90% reduction in torsional strength.

2. Fifty percent cortical defect (centered) = 60% bending strength reduction.

3. Fifty percent cortical defect (eccentric) = >90% bending strength reduction.

IV. Impending Fractures/Prophylactic Fixation

A. Indications for fixation

1. Snell/Beals criteria

   a. A 2.5-cm lytic bone lesion

   b. Fifty percent cortical involvement

   c. Pain persisting after radiation

   d. Peritrochanteric lesion

2. Mirels scoring system (**Table 3**)

   a. Four factors are scored: radiographic appearance, size (proportion of bone diameter occupied by the lesion), site, and pain.

   b. Prophylactic fixation is recommended for a score ≥9 (33% fracture risk).

4: Orthopaedic Oncology/Systemic Disease

3. Spinal lesions—impending fracture/collapse

   a. Thoracic

   - Risk of fracture/collapse exists when 50% to 60% of the vertebral body is involved (without other abnormalities).

   - Risk of fracture/collapse exists when only 20% to 30% of the vertebral body is involved if there is also costovertebral joint involvement.

   b. Lumbar

   - Risk of fracture/collapse exists when 35% to 40% of the vertebral body is involved (without other abnormalities).

   - Risk of fracture/collapse exists when 25% of vertebral body is involved if there is also pedicle/posterior element involvement.

B. Other factors to consider

   1. Scoring systems are not exact and cannot predict all human factors.

   2. Histology of primary lesion

   3. Expected lifespan, comorbid conditions, and activity level

   4. Most surgical decisions can be based on plain radiographs (MRI not needed for extremity lesions).

   5. Prophylactic fixation compared with fixation of actual pathologic fracture

      a. Decreased perioperative morbidity/pain

      b. Shorter operating room time

      c. Faster recovery/shorter hospital stay

      d. Ability to coordinate care with medical oncology

V. Nonsurgical Treatment

A. Indications

   1. Nondisplaced fractures (depending on location)

   2. Non–weight-bearing bones (**Figure 4**)

   3. Poor medical health/shortened lifespan

B. Observation/pain management/bracing

   1. Observation or activity modifications are used for patients with very small lesions or advanced disease.

   2. Functional bracing can be used in the upper and lower extremities and spine.

   3. Pain management is important in all symptomatic patients.

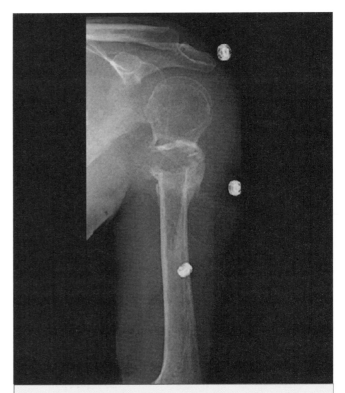

Figure 4   AP radiograph shows the left humerus of a 59-year-old woman with metastatic thyroid cancer that caused a pathologic fracture. She was not a safe surgical candidate and was therefore treated nonsurgically. Note the callus formation about the fracture site.

   a. Opioids

   b. Nonopioids: NSAIDs, tricyclic antidepressants, muscle relaxants, steroids

   c. A bowel program is necessary to prevent severe constipation.

C. Medical

   1. Cytotoxic chemotherapy

   2. Hormonal treatment (prostate, breast metastasis)

   3. Growth factor receptor inhibitors (lung, renal cell metastasis)

   4. Bisphosphonates

      a. Inhibit osteoclast activity by inducing apoptosis

      b. Inhibit protein prenylation and act on the mevalonate pathway

      c. Significant decrease in skeletal events (breast, prostate, lung)

      d. Reduced pain

      e. Used commonly in metastatic bone disease (intravenous zoledronic acid)—but denosumab is

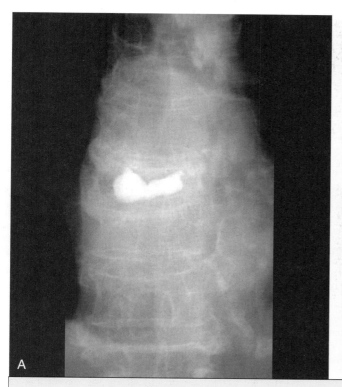
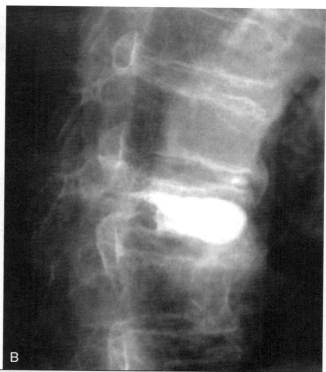

Figure 5 AP (**A**) and lateral (**B**) radiographs of the spine of a woman with metastatic lung cancer to the thoracic vertebra, causing painful collapse. The patient was treated with vertebroplasty and experienced marked pain relief.

now becoming the treatment of choice to inhibit bone destruction

 f. Complications: Osteonecrosis of the jaw and occasional nephrotoxicity

5. Denosumab—Human monoclonal antibody to RANKL.

 a. Subcutaneous injection

 b. Does not require monitoring of renal function

 c. Superior to zoledronic acid in delaying time to first skeletal-related event (in metastatic breast cancer patients)

 d. Greater reduction of bone turnover markers compared with zoledronic acid (metastatic breast cancer)

 e. No difference between denosumab and zoledronic acid in terms of survival or disease progression (metastatic breast cancer)

 f. Complications: Hypocalcemia and osteonecrosis of the jaw

D. Radiation

 1. External beam radiation

  a. Indications: pain, impending fracture, neurologic symptoms

  b. Dose: usually 30 Gy in 10 fractions to bone lesion (but can use higher dose/less fractions)

  c. Pain relief in 70% of patients

  d. Postoperatively, the entire implant should be irradiated after 2 weeks to decrease fixation failure and improve local control.

  e. Should be used for patients with radiosensitive tumors of the spine who have pain or tumor progression without instability or myelopathy

 2. Radiopharmaceuticals

  a. Samarium Sm-153 or strontium chloride 89

  b. Delivery of radiation to the entire skeleton (bone scan concept)

  c. Palliation of pain—may delay progression of lesions

  d. Use requires normal renal function and blood counts.

  e. Iodine-131 is used to treat metastatic thyroid cancer.

E. Minimally invasive techniques

 1. Radiofrequency ablation or cryoablation—Used for palliative pain control (commonly used in pelvis/acetabulum).

 2. Kyphoplasty/vertebroplasty (**Figure 5**)

  a. Pain relief in patients with vertebral compression fractures from metastasis

4: Orthopaedic Oncology/Systemic Disease

b. The risk of cement leakage in vertebroplasty (35% to 65%) is usually not clinically relevant.

c. Vertebroplasty is not indicated for osteoporotic spinal compression fractures, but it is still used for metastatic disease and multiple myeloma affecting the spine.

VI. Surgical Treatment/Outcome

A. Overview

1. Goals of surgical treatment

   a. Relieve pain

   b. Improve function

   c. Restore skeletal stability

2. Considerations before surgery

   a. Patient selection (functional status, activity level, comorbidities)

   b. Stability/durability of planned construct (withstand force of six times body weight around hip)

   c. Addressing all areas of weakened bone

   d. Preoperative embolization for highly vascular lesions (renal, thyroid metastasis)

   e. Extensive use of methylmethacrylate (cement) to improve stability of construct

   f. Cemented (rather than uncemented) joint prostheses are more widely used in patients with bone metastasis.

B. Upper extremity

1. Overview

   a. Upper extremity metastases affect activities of daily living, use of external aids, bed-to-chair transfers.

   b. Much less common (20%) than lower extremity metastases

2. Scapula/clavicle—Usually nonsurgical treatment/radiation.

3. Proximal humerus

   a. Resection and proximal humeral replacement (megaprosthesis); excellent pain relief but poor shoulder function

   b. Intramedullary locked device (closed versus open with curettage/cement) if bone quality allows (**Figure 6**)

4. Humeral diaphysis

   a. Intramedullary fixation: closed versus open with curettage/cement

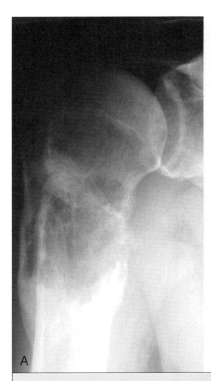
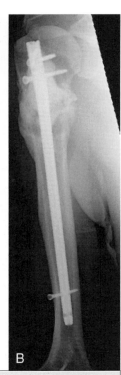

Figure 6   Radiographs of the upper extremity of a 67-year-old right-handed man with metastatic renal carcinoma that caused pain at rest and with activity. **A,** AP radiograph shows the osteolytic lesion in the right proximal humerus. **B,** Postoperative radiograph obtained after placement of a locked right humeral intramedullary rod. This lesion was curetted and cemented during the surgery and received radiation after 2 weeks.

b. Intercalary metal spacer: selected indications for extensive diaphyseal destruction or failed prior implant

5. Distal humerus

   a. Flexible crossed nails can be supplemented with cement and extend the entire length of bone (insert at elbow).

   b. Orthogonal plating—Combine with curettage/cement (**Figure 7**).

   c. Resection and modular distal humeral prosthetic reconstruction

6. Distal to elbow—Individualize treatment with plates or intramedullary devices versus nonsurgical treatment.

C. Lower extremity

1. Overview

   a. Common location for bone metastasis

   b. Surgical treatment if patient has ≥3 months to live (but displaced femoral diaphyseal fractures may be fixed in patients with less time to live)

2. Pelvis (**Figure 8**)

   a. Treat non–weight-bearing areas with radiation or minimally invasive techniques.

   b. Resection or curettage in selected cases

3. Acetabulum (**Figure 9, A and B**)

   a. Surgical treatment requires extensive preoperative planning (cross-sectional imaging, embolization for vascular lesions).

   b. Extent of bone destruction delineates treatment options (standard total hip arthroplasty, acetabular mesh/cage, rebar reconstruction to transmit stresses from acetabulum to unaffected ilium/sacrum).

   c. Girdlestone procedure is appropriate in patients with end-stage disease, severe pain, and substantial periacetabular bone loss (**Figure 9, C**).

4. Femoral neck (**Figure 10**)

   a. Pathologic fractures or impending fractures require prosthetic reconstruction.

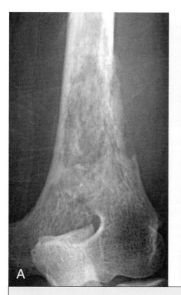
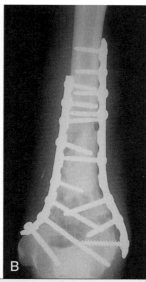

Figure 7 Radiographs of the distal humerus of a 56-year-old woman with metastatic endometrial cancer. **A,** AP view demonstrates the permeative appearance of the lesion. The patient had persistent pain after radiation of the metastasis. **B,** Postoperative AP view obtained after curettage, cementation, and double plating of the lesion.

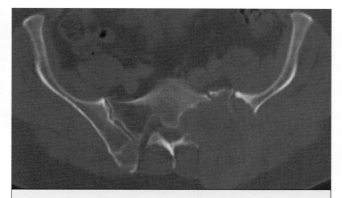

Figure 8 Axial CT scan of the pelvis of a 47-year-old man with metastatic thyroid cancer defines a large, destructive lesion in the left sacroiliac region.

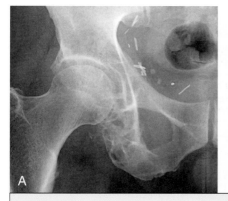
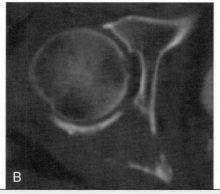
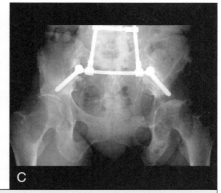

Figure 9 Imaging studies in patients with metastatic disease to the acetabulum. **A,** AP radiograph of the right pelvis in a 71-year-old man with metastatic renal cell carcinoma to the right acetabulum and ischium. The acetabular disease is not well defined on plain radiographs. **B,** CT scan of the right acetabulum of the patient shown in panel A defines the destruction of the posterior acetabulum, placing the patient at risk for a displaced fracture. Acetabular reconstruction may require a reinforced ring or cage device or tantalum acetabular component to prevent protrusion with disease progression. **C,** AP radiograph of the pelvis in a 59-year-old woman with widely metastatic thyroid cancer and multiple comorbidities shows destruction of the left acetabulum. Nonsurgical treatment with immobilization in a wheelchair or a Girdlestone procedure for pain relief would be reasonable options.

4: Orthopaedic Oncology/Systemic Disease

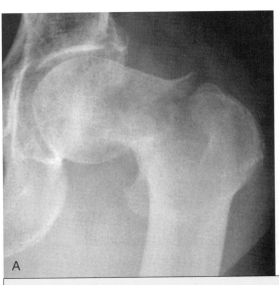 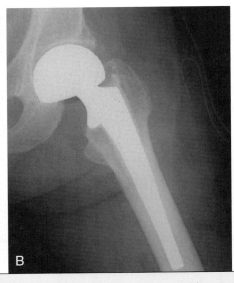 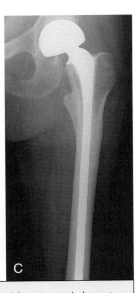

Figure 10 Metastases to the femoral neck. **A,** AP radiograph of the left hip in a 70-year-old woman with metastatic breast cancer reveals a pathologic femoral neck fracture. No other lesions were noted throughout the femur. **B,** AP radiograph obtained after a cemented bipolar hip reconstruction. Most patients with femoral neck disease do not require acetabular components. Internal fixation of a pathologic hip fracture is not indicated. **C,** AP radiograph of a hip obtained after implantation of a long-stemmed femoral component, which can be used to prevent pathologic fractures in the femoral diaphysis. Patients with long-stemmed prostheses have a higher risk of cardiopulmonary complications due to intraoperative/postoperative thromboembolic events.

  b. Internal fixation with cement has an unacceptably high failure rate because of the likelihood of disease progression.

  c. Usually a bipolar cup is satisfactory; a total hip arthroplasty should be performed only if the acetabulum is involved with metastatic disease or the patient has extensive degenerative joint disease.

5. Intertrochanteric (**Figure 11**)

  a. Intramedullary reconstruction nail (open versus closed) protects the entire femur (**Figure 11**).

  b. Calcar replacement prosthesis for lesions with extensive bone destruction

6. Subtrochanteric

  a. Intramedullary locked reconstruction nail (**Figure 12**)

  b. Resection and prosthetic replacement (megaprosthesis)

   • Patients with periarticular bone destruction that does not allow rigid fixation

   • Displaced pathologic fracture through large osteolytic lesion

   • Radioresistant lesion (large renal cell metastasis)

   • Solitary lesion (some series indicate improved survival for resection of solitary metastasis from renal carcinoma)

   • Salvage of failed fixation devices (**Figure 13**)

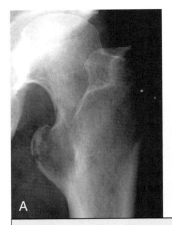 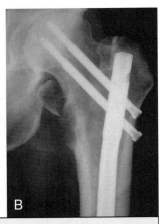

Figure 11 Intertrochanteric lesions. **A,** AP radiograph of the hip of a patient with metastatic thyroid cancer. A lesser trochanter avulsion or osteolytic lesion indicates a pathologic process in the older patient. **B,** AP radiograph obtained after the patient was treated prophylactically with a locked femoral reconstruction nail.

7. Femoral diaphysis: intramedullary locked reconstruction nail (**Figure 14**)

8. Distal femur

  a. Locking plate/screws/cement

  b. Retrograde intramedullary device (less ideal because of tumor reaming in knee joint and stress riser at tip of rod in proximal femur)

c. Resection and distal femoral replacement

9. Distal to knee

   a. Individualize treatment with prostheses, intramedullary devices, plates/screws/cement (**Figure 15**).

   b. Avoid amputation if possible.

D. Spine

   1. Risk factors for progressive neurologic deficit

      a. Osteolytic lesions

      b. Pedicle involvement ("winking owl" sign on AP radiograph)

      c. Posterior column involvement

   2. Indications for surgical treatment

      a. Significant or progressive neurologic deficit

      b. Intractable pain

      c. Progression of deformity

   3. Surgical options

      a. Anterior vertebrectomy

      b. Posterior decompression/instrumentation

      c. Anterior/posterior combination approach (**Figure 16**)

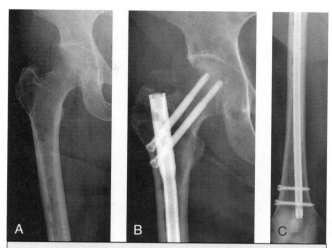

Figure 12   Radiographs of the right femur of a 78-year-old woman with metastatic endometrial cancer. **A**, AP view reveals multiple osteolytic lesions. The lesion in the greater trochanter placed the patient at increased risk of pathologic fracture. Postoperative AP radiographs of the proximal (**B**) and distal (**C**) femur show stabilization of the entire femur with an intramedullary reconstruction nail.

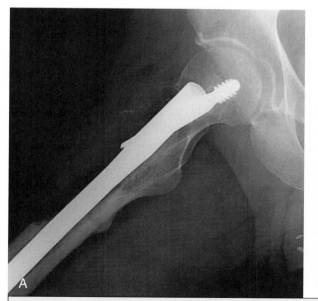
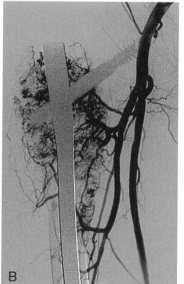
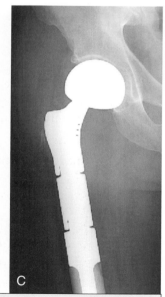

Figure 13   Imaging studies of a 49-year-old man with metastatic renal cell carcinoma and painful progression of disease after placement of an intramedullary reconstruction nail in the right femur. **A**, Lateral radiograph demonstrates the loss of anterior cortex proximally. **B**, Prior to salvage of the impending hardware failure, embolization of the feeding vessels is performed, as shown in this angiogram. This should be done routinely for patients with metastatic renal carcinoma unless a tourniquet can be used for surgery. **C**, AP radiograph obtained after the proximal femur was resected shows the defect reconstructed with a cemented megaprosthesis using a bipolar acetabular component.

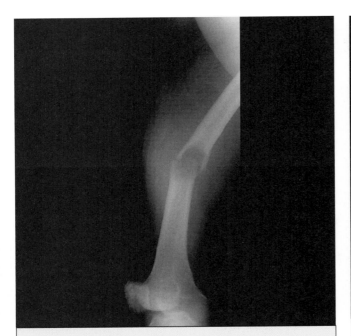

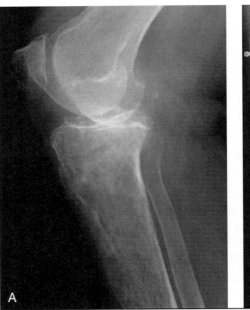

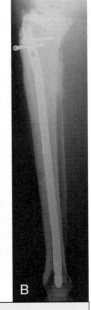

Figure 14   Radiograph of the right femur of a 60-year-old woman demonstrates a pathologic fracture. A staging workup did not reveal a primary site of disease, but a biopsy of the femoral lesion showed carcinoma. The patient should be treated with a femoral reconstruction nail.

Figure 15   Radiographs of the right knee of a 67-year-old woman with metastatic breast cancer to the tibia. **A,** Lateral radiograph demonstrates the destruction of the tibia with concomitant severe osteopenia. This extends throughout the length of the bone. **B,** Lateral radiograph obtained after 18 months reveals a locked intramedullary tibial rod in good position. With postoperative radiation, bisphosphonates, and hormonal treatment, the bone quality greatly improved.

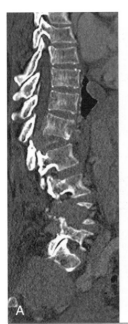

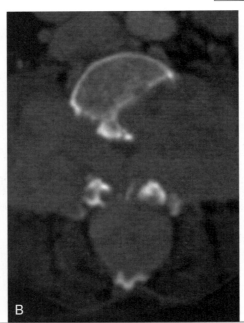

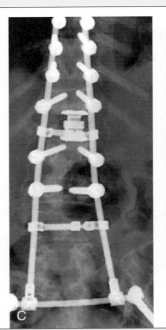

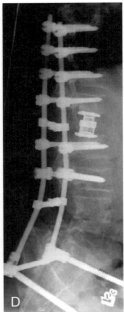

Figure 16   Images of the spine of a 57-year-old woman with metastatic thyroid cancer. **A,** A CT sagittal reconstruction of the thoracolumbar spine demonstrates complete destruction and collapse of L1, with severe central canal obstruction at this level. Note also the extensive disease at L4 and S2. **B,** Axial CT image at L4 demonstrates the canal compromise at this level and the extent of the soft-tissue mass. AP **(C)** and lateral **(D)** radiographs obtained after L1 corpectomy, partial L4 corpectomy, and posterior thoracic-lumbar-pelvic fixation with pedicle screws, rods, and a transiliac bar. A distractible cage is shown at L1.

Top Testing Facts

1. The most common diagnosis of a lytic, destructive lesion in a patient older than 40 years is bone metastasis.

2. The most common primary sites that metastasize to bone are breast, prostate, lung, kidney, and thyroid.

3. Careful history, physical examination, and radiographic staging will identify 85% of primary lesions; biopsy is needed when the primary lesion has not been identified.

4. The histologic features of metastatic carcinoma include epithelial cells in a fibrous stroma.

5. Breast carcinoma cells secrete PTHrP, which signals osteoblasts to release RANKL, which causes osteoclast activation and further bone resorption.

6. Osteolytic lesions have a greater likelihood of pathologic fracture than osteoblastic lesions.

7. Bisphosphonates cause osteoclast apoptosis by inhibiting protein prenylation and act via the mevalonate pathway.

8. External beam radiation is helpful for pain control and is important in maintaining local control postoperatively.

9. Pathologic femoral neck lesions require prosthetic replacement, not in situ fixation.

10. Locked intramedullary fixation is used for impending or actual diaphyseal fractures. (Femoral rods must extend into the femoral neck.)

Bibliography

Biermann JS, Holt GE, Lewis VO, Schwartz HS, Yaszemski MJ: Metastatic bone disease: Diagnosis, evaluation, and treatment. *J Bone Joint Surg Am* 2009;91(6):1518-1530.

Damron TA, Morgan H, Prakash D, Grant W, Aronowitz J, Heiner J: Critical evaluation of Mirels' rating system for impending pathologic fractures. *Clin Orthop Relat Res* 2003;415(415, suppl):S201-S207.

D'angelo G, Sciuto R, Salvatori M, et al: Targeted "bone-seeking" radiopharmaceuticals for palliative treatment of bone metastases: A systematic review and meta-analysis. *Q J Nucl Med Mol Imaging* 2012;56(6):538-543.

Frassica DA: General principles of external beam radiation therapy for skeletal metastases. *Clin Orthop Relat Res* 2003; 415(415, suppl):S158-S164.

Harrington KD: The management of acetabular insufficiency secondary to metastatic malignant disease. *J Bone Joint Surg Am* 1981;63(4):653-664.

Lutz ST, Lo SS, Chang EL, et al: ACR Appropriateness Criteria® non-spine bone metastases. *J Palliat Med* 2012;15(5): 521-526.

Patchell RA, Tibbs PA, Regine WF, et al: Direct decompressive surgical resection in the treatment of spinal cord compression caused by metastatic cancer: A randomised trial. *Lancet* 2005;366(9486):643-648.

Roodman GD: Mechanisms of bone metastasis. *N Engl J Med* 2004;350(16):1655-1664.

Rosenthal D, Callstrom MR: Critical review and state of the art in interventional oncology: Benign and metastatic disease involving bone. *Radiology* 2012;262(3):765-780.

Rougraff BT: Evaluation of the patient with carcinoma of unknown origin metastatic to bone. *Clin Orthop Relat Res* 2003;415(415, suppl):S105-S109.

Stopeck AT, Lipton A, Body J-J, et al: Denosumab compared with zoledronic acid for the treatment of bone metastases in patients with advanced breast cancer: A randomized, double-blind study. *J Clin Oncol* 2010;28(35):5132-5139.

Thai DM, Kitagawa Y, Choong PF: Outcome of surgical management of bony metastases to the humerus and shoulder girdle: A retrospective analysis of 93 patients. *Int Semin Surg Oncol* 2006;3:5.

Ward WG, Holsenbeck S, Dorey FJ, Spang J, Howe D: Metastatic disease of the femur: Surgical treatment. *Clin Orthop Relat Res* 2003;415(415, suppl):S230-S244.

Chapter 52

Metabolic Bone and Inflammatory Joint Disease

Frank J. Frassica, MD

I. Osteopetrosis (Albers-Schönberg Disease)

A. Definition and demographics

1. Osteopetrosis is a rare disorder characterized by deficient formation or function of osteoclasts with resultant dense bone and no medullary cavity.

2. Autosomal recessive forms are diagnosed in children; the delayed type is more common and often is not diagnosed until adulthood.

B. Genetics/etiology

1. The lethal form is autosomal recessive.

2. The delayed type is autosomal dominant.

3. When osteopetrosis occurs with renal tubular acidosis and cerebral calcification, an associated carbonic anhydrase II deficiency is present.

4. Deactivating mutations in multiple genes have been found. Major sites of the defects include:

   a. Carbonic anhydrase II (CA II)

   b. *TCIRG1* (*ATP6i*) gene mutation

   c. Chloride channel 7

C. Clinical presentation

1. Fracture (long bones, ribs, acromion)

2. Complications following tooth extraction due to poor tooth quality

3. Pancytopenia

4. Central nervous system and eye problems (Lack of bone remodeling results in cranial nerve compression.)

5. Short stature (in childhood form)

6. Hypocalcemia

7. Respiratory compromise

D. Radiographic appearance (**Figure 1**)

1. Symmetric increase in bone mass

2. Thickened cortical and trabecular bone

3. Often alternating sclerotic and lucent bands

4. Widened metaphyses (Erlenmeyer flask deformity)

E. Pathology

1. Islands or bars of calcified cartilage within mature trabeculae

2. Osteoclasts without ruffled borders

F. Treatment

1. Bone marrow transplantation for infantile form

2. Interferon gamma-1β for delayed type

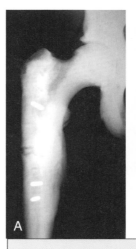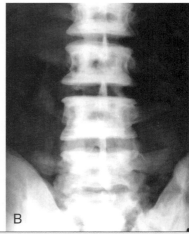

Figure 1 Osteopetrosis. **A,** AP radiograph of the hip in a patient with osteopetrosis. The medullary cavity is intensely sclerotic and is absent in the periacetabular region. **B,** AP view of the spine of a patient with osteopetrosis demonstrates the dense sclerosis at the superior and inferior end plates of the vertebral bodies.

4: Orthopaedic Oncology/Systemic Disease

II. Oncologic Osteomalacia (Tumor-Induced Osteomalacia)

A. Definition and demographics

1. Oncologic osteomalacia is a rare paraneoplastic syndrome of renal phosphate wasting caused by a bone or soft-tissue tumor that secretes a substance that leads to osteomalacia.

2. Tumor-overexpressed fibroblast growth factor-23 (FGF23), a phosphatonin, is responsible for hypophosphatemia and osteomalacia.

3. A long delay in detecting the tumor, which may be very small, is common.

B. Genetics/etiology—Common bone and soft-tissue tumors that cause oncologic osteomalacia:

1. Phosphaturic mesenchymal tumor, mixed connective tissue type (majority)

2. Hemangioma

3. Hemangiopericytoma

4. Giant cell tumor

5. Osteoblastoma

6. Sarcomas

C. Clinical presentation

1. Progressive bone and muscle pain

2. Weakness and fatigue

3. Fractures of the long bones, ribs, and vertebrae

D. Imaging appearance

1. Radiographs: diffuse osteopenia, pseudofractures

2. Octreotide scan (indium-111–pentetreotide scintigraphy, radiolabeled somatostatin analog): tumors can be detected

E. Laboratory features

1. Hypophosphatemia

2. Phosphaturia due to low proximal tubular reabsorption

3. Low or normal serum 1,25-dihydroxyvitamin D level

4. Elevated serum alkaline phosphatase level

F. Treatment

1. Removal of the tumor

2. Phosphate supplementation with 1,25-dihydroxyvitamin D

III. Hypercalcemia of Malignancy

A. Definition and demographics

1. Hypercalcemia may develop in 10% to 30% of patients with cancer and is a poor prognostic sign.

a. Hypercalcemia with diffuse lytic metastases (20% of cases) is commonly associated with the following:

- Breast cancer

- Hematologic malignancies (eg, multiple myeloma, lymphoma, leukemia)

b. Hypercalcemia without diffuse lytic metastases (80% of cases) is commonly associated with the following:

- Squamous cell carcinoma

- Renal or bladder carcinoma

- Ovarian or endometrial cancer

- Breast cancer

B. Genetics/etiology

1. Humoral hypercalcemia due to secreted factors such as parathyroid-related hormone

2. Local osteolysis due to tumor invasion of bone

3. Absorptive hypercalcemia due to excessive vitamin D produced by malignancies

C. Clinical presentation

1. Neurologic: difficulty concentrating, sleepiness, depression, confusion, coma

2. Gastrointestinal: constipation, anorexia, nausea, vomiting

3. Genitourinary: polyuria, dehydration

4. Cardiac: shortening of QT interval, bradycardia, first-degree block

D. Radiographic appearance—Diffuse lytic metastases may be present.

E. Laboratory features

1. Hypercalcemia

2. Normal or high serum phosphorus level

3. Low parathyroid hormone level

F. Pathology—Osteoclastic bone resorption.

G. Treatment

1. Aggressive volume expansion with intravenous saline solution

2. Diphosphonate therapy to halt osteoclastic bone resorption

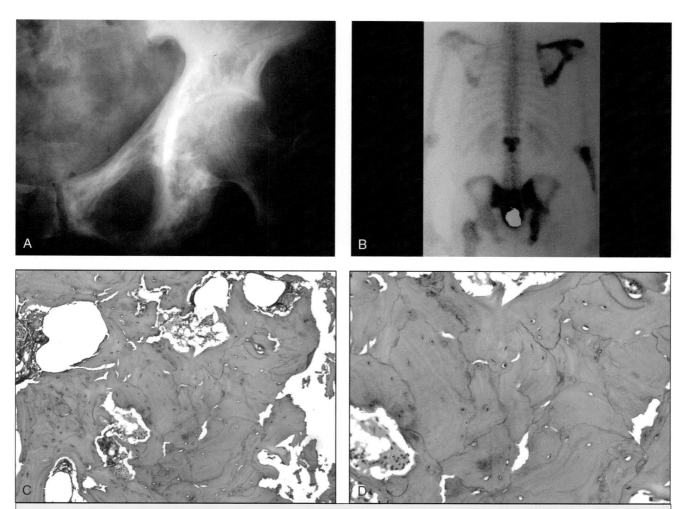

Figure 2 Paget disease. **A,** AP view of the pelvis in a patient with Paget disease. Note the coarsened trabeculae from the pubis to the supra-acetabular area and marked thickening of the iliopectineal line. **B,** Technetium Tc 99m bone scan of a patient with Paget disease. Note the intense uptake in the scapula, lumbar vertebral body, right ilium, and right ulna. **C** and **D,** Hematoxylin and eosin stain of pagetic bone. Note the disordered appearance of the bone and the multiple cement lines (curved blue lines).

3. Loop diuretics

4. Combination therapy (chemotherapy and radiation) to kill the cancer cells

IV. Paget Disease

A. Definition and demographics

1. Paget disease is a remodeling disease characterized initially by increased osteoclast-mediated bone resorption and then disordered bone turnover.

2. Usually occurs in patients older than 50 years

B. Genetics/etiology

1. Caused by dysregulation of osteoclast differentiation and function

2. Possibly caused by a slow viral infection (paramyxovirus, respiratory syncytial virus)

3. Most common in Caucasians of Anglo-Saxon descent

4. Strong genetic tendency (autosomal dominant)—Most important predisposing gene is *SQSTM1*, which harbors mutations that cause osteoclast activation in 5% to 20% of patients.

C. Clinical presentation

1. No sex predilection

2. May be monostotic or polyostotic; the number of sites remains constant.

3. Common sites: femur, pelvis, tibia, skull, spine (**Figure 2**)

4. Often asymptomatic and found incidentally on a bone scan, chest radiograph, or in patients with elevated alkaline phosphatase levels

5. Progresses through three phases

   a. Lytic phase

      • Profound resorption of the bone

      • Purely lucent on radiographs, with expansion and thinned but intact cortices

   b. Mixed phase: combination of osteolysis and bone formation with coarsened trabeculae

   c. Sclerotic phase: enlargement of the bone with thickened cortices and both sclerotic and lucent areas

6. Bone pain may be present, possibly caused by increased vascularity and warmth or by stress fractures.

7. Bowing of the femur or tibia

8. Fractures, most commonly femoral neck

9. Arthritis of the hip and knee

10. Lumbar spinal stenosis

11. Deafness

12. Malignant degeneration

   a. Occurs in 1% of patients

   b. Most common locations: pelvis, femur, humerus

   c. Patients often note a marked increase in constant pain.

D. Laboratory features

   1. Increased alkaline phosphatase level

   2. Increased urinary markers of bone turnover

      a. Collagen cross-links

      b. N-telopeptide, hydroxyproline, deoxypyridinoline

   3. Normal calcium level

E. Imaging

   1. Appearance on plain radiographs (**Figure 2, A**)

      a. Coarsened trabeculae

      b. Cortical thickening

      c. Lucent advancing edge ("blade of grass" or "flame-shaped") in active disease

      d. Loss of distinction between the cortices and medullary cavity

      e. Enlargement of the bone

2. Technetium Tc 99m bone scans—Increased uptake accurately marks sites of disease (**Figure 2, B**).

   a. Intense activity, which often outlines the shape of the bone, during the active phase

   b. Mild to moderate activity in the sclerotic phases

3. Appearance on CT scans

   a. Cortical thickening

   b. Coarsened trabeculae

F. Pathology

   1. Profound osteoclastic bone resorption

   2. Abnormal bone formation: mosaic pattern

      a. Woven bone and irregular sections of thickened trabecular bone

      b. Numerous cement lines

G. Treatment

   1. Therapy is aimed at stopping the osteoclasts from resorbing bone.

   2. Bisphosphonates

      a. Oral agents: alendronate and risedronate

      b. Intravenous agents: pamidronate and zoledronic acid

   3. Calcitonin—Salmon calcitonin is administered subcutaneously or intramuscularly.

V. Osteonecrosis

A. Osteonecrosis is the death of bone cells and bone marrow secondary to a loss of blood supply.

B. Genetics/etiology

   1. Four mechanisms have been proposed.

      a. Mechanical disruption of the blood vessels (trauma, such as a hip dislocation)

      b. Arterial vessel occlusion: nitrogen bubbles (bends), sickle cell disease, fat emboli

      c. Injury or pressure on the blood vessel wall: marrow diseases (such as Gaucher), vasculitis, radiation injury

      d. Venous outflow obstruction

   2. Associated with hypercoagulable states

      a. Decreased anticoagulants—proteins C, S

      b. Increased procoagulants

C. Clinical presentation—The patient may present with a dull pain in the joint or severe arthritic pain with collapse of the joint, or may be asymptomatic.

4: Orthopaedic Oncology/Systemic Disease

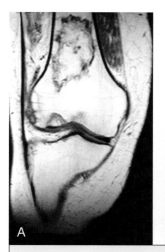
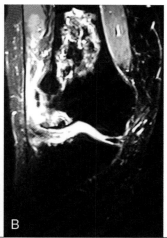
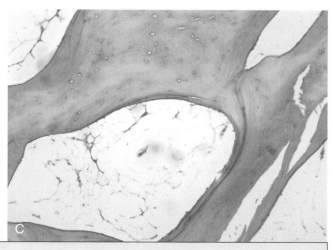

Figure 3   Osteonecrosis. **A,** T1-weighted coronal MRI of the knee of a patient with osteonecrosis shows a large metaphyseal lesion and a wedge-shaped area of necrosis at the subchondral region of the lateral femoral condyle. **B,** T2-weighted coronal MRI of the knee of a patient with osteonecrosis demonstrates a large metaphyseal lesion with a large subchondral wedge-shaped lesion in the lateral femur. **C,** Hematoxylin and eosin stain demonstrates the complete loss of the bone marrow and an absence of osteocytes in the trabecular lacunae.

D. Imaging

  1. Appearance on radiographs

    a. Initially normal

    b. Sclerosis and cyst formation

    c. Subchondral fracture (crescent sign), subchondral collapse

    d. Arthritic changes: osteophytes, loss of joint space

  2. Appearance on MRI: characteristic marrow changes in the metaphyseal marrow and subchondral locations (**Figure 3**)

E. Pathology

  1. Osteocyte death (no cells in the bone lacunae)

  2. Marrow necrosis

  3. Loss of the vascular supply

F. Treatment

  1. Core decompression or vascularized bone graft if the joint surfaces remain intact (no collapse)

  2. Arthroplasty or osteotomy for joint collapse

VI. Rheumatoid Arthritis

A. Definition and demographics

  1. Rheumatoid arthritis is a systemic inflammatory disease of the synovium.

  2. Twice as common in females as in males

  3. According to the American College of Rheumatology revised criteria (2010), the patient must score at least 6 points based on joint distribution, serology, symptom duration, and presence of acute phase reactants (**Table 1**). Radiographs are no longer required for diagnosis.

B. Genetics/etiology

  1. Genetic marker human leukocyte antigen (HLA)-DR4 (in patients of northern European descent)

  2. Monozygotic twins have a concordance rate of 12% to 15%.

C. Clinical presentation

  1. Morning stiffness, pain

  2. Joint swelling (most prominent in small joints of the hands and feet)

    a. Effusions

    b. Synovial proliferation

  3. Hand deformities: metacarpophalangeal joint, subluxation, ulnar drift of the fingers, swan-neck deformity, boutonnière deformity

D. Imaging appearance (**Figure 4**)

  1. Periarticular osteopenia

  2. Juxta-articular erosions

  3. Joint space narrowing

E. Laboratory features

  1. Approximately 90% of patients are positive for rheumatoid factor.

Table 1

2010 ACR-EULAR Classification Criteria for Rheumatoid Arthritis

	Score
Target population (Who should be tested?): Patients who 1. have at least 1 joint with definite clinical synovitis (swelling)[a] 2. with the synovitis not better explained by another disease[b]	
Classification criteria for RA (score-based algorithm: add score of categories A–D; a score of ≥ 6/10 is needed for classification of a patient as having definite RA)[c]	
A. Joint involvement[d]	
1 large joint[e]	0
2–10 large joints	1
1–3 small joints (with or without involvement of large joints)[f]	2
4–10 small joints (with or without involvement of large joints)	3
>10 joints (at least one small joint)[g]	5
B. Serology (at least one test result is needed for classification)[h]	
Negative RF *and* negative ACPA	0
Low-positive RF *or* low-positive ACPA	2
High-positive RF *or* high-positive ACPA	3
C. Acute-phase reactants (at least one test result is needed for classification)[i]	
Normal CRP *and* normal ESR	0
Abnormal CRP *or* abnormal ESR	1
D. Duration of symptoms[j]	
< 6 weeks	0
≥ 6 weeks	1

ACR-EULAR = American College of Rheumatology/European League Against Rheumatism, ACPA = anticitrullinated protein antibody, CRP = C-reactive protein, ESR = erythrocyte sedimentation rate, RA = rheumatoid arthritis, RF = rheumatoid factor

[a]The criteria are aimed at classification of newly presenting patients. In addition, patients with erosive disease typical of RA with a history compatible with prior fulfillment of the 2010 criteria should be classified as having RA. Patients with long-standing disease, including those whose disease is inactive (with or without treatment) and who, based on retrospectively available data, have previously fulfilled the 2010 criteria should be classified as having RA.

[b]Differential diagnoses vary among patients with different presentations, but may include conditions such as systemic lupus erythematosus, psoriatic arthritis, and gout. If it is unclear about the relevant differential diagnoses to consider, an expert rheumatologist should be consulted.

[c]Although patients with a score of < 6/10 are not classifiable as having RA, their status can be reassessed and the criteria might be fulfilled cumulatively over time.

[d]Joint involvement refers to any swollen or tender joint on examination, which may be confirmed by imaging evidence of synovitis. Distal interphalangeal joints, first carpometacarpal joints, and first metatarsophalangeal joints are excluded from assessment. Categories of joint distribution are classified according to the location and number of involved joints, with placement into the highest category possible based on the pattern of joint involvement.

[e]"Large joints" refers to shoulders, elbows, hips, knees, and ankles.

[f]"Small joints" refers to the metacarpophalangeal joints, proximal interphalangeal joints, second through fifth metatarsophalangeal joints, thumb interphalangeal joints, and wrists.

[g]In this category, at least one of the involved joints must be a small joint; the other joints can include any combination of large and additional small joints, as well as other joints not specifically listed elsewhere (eg, temporomandibular, acromioclavicular, sternoclavicular, etc.).

[h]Negative refers to IU values that are less than or equal to the upper limit of normal (ULN) for the laboratory and assay; low-positive refers to IU values that are higher than the ULN but ≤ 3 times the ULN for the laboratory and assay; high-positive refers to IU values that are > 3 times the ULN for the laboratory and assay. Where RF information is only available as positive or negative, a positive result should be scored as low-positive for RF.

[i]Normal/abnormal is determined by local laboratory standards.

[j]Duration of symptoms refers to patient self-report of the duration of signs or symptoms of synovitis (eg, pain, swelling, tenderness) of joints that are clinically involved at the time of assessment, regardless of treatment status.

Adapted from American College of Rheumatolgy: 2010 rheumatoid arthritis classification. www.rheumatology.org/practice/clinical/classification/ra/ra_2010.asp. Accessed November 1, 2013.

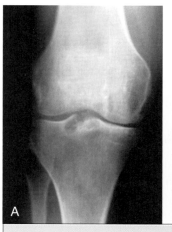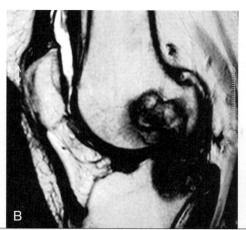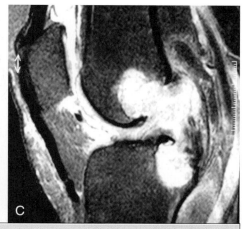

Figure 4 Rheumatoid arthritis. **A,** AP radiograph of the knee shows a subchondral cyst in the proximal tibia with narrowing of the medial compartment of the knee. **B,** T1-weighted sagittal MRI of the knee shows a large subchondral lesion in the distal femur and proximal tibia and an erosion on the tibial condylar surface. **C,** T2-weighted sagittal MRI of the knee demonstrates a large erosion on the distal femur and proximal tibia, an effusion, and diffuse synovial thickening.

2. Elevation of acute-phase reactants: erythrocyte sedimentation rate (ESR), C-reactive protein (CRP) level

F. Pathology—Inflammatory infiltrate destroys cartilage, ligaments, and bone.

G. Treatment

1. Nonsteroidal anti-inflammatory drugs

2. Aspirin

3. Disease-modifying antirheumatic drugs (DMARDs)

   a. Methotrexate (current treatment of choice)

   b. Others (D-penicillamine, sulfasalazine, gold, antimalarials)

4. Cytokine-neutralizing

   a. Etanercept (soluble p75 tumor necrosis factor [TNF] receptor immunoglobulin G–fusion protein)

   b. Infliximab (chimeric monoclonal antibody to TNF-α)

   c. Rituximab (monoclonal antibody to CD20 antigen; inhibits B-cells)

5. Physical therapy—To maintain joint motion and muscle strength.

VII. Ankylosing Spondylitis (Marie-Strumpell Disease)

A. Definition and demographics

1. Inflammatory disorder that affects the spine, sacroiliac joints, and large joints (hip) in young adults

2. Male-to-female ratio = 3:1

B. Genetics/etiology

1. Ninety percent of patients have HLA-B27.

2. Autoimmune disorder

   a. High levels of TNF are found.

   b. CD4+, CD8+ T-cells are present

C. Clinical presentation

1. Young adults

2. Low back and pelvic pain

3. Morning stiffness

4. Hip arthritis in approximately one third of patients

5. Uveitis: pain, light sensitivity

6. Heart involvement

   a. Aortic valve insufficiency

   b. Third-degree heart block

D. Radiographic appearance

1. Sacroiliac joint inflammation

   a. Blurring of subchondral margins

   b. Erosions

   c. Bony bridging

2. Lumbar spine involvement (**Figure 5**)

   a. Loss of lumbar lordosis

   b. Squaring of the vertebrae

   c. Osteophytes bridging the vertebrae

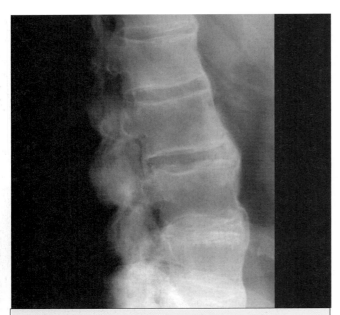

Figure 5 Lateral radiograph of the spine of a patient with ankylosing spondylitis. Note the anterior osteophytes bridging all the lumbar vertebrae.

E. Pathology

   1. Laboratory findings

      a. HLA-B27 in 90% of patients

      b. Elevated ESR and CRP level

   2. Inflammation of ligamentous attachment sites

      a. Erosions, subchondral inflammation

      b. Ossification of joints (sacroiliac joint)

   3. Arthritis—Pannus formation with lymphoid infiltration.

F. Treatment: anti-TNF therapy

   1. Infliximab (chimeric monoclonal antibody to TNF-α)

   2. Etanercept (soluble p75 TNF receptor immunoglobulin G–fusion protein)

VIII. Reactive Arthritis

A. Reactive arthritis (formerly called Reiter syndrome) is a type of inflammatory arthritis that occurs after an infection at another site in the body.

B. Genetics/etiology—Affected individuals are genetically predisposed (high incidence of HLA-B27).

C. Clinical presentation

   1. An infection will have occurred 1 to 8 weeks before the onset of the arthritis.

   2. Common extraskeletal involvement

      a. Urethritis, prostatitis

      b. Uveitis

      c. Mucocutaneous involvement

   3. Systemic symptoms: fatigue, malaise, fever, weight loss

   4. Arthritis is asymmetric.

   5. Common sites include the knee, ankle, subtalar joint, and metatarsophalangeal and interphalangeal joints.

   6. Tendinitis/fasciitis (common)

      a. Achilles tendon insertion

      b. Plantar fascia

   7. Recurrent joint symptoms and tendinitis are common even after treatment.

D. Radiographic appearance

   1. Juxta-articular erosions

   2. Joint destruction

E. Pathology

   1. Synovial inflammation

   2. Enthesitis

F. Treatment: indomethacin

IX. Systemic Lupus Erythematosus

A. Systemic lupus erythematosus (SLE) is an autoimmune disorder in which autoimmune complexes damage joints, skin, kidneys, lungs, heart, blood vessels, and nervous system.

B. Genetics/etiology

   1. Multiple genes

   2. HLA class II, HLA class III, HLA-DR, HLA-DQ are associated

C. Clinical presentation

   1. Multiple joint involvement

   2. Osteonecrosis of the hips (common, especially in patients taking glucocorticoids)

D. Radiographic appearance

   1. Erosions or joint destruction (uncommon)

   2. Osteonecrosis may be seen as a result of corticosteroid treatment.

E. Pathology—Antinuclear antibodies are present in 95% of patients.

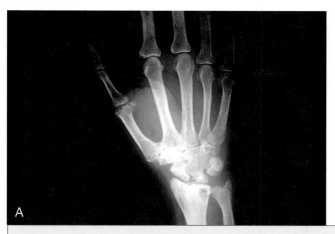
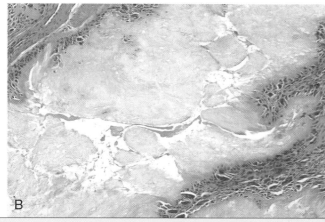

Figure 6   Gout. **A,** PA radiograph of the hand of a patient with gout shows a lucent lesion in the distal radius and erosive changes in the carpal bones. **B,** Hematoxylin and eosin stain of a lesion in a patient with gout. Note that the tophaceous areas are amorphous and white and are bordered by inflammatory cells.

F. Treatment

1. Analgesics

2. Antimalarials

X. Gout

A. Definition and demographics

1. Gout is a metabolic disorder manifested by uric acid crystals in the synovium.

2. Affects older men and postmenopausal women

3. Prevalence is increasing

B. Clinical presentation

1. Involvement of a single joint is common.

2. Gout is often polyarticular in men with hypertension and alcohol abuse.

3. Involved joints are intensely painful, swollen, and erythematous.

C. Radiographic appearance (**Figure 6, A**)

1. Periarticular erosions

2. The peripheral margin of the erosion often has a thin overlying rim of bone (cliff sign).

D. Pathology

1. Joint aspiration is the only definitive diagnostic procedure. Needle- and rod-shaped crystals with negative birefringence are seen.

2. Joint white blood cell count is usually less than 50,000 to 60,000/μL.

3. Serum uric acid level is often elevated (but not always).

4. Hematoxylin and eosin staining shows amorphous material and inflammatory cells (**Figure 6, B**).

E. Treatment

1. Nonsteroidal anti-inflammatory drugs

2. Colchicine

3. Hypouricemic therapy: allopurinol, probenecid

XI. Osteoporosis

A. Definition and demographics

1. Characteristics

a. Low bone mass

b. Microarchitectural deterioration

c. Fractures

2. Bone mass is acquired between 2 and 30 years of age; failure to attain adequate bone mass during this period is one of the main determinants in the development of osteoporosis.

3. World Health Organization definition

a. Normal: within 1 SD of peak bone mass (T-score = 0 to −1.0)

b. Low bone mass (osteopenia): 1.0 to 2.5 SDs below peak bone mass (T-score = −1.0 to −2.5)

c. Osteoporosis: more than 2.5 SDs below peak bone mass (T-score < −2.5)

B. Genetics/etiology

1. Causes are multifactorial.

2. Withdrawal of estrogen is one of the main causes in women; this deficiency results in an increase in

receptor activator of nuclear factor κB ligand expression.

3. Genetic predisposition is important.

4. Genes associated with the development of osteoporosis

   a. *COL1A1*

   b. Vitamin D receptor

   c. *LRP5* (codes for low-density lipoprotein receptor-related protein)

C. Clinical presentation

1. Patient usually presents with a fracture following minor trauma.

2. Low bone mineral density (found on routine screening)

3. Most important risk factors

   a. Increasing age (geriatric patient)

   b. Female sex

   c. Early menopause

   d. Fair-skinned

   e. Maternal/paternal history of hip fracture

   f. Low body weight

   g. Cigarette smoking

   h. Glucocorticoid use

   i. Excessive alcohol use

   j. Low protein intake

   k. Anticonvulsant or antidepressant use

D. Radiographic appearance

1. Osteopenia

2. Thinning of the cortices

3. Loss of trabecular bone

E. Pathology

1. Loss of trabecular bone

2. Loss of continuity of the trabecular bone

F. Treatment

1. Adequate calcium and vitamin D intake

2. Antiresorptive therapy for patients with osteoporosis

3. Bisphosphonates (analogs of pyrophosphate). The potency of bisphosphonates is related to their chemical structure.

   a. Actions: cause apoptosis of the osteoclast and withdrawing of the osteoclast from the bone surface (hence, bone resorption is halted).

   b. Mechanism

     • Inhibit protein prenylation

     • Act via the mevalonate pathway

     • Specifically inhibit farnesyl pyrophosphate

     • Disrupt the ruffled border of osteoclasts

   c. Side effects

     • Myalgias, bone pain, or weakness (up to one third of patients)

     • Gastric irritation

     • Osteonecrosis of the jaw (occurs in patients on long-term therapy)

     • Atypical fractures of the subtrochanteric and diaphyseal areas of the femur (stress fractures)

4. Anabolic therapy with parathyroid hormone 1-34 (PTH [1-34]) (teriparatide).

   a. Indications: Intermittent PTH at a low dose is an anabolic factor in the treatment of osteoporosis. Teriparatide is approved for the treatment of osteoporosis in women and men at high risk for fracture (T-score less than −3.0 with or without a history of previous fragility fracture). The maximum period of administration is 2 years.

   b. Mechanism: The precise mechanism is unknown, although PTH most likely has direct and indirect effects positive for osteoblast differentiation, function, and survival.

   c. Side effects: mild hypercalcemia

   d. Contraindications: children, active Paget disease, hypercalcemia, previous history of irradiation (risk of development of osteosarcoma)

Top Testing Facts

1. Osteopetrosis is a rare disorder characterized by a failure of osteoclastic resorption with resultant dense bone with no medullary cavity (prone to fracture).

2. Oncologic osteomalacia is a paraneoplastic syndrome characterized by renal phosphate wasting. It is caused by a variety of bone and soft-tissue tumors (osteoblastoma, hemangiopericytoma, and phosphaturic mesenchymal tumor).

3. Hypercalcemia may occur as a complication of breast cancer, multiple myeloma, lymphoma, and leukemia.

4. Paget disease is a remodeling disease characterized by disordered bone formation; it is treated with bisphosphonates.

5. Rheumatoid arthritis is a systemic inflammatory disorder characterized by morning stiffness and joint pain; approximately 90% of patients are positive for rheumatoid factor.

6. Ankylosing spondylitis is an inflammatory disorder of the spine and sacroiliac joints characterized by HLA-B27 positivity; it is treated with anti-TNF therapy.

7. Gout is a metabolic disorder caused by uric acid crystals in the synovium resulting in periarticular erosions.

8. Osteoporosis is characterized by low bone mass (>2.5 SDs below the mean) and an increased risk of fracture.

9. The action of bisphosphonates is through inhibition (apoptosis) of osteoclasts through protein prenylation. The specific enzyme inhibited is farnesyl pyrophosphate.

10. Possible side effects of bisphosphonate therapy: atypical stress fractures of the subtrochanteric and diaphyseal region of the femur.

11. Intermittent PTH (teriparatide) is approved for patients at high risk for osteoporotic fractures.

Bibliography

Bukata SV, Tyler WK: Metabolic bone disease, in O'Keefe RJ, Jacobs JJ, Chu CR, Einhorn TA, eds: *Orthopaedic Basic Science: Foundations of Clinical Practice*, ed 4. Rosemont, IL, American Academy of Orthopaedic Surgeons, 2013, pp 331-333.

Canalis E, Giustina A, Bilezikian JP: Mechanisms of anabolic therapies for osteoporosis. *N Engl J Med* 2007;357(9):905-916.

Fauci AS, Langford CA, eds: *Harrison's Rheumatology*. New York, NY, McGraw-Hill, 2010.

Favus MJ: Bisphosphonates for osteoporosis. *N Engl J Med* 2010;363(21):2027-2035.

Jiang Y, Xia WB, Xing XP, et al: Tumor-induced osteomalacia: An important cause of adult-onset hypophosphatemic osteomalacia in China. Report of 39 cases and review of the literature. *J Bone Miner Res* 2012;27(9):1967-1975.

Ralston SH, Layfield R: Pathogenesis of Paget disease of bone. *Calcif Tissue Int* 2012;91(2):97-113.

Rosen CJ, ed: *Primer on the Metabolic Bone Diseases and Disorders of Mineral Metabolism*, ed 8. Washington, DC, American Society for Bone and Mineral Research, 2013.

Rosner MH, Dalkin AC: Onco-nephrology: The pathophysiology and treatment of malignancy-associated hypercalcemia. *Clin J Am Soc Nephrol* 2012;7(10):1722-1729.

Siris ES, Roodman GD: *Paget's Disease of Bone*, ed 6. Washington, DC, American Society for Bone and Mineral Research, 2006, pp 320-329.

Steward CG: Hematopoietic stem cell transplantation for osteopetrosis. *Pediatr Clin North Am* 2010;57(1):171-180.

4: Orthopaedic Oncology/Systemic Disease

Section 5

Pediatrics

Section Editors:
Lisa Berglund, MD
Steven L. Frick, MD

Chapter 53

Skeletal Dysplasias and Mucopolysaccharidoses

Samantha Spencer, MD

I. Skeletal Dysplasias

A. Achondroplasia (**Table 1**)

1. Overview

   a. Short-limbed dwarfism with abnormal facial features

   b. The most common skeletal dysplasia

   c. An autosomal dominant trait, but 90% of instances arise from new mutations rather than inheritance

2. Pathoanatomy

   a. The mutation responsible is a single amino acid substitution (glycine→arginine) that causes a defect in the fibroblast growth factor receptor-3 (*FGFR-3*) gene.

   b. The mutation results in inhibition of chondrocyte profileration and differentiation, and therefore in growth retardation of the long bones formed by endochondral ossification.

   c. The growth plates with the greatest growth during development (proximal humerus/distal femur) are most affected, resulting in rhizomelic (more proximal than distal) short stature.

3. Evaluation

   a. Features include rhizomelic shortening of limbs, frontal bossing, button nose, trident hands (inability to approximate the middle and ring fingers), increased lumbar lordosis, posterior dislocation of the radial head, a "champagne glass" pelvic outlet, and genu varum (**Figure 1**).

   b. Abnormalities of the lumbar spine include thoracolumbar kyphosis (which usually resolves with ambulation), decreased interpedicular distances from L1 to L5, and lumbar stenosis with lordosis and short pedicles.

   c. Stenosis of the foramen magnum and upper cervical spine may be present and cause central apnea and weakness in the first few years of life. Sudden death may occur.

4. Treatment

   a. Thoracolumbar kyphosis present in infancy may be treated nonsurgically. Avoidance of unsupported sitting and bracing may be helpful.

   b. Genu varum is treated with osteotomies if symptomatic or if severe deformity exists.

   c. Screening for stenosis of the foramen magnum or upper cervical spine should be performed; decompression may be required if cord compression is present.

   d. The main issue in adults with achondroplasia is lumbar stenosis, sometimes requiring decompression and/or spinal fusion. Osteoarthritis is not common.

   e. Limb lengthening is controversial and does not treat the other dysmorphic features; if lower limb lengthening is performed, humeral lengthening is indicated as well.

   f. Growth hormone is not effective for increasing stature in achondroplasia.

B. Pseudoachondroplasia (**Table 1**)

1. Overview

   a. Short-limbed rhizomelic dwarfism with normal facial features

   b. Development is normal up to 2 years of age

2. Pathoanatomy

   a. An autosomal dominant trait

   b. The causative mutation is in cartilage oligomeric matrix protein (COMP) on chromosome 19.

Dr. Spencer or an immediate family member serves as a board member, owner, officer, or committee member of the American Academy of Orthopaedic Surgeons, the Massachusetts Orthopaedic Association, and the Pediatric Orthopaedic Society of North America.

5: Pediatrics

Table 1

Skeletal Dysplasias: Genetics and Features

Name	Genetics	Features
Achondroplasia	*FGFR-3*; autosomal dominant; 90% sporadic mutations; affects proliferative zone of physis	Rhizomelic shortening with normal trunk, frontal bossing, button nose, trident hands (cannot approximate long and ring fingers), thoracolumbar kyphosis (usually resolves with sitting), lumbar stenosis and lordosis, radial head subluxations, champagne glass pelvic outlet, genu varum
Hypochondroplasia	*FGFR-3* in a different area than achondroplasia; autosomal dominant	Milder than achondroplasia; short stature, lumbar stenosis, genu varum
Thantophoric dysplasia	*FGFR-3*	Rhizomelic shortening, platyspondyly, protuberant abdomen, small thoracic cavity Death by age 2 years
SED congenita	Type II collagen mutation in *COL2A1;* autosomal dominant but usually sporadic mutation; affects proliferative zone of physis	Short stature, trunk, and limbs; abnormal epiphyses including spine; atlantoaxial instability/odontoid hypoplasia; coxa vara and DDH; genu valgum; early OA; retinal detachment/myopia; sensorineural hearing loss
SED tarda	Unidentified mutation likely in type II collagen, X-linked recessive	Late onset (age range, 8 to 10 years), premature OA, associated with DDH but not lower extremity bowing
Kniest dysplasia	Type II collagen mutation in *COL2A1;* autosomal dominant	Joint contractures (treat with early physical therapy), kyphosis/scoliosis, dumbbell-shaped femora, respiratory problems, cleft palate, retinal detachment/myopia, otitis media/hearing loss, early OA
Cleidocranial dyplasia	Defect in CBFA-1, a transcription factor that activates osteoblast differentiation; autosomal dominant; affects intramembranous ossification	Aplasia/hypoplasia of clavicles (no need to treat), delayed skull suture closure, frontal bossing, coxa vara (osteotomy if neck-shaft angle <100°), delayed ossification pubis, genu valgum, shortened middle phalanges of third through fifth rays
Nail-patella syndrome (osteo-onycho-dysplasia)	Mutation in LIM homeobox transcription factor 1-β also expressed in eyes/kidneys; autosomal dominant	Aplasia/hypoplasia of the patellae and condyles, dysplastic nails, iliac horns, posterior dislocation of the radial head; 30% will experience renal failure and glaucoma as adults
Diastrophic dysplasia	Mutation in sulfate transporter gene affects proteoglycan sulfate groups in cartilage; autosomal recessive; 1 in 70 mutated sulfate transporter gene in Finland; very rare elsewhere	Short stature; rhizomelic shortening, cervical kyphosis, kyphoscoliosis, hitchhiker thumbs, cauliflower ears, rigid clubfoot, skewfoot, severe OA, joint contractures
Mucopolysaccharidoses	All defects in enzymes that degrade glycosaminoglycans in lysosomes. The incomplete degradation products accumulate in various organs and cause dysfunction. All autosomal recessive except Hunter syndrome (X-linked recessive).	Visceromegaly, corneal clouding, cardiac disease, deafness, short stature, mental retardation (except Morquio syndrome, which has normal intelligence); C1-C2 instability is common, as is hip dysplasia and abnormal epiphyses; Hurler syndrome is the most severe; bone marrow transplantation improves life expectancy but does not alter orthopaedic manifestations
Metaphyseal dysplasia: Schmid type	Type X collagen mutation in *COL10A1;* autosomal dominant; affects proliferative/hypertrophic zones	Milder; coxa vara, genu varum
Metaphyseal dyplasia: Jansen type	Mutation in parathyroid hormone receptor (affects parathyroid hormone-related protein), which regulates chondrocyte differentiation; affects proliferative/hypertrophic zones; autosomal dominant	Wide eyes, squatting stance, hypercalcemia, bulbous metaphyseal expansion of long bones, and extremity malalignment *(continued on the next page)*

Table 1

Skeletal Dysplasias: Genetics and Features (continued)

Name	Genetics	Features
Metaphyseal dysplasia: McKusick type	Mutation in *RMRP* (ribosomal nucleic acid component of mitochondrial ribosomal nucleic acid processing endoribonuclease); affects proliferative/hypertrophic zones	C1-C2 instability, hypoplasia of cartilage, small-diameter "fine" hair, intestinal malabsorbtion and megacolon, increased risk of viral infections and malignancies (immune dysfunction), ligamentous laxity, pectus abnormalities, genu varum and ankle deformities due to fibular overgrowth
Pseudoachondroplasia	Mutation in *COMP* on chromosome 19, which is an extracellular matrix glycoprotein in cartilage; autosomal dominant	C1-C2 instability caused by odontoid hypoplasia, normal facies, metaphyseal flaring, delayed epiphyses, lower extremity malalignment, DDH, scoliosis, early OA
MED	Mutations in *COMP, COL9A2*, or *COL9A3* genes (collagen IX, which is a linker for collagen II in cartilage); autosomal dominant	Short stature, epiphyseal dysplasia, genu valgum, hip osteonecrosis and dysplasia, early OA; spine not involved; short metacarpals/metatarsals, double-layer patella
EVC syndrome/ chondroectodermal dysplasia	Mutation in the *EVC* gene; autosomal recessive	Acromesomelic shortening (distal and middle limb segments), postaxial polydactyly, genu valgum, dysplastic nails/teeth, medial iliac spikes, fused capitate/hamate, 60% have congenital heart disease
Diaphyseal dysplasia (also known as Camurati-Engelmann syndrome)	Autosomal dominant	Symmetric cortical thickening of long bones most commonly seen in tibia, femur, humerus; treat with NSAIDs; watch for limb-length discrepancy
Leri-Weil dyschondrosteosis	*SHOX* gene tip of sex chromosome; autosomal dominant	Mildly short stature, mesomelic shortening, Madelung deformity
Menke syndrome and occipital horn syndrome	Both are copper transporter defects; Menke syndrome is X-linked recessive	Menke syndrome: kinky hair Occipital horn syndrome: bony projections from the occiput

DDH = developmental dysplasia of the hip, EVC = Ellis-van Creveld, MED = multiple epiphyseal dysplasia, OA = osteoarthritis, SED = spondyloepiphyseal dysplasia.

c. Epiphyseal closure is delayed and abnormal, metaphyseal flaring is present, and early-onset osteoarthritis is common.

3. Evaluation

a. Cervical instability is common, and flexion-extension radiographs should be obtained (**Figure 2, A** and **B**).

b. Valgus, varus, or windswept bowing of the lower extremities may be present.

c. Joints may demonstrate hyperlaxity early in life but later develop flexion contractures and early osteoarthritis.

d. Platyspondyly is always present, but is not associated with spinal stenosis.

4. Treatment

a. Cervical instability should be stabilized (**Figure 2, C**).

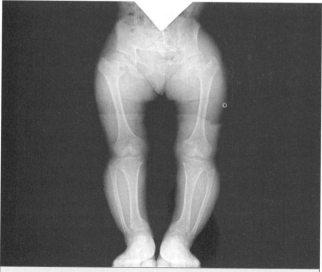

Figure 1   Weight-bearing hip-to-ankle AP radiograph of a child with achondroplasia demonstrates the classic lower extremity features of a "champagne glass" pelvic outlet and genu varum.

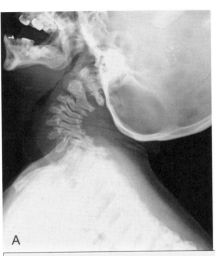
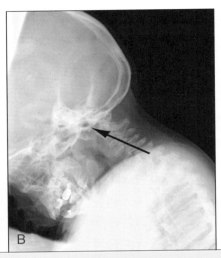
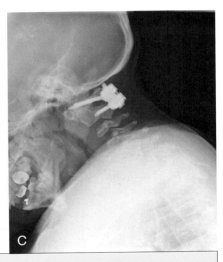

Figure 2 Radiographs of the cervical spine of a patient with Hurler syndrome who had cervical instability that was corrected surgically. **A,** Lateral extension view demonstrates cervical instability. **B,** Lateral flexion view shows the widened atlanto-dens interval (arrow). **C,** Postoperative lateral flexion view shows a stable atlanto-dens interval.

   b. Symptomatic limb bowing should be surgically corrected, but its recurrence is common and osteoarthritis is progressive.

C. Diastrophic dysplasia (**Table 1**)

   1. Overview—Short-limbed dwarfism is apparent from birth. Other common findings include cleft palate, clubfoot, hip dysplasia, cauliflower ears, and hitchhiker thumbs (**Figure 3**).

   2. Pathoanatomy

     a. An autosomal recessive trait

     b. Caused by a mutation in sulfate transport protein that primarily affects cartilage matrix. Present in 1 in 70 Finnish citizens.

   3. Evaluation

     a. Cleft palate is present in 60% of affected individuals.

     b. Cauliflower ears are present in 80% of affected individuals and develop after birth from cystic swellings in the ear cartilage (**Figure 4, A**).

     c. Cervical kyphosis and thoracolumbar scoliosis are often present.

     d. Joint contractures (hip flexion, genu valgum with dislocated patellae) and rigid clubfoot or skewfoot are often present.

   4. Treatment

     a. Surgery is indicated for progressive spinal deformity or cord compromise; the cervical kyphosis in diastrophic dysplasia often resolves spontaneously.

     b. Surgery is also indicated for progressive, symp-

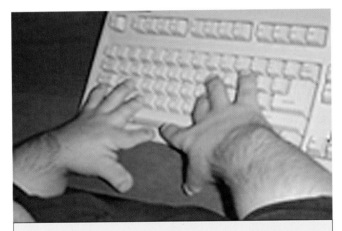

Figure 3 Photograph of the hands of a child with diastrophic dysplasia. Note the hitchhiker thumbs. (Courtesy of Ms. Vita Gagne, from the *2004 Diastrophic Dysplasia* booklet.)

tomatic lower-extremity deformity; however, recurrence of deformity after surgery is common.

     c. Compressive wrapping is used for cystic swelling of the ears (**Figure 4, B**).

D. Cleidocranial dysostosis (**Table 1**)

   1. Overview—Proportionate dwarfism characterized by mildly short stature, a broad forehead, and absent clavicles

   2. Pathoanatomy

     a. An autosomal dominant trait

     b. Caused by a defect in core-binding factor α 1 (CBFA-1), which is a transcription factor for

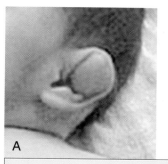
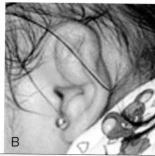

Figure 4 Photographs of the ear of a child with diastrophic dysplasia. **A,** The classic cauliflower ear appearance is observed in the neonate. **B,** The same ear several years later, after early treatment with compression bandages. (Courtesy of Ms. Vita Gagne, from the *2004 Diastrophic Dysplasia* booklet.)

osteocalcin; additionally, the *RUNX2* gene is abnormal.

  c. Affects intramembranous ossification of the skull, clavicles, and pelvis.

3. Evaluation

  a. Manifestations include delayed closure of the cranial sutures with frontal bossing, and delayed eruption of the permanent teeth.

  b. Aplasia of the clavicles is present, with ability to appose the shoulders in front of the chest.

  c. The symphysis pubis is widened.

  d. Coxa vara may be present.

  e. Shortening of the middle phalanges of the long, ring, and little fingers is seen.

4. Treatment

  a. Progressive and/or symptomatic coxa vara is treated with valgus intertrochanteric osteotomy.

  b. The other features of cleidocranial dysostosis are treated supportively.

E. Multiple epiphyseal dysplasia (MED) (**Table 1**)

1. Overview

  a. Proportionate dwarfisim with involvement of multiple epiphyses but without spinal involvement.

  b. Often diagnosed in midchildhood

2. Pathoanatomy

  a. An autosomal dominant trait

  b. Genes identified as causing MED include the gene; the gene for collagen type IX, alpha 2 (*COL9A2*), which encodes a chain for type IX collagen (a link protein for type II collagen);

and a similar, recently discovered gene, *COL9A3*.

3. Evaluation

  a. Manifestations include multiple abnormal epiphyses.

  b. Shortened metacarpals and metatarsals are present.

  c. Valgus knees with a double-layer patella are found (**Figure 5, A**).

  d. Mild to severe epiphyseal involvement may be present; the long-term prognosis ranges from mild joint problems to end-stage osteoarthritis with severe joint contractures at a young age.

  e. No spinal involvement

  f. Multiple epiphyseal dysplasia must be ruled out for or any patients with bilateral Legg-Calvé-Perthes disease.

4. Treatment

  a. Progressive genu valgum can be managed by growth modulation or osteotomy (**Figure 5, B**).

  b. Painful, stiff joints are managed with physical therapy and NSAIDs; end-stage osteoarthritis is treated with joint arthroplasty.

F. Spondyloepiphyseal dysplasia (SED)

1. Overview—Proportionate dwarfism with spinal involvement and a barrel chest

2. Pathoanatomy

  a. The most common autosomal dominant form of SED is congenital SED, which is apparent from birth and caused by mutations in the *COL2A1* gene, which encodes type II collagen, found in articular cartilage and the vitreous humor of the eyes. The proliferative zone of the growth plates is affected.

  b. A rarer, X-linked recessive form of SED is SED tarda (**Table 1**), which is more mild than congenital SED, has a later onset (ages 8 to 10 years), and is thought to involve the gene for SED tarda (*SEDL*).

3. Evaluation

  a. Cervical instability is common in both congenital SED and SED tarda, and flexion-extension radiographs of the cervical spine should be used to examine for its presence.

  b. Platyspondyly and delayed epiphyseal ossification, as well as premature osteoarthritis, are present in both congenital SED and SED tarda.

  c. Congenital SED is also marked by the presence of coxa vara, genu valgum, planovalgus feet,

5: Pediatrics

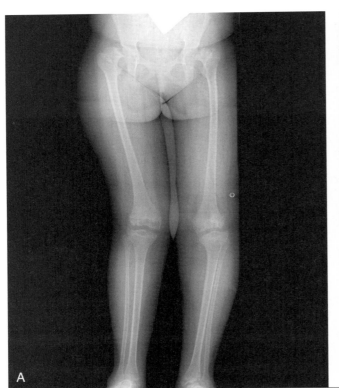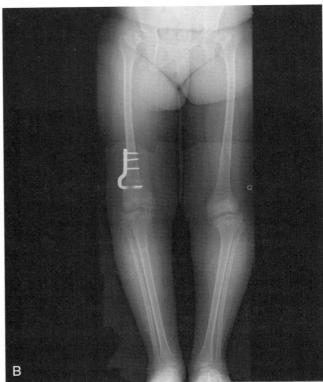

Figure 5   Radiographs of a patient with spondyloepiphyseal dysplasia. **A,** Preoperative AP weight-bearing hip-to-ankle radiograph demonstrates classic epiphyseal irregularities and substantial right genu valgum. **B,** Postoperative AP weight-bearing hip-to-ankle radiograph of the same patient following distal femoral osteotomy to correct varus deformity.

retinal detachment, myopia, and hearing loss.

   d. No bowing of the lower limb is present in SED tarda, but dislocated hips are sometimes seen.

4. Treatment

   a. Cervical instability should be stabilized.

   b. Progressive, symptomatic deformity of the lower extremities should be corrected with osteotomy, with care taken to assess the entire limb for deformities in joints above and below the affected joints, and recognition that treatment for early osteoarthritis and joint arthroplasty are likely to be needed.

II. Mucopolysaccharidoses

A. Overview

1. The mucopolysaccharidoses (MPS) (**Table 2**) disorders have a wide clinical spectrum of manifestations, with initial normal development followed by the development of cognitive and /or somatic manifestations.

2. All patients with MPS have short stature; additional features vary but often include corneal clouding, an enlarged skull, bullet-shaped phalanges, mental retardation, visceromegaly, upper-airway obstruction, cardiac disorders, cervical instability, genu valgum, and late-onset developmental dysplasia of the hip.

B. Pathoanatomy

1. MPS disorders are lysosomal storage diseases that result in the intracellular accumulation of mucopolysaccharides in multiple organs.

2. All are autosomal recessive traits except MPS II (Hunter syndrome), which is an X-linked recessive trait.

C. Evaluation

1. Urine screening can determine which MPS breakdown products are present.

2. If MPS is clinically suspected, a skeletal survey may be performed.

3. The diagnosis of MPS is confirmed by an assay for enzyme activity in skin fibroblast culture or white blood cells.

4. Prenatal screening (chorionic villous sampling) should be performed if a sibling has a known gene mutation.

Table 2		
Mucopolysaccharidoses Subtypes		
Subtype	**Cause**	**Prognosis**
Type I H (Hurler syndrome) Type I HS (Hurler-Scheie syndrome) Type I S (Scheie syndrome)	Alpha-L-iduronidase deficiency	Type I H: death in first decade of life Type I HS: death in third decade of life Type I S: good survival
Type II (Hunter syndrome)	Sulpho iduronate sulphatase deficiency	Death in second decade of life
Type III (Sanfilippo syndrome)	Multiple enzyme deficiency	Death in second decade of life
Type IV (Morquio syndrome)	Type A (galactosamine-6-sulfate sulphatase deficiency) Type B (beta-galactosidase deficiency)	More severe involvement in patients with type IV A than in those with type IV B; survival into adulthood is possible
Type VI (Maroteaux-Lamy syndrome)	Arylsulphatase B deficiency	Poor survival with severe form
Type VII (Sly syndrome)	Beta-glycuronidase deficiency	Poor survival

Reproduced from Mackenzie WG, Ballock RT: Genetic diseases and skeletal dysplasias, in Vaccaro AR, ed: *Orthopaedic Knowledge Update,* ed 8. Rosemont, IL American Academy of Orthopaedic Surgeons, 2005, pp 663-675.

D. Treatment

1. Medical management

    a. Hematopoietic stem cell transplantation is used to treat MPS I (Hurler syndrome).

    b. Intravenous enzyme replacement therapy is used to treat attenuated MPS I and also shows promise in MPS II and MPS VI, although it does not affect neurocognitive function.

2. Surgical management

    a. Surgical stabilization is indicated for cervical instability (often atlantoaxial) and progressive gibbus deformity (in MPS I).

    b. Hip dysplasia is present in several types of MPS and typically requires surgical management that includes pelvic osteotomies with possible proximal femoral osteotomies.

    c. Genu valgum may respond to early growth modulation, although osteotomies are often necessary in patients with limited growth potential (**Figure 2, C**).

    d. Carpal tunnel syndrome is common in MPS and often requires carpal tunnel release with tenosynovectomy and A1 pulley releases if trigger digits present.

5: Pediatrics

Top Testing Facts

1. Achondroplasia is the most common skeletal dysplasia.

2. Achondroplasia is caused by an autosomal dominant mutation in *FGFR-3*; 90% of these mutations are sporadic.

3. The most common disabling feature of achondroplasia in the adult is lumbar stenosis caused by a decreased interpedicular distance and shortened pedicles.

4. The most serious complications of achondroplasia in the infant and toddler are stenosis of the cervical spine and foramen magnum, which may cause apnea, weakness, and sudden death.

5. Achondroplasia affects the proliferative zone of the physis.

6. Pseudochondroplasia is associated with a mutation in *COMP* on chromosome 19; phenotypic features of this disorder are similar to those in achondroplasia but with normal facies.

7. Atlantoaxial instability is common in pseudoachondroplasia, SED, MPS, trisomy 21, and McKusick-type metaphyseal dysplasia.

8. Cauliflower ears, clubfoot, and hitchhiker thumbs are characteristic of diastrophic dysplasia.

9. Subluxation of the radial head is common in both achondroplasia and nail-patella syndrome.

10. Almost one-third of adults with nail-patella syndrome develop renal failure and glaucoma.

11. Patients with mucopolysaccharidoses (MPS disorders) often have upper cervical instability and progressive kyphosis.

12. Patients with MPS disorders have progressive orthopaedic deformity, including late-onset developmental dysplasia of the hip, and progressive organ dysfunction, including cardiac arrhythmias that are not present at birth.

Bibliography

Ain MC, Chaichana KL, Schkrohowsky JG: Retrospective study of cervical arthrodesis in patients with various types of skeletal dysplasia. *Spine (Phila Pa 1976)* 2006;31(6): E169-E174.

Aldegheri R, Dall'Oca C: Limb lengthening in short stature patients. *J Pediatr Orthop B* 2001;10(3):238-247.

Beguiristáin JL, de Rada PD, Barriga A: Nail-patella syndrome: Long term evolution. *J Pediatr Orthop B* 2003;12(1): 13-16.

Bethem D, Winter RB, Lutter L, et al: Spinal disorders of dwarfism: Review of the literature and report of eighty cases. *J Bone Joint Surg Am* 1981;63(9):1412-1425.

Cooper SC, Flaitz CM, Johnston DA, Lee B, Hecht JT: A natural history of cleidocranial dysplasia. *Am J Med Genet* 2001;104(1):1-6.

Carten M, Gagne V: Diastrophic dysplasia. 2004. http://pixelscapes.com/ddhelp/Diastrophic-Dysplasia.pdf. Accessed June 29, 2007.

Fassier F, Hamdy RC: Arthogrypotic syndromes and osteochondrodysplasias, in Abel MF, ed: *Orthopaedic Knowledge Update: Pediatrics*, ed 3. Rosemont, IL, American Academy of Orthopaedic Surgeons, 2006, pp 137-151.

Goldberg MJ: *The Dysmorphic Child: An Orthopedic Perspective*. New York, NY, Raven Press, 1987.

Mackenzie WG, Ballock RT: Genetic diseases and skeletal dysplasias, in Vaccaro AR, ed: *Orthopaedic Knowledge Update*, ed 8. Rosemont, IL, American Academy of Orthopaedic Surgeons, 2005, pp 663-675.

Sponseller PD, Ain MC: The skeletal dysplasias, in Morrissy RT, Weinstein SL, eds: *Lovell and Winter's Pediatric Orthopaedics*, ed 6. Philadelphia, PA, Lippincott Williams & Wilkins, 2006, pp 205-250.

Taybi H, Lachman RS: *Radiology of Syndromes, Metabolic Disorders, and Skeletal Dysplasias*, ed 4. St. Louis, MO, Mosby-Year Book, 1996.

Unger S: A genetic approach to the diagnosis of skeletal dysplasia. *Clin Orthop Relat Res* 2002;401:32-38.

Chapter 54

Pediatric Musculoskeletal Disorders and Syndromes

Samantha Spencer, MD

I. Neurofibromatosis

A. Overview

1. Neurofibromatosis (NF) occurs in two forms: NF1 and NF2.

2. NF is a common single-gene disorder (1 in 3,000 births).

B. Pathoanatomy

1. The mutation in NF is in the neurofibromin gene.

2. Neurofibromin regulates cell growth by modulating Ras signaling, which mediates the activation of genes involved in cell growth, differentiation, and survival.

3. The malignant transformation of NF to neurofibrosarcoma is possible if there is a second mutation in the normal allele of an NF gene pair.

C. Evaluation and diagnostic criteria (**Table 1**)

D. Treatment

1. Anterolateral bowing of the tibia (**Figure 1**) is often treated with prophylactic bracing with a total contact orthosis to prevent pseudarthrosis. Fifty percent of children with anterolateral bowing of the tibia have NF, although such bowing is present in only 10% of children with NF.

2. Pseudarthrosis in patients with NF may be treated with bone grafting and intramedullary rodding; some patients will later require a vascularized bone graft or bone transport through distraction osteogenesis. Amputation is sometimes necessary.

3. Plexiform neurofibromas (in 40% of patients with NF1) may cause limb overgrowth. Limb equalization procedures are indicated for children with projected limb-length discrepancies exceeding 2 cm.

4. Scoliosis

a. Scoliosis is common in patients with NF.

b. Nondystrophic scoliosis in NF is treated in the same way as adolescent idiopathic scoliosis.

c. Dystrophic scoliosis is short (involving four to six levels of the spine), has sharp curves, and often occurs in children younger than 6 years.

- It is characterized by the scalloping of vertebral end plates, foraminal enlargement, and penciling of ribs.

- When three or more ribs are penciled, 87% of scoliosis curves progress rapidly.

- Dystrophic scoliosis in NF is resistant to treatment by bracing and is treated with early anterior and posterior fusion.

- A preoperative MRI should be obtained in patients with NF to rule out dural ectasia and intraspinal neurofibromas.

Table 1

Diagnostic Criteria for Neurofibromatosis Type 1

Six or more café-au-lait spots, with greatest diameter 5 mm in prepubertal and 15 mm in postpubertal patients

Two or more neurofibromas of any type or one plexiform neurofibroma

Axillary freckling

Optic glioma

Two or more Lisch nodules (iris hamartomas)

A distinctive osseous lesion

A first-degree relative with neurofibromatosis type 1

Reproduced from Mackenzie WG, Ballock RT: Genetic diseases and skeletal dysplasias, in Vaccaro AR, ed: *Orthopaedic Knowledge Update*, ed 8. Rosemont, IL, American Academy of Orthopaedic Surgeons, 2005, pp 663-675.

Dr. Spencer or an immediate family member serves as a board member, owner, officer, or committee member of the American Academy of Orthopaedic Surgeons, the Massachusetts Orthopaedic Association, and the Pediatric Orthopaedic Society of North America.

5: Pediatrics

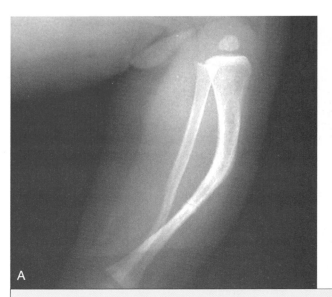
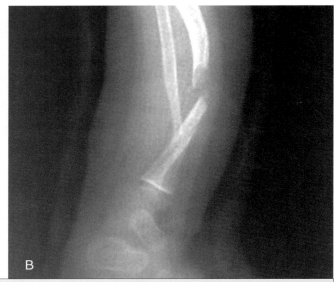

Figure 1   Lateral radiographs of congenital pseudarthrosis of the tibia. **A,** View of the tibia and fibula in a child with neuro-fibromatosis demonstrating anterolateral bowing of a dystrophic tibia. **B,** View of the same child after the bowing of the tibia has progressed to true pseudarthrosis. (Reproduced from Mackenzie WG, Ballock RT: Genetic diseases and skeletal dysplasias, in Vaccaro AR, ed: *Orthopaedic Knowledge Update*, ed 8. Rosemont, IL, American Academy of Orthopaedic Surgeons, 2005, pp 663-675.)

II. Connective Tissue Diseases

A. Marfan syndrome

1. Overview

   a. Marfan syndrome (**Table 2**) is a disorder of connective tissue that affects its elasticity and results in joint laxity, scoliosis, and cardiac valve and aortic dilatation, among other effects.

   b. Its incidence is 1 in 10,000, without any ethnic or sex predilections.

2. Pathoanatomy

   a. Marfan syndrome can result from a mutation in the fibrillin-1 gene (*FBN1*) on chromosome 15q21; multiple mutations have been identified.

   b. Twenty-five percent of occurrences result from new mutations.

3. Evaluation

   a. Affected individuals are often tall and thin, with long limbs (dolichostenomelia), spider-like fingers (arachnodactyly), and joint hypermobility.

   b. Positive wrist sign (Walker sign)—The thumb and little finger overlap when used to encircle the opposite wrist.

   c. Positive thumb sign (Steinberg sign)—When adducted across the fisted hand, the thumb

protrudes on the ulnar side of the hand.

   d. The arm span–to-height ratio exceeds 1.05.

   e. Cardiac defects, especially dilatation and later dissection of the aortic root, are common; accordingly, if Marfan syndrome is suspected, an echocardiogram and a cardiology consultation should be obtained.

   f. Scoliosis is seen in 60% to 70% of patients with Marfan syndrome and is difficult to brace. Because dural ectasia is common (> 60% of patients), MRI should be obtained before surgery (**Figure 2**).

   g. Pectus excavatum and spontaneous pneumothoraces can occur (**Figure 3**).

   h. Superior dislocation of the lens (ectopia lentis) and myopia are common. (Inferior dislocation of the lens is seen in homocysteinuria.)

   i. Protrusio acetabuli and severe pes planovalgus are seen in the lower extremities.

4. Classification

   a. The Ghent system of classification for Marfan syndrome requires the presence of one major diagnostic criterion in each of two different organ systems and involvement of a third organ system.

   b. Patients with the MASS (mitral valve prolapse, aortic root diameter at upper limits of normal, stretch marks, and skeletal manifestations of Marfan syndrome) phenotype do not have ec-

Table 2

Marfan Syndrome

System	Major Criteria	Minor Criteria
Musculoskeletal[a]	Pectus carinatum; pectus excavatum requiring surgery; dolichostenomelia; wrist and thumb signs; scoliosis greater than 20° or spondylolisthesis; reduced elbow extension; pes planus; protrusio acetabuli	Moderately severe pectus excavatum; joint hypermobility; highly arched palate with crowding of teeth; facies (dolichocephaly, malar hypoplasia, enophthalmos, retrognathia, downslanting palpebral fissures)
Ocular[b]	Ectopia lentis	Abnormally flat cornea; increased axial length of globe; hypoplastic iris or hypoplastic ciliary muscle causing decreased miosis
Cardiovascular[c]	Dilatation of ascending aorta ± aortic regurgitation, involving sinuses of Valsalva; dissection of ascending aorta	Mitral valve prolapse ± regurgitation
Family/Genetic history[d]	Parent, child, or sibling meets diagnostic criteria; mutation in *FBN1* known to cause Marfan syndrome; inherited haplotype around *FBN1* associated with Marfan syndrome in family	None
Skin and integument[e]	None	Stretch marks not associated with pregnancy, weight gain, or repetitive stress; recurrent incisional hernias
Dura[d]	Lumbosacral dural ectasia	None
Pulmonary[e]	None	Spontaneous pneumothorax or apical blebs

[a]Two or more major or one major plus two minor criteria required for involvement.

[b]At least two minor criteria required for involvement.

[c]One major or minor criterion required for involvement.

[d]One major criterion required for involvement.

[e]One minor criterion required for involvement.

Adapted from Miller NH: Connective tissue disorders, in Koval KJ, ed: *Orthopaedic Knowledge Update*, ed 7. Rosemont, IL, American Academy of Orthopaedic Surgeons, 2002, pp 201-207.

topia lentis or aortic dissection and have a better prognosis; they are not considered to have true Marfan syndrome.

5. Treatment

   a. Nonsurgical

   - Beta blockers are used to treat mitral valve prolapse and aortic dilatation in Marfan syndrome.

   - Bracing is used to treat early scoliosis and pes planovalgus.

   b. Surgical

   - For progressive scoliosis, long scoliosis fusion is indicated to treat junctional problems (with a preoperative cardiac workup and preoperative MRI to assess dural ectasia). However, this procedure is followed by a high rate of pseudarthrosis.

   - For progressive protrusio acetabuli, closure of the triradiate cartilage has been described.

   - For progressive, symptomatic pes planovalgus, corrective surgery is indicated.

B. Ehlers-Danlos syndrome (**Table 3**)

   1. Ehlers-Danlos syndrome (EDS) is a connective tissue disorder in which there is hypermobility of the skin and joints.

   2. Pathoanatomy

   a. From 40% to 50% of patients with EDS have a mutation in *COL5A1* or *COL5A2*, both of which encode type V collagen, which is important for the proper assembly of collagen fibrils in the skin matrix and the basement membranes of tissues. These mutations are responsible for the classic form of EDS and are autosomal dominant.

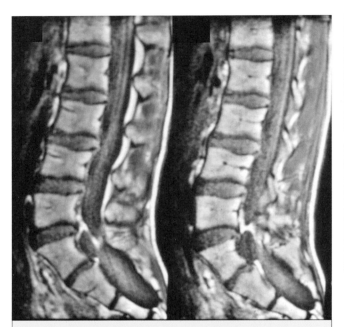

Figure 2 Lateral MRI of the lower spine in a patient with Marfan syndrome demonstrates dural ectasia of the lumbosacral junction. (Courtesy of M. Timothy Hresko, MD, Boston, MA.)

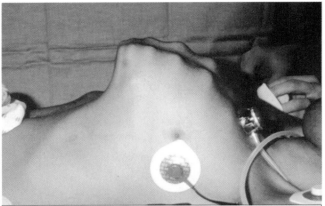

Figure 3 Photograph demonstrates pectus deformity in a patient with Marfan syndrome. (Courtesy of M. Timothy Hresko, MD, Boston, MA.)

b. EDS, characterized by a defect in type VI collagen, is an autosomal recessive condition that results from a mutation in the gene for lysyl hydroxylase, an enzyme important in the cross-linking of collagen. Severe kyphoscoliosis is characteristic of this form of EDS.

c. The form of EDS syndrome characterized by a defect in type IV collagen is an autosomal dominant condition that results from a mutation in *COL3A1* that generates abnormal collagen III. Arterial, intestinal, and uterine rupture are seen in this form of EDS.

3. Evaluation

a. The skin of patients with EDS is velvety and fragile. Severe scarring from minor trauma is common.

b. The joints are hypermobile, particularly the shoulders, patellae, and ankles.

c. Up to one-third of patients have aortic root dilatation; therefore, an echocardiogram and a cardiac evaluation are advised.

d. Patients with the vascular subtype of EDS can have spontaneous visceral or arterial ruptures.

4. Treatment

a. Lax joints should not be treated surgically; soft-tissue procedures are unlikely to be effective.

b. Scoliosis is most common in type VI EDS (Figure 4) and is usually progressive. Surgery is indicated for progressive curves, and longer fusions are necessary to prevent junctional problems.

c. Chronic musculoskeletal pain is present in more than 50% of patients with EDS and should be treated supportively if at all possible.

III. Arthritides

A. Rheumatoid (seropositive) arthritis (RA; **Table 4**)

1. Overview—RA is an autoimmune inflammatory arthritis that causes joint destruction at a younger age than does osteoarthritis (OA).

2. Pathoanatomy

a. In RA, the synovium thickens and fills with B cells, T cells, and macrophages, which erode the joint cartilage.

b. The disease process is autoimmune and systemic.

3. Evaluation

a. Rheumatoid factor (RF) is found in only one-half of patients with RA and in 5% of the general population; however, it may help identify more aggressive cases of RF.

b. The prevalence of RA in the general US population is 0.5% to 1.0%, and the lifetime risk of acquiring RA is 4% in women and 3% in men. The concordance for RA in monozygotic twins is only 12% to 15%.

c. The physical examination of patients with RA reveals multiple hot, swollen, and stiff joints. Subcutaneous calcified nodules and iridis may be present.

Table 3

Ehlers-Danlos Syndrome Classification

Villefranche Classification (1998)	Berlin Classification (1988)	Genetics	Major Symptomatic Criteria	Biochemical Defects (Minor Criteria)
Classic	Type I (gravis) Type II (mitis)	AD	Hyperextensible skin, atrophic scars, joint hypermobility	*COL5A1, COL5A2* mutations (40% to 50% of families); mutations in type V collagen
Hypermobility	Type III (hypermobile)	AD	Velvety soft skin, small and large joint hypermobility; tendency for dislocation, chronic pain, scoliosis	Unknown
Vascular	Type IV (vascular)	AD (rarely) AR	Arterial, intestinal, and uterine fragility; rupture; thin translucent skin; extensive bruising	*COL3A1* mutation, abnormal type III collagen structure of synthesis
Kyphoscoliosis	Type VI (ocular scoliotic)	AR	Severe hypotonia at birth, progressive infantile scoliosis, generalized joint laxity, scleral fragility, globe rupture	Lysyl hydroxylase deficiency, mutations in *PLOD* gene
Arthrochalasis	Type VIIA, VIIB	AD	Congenital bilateral hip dislocation, hypermobility, soft skin	Deletion of type I collagen exons that encode for N-terminal propeptide (*COL1A1, COL1A2*)
Dermatosparaxis	Type VIIIC	AR	Severe sagging or redundant skin	Mutations in type I collagen N peptidase

AD = autosomal dominant, AR = autosomal recessive.

Reproduced from D'Astous JL, Carroll KL: Connective tissue disorders, in Vaccaro AR, ed: *Orthopaedic Knowledge Update*, ed 8. Rosemont, IL, American Academy of Orthopaedic Surgeons, 2005, p 246.

   d. Radiographic findings include symmetric joint space narrowing, periarticular erosions, and osteopenia.

4. Treatment

   a. Nonsurgical—Most treatment of RA is now medical and provided by rheumatologists, with a combination of NSAIDs and disease-modifying antirheumatic drugs (DMARDs). Most DMARDs are immunosuppressive and should be stopped before orthopaedic procedures are undertaken, and the patient's cell count should be checked to avoid neutropenia.

   b. Surgical—The surgical treatment of RA involves synovectomy and joint realignment early in the disease and joint arthroplasty in the later stages.

B. Juvenile idiopathic arthritis (JIA, previously known as juvenile rheumatoid arthritis [JRA])

   1. Definition—JIA is an autoimmune inflammatory arthritis of the joints of children that lasts for more than 6 weeks.

   2. Pathoanatomy

   a. As in adult RA, autoimmune erosion of cartilage occurs in JIA.

   b. Positive test results for RF and antinuclear antibody (ANA) may indicate a more aggressive course of JIA.

   3. Types of JIA

   a. Systemic JIA/JRA (Still disease)

   • A rash, high fever, multiple inflamed joints, and an acute presentation are typical.

   • Anemia and/or a high white blood cell count may be present; platelets, erythrocyte sedimentation rate, and C-reactive protein level are elevated.

   • Serositis, hepatosplenomegaly, lymphade-

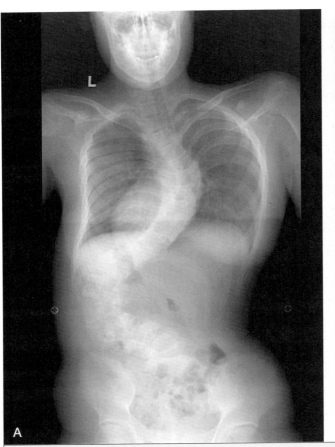
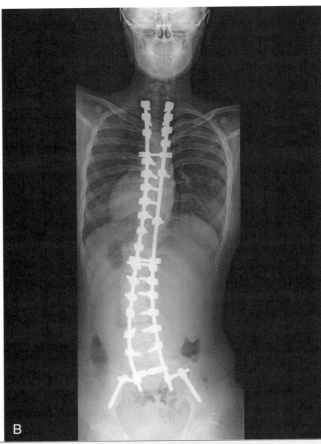

Figure 4   PA radiographs of the spine in a patient with type VI Ehlers-Danlos syndrome. **A,** Preoperative view demonstrates severe scoliosis. **B,** Postoperative view demonstrates the long fusion needed to treat connective tissue syndromes.

nopathy, and pericarditis may be present.

- Infection must be ruled out.

- The disease usually presents at age 5 to 10 years; girls and boys are affected equally.

- Has the poorest long-term prognosis of any form of JIA

- Is the least common type of JIA (comprising 10% to 15% of all cases)

b. Oligoarticular JIA (previously known as pauci-articular JRA)

- Is the most common type of JIA (comprising 30% to 40% of all JIA)

- Four or fewer joints are involved; usually large joints, commonly the knees and ankles

- The peak age of occurrence is 2 to 3 years; the disease is four times more common in girls.

- A limp that improves during the day is typical.

- Uveitis is present in 20% of patients. An

ophthalmologic evaluation is needed every 4 months for patients who are ANA-positive, and every 6 months for those who are ANA-negative.

- Limb-length discrepancy is an effect of oligoarticular JIA, with the affected side often longer than the unaffected side.

- Oligoarticular JIA has the best prognosis of any form of JIA for long-term remission (70%).

c. Polyarticular JIA/polyarticular JRA

- Five or more joints are involved; often, small joints (hand/wrist) are affected.

- Uveitis is sometimes present but is less common than in oligoarticular JIA.

- Polyarticular disease is more common in girls than in boys.

- The prognosis is good, with a 60% frequency of remission.

4. Treatment

Table 4

Differentiating Osteoarthritis From Rheumatoid Arthritis

	Osteoarthritis	Rheumatoid Arthritis
Age	Older	Younger
Physical findings	IP joints affected in hands, gradual stiffness/loss of motion in affected joints (most common in knees/hips), oligoarticular	MCP joints affected in hands with ulnar deviation, polyarticular arthritis, joint effusions, warmth; rheumatoid nodules on extensor surfaces
Pathology	Cartilage fibrillation, increased water content of the cartilage, increased collagen I/II ratio, higher friction and lower elasticity	Thickened synovial pannus that cascades over the joint surface; numerous T cells and B cells and some plasma cells seen
Radiographic findings	Osteophytes, subchondral sclerosis, subchondral cyst formation; superolateral joint space narrowing in the hip and the medial compartment of the knee commonly seen	Symmetric joint space narrowing with osteopenia and periarticular erosions; protrusio in the hip
Pathophysiology	Chondrocytes release matrix metalloproteinases that degrade the extracellular matrix; cytokines such as IL-1 and TNF-α also are found in the joint fluid. These cause prostaglandin release, which may cause pain.	Autoimmune arthritis in which the joint synovium triggers a T cell–mediated attack resulting in release of IL-1 and TNF-α, which degrade cartilage
Associated findings	Obesity is associated with an increased risk of knee (but not hip) and hand OA, particularly in women.	Basilar invagination, eye involvement, entrapment neuropathies, pleural/pericardial effusions

IL = interleukin, IP = interphalangeal, MCP = metacarpophalangeal, TNF = tumor necrosis factor.

a. Limb-length discrepancy may require epiphysiodesis; arthroplasty may be needed in adulthood for destroyed joints.

b. Medical management by a rheumatologist, with NSAIDs or DMARDs, is common in JIA.

c. An arthrocentesis or synovial biopsy may be needed for diagnosis.

d. Steroid injections and synovectomy may prove beneficial if medical management fails.

C. Seronegative spondyloarthopathies

1. Definition—Autoimmune arthropathies in which RF is absent.

2. Types of seronegative spondyloarthropathies

a. Ankylosing spondylitis

- Age of onset is 15 to 35 years, with males more commonly affected than females; seronegative spondyloarthropathies are characterized by morning stiffness and low back pain.

- Sacroiliitis and progressive fusion of the spine ("bamboo spine") are typical.

- Peripheral joint arthritis, usually unilateral, is common.

- Uveitis occurs in up to 40% of patients; cardiac and pulmonary disease also can occur.

Oral aphthous ulcers and fatigue are common.

- Aggressive physical therapy and NSAIDs are indicated for treatment.

- Spinal fractures are highly unstable and accompanied by high rates of neurologic injury.

- HLA-B27 is found in 95% of white and 50% of African American patients with ankylosing spondylitis, although less than 5% of all HLA-B27–positive individuals have ankylosing spondylitis.

b. Psoriatic arthritis

- Typical psoriatic skin plaques (scaly extensor surface, silvery plaques) usually precede the development of arthritis, but in 20% of patients, the arthritis occurs first.

- A common radiographic finding is a "pencil-in-cup" deformity of the hand, which is an X-linked recessive trait.

- Nail pitting and dactylitis are common.

c. Reactive arthritis (Reiter syndrome)

- Reactive arthritis is triggered by an infectious disease, such as a bacterial infection with *Chlamydia, Yersinia, Salmonella, Campylobacter,* or *Shigella,* that causes the deposition of an autoimmune complex in

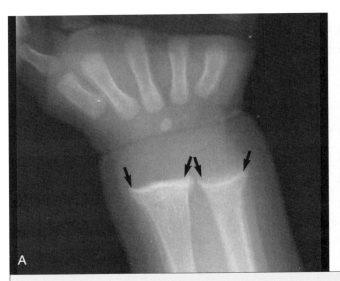
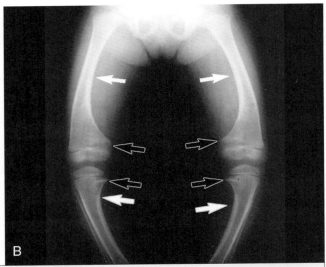

Figure 5 Radiographic features of rickets. **A,** PA view of the wrist in a child with rickets shows radial and ulnar metaphyseal fraying and cupping (arrows). **B,** AP view of the lower extremities in a child with rickets demonstrates bowing of the femora and tibiae (white arrows), as well as metaphyseal widening and irregularity (black arrows). (Reproduced from Johnson TR: General orthopaedics, in Johnson TR, Steinbach LS, eds: *Essentials of Musculoskeletal Imaging.* Rosemont, IL, American Academy of Orthopaedic Surgeons, 2004, p 78.)

the joints (commonly the knee), which results in painful swelling.

- The mnemonic "Can't see, can't pee, can't climb a tree" is useful for remembering the conjunctivitis and dysuria associated with reactive arthritis. The disease may cause oral ulcers and a rash on the hands and feet.

- The condition underlying the arthritic reaction should be treated, and the arthritis should be managed supportively.

d. Enteropathic arthropathies—Arthropathies associated with inflammatory bowel disease, such as Crohn disease or ulcerative colitis.

- These arthropathies occur in 20% of patients with inflammatory bowel disease.

- They should be managed supportively.

IV. Other Conditions With Musculoskeletal Involvement

A. Rickets

1. Overview

    a. Results from defective mineralization in growing bone from a variety of causes.

    b. The most common form of rickets in North America is hypophosphatemic rickets.

2. Pathoanatomy

    a. Calcium/phosphate homeostasis is disturbed,

resulting in poor calcification of the cartilage matrix of growing long bones.

    b. Radiographic features (**Figure 5**) include widened osteoid seams, metaphyseal cupping, prominence of the rib heads (osteochondral junction [rachitic rosary]), bowing (particularly genu varum), and fractures.

    c. Microscopically, the zone of cartilage proliferation in the growth plate is disordered and elongated.

3. Evaluation

    a. Serum Ca^{2+}, phosphorus, alkaline phosphatase, parathyroid hormone, 25-hydroxyvitamin D, and 1,25-dihydroxyvitamin D must be checked to assess the cause of a particular case of rickets.

    b. A history of breastfeeding with little sun exposure is the most likely setting for vitamin D–deficient rickets.

4. Classification/treatment (**Table 5**)

5. Surgery is indicated for lower-limb bowing that does not resolve after medical treatment of rickets; hemiepiphysiodesis or osteotomy may be indicated.

B. Trisomy 21

1. Trisomy 21 (Down syndrome) is the most common chromosomal abnormality in the United States, with an incidence of 1 in 700 live births. Its incidence increases with advanced maternal age; however, as a result of increased screening

Table 5

Most Common Types of Rickets With Associated Genetics, Features, and Treatment

Condition	Genetics	Serum Values	Associated Features	Treatment
Hypophosphatemic rickets	X-linked dominant, impaired renal phosphate absorption	Decreased phosphate; normal calcium, PTH, and vitamin D; increased alkaline phosphatase	Most common type in North America	No established medical therapy
Vitamin D–deficient rickets	Nutritional	Decreased vitamin D, calcium, and phosphate; increased PTH and alkaline phosphatase		Vitamin D replacement
Vitamin D–dependent rickets, type 1	Autosomal recessive; defect in renal 25-hydroxyvitamin D 1-α-hydroxylase	Low calcium and phosphate; normal 25-hydroxyvitamin D, very low 1,25-dihydroxyvitamin D; high alkaline phosphatase and PTH		1,25-dihydroxyvitamin D replacement
Vitamin D–dependent rickets, type 2	Defect in the intracellular receptor for 1,25-dihydroxyvitamin D	Low calcium and phosphate; high alkaline phosphatase and PTH; very high 1,25-dihydroxyvitamin D levels	Alopecia	High-dose 1,25-dihydroxy-vitamin D, calcium
Hypophosphatasia	Autosomal recessive, deficient or nonfunctional alkaline phosphatase	Increased calcium and phosphate levels; very low alkaline phosphatase levels; normal PTH and vitamin D levels	Early loss of teeth	No established medical therapy

PTH = parathyroid hormone.

and selective termination in advanced maternal age, most affected children are born to younger women.

2. Pathoanatomy—Trisomy 21 usually results from a duplication of maternal chromosome 21, with three copies of this chromosome rather than the normal diploid number.

3. Evaluation

   a. Phenotypic features include a flattened face, upward-slanting eyes with epicanthal folds, a single palmar crease, mental retardation (varies), congenital heart disease (endocardial cushion defects in 50% of patients), duodenal atresia, hypothyroidism, hearing loss, ligamentous laxity, a high incidence of leukemia/lymphoma, and diabetes and Alzheimer disease in later adult life.

   b. Spine

      • Atlantoaxial instability is present in 9% to 22% of patients with trisomy 21; it is controversial whether flexion-extension views of the cervical spine are needed before a patient with trisomy 21 can participate in sports.

      • Scoliosis in present in up to 50% of patients.

      • Spondylolisthesis is present in up to 6% of patients.

   c. Metatarsus primus varus, pes planovalgus, and hallux valgus are seen; almost 50% of patients have pes planus and 25% have hallux valgus. Management is with supportive orthotics unless very severe.

   d. Patellar dislocation, pain, and instability are common.

   e. Hip instability (often late) can occur, sometimes with only mild bone abnormality.

4. Treatment

   a. Supportive bracing is indicated for the feet (supramalleolar or University of California at Berkeley Laboratory orthoses for pes planovalgus), the knees (patellar stabilizing braces), and the hips (hip abduction braces) when clinically indicated.

   b. An atlanto-dens interval (ADI) of 5 mm or less is normal.

   c. The need for treatment of an asymptomatic ADI of 5 to 10 mm is controversial; many practitioners observe and obtain an MRI to determine whether the spinal cord is compromised.

   d. Fusion is indicated if cord compromise is seen on MRI or if the ADI exceeds 5 mm and the patient has symptoms; however, fusion has a

5: Pediatrics

high (up to 50%) complication rate.

e. Soft-tissue procedures are ineffective for correcting the orthopaedic abnormalities in trisomy 21 because of ligamentous laxity and hypotonia; therefore, if surgery is performed, bone realignment is indicated (such as periacetabular osteotomy for hip dislocation and osteotomy of the tibial tubercle for lateral patellar dislocation).

C. Osteogenesis imperfecta (OI; **Tables 6** and **7**)

1. Overview

a. The weak organic bone matrix in OI results in frequent fractures and severe bowing and deformity of the legs in the more severe types of the disease.

b. Intelligence is normal.

2. Pathoanatomy

a. Approximately 85% of OI cases result from mutations in *COL1A1* and *COL1A2* that encode type I collagen, the mainstay of the organic bone matrix. Phenotypically, these types of OI are still described using the modified Sillence classification; the mildest type I comprises 50% of patients.

- The result is bone that has a decreased number of trabeculae and decreased cortical thickness (wormian bone).

- Specific mutations in *COL1A1* and *COL1A2* are identified via the analysis of DNA in blood.

Table 6

Clinical Classification of Osteogenesis Imperfecta

Type	Features	Inheritance
I (dominant, blue sclerae)	IA: bone fragility, blue sclerae, and normal teeth IB: same as IA but with dentinogenesis imperfecta IC: more severe than IB but with normal teeth	Autosomal dominant
II (lethal, perinatal)	IIA: broad, crumpled long bones and beaded rib; generally perinatal death IIB: broad, crumpled long bones, but ribs show minimal or no beading; death variable from perinatal to several years IIC: thin, fractured, cylindrical, dysplastic long bones and thin beaded ribs; very low birth rate; stillbirth or perinatal death IID: severely ostepenic with generally well-formed skeleton; normally shaped vertebrae and pelvis; perinatal death	Autosomal dominant
III (progressive, deforming)	Multiple fractures at birth with progressive deformities, normal sclerae, and dentinogenesis imperfecta	Autosomal recessive
IV (dominant, white sclerae)	IVA: bone fragility, white sclerae, and normal teeth IVB: similar to IVA but with dentinogenesis imperfecta	Autosomal dominant

Reproduced with permission from Cole WG: The molecular pathology of osteogenesis imperfecta. *Clin Orthop* 1997;343:235-248.

Table 7

Biochemical Classification of Type I Collagen Mutations in Osteogenesis Imperfecta

Protein Feature	Category of Mutation	Clinical Phenotype
Moderate reduction of normal type I collagen in tissues	Haploinsufficiency	OI-IA
Mixture of normal and mutant type I collagen molecules in tissues	Dominant negative	OI-IB:IIA-IIC:III:IVB
Severe reduction of normal type I collagen in tissues	Dominant negative	OI-IC
Very severe reduction of normal type I collagen in tissues	Dominant negative	OI-IID

OI = osteogenesis imperfecta.

Reproduced with permission from Cole WG: The molecular pathology of osteogenesis imperfecta. *Clin Orthop* 1997;343:235-248.

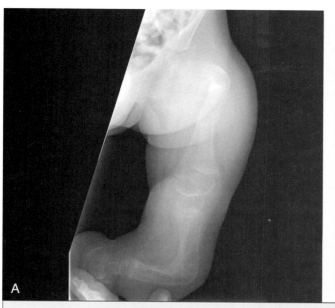
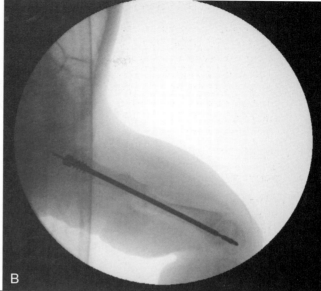

Figure 6 Images of the femur in a patient with type III osteogenesis imperfecta. **A,** Preoperative frog-lateral hip-to-ankle radiograph demonstrates femoral deformity. **B,** Postoperative frog-lateral fluoroscopic image shows osteotomies and fixation using a telescoping rod.

b. Other noncollagenous types of OI do not have mutations affecting type I collagen but are phenotypically similar to and have similar bone abnormalities seen on microscopy to those in OI types I through IV. Genetic testing can be performed for some but not all of these types.

3. Evaluation

a. Child abuse should not be ruled out in patients with OI; conversely, OI should not be ruled out in a workup for child abuse.

b. Basilar invagination and severe scoliosis may occur in OI types II and III in particular.

c. Apophyseal avulsion fractures of the olecranon are characteristic of OI; children presenting with these should be evaluated for OI.

d. Associated dentinogenesis imperfecta, hearing loss, blue sclerae, joint hyperlaxity, and wormian skull bones (a "puzzle-piece" appearance of the skull after closure of the fontanelles) are seen.

4. Treatment

a. Manage fractures with light splints and short immobilization times.

b. Bisphosphonates are used to inhibit osteoclasts, yielding increased cortical thickness with decreased fracture rates and pain.

c. For severe bowing of the limbs or recurrent fracture, intramedullary fixation is indicated as

needed. Newer fixation devices have telescoping rods to allow bone growth (**Figure 6**).

d. Progressive scoliosis/basilar invagination is treated with spinal fusion.

D. Gaucher disease

1. Overview—A disease in which an enzymatic defect results in an overaccumulation of glucocerebrosides (lipids) in many organ systems, including bone marrow and the spleen.

2. Pathoanatomy

a. A defect in the *GBA* gene encoding β-glucocerebrosidase, which breaks down glucocerebrosides, results in the accumulation of glucocerebrosides in macrophages in many organ systems.

b. An autosomal recessive condition with more than 200 mutations, although 3 alleles comprise most cases.

c. Genotype does not predict phenotype well; penetrance is highly variable.

3. Evaluation

a. Glucocerebrosidase enzyme activity in peripheral white blood cells is the most common diagnostic test; less than 30% of normal activity confirms the diagnosis. Cultured skin fibroblasts or urine also can be tested for enzyme activity. Genetic testing can be performed to assess for mutations.

b. Three forms of Gaucher disease have been

5: Pediatrics

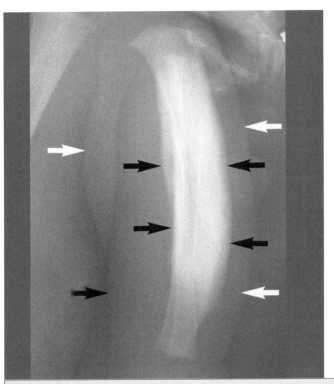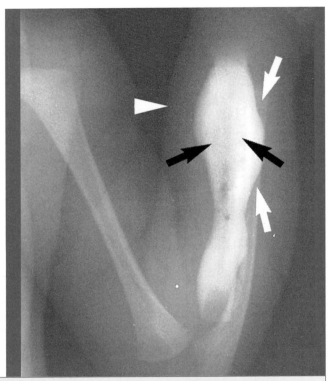

Figure 7 Radiographic features of Caffey disease. **A,** Lateral view of the tibia shows increased bone formation throughout the diaphysis (black arrows) with an increased diameter and soft-tissue swelling (white arrows). **B,** Lateral view of the forearm shows an increased diameter of the diaphysis of the radius (black arrows), extensive periosteal reaction (white arrows), and soft-tissue swelling (arrowhead). (Reproduced from Sarwark JF, Shore RM: Pediatric orthopaedics, in Johnson TR, Steinbach LS, eds: *Essentials of Musculoskeletal Imaging.* Rosemont, IL, American Academy of Orthopaedic Surgeons, 2004, p. 814.)

identified, based on age of onset. Types 2 and 3 have neurologic involvement.

- Type 1 (adult) disease is marked by easy bruising (thrombocytopenia), anemia, enlarged liver and/or spleen, and bone pain and/or fractures.

- Type 2 (infantile) disease is marked by an enlarged spleen and/or liver by age 3 months and brain involvement; this form of the disease is lethal by age 2 years.

- Type 3 (juvenile) disease onset occurs in adolescence and is marked by thrombocytopenia, anemia, enlargement of the liver and/or spleen, bone pain and/or fractures, and gradual, mild brain involvement.

   c. Radiographic findings include an Erlenmeyer flask appearance of the distal femurs (also seen in osteopetrosis), osteonecrosis of the hips and/or femoral condyles, and thinning of cortical bone.

4. Treatment

   a. Enzyme replacement therapy is now available for Gaucher disease and works well for treat-

ing all but neurologic symptoms.

   b. Bone-marrow transplantation can be curative if performed at an early stage of disease.

E. Caffey disease (cortical hyperostosis)

1. Definition—A cortical hyperostosis of infancy (mean age of onset, younger than 9 weeks) that is self-resolving and is a diagnosis of exclusion.

2. Pathoanatomy

   a. The erythrocyte sedimentation rate and serum alkaline phosphatase concentration are elevated, but cultures for microbial pathogens are negative.

   b. Pathology shows hyperplasia of collagen fibers and fibrinoid degeneration.

3. Evaluation

   a. Bones of the jaw (mandible) and forearm (ulna) are most commonly affected, with diffuse cortical thickening, but any bone except the vertebrae and phalanges may be affected (**Figure 7**).

   b. Caffey disease is marked by fever with hyperirritability, swelling of the soft tissues, and cortical thickening of bone.

4. Treatment is supportive, with glucocorticoids sometimes used.

F. Arthrogryposis

1. Overview

a. The term arthrogryposis represents a large group of disorders that include contractures of joints present at birth.

b. Occurs in 1 out of every 3000 live births

c. Intellect is typically normal.

d. Etiology is multifactorial; decreased fetal movement is a common element.

e. Amyoplasia describes conditions in which all four extremities demonstrate joint contractures.

f. Distal arthrogryposes include those disorders that predominantly or exclusively involve the hands and feet.

   • Various subtypes of distal arthrogryposis exist.

   • Gordon and Freeman-Sheldon syndromes have craniofacial involvement and autodomal dominant inheritance patterns.

2. Pathoanatomy

a. Histologic analysis has revealed decreased muscle mass with fibrosis and fat between muscle fibers.

b. Periarticular soft tissues are thickened and fibrotic.

3. Evaluation

a. A thorough birth history and family history should be obtained.

b. Examination

   • Patient may demonstrate loss of skin creases and deep dimples over joints.

   • Muscle mass may be reduced, though subcutaneous tissue is often abundant.

   • Each joint should be examined; active and passive motion should be noted, as well as degree of contracture.

   • Upper extremities often demonstrate adducted, internally rotated shoulders with elbows often extended and wrist flexed with ulnar deviation.

   • Lower extremities may demonstrate hip flexion contractures, knee contractures and clubfeet.

      ○ Hips are dislocated in 40% of patients; an

ultrasonography and/or a pelvic radiograph may be necessary to evaluate the status of the hip joints.

      ○ Knee abnormalities are present in 70% of patients and may be either flexion or extension contractures.

      ○ Clubfoot occurs in 90% of patients.

   • Scoliosis may occur in up to 30% of patients with amyoplasia.

c. Diagnostic work up

   • Initial radiographs are normal, although adaptive changes may occur with time.

   • Electromyographic testing and muscle biopsy are of questionable diagnostic value.

4. Treatment

a. Goals of treatment in the upper extremity are to obtain motion and function for self care. Lower extremity goals are limb alignment and stability for ambulation.

b. Intervention may be necessary before adaptive changes occur in the joints.

c. A multidisciplinary team including a geneticist, physical and occupational therapists, and a physiatrist should assist in the treatment of patients with arthrogryposis.

d. Upper extremity

   • Stretching and range-of-motion exercises may be initiated during infancy, and may decrease the need for surgery.

   • Humeral derotational osteotomy may be necessary if fixed internal rotation is present.

   • If fixed elbow extension exists, posterior elbow release and tricepsplasty may be needed.

   • Wrist deformity may require proximal row carpectomy and soft-tissue balance to preserve wrist motion and prevent recurrence of deformity.

   • Thumb adductor may require release and opponensplasty.

e. Lower extremity

   • Unilateral dislocations should be treated with open reduction. Treatment of bilateral dislocations is controversial.

   • Hip flexor contractures may require iliopsoas release.

   • Mild knee contractures may be treated with stretching and bracing, but more severe

5: Pediatrics

deformity may require an osteotomy. Growth modulation has also been described.

- Treatment of knee contractures can change but not increase the arc of motion.

- The Ponseti method has been described for arthrygrypotic clubfoot, although more often it may need to be augmented with open surgical releases and prolonged bracing to maintain corrected position. Recurrences are frequent.

- Clubfoot associated with amyoplasia may require circumferential release.

- Severe or recurrent deformity may be addressed by talectomy.

- Treatment with osteotomies and circular external fixator has also been described.

G. Larsen syndrome

1. Overview

a. Features of Larsen syndrome include multiple congenital joint dislocations, ligamentous laxity, and abnormal facies.

b. Airway issues and congenital cardiac defects result in increased mortality in the first year of life.

c. Inheritance may be autosomal dominant or recessive, although many cases are sporadic.

2. Evaluation

a. Bilateral knee dislocations and clubfoot should prompt evaluation for Larsen syndrome.

b. Hip ultrasonography should be obtained to evaluate for dislocation.

c. Bilateral radial head dislocations may be present.

d. Cervical spine films should be obtained in the first year of life to identity kyphosis secondary to hypoplasia of vertebral bodies because this deformity may result in neurologic compromise.

3. Treatment

a. Knee dislocations may require surgery and long-term bracing.

b. Hip dislocations and clubfoot are treated in a similar manner as that associated with arthrogryposis (see IV.A.4).

c. If cervical kyphosis is present, posterior fusion should be performed during the first 18 months of life.

H. Pterygia syndromes

1. Multiple pterygia syndrome (Escobar syndrome) is a rare disorder characterized by webs across flexion creases in the extremities and the neck, vertical talus, and spinal abnormalities.

2. Popliteal pterygia syndrome is characterized by facial abnormalities, popliteal webbing, and genital involvement.

3. The popliteal web is addressed before adaptive changes occur with Z-plasty and femoral shortening/extension osteotomy.

Top Testing Facts

Neurofibromatosis

1. Many patients have café-au-lait spots. Six or more (of the noted size) are required as a criterion for a diagnosis of NF.

2. Although 50% of cases of anterolateral bowing of the tibia are the result of NF, only 10% of patients with NF have such anterolateral bowing.

3. Scoliosis in patients with NF is often dystrophic (a short, sharply angular scoliotic curve). Surgical success is much greater with combined anterior and posterior fusions.

4. When three or more ribs are penciled, 87% of scoliotic curves progress rapidly.

5. A preoperative MRI should be obtained to rule out dural ectasia and intraspinal neurofibromas.

Connective Tissue Diseases

1. Dural ectasia is commonly seen in Marfan syndrome and may cause back pain and complicate surgery for scoliosis; preoperative MRI is mandatory.

2. Ectopia lentis associated with Marfan syndrome consists of a superior dislocation of the lens; with homocysteinuria, the lens has an inferior dislocation.

3. Patients with the MASS phenotype never have ectopia lentis or aortic dissection.

4. Marfan syndrome is caused by a mutation in the fibrillin-1 gene (*FBN1*).

Arthritides

1. IIA is commonly associated with uveitis, for which screening should be performed, and may be associated with limb-length discrepancy.

Other Conditions With Musculoskeletal Involvement

1. The most common form of rickets in North America is hypophosphatemic rickets, which is an X-linked dominant condition.

2. The most common chromosomal abnormality in the United States is trisomy 21.

3. Apophyseal avulsion fractures of the olecranon are characteristic of OI.

4. Erlenmyer flask deformities of the femora are seen in Gaucher disease and osteopetrosis.

5. Gaucher disease is associated with a defect in the gene encoding β-glucocerebrosidase.

6. Arthrogryposis results in joint contractures present in 1 of every 3,000 live births. They are characterized by decreased muscle mass, with fibrosis and fat between muscle fibers, and the periarticular soft tissues are thickened and fibrotic.

7. Larsen syndrome can result in multiple congenital joint dislocations, ligamentous laxity, and abnormal facies, with airway issues and congenital cardiac defects increasing mortality in the first year of life.

8. Multiple pterygia syndrome is rare, and characterized by webs across flexion creases in the extremities and neck, and well as vertical talus and spinal abnormalities. Popliteal pterygia syndrome is characterized by facial abnormalities, popliteal webbing, and genital involvement.

Bibliography

Aldegheri R, Dall'Oca C: Limb lengthening in short stature patients. *J Pediatr Orthop B* 2001;10(3):238-247.

Alman BA, Goldberg MJ: Syndromes of Orthopaedic Importance, in Morrissy RT, Weinstein SL, eds: *Lovell and Winter's Pediatric Orthopaedics*, ed 6. Philadelphia, PA, Lippincott Williams & Wilkins, 2006, pp 250-303.

Bevan WP, Hall JG, Bamshad M, Staheli LT, Jaffe KM, Song K: Arthrogryposis multiplex congenita (amyoplasia): An orthopaedic perspective. *J Pediatr Orthop* 2007;27(5):594-600.

Caird MS, Wills BP, Dormans JP: Down syndrome in children: The role of the orthopaedic surgeon. *J Am Acad Orthop Surg* 2006;14(11):610-619.

Crowson CS, Matteson EL, Myasoedova E, et al: The lifetime risk of adult-onset rheumatoid arthritis and other inflammatory autoimmune rheumatic diseases. *Arthritis Rheum* 2011; 63(3):633-639.

D'Astous JL, Carroll KL: Connective tissue diseases, in Vaccaro AR, ed: *Orthopaedic Knowledge Update*, ed 8. Rosemont, IL, American Academy of Orthopaedic Surgeons, 2005, pp 245-254.

Fassier F, Hamdy RC: Arthogrypotic syndromes and osteochondrodysplasias, in Abel MF, ed: *Orthopaedic Knowledge Update: Pediatrics*, ed 3. Rosemont, IL, American Academy of Orthopaedic Surgeons, 2006, pp 137-151.

5: Pediatrics

Goldberg MJ: *The Dysmorphic Child: An Orthopedic Perspective.* New York, NY, Raven Press, 1987.

Judge DP, Dietz HC: Marfan's syndrome. *Lancet* 2005; 366(9501):1965-1976.

Morris CD, Einhorn TA: Bisphosphonates in orthopaedic surgery. *J Bone Joint Surg Am* 2005;87(7):1609-1618.

Silman AJ, Hochberg MC: *Epidemiology of the Rheumatic Diseases,* ed 2. New York, NY, Oxford University Press, 2001.

Sponseller PD, Ain MC: The skeletal dysplasias, in Morrissy RT, Weinstein SL, eds: *Lovell and Winter's Pediatric Orthopaedics,* ed 6. Philadelphia, PA, Lippincott Williams & Wilkins, 2006, pp 205-250.

Stanitski DF, Nadjarian R, Stanitski CL, Bawle E, Tsipouras P: Orthopaedic manifestations of Ehlers-Danlos syndrome. *Clin Orthop Relat Res* 2000;376:213-221.

Taybi H, Lachman RS: *Radiology of Syndromes, Metabolic Disorders, and Skeletal Dyplasias,* ed 4. St. Louis, MO, Mosby-Year Book Inc, 1996.

Unger S: A genetic approach to the diagnosis of skeletal dysplasia. *Clin Orthop Relat Res* 2002;401:32-38.

van Bosse HJ, Marangoz S, Lehman WB, Sala DA: Correction of arthrogrypotic clubfoot with a modified Ponseti technique. *Clin Orthop Relat Res* 2009;467(5):1283-1293.

Zeitlin L, Fassier F, Glorieux FH: Modern approach to children with osteogenesis imperfecta. *J Pediatr Orthop B* 2003; 12(2):77-87.

Chapter 55

Pediatric Neuromuscular Disorders

M. Siobhan Murphy Zane, MD

I. Cerebral Palsy

A. Epidemiology

1. The incidence of cerebral palsy (CP) is from 1 to 3 per 1,000 live births.

2. Prematurity and low birth weight (<1,500 g) increase the incidence to 90 per 1,000 live births.

B. Pathoanatomy

1. CP is a static encephalopathy: a nonprogressive, permanent injury to the brain caused by damage, defectiveness, or illness.

2. CP can affect childhood motor development, speech, cognition, and sensation.

3. Although the brain injury in CP is static, the peripheral manifestations (for example, contractures and bone deformities) of CP are often not static.

4. Ongoing seizures may contribute to loss of function in CP.

C. The risk factors for CP are listed in **Table 1**.

1. CP is not a genetic condition; familial spastic paraparesis, which is manifested by progressive weakness and stiffness of the lower extremities resembling that in CP, is a hereditary condition and should be considered as a diagnostic possibility if there is a family history of CP.

D. Developmental evaluation

1. In normal development, children should

   a. Sit independently by age 6 to 9 months

   b. Cruise, or walk while holding onto furniture, by age 14 months

   c. Walk independently by age 18 months

2. Positive predictive factors for walking include pulling up to a standing position and sitting independently by age 2 years.

3. Poor prognostic indicators for walking are listed in **Table 2**.

E. Classification—Several classification systems are useful in treating CP.

1. Physiologic—The location of the brain injury in CP will cause different types of motor dysfunction.

   a. Patients with spastic-type (pyramidal) CP exhibit increased tone or rigidity with rapid stretching, which can lead to disturbances in gait and limb-muscle contracture. These patients most often benefit from orthopaedic interventions.

   b. Patients with dyskinetic (extrapyramidal) or choreoathetoid CP exhibit involuntary movements, athetosis, and dystonia. This type of CP has been less frequently seen than pyramidal CP with the administration of Rh-immune globulin to pregnant women to prevent Rh incompatibility between mothers and their infants.

   c. Patients with ataxia (cerebellar) exhibit disturbed balance and coordination.

   d. Patients with mixed types of CP show spasticity and dyskinesia.

Table 1

Risk Factors for Cerebral Palsy

Prematurity
Low birth weight
Multiple births
TORCH (toxoplasmosis, other infections [syphilis and so forth], rubella, cytomegalovirus, herpes) infections
Chorioamnionitis
Placental complications
Third-trimester bleeding
Maternal epilepsy
Toxemia
Low Apgar scores
Anoxia
Intraventricular hemorrhage
Infection
Maternal drug and alcohol use
Teratogens

5: Pediatrics

Table 2

Poor Prognostic Indicators for Walking

Persistence of two or more of the following primitive reflexes at 1 year of age

Moro: with the child in the supine position, sudden extension of the neck causes arm abduction with finger extension, followed by an embrace

Asymmetric tonic neck: turning of the head to the side causes a "fencer's pose"

Symmetric tonic neck: Flexion of the neck causes flexion of the arm and extension of the leg.

Neck righting: when the child turns his or her head to the side, the trunk and limbs follow

Extensor thrust (abnormal reflex): touching of the child's feet to the floor causes extension of all joints

Absence of the following postural reflexes at 1 year of age

Parachute: with the child in the upright position, sudden forward rotation of the child's body causes the arms to extend to break a perceived fall

Foot placement: with support, touching the child's feet to a surface will elicit walking motion

Not sitting by 5 years of age

Not walking by 8 years of age

Table 3

Anatomic Classification of Cerebral Palsy

Type	Area Affected
Quadriplegia	Four limbs
Whole body	Four limbs and bulbar problems (for example, swallowing)
Hemiplegia	One side of the body
Diplegia	Lower extremities, but can have some upper extremity posturing

2. Anatomic (**Table 3**).

3. Functional—Gross Motor Function Classification System (GMFCS). The patient is assigned a grade from I to V, representing the highest to lowest level of function (**Figure 1**).

F. Gait assessment is central to the orthopaedic care of patients with CP and meningomyelocele.

1. Perry/Gage criteria—Five essential factors for normal gait:

   a. Symmetric step length

   b. Stance stability

   c. Swing clearance

   d. Adequate foot position before initial contact

   e. Energy conservation

2. Normal gait (**Figure 2**)

   a. A complete gait cycle is from one foot strike to the next foot strike on the same side of the body.

   b. Stance is the first 62% of the cycle.

   c. Swing is the final 38% of the cycle.

3. The physical examination of gait includes the range of motion (ROM) of the hip, knee, and ankle.

4. Test for spasticity—The "catch" test shows a velocity-dependent difference in muscle tightness, in which a quick passive motion elicits a rapid tightening of the muscles used in walking.

   a. On the Modified Ashworth Scale of tone in response to passive stretching of a limb, grade 1 is resistance to stretch without a catch, grade 2 is a clearly evident catch, and grade 5 is a rigid joint.

5. Tests for contractures and spasticity

   a. Duncan-Ely test (for spasticity of the rectus femoris muscle)—With the child in the prone position, the knee is flexed. If the ipsilateral hip rises, there is spasticity of the rectus femoris.

   b. Thomas test (for contracture on hip flexion)—With the child in the supine position, the knee of one leg is flexed and brought up toward the chest while the other leg remains extended. The degree of hip flexion on the side of the extended leg is the degree of contracture and deformity in hip flexion.

   c. Silfverskiöld test (for ankle equinus)—Ankle dorsiflexion is assessed with the knee in both extension and flexion. Should be performed with the foot in the supine position to lock the midfoot and prevent midfoot break and false appearance of dorsiflexion. If an equinus contracture resolves with the knee flexed, the contracture is caused by the gastrocnemius muscle alone. If the equinus contracture remains with the knee flexed, the contracture involves both the gastrocnemius and soleus muscles.

6. Muscle weakness or pain, athetosis or ataxia, scoliosis, and bony malalignment should be noted when examining a patient's gait.

7. Observation of gait should be made in the following three dimensions:

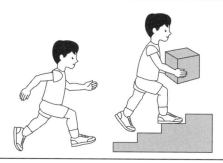

GMFCS Level I

Children walk indoors and outdoors and climb stairs without limitation. Children perform gross motor skills, including running and jumping, but speed, balance, and coordination are impaired.

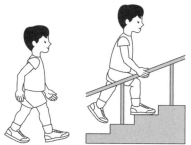

GMFCS Level II

Children walk indoors and outdoors and climb stairs holding onto a railing but experience limitations walking on uneven surfaces and inclines and walking in crowds or confined spaces.

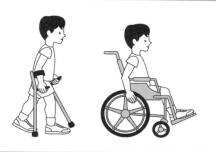

GMFCS Level III

Children walk indoors or outdoors on a level surface with an assistive mobility device. Children may climb stairs holding onto a railing. Children may propel a wheelchair manually or are transported when traveling for long distances or outdoors on uneven terrain.

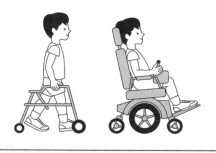

GMFCS Level IV

Children may continue to walk for short distances on a walker or rely more on wheeled mobility at home and school and in the community.

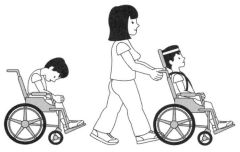

GMFCS Level V

Physical impairment restricts voluntary control of movement and the ability to maintain antigravity head and trunk postures. All areas of motor function are limited. Children have no means of independent mobility and are transported.

Figure 1   Gross Motor Function Classification System (GMFCS) for children age 6 to 12 years. (Reproduced with permission from Palisano RJ, Rosenbaum P, Walter S, Russell D, Wood E, Galuppi B: Development and reliability of a system to classify gross motor function in children with cerebral palsy. *Dev Med Child Neurol* 1997;45:113-120. Illustrated by Kerr Graham and Bill Reid, The Royal Children's Hospital, Melbourne.)

5: Pediatrics

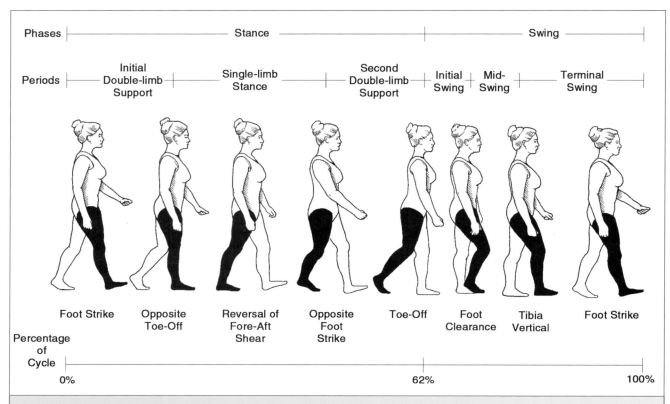

Phases	Stance				Swing		
Periods	Initial Double-limb Support	Single-limb Stance	Second Double-limb Support		Initial Swing	Mid-Swing	Terminal Swing

Foot Strike — Opposite Toe-Off — Reversal of Fore-Aft Shear — Opposite Foot Strike — Toe-Off — Foot Clearance — Tibia Vertical — Foot Strike

Percentage of Cycle

0%   62%   100%

Figure 2   Typical normal gait cycle. (Reproduced from Chambers HG, Sutherland DH: A practical guide to gait analysis. *J Am Acad Orthop Surg* 2002;10[3]:222-231.)

a. Coronal (patient walking away and toward the examiner)—Trendelenberg gait, pelvic obliquity, and equinus should be noted.

b. Sagittal (patient walking back and forth in front of the examiner)—Flexion/extension of hip, knee, and ankle should be noted, as well as step length.

c. Axial (looking vertically downward from above)—Internal and external rotation of the femur, tibia, or foot should be noted.

G. A gait analysis of a patient's crouch gait should be performed (**Figure 3**).

H. Nonsurgical treatment

1. Physical therapy addresses the development of gait and functional mobility with gait trainers, walkers, or crutches, as well as the prevention of contracture through stretching, bracing, and standing programs. The efficacy of frequent physical therapy sessions for improving gait has not been shown, but strength training helps with limb-muscle strength and gait.

2. Occupational therapy addresses fine motor function, activities of daily living, self-feeding, self-dressing, and communication through speech or adaptive equipment.

3. Speech and swallowing therapy are often needed for patients with CP, particularly for children with substantial bulbar involvement.

4. Splinting or serial casting may prevent or reduce spasticity and contracture.

5. Bracing is often used to improve joint or limb position in standing or ambulation, or to prevent deformity.

a. Supramalleolar orthoses may be used to control deformities of the foot and ankle in the coronal plane (pronation or supination), but do not address deformities in the sagittal plane (equinus or calcaneus).

b. Ankle-foot orthoses (AFOs) may be used to stabilize the ankle joint.

- Solid-ankle AFOs may be used to prevent equinus or a crouched stance caused by uncontrolled dorsiflexion at the ankle. Prevention of equinus and calcaneus has been shown to improve walking speed and stride length for most children with CP.

- Hinged AFOs may be used to allow dorsiflexion while preventing equinus during gait.

- Floor-reaction AFOs cause extension of the

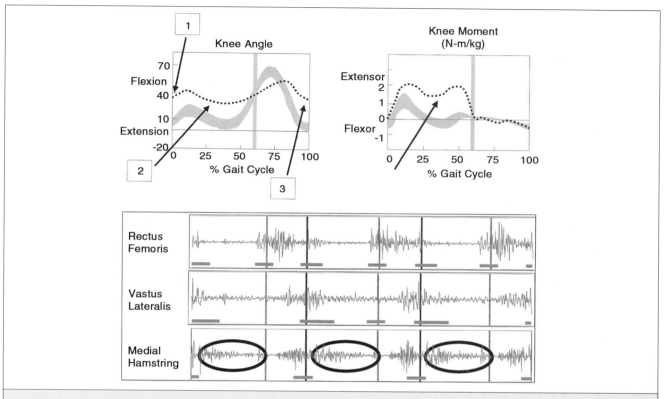

Figure 3 Findings on quantitative gait analysis that serve as indicators of medial hamstring lengthening. (Reproduced from Davids JR, Ounpuu S, DeLuca PA, Davis RB: Optimization of walking ability of children with cerebral palsy. *Inst Course Lect* 2004;53:511-522.)

knee that may improve crouched gait caused by excessive ankle dorsiflexion with weak ankle plantar flexion.

c. Knee-ankle-foot orthoses (KAFOs) stabilize the knee and are useful for maintaining knee position in children who walk very limited distances or only stand.

6. Antispasticity medicines

a. Baclofen—An analogue of gamma-aminobutyric acid (GABA) that binds to neuronal GABA receptors in the spinal cord, blocking the effect of GABA and decreasing the release of excitatory neurotransmitters.

- Oral administration of baclofen is common, but the dosage needs to be adjusted if relaxation is accompanied by an unacceptable degree of sedation.

- Intrathecal baclofen (ITB) is administered with an intrathecal pump and is associated with less sedation than orally administered baclofen. Potential recipients of ITB are nonambulatory patients with moderate to severe spasticity and patients in whom dystonia is a component of CP.

b. Diazepam (Valium) is given orally but, like ba-

clofen, it can also cause substantial sedation before producing sufficient muscle relaxation for ambulation.

c. Botulinum toxin produces muscle relaxation by irreversibly binding to synaptic proteins at the neuromuscular junction to block the presynaptic release of acetylcholine, which depolarizes muscle fibers and can ultimately cause muscle contraction.

- Botulinum toxin A is the form commonly used in the United States for inducing muscle relaxation in children with CP. In CP, the intramuscular injection of botulinum toxin results in 3 to 6 months of relaxation of spastic muscles; it is commonly used in conjunction with physical therapy, stretching, casting, or bracing. However, botulinum toxin is not FDA-approved for use in patients younger than 18 years. Its use is off-label and in particular should not be used in children younger than 2 years. In adults, it is FDA-approved only for upper extremity spasticity.

- Botulinum toxin is useful only for treating dynamic spasticity, not for fixed contractures.

I. Surgical treatment

Table 4

Surgical Treatment of Common Gait Disturbances in Cerebral Palsy

Gait Disturbance	Problem	Recommended Surgery
Scissoring	Tight adductors	Adductor tenotomy
Toe-walking	Tight gastrocnemius-soleus (equinus deformity)	Gastrocnemius-soleus intramuscular aponeurotic recession or Achilles lengthening if > 30° of fixed plantar flexion (Do not overlengthen!)
	Apparent equinus with crouched gait because of hip and/or knee deformities (ankle is actually neutral)	Do not lengthen gastrocnemius-soleus; address hip and knee contractures!
Back-knee gait	Tight gastrocnemius-soleus (equinus deformity)	Gastrocnemius or Achilles lengthening (Do not overlengthen!)
	Iatrogenic overlengthening of the hamstrings without distal RF transfer	Distal RF transfer may be helpful
Decreased knee flexion in swing phase (even without crouched gait)	Overactive RF	Distal RF transfer (to semitendinosis if possible)
Crouched gait	Tight hip flexors	Intramuscular psoas lengthening
	Tight hamstrings	Mild or moderate: hamstring lengthenings Severe: extension distal femoral osteotomy with patellar tendon shortening or advancement
	Excessively loose heel cords (which can then cause tight hip flexors and hamstrings)	None (Achilles tendon shortening and proximal calcaneal slide have mixed results; usually need to go to solid AFOs)
	Lever arm dysfunction	See intoeing and pes valgus
Intoeing	Increased femoral anteversion	Femoral rotational osteotomy
	Internal tibial torsion	Tibial rotational osteotomy
	Varus foot	Varus foot correction (see equinovarus foot)
Pes valgus, common in patients with diplegia and quadriplegia	Spastic gastrocnemius-soleus and peroneal muscles with tibialis posterior weakness	Calcaneal lengthening (best after age 6 years) Calcaneal medial sliding osteotomy, possibly with midfoot osteotomies
Equinovarus foot	Spastic tibialis anterior and/or tibialis posterior overpower the peroneal muscles, with gastrocnemius-soleus equinus	Treat equinus as noted for toe-walking Split anterior tendon transfer if anterior tibialis causative Posterior tibialis lengthening or split transfer if posterior tibialis causative Must add calcaneal osteotomy if hindfoot deformity is rigid

AFO = ankle foot orthosis, RF = rectus femoris

1. Surgical intervention is generally undertaken when a plateau or worsening of function and/or deformity has occurred in a patient with CP despite nonsurgical interventions.

2. Single-event multilevel surgery is preferred and is most successful in patients with mild hemiplegia.

3. **Table 4** lists the recommended surgical interventions for common gait disturbances associated with CP.

4. Selective dorsal rhizotomy (SDR) reduces spastic-ity by selectively severing dorsal nerve rootlets between L1 and S1.

   a. SDR may be indicated in ambulatory patients between ages 3 and 8 years who have diplegia in the presence of good selective motor control and minimal cognitive delay.

   b. Complications of SDR include scoliosis (44%), spondylolisthesis (19%), risk of bowel/bladder incontinence, dysesthesias, and increasing weakness by adolescence.

J. Scoliosis associated with CP

1. Incidence and severity are related to the severity of CP.

2. Progression of scoliosis is common after skeletal maturity in patients with quadriplegia.

3. Bracing is typically ineffective in treating neuromuscular scoliosis, but it may be used to aid with seating in patients with flexible curves.

4. Spinal fusion from the upper thoracic spine to the pelvis in nonambulatory patients may be indicated for large curves that cause pain and/or interfere with sitting.

   a. Curves exceeding 90° may require anterior release with a posterior fusion, as a single-step or two-step procedure.

   b. Quality of life seems to improve after surgery.

   c. Growing rods have a 27% rate of infection.

K. Hip subluxation/dislocation associated with CP

1. Overview

   a. Subluxation is less common in the ambulatory patient, but will develop in 50% of quadriplegic patients with CP.

   b. Subluxation (usually posterosuperior) results from spasticity of the adductor and iliopsoas muscles and non–weight-bearing status.

   c. From 50% to 75% of dislocated hips will become painful.

2. Treatment

   a. Goals are to prevent subluxation and dislocation of the hip, maintain comfort in seating, and facilitate care and hygiene.

   b. Treatment is based on radiologic assessment and use of the Reimer migration index of hip subluxation (**Figure 4**).

   c. Surgical management is appropriate when subluxation progresses to 50% or more according to the Reimer index. Regardless of treatment, patients at GMFCS levels IV and V have a higher rate of migration than those at GMFCS levels I, II, or III.

      • Children younger than 8 years and with less than 60% subluxation can be treated with adductor and gracilis tenotomy, and with iliopsoas release when hip flexion exceeds 20°. For patients at GMFCS level V, some centers recommend phenolization of the obturator nerve (anterior branch).

      • Children younger than 8 years and with more than 60% subluxation should be treated with a proximal femoral osteotomy (varus derotational osteotomy [VDRO]) and

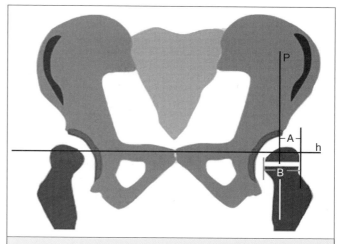

Figure 4 Illustration shows how the Reimer migration percentage is measured using an AP radiograph. The Hilgenreiner (h) and Perkin (P) lines are drawn. Distance A (the distance from P to the lateral border of the femoral epiphysis) is divided by distance B (the width of the femoral epiphysis) and multiplied by 100 to calculate the Reimer migration percentage (A/B × 100). (Reproduced with permission from Miller F: Hip, in Dabney K, Alexander M, eds: *Cerebral Palsy.* New York, NY, Springer, 2005, p 532.)

a possible pelvic osteotomy (Dega or Albee type).

• Children older than 8 years and with more than 40% subluxation should be treated with a proximal femoral osteotomy (VDRO) and a possible pelvic osteotomy (Dega or Albee type).

• Older children with closed triradiate cartilage or those with recurrent subluxation may benefit from a Ganz or Chiari pelvic osteotomy or a Staheli shelf with a VDRO.

• Children with a failed hip reconstruction or older children with arthritis, even if they have not undergone previous surgery, may require salvage procedures, such as a resection arthroplasty (Castle procedure) for pain relief.

L. Hip adduction contracture

1. Scissoring (caused by adductor tightness) at the hip joint can interfere with gait and hygiene and is treated with proximal release of the adductor muscles.

2. An obturator neurectomy should not be performed.

M. Contracture on hip flexion is treated with intramuscular lengthening of the iliopsoas muscle.

N. Lever-arm dysfunction associated with CP

Table 5

Causes of Anterior Knee Pain in Cerebral Palsy

Patella alta
Weak quadriceps
Tight hamstrings
Femoral anteversion
External tibial torsion
Pes valgus
Genu valgum
Patellar instability (may sometimes be asymptomatic)

1. Lever-arm dysfunction results in posterior displacement of the ground-reaction force relative to the knee and often results in crouch and power abnormalities in gait.

2. Intoeing from femoral anteversion can be treated with femoral rotational osteotomies.

3. Intoeing from internal tibial torsion can be treated with supramalleolar tibial osteotomies (a concurrent fibular osteotomy is not needed if correction is less than 25°).

4. Pes planus (pes valgus)—See section I.P.4.

O. Knee problems specific to CP

1. Crouched gait

a. Most common cause is spastic or contracted hamstrings, although crouch may result from excessive dorsiflextion of the ankle or ankle equinus.

b. Nonsurgical treatment includes physical therapy, bracing (such as the use of knee immobilizers at night), and spasticity management.

c. Mild crouch—If sustained and complete nonsurgical management fails, surgical treatment consists of medial (and possibly lateral) lengthening of the hamstring muscles, with concomitant posterior transfer of the rectus femoris. Lengthening of the medial and lateral hamstrings in an ambulatory patient carries an increased risk of recurvatum in stance.

d. Severe crouch or fixed deformity—Excellent results have been found with extension distal femoral osteotomy with an anterior closing wedge (fixed with a blade plate, fixed-angle plate, or wires) with shortening or advancement of the patellar tendon.

2. Stiff-knee gait (Table 5)

3. Knee contracture—In a nonambulatory patient, hamstring release may be useful for maintaining leg position in a program to improve standing.

P. Foot and ankle—Abnormal position or ROM at the foot and ankle cause abnormalities of gait and decreased push-off power. Goals of treatment include a painless, plantigrade (stable) foot.

1. Equinus deformity (the most common foot problem in CP) results from spasticity of the gastrocnemius-soleus muscle complex. It can result in toe-walking or a back-knee (genu recurvatum) gait.

a. Nonsurgical treatment includes stretching, physical therapy for ROM, the use of AFOs, and spasticity management.

b. Surgical treatment should be considered only for patients with fixed contractures and is typically deferred until the patient is at least 6 years of age.

• The Silverskiöld test (section I.F.5.c), performed with anesthesia, helps to determine whether a gastrocnemius recession and/or a soleus recession is appropriate. If the ankle rises above neutral with the knee flexed (gastrocnemius relaxed), a gastrocnemius recession should be performed. If the ankle is in equinus with the knee flexed and extended, the soleus is also tight, and a soleus recession should be performed. Lengthening of the Achilles tendon has been used to relieve tightness of the gastrocnemius-soleus complex.

• Overlengthening of the heel cord may cause a crouched gait and calcaneus foot position, resulting in poor push-off power. This is less of a problem with a gastrocnemius–soleus recession than with a lengthening of the Achilles tendon.

2. Equinovarus deformity of the foot can cause painful weight bearing over the lateral border of the foot and instability in the stance phase of gait.

a. Generally, isolated forefoot supination is the result of excessive tension of the tibialis anterior muscle, whereas hindfoot varus comes from excessive tension of the tibialis posterior muscle.

b. The tibialis anterior and the tibialis posterior muscles (the invertor muscles) overpower the peroneal muscles (the evertor muscles), whereas a tight gastrocnemius-soleus muscle complex causes equinus.

c. Dynamic electromyography (EMG) is useful in determining whether the anterior tibialis and/or the posterior tibialis is causing a varus deformity of the foot.

d. Clinically, the tibialis anterior muscle can be assessed using the confusion test.

• The patient sits on the edge of the examining table and flexes the hip actively.

- The tibialis anterior muscle will activate and contract.

- If the forefoot supinates as it dorsiflexes, a varus deformity of the foot is at least partly the result of overactivity of the tibialis anterior muscle.

e. Clinically, the posterior tibialis muscle is assessed by tightness when the hindfoot is positioned in valgus.

f. Split tendon transfers of the anterior tibialis muscle and/or posterior tibialis muscle are recommended for the correction of varus deformity of the foot in CP, rather than full tendon transfers, because the latter may cause overcorrection.

g. Lengthening of the tibialis posterior muscle is helpful in less severe deformities caused by this muscle.

h. In the case of a rigid varus deformity, both soft-tissue and bony procedures (calcaneal osteotomy) are necessary.

3. Equinovalgus arises from spasticity of the gastrocnemius-soleus muscle complex and peroneus muscle with weakness of the tibialis posterior muscle.

a. Weight-bearing AP radiographs of the ankles must be obtained in cases of equinovalgus because valgus may contribute to ankle deformity.

b. Nonsurgical treatment of equinovalgus includes bracing with a supramalleolar orthosis or AFO, physical therapy for ROM, and may include injection of botulinum toxin.

c. Surgical treatment—Calcaneal osteotomies preserve ROM and are preferred when feasible.

- Moderate deformity—Calcaneal lengthening with lengthening of the peroneus brevis muscle is preferred because it can restore the anatomy of the foot and ankle. Lengthening of the peroneus longus should be avoided because it can increase dorsiflexion of the first ray.

- Severe deformity—A medial calcaneal sliding osteotomy brings the calcaneus into line with the weight-bearing axis of the tibia. It is performed concomitantly with medial closing wedge osteotomy of the cuneiform bone, opening wedge osteotomy of the cuboid bone, and lengthening of the Achilles tendon.

- Arthrodesis should be considered if the patient has poor selective control of the muscles crossing the joint and if deformity is severe.

- Subtalar arthrodesis is sometimes needed but may be necessary in the presence of marked deformity or ligamentous laxity.

- Triple arthrodesis is rarely required.

4. Pes valgus/pes planus

a. Pes planus is common in patients with diplegia and quadriplegia.

b. The foot is externally rotated by spasticity of the gastrocnemius, soleus, and peroneal muscles, with weak function of the tibialis posterior muscle.

c. Patients bear weight on the medial border of the foot, on the talar head.

d. The foot is unstable in push-off.

e. Treatment

- Feet with mild planovalgus can be treated with supramalleolar orthoses or AFOs.

- Moderate to severe deformities can be treated with a calcaneal osteotomy.

  ○ A calcaneal lengthening osteotomy (best undertaken after age 6 years) can restore normal anatomy and is combined with lengthening of the peroneus brevis muscle and tightening of the medial talonavicular joint capsule and/or the posterior tibial tendon. Note that the peroneus longus muscle should be not routinely lengthened because this exacerbates dorsiflexion of the first ray.

  ○ A medial calcaneal sliding osteotomy with plantar flexion closing-wedge osteotomies of the cuneiform bones and an opening wedge osteotomy of the cuboid bone can also improve foot alignment.

- Severe deformities can be treated with subtalar fusion, although this is usually needed only in very large children and/or those with extreme laxity. (Triple arthrodesis is almost never required.)

- Compensatory midfoot supination can be treated with plantar flexion osteotomy of the first ray, often with lengthening of the peroneus brevis muscle.

5. Hallux valgus deformity occurs frequently with pes valgus, equinovalgus, and equinovarus feet.

a. Toe straps added to AFOs or nighttime splinting of hallux valgus may be helpful.

b. Severe hallux valgus should be treated with fusion of the first metatarsophalangeal (MTP) joint.

c. Pes valgus must be simultaneously corrected to

5: Pediatrics

avoid recurrence.

    d. Pitfalls—At the time of correction of hallux valgus, the patient also will often have valgus interphalangeus, which should be treated with proximal phalanx (Akin) osteotomy.

6. A dorsal bunion is a deformity in which the great toe is flexed in relation to an elevated metatarsal bone, causing a prominence over the uncovered metatarsal head, which can be painful with the wearing of shoes.

    a. Dorsal bunions may be iatrogenic, occurring after surgery to balance the foot. The deformation may be caused either by an overpowering tibialis anterior muscle or an overpowering flexor hallucis longus (FHL) muscle.

    b. Treatment

- Nonsurgical treatment of a dorsal bunion is done with shoes having soft, deep toe boxes.

- Surgical treatment is needed in recalcitrant cases. Flexible deformities are treated with lengthening or split transfer of the anterior tibialis muscle and transfer of the FHL muscle to the plantar aspect of the first metatarsal head. Rigid deformities require fusion of the first MTP joint and lengthening or split transfer of the anterior tibialis.

Q. Upper-extremity problems specific to CP

1. General information—Involvement of the upper extremities is typical in patients with hemiplegia and quadriplegia as effects of CP. Commonly, the hand is in a fist, the thumb is in the palm, the forearm is flexed and pronated, the wrist is flexed, and the shoulder is internally rotated.

2. Nonsurgical treatment

    a. Occupational therapy for patients with upper extremity problems is useful in early childhood for activities of daily living, stretching, and splinting.

    b. Botulinum toxin is useful for treating dynamic deformities.

    c. Constraint-induced therapy (splinting of the uninvolved upper extremity to encourage use of the involved arm) in patients with hemiplegia is becoming common but does not have extensive data.

3. Surgical treatment

    a. Surgical treatment is undertaken primarily for functional concerns, hygiene, and sometimes appearance.

    b. Adduction of the shoulder and contractures on internal rotation may be treated with release of the subscapularis muscle and lengthening of the pectoralis major muscle. A proximal humeral derotational osteotomy is rarely necessary.

    c. Contractures on elbow flexion may be treated with resection of the lacertus fibrosis (bicipital aponeurosis), lengthening of the biceps and brachialis muscles, and release of the brachioradialis muscle at its origin.

    d. Contractures on elbow pronation

- Release or rerouting of the pronator teres should be considered. Transfer of the pronator teres to an anterolateral position (to act as a supinator) may cause a supination deformity, which is not preferable to pronation.

- Transfer of the flexor carpi ulnaris (FCU) to the extensor carpi radialis brevis may also ease supination.

    e. Dislocation of the head of the radius is uncommon and, if symptomatic, may be treated with excision of the radial head when the patient reaches maturity.

    f. Wrist deformities usually include flexion contracture with ulnar deviation and are associated with weak wrist extension and a pronated forearm.

- If finger extension is good and there is little spasticity on flexion of the wrist, the FCU or the flexor carpi radialis (FCR) muscle should be lengthened.

- Releasing the wrist and finger flexors and the pronator teres from the medial epicondyle of the humerus weakens wrist and finger flexion but is nonselective.

- In severe spasticity, an FCU transfer is recommended.

    ○ If grasp is good, release is weak, and the FCU is active in release, it should be transferred to the extensor digitorum communis muscle.

    ○ If grasp is weak, release is good, and the FCU is active in grasp, it should be transferred to the extensor carpi radialis brevis (ECRB) muscle.

    ○ A concurrent release of the FCR can excessively weaken flexion of the wrist and should not be done.

4. Hand deformities

    a. Thumb-in-palm deformity can be treated with release of the adductor pollicis muscle, transfer of tendons to improve extension, and stabilization of the metacarpophalangeal (MCP) joint.

b. Clawing of the fingers, with wrist flexion and hyperextension at the MCP joint, can be treated with transfer of the FCR or FCU muscle to the ECRB.

c. Contraction on finger flexion is treated with lengthening or tenotomy of the flexor digitorum sublimis (FDS) and flexor digitorum longus (FDL) muscles.

d. Swan neck deformities of the fingers are a result of intrinsic muscle tightness and extrinsic overpull of the finger extensor muscles. These deformities are sometimes caused by wrist flexion or weak wrist extensors and can sometimes be helped by correcting deformity in wrist flexion.

R. Fractures specific to CP

1. Nonambulatory patients are at risk for fracture because of low bone-mineral density (BMD), which may be exacerbated by nonweight bearing, poor calcium intake, or antiseizure medications.

2. Intravenous pamidronate should be considered for children with three or more fractures and a dual-energy X-ray absorptiometry Z-score of less than 2 SD.

II. Myelomeningocele

A. Overview/epidemiology

1. Myelodysplasia/spina bifida disorders comprise a spectrum of congenital malformation of the spinal column and spinal cord resulting from failure of closure of the neural crests (neural tube) at 3 to 4 weeks after fertilization. Spina bifida occulta is the failure of posterior bony spinal elements to fuse but causes no neurologic impairment. In a meningocele, the dura and tissue overlying the spinal cord pouch out through the bony defect, but the spinal cord remains within the spinal canal, frequently causing little neurologic impairment. In a myelomeningocele, overlying tissues and the spinal cord are not contained by the unfused posterior bony spine elements. The neural elements can be found covered in a pouch of skin, or with only dura, or entirely exposed. This can cause major motor and sensory deficits.

2. Myelomeningocele is the most common major birth defect, occurring in 0.9 per 1,000 live births.

3. Prenatal diagnosis made through assay of the α-fetoprotein concentration in maternal serum is 60% to 95% accurate.

4. The diagnosis also can be made with ultrasonography or by amniocentesis.

5. Women of childbearing age should be encouraged to have a diet with adequate folic acid intake. Supplementation with folic acid decreases the risk of spina bifida, but only if done in the first weeks after conception. Supplemental intake of folic acid also has been addressed by adding folic acid to many foods, such as breads and cereals.

B. Risk factors

1. History of a previously affected pregnancy

2. Low folic acid intake

3. Pregestational maternal diabetes

4. In utero exposure to valproic acid or carbamazepine

C. Classification

1. Motor level and functional status are given in **Table 6**.

2. Spinal functional integrity at the L4 level or lower (active quadriceps muscle function) is considered necessary for ambulation in the community.

D. Treatment—The long-term medical and skeletal issues associated with myelomeningocele are often best addressed by multidisciplinary teams.

1. Nonsurgical treatment

a. Frequent skin checks for pressure sores, and well-fitting braces and wheelchairs, are important in the management of myelomeningocele because those it affects often have substantial sensory deficits.

b. Urologic and gastrointestinal issues, including detrusor malfunction and abnormal sphincter tone, make early catheterization and bowel regimens important. Kidney reflux and pyelonephritis cause substantial morbidity and mortality in patients with myelomeningocele.

c. Late issues requiring neurosurgery are common (tethering, syrinx, and shunts), making carefully recorded neurologic examinations important.

d. Latex allergies are common in patients with myelomeningocele, necessitating precautions against contact with latex for all patients with this condition.

e. Rehabilitation efforts should include early mobilization, physical therapy, bracing, and wheelchair fitting for optimal physical function.

f. Bracing

• Hip-knee-ankle-foot orthoses, KAFOs, or AFOs are frequently used to support stance and/or prevent contracture in patients with myelomeningocele.

• As the child grows, bracing and crutch

5: Pediatrics

Table 6

Motor Level and Functional Status for Myelomeningocele

Group	Lesion Level	Muscle Involvement	Function	Ambulation
1	Thoracic/high lumbar	No quadriceps function	Sitter Possible household ambulatory with RGO	Some degree until age 13 years with HKAFO, RGO 95% to 99% wheelchair dependent as adults
2	Low lumbar	Quadriceps and medial hamstring function, no gluteus medius or maximus	Household/community ambulator with KAFO or AFO	Require AFO and crutches, 79% community ambulators as adults, wheelchair for long distances; substantial difference between L3 and L4 level, medial hamstring needed for community ambulation
3	Sacral	Quadriceps and gluteus medius function	Community ambulator with AFO, UCBL, or none	94% retain walking ability as adults
	High sacral	No gastrocnemius-soleus strength	Community ambulator with AFO, UCBL, or none	Walk without support but require AFO; have gluteus lurch and excessive pelvic obliquity and rotation during gait
	Low sacral	Good gastrocnemius-soleus strength, normal gluteus medius and maximus		Walk without AFO; gait close to normal

AFO = ankle-foot orthosis, HKAFO = hip-knee-ankle-foot orthosis, KAFO = knee-ankle-foot orthosis, RGO = reciprocating gait orthosis, UCBL = University of California/Berkeley Lab (orthosis).

Reproduced from Sarwark JF, Aminian A, Westberry DE, Davids JR, Karol LA: Neuromuscular disorders in children, in Vaccaro AR, ed: *Orthopaedic Knowledge Update*, ed 8. Rosemont, IL, American Academy of Orthopaedic Surgeons, 2005, p 678.

requirements may decrease with gains in skills or may increase if there is weight gain or development of deformity.

E. The spine

1. Delivery of infants with myelomeningocele is done by cesarean section to avoid further neurologic damage. Neurosurgical closure of myelomeningocele is done within 48 hours after delivery, with a shunt used to treat hydrocephalus. Closure of myelomeningocele also can be done prenatally.

2. Tethering of the spinal cord in a child with myelomeningocele can cause progressive scoliosis, alter the child's functional capabilities, or cause spasticity.

3. Syrinx, shunt problems, or new hydrocephalus can cause new symptoms affecting the upper extremities, such as weakness or increasing spasticity.

4. An Arnold-Chiari malformation is often addressed with shunting in infancy to control hydrocephalus but may later require decompression. Later symptoms may include spasticity or weakness of the lower extremities, problems with swallowing, and absence of the cough reflex.

5. Scoliosis and kyphosis may be progressive in myelomeningocele.

a. Kyphectomy and posterior fusion may be needed in 90% of patients with thoracic myelomeningocele; surgery may be needed in 10% of patients with myelomeningocele at L4.

b. Prior to kyphectomy, it is important to check shunt function because shunt failure can result in acute hydrocephalus and death when the spinal cord is tied off during kyphectomy.

F. The hip

1. Flexion contractures are common in patients with myelomeningocele but are often not severe. Contracture exceeding 40° in patients with involvement at the lower lumbar level may require flexor muscle release.

2. Dysplasia and/or dislocation of the hip occurs in 80% of patients with involvement at the midlumbar level.

a. These patients have medial hamstring and quadriceps muscle function and poor hip extensor and abductor function, causing muscle imbalance that results in hip dysplasia and instability.

b. Currently, the trend in treatment is not to reduce a dislocated hip in any child with myelomeningocele.

c. The exception to nontreatment for hip dislocation in children with myelomeningocele may be a unilateral dislocation of the hip in a child with a low-level lesion (that is, a community ambulator). However, the rate of recurrence of dislocation is high, and the procedure is controversial.

G. The knee

1. Flexion contracture of the knee exceeding 20° should be treated with hamstring lengthening, capsular release, growth modulation of the anterior distal femoral physis, and/or distal femoral extension osteotomy. There is, however, a substantial rate of recurrence of flexion contracture after extension osteotomy in growing children.

2. Extension contracture of the knee can be treated with serial casting or V-Y quadriceps lengthening.

3. Knee valgus, often with associated external tibial torsion and femoral anteversion, is common in patients with midlumbar level involvement by myelomeningocele because they lack functional hip abductors and have a substantial trunk shift when walking with AFOs. This can be addressed with the use of KAFOs or crutches with AFOs.

4. External tibial torsion can be addressed with a distal tibial derotational osteotomy.

H. The foot

1. About 30% of children with myelomeningocele have a rigid clubfoot.

2. With surgical treatment, portions of the tendons of the foot (for example, Achilles, tibialis posterior, FHL, flexor digitorum communis) may be resected rather than lengthened to decrease the risk of recurrence of clubfoot.

3. Equinus contracture is common in patients with thoracic and high lumbar level involvement by myelomeningocele.

4. Calcaneus foot position can occur with unopposed contraction of the anterior tibialis muscle (myelomeningocele affecting the L3-L4 level of the spine).

5. Equinovarus, equinus, and calcaneal foot deformities are often best treated with a simple tenotomy rather than tendon transfer, achieving a flail but braceable foot.

6. Valgus foot deformities are common in patients with myelomeningocele at the L4-L5 level. If surgery is necessary to achieve a plantigrade foot, fusion should be avoided to maintain foot flexibility and decrease the risk of pressure sores.

I. Fractures in children

1. In children without sensation, fractures often present with erythema, warmth, and swelling.

2. A child with myelomeningocele who presents with

a red, hot, and swollen leg should be suspected of having a fracture until proven otherwise.

III. Muscular Dystrophies

A. Overview

1. Muscular dystrophies are muscle diseases of genetic origin that cause progressive weakness (Table 7).

2. Although muscular dystrophies are genetically based, new mutations causative of these diseases are frequent; thus, for example, one-third of cases of Duchenne muscular dystrophy (DMD) are the result of new mutations that arise during spermatogenesis on the patient's mother's paternal side.

B. Duchenne muscular dystrophy

1. DMD has an incidence of 1 in 3,500 male births and is an X-linked recessive disorder. The involved gene encodes dystrophin, a protein that stabilizes the muscle cell membrane. In DMD, dystrophin is absent, whereas its presence in the less severe Becker dystrophy is subnormal.

2. DMD presents between ages 3 and 6 years with toe-walking or flatfootedness, difficulty in running or climbing stairs, and the classic calf pseudohypertrophy, which is seen in 85% of patients (Figure 5).

3. Weakness in DMD presents proximally, first in the gluteus maximus muscle and then in the quadriceps and hip abductors. The gower sign describes patients' use of their hands to push their legs into extension.

4. With age, DMD in male children continues to worsen, causing shoulder weakness and scoliosis. Ambulation is often limited by age 10 years.

5. Nonsurgical management

a. Corticosteroid therapy

• Prolongs ambulation, slows progression of scoliosis, and slows the deterioration of forced vital capacity.

• The optimum age for beginning therapy is 5 to 7 years.

• Treatment is associated with a high risk of complications and side effects, including osteonecrosis, obesity, Cushingoid appearance, gastrointestinal symptoms, mood swings, headaches, short stature, and cataracts.

b. Nighttime ventilation substantially prolongs survival.

c. Rehabilitation includes physical therapy for ROM, the use of adaptive equipment and

Table 7			

Muscular Dystrophies

Type	Frequency	Inheritance	Gene Defect
Duchenne (DMD)	1/3,500 males	X-linked recessive	Xp21 dystrophin, point deletion, nonsense mutation, no dystrophin protein produced
Becker	1/30,000 males	X-linked recessive	Xp21 dystrophin in noncoding region with normal reading frame, lesser amounts of truncated dystrophin produced
Emery-Dreifuss	Uncommon	X-linked recessive but seen mildly in females	Xq28
Limb girdle	1/14,500	Heterogeneous, mostly AR	AD 5q AR 15q
Adult fascioscapular humeral dystrophy	Rare	AD	4q35
Infantile fascioscapular humeral dystrophy	Rare	AR	Unknown
Myotonic	13/100,000 adults (most common neuromuscular disease in adults)	AD	C9 near myotin protein kinase gene Severity increases with amplification (number of trinucleotide repeats increases with oogenesis) Mildly affected mothers may have severely affected children

AD = autosomal dominant, AR = autosomal recessive, CPK = creatine phosphokinase, DMD = Duchenne muscular dystrophy, EMG = electromyography.

power wheelchairs, and nighttime bracing.

6. Surgical management

   a. Surgery on the lower extremities is controversial in children with DMD.

      - If surgery is performed, the focus should be on early postoperative mobilization and ambulation to prevent deconditioning and deterioration.

      - If surgery is performed, it should include the release of contractures (with lengthening of the hip abductors, hamstrings, Achilles tendon, tibialis posterior muscles) while a child is still ambulatory.

   b. Spine—Scoliosis develops in 95% of patients with DMD after they transition to a wheelchair (usually around age 12 years).

      - Bracing is ineffective and not recommended.

      - Early posterior instrumented fusion (for spinal curvature of 20° or more) is recommended before loss of forced vital capacity from respiratory muscle weakness and progressively decreasing cardiac output.

      - Stiff curves may require anterior and posterior fusion.

   c. Patients with DMD are at risk for malignant hyperthermia and may be pretreated with dantrolene.

Table 7

Muscular Dystrophies (continued)

Diagnostic Features	EMG/Biopsy	Clinical Course
Two of three diagnosed by DNA, CPK 10 to 200× normal Delayed walking, waddling gait, toe-walking, Gower sign, calf pseudohypertrophy Present deep tendon reflexes, lumbar hyperlordosis, often with static encephalopathy	EMG: myopathic, decreased amplitude, short duration, polyphasic motor Biopsy: fibrofatty muscle replacement	Decreasing ambulation by age 6 to 8 years, transitions to wheelchair about age 12 years. Progressive scoliosis and respiratory illness, cardiac failure, death toward end of second decade
CPK less elevated than in DMD, similar physical findings but later onset and less progressive	Similar to DMD, but some dystrophin present by biopsy	Onset after age 7 years, slower progression Walks into teens Cardiac and pulmonary symptoms present but less severe Equinus frequent
Mildly elevated CPK, toe-walking Distinctive clinical contractures of Achilles, elbows, and neck extension occur in late childhood	Myopathic	Slowly progressive; walks into sixth decade
CPK mildly elevated, mild DMD symptoms, muscle weakness in the muscles around the shoulder and hip	Dystrophic muscle biopsy	Begins in second or third decade; death before age 40 years
CPK normal Face, shoulder, upper arm affected		Weak shoulder flexion and abduction Normal life expectancy
Face, shoulder, upper arm affected; weak gluteus maximus muscle leading to substantial lumbar lordosis		Lumbar lordosis leads to wheelchair dependency and fixed hip flexion contractures
Often severe hypotonia at birth Weakness is worse distally than proximally (unlike DMD)	EMG demonstrates classic "dive bomber" response	75% survive at birth, growing stronger with age, walk by age 5 years Equinus deformities and distal weakness are common "Drooping face" appearance Cardiomyopathy and conduction problems frequent, very sensitive to anesthesia

IV. Spinal Muscular Atrophy

A. Overview

1. Spinal muscular atrophy (SMA) is the genetic disease that is most commonly fatal during childhood. It has an incidence of 1 in 10,000 live births.

2. The inheritance pattern of SMA is autosomal recessive.

3. Progressive weakness starts proximally and moves distally through the body.

B. Classification

1. SMA type I (Werdnig-Hoffmann disease) onset occurs at birth, with severe involvement of the spinal muscles. Death from respiratory failure occurs by age 2 years.

2. SMA type II onset occurs at age 6 to 18 months and causes diminishing function with time.

   a. Hip dislocations, scoliosis, and joint contractures are common.

   b. Life expectancy is 15+ years.

3. SMA type III onset occurs after age 18 months, with physical manifestations similar to those of SMA type II, but patients with type III can stand independently. Life expectancy is normal.

C. Pathoanatomy

1. Mutations in the survival motor neuron (SMN) gene on chromosome 5 cause deficiency of the SMN protein, resulting in progressive loss of alpha-motor neurons in the anterior horn of the

5: Pediatrics

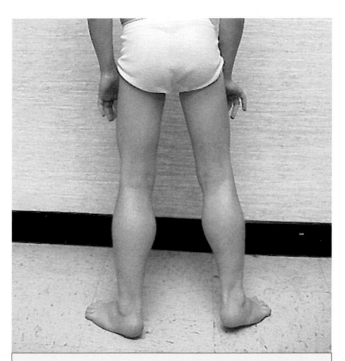

Figure 5 Photograph of a 5-year-old boy with Duchenne muscular dystrophy (DMD). The marked pseudohypertrophy of the calves is a common physical finding in DMD. (Reproduced from Sussman M: Duchenne muscular dystrophy. *J Am Acad Orthop Surg* 2002;10[2]:138-151.)

spinal cord and progressive weakness.

2. Two genes, SMN I and SMN II, both at 5q13, are involved in the occurrence of SMA. They both code for the SMN protein, but SMN II codes for a less functional SMN protein.

a. All patients with SMA lack both copies of SMN I.

b. The severity of SMA is determined by the number of functional copies of the SMN II gene. Healthy individuals have two SMA II gene copies. In patients with SMA, the mutation in SMN I can functionally convert it to SMN II. Patients with SMA can have up to four functional copies. The more functional copies of SMA II they have, the better they do.

D. Treatment—No effective medical treatment (such as steroids) is available for SMA.

1. Scoliosis is very common in SMA, occurring by age 2 to 3 years, and is progressive.

a. A thoracolumbosacral orthosis improves sitting balance in patients with SMA but does not stop progression of the disease.

b. A vertical expandable prosthetic titanium rib for thoracic insufficiency in young patients with SMA II who have spinal curves exceeding

50° has produced good results.

c. Posterior spinal fusion with fixation to the pelvis is performed when the spinal curvature exceeds 40° and forced vital capacity is more than 40% of normal. Fusion may cause an ambulatory child to lose the ability to walk (and may cause temporary loss of upper extremity function) because of loss of trunk motion.

2. Hip dislocation

a. May be unilateral or bilateral

b. Treatment of hip dysplasia and instability in SMA is controversial

c. The presence of pain should be the main indication for treatment and may require release of the hip adductor and flexor and/or osteotomies to maintain reduction of hip dislocation and minimize symptoms.

3. Contractures of the lower extremities are common in SMA.

a. Hip and knee contractures exceeding 30° to 40° are not generally treated surgically. Hamstring lengthening may sometimes be considered for contractures smaller than this in patients who are strong enough and have a strong motivation to walk.

b. Foot deformities such as equinovarus occur commonly in SMA. Rarely, if the patient is ambulatory and retains strength, tenotomy of the gastrocnemius-soleus, posterior tibialis, FDL, and FHL tendons may be done to maintain standing and walking.

V. Hereditary Motor Sensory Neuropathies

A. Hereditary motor sensory neuropathies (HMSNs) are chronic progressive peripheral neuropathies. They are common causes of cavus feet in children but may not be diagnosed before age 10 years. The distal hands and feet are affected first. Weakness of the proximal muscles is rare in Charcot-Marie-Tooth (CMT) disease, except in the most severe cases.

B. Classification

1. HMSN type I (CMT type I)

a. Is the most common type of HMSN, with an incidence of 1 in 2,500 children.

b. Peripheral myelin degeneration occurs with decreased motor nerve conduction.

c. Commonly caused by duplication of the gene at 17p11 (*PMP-22*) and mutations in X-linked connexin 32.

d. Autosomal dominant inheritance is the most common mode of inheritance of HMSN I, but

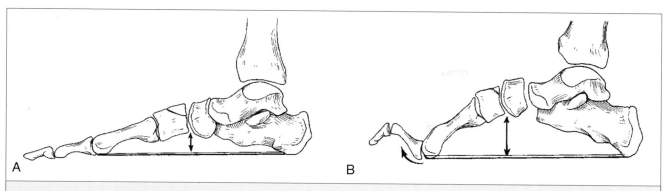

Figure 6   Illustrations show a normal foot and a cavus foot. **A,** Normal foot with normal arch height (double arrow) during standing. **B,** Cavus foot with increased arch height (double arrow) as a result of metatarsophalangeal joint hyperextension (curved arrow), such as occurs at toe-off and as seen in the windlass effect of the plantar fascia. (Reproduced from Schwend RM, Drennan JC: Cavus foot deformity in children. *J Am Acad Orthop Surg* 2003;11[3]: 201-211.)

its inheritance also can be autosomal recessive, X-linked, or sporadic.

   e. The onset of HMSN I occurs in the first to second decade of life.

   f. HMSN I (CMT I) shows slowed nerve conduction velocity (by definition <38 m/s) in upper limb motor nerves.

2. HMSN type II (CMT type II)

   a. The myelin sheath is intact, but wallerian axonal degeneration occurs, with decreased motor and sensory conduction.

   b. Autosomal dominant inheritance is the most common mode of inheritance of HMSN II, but it also can be inherited in an autosomal recessive, X-linked, or sporadic manner.

   c. The age at onset of HMSN II is the second decade of life or later.

   d. EMG shows a normal or slightly prolonged duration of the muscle action potential.

3. HMSN type III (Dejerine-Sottas disease)

   a. This type of HMSN is characterized by peripheral-nerve demyelination with severely decreased motor nerve conduction.

   b. An autosomal recessive mode of inheritance is common for HMSN III, with the causative mutation for the disease occurring in the myelin protein zero (*MPZ*) gene.

   c. HMSN III presents in infancy.

   d. HMSN III is characterized by enlarged peripheral nerves, ataxia, and nystagmus. The patient stops walking by maturity.

4. Other peripheral-nerve abnormalities in HMSN III include polyneuritis and atrophy of the small muscles of the hands.

C. Treatment

1. HMSN commonly presents as distal weakness, affecting intrinsic and extrinsic muscles.

2. Decreased sensation and areflexia also may be present.

3. Hip dysplasia (occurring in 5% to 10% of patients) results from weak hip abductor and extensor muscles.

   a. Hip dysplasia requires treatment, even if not symptomatic.

   b. Acetabular reconstruction is usually performed before VDRO.

4. Cavus foot (**Figure 6**)

   a. Cavus foot in HMSN results from contracted plantar fascia, weak anterior tibialis and peroneal muscles, and tightness of intrinsic muscles of the foot with normal FDL and FHL.

   b. The peroneus longus muscle is generally somewhat stronger than the peroneus brevis and anterior tibialis muscles.

   c. Surgery for cavus feet is performed to balance the muscle forces in the feet and maintain flexibility.

   • Surgery typically involves plantar release and posterior tibial tendon transfer to the dorsum or split posterior tibial tendon transfer.

   • Forefoot equinus should be corrected with plantar release and possibly midfoot osteotomies.

   • Lengthening of the Achilles tendon is occasionally needed, but only if there is true hindfoot equinus.

   • Osteotomies to correct bony deformities in

5: Pediatrics

adolescence include a calcaneal osteotomy (Dwyer) for fixed hindfoot varus (as determined with the Coleman block test).

- Fusion should be avoided to preserve flexibility.

5. Claw toes may become rigid and require treatment, such as interphalangeal fusion, often in conjunction with Jones transfers of the extensor tendons to the metatarsal heads.

6. Scoliosis or kyphoscoliosis is seen in 15% to 37% of children with HMSN and in up to 50% of patients with HMSN who are skeletally mature; it is more common in children with HMSN I and in girls.

    a. Bracing arrests the progression of scoliosis or kyphoscoliosis in a few cases.

    b. Surgery using posterior fusion is effective.

    c. Intraoperative somatosensory cortical evoked potentials may show a lack of signal transmission in patients with HMSN.

7. Intrinsic muscles of the hand and the thenar and hypothenar muscles may show wasting, limiting thumb abduction, and compromising pinch power. Surgically, transfer of the FDS, nerve decompression, release of contractures, and joint arthrodesis may be helpful.

VI. Friedreich Ataxia

A. Overview

1. Friedreich ataxia (FA) is the most common form of the uncommon spinocerebellar degenerative diseases. It occurs in 1 in 50,000 births.

2. The onset of FA occurs before age 25 years, with ataxia, areflexia, a positive extensor plantar response, and weakness. Often, the gluteus maximus is the first muscle involved.

3. Death usually occurs by the fourth or fifth decade of life.

4. Nerve conduction velocity is decreased in the upper extremities.

B. Pathoanatomy

1. The genetic mutation responsible for FA is multiple repetition of the base sequence guanine-adenine-adenine (GAA) in the frataxin (FXN) gene on chromosome 9q13, causing a lack of the protein frataxin, which is encoded by this gene and required for normal regulation of cellular iron homeostasis.

2. The age of onset of FA is related to the number of GAA repeats, with a greater number of repeats

associated with an earlier age of onset of the disease.

C. Treatment

1. The pes cavovarus in FA is progressive, rigid, and resistant to bracing.

    a. Ambulatory patients may be treated with tendon lengthenings and transfers.

    b. For rigid deformities, arthrodesis is needed to achieve a plantigrade foot.

2. Scoliosis occurs frequently in FA and will usually progress if the onset of the disease occured before age 10 years and the scoliosis began before age 15 years.

3. Posterior instrumented spinal fusion is effective for treating scoliosis in FA and does not need to extend to the pelvis.

VII. Rett Syndrome

A. Overview

1. Rett syndrome (RTT) is a neurodevelopmental disorder affecting the gray matter of the brain. The syndrome has an X-linked dominant pattern of inheritance and is generally caused by a de novo mutation. The affected gene encodes the methyl-CpG-binding protein-2 (MECP2), which methylates DNA.

2. Because it is X-linked dominant, RTT is generally lethal in affected male fetuses. Those carried to term frequently die of neonatal encephalopathy by 2 years of age. Males with RTT may result from Klinefelter syndrome, in which the male has an XXY karyotype.

3. The incidence of RTT is 1 in 10,000 births.

B. Clinical presentation

1. Development is normal until 6 to 18 months of age, after which it causes developmental regression.

2. Regression, with signs of mental retardation, autism, and ataxia, is rapid until age 3 years, and is followed by a more stable phase until age 10 years.

3. Seizures are common (80%).

4. Behavioral abnormalities include hand-wringing and hand-mouthing, lack of purposeful hand function, screaming and crying, loss of speech, and grinding of the teeth.

5. One-half of children with RTT become unable to walk after age 10 years as the result of deterioration of motor funciton. Most have ataxia and spasticity.

6. Gastrointestinal disorders, especially constipation, are common. Swallowing problems are common.

C. Orthopaedic concerns

1. Scoliosis occurs in more than 50% of patients with RTT.

   a. Long, neuromuscular-type thoracolumbar spinal curves develop at about age 10 years.

   b. Bracing is ineffective.

   c. Posterior spinal fusion is indicated when curves interfere with sitting or balance.

2. Spasticity frequently causes contractures, particularly equinus, in children with RTT.

3. Coxa valga occurs frequently, with hip instability, and should be treated to optimize function and/or decrease pain.

Top Testing Facts

Cerebral Palsy

1. The damage to the brain in CP is static, but the peripheral manifestations of CP often change over time.

2. Botulinum toxin blocks the presynaptic release of acetylcholine and generally relaxes the muscles into which it is injected for 3 to 6 months.

3. Progression of scoliosis is common after skeletal maturity in patients with quadriplegic CP.

4. Isolated supination of the forefoot in CP results from excessive tension of the anterior tibialis, whereas hindfoot varus comes from excessive tension of the posterior tibialis muscle.

5. Dynamic EMG helps determine whether the anterior or posterior tibialis muscle is causing a varus deformity of the foot in CP.

6. Calcaneal lengthening osteotomy (best undertaken in patients older than 6 years) can restore normal anatomy in patients with CP and is combined with lengthening of the peroneus brevis muscle and tightening of the medial talonavicular joint capsule and/or the posterior tibial tendon.

7. Swan neck deformities of the fingers in CP are a result of intrinsic muscle tightness and extrinsic overpull of the finger extensor muscles.

8. Nonambulatory patients with CP are at risk for fracture because of low BMD), which may be exacerbated by no weight bearing, poor calcium intake, or antiseizure medications.

Myelomeningocele

1. Prenatal diagnosis of myelomeningocele is made through assay of the α-fetoprotein concentration in maternal serum and is 60% to 95% accurate.

2. Urologic and gastrointestinal issues, including detrusor malfunction and abnormal sphincter tone, make early catheterization and bowel regimens important in patients with myelomeningocele.

3. Latex allergies are common in patients with myelomeningocele, necessitating precautions against contact with latex for all patients with this condition.

4. Hip-knee-ankle-foot orthoses, KAFOs, or AFOs are frequently used to support stance and/or prevent contracture in patients with myelomeningocele.

5. Dysplasia and/or dislocation of the hip occur in 80% of patients with involvement by myelomeningocele at the midlumbar level.

6. Flexion contracture of the knee exceeding 20° in a patient with myelomeningocele should be treated with hamstring lengthening, capsular release, growth modulation of the anterior distal femoral physis, and/or a distal femoral extension osteotomy.

7. In children without sensation, fractures often present with erythema, warmth, and swelling.

Muscular Dystrophies

1. DMD presents between ages 3 and 6 years with toe-walking or flatfootedness, difficulty in running or climbing stairs, and the classic calf pseudohypertrophy (seen in 85% of patients).

2. With increasing age, DMD in male children continues to worsen, causing shoulder weakness and scoliosis. Ambulation is often limited by age 10 years.

3. Nighttime ventilation substantially prolongs survival.

4. Early posterior instrumented fusion (for spinal curvature of 20° or more) is recommended before loss of forced vital capacity from respiratory-muscle weakness and progressively decreasing cardiac output.

5. Patients with DMD are at risk for malignant hyperthermia and may be pretreated with dantrolene.

Spinal Muscle Atrophy

1. SMA is the genetic disease that is most commonly fatal during childhood. It has an incidence of 1 in 10,000 live births.

2. SMA type I (Werdnig-Hoffmann disease) onset occurs at birth, with severe involvement of the spinal muscles. Death from respiratory failure occurs by age 2 years.

3. SMA type III onset occurs after 18 months of age, with physical manifestations similar to those of SMA type II, but patients with type III can stand independently. Life expectancy is normal.

4. Hip and knee contractures exceeding 30° to 40° are not generally treated surgically.

Top Testing Facts

Hereditary Motor Sensory Neuropathies

1. HMSNs are chronic progressive peripheral neuropathies.

2. HMSN I (CMT I) is the most common type of HMSN, with an incidence of 1 in 2,500 children.

3. Scoliosis or kyphoscoliosis is seen in 15% to 37% of children with HMSN and in up to 50% of patients with HMSN who are skeletally mature; it is more common in children with HMSN I and in girls.

Friedreich Ataxia

1. The onset of FA is before age 25 years, with ataxia, areflexia, a positive extensor plantar response, and weakness. Often the gluteus maximus is the first muscle involved.

2. The genetic mutation responsible for FA is multiple repetition of the base sequence GAA in the *FXN* gene on chromosome 9q13, causing a lack of the protein frataxin, which is encoded by this gene and required for normal regulation of cellular iron homeostasis.

3. Posterior instrumented spinal fusion is effective for treating scoliosis in FA and does not need to extend to the pelvis.

Rett Syndrome

1. RTT is a neurodevelopmental disorder affecting the gray matter of the brain.

2. Development is normal in children with RTT until 6 to 18 months of age, after which the syndrome causes developmental regression.

3. Behavioral abnormalities include hand-wringing and hand-mouthing, lack of purposeful hand function, screaming and crying, loss of speech, and grinding of the teeth.

4. Scoliosis occurs in more than 50% of patients with RTT.

Bibliography

Alman BA, Raza SN, Biggar WD: Steroid treatment and the development of scoliosis in males with duchenne muscular dystrophy. *J Bone Joint Surg Am* 2004;86(3):519-524.

Beaty JH, Canale ST: Orthopaedic aspects of myelomeningocele. *J Bone Joint Surg Am* 1990;72(4):626-630.

Boyd RN, Dobson F, Parrott J, et al: The effect of botulinum toxin type A and a variable hip abduction orthosis on gross motor function: A randomized controlled trial. *Eur J Neurol* 2001;8(suppl 5):109-119.

Chambers HG, Sutherland DH: A practical guide to gait analysis. *J Am Acad Orthop Surg* 2002;10(3):222-231.

Chan G, Bowen JR, Kumar SJ: Evaluation and treatment of hip dysplasia in Charcot-Marie-Tooth disease. *Orthop Clin North Am* 2006;37(2):203-209, vii.

Dabney KW, Miller F: Cerebral palsy, in Abel MF, ed: *Orthopaedic Knowledge Update: Pediatrics*, ed 3. Rosemont, IL, American Academy of Orthopaedic Surgeons, 2006, pp 93-109.

Davids JR, Rowan F, Davis RB: Indications for orthoses to improve gait in children with cerebral palsy. *J Am Acad Orthop Surg* 2007;15(3):178-188.

Flynn JM, Miller F: Management of hip disorders in patients with cerebral palsy. *J Am Acad Orthop Surg* 2002;10(3):198-209.

Gabrieli AP, Vankoski SJ, Dias LS, et al: Gait analysis in low lumbar myelomeningocele patients with unilateral hip dislocation or subluxation. *J Pediatr Orthop* 2003;23(3):330-334.

Gage JR: *Gait Analysis in Cerebral Palsy*. London, United Kingdom, Mac Keith Press, 1991.

Gage JR, DeLuca PA, Renshaw TS: Gait analysis: Principle and applications with emphasis on its use in cerebral palsy. *Instr Course Lect* 1996;45:491-507.

Hensinger RN, MacEwen GD: Spinal deformity associated with heritable neurological conditions: Spinal muscular atrophy, Friedreich's ataxia, familial dysautonomia, and Charcot-Marie-Tooth disease. *J Bone Joint Surg Am* 1976;58(1):13-24.

Karol LA: Surgical management of the lower extremity in ambulatory children with cerebral palsy. *J Am Acad Orthop Surg* 2004;12(3):196-203.

Kerr Graham H, Selber P: Musculoskeletal aspects of cerebral palsy. *J Bone Joint Surg Br* 2003;85(2):157-166.

McCarthy JJ, D'Andrea LP, Betz RR, Clements DH: Scoliosis in the child with cerebral palsy. *J Am Acad Orthop Surg* 2006;14(6):367-375.

Perry J: Normal and pathologic gait, in Bunch WH, ed: *Atlas of Orthotics*. St. Louis, MO, Mosby, 1985.

Renshaw TS, DeLuca PA: Cerebral palsy, in Morrissey RT, Weinstein WL, eds: *Lovell and Winter's Pediatric Orthopaedics*, ed 6. Philadelphia, PA, Lippincott Williams & Wilkins, 2006, pp 551-604.

Rodda JM, Graham HK, Nattrass GR, Galea MP, Baker R, Wolfe R: Correction of severe crouch gait in patients with spastic diplegia with use of multilevel orthopaedic surgery. *J Bone Joint Surg Am* 2006;88(12):2653-2664.

Sarwark JF, Aminian A, Westberry DE, Davids JR, Karol LA: Neuromuscular disorders in children, in Vaccaro AR, ed: *Orthopaedic Knowledge Update*, ed 8. Rosemont, IL, American Academy of Orthopaedic Surgeons, 2005, pp 677-689.

Scher DM, Mubarak SJ: Surgical prevention of foot deformity in patients with Duchenne muscular dystrophy. *J Pediatr Orthop* 2002;22(3):384-391.

Schwend RM, Drennan JC: Cavus foot deformity in children. *J Am Acad Orthop Surg* 2003;11(3):201-211.

Stout JL, Gage JR, Schwartz MH, Novacheck TF: Distal femoral extension osteotomy and patellar tendon advancement to treat persistent crouch gait in cerebral palsy. *J Bone Joint Surg Am* 2008;90(11):2470-2484.

Sussman M: Duchenne muscular dystrophy. *J Am Acad Orthop Surg* 2002;10(2):138-151.

Sussman M: Progressive neuromuscular diseases, in Abel MF, ed: *Orthopaedic Knowledge Update: Pediatrics*, ed 3. Rosemont, IL, American Academy of Orthopaedic Surgeons, 2006, pp 123-135.

Thompson GH, Bereson FR: Other neuromuscular diseases, in Morrissy RT, Weinstein SL, eds: *Lovell and Winter's Pediatric Orthopaedics*, ed 5. Philadelphia, PA, Lippincott Williams & Wilkins, 2001, pp 634-676.

Thompson JD: Myelomeningocele, in Abel MF, ed: *Orthopaedic Knowledge Update: Pediatrics*, ed 3. Rosemont, IL, American Academy of Orthopaedic Surgeons, 2006, pp 111-122.

Westberry DE, Davids JR: Cerebral palsy, in Song KM, ed: *Orthopaedic Knowledge Update: Pediatrics*, ed 4. Rosemont IL, American Academy of Orthopaedic Surgeons, 2011, pp 95-104.

5: Pediatrics

Chapter 56

Osteoarticular Infection

Howard R. Epps, MD   Scott B. Rosenfeld, MD

I. Osteomyelitis

A. Overview

1. Usually occurs in the first decade of life and affects 1 in 5,000 children younger than 13 years.

2. Is 2.5 times more common in boys than in girls

3. Management has become more complex with the emergence of more resistant, virulent strains of bacteria.

4. Often affects otherwise healthy children

5. Acute hematogenous osteomyelitis (AHO) is the most common type.

6. Risk factors include diabetes mellitus, chronic renal disease, hemoglobinopathies, rheumatoid arthritis, concurrent varicella infection, immunocompromise, sickle cell trait, and prematurity.

7. A child with bone pain and fever should be assumed to have osteomyelitis until a definitive diagnosis is made.

B. Pathophysiology

1. Acute hematogenous osteomyelitis

a. Bacteremia may result from a violation of the skin, a concurrent infection, or an event as simple as brushing the teeth.

b. Slow blood flow in the capillaries of the metaphysis allows bacteria to exit the vessel walls.

c. Infection occurs when bacteria lodge in the bone in sufficient numbers to overwhelm local defenses.

d. Osteoblast necrosis, activation of osteoclasts, release of inflammatory mediators, recruit-

ment of inflammatory cells, and blood vessel thrombosis cause a purulent exudate.

e. A subperiosteal abscess forms when the purulent exudate penetrates the porous metaphyseal cortex.

f. In bones with an intra-articular metaphysis (hip, shoulder, elbow, ankle), the purulent exudate can enter the joint and cause septic arthritis.

g. Local trauma has been associated with the development of AHO because it renders the bone more susceptible to bacterial seeding.

2. Chronic osteomyelitis

a. Periosteal elevation may deprive the underlying cortical bone of its blood supply, creating a necrotic fragment of bone (sequestrum).

b. The periosteum may form an outer layer of new bone (involucrum).

C. Bacteriology (**Table 1**)

1. *Staphylococcus aureus* is the most common cause of AHO.

2. A marked increase has occurred in infection by community-acquired methicillin-resistant *S aureus* (CA-MRSA).

a. Some strains of CA-MRSA harbor genes that encode the cytotoxin Panton-Valentine leukocidin (PVL).

b. PVL-positive strains of CA-MRSA are associated with complex infections, a greater incidence of multifocal infections, prolonged fever, myositis, pyomyositis, intraosseous or subperiosteal abscesses, chronic osteomyelitis, deep vein thrombosis (DVT), septic emboli, sepsis, and multisystem organ failure (**Figure 1**).

3. MRSA is responsible for more than half of staphylococcal infections in most communities, thus clindamycin is an appropriate choice for empiric antibiotic therapy. If/when cultures demonstrate MSSA, then antibiotics can be switched appropriately, typically to a first-generation cephalosporin.

4. *Kingella kingae* is a gram-negative aerobe that

Dr. Epps or an immediate family member serves as a board member, owner, officer, or committee member of the American Orthopaedic Association, the Pediatric Orthopaedic Society of North America, and the Texas Orthopaedic Association. Neither Dr. Rosenfeld nor any immediate family member has received anything of value from or has stock or stock options held in a commercial company or institution related directly or indirectly to the subject of this chapter.

5: Pediatrics

Table 1

Empiric Antibiotic Recommendations for Pediatric Musculoskeletal Infection

Age Group	Antibiotic	Dose (mg/kg)	Route	Frequency
Pediatric and adolescent	Clindamycin	10	IV	Every 6 h
	Clindamycin	8	Oral	Every 8 h
	Vancomycin[a]	15	IV	Every 6 h, intitally[b,c]
	Rifampin[d]	10	IV or oral	Every 24 h
Neonatal (age < 1 mo)	Ampicillin/sulbactam	150	IV	Every 6 h
	Gentamycin[e]	2	IV	every 8 h[b]
Neonatal (age 1-3 mo)	Vancomycin[e]	15	IV	Every 6 h, initially[b,c]
	Ceftriaxone[e]	100	IV	Every 24 h

[a]Recommended for suspected sepsis/severe infection

[b]Peak and trough measured after third dose

[c]Targe peak, 45 µg/mL; target trough, 15 µg/mL

[d]Used in conjunction with vancomycin in cases of osteomyelitis

[e]Recommended in combination

IV = intravenous.

Reproduced from Copley LA: Pediatric musculoskeltal infection: Trends and antibiotic recommendations. *J Am Acad Orthop Surg* 2009;17(10):618-626.

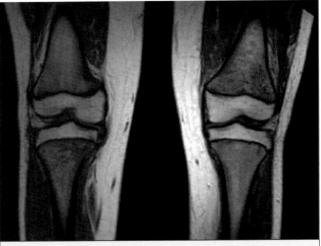

Figure 1 Coronal MRI from a girl with osteomyelitis of the left distal femur and the right proximal tibia caused by methicillin-resistant *Staphylococcus aureus*. The patient also had gluteal myositis and septic arthritis of the ankle.

has emerged as a leading cause of musculoskeletal infection in children 6 to 48 months of age.

a. Infections are characterized by mild to moderate clinical and laboratory signs of inflammation.

b. Patients can present with a low-grade or no fever, and in some series, the C-reactive protein (CRP) level concentration, the erythrocyte sedimentation rate (ESR), and the white blood cell (WBC) count in infected patients have all been substantially lower than in infections caused by other pathogens.

c. A fluid specimin placed in a blood culture bottle increases the probability of identifying *K kingae* in a joint in which infection is suspected, but the polymarase chain reaction has been shown to be the most sensitive method for identifying the pathogen.

5. Anaerobic bacteria are a rare cause of pediatric osteomyelitis and usually do this by spreading from infection at a contiguous site, as in conditions such as mastoiditis, otitis media, sinusitis, periodontal abscess, human bites, or decubitus ulcers.

D. Evaluation

1. History

a. The history of suspected osteomyelitis in a child should cover fever, pain, limp, refusal to bear weight, and recent local trauma or infections.

b. An immunization history must be obtained, particularly with regard to vaccination against *Haemophilus influenzae*.

c. Antibiotics may mask symptoms of osteomyelitis.

2. Examination

a. Temperature and vital signs should be measured to rule out hemodynamic instability.

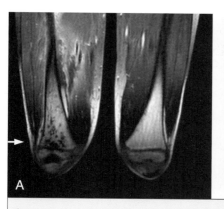
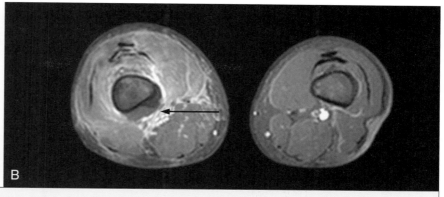

Figure 2   Coronal (**A**) and axial (**B**) MRIs in a child show osteomyelitis of the right distal femur with a posteromedial subperiosteal abscess (arrows).

b. The patient should specifically be examined for general appearance, the ability to bear weight, point tenderness, range of motion of adjacent joints (including the spine), and localized warmth, edema, and erythema.

3. Laboratory findings

   a. Initial blood work should include assay for CRP, ESR, blood cultures, and WBC count with differential count.

   b. The CRP is elevated in 98% of patients with AHO and becomes abnormal within 6 hours of infection.

   c. The ESR becomes elevated in 90% of patients with osteomyelitis and peaks in 3 to 5 days.

   d. Blood cultures may yield an organism in 30% of cases.

   e. The WBC count is elevated in only 25% of patients.

4. Diagnostic imaging

   a. Plain radiographs do not show bone changes for 7 days after infection but can demonstrate deep soft-tissue swelling and loss of tissue planes.

   b. Technetium Tc-99m bone scanning can help localize the focus of infection and will demonstrate a multifocal infection.

      • The overall accuracy is 92%.

      • A "cold" bone scan is associated with more aggressive infections, possibly requiring surgical treatment.

   c. MRI

      • Has a sensitivity of 88% to 100% for osteomyelitis

      • Detects the marrow and soft-tissue edema seen early in infection as well as abscesses

requiring surgical drainage (**Figure 2**)

      • Gadolinium-enhanced MRI increases diagnostic sensitivity and may show areas of involvement in nonossified growth cartilage.

      • Assists with preoperative planning

   d. CT demonstrates abscess formation and bony changes such as sequestra but is most helpful in the evaluation of chronic osteomyelitis.

5. Differential diagnosis—The differential diagnosis of AHO includes cellulitis, septic arthritis, toxic synovitis, fracture, thrombophlebitis, rheumatic fever, bone infarction, Gaucher disease, and malignancy (including leukemia).

E. Treatment

1. Aspiration—Aspiration of the suspected area is critical in both diagnosis and management.

   a. Performed before initiating antibiotics if the clinical condition of the patient allows

   b. Diagnostic aspiration helps guide medical management when the organism is identified (50% of cases).

   c. Antibiotic susceptibilities and the incidence of CA-MRSA vary by community, increasing the importance of specimen cultures.

   d. A large-bore needle is used to aspirate both the subperiosteal space and the intraosseous space.

   e. After aspiration, antibiotics may be started according to the guidelines in **Table 1**.

2. Nonsurgical

   a. If no purulent material is aspirated, the patient should be admitted for intravenous administration of antibiotics. Because of its frequency, CA-MRSA should be covered in most (if not all) cases.

   b. Intravenous antibiotics can be replaced by oral

5: Pediatrics

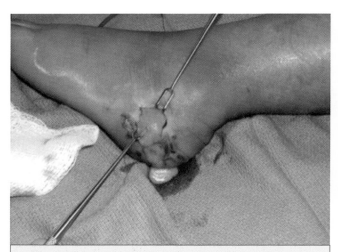

Figure 3 Photograph of surgical drainage of osteomyelitis of the calcaneus.

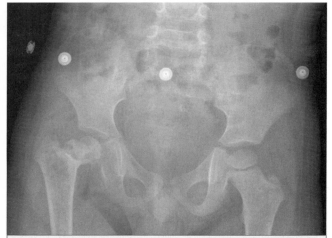

Figure 4 AP radiograph of the pelvis shows a pathologic fracture of the right femoral neck following osteomyelitis of the proximal femur.

antibiotics after improvement of clinical and laboratory findings is confirmed.

   c. For nonresistant organisms, antibiotics are usually given for at least 3 weeks and/or until the patient's ESR and CRP have normalized.

   d. For osteomyelitis caused by MRSA, antibiotics should be given for at least 8 weeks.

3. Surgical

   a. Indications for surgical drainage are aspiration of pus, abscess formation seen on imaging studies, and failure to respond adequately to nonsurgical treatment.

   b. Hemodynamic instability is a contraindication to emergent surgery; the patient should first be stabilized.

   c. Surgical drainage requires evacuation of all purulent material, débridement of devitalized tissue, drilling of the cortex, and débridement of intraosseous collections (**Figure 3**).

   d. Samples should be sent for culture and histology to rule out neoplasm.

   e. The wound can be either closed over drains if deemed to be adequately débrided or packed and débrided again after 2 to 3 days before closure over drains.

   f. More aggressive débridement may be needed in chronic osteomyelitis, sometimes including excision of a sequestrum.

F. Complications of AHO

   1. Meningitis

   2. Chronic osteomyelitis

   3. Septic arthritis

   4. Growth disturbance

   5. Pathologic fracture (**Figure 4**)

   6. Limb-length discrepancy

   7. Gait abnormality

   8. DVT and pulmonary embolism

   9. Sepsis and multiorgan failure

G. Subacute osteomyelitis

   1. Subacute osteomyelitis is an uncommon osseous infection characterized by bone pain and radiographic changes without systemic signs such as fever.

   2. The presentation is similar to that of a bony neoplasm, which should be included in the differential diagnosis.

   3. Its difference in presentation from that of AHO results from increased host resistance, less virulent pathogens, prior antibiotic exposure, or a combination of these factors.

   4. *S aureus* is the pathogen in most cases.

   5. Laboratory findings are usually unhelpful. The WBC count is usually normal or slightly elevated, the ESR is slightly elevated, the CRP is normal, and blood cultures are negative.

   6. Plain radiographs show changes ranging from a well-circumscribed radiolucency in the metaphysis or epiphysis to periosteal new bone formation resembling that in an aggressive malignancy (**Figure 5**). Subacute osteomyelitis lesions often cross the physis in contrast with those of AHO.

   7. Treatment is based on radiographic classification (**Figure 6**).

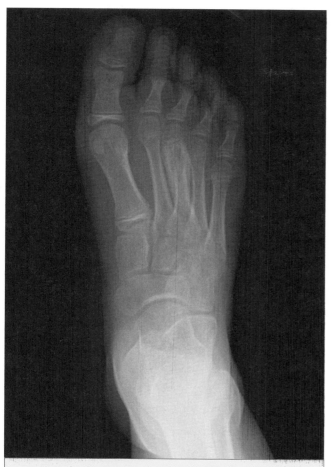

Figure 5 AP radiograph of the foot shows subacute osteomyelitis of the third metatarsal. The only symptom was activity-related pain.

a. If radiographic features of subacute osteomyelitis are present, a biopsy is needed to rule out malignancy.

b. Nonsurgical treatment is reserved for lesions without malignant features and that may respond to antibiotic therapy covering *S aureus*.

c. Débridement/curettage and treatment with appropriate antibiotics are indicated whenever radiographs show aggressive features (types II, III, and IV).

8. Complications include chronic osteomyelitis. Growth disturbance is unusual in subacute osteomyelitis.

II. Septic Arthritis

A. Overview

1. Septic arthritis is a surgical emergency. Delay in diagnosis and/or treatment may result in perma-

nent joint damage, deformity, and long-term disability.

2. The incidence of septic arthritis peaks in the first few years of life.

a. One-half of cases of septic arthritis occur in children younger than 2 years.

b. Large joints such as the hip (35%) and knee (35%) are most commonly involved.

B. Pathophysiology

1. Most cases of septic arthritis result from bacteremic seeding of a joint, direct inoculation of a joint (trauma or surgery), or contiguous spread from adjacent osteomyelitis.

2. Release of proteolytic enzymes from inflammatory cells, synovial cells, cartilage, and bacteria may damage the articular cartilage within 8 hours.

3. Increased joint pressure in the hip may cause osteonecrosis of the femoral head if not promptly relieved.

C. Bacteriology (**Table 1**)

1. Similar to that listed for osteomyelitis (see section I.C.)

2. The incidence of septic arthritis caused by *H influenzae* has decreased markedly since the advent of *H influenzae* vaccine.

D. Evaluation

1. The history should include the points listed in section I for osteomyelitis.

2. Physical examination

a. Patients may have fever and often show toxicity.

b. Patients do not use the affected extremity or refuse to bear weight on it.

c. Septic joints have an associated effusion, tenderness, and warmth; any motion causes severe pain.

d. The extremity is kept in the position that maximizes the volume of the joint; for the hip, this results in hip flexion, abduction, and external rotation (FABER).

3. Laboratory findings

a. The WBC count is elevated (leukocytosis) in 30% to 60% of patients, with a left shift in 60% of them.

b. The ESR is often elevated but may be normal early in the course of infection.

c. An elevated CRP level is the most helpful laboratory finding.

d. Blood cultures should be performed because

5: Pediatrics

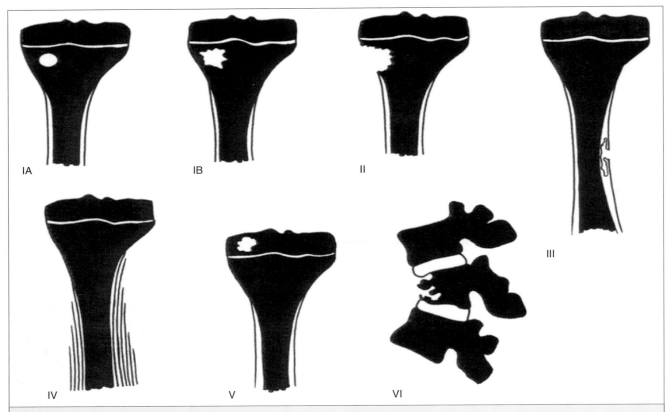

Figure 6 Radiographic classification of subacute osteomyelitis. Types IA and IB indicate lucency; type II, metaphyseal disease with loss of cortical bone; type III, diaphyseal disease; type IV, onion skinning; type V, epiphyseal disease; and type VI, disease of the spine. (Reproduced from Dormans JP, Drummond DS: Pediatric hematogenous osteomyelitis: New trends in presentation, diagnosis, and treatment. *J Am Acad Orthop Surg* 1994;2:333-341.)

they are often positive, even when local cultures are negative.

4. Diagnostic imaging

   a. Plain radiographs may show joint space widening and are needed to identify any possible bone involvement.

   b. Ultrasonography confirms a hip effusion and can be used to guide joint aspiration; it cannot differentiate septic from sterile effusions.

   c. MRI detects a joint effusion and can be used to assess for adjacent osseous involvement, but it can be difficult to perform expeditiously.

5. Aspiration

   a. Joint aspiration is necessary for the diagnosis of septic arthritis.

   b. Fluid samples should be taken for WBC count with differential (**Table 2**), Gram stain, and culture.

6. Differential diagnosis

   a. The differential diagnosis includes osteomyelitis, toxic synovitis, rheumatologic disorders, tuberculosis (TB), Lyme disease, poststreptococcal arthritis, reactive arthritis, villonodular synovitis, leukemia, sickle cell disease, hemophilia, serum sickness, and Henoch-Schönlein purpura.

   b. Septic arthritis of the hip can be differentiated from toxic synovitis through findings on physical examination and laboratory tests, although joint aspiration may be needed to confirm the diagnosis.

E. Diagnosis—Accurate diagnosis requires combined assessment of the clinical findings, laboratory studies, results of imaging, and clinical judgment.

1. If all four of the following are present, the probability of septic arthritis ranges from 59.0% to 99.6% in various series:

   a. Fever higher than 38.5°C

   b. Inability to bear weight

   c. ESR greater than 40 mm/h

   d. WBC count greater than 12,000/µL

2. A CRP level greater than 2.0 mg/dL is an independent risk factor for septic arthritis.

Table 2

Synovial Fluid Analysis

Disease	Leukocytes (cells/mL)	Polymorphonucleocytes (%)
Normal	<200	<25
Traumatic effusion	<5,000, with many erythrocytes	<25
Toxic synovitis	5,000-15,000	<25
Acute rheumatic fever	10,000-15,000	50
Juvenile rheumatoid arthritis	15,000-80,000	75
Lyme arthrtitis	40,000-140,000	> 75
Septic arthritis	>50,000	>75

Adapted with permission from Stans A: Osteomyelitis and septic arthritis, in Morrissy R, Weinstein S, eds: *Lovell and Winter's Pediatric Orthopaedics*, ed 6. Philadelphia, PA, Lippincott Williams & Wilkins, 2006, pp 439-492.

3. The order of importance of predictors is fever higher than 38.5°C, elevated CRP level, elevated ESR, refusal to bear weight, and elevated WBC count.

F. Treatment

1. Initial

   a. Treatment starts with joint aspiration, preferably before empiric administration of antibiotics (**Table 1**).

   b. Intravenous antibiotics are started after samples are sent for culture and are usually continued for 3 weeks. The patient's immunization status should be checked to determine whether empiric antibiotics should provide coverage of *H influenzae*.

2. Nonsurgical

   a. Nonsurgical treatment rarely has a role in septic arthritis, although some authors advocate intravenous antibiotics and serial aspirations for accessible joints.

   b. Recent data support the use of shorter courses of antibiotics, but the treatment plan should be made in concert with an infectious disease specialist familiar with the prevalence and virulence of local strains of pathogens.

3. Surgical

   a. Indications—Surgical drainage by arthrotomy and irrigation is the standard of care for almost all septic joints to remove damaging enzymes. In possible septic arthritis of the hip, it is better to err on the side of surgical drainage, which is associated with a much lower morbidity than a neglected septic hip.

   b. Contraindications—Surgical treatment is con-

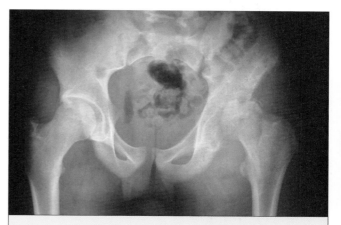

Figure 7 AP radiograph of the pelvis shows osteonecrosis of the left hip following septic arthritis with osteomyelitis of the pelvis.

traindicated when the patient's clinical status prevents it.

c. Procedures

   • Arthrotomy is performed to remove all purulent fluid and irrigate the joint.

   • In the case of an infected hip, an anterolateral or medial approach is performed emergently to decrease the risk of osteonecrosis.

   • Drainage of the shoulder, elbow, knee, and ankle can be open or arthroscopic.

G. Complications of septic arthritis are joint contracture, hip dislocation, growth disturbance, limb-length discrepancy, joint destruction, gait disturbance, and osteonecrosis (**Figure 7**).

5: Pediatrics

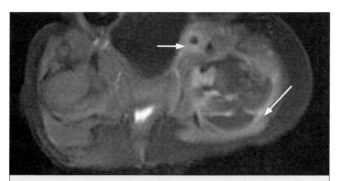

Figure 8 Coronal MRI of an 18-day-old premature neonate with septic arthritis of the hip and osteomyelitis of the left proximal femur. Note the deep vein thrombosis at the 1 o'clock position (short arrow) and the large intramuscular abscess at the 4 o'clock position (long arrow).

III. Specific Infections

A. Neonatal infections

1. Overview

   a. Neonates younger than 8 weeks deserve special consideration because their immune systems are immature.

   b. Neonates are more susceptible to infection than older children and often do not show the symptoms and signs that normally assist in the diagnosis of bone or joint infection.

2. Patient groups

   a. Infants in the neonatal intensive care unit

   • Are at risk for infection via sites of phlebotomy, indwelling catheters, invasive monitoring, peripheral alimentation, and intravenous drug administration

   • Those with musculoskeletal infections, which are typically caused by *S aureus* or gram-negative organisms, have multiple sites of infection in 40% of cases (**Figure 8**).

   b. Otherwise healthy infants 2 to 4 weeks of age who develop an infection at home

   • Group B streptococcus is usually the causative organism.

   • Usually, only a single site is involved.

3. Anatomy

   a. Before the secondary center of ossification appears, the metaphyseal vessels also supply the epiphysis, often (76% of cases) causing the spread of osteomyelitis in the metaphysis to the epiphysis and the adjacent joint.

   b. Growth disturbance and physeal arrest can occur.

4. Diagnosis—Diagnosis of bone or joint infections in the neonate can be difficult.

   a. Fever is usually absent.

   b. Early signs are pain with motion, decreased use of the affected extremity, pseudoparalysis, difficulty in feeding, and temperature instability.

   c. Tenderness, swelling, and erythema occur later.

5. Laboratory findings

   a. The WBC count is usually normal.

   b. Blood cultures are positive in 40% of cases, and the ESR may be elevated.

6. Treatment

   a. Neonates with documented sepsis should have aspiration and culture of all suspicious areas.

   b. Areas with sepsis should be surgically drained, with care taken to avoid additional damage to growth centers.

B. Shoe puncture

1. Superficial infections occur in 10% to 15% of children with shoe-puncture wounds, and deep infections occur in approximately 1%.

2. *Pseudomonas* is an organism of concern, although infection by *S aureus* is more common.

3. Tetanus immunization should be documented and provided if not already given.

4. Radiography should be performed to investigate for a retained foreign body.

5. Initial treatment consists of soaks, elevation, rest, and antibiotics that cover both *S aureus* and *Pseudomonas*.

6. Bone scanning or MRI can help identify more complex infections requiring surgical débridement.

7. Surgery is indicated for a foreign body, abscess, or septic arthritis or in cases of failure to respond to antibiotics.

8. More than 90% of late, deep infections are caused by *Pseudomonas*.

C. Diskitis

1. Usually occurs in children younger than 5 years

2. Begins in the vertebral end plates and moves to the disk through vascular channels

3. *S aureus* is the most common cause.

4. Blood cultures should be performed; local cultures are not routinely needed.

5. Patients present with low-grade fever, a limp, or

refusal to bear weight; the child refuses to move the spine.

6. Plain radiographs are normal for the first 2 to 3 weeks but may show loss of normal sagittal spinal contour early; bone scanning or MRI confirms the diagnosis earlier than plain radiography.

7. Antibiotic treatment is effective in most cases; patients who do not respond to antibiotics should have a biopsy.

D. Vertebral osteomyelitis

1. Affects older children

2. Usually causes more constitutional symptoms than does diskitis and more focal tenderness on examination

3. MRI or bone scanning is sensitive early in the disease process; plain radiography shows bone destruction later.

4. Treatment with antistaphylococcal agents is typically curative.

E. Sacroiliac infections

1. Infections of the sacroiliac joint cause fever, pain, and a limp.

2. Patients have pain with lateral compression of the pelvis, a positive FABER test, and tenderness over the sacroiliac joint.

3. MRI is the most sensitive diagnostic procedure.

4. Initial antibiotic treatment should cover *S aureus*, which is the most common pathogenic agent.

5. If needed, aspiration or drainage can usually be performed with CT guidance.

F. Sickle cell disease

1. Affected children are at increased risk for both septic arthritis and osteomyelitis.

2. The frequent bone infarcts, sluggish circulation, and decreased opsonization of bacteria in the disease increase the susceptibility to bone or joint infection.

3. Because *S aureus* and *Salmonella* are the most common pathogens, initial antibiotic treatment should cover both.

4. Differentiation between sickle cell crisis and infection can be challenging.

   a. Both entities may cause fever, pain, tenderness, swelling, and warmth.

   b. The WBC count, CRP level, and ESR may be elevated in both conditions.

   c. Bone scanning and MRI are often not specific.

5. Osteoarticular infection is present in only about 2% of children with sickle cell disease who are

hospitalized with musculoskeletal pain.

6. A positive blood culture or positive osteoarticular aspirate is diagnostic.

G. Notable diseases

1. Tuberculosis

   a. The incidence of TB has increased in developed countries in the past 30 years because of immunocompromised patients and the emergence of multidrug-resistant strains.

   b. Bone and/or joint involvement occurs in 2% to 5% of children with TB, most commonly involving the spine (50%), large joints (25%), and long bones (11%). Polyostotic involvement has been reported in 12% of children.

   c. Patients can present with fever, night sweats, weight loss, and pain. Patients with skeletal infections may have more subtle manifestations.

   d. In the spine, TB usually involves the anterior one-third of the vertebral body, most often in the region of the thoracolumbar junction; a paravertebral abscess may cause neurologic deficits.

   e. Long bone lesions are radiolucent, with poorly defined margins and surrounding osteopenia.

   f. The hip and knee are the most commonly affected joints. Involved joints have diffuse osteopenia and subchondral erosions.

   g. Laboratory findings—The WBC count is normal, the ESR is usually elevated, and the purified protein derivative test is usually positive.

   h. A biopsy with staining and culture showing acid-fast bacilli is diagnostic.

   i. Treatment is usually medical and is given for at least 1 year.

      • Surgical débridement of long bone lesions may hasten the resolution of constitutional symptoms, but incisions should be closed to avoid chronic sinus formation.

      • Drainage and stabilization of spinal lesions are indicated for neurologic deficits, spinal instability, progressive kyphosis, or failure of medical therapy.

2. Lyme disease

   a. Caused by *Borrelia burgdorferi*, which can induce erythema migrans, intermittent reactive arthritis, neuropathies, cardiac arrhythmias, and acute arthritis

   b. Infection is caused by a bite from the deer tick, which is prevalent in New England and the upper Midwest region of the United States.

   c. Patients can present with fever and a swollen,

irritable joint but will typically still bear weight.

   d. Infection with *B burgdorferi* typically causes erythema migrans, an expanding, red "bulls-eye" rash, although this rash is not always present.

   e. Laboratory workup should include an enzyme-linked immunosorbent assay for antibodies to *B burgdorferi* and a confirmatory Western blot assay. The WBC count may be normal or elevated; the ESR and the CRP level are usually elevated.

   f. Lyme arthritis is treated with antibiotics, including doxycycline, amoxicillin, and cefuroxime.

3. Gonococcal arthritis

   a. Caused by infection with *Neisseria gonorrhoeae,* it affects sexually active adolescents, sexually abused children, and neonates of infected mothers.

   b. Because of its association with sexual abuse, children with suspected gonococcal arthritis should have cultures of specimens from all mucous membranes.

   c. The knee is the most commonly involved joint, but the infection is polyarticular in 80% of cases.

   d. Because *N gonorrhoeae* is difficult to culture, synovial aspirates should be cultured on chocolate blood agar.

   e. Arthrotomy is required for treating hip infections; other joints can be observed or treated with serial aspiration.

   f. Ceftriaxone or cefixime are antibiotics of choice.

4. Coccidioidomycosis

   a. Caused by *Coccidioides immitis*, a fungus endemic to the southwestern United States

   b. Manifests as an upper respiratory infection but can progress to disseminated disease resulting in polyostotic osteomyelitis

   c. Both antifungal medical therapy and surgical débridement are usually required for cure.

IV. Chronic Recurrent Multifocal Osteomyelitis

A. Overview

1. Chronic recurrent multifocal osteomyelitis (CRMO), an idiopathic inflammatory disease of the skeleton, is a diagnosis of exclusion.

2. CRMO is characterized by a prolonged course with periodic exacerbations.

3. When there is associated synovitis, acne, pustulosis, hyperostosis, and osteitis, the condition is known as the SAPHO syndrome.

4. Periods of exacerbation characterize CRMO, but it usually goes into remission after 3 to 5 years.

5. The incidence is unknown.

6. CRMO occurs primarily in children and adolescents and is more common in girls; the peak age of onset is 10 years.

7. The metaphyses of long bones are most commonly involved, but CRMO also may involve the clavicle and the spine.

B. Pathoanatomy

1. The pathophysiology of CRMO is unknown.

2. Theories include infection by an organism with fastidious growth requirements or an autoimmune disorder.

C. Evaluation

1. Patients with CRMO have an episodic fever of insidious onset, malaise, local pain, tenderness, and swelling.

2. Laboratory findings

   a. The WBC count is usually normal.

   b. The ESR and the CRP level may be elevated.

   c. Biopsy and bone cultures are negative.

3. Diagnostic imaging

   a. Plain radiography shows eccentric metaphyseal lesions with sclerosis, osteolysis, and new bone formation that is often symmetric.

   b. Bone scanning helps identify all sites of involvement.

   c. Because of the shared characteristics of CRMO and malignancy, MRI helps the differential diagnosis by revealing the extent and soft-tissue involvement of the lesion.

D. Treatment

1. Nonsurgical

   a. Scheduled NSAIDs during exacerbations successfully manage the symptoms of CRMO in 90% of patients.

   b. Pamidronate therapy has been shown to provide symptomatic improvement and stimulate vertebral remodeling.

2. Surgical—Surgery is indicated only when a biopsy is needed to establish the diagnosis.

Top Testing Facts

1. A child with bone pain and fever should be assumed to have osteomyelitis until a definitive diagnosis is made.

2. PVL-positive strains of CA-MRSA are associated with complex infections, a greater frequency of multifocal infections, prolonged fever, myositis, pyomyositis, intraosseous or subperiosteal abscesses, chronic osteomyelitis, DVT, septic emboli, sepsis, and multisystem organ failure.

3. Biopsy is required to rule out malignancy in cases of subacute osteomyelitis.

4. Patients with subacute osteomyelitis may present without fever and with a normal WBC count and CRP level.

5. When managing the hip in septic arthritis, drainage should be more strongly considered in equivocal cases; the morbidity of arthrotomy is minimal compared with the sequelae of a neglected septic hip.

6. *Pseudomonas* is responsible for more than 90% of late deep infections following nail puncture through sneakers.

7. In diskitis, the infection begins in the vertebral end plates and moves to the disk through vascular channels.

8. *S aureus* and *Salmonella* are the most common infecting organisms in children with sickle cell anemia and musculoskeletal infection.

9. In children with TB, the most common sites of musculoskeletal infection are the spine (50%), large joints (25%), and long bones (11%). Polyostotic involvement occurs in 12% of children with TB.

10. A fluid specimen collected by arthrocentesis from a joint with suspected sepsis should be placed in a blood culture bottle to evaluate for *K kingae* infection in a young patient.

Bibliography

Belthur MV, Birchansky SB, Verdugo AA, et al: Pathologic fractures in children with acute Staphylococcus aureus osteomyelitis. *J Bone Joint Surg Am* 2012;94(1):34-42.

Browne LP, Guillerman RP, Orth RC, Patel J, Mason EO, Kaplan SL: Community-acquired staphylococcal musculoskeletal infection in infants and young children: Necessity of contrast-enhanced MRI for the diagnosis of growth cartilage involvement. *AJR Am J Roentgenol* 2012;198(1):194-199.

Ceroni D, Cherkaoui A, Combescure C, François P, Kaelin A, Schrenzel J: Differentiating osteoarticular infections caused by Kingella kingae from those due to typical pathogens in young children. *Pediatr Infect Dis J* 2011;30(10):906-909.

Copley LA: Pediatric musculoskeletal infection: Trends and antibiotic recommendations. *J Am Acad Orthop Surg* 2009;17(10):618-626.

Espinosa CM, Davis MM, Gilsdorf JR: Anaerobic osteomyelitis in children. *Pediatr Infect Dis J* 2011;30(5):422-423.

Gleeson H, Wiltshire E, Briody J, et al: Childhood chronic recurrent multifocal osteomyelitis: Pamidronate therapy decreases pain and improves vertebral shape. *J Rheumatol* 2008;35(4):707-712.

Kocher M, Dolan M: Weinberg J: Pediatric orthopaedic infections, in Abel M, ed: *Orthopaedic Knowledge Update: Pediatrics*, ed 3. Rosemont, IL, American Academy of Orthopaedic Surgeons, 2006, pp 57-73.

Liu C, Bayer A, Cosgrove SE, et al: Clinical practice guidelines by the infectious diseases society of america for the treatment of methicillin-resistant *Staphylococcus aureus* infections in adults and children: Executive summary. *Clin Infect Dis* 2011;53(3):285-292.

Martínez-Aguilar G, Avalos-Mishaan A, Hulten K, Hammerman W, Mason EO Jr, Kaplan SL: Community-acquired, methicillin-resistant and methicillin-susceptible Staphylococcus aureus musculoskeletal infections in children. *Pediatr Infect Dis J* 2004;23(8):701-706.

McCarthy JJ, Dormans JP, Kozin SH, Pizzutillo PD: Musculoskeletal infections in children: Basic treatment principles and recent advancements. *Instr Course Lect* 2005;54:515-528.

Moran GJ, Krishnadasan A, Gorwitz RJ, et al: Methicillin-resistant S. aureus infections among patients in the emergency department. *N Engl J Med* 2006;355(7):666-674.

Pääkkönen M, Kallio MJ, Peltola H, Kallio PE: Pediatric septic hip with or without arthrotomy: Retrospective analysis of 62 consecutive nonneonatal culture-positive cases. *J Pediatr Orthop B* 2010;19(3):264-269.

Peltola H, Pääkkönen M, Kallio P, Kallio MJ; Osteomyelitis-Septic Arthritis (OM-SA) Study Group: Prospective, randomized trial of 10 days versus 30 days of antimicrobial treatment, including a short-term course of parenteral therapy, for childhood septic arthritis. *Clin Infect Dis* 2009;48(9):1201-1210.

Singhal R, Perry DC, Khan FN, et al: The use of CRP within a clinical prediction algorithm for the differentiation of septic arthritis and transient synovitis in children. *J Bone Joint Surg Br* 2011;93(11):1556-1561.

5: Pediatrics

Stans A: Osteomyelitis and septic arthritis, in Morrissy R, Weinstein S, eds: *Lovell and Winter's Pediatric Orthopaedics*, ed 6. Philadelphia, PA, Lippincott Williams & Wilkins, 2006, pp 439-491.

Vaz A, Pineda-Roman M, Thomas AR, Carlson RW: Coccidioidomycosis: An update. *Hosp Pract* 1995;1998(33): 105-108, 113-115, 119-120.

Williams DJ, Cooper WO, Kaltenbach LA, et al: Comparative effectiveness of antibiotic treatment strategies for pediatric skin and soft-tissue infections. *Pediatrics* 2011;128(3): e479-e487.

Willis AA, Widmann RF, Flynn JM, Green DW, Onel KB: Lyme arthritis presenting as acute septic arthritis in children. *J Pediatr Orthop* 2003;23(1):114-118.

Yagupsky P, Porsch E, St Geme JW III: Kingella kingae: An emerging pathogen in young children. *Pediatrics* 2011; 127(3):557-565.

Chapter 57
The Pediatric Hip

Paul D. Choi, MD

I. Developmental Dysplasia of the Hip

A. Overview

1. Definition

   a. Developmental dysplasia of the hip (DDH) refers to the spectrum of pathologic conditions involving the developing hip, ranging from acetabular dysplasia to complete dislocation of the hip.

   b. Teratologic dislocation of the hip occurs in utero and is irreducible on neonatal examination. A pseudoacetabulum is usually present. This condition always accompanies other congenital anomalies or neuromuscular conditions, most often arthrogryposis and myelomeningocele.

2. Epidemiology

   a. DDH is the most common disorder of the hip in children. One in 1,000 children (0.1%) is born with a dislocated hip; 10 in 1,000 children (1%) are born with hip subluxation or dysplasia.

   b. Eighty percent of affected children are female.

   c. The left hip is more commonly involved (60%) than the right; bilateral involvement occurs in 20% of cases.

   d. The condition is more common in Native Americans and people of northern Finnish descent than in those of other ethnic backgrounds; DDH is rarely seen in African Americans.

   e. The etiology of DDH is unknown but is thought to be multifactorial (genetic, hormonal, and mechanical).

B. Pathoanatomy

1. Risk factors for DDH

   a. Female sex, first born child, breech presentation

   b. Disorders of intrauterine packing phenomenon, such as congenital dislocation of the knee, congenital muscular torticollis, and metatarsus adductus

   c. In affected children, 12% to 33% have a family history of DDH. The risk is 6% with one affected sibling, 12% with one affected parent, and 36% with a parent and sibling affected.

C. Evaluation

1. Clinical presentation

   a. Clinical presentation varies with age. In the neonatal period, the key clinical finding is instability of the hip.

   b. Hip clicks are nonspecific physical findings.

   c. Asymmetric skin folds are an unreliable and nonspecific finding.

   d. In infants older than 6 months, common findings are limitation of motion and apparent limb shortening.

   e. In toddlers, restricted motion may be accompanied by a limb-length discrepancy, a limp, or a waddling gait.

   f. Adolescents may manifest all of the above signs and symptoms in addition to fatigue and pain in the hip, thigh, or knee.

2. Physical examination—Accuracy of the physical examination requires that the patient be relaxed.

   a. The Galeazzi test is performed with the patient in the supine position with the hips and knees flexed to 90°. The test is positive when the knee on the involved side is lower than the contralateral knee. It is positive only in unilateral subluxation or dislocation of the hip.

   b. The Barlow test is performed by applying a posterolateral force to the leg with the hip in a flexed and adducted position (**Figure 1**). The test is positive when the hip on the affected side subluxates or dislocates.

   c. The Ortolani test is performed by abducting and lifting the proximal femur anteriorly (**Fig-**

5: Pediatrics

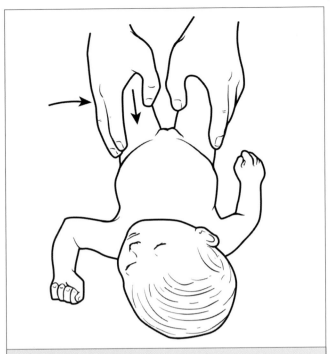

Figure 1 Illustration shows the Barlow test. The test is positive when the hip subluxates or dislocates. (Reproduced from Sarwark JF, ed: *Essentials of Musculoskeletal Care*, ed. 4. Rosemont, IL, American Academy of Orthopaedic Surgeons, 2010, p 1051.)

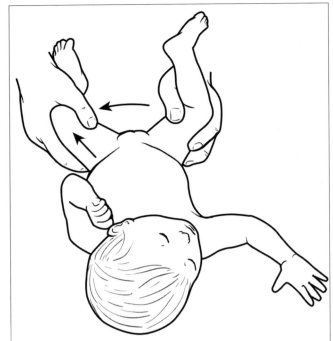

Figure 2 Illustration shows the Ortolani test. The test is positive when the dislocated hip is reducible. (Reproduced from Sarwark JF, ed: *Essentials of Musculoskeletal Care*, ed. 4. Rosemont, IL, American Academy of Orthopaedic Surgeons, 2010, p 1051.)

ure 2). The test is positive when the dislocated hip is reducible.

   d. Range of motion (ROM) testing of the hip is important; a decrease in abduction is the most sensitive test result for DDH. ROM will be normal in children younger than 6 months, however, because contractures will not yet have developed.

D. Diagnostic tests

  1. Ultrasonography

   a. In the first 4 to 6 months of life, when plain radiographic evaluation is unreliable because the femoral epiphysis has not yet ossified, ultrasonography can help confirm a diagnosis of DDH. Ultrasonography can also document reducibility and stability of the hip in an infant being treated with a Pavlik harness or brace.

   b. Reference parameters (**Figure 3**):

     • At age 4 to 6 weeks, a normal α angle is greater than 60°; a normal β angle is less than 55°. (The α angle is formed by a vertical reference line through the iliac bone and a line along the osseous roof of the acetabulum; the β angle is formed by a line drawn through the labrum and the vertical iliac reference line and represents the cartilaginous roof of the acetabulum.)

     • The acetabulum should cover more than 50% of the femoral head.

  2. Plain radiography—**Figure 4** shows the reference lines and angles used on the AP view of the pelvis (**Figure 5**).

   a. The Hilgenreiner line is drawn horizontally through each triradiate cartilage.

   b. The Perkin line is drawn perpendicular to the Hilgenreiner line at the lateral edge of the acetabulum.

   c. The Shenton line is a continuous arch drawn along the medial border of the femoral neck and superior border of the obturator foramen.

   d. The acetabular index is the angle formed by an oblique line (through the outer edge of the acetabulum and triradiate cartilage) and the Hilgenreiner line. The acetabular index should be less than 25° at age 12 months and less than 20° at age 24 months.

   e. The center-edge angle of Wiberg is the angle formed by a vertical line through the center of the femoral head and an oblique line through

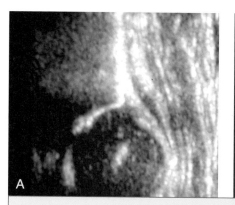
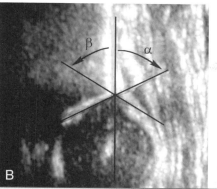
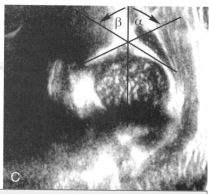

Figure 3 Ultrasonographic images of a normal hip and a hip with developmental dysplasia of the hip. **A,** Ultrasonographic image of a normal hip. **B,** The same ultrasonographic image as in A, with the α and β angles drawn. In a normal hip, femoral head coverage should be greater than 50%. The α angle should be greater than 60°. **C,** Ultrasonographic image of a dysplastic hip reveals approximately 30% femoral head coverage, an α angle of 50°, a β angle of 90°, and an echogenic labrum. (Reproduced from DeLuca PA: Developmental dysplasia of the hip and congenital coxa vara, in Abel MF, ed: *Orthopaedic Knowledge Update: Pediatrics*, ed 3. Rosemont, IL, American Academy of Orthopaedic Surgeons, 2006, p 181.)

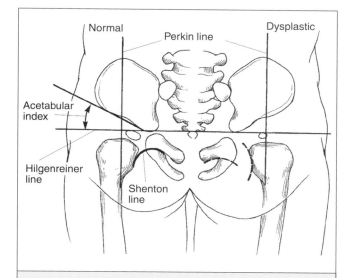

Figure 4 Illustration shows reference lines and angles used in the evaluation of developmental dysplasia of the hip.

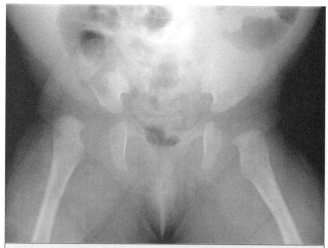

Figure 5 Plain AP radiograph of the pelvis demonstrates a dislocated right hip. The proximal femoral ossific nucleus is not yet present. Also note that the Shenton line is disrupted.

the outer edge of the acetabulum and the center of the femoral head (**Figure 6**). An angle less than 20° is considered abnormal. The center-edge angle of Wiberg is reliable only in patients older than 5 years.

3. Arthrography of the hip is performed to dynamically assess the quality of a closed reduction.

4. CT or MRI may be performed to confirm acceptable reduction for a patient in a spica cast following a closed or open procedure.

E. Neonatal screening

1. Ultrasonographic screening of all newborn hips remains controversial.

2. Routine ultrasonographic screening should be performed for infants with risk factors for DDH (for example, breech, family history). The screening should be delayed until age 4 to 6 weeks (or corrected age for premature infants) because ultrasonography is associated with poor specificity in the early newborn period.

F. Treatment—Treatment of DDH is based on age, stability, and severity of dysplasia. The goal is a stable, concentric reduction of the femoral head in the true acetabulum (**Table 1**).

1. Newborns and infants younger than 6 months

   a. Closed reduction and immobilization in a Pavlik harness is the treatment of choice for

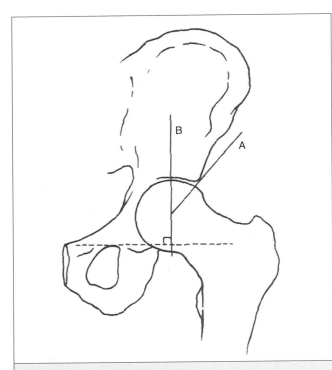

Figure 6 Illustration demonstrates the center-edge angle of Wiberg, which is formed by two lines passing through the center of the femoral head; one extends to the lateral edge of the sourcil (**A**), and the other is perpendicular to the inter-teardrop line (**B**). (Reproduced with permission from MacDonald SJ, Hersche O, Ganz R: Periacetabular osteotomy in the treatment of neurogenic acetabular dysplasia. *J Bone Joint Surg Br* 1999;81:975-978.)

Table 1		
Treatment of Developmental Dysplasia of the Hip		
Age (months)	**Initial Treatment**	
0–6	Pavlik harness	
6–18	Closed or open reduction (closed reduction is preferred if the hip has a small medial dye pool and is stable with < 60° of abduction.)	
> 18[a]	Open reduction Femoral shortening osteotomy is indicated in high-riding dislocations (typically, in children ≥ 2 years old) Pelvic osteotomy is indicated for significant dysplasia (often in children ≥ 18–24 months old)	

[a]Open treatment is generally indicated for children with unilateral dislocations up to age 8 years at the time of initial presentation and for those with bilateral dislocations presenting at up to 6 years of age.

dysplasia, subluxation, or complete dislocation of the hip.

b. Proper positioning of the Pavlik harness is critical.

- The hips should be flexed to 100° with mild abduction.

- Excessive flexion should be avoided to reduce the risk of femoral nerve palsy.

- Excessive abduction should be avoided to reduce the risk of osteonecrosis.

c. The duration of treatment varies. Most authors recommend uninterrupted treatment for 6 to 12 weeks after clinical stability is achieved.

d. Frequent (every 1 to 2 weeks) clinical examination and ultrasonographic examination are needed to evaluate reduction and stability of the hip or hips.

e. Pavlik harness treatment should be discontinued if the dislocated hip does not reduce within 3 to 4 weeks, to avoid "Pavlik harness disease"

(erosion of the posterosuperior acetabular rim). Success rates greater than 90% have been reported with use of the Pavlik harness in treating hips with a positive Ortolani test result (that is, dislocated hips).

f. Because the rate of recurrence is 10%, follow-up until maturity is necessary.

g. When a Pavlik harness is ineffective, a trial of a hip abduction orthosis may be successful in stabilizing a dysplastic hip.

2. Children 6 to 18 months of age

a. Closed reduction under general anesthesia is the preferred treatment.

b. The evidence for preliminary traction is equivocal. Given this fact and the possible complications of skin sloughing and leg ischemia, most centers have abandoned preliminary traction.

c. Hip arthrography is used intraoperatively to confirm adequacy of reduction. Less than 5 mm of medial pooling of contrast material should be seen between the femoral head and acetabulum.

d. The safe and stable zones for abduction/adduction, flexion/extension, and internal/external rotation should be established.

e. Adductor tenotomy is often necessary to widen the safe zone.

f. A spica cast is applied with the hip maintained in the "human position" (hip flexion of 90° to 100° and abduction). Hip abduction should be less than 60° to minimize the risk of osteonecrosis.

g. Open reduction is indicated when concentric closed reduction cannot be achieved or when excessive abduction (> 60°) is required to maintain reduction.

h. The reduction of the hip in the cast must be confirmed with either CT or MRI.

i. Cast immobilization is continued for 3 to 4 months; an abduction brace may then be used until the acetabulum normalizes.

3. Children older than 18 months

a. Open reduction is the preferred treatment.

b. Surgical treatment is generally indicated for children up to 8 years of age with a unilateral dislocation. After 8 years of age, the risks of surgery outweigh the benefits. The upper age limit for surgical treatment of DDH in children with bilateral dislocations is typically 5 to 6 years.

c. The goal of open reduction is to remove the obstacles to reduction and/or safely increase its stability (**Table 2**). Impediments to congruent reduction are the iliopsoas muscle, hip adductors, joint capsule, ligamentum teres, pulvinar, and transverse acetabular ligament. An infolded labrum may be an impediment in some cases.

d. The most commonly used approaches are anterior and medial (or anteromedial) (**Table 3**).

e. Femoral shortening osteotomy is indicated in children with high-riding dislocations, to achieve and maintain reduction and minimize the risk of osteonecrosis. This is necessary in most but not all children 2 years of age or older.

f. Pelvic osteotomy is needed for substantial acetabular dysplasia (typical in children older than 18 to 24 months of age). Osteotomy notably reduces the rate of reoperation when performed at the time of initial surgery in children in this age group.

4. Residual dysplasia after closed or open treatment

a. Pelvic osteotomy may be indicated for persistent acetabular dysplasia and hip instability. Clinical practice varies considerably with regard to pelvic osteotomy in children older than 2 years.

b. The two general types of pelvic osteotomy are reconstructive and salvage (**Table 4**).

c. Reconstructive pelvic osteotomies redirect or reshape the roof of the acetabulum, with its

---

Table 2

Obstacles to a Concentric Reduction in Developmental Dysplasia of the Hip

Extra-articular	Intra-articular
Tight psoas tendon	Constricted joint capsule
Tight adductor muscles	Pulvinar
	Hypertrophied ligamentum teres
	Infolded labrum
	Hypertrophied transverse acetabulum ligament

Adapted from Vitale MG, Skaggs DL: Developmental dysplasia of the hip from six months to four years of age. *J Am Acad Orthop Surg* 2001;9:401-411.

Table 3

Advantages and Disadvantages of Anterior Versus Medial or Anteromedial Approaches for Developmental Dysplasia of the Hip

Approach	Advantages	Disadvantages
Anterior	Capsulorrhaphy and pelvic osteotomy possible through the same incision Acetabulum (including labrum) directly accessible Lower reported risk of osteonecrosis Shorter duration of spica casting (6 weeks) Familiar surgical approach	Postoperative stiffness Potential blood loss Potential injury to the lateral femoral cutaneous nerve
Medial or anteromedial	Allows direct access to medial structures blocking reduction (pulvinar, ligamentum teres, transverse acetabular ligament) Avoids splitting iliac crest apophysis Avoids damage to hip abductors Less invasive, minimal dissection Cosmetically acceptable scar	Capsulorrhaphy and pelvic osteotomy not possible through this incision Poor visualization of acetabulum; labrum not accessible Higher risk of osteonecrosis Longer duration of cast immobilization (3–4 months)

Table 4

Pelvic Osteotomies for the Treatment of Developmental Dysplasia of the Hip

	Reconstructive	Salvage
Redirectional	**Reshaping**	
Single innominate (Salter)	Pemberton	Chiari osteotomy
Triple innominate	Dega	Shelf arthroplasty
Periacetabular (for example, Ganz)		

Adapted from Gillingham BL, Sanchez AA, Wenger DR: Pelvic osteotomies for the treatment of hip dysplasia in children and young adults. *J Am Acad Orthop Surg* 1999;7:325-337.

normal hyaline cartilage, into a more appropriate weight-bearing position. A prerequisite for reconstructive pelvic osteotomy is a hip that can be reduced concentrically and congruently. The hip must also have near-normal ROM.

- Redirectional pelvic osteotomies (**Figure 7**) include the single innominate (Salter), triple innominate, and periacetabular (for example, Ganz) osteotomies.

- Reshaping pelvic osteotomies (acetabuloplasties) include the Pemberton, Dega, Pembersal, and San Diego osteotomies.

d. Salvage osteotomies increase weight-bearing coverage by using the joint capsule as a structure interposed between the femoral head and bone above it. Salvage osteotomies rely on fibrocartilaginous metaplasia of the interposed joint capsule to provide an increased articulating surface. The intent of these osteotomies is to reduce point loading at the edge of the acetabulum.

- Salvage osteotomies are typically indicated for adolescents with severe dysplasia in whom acetabular deficiency precludes a reconstructive osteotomy.

- Salvage osteotomies include the Chiari (**Figure 8**) and shelf osteotomies.

II. Legg-Calvé-Perthes Disease

A. Overview

1. Legg-Calvé-Perthes (LCP) disease is an idiopathic osteonecrosis of the femoral head in children.

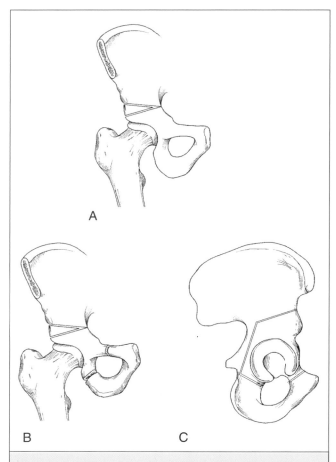

Figure 7 Illustrations show redirectional pelvic osteotomy options. **A,** Single innominate (Salter). **B,** Triple innominate. **C,** Periacetabular.

2. Epidemiology

a. LCP disease affects 1 in 1,200 children.

b. It affects boys between four and five times more commonly than girls.

c. Bilateral hip involvement is present in 10% to 15% of patients.

d. LCP disease is more commonly diagnosed in urban than in rural communities.

e. A predilection appears to exist for certain populations, with an above-average incidence in Asians, the Inuit, and central Europeans. The incidence is below average in native Australians, Native Americans, Polynesians, and African Americans.

B. Etiology

1. The exact etiology of LCP disease is unknown, but it is probably caused by a combination of genetic and environmental factors.

2. Historically, the cause was thought to be inflammatory or infectious, with transient synovitis as a

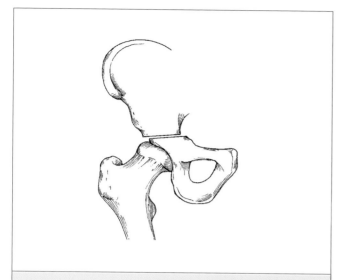

Figure 8 Illustration shows salvage pelvic osteotomy using a Chiari medial displacement osteotomy.

possible precursor. Trauma was once also believed to be causative.

3. Proposed etiologies include mutations in type II collagen, abnormal insulin-like growth factor-1 action pathways, and various types of thrombophilia.

4. The role of thrombophilia as a cause of LCP disease is controversial. Some studies have reported a 50% to 75% association between LCP disease and a coagulation abnormality; other studies have not shown any such association.

5. Associated factors

a. A family history is found in 1.6% to 20.0% of cases.

b. LCP disease is associated with attention deficit hyperactivity disorder in 33%.

c. Patients are commonly skeletally immature, with bone age delayed in 89%.

C. Pathoanatomy

1. Current theories propose that a disruption of the vascularity of the femoral head serves as the key pathogenic event in LCP disease, resulting in ischemic necrosis and subsequent revascularization.

2. The abnormal femoral head (weakened by ischemia) can deform when its mechanical strength is surpassed by loading forces on the hip joint. This deformity may eventually remodel with healing and revascularization.

3. The articular cartilage, capital epiphysis, physis, and metaphysis of the hip joint are histologically abnormal in LCP disease, with disorganized cartilaginous areas of hypercellularity and fibrillation.

D. Evaluation

1. LCP disease is a diagnosis of exclusion. Other causes of osteonecrosis (for example, septic arthritis, sickle cell disease, corticosteroid therapy) and mimicking conditions (for example, skeletal dysplasias, mucopolysaccharidoses) must be ruled out.

2. Clinical presentation

a. LCP disease occurs most often in children 4 to 8 years of age (range, 2 years to late teens).

b. The onset is insidious; children with LCP disease commonly have a limp and pain in the groin, hip, thigh, or knee regions.

c. Occasionally, children with LCP disease have a history of recent or remote viral illness.

3. Physical examination

a. Examination may reveal an abnormal gait (antalgic and/or Trendelenburg).

b. Limitation of hip motion depends on the stage of disease. ROM testing often reveals decreased abduction and internal rotation. Hip flexion contractures are seen rarely.

c. Limb-length discrepancy, if present, is mild and a result of femoral head collapse. Hip contractures may make the limb-length discrepancy seem greater than it actually is.

E. Diagnostic tests

1. Plain radiographs

a. A standard AP view of the pelvis and lateral view of the proximal femur are critical in making the initial diagnosis and assessing the subsequent clinical course.

2. LCP disease typically proceeds through four radiographic stages (described by Waldenström).

a. Initial stage—Early radiographic findings are a sclerotic, smaller proximal femoral ossific nucleus (because of failure of the epiphysis to increase in size) and widened medial clear space (distance between the teardrop and femoral head).

b. Fragmentation stage (mean duration = 1 year)—Segmental collapse (resorption) of the capital femoral epiphysis, with increased density of the epiphysis.

c. Reossification or reparative stage (mean duration = 3 to 5 years)—Necrotic bone is resorbed, with subsequent reossification of the capital femoral epiphysis.

d. Remodeling stage—Remodeling begins when the capital femoral epiphysis is completely reossified.

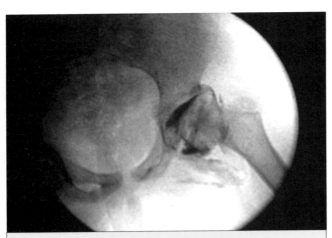

Figure 9 Arthrogram of the left hip shows hinge abduction. With the hip abducted, the lateral edge of the epiphysis hinges on the lateral acetabulum, with concomitant medial dye pooling. (Reproduced from Matheney T: Legg-Calvé Perthes disease, in Song KM, ed: *Orthopaedic Knowledge Update: Pediatrics*, ed 4. Rosemont, IL, American Academy of Orthopaedic Surgeons, 2011, p 183.)

3. MRI—The role of MRI in LCP disease is evolving.

   a. MRI can aid in the early diagnosis of LCP disease.

   b. Enhanced MRI techniques may provide information about the vascular status of the femoral head.

4. Arthrography is useful for assessing coverage and containment of the femoral head.

   a. Dynamic arthrography is often used at the time of surgery to confirm the degree of correction that femoral and/or pelvic osteotomies need to provide.

   b. Dynamic arthrography may also be used to identify hips with severe deformity and hinge abduction (**Figure 9**).

F. Classification

   1. The lateral pillar (Herring) classification of LCP disease (**Figure 10**) is based on the height of the lateral 15% to 30% of the epiphysis (that is, the lateral pillar) on an AP view of the pelvis. The groups in this classification are described below.

      a. Group A—No involvement of the lateral pillar, with no changes in its density and no loss of its height.

      b. Group B—More than 50% of the height of the lateral pillar is maintained.

      c. Group C—Less than 50% of the height of the lateral pillar is maintained.

   d. B/C border groups—These groups were later added to the original three-category Herring classification. In these groups, the lateral pillar is narrow (2 to 3 mm wide) or poorly ossified, or exactly 50% of the lateral pillar height is maintained.

   e. The advantage of the Herring classification is that it strongly correlates with the prognosis in LCP disease. Its limitation is that the final classification cannot be determined at the time of initial presentation.

2. The Catterall classification defines the extent of involvement of the femoral head in LCP disease (**Figure 11**). Although commonly used in the past, it has more recently been criticized for its poor interobserver reliability.

   a. Group I—Involvement is limited to the anterior head.

   b. Group II—The anterior and central parts of the head are involved.

   c. Group III—Most of the head is involved, with sparing of the posteromedial corner of the epiphysis.

   d. Group IV—The entire head is involved.

3. Catterall also described four signs of risk that indicate a more severe course of disease:

   a. The Gage sign (radiolucency in the shape of a V in the lateral portion of the epiphysis)

   b. Calcification lateral to the epiphysis

   c. Lateral subluxation of the femoral head

   d. A horizontal physis

4. None of the existing classifications of LCP disease are sufficiently prospective to provide a prognosis before the onset of deformity.

G. Treatment

   1. The treatment of LCP disease is highly controversial.

   2. Current treatments are largely based on containing the femoral head in the acetabulum, which optimizes molding of the soft femoral head and minimizes deformity of the head.

   3. The aim of treatment is to achieve a spherical femoral head and congruent joint to minimize the risk of osteoarthritis.

   4. Treatment is based on the patient's age at disease onset and the severity of involvement of the femoral head (defined by the lateral pillar classification).

      a. Patients younger than 6 years without complete collapse of the lateral pillar can generally be treated nonsurgically. Most patients achieve

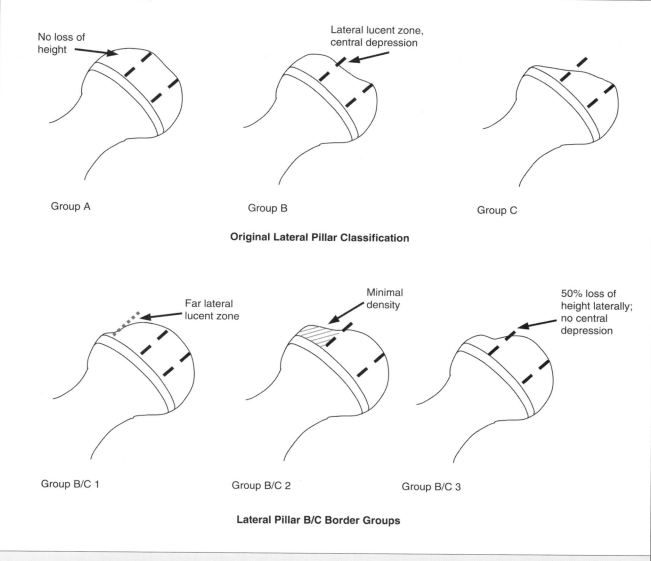

Figure 10   Illustrations show the lateral pillar (Herring) classification for Legg-Calvé-Perthes disease. Group A hips have no loss of height of the lateral pillar (lateral third of the epiphysis). Group B hips have less than 50% loss of lateral pillar height. Group C hips have more than 50% loss of lateral pillar height. In B/C border group hips, the lateral pillar is narrow (2 to 3 mm wide; group B/C 1) or poorly ossified (group B/C 2), or exactly 50% of the height of the lateral pillar is maintained without central depression (group B/C 3). (Reproduced from Matheney T: Legg-Calvé Perthes disease, in Song KM, ed: *Orthopaedic Knowledge Update: Pediatrics*, ed 4. Rosemont, IL, American Academy of Orthopaedic Surgeons, 2011, p 181.)

Stulberg I/II hips at maturity, with 80% achieving a good outcome.

b. Patients older than 8 years appear to benefit from surgically provided containment of the femoral head. This is particularly true for hips in the lateral pillar B and B/C border groups.

c. Patients with lateral pillar group C hips tend to do poorly regardless of treatment and age at onset.

d. For patients age 6 to 8 years at onset, evidence is not clear regarding potential advantages of a specific surgical procedure in lateral pillar classification.

5. Nonsurgical treatment

a. Containment of the femoral head may be achieved nonsurgically by casting or bracing with the hip in an abducted and internally rotated position.

b. Petrie casts and a variety of abduction orthoses have been used.

c. Protected weight bearing has also been recom-

5: Pediatrics

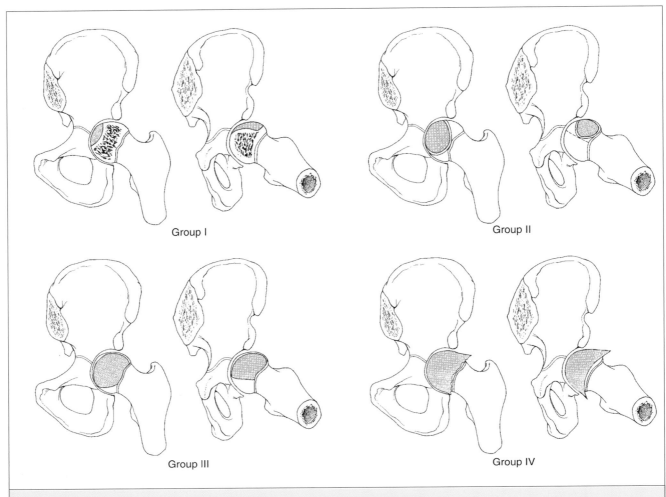

Group I

Group II

Group III

Group IV

Figure 11　Illustration shows the Catterall classification for Legg-Calvé-Perthes disease.

mended, especially before the reossification stage.

　d. The use of bisphosphonates, which inhibit bone resorption and thereby prevent deformity of the femoral head, is under investigation for LCP disease.

6. Surgical treatment

　a. Surgical containment of the femoral head may be approached from the femoral side, the acetabular side, or both, according to the surgeon's preference. These procedures produce comparable outcomes.

　b. Containment of the femur is achieved with a proximal femoral varus osteotomy.

　c. Containment by the acetabulum is achieved with a redirectional osteotomy (Salter, triple innominate), acetabuloplasty (Dega, Pemberton), or acetabular augmentation procedure (shelf arthroplasty).

　d. For improved outcomes, the hips must be con-

tainable; that is, they must have a relatively full ROM with congruency between the femoral head and the acetabulum.

　e. To allow maximal remodeling, the earliest possible initiation of treatment (before or during the early fragmentation stage of LCP disease) should be strongly considered.

　f. Bracing/casting and physical therapy may be used to improve preoperative joint mobility.

　g. Hip arthrodiastasis (via an external fixator) for 4 to 5 months has also been advocated in some centers.

7. Salvage treatment

　a. Salvage is used when the hip has poor congruency or is no longer containable. The goals of treatment are to relieve symptoms and restore stability.

　b. Hinge abduction, in which lateral extrusion of the femoral head results in its impinging on the edge of the acetabulum with abduction

Table 5

Stulberg Radiographic Classification of Legg-Calvé-Perthes Disease and Evidence of Osteoarthritis[a]

Class	Descriptive Features	Radiographic Signs of Osteo-arthritis (%)	Radiographic Evidence of Joint Space Narrowing (%)
I	Normal hip joint	0	0
II	Spherical head with enlargement, short neck, or steep acetabulum	16	0
III	Nonspherical head (that is, ovoid, mushroom-shaped, umbrella-shaped)	58	47
IV	Flat head	75	53
V	Flat head with incongruent hip joint	78	61

[a]At mean 40-year follow-up.

(**Figure 9**), may be present. Management possibilities are the following:

- An abduction-extension proximal femoral osteotomy

- Pelvic osteotomy procedures, such as a Chiari osteotomy, shelf arthroplasty, and shelf acetabuloplasty (labral support procedure) may also be beneficial.

8. Residual deformities

a. Deformity of the femoral head may result in femoroacetabular impingement (FAI). FAI may be treated with surgical dislocation and proximal femoral osteochondroplasty.

b. An overriding greater trochanter and short femoral neck also may result in FAI. Management options include intertrochanteric valgus osteotomy and surgical dislocation with relative lengthening of the femoral neck.

c. Accommodative acetabular dysplasia that is severe and/or causes instability may require periacetabular osteotomy.

d. The possibility of proximal femoral physeal arrest requires monitoring of leg lengths until skeletal maturity.

e. Osteochondritis dissecans after LCP disease may require treatment if it is symptomatic or if the lesion becomes unstable.

H. Outcome

1. Prognosis is related to patient age at disease onset. Age younger than 6 years at disease onset is more predictive of a good outcome.

2. Deformity of the femoral head also correlates with long-term outcome. The severity of this deformity and the degree of hip joint congruence at maturity (as defined by Stulberg) corre-

late with the risk of premature osteoarthritis (**Table 5**).

a. The risk of osteoarthritis of the hip is low (0% to 16%) when the femoral head is spherical (classes I and II).

b. The risk of osteoarthritis of the hip is high (58% to 78%) when the femoral head is nonspherical (classes III through V).

3. Longer follow-up (> 45 years) reveals substantial deterioration in hip function, with only 40% of patients maintaining good function and the remaining 60% requiring arthroplasty, having severe pain, or having poor function.

III. Slipped Capital Femoral Epiphysis

A. Overview

1. Definition

a. Slipped capital femoral epiphysis (SCFE) is a disorder of the hip in which the femoral neck displaces anteriorly and superiorly relative to the femoral epiphysis.

b. Displacement occurs through the proximal femoral physis.

c. Uncommonly, the femoral neck displaces posteriorly or medially relative to the femoral epiphysis (valgus SCFE).

2. Epidemiology

a. SCFE is the most common disorder of the hip in adolescents.

b. Males are more commonly affected than females (2:1). The cumulative risk in males is 1 per 1,000 to 2,000; the risk in females is 1 per 2,000 to 3,000.

c. Unilateral involvement is more common (80%) than bilateral involvement at the time of presentation. Ultimately, the hips are involved bilaterally in 10% to 60% of cases.

d. SCFE occurs most commonly in Hispanic, Polynesian, and African American populations.

B. Etiology

1. The precise etiology of SCFE is unknown.

2. In general, SCFE is thought to result from insufficient mechanical ability of the proximal femoral physis to resist loading. This can result either from physiologic loads across an abnormally weak physis or from abnormally high loads across a normal physis.

a. Conditions that weaken the physis include endocrinopathies such as hypothyroidism, panhypopituitarism, growth hormone abnormalities, hypogonadism, and hyper- or hypoparathyroidism; systemic diseases such as renal osteodystropy; and prior radiation therapy to the proximal femur.

b. Several mechanical factors that can increase the load across the physis are associated with SCFE, including obesity, relative or absolute femoral retroversion, a decreased femoral neck-shaft angle, and increased physeal obliquity.

C. Pathology—The physis in SCFE is abnormally widened, with irregular organization. The slip occurs through the proliferative and hypertrophic zones of the physis.

D. Evaluation

1. Clinical presentation

a. SCFE is most common in children 10 to 16 years of age.

- In boys, the age at presentation is from age 12 to 16 years (mean, 13.5 years).

- In girls, the age at presentation is from age 10 to 14 years (mean, 11.5 years).

b. Children with SCFE commonly have a limp and localized pain in the groin, hip, thigh, or knee.

c. Symptoms may be present for weeks to months before a diagnosis is made.

2. Physical examination

a. Common physical findings include an abnormal gait (antalgic and/or Trendelenburg), decreased ROM (in particular, decreased hip flexion and decreased internal rotation), and mild limb-length discrepancy.

b. Testing of the ROM of the hip may reveal ob-

ligate external rotation (external rotation of the hip as the hip is brought into flexion).

c. The foot and knee progression angles are usually externally rotated.

E. Diagnostic tests

1. Plain radiographs—Standard AP and frog-leg lateral views of the pelvis are recommended. Both hips should be visualized. For patients who cannot be positioned for the frog-leg lateral view, alternate lateral views (for example, cross-table, Dunn lateral) may be warranted.

a. In a normal hip, the Klein line, a line tangential to the superior border of the femoral neck on the AP view, intersects the proximal femoral epiphysis. In a hip with SCFE, the Klein line may fail to intersect the proximal femoral epiphysis, or will be asymmetrical in the two hips (**Figure 12, A**).

b. Lateral radiographs are more sensitive than other views in detecting SCFE (**Figure 12, B**).

c. Other radiographic findings in SCFE include a widened, blurred physis and the metaphyseal blanch sign, in which the posteriorly displaced epiphysis is superimposed on the femoral neck on the AP view.

2. MRI may be useful in identifying a hip at risk for SCFE before it occurs. An abnormally widened physis with surrounding edematous changes on MRI is suggestive of such a hip.

F. Classification

1. The weight-bearing or Loder classification is the preferred and most widely used system. It defines the SCFE as stable or unstable based on the patient's ability to bear weight (**Table 6**).

a. The SCFE is stable when the patient can bear weight on the involved extremity (with or without crutches).

b. The SCFE is unstable when the patient cannot bear weight on the involved extremity.

c. The value of this stability classification is its superior ability to predict osteonecrosis. In a single study, the risk of osteonecrosis in unstable hips was reported as 47% and that in stable hips as zero.

d. Most cases of SCFE are stable slips (> 90%).

2. The traditional classification was based on duration of symptoms, but it has largely been replaced by the stability classification because of its better prognostic value. This traditional classification used the following categories:

a. Chronic SCFE: symptoms have been present for more than 3 weeks.

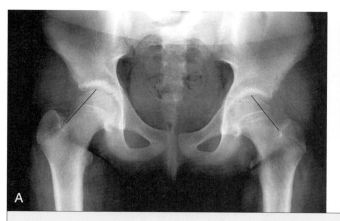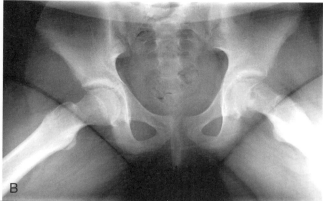

Figure 12 Radiographs of a 10-year-old girl with a stable slipped capital femoral epiphysis (SCFE) on the left. **A,** On the AP view, the Klein line intersects the epiphysis bilaterally. **B,** A frog-leg lateral view of the same patient as in A more clearly demonstrates the left SCFE.

b. Acute SCFE: symptoms have been present for less than 3 weeks.

c. Acute-on-chronic SCFE: an acute exacerbation of symptoms follows a prodrome of at least 3 weeks.

3. Radiographic classification

a. An SCFE slip is graded according to the percentage of epiphyseal displacement relative to the metaphyseal width of the femoral neck on AP or lateral radiographs. The grades are mild (< 33%), moderate (33% to 50%), and severe (> 50%).

b. The Southwick angle (femoral head-shaft angle) is the angle formed by the proximal femoral physis and the femoral shaft on lateral radiographs. An SCFE may also be graded on the basis of the difference in the Southwick angle between the involved and uninvolved sides of the hip, with the respective grades of mild (< 30° difference), moderate (30° to 50° difference), or severe (> 50° difference).

G. Surgical treatment

1. The goal of treatment is to prevent progression of the slip. SCFE should be treated surgically as soon as it is recognized.

2. Stable SCFE—In situ screw fixation is the preferred initial treatment (**Figure 13**).

3. Unstable SCFE—Management is controversial.

a. The timing of treatment is debated (emergent versus urgent [within 24 hours]).

b. Most centers continue to favor in situ screw fixation for unstable SCFE.

c. Some centers have moved toward open reduction through an anterior approach (Smith-

Table 6

Classification of SCFE

Type of SCFE	Able to Bear Weight?	Risk of Osteonecrosis
Stable	Yes	0%
Unstable	No	47%

Adapted with permission from Loder RT: Unstable slipped capital femoral epiphysis. *J Pediatr Orthop* 2001;21:694-699.

Petersen) or through a surgical hip dislocation approach (modified Dunn procedure).

d. Decompression of the intracapsular hematoma in SCFE via a capsulotomy (open or percutaneous) may be recommended to decrease the risk of osteonecrosis.

e. Forceful manipulation is never indicated because it is associated with an increased risk of complications, including osteonecrosis.

f. Serendipitous or gentle reduction does not appear to adversely affect patient outcomes.

4. Technical points of in situ screw fixation

a. Large (≥ 6.5 mm), fully threaded, cannulated screw systems are preferred.

b. A single-screw construct is usually adequate for a stable SCFE. For an unstable SCFE, the use of two screws is recommended for added stability.

c. The screw or screws are started on the anterior femoral neck to allow them to be targeted to the center position of the femoral head and perpendicular to the physis.

5: Pediatrics

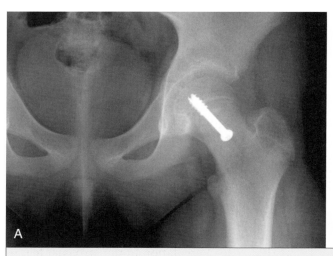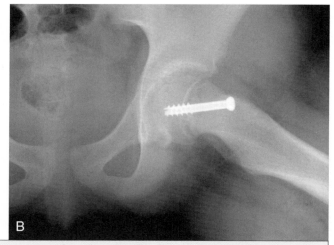

Figure 13   Postoperative AP (**A**) and frog-leg lateral (**B**) views show in situ screw fixation of a stable slipped capital femoral epiphysis.

d. Screw heads should be lateral to the intertrochanteric line to minimize the risk of the screw head impinging on the acetabular rim.

5. Indications for prophylactic fixation of the contralateral hip include age younger than 10 years for girls and younger than 12 years for boys, and associated risk factors such as endocrinopathies, renal osteodystrophy, and history of radiation therapy. If prophylactic fixation is not performed, the contralateral hip should be monitored radiographically every 6 months.

6. Rehabilitation—Weight bearing is usually protected postoperatively.

H. Management of residual deformity

1. Moderate to severe posteroinferior displacement of the epiphysis relative to the metaphysis can result in substantial proximal femoral deformities, particularly decreased femoral head-neck offset, excessive retroversion of the femoral head, and metaphyseal prominence. These deformities can lead to FAI and pain, stiffness, and premature osteoarthritis of the hip.

2. Moderate to severe SCFE deformities can be corrected to relieve pain and improve function.

   a. Osteotomy of the proximal femur can be performed at the subcapital, femoral neck, or intertrochanteric (Southwick, Imhäuser) level.

   b. Osteotomy at the subcapital level or level of the femoral neck can provide the greatest correction but may be associated with higher rates of complication.

   c. Surgical dislocation of the hip with concomitant osteoplasty and/or modified Dunn osteotomy (correction through the physis) has been safely adopted at select centers.

I. Complications

1. Osteonecrosis—Unstable SCFE is the greatest risk factor for osteonecrosis, but hardware placement in the posterior and superior femoral neck can disrupt the interosseous blood supply and also lead to osteonecrosis.

2. Chondrolysis—Chondrolysis is usually caused by unrecognized screw penetration of the articular surface. If penetration is recognized and corrected at the time of surgery, chondrolysis does not occur.

3. Slip progression—Progression occurs in 1% to 2% of cases following in situ single-screw fixation.

4. Fracture—The risk of fracture is increased with entry sites through the lateral cortex and those at or distal to the lesser trochanter.

IV. Coxa Vara

A. Overview

1. Definition—Coxa vara is an abnormally low femoral neck-shaft angle (< 120°).

2. Classification—Coxa vara is classified as congenital, acquired, or developmental.

   a. Congenital coxa vara is characterized by a primary cartilaginous defect in the femoral neck. It is commonly associated with a congenitally short femur, a congenitally bowed femur, and proximal femoral focal deficiency (also known as partial longitudinal deficiency of the femur).

   b. Acquired coxa vara can result from numerous conditions, including trauma, infection, patho-

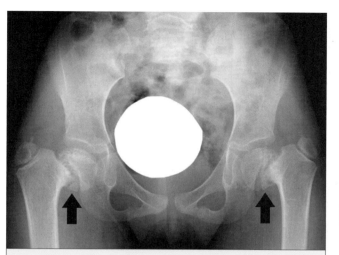

Figure 14   The inverted Y sign (arrows), formed by a triangular metaphyseal fragment in the inferior femoral neck, is pathognomonic for coxa vara.

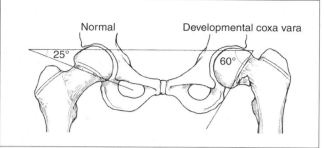

Figure 15   The Hilgenreiner-epiphyseal (H-E) angle is formed by a line through the physis and the Hilgenreiner line. A normal H-E angle is approximately 25°.

logic bone disorders (for example, osteopetrosis), SCFE, LCP disease, and skeletal dysplasias (cleidocranial dysostosis, metaphyseal dysostosis, and some types of spondylometaphyseal dysplasia).

  c. Developmental coxa vara occurs in early childhood, with classic radiographic changes (including the inverted Y sign) and no other skeletal manifestations. The remainder of this section focuses on developmental coxa vara.

3. Epidemiology

  a. Coxa vara occurs in 1 in 25,000 live births worldwide.

  b. Boys and girls are affected equally.

  c. Right-side or left-side involvement occurs with equal frequency.

  d. Bilateral involvement occurs in 30% to 50% of cases.

  e. The incidence does not vary significantly by race.

B. Etiology

1. The precise cause of coxa vara is unclear.

2. A genetic predisposition appears to exist, with an autosomal dominant pattern and incomplete penetrance.

3. Coxa vara may result from a primary defect in endochondral ossification in the medial part of the femoral neck.

  a. Bone along the medial inferior aspect of the femoral neck fatigues with weight bearing, resulting in a progressive varus deformity.

  b. The vertical orientation of the proximal femoral physis transforms normal compressive forces across the physis into an increasing shear force. Additionally, compressive forces across the medial femoral neck are increased.

C. Evaluation

1. Clinical presentation

  a. The patient usually presents after walking has begun and before 6 years of age.

  b. Pain is uncommon.

  c. An apparent limb shortening or a painless limp may be present in cases of unilateral coxa vara. A waddling gait is more characteristic in cases of bilateral coxa vara.

2. Physical examination

  a. Findings include a prominent greater trochanter, which may also be more proximal than the contralateral greater trochanter.

  b. With unilateral involvement, limb-length discrepancy (usually minor, < 3 cm) may be present.

  c. Abductor muscle weakness is common. Consequently, Trendelenburg gait may be present, and the Trendelenburg sign may be positive.

  d. ROM testing may demonstrate a decrease in abduction and internal rotation.

  e. With bilateral involvement, lumbar lordosis may be increased.

3. Plain radiographs—AP and frog-leg lateral views of the pelvis are recommended. Radiographic findings include the following:

  a. A decreased femoral neck-shaft angle (mean femoral neck-shaft angle = 148° at 1 year of age, gradually decreasing to 120° in the adult)

  b. The inverted Y sign (resulting from a triangular metaphyseal fragment in the inferior

5: Pediatrics

femoral neck), which is pathognomonic (**Figure 14**)

    c. Vertical orientation of the physis, a shortened femoral neck, and decreased femoral anteversion

    d. An abnormal Hilgenreiner-epiphyseal (H-E) angle (angle formed by a line through the proximal femoral physis and the Hilgenreiner line) (**Figure 15**)

D. Natural history—The H-E angle correlates with the risk of progression of coxa vara.

    1. Hips with an H-E angle less than 45° typically remain stable or improve.

    2. An H-E angle of 45° to 60° is associated with an indeterminate risk of progression.

    3. An H-E angle greater than 60° is associated with a significantly high risk of progression.

E. Treatment—Recommendations are based on the severity of the H-E angle and the presence of symptoms.

    1. Nonsurgical treatment

        a. Asymptomatic patients with an H-E angle less than 45° should be observed.

        b. Asymptomatic patients with an H-E angle between 45° and 59° also can be observed. Serial radiographs are critical to assess for disease progression.

    2. Surgical treatment

        a. Indications—Surgery is indicated for the following:

          • Patients with a Trendelenburg gait and/or fatigue pain in the hip abductors and an H-E angle of 45° to 59° or patients with evidence of progression

          • Patients with an H-E angle greater than 60°

          • Patients with a progressive decrease in the femoral neck-shaft angle to 100° or less

        b. Procedures

          • The standard procedure for coxa vara is a proximal femoral valgus derotational osteotomy.

          • The osteotomy can be performed at the intertrochanteric or subtrochanteric level, as described by Borden (intertrochanteric), Pauwel (Y-shaped intertrochanteric), and Keetley (subtrochanteric).

          • Osteotomy at the level of the femoral neck should be avoided because of reportedly high morbidity rates and poor clinical results.

        c. The ultimate goal of surgery is valgus overcorrection of the femoral neck-shaft angle (H-E angle < 38°).

        d. Adductor tenotomy is often necessary.

        e. Epiphysiodesis of the greater trochanter may be necessary in conjunction with valgus osteotomy to prevent recurrence of varus deformity.

    3. Complications

        a. Varus deformity recurs after valgus osteotomy in up to 50% of cases. The risk of recurrence may be decreased by valgus overcorrection.

        b. Premature closure of the proximal femoral physis has been reported in up to 89% of cases. Premature closure is usually noted within the first 12 to 24 months after surgery. Premature closure may lead to limb-length discrepancy and/or trochanteric overgrowth.

    4. Rehabilitation—Spica cast immobilization is recommended for 6 to 8 weeks after surgery.

Top Testing Facts

Developmental Dysplasia of the Hip

1. Because the ossific nucleus of the femoral head does not appear until 4 to 6 months of age, ultrasonography is better than plain radiography for confirming DDH in the first 4 to 6 months of life.

2. If a dislocated hip does not relocate within 3 to 4 weeks, use of a Pavlik harness should be discontinued to avoid Pavlik harness disease.

3. Excessive hip flexion in the Pavlik harness increases the risk of femoral nerve palsy.

4. Excessive hip abduction in the Pavlik harness increases the risk of osteonecrosis of the femoral head.

5. The Galeazzi test is positive in unilateral but not bilateral dislocation of the hip in DDH.

6. Hip abduction does not become limited in DDH until approximately 6 months of age.

Legg-Calvé-Perthes Disease

1. The most important prognostic factors are patient age at disease onset and the shape of the femoral head and its congruency at skeletal maturity. Stulberg correlated poorer long-term outcomes with greater deformities of the femoral head at maturity.

2. The lateral pillar (Herring) classification, based on preservation of the height and integrity of the lateral pillar of the femoral head, is the most reliable classification scheme for LCP disease and is related to prognosis. Its limitation is that it cannot provide a final classification at the time of presentation.

Slipped Capital Femoral Epiphysis

1. Thigh or knee pain in an adolescent mandates a workup to rule out an SCFE.

2. The frog-leg lateral radiograph is the most sensitive view for detecting an SCFE.

3. The most accurate predictor of osteonecrosis is the stability of the hip at presentation; an unstable SCFE is associated with a risk of osteonecrosis as high as 47%.

4. Chondrolysis is a consequence of unrecognized screw penetration. If screw penetration is noted and corrected at the time of surgery, there is no increased risk of chondrolysis.

5. A SCFE should be stabilized as soon as it is recognized. If prophylactic pinning of the contralateral hip is not performed, radiographs should be repeated every 4 to 6 months to monitor for a contralateral slip.

Coxa Vara

1. The inverted Y sign on radiographs is pathognomonic for coxa vara.

2. The H-E angle is prognostic and critical in selecting treatment for coxa vara. Surgery is indicated for an angle greater than 60° and observation for an angle less than 45°. Hips with angles between 45° and 60° require observation for potential progression.

3. A successful outcome following surgery for coxa vara depends on valgus overcorrection of the proximal femoral deformity.

Bibliography

Aronsson DD, Loder RT, Breur GJ, Weinstein SL: Slipped capital femoral epiphysis: Current concepts. *J Am Acad Orthop Surg* 2006;14(12):666-679.

Beals RK: Coxa vara in childhood: Evaluation and management. *J Am Acad Orthop Surg* 1998;6(2):93-99.

Carney BT, Weinstein SL, Noble J: Long-term follow-up of slipped capital femoral epiphysis. *J Bone Joint Surg Am* 1991;73(5):667-674.

Herring JA, Kim HT, Browne R: Legg-Calve-Perthes disease: Part I. Classification of radiographs with use of the modified lateral pillar and Stulberg classifications. *J Bone Joint Surg Am* 2004;86(10):2103-2120.

Herring JA, Kim HT, Browne R: Legg-Calve-Perthes disease: Part II. Prospective multicenter study of the effect of treatment on outcome. *J Bone Joint Surg Am* 2004;86(10):2121-2134.

Kim HK: Legg-Calvé-Perthes disease. *J Am Acad Orthop Surg* 2010;18(11):676-686.

Loder RT: Unstable slipped capital femoral epiphysis. *J Pediatr Orthop* 2001;21(5):694-699.

Skaggs DL, Tolo VT: Legg-Calve-Perthes disease. *J Am Acad Orthop Surg* 1996;4(1):9-16.

Vitale MG, Skaggs DL: Developmental dysplasia of the hip from six months to four years of age. *J Am Acad Orthop Surg* 2001;9(6):401-411.

Weinstein SL, Mubarak SJ, Wenger DR: Developmental hip dysplasia and dislocation: Part I. *Instr Course Lect* 2004;53:523-530.

Weinstein SL, Mubarak SJ, Wenger DR: Developmental hip dysplasia and dislocation: Part II. *Instr Course Lect* 2004;53:531-542.

5: Pediatrics

Chapter 58

Pediatric Foot Conditions

Anthony A. Scaduto, MD   Nathan L. Frost, MD

I. Clubfoot (Talipes Equinovarus)

A. Overview

1. Clubfoot is a congenital foot deformity consisting of hindfoot equinus and varus as well as midfoot and forefoot adduction and cavus.

2. It is more common in males.

3. One-half of cases are bilateral.

4. Unaffected parents with an affected child have a 2.5% to 6.5% chance of having another child with clubfoot.

5. Potential etiologies include abnormal fibrosis, neurologic abnormalities, and arrested embryologic development.

B. Pathoanatomy

1. The four basic deformities are cavus, adductus, varus, and equinus.

2. The forefoot deformity results from medial and plantar subluxation of the navicular bone on the talar head.

3. The hindfoot is adducted and inverted under the talus.

4. The entire foot appears supinated; however, the forefoot is pronated relative to the hindfoot, leading to the cavus deformity.

5. The muscles and tendons of the gastrocnemius-soleus complex, the posterior tibialis, and the long toe flexors are shortened.

C. Evaluation

1. Common clinical findings are a small foot, a small calf, a slightly shortened tibia, and skin creases medially and posteriorly.

2. Clubfeet associated with arthrogryposis, myelomeningocele, diastrophic dysplasia, and amniotic band syndrome are more challenging to treat and more prone to relapse.

3. Radiographs are of limited use.

4. On both the AP and lateral views of a clubfoot, the talus and calcaneus are less divergent and more parallel (smaller talocalcaneal angle) than normal.

D. Classification—The Dimeglio-Bensahel and Catterall-Pirani classification systems are based on the severity of the clinical findings and the correctability of the deformity.

E. Treatment

1. Ponseti method

   a. The outcome is much better than with historic casting techniques (80% to 90% success rate versus 10% to 50%).

   b. The sequence of deformity correction is cavus, adductus, varus, and equinus.

   c. Long leg casts are changed weekly.

   d. The initial cast places the forefoot in supination to correct forefoot cavus.

   e. Counter pressure is applied to the lateral aspect of the talar head only, not the calcaneus.

   f. Percutaneous Achilles tenotomy is frequently required before final cast application to treat residual equinus (up to 90% of feet).

   g. Foot abduction orthoses, such as the Denis-Brown splint, are used to prevent recurrence. The recommended use is 23 hours per day for 3 months after casting and then during naps and overnight for 2 to 3 years.

   h. Recurrences are typically managed with repeat manipulation and casting followed by resumption of bracing.

   i. Tibialis anterior tendon transfer may be required in patients with dynamic swing phase supination.

2. French method

   a. Daily manipulations are required for clubfeet

5: Pediatrics

Table 1

Treatment of Residual Clubfoot Deformity

Residual/Recurrent Deformity	Corrective Surgery
Supination	Transfer of tibialis anterior tendon
Varus	Revision posteromedial release versus calcaneal osteotomy. (Osteotomy is needed for rigid deformity.)
Adductus	Medial column lengthening/lateral column shortening osteotomies
Internal rotation of foot	Supramalleolar tibial osteotomy
Planovalgus	Calcaneal neck lengthening or medial calcaneal slide
Severe multiplanar residual clubfoot deformity	Multiplanar osteotomies of midfoot and/or hindfoot Triple arthrodesis if not amenable to joint-sparing osteotomies

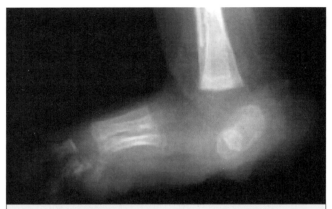

Figure 1   Lateral forced plantar flexion radiograph shows a foot with congenital vertical talus. The first metatarsal (and unossified navicular) remain dorsally dislocated relative to the talus. (Reproduced from Sullivan JA: Pediatric flatfoot: Evaluation and management. *J Am Acad Orthop Surg* 1999;7[1]:44-53.)

in newborns, typically performed and directed by a physical therapist.

   b. The feet are taped, not casted, in position following manipulations.

   c. Continuous passive motion devices are used in the first 12 weeks of treatment.

   d. Therapy sessions are continued until the child is walking or the deformity is stable.

3. Surgical management

   a. Surgery is reserved for feet that are refractory to manipulations/casting, syndrome-associated clubfoot, and delayed presentation (children older than 1 to 2 years).

   b. The surgical plan should be individualized for each patient. Releases of the posteromedial structures are performed as needed (the "a la carte" approach).

   c. Residual deformities may require surgical intervention (**Table 1**).

II. Congenital Vertical Talus

A. Overview

1. Congenital vertical talus is an irreducible dorsal dislocation of the navicular on the talus.

2. Rare condition (1 in 150,000 births); commonly (approximately 50%) associated with neuromus-

cular disease (myelomeningocele, arthrogryposis, diastematomyelia) or chromosomal abnormalities

B. Pathoanatomy

1. The navicular is dislocated dorsolaterally.

2. The deformity also includes eversion of the calcaneus, contracture of the dorsolateral muscles and Achilles tendon, and attenuation of the spring ligament.

C. Evaluation

1. Clinically, the foot has a rigid convex plantar surface with a prominent talar head (rocker bottom).

2. Unlike flexible flatfoot, the arch does not reconstitute standing on the toes or hyperextending with the great toe.

3. An awkward, calcaneal-type gait pattern results from limited push-off power, limited forefoot contact, and excessive heel contact.

4. Radiographs—The lateral view with the foot in forced plantar flexion is diagnostic for a vertical talus (**Figure 1**).

   a. The navicular remains dorsally dislocated in this view. This differs from oblique talus, in which the navicular reduces on this view.

   b. Prior to ossification of the navicular at age 3 years, the first metatarsal is used as a proxy for the dorsal alignment of the navicular on the lateral view.

D. Treatment

1. Manipulation and casting (reverse Ponseti method)

   a. Entails serial manipulation and casting to re-

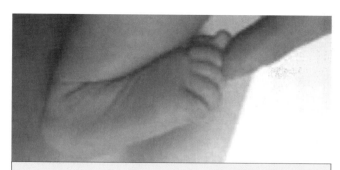

Figure 2 Clinical photograph shows a calcaneovalgus foot in a newborn. Note the characteristic hyperdorsiflexion and hindfoot valgus. (Reproduced from Sullivan JA: Pediatric flatfoot: Evaluation and management. *J Am Acad Orthop Surg* 1999;7[1]:44-53.)

duce the dorsal dislocation of the navicular on the talus and stretch dorsolateral soft tissues

b. Counter pressure is applied to the talar head while the foot is stretched into plantar flexion and inversion.

c. After passive reduction of the talus is achieved and confirmed with a lateral radiograph, surgical release and pinning of the talonavicular joint and percutaneous Achilles tenotomy are performed to complete the correction.

d. More extensive surgical release may be required in cases of incomplete correction.

2. Surgical

a. A traditional pantalar release is usually performed between 12 and 18 months of age.

b. Surgical treatment includes pantalar release with lengthening of the Achilles, toe extensors, and peroneal tendons and pinning of the talonavicular joint. The tibialis anterior is generally transferred to the neck of the talus.

c. The outcome of reconstruction in children older than 3 years is less predictable. Triple arthrodesis is rarely needed as a salvage procedure.

III. Oblique Talus

A. May have clinical appearance similar to vertical talus

B. The plantar flexion lateral radiograph demonstrates reducible talonavicular subluxation.

C. Treatment is controversial. Many authors propose observation, whereas others advocate for manipulation and/or casting similar to that described for congenital vertical talus.

IV. Calcaneovalgus Foot

A. Overview

1. Calcaneovalgus foot is a positional deformity in infants in which the foot is hyperdorsiflexed secondary to intrauterine positioning (**Figure 2**).

2. It is more common in first-born females.

B. Pathoanatomy

1. A calcaneovalgus foot in newborns is a soft-tissue contracture problem.

2. No dislocation or bony deformity of the foot exists.

C. Evaluation

1. The deformity should be passively correctable to neutral.

2. May be associated with posteromedial bowing of the tibia; however, isolated posteromedial tibial bowing may be misdiagnosed as a calcaneovalgus foot.

D. Treatment

1. The deformity typically resolves without intervention.

2. Stretching may expedite resolution.

V. Pes Cavus

A. Overview

1. A pes cauus (cavus foot) has an elevated medial longitudinal arch secondary to forefoot plantar flexion or, less frequently, as a result of excessive calcaneal dorsiflexion (calcaneus hindfoot).

2. Two-thirds of patients with a cavus foot have an underlying neurologic disorder, most commonly Charcot-Marie-Tooth disease.

B. Pathoanatomy

1. The primary structural problem is forefoot plantar flexion. The first ray is often more markedly plantarflexed, which results in forefoot pronation.

2. For the lateral half of the foot to be in contact with the ground, the hindfoot must deviate into varus (**Figure 3**).

3. First ray plantar flexion may result from a weak tibialis anterior relative to the peroneus longus, but it is more commonly caused by intrinsic weakness and contracture.

4. Over time, the plantar fascia contracts, and the hindfoot varus deformity becomes more rigid.

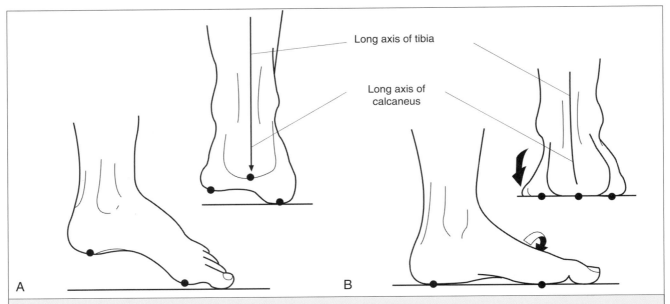

Figure 3   Illustrations show the tripod effect in a cavus foot. **A,** Posterior and lateral views show a cavus foot in the non–weight-bearing position. The long axes of the tibia and the calcaneus are parallel, and the first metatarsal is pronated. Dots indicate the three major weight-bearing plantar areas, the heel and the first and fifth metatarsals. **B,** Posterior and lateral views show a cavus foot in the weight-bearing position. The long axes of the tibia and the calcaneus are not parallel. During weight bearing, a rigid equinus forefoot deformity forces the flexible hindfoot into varus. This is the tripod effect. (Adapted with permission from Paulos L, Coleman SS, Samuelson KM: Pes cavovarus: Review of a surgical approach using selective soft-tissue procedures. *J Bone Joint Surg Am* 1980;62: 942-953.)

C. Evaluation

1. Patients may report instability (ankle sprains).

2. A neurologic examination and a family history are essential.

3. Unilateral involvement suggests a focal diagnosis (for example, spinal cord anomaly or nerve injury).

4. Bilateral involvement and a positive family history are common with Charcot-Marie-Tooth disease. Despite bilateral involvement, asymmetry may be seen in Charcot-Marie-Tooth disease.

5. Hindfoot flexibility is assessed by placing a 1-inch block under the lateral border of the foot (Coleman block test).

6. Radiographs—Weight-bearing views are required.

   a. Increased Meary angle—The long axis of the talus will intersect the long axis of the first metatarsal dorsally on the lateral view of the foot. The normal value is 0° to 5°.

   b. Increased calcaneal pitch—Intersection of a line running along the undersurface of the calcaneus and the floor. Calcaneal pitch greater than 30° indicates a calcaneocavus foot.

7. MRI of the spine is indicated with unilateral involvement.

D. Treatment

1. Joint-sparing procedures are preferred whenever possible.

2. A key to surgical decision making is the flexibility of the hindfoot. Some general guidelines exist (**Table 2**).

3. Percutaneous plantar fascia release is insufficient to correct a cavus foot. At minimum, an open release and soft-tissue rebalancing are needed.

4. Achilles tendon lengthening should not be performed concomitantly with plantar fasciotomy. An intact Achilles tendon provides the resistance necessary to stretch the contracted plantar tissues and correct the cavus deformity.

VI. Pes Planovalgus

A. Overview

1. Pes planovalgus (flexible flatfoot) is a physiologic variation of normal.

2. It is defined by a decreased longitudinal arch and a valgus hindfoot during weight bearing.

3. It is rarely symptomatic, is common in childhood, and resolves spontaneously in most cases.

Table 2		
Treatment of Pes Cavus		
Severity of Deformity	**Examination and History**	**Corrective Treatment**
Mild	Flexible, painless	Heel cord stretching, eversion/dorsiflexion strengthening program
Mild	Progressive or symptomatic	Plantar release ± peroneus longus to brevis transfer
	Varus because of peroneal weakness	Add tibialis anterior and/or posterior tendon transfer to the peroneal muscles
Moderate	Rigid medial cavus	Dorsiflexion osteotomy of either first metatarsal or cuneiform
	Rigid medial and lateral cavus	Dorsiflexion osteotomies of the cuboid and cuneiforms
	Rigid hindfoot varus	Closing/sliding calcaneal osteotomy
	Clawing of hallux	Add EHL transfer to first metatarsal (Jones)
Severe	Not correctable to plantigrade with other procedures	Triple arthrodesis is rarely needed and should be avoided whenever possible.

EHL = extensor hallucis longus.

4. Flexible flatfoot is present in 20% to 25% of adults.

B. Pathoanatomy

1. Generalized ligamentous laxity is common.

2. Approximately one-fourth of flexible flatfeet have a contracture of the gastrocnemius-soleus complex. These cases may be associated with disability.

C. Evaluation

1. An arch should be evident when toe-standing, during dorsiflexion of the hallux, or when not bearing weight.

2. Subtalar motion should be full and painless as evidenced by heel swing from valgus to varus with toe-standing.

3. On a lateral radiograph, the talus is plantarflexed relative to the first metatarsal (decreased Meary angle).

4. Apparent hindfoot valgus may actually be caused by ankle valgus (particularly in children with myelodysplasia). If any suspicion of ankle valgus is present, ankle radiographs should be obtained.

5. The differential of flatfoot includes tarsal coalition, congenital vertical talus, and accessory navicular.

D. Treatment

1. No treatment is indicated for asymptomatic patients.

2. Nonsurgical

a. Shoes or orthoses do not promote arch development.

b. Athletic shoes with arch and heel support can help relieve pain.

c. The University of California Biomechanics Laboratory orthosis is a rigid orthotic insert designed to support the arch and control the hindfoot. A soft molded insert is an alternative but may be inadequate to control hindfoot valgus.

d. Stretching exercises are recommended if the patient is symptomatic and an Achilles contracture is present.

3. Surgical

a. Surgery is reserved for rare cases in which pain is recalcitrant to nonsurgical treatment.

b. A calcaneal neck lengthening with soft-tissue balancing is the treatment of choice. It corrects deformity while preserving motion and growth. Arthrodesis is rarely indicated.

VII. Metatarsus Adductus

A. Overview

1. Metatarsus adductus is a medial deviation of the forefoot with normal alignment of the hindfoot.

2. It occurs in up to 12% of newborns.

B. Pathoanatomy—Intrauterine positioning of the foot is thought to be one possible cause.

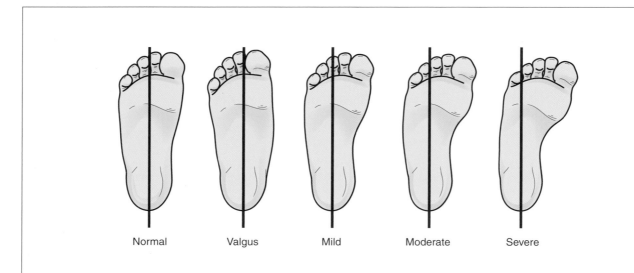

Normal   Valgus   Mild   Moderate   Severe

Figure 4   Illustrations depict the heel bisector line, which defines the relationship of the heel to the forefoot. Normal foot: line bisects the second and third toes; valgus: line bisects the great and second toes; mild metatarsus adductus: line bisects the third toe; moderate metatarsus adductus: line bisects the third and fourth toes; and severe metatarsus adductus: line bisects the fourth and fifth toes.

C. Evaluation

1. The foot has a kidney-bean shape (convex lateral border), and the hindfoot is in a neutral position.

2. The amount of active correction is assessed by tickling the foot.

3. The Bleck classification system grades the severity of the deformity based on flexibility. A flexible forefoot is one that could be abducted beyond the midline heel-bisector angle, a partially flexible forefoot could be abducted to the midline, and a rigid forefoot could not be abducted to the midline (**Figure 4**).

4. Must be distinguished from metatarsus primus varus, in which the lateral border of the foot is normal, but a medial crease is present secondary to isolated varus alignment of the first ray. This deformity is typically rigid, requires early casting, and may result in hallux valgus.

D. Prognosis and treatment

1. Nonsurgical

a. Spontaneous resolution of metatarsus adductus occurs in 90% of children by age 4 years.

b. Passive stretching is recommended for a flexible deformity but may not improve the final outcome.

c. Serial casting between 6 and 12 months of age is useful in children with deformity that has a rigid component.

2. Surgical

a. Surgery is indicated only in children older than 7 years with severe residual deformity that produces problems with shoe wear and pain.

b. A medial column lengthening (opening wedge osteotomy of cuneiform) combined with lateral column shortening (closing wedge of the cuboid)

VIII. Skewfoot

A. Definition—Skewfoot deformity consists of an adducted forefoot and hindfoot valgus with plantar flexion of the talus.

B. Evaluation

1. Patients may become symptomatic at the talar head or the base of the fifth metatarsal.

2. Clinical examination and weight-bearing radiographs confirm the diagnosis.

C. Treatment—Surgery (combined opening wedge medial cuneiform osteotomy and calcaneal osteotomy) is limited to patients who have persistent pain.

IX. Idiopathic Toe Walking

A. Overview

1. Can occur normally as a child develops the gait pattern; toe walking beyond 2 years of age requires investigation to rule out neuromuscular or developmental abnormalities.

Table 3

Imaging Evaluation of Tarsal Coalitions

Type of Coalition	Imaging View	Findings Suggestive of Coalition
Calcaneonavicular	Oblique radiograph	Elongated dorsal process of calcaneus (anteater's nose)
Talocalcaneal	Lateral radiograph	C-shaped line that extends from talar dome to sustentaculum tali (C sign of Lefleur)
	CT scan	Absent or vertically oriented middle facet

2. The etiology is largely unknown, although proposed causes include defects in sensory processing, abnormalities of underlying muscle fibers, and a possible genetic component.

B. Evaluation

1. A thorough history and physical examination should be performed to rule out neurologic and developmental causes of toe walking.

2. Patients may or may not be able to walk flat-footed, depending on the degree of equinus contracture present.

3. If limited ankle dorsiflexion is present, it is important to determine whether contracture is caused by the gastrocnemius alone or the entire gastrocnemius-soleus complex. Persistent limitation of dorsiflexion with knee extension and flexion likely is secondary to contracture of the gastrocnemius-soleus complex, whereas equinus that improves with knee flexion indicates gastrocnemius contracture.

C. Treatment

1. Nonsurgical methods are most successful in children with dorsiflexion beyond 0°.

2. Stretching, bracing, and/or casting should be attempted in children older than 2 years who are able to dorsiflex beyond 0°.

3. Children older than 2 years with fixed equinus contracture are candidates for tendon lengthening. Patients with fixed contracture in knee flexion/extension should undergo lengthening of the entire gastrocnemius-soleus complex, whereas patients with contracture that resolves with knee flexion can undergo lengthening of the gastrocnemius tendon alone.

X. Tarsal Coalition

A. Overview

1. An osseous, cartilaginous, or fibrous connection between the tarsal bones

2. Occurs in 1% to 6% of the population

3. May be asymptomatic

4. Of patients with tarsal coalitions, 10% to 20% have multiple coalitions, and 50% are bilateral.

5. Calcaneonavicular coalitions are the most common type and occur in children 8 to 12 years of age.

6. Talocalcaneal coalitions are the second most common type, occurring in children between 12 and 15 years of age. They can occur at any of the three facets of the subtalar joint, with the middle facet being most common.

7. Multiple coalitions are common with fibular deficiency and Apert syndrome.

B. Pathoanatomy—The cause of symptoms is not precisely known but may be related to the transition of a cartilaginous coalition to bone during late childhood and early adolescence.

C. Evaluation

1. Patients often present with a symptomatic flatfoot.

2. Pain is typically in the sinus tarsi or along the medial longitudinal arch.

3. Limited subtalar motion may present as difficulty with movement on uneven ground and/or frequent ankle sprains.

4. Radiographs should include weight-bearing AP, lateral, internal oblique, and Harris views (**Table 3** and **Figure 5**).

   a. Lateral radiographs may demonstrate dorsal talar beaking, which is a nonspecific finding associated with many coalitions. It is not a sign of degenerative arthrosis.

   b. Harris axial radiographs have a high false-positive rate for tarsal coalition. If the view is slightly oblique to the posterior or middle facet, a coalition will appear to be present when it is not.

5. CT helps delineate the coalition and clarify whether a child has multiple coalitions in the foot. It is helpful in surgical planning.

6. MRI may help identify a fibrous coalition.

D. Treatment

1. Asymptomatic coalitions may be observed.

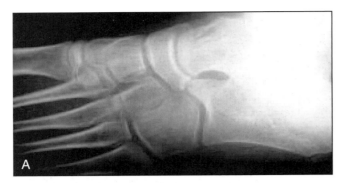

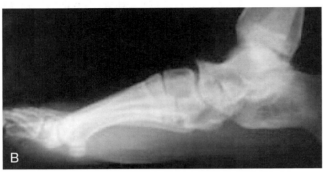

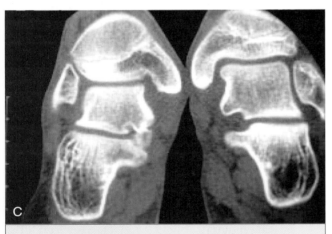

Figure 5 Images demonstrate calcaneonavicular and talocalcaneal coalitions. **A,** This 45° oblique radiograph demonstrates a calcaneonavicular coalition. **B,** Non–weight-bearing lateral radiograph depicts a talocalcaneal coalition. Talar beaking and loss of definition of the subtalar joint space are present. **C,** CT scan illustrates a talocalcaneal coalition in the left foot as viewed from posterior. (Reproduced from Sullivan JA: Pediatric flatfoot: Evaluation and management. *J Am Acad Orthop Surg* 1999;7[1]:44-53.)

2. Nonsurgical

    a. Initial management of symptomatic patients includes NSAIDs, activity modification, shoe orthoses, and cast immobilization.

    b. Of the total, 30% of patients have resolution of pain after cast immobilization.

3. Surgical

    a. Calcaneonavicular coalition

      • Coalition resection and interposition of extensor digitorum brevis or fat is effective in most cases.

      • Contraindications to resection are advanced degenerative changes in adjacent joints or multiple coalitions.

    b. Talocalcaneal coalition

      • Resection has traditionally been limited to small coalitions (<50% of middle facet) with minimal hindfoot valgus (<20°) and no degenerative arthrosis. More recent studies call these recommendations into question.

      • If severe valgus is present at the time of coalition excision, a calcaneal osteotomy (either a calcaneal neck lengthening or a medial slide) generally improves the clinical outcome and reduces the risk of recurrent symptoms.

    c. Triple arthrodesis or limited subtalar arthrodesis may be indicated when degenerative arthrosis or multiple coalitions are present or when coalition resection fails to relieve symptoms.

XI. Accessory Navicular

A. Overview

1. Accessory navicular is an accessory ossicle of the plantar medial aspect of the navicular.

2. The extra bone may be completely separate or in continuity with the true navicular.

3. It occurs in up to 12% of the population; most are asymptomatic.

B. Pathoanatomy

1. The accessory navicular usually does not ossify until after 8 years of age. In approximately one-half of patients, the ossicle fuses to the true navicular.

2. Pain is secondary to repeated microfracture or an inflammatory response.

C. Evaluation

1. Often associated with flat feet

2. A firm, tender prominence on the plantar medial midfoot (distal to the talar head) is typically present.

3. Often, the ossicle is evident on weight-bearing AP radiographs. An external oblique view (not the commonly used internal oblique) may best identify an accessory navicular (**Figure 6**).

D. Treatment

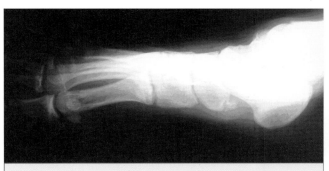

Figure 6 External oblique radiograph of a foot shows an accessory navicular.

1. Nonsurgical

    a. Doughnut-shaped pads and orthotic devices that reduce direct pressure on the prominence may be effective.

    b. A period of immobilization also may relieve symptoms.

2. Surgical—Simple excision of the ossicle and any navicular prominence via a tendon-splitting approach (without tendon advancement) has been shown to be effective 90% of the time.

XII. Köhler Disease

A. Overview

    1. Köhler disease is a self-limiting, painful osteochondrosis of the navicular in young children.

    2. It occurs more commonly in boys than in girls (4:1) and is frequently bilateral.

B. Pathoanatomy—The navicular is the last tarsal bone to ossify; therfore, it is more susceptible to direct mechanical compression injury.

C. Evaluation

    1. Children with Köhler disease typically walk with an antalgic gait on the lateral border of the foot.

    2. Radiographs confirm the diagnosis with flattening, sclerosis, and fragmentation of the navicular (**Figure 7**).

    3. Irregular ossification of the navicular is common during early ossification.

D. Treatment

    1. Symptoms resolve spontaneously within 6 to 15 months.

    2. The navicular reconstitutes in 6 to 48 months.

    3. No residual deformity or disability occurs in adulthood.

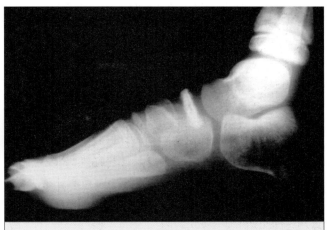

Figure 7 Lateral radiograph shows the foot of a child with Köhler bone disease. Note the sclerosis and flattening of the navicular bone. (Reproduced from Olney BW: Conditions of the foot, in Abel MF, ed: *Orthopaedic Knowledge Update: Pediatrics*, ed 3. Rosemont, IL, American Academy of Orthopaedic Surgeons, 2006, p 239.)

    4. Casting for 4 to 8 weeks with a short leg walking cast will decrease the duration of symptoms.

    5. Surgery is never indicated.

XIII. Toe Disorders

A. Atavistic great toe

    1. Adduction deformity of the great toe that usually presents after walking age

    2. It is thought to be secondary to an imbalance between the great toe abductor and the adductor musculature.

    3. Typically resolves with age; resistant cases may require release of the abductor hallucis longus muscle.

B. Polydactyly

    1. Toe polydactyly occurs in 1 in 500 births.

    2. Postaxial polydactyly is most common.

    3. Of affected patients, 30% have a family history; typically demonstrates an autosomal dominant inheritance pattern

    4. Surgery is indicated to facilitate shoe wear and prevent toe deformities.

C. Syndactyly

    1. Occurs approximately 1 in 2,000 births and is often familial.

    2. Characterized as either simple (fusion of soft tissues) or complex (fusion of bones).

5: Pediatrics

3. Most frequently occurs between the second and third toes

4. Simple syndactyly is an esthetic deformity that rarely requires surgical intervention.

D. Overlapping fifth toe

1. A dorsal adduction deformity of the fifth toe

2. It is typically familial and bilateral.

3. The extensor digitorum longus tendon is contracted.

4. Treatment is indicated when pain or shoe-wear

problems arise. The Butler procedure involves a double racket-handle incision and release of the extensor digitorum longus.

E. Curly toe(s)

1. A malrotation and flexion deformity of one or more toes

2. A contracture of the flexor digitorum longus or flexor digitorum brevis is the most common cause.

3. Treatment involves flexor digitorum longus tenotomy at age 3 to 4 years.

Top Testing Facts

1. The sequence of deformity correction with the Ponseti technique is cavus, adductus, varus, and equinus.

2. Up to 90% of clubfeet treated with the Ponseti method require percutaneous Achilles tenotomy at the time of final cast application.

3. Tibialis anterior tendon transfer (split or whole transfer) is needed in one-third of clubfeet treated with the Ponseti method.

4. Congenital vertical talus is associated with neuromuscular disease and/or genetic syndromes in up to 50% of children.

5. The diagnostic radiographic view for congenital vertical talus is the forced plantar flexion lateral view.

6. Unless proven otherwise, a child with pes cavus should be assumed to have an underlying neurologic condition causing the deformity. Charcot-Marie-Tooth disease is the most common etiology of pes cavus in children.

7. Simultaneous plantar fascia release should be avoided with an Achilles tendon lengthening. An intact Achilles

tendon provides the resistance necessary to stretch the divided plantar tissues.

8. Percutaneous plantar fascia release is insufficient to correct a cavus foot.

9. Apparent hindfoot valgus may actually be the result of ankle valgus. If any suspicion of ankle valgus exists, radiographic views of the ankle should be obtained.

10. Severe forefoot adductus combined with hindfoot valgus is a condition known as skewfoot. Although rare, it is important to recognize because correction requires both hindfoot and midfoot osteotomies.

11. Calcaneonavicular coalitions are the most common form of tarsal coalition.

12. Harris axial radiographs have a high false-positive rate for tarsal coalition. If the view is slightly oblique to the posterior or middle facet, a coalition will appear to be present when it is not.

13. Preoperative CT assessment is helpful before tarsal coalition excision because multiple coalitions are present in 10% to 20% of feet with tarsal coalition.

Bibliography

Bleck EE: Metatarsus adductus: Classification and relationship to outcomes of treatment. *J Pediatr Orthop* 1983; 3(1):2-9.

Hoffinger SA: Evaluation and management of pediatric foot deformities. *Pediatr Clin North Am* 1996;43(5):1091-1111.

Katz MM, Mubarak SJ: Hereditary tendo Achillis contractures. *J Pediatr Orthop* 1984;4(6):711-714.

Levine MS: Congenital short tendo calcaneus: Report of a family. *Am J Dis Child* 1973;125(6):858-859.

Mosca VS: Skewfoot deformity in children: Correction by calcaneal neck lengthening and medial cuneiform opening wedge osteotomies. *J Pediatr Orthop* 1993;13:807.

Oetgen ME, Peden S: Idiopathic toe walking. *J Am Acad Orthop Surg* 2012;20(5):292-300.

Scher DM, Georgopoulos G: Congenital disorders of the foot, in Song KM, ed: *Orthopaedic Knowledge Update: Pediatrics*, ed 4. Rosemont, IL, American Academy of Orthopaedic Surgeons, 2011, pp 203-218.

Schwend RM, Drennan JC: Cavus foot deformity in children. *J Am Acad Orthop Surg* 2003;11(3):201-211.

Sullivan JA: Pediatric flatfoot: Evaluation and management. *J Am Acad Orthop Surg* 1999;7(1):44-53.

Chapter 59

Pediatric Lower Extremity Deformities and Limb Deficiencies

Anthony A. Scaduto, MD   Nathan L. Frost, MD

I. Limb-Length Discrepancy

A. Epidemiology—Small (up to 2 cm) limb-length discrepancies (LLDs) are common, occurring in up to two thirds of the general population.

B. Secondary problems from LLD

1. The prevalence of back pain may be higher with large discrepancies (>2 cm).

2. During double-limb stance, the hip on the long side is relatively less covered by the acetabulum. This may predispose patients to hip arthropathy on the long-leg side.

3. LLD increases the incidence of structural scoliosis to the short side. In up to one third of cases, the scoliosis is in a noncompensatory direction.

C. Evaluation

1. The discrepancy is measured by placing blocks under the short leg to level the pelvis.

2. Hip, knee, and ankle contractures will affect the apparent limb length and must be ruled out. A hip adduction contracture causes an apparent shortening of the adducted side.

3. The advantages and disadvantages of various imaging techniques are listed in **Table 1**.

4. Up to 6% of patients with LLD from hemihypertrophy develop embryonal cancers (for example, Wilms tumor). Routine abdominal ultrasonography is recommended until age 6 years.

D. Prediction methods

1. Arithmetic or rule-of-thumb method

   a. Assumes growth ends at chronologic age 14 years for girls and 16 years for boys

   b. Estimates the annual contribution to leg length of each physis near skeletal maturity (during the last 4 years of growth)

   • Proximal femoral physis—3 mm

   • Distal femoral physis—9 mm

   • Proximal tibial physis—6 mm

   • Distal tibial physis—3 mm

2. Growth remaining method

   a. LLD prediction based on Green and Anderson tables of extremity length for a given age

   b. Uses skeletal age for predicting discrepancy

3. Mosley straight-line graph method

   a. This method improves the accuracy of the Green and Anderson prediction by reformatting the data in graph form.

   b. It minimizes errors of arithmetic or interpretation by averaging serial measurements.

4. Multiplier method

   a. This method predicts final limb length by multiplying the current discrepancy by a sex-specific and age-specific factor.

   b. It is most accurate for discrepancies that are constantly proportional (for example, congenital).

E. Classification

1. Causes of LLD include congenital conditions, infection, paralytic conditions, tumors, trauma, and osteonecrosis.

   a. In congenital conditions, the absolute discrepancy increases but the relative percentage remains constant (for example, a short limb that is 70% of the long side at birth will be 70% of the long side at maturity).

   b. Children with paralysis usually have

Dr. Scaduto or an immediate family member serves as a board member, owner, officer, or committee member of the American Academy of Orthopaedic Surgeons and the Pediatric Orthopaedic Society of North America. Neither Dr. Frost nor any immediate family member has received anything of value from or has stock or stock options held in a commercial company or institution related directly or indirectly to the subject of this chapter.

5: Pediatrics

Table 1

Assessment of Limb-Length Discrepancy Using Imaging Techniques

Technique	Description	Advantages	Disadvantages
Teleoradiograph	Single exposure of entire leg on a long cassette	Can assess angular deformity	Magnification error
Orthoradiograph	Three separate exposures (hip, knee, and ankle) on a long cassette	Eliminates magnification error	Cannot assess angular deformity Movement error may occur
Scanogram	Three separate exposures on a small cassette	Eliminates magnification error Small cassette	Cannot assess angular deformity Movement error may occur
CT scanogram	CT scan through hip, knee, and ankle to assess length	Accurate length measurement possible in the presence of joint contractures	Cannot assess angular deformity

Table 2

Treatment Algorithm for Limb-Length Discrepancy

Discrepancy	Treatment Options
0–2 cm	No treatment if asymptomatic. May use shoe lift if symptomatic.
2–5 cm	Shoe lift, epiphysiodesis, shortening, lengthening
5–15 cm	Lengthening(s). May be combined with epiphysiodesis/shortening procedure(s).
>15 cm	Lengthenings plus epiphysiodesis/shortening versus prosthesis

shortening of the more severely affected side.

2. Static discrepancies (for example, a malunion of the femur in a shortened position) must be differentiated from progressive discrepancies (for example, physeal growth arrest).

F. Treatment (**Table 2**)

1. Surgical correction must address the projected LLD at skeletal maturity.

2. Goals of treatment include a level pelvis and equal limb lengths.

   a. In paralytic conditions or in patients with a stiff knee, it is often best to leave the LLD undercorrected to facilitate foot clearance of the weak leg.

   b. In patients with fixed pelvic obliquity, functional limb-length equality should be the goal of treatment.

3. Nonsurgical management with or without a shoe lift is typically reserved for a projected LLD of less than 2 cm.

4. Shortening techniques

   a. Epiphysiodesis is the treatment of choice for skeletally immature patients with discrepancies of 2 to 5 cm because of the low complication rate. If proximal tibial epiphysiodesis is performed, concomitant proximal fibular epiphysiodesis should also be performed if more than 2 to 3 years of growth remain.

   b. Acute osseous shortening, typically of the femur, is used for skeletally mature patients with discrepancies of 2 to 5 cm.

5. Lengthening techniques

   a. Limb lengthening is typically reserved for LLD greater than 5 or 6 cm.

   b. Modern techniques involve osteotomy or corticotomy and incremental distraction using a uniplanar or multiplanar external fixator, often over an intramedullary nail to reduce the time spent in the fixator during the consolidation phase.

   c. Technical considerations for lengthening include making the corticotomy at the metaphyseal level when possible and delaying distraction for 5 to 7 days after the corticotomy.

   d. The typical rate of distraction is 1 mm/d (0.25 mm four times daily).

   e. Complications of limb lengthening include pin site infection, hardware failure, regenerate deformity or fracture, delayed union, premature union at corticotomy, and joint subluxation/dislocation.

II. Angular Deformities

A. Overview

1. Normal physiologic knee alignment includes periods of "knock knees" and "bowed legs" (**Figure 1**).

2. Children older than 2 years with bowed legs may require further evaluation.

B. Blount Disease (tibia vara)

1. Overview

   a. The most common cause of pathologic genu varum is Blount disease.

   b. Progressive tibia vara can occur in infants and adolescents (**Table 3**).

2. Pathoanatomy

   a. In infantile Blount disease, excess medial pressure (such as obese, early walkers who are in physiologic varus alignment) produces an osteochondrosis of the physis and adjacent epiphysis that can progress to physeal bar.

   b. In adolescent Blount disease, a varus moment at the knee during the stance phase of gait further inhibits medial physeal growth according to the Hueter-Volkmann principle (compression = decreased growth of the physis).

3. Evaluation

   a. Clinical findings suggestive of pathologic bowing include localized bowing at the proximal tibia, severe deformity, progression, and lateral thrust during gait.

   b. Full-length standing radiographs should be performed on children older than 18 months with the aforementioned findings.

c. If the metaphyseal-diaphyseal (MD) angle (**Figure 2**) is less than 10°, there is a 95% chance the bowing will resolve.

d. If the MD angle is greater than 16°, there is a 95% chance the bowing will progress. For MD angles between 11° and 16°, monitoring is required.

4. Classification—Langenskiöld described six radiographic stages that can develop over 4 to 5 years.

   a. Early changes include metaphyseal beaking

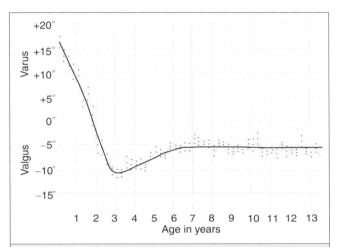

Figure 1 Graph illustrates the development of the tibiofemoral angle in children during growth, based on measurements from 1,480 examinations of 979 children. Of the lighter lines, the middle one represents the mean value at a given point in time, and the other two represent the deviation from the mean. The darker line represents the general trend. (Adapted with permission from Salenius P, Vankka E: The development of the tibiofemoral angle in children. *J Bone Joint Surg Am* 1975;57:259-261.)

Table 3						

Infantile Versus Adolescent Blount Disease

Condition	Age (Years)	Typical History	Location of Deformity	Other Angular Deformities	Laterality	Treatment
Infantile Blount	1 to 3	Early walker, obese	Epiphysis/physis; joint depression in advanced stages	None	Often bilateral	Bracing (limited effectiveness) Proximal tibia/fibula osteotomy
Adolescent Blount	9 to 11	Morbid obesity	Proximal tibia; no joint depression	Distal femur and distal tibia common	Unilateral more common	Bracing not effective Hemiepiphysiodesis if growth remaining Proximal tibia/fibula osteotomy ± femoral and distal tibia osteotomies

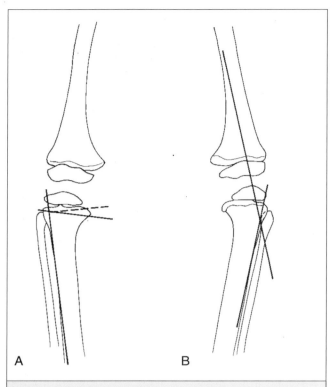

Figure 2 Illustration shows the assessment of the metaphyseal-diaphyseal (**A**) and tibial-femoral (**B**) angles. (Reproduced from Brooks WC, Gross RH: Genu varum in children: Diagnosis and treatment. *J Am Acad Orthop Surg* 1995;3[6]:326-336.)

and sloping.

b. Advanced changes include articular depression and medial physeal closure.

5. Nonsurgical treatment of infantile Blount disease

a. The efficacy of bracing is controversial.

b. Bracing with a knee-ankle-foot orthosis may be indicated in patients 2 to 3 years of age with mild disease (stage 1 to 2).

c. Poor results are associated with obesity and bilaterality.

d. Improvement should occur within 1 year, although treatment must be continued until the bony changes resolve, which usually takes 1.5 to 2.0 years.

6. Surgical treatment of infantile Blount disease

a. Patients older than 3 years require proximal tibial osteotomy.

b. To avoid undercorrection, the distal fragment is fixed in slight valgus, lateral translation, and external rotation.

c. Performing an anterior compartment fasciot-

omy at the time of surgery reduces the postoperative risk of compartment syndrome.

d. The risk of recurrence is much less if the surgery is performed in children younger than 4 years.

e. If a bony bar is present, a bar resection with interposition of methylmethacrylate (epiphysiolysis) is performed concomitantly.

7. Surgical treatment of adolescent Blount disease

a. Temporary or permanent hemiepiphysiodesis of the proximal lateral tibia prevents deformity progression and may allow some correction in adolescents with mild to moderate Blount disease in whom at least 15 to 18 months of growth remain.

b. Severe deformities and/or deformities in skeletally mature patients require proximal tibial osteotomy.

c. Correction of deformity may be performed acutely or gradually using an external fixator.

d. Patients should be carefully assessed for distal femoral varus, which can be treated similarly with a hemiepiphysiodesis in immature patients or distal femoral osteotomy in severe cases or in mature patients.

C. Genu valgum

1. Overview

a. Children age 3 to 4 years typically have up to 20° of genu valgum.

b. Genu valgum should not increase after 7 years of age.

c. After age 7 years, valgus should not exceed 12°, and the intermalleolar distance should be less than 8 cm.

2. Pathoanatomy

a. The deformity is usually in the distal femur but may also arise in the proximal tibia.

b. The degree of deformity necessary to lead to degenerative changes in the knee is not known.

3. Etiology (**Table 4**)

4. Treatment

a. There is no role for bracing in genu valgum.

b. Genu valgum following proximal tibial metaphyseal fractures (Cozen phenomenon) typically remodels spontaneously and should be observed.

c. Correction is indicated if the mechanical axis (represented by a line drawn from the center of the femoral head to the center of the distal tibial plafond) falls in the outer quadrant of the

Table 4

Common Causes of Genu Valgum

Bilateral
Physiologic genu valgum
Rickets
Skeletal dysplasia (for example, chondroctodermal dysplasia, spondyloepiphyseal, Morquio syndrome)

Unilateral
Physeal injury (trauma, infection, or vascular)
Proximal tibial metaphyseal (Cozen) fracture
Benign tumors (for example, fibrous dysplasia, Ollier disease, osteochondroma)

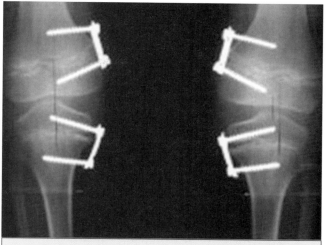

Figure 3 Radiographs demonstrate hemiphyseal tethering with a plate-screw construct. (Courtesy of Orthofix, Lewisville, TX.)

tibial plateau (or beyond) in children older than 10 years.

d. In skeletally immature patients, hemiepiphysiodesis or temporary physeal tethering may be performed with staples, transphyseal screws, or plate/screw devices (**Figure 3**).

e. Varus-producing osteotomies are necessary when insufficient growth remains or the site of the deformity is away from the physis. To reduce the risk of peroneal injury, gradual correction, preemptive peroneal nerve release, or a closing-wedge technique should be considered.

III. Rotational Deformities

A. Femoral anteversion

1. Overview

a. Normal anteversion is 30° to 40° at birth and decreases to 15° by skeletal maturity.

b. Intoeing from femoral anteversion is most evident between 3 and 6 years of age.

c. Increased femoral anteversion occurs more commonly in girls than in boys (2:1 ratio) and often is hereditary.

2. Pathoanatomy

a. Rotation variations have not been directly correlated to degenerative changes of the hip or knee.

b. Patellofemoral pain can arise with increasing femoral anteversion, but a pathologic threshold has not been identified.

3. Evaluation

a. Intoeing gait with medially rotated patellae is indicative of femoral anteversion.

b. Rotational profile assessment should include the knee-progression and foot-progression an-

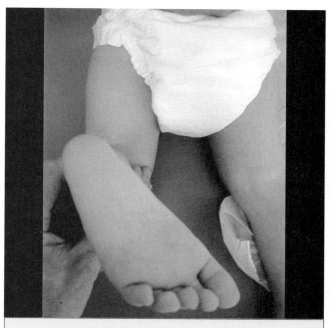

Figure 4 Photograph depicts the measuring of the thigh-foot axis, which is best performed with the child in the prone position. (Reproduced from Lincoln TL, Suen PW: Common rotational variations in children. *J Am Acad Orthop Surg* 2003;11[5]:312-320.)

gles during gait, the thigh-foot angle, and the maximum hip internal and external rotation (**Figure 4**). After age 10 years, internal rotation greater than 70° and external rotation less than 20° suggests excessive femoral anteversion.

c. Femoral anteversion is estimated by measuring the degree of internal hip rotation necessary to make the greater trochanter most prominent

5: Pediatrics

Table 5

Types of Tibial Bowing

	Anterolateral Bowing	Posteromedial Bowing	Anteromedial Bowing
Associated Conditions	Neurofibromatosis	Calcaneal valgus foot	Fibular deficiency
Prognosis	1. Progressive bowing 2. Pseudarthrosis	1. Spontaneous improvement in bowing (rarely complete) 2. Limb-length discrepancy	Varies with severity of shortening and foot function
Treatment	1. Bracing to prevent fracture 2. Osteotomy contraindicated	Observation versus epiphysiodesis for limb-length discrepancy	Osteotomy with lengthening versus amputation

laterally (trochanteric prominence angle test).

   d. CT or MRI can quantify anteversion accurately but are unnecessary in most cases.

   e. Differential diagnoses of intoeing include internal tibial torsion and metatarsus adductus.

4. Treatment

   a. Shoes and orthoses are ineffective.

   b. Children older than 8 years with unacceptable gait or pain and less than 10° external hip rotation are candidates for a derotational osteotomy.

   c. The amount of rotation to correct excessive anteversion = (prone internal rotation − prone external rotation)/2.

B. Internal tibial torsion

1. Epidemiology

   a. Most evident between ages 1 and 2 years

   b. Usually resolves by age 6 years

2. Evaluation

   a. The transmalleolar axis—the angular difference between the bimalleolar axis at the ankle and the bicondylar axis of the knee—is determined; normal is 20° of external rotation.

   b. Measurement of the thigh-foot axis in the prone position; by 8 years, normal is 10° of external rotation.

3. Treatment

   a. Parent education is the primary treatment.

   b. Special shoes and braces do not change outcome.

   c. Derotational osteotomy is rarely indicated and should be reserved for children older than 8 years with marked functional and/or esthetic deformity.

IV. Tibial Bowing

A. Overview—Three types of tibial bowing exist in children, with considerable differences in prognosis and treatment (**Table 5**).

B. Anterolateral bowing

1. Epidemiology

   a. Of patients with anterolateral bowing, 50% have neurofibromatosis.

   b. Of patients with neurofibromatosis, 10% have anterolateral bowing.

2. Classification—The presence of sclerosis, cysts, fibular dysplasia, and narrowing are the basis of the Boyd and Crawford classification (**Figure 5**).

3. Natural history

   a. Spontaneous resolution is unusual.

   b. Good prognostic signs include a duplicated hallux and a delta-shaped osseous segment in the concavity of the bow.

   c. Fracture risk decreases at skeletal maturity.

4. Treatment

   a. The initial goal of treatment is prevention of pseudarthrosis with a clam-shell total contact brace.

   b. Osteotomies to correct bowing are contraindicated because of the risk of pseudarthrosis of the osteotomy site.

   c. If pseudarthrosis develops, all treatment options have limited success.

   d. Treatment options of pseudarthrosis include

   • Intramedullary rod and bone grafting

   • Circular fixator with bone transport

   • Vascularized fibular graft

   • Adjunctive use of bone morphogenetic proteins is gaining support.

e. Amputation may be considered for persistent pseudarthrosis (usually after two or three failed surgeries).

C. Posteromedial bowing

1. Congenital posteromedial bowing is often associated with a calcaneovalgus foot. The dorsum of the foot may be in contact with the anterior tibia in this condition.

2. The bow improves in the first years of life, but it rarely resolves completely.

3. Monitoring for LLD is a must—LLDs at maturity are usually in the 3 to 8 cm range (mean, 4 cm) and are treated as described above in section I.

D. Anteromedial bowing—See fibular deficiency in section V.

V. Limb Deficiencies

A. General principles for amputation, when indicated

1. The optimal age for amputation for limb deficiency is 10 months to 2 years.

2. Early amputation is avoided if severe upper extremity deficiencies require use of the feet for activities of daily living.

3. Syme versus Boyd amputation

a. The Syme amputation (ankle disarticulation) is simple and accommodates a tapered prosthesis at the ankle for optimal cosmesis.

b. The Boyd amputation, in which the calcaneus is retained and fused to the distal tibia, prevents heel pad migration, aids prosthesis suspension, and may provide better end bearing. It also may limit prosthetic foot options because of its greater length.

B. Proximal femoral focal deficiency (PFFD) and congenital short femur

1. Overview

a. The spectrum of femoral hypoplasia ranges from congenital short femur to complete absence of the proximal femur.

b. Bilateral involvement is seen in 15% of cases. Ipsilateral foot and lower-limb anomalies are present up to 70% of the time.

c. Fibular deficiency occurs in 50% of patients with PFFD.

2. Pathoanatomy (**Table 6**)

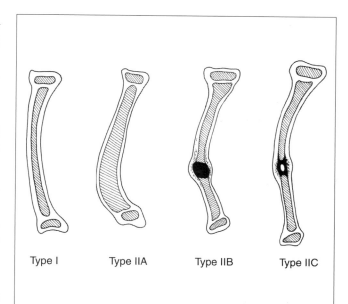

| Type I | Type IIA | Type IIB | Type IIC |

Figure 5 Illustrations show the Boyd and Crawford classification of congenital tibial dysplasia. Type I is characterized by anterior lateral bowing with increased cortical density and a narrow but normal medullary canal; type IIA, by anterior lateral bowing with failure of tubularization and a widened medullary canal; type IIB, by anterior lateral bowing with a cystic lesion before fracture or canal enlargement from a previous fracture; and type IIC, by frank pseudarthrosis and bone atrophy with "sucked candy" narrowing of the ends of the two fragments. (Reproduced from Crawford AH, Schorry EK: Neurofibromatosis in children: The role of the orthopaedist. *J Am Acad Orthop Surg* 1999; 7[4]:217-230.)

Table 6

Spectrum of Problems Associated With Proximal Femoral Focal Deficiency

Condition	Acetabulum	Proximal Femur	Knee	Lower Leg
Mild PFFD	Normal	Delayed ossification and varus	Anterior-posterior laxity	Normal
Moderate PFFD	Dysplastic	Pseudarthrosis	Cruciate deficiency	Fibular deficiency
Severe PFFD	Absent	Complete absence	Flexion contracture	Severe fibular and foot deficiency

PFFD = proximal femoral focal deficiency.

5: Pediatrics

Type		Femoral Head	Acetabulum	Femoral Segment	Relationship Among Components of Femur and Acetabulum at Skeletal Maturity
A	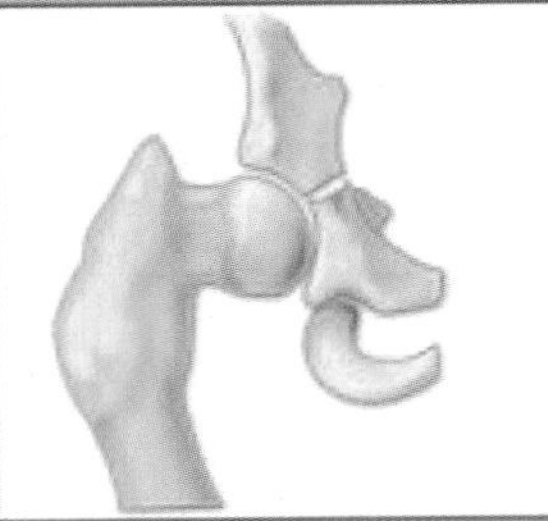	Present	Normal	Short	Bony connection between components of femur Femoral head in acetabulum Subtrochanteric varus angulation, often with pseudarthrosis
B	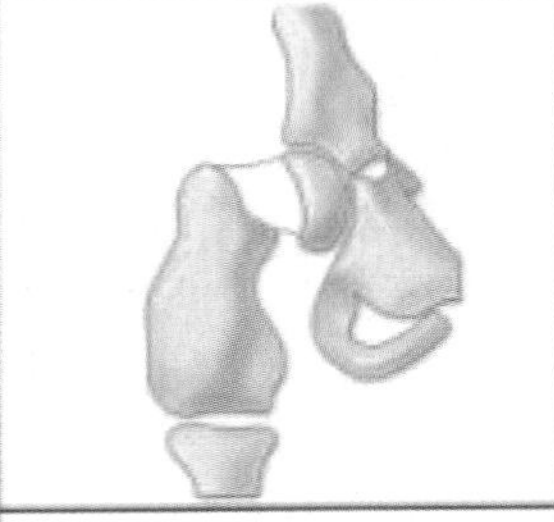	Present	Adequate or moderately dysplastic	Short, usually proximal bony tuft	No osseous connection between head and shaft Femoral head in acetabulum
C	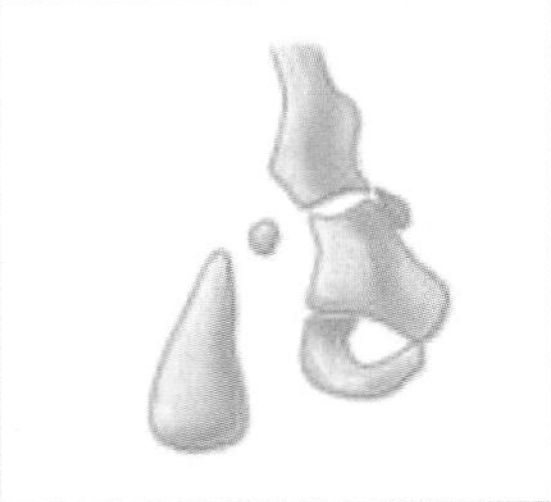	Absent or represented by ossicle	Severely dysplastic	Short, usually proximally tapered	May be osseous connection between shaft and proximal ossicle No articular relation between femur and acetabulum
D	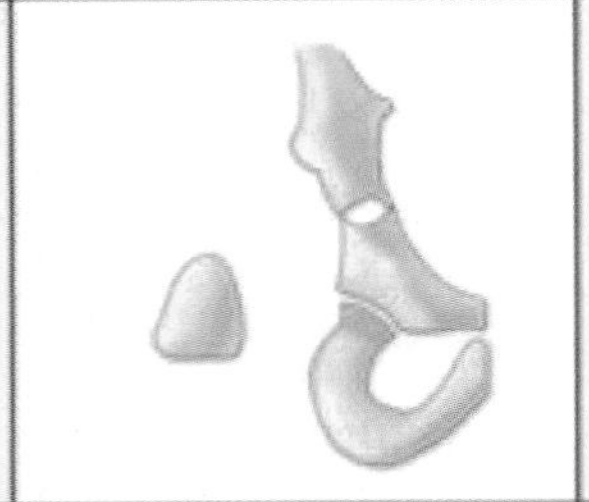	Absent	Absent Obturator foramen enlarged Pelvis squared in bilateral cases	Short, deformed	None

Figure 6   Diagram describes the Aitken classification for proximal focal femoral deficiency. (Adapted with permission from Herring JA: *Pediatric Orthopaedics*, ed 4. Philadelphia, PA, WB Saunders, 2007.)

a. In a congenitally short femur, the primary defect is a longitudinal deficiency of the femur.

b. In PFFD, the Aitken classification outlines the varying deformities of the proximal femur and hip joint, including coxa vara, proximal femoral pseudarthrosis, and acetabular dysplasia (**Figure 6**).

c. Associated ipsilateral limb anomalies include knee laxity with deficiency of the cruciate ligaments, fibular hemimelia, and absent lateral rays.

3. Evaluation

a. Patients with a congenitally short femur have an externally rotated limb secondary to femo-

ral retroversion.

b. In PFFD, the thigh is short, flexed, abducted, and externally rotated (**Figure 7**).

c. The entire lower extremity should be carefully evaluated for the associated anomalies listed previously.

4. The treatment of congenital short femur consists of treating the associated LLD, as described previously.

5. Treatment of PFFD

a. Treatment should parallel development; thus initial prosthesis fitting should occur when the patient is pulling to stand.

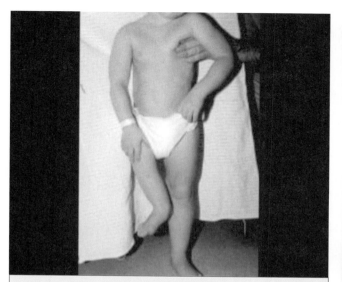

Figure 7 Photograph shows a child with proximal femoral focal deficiency. The ankle of the affected extremity is almost at the level of the contralateral knee. The foot on the affected side is almost normal. This child would be a good candidate for knee fusion and rotationplasty. (Reproduced from Krajbich JI: Lower-limb deficiencies and amputations in children. *J Am Acad Orthop Surg* 1998;6[6]:358-367.)

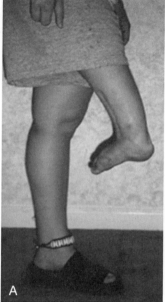
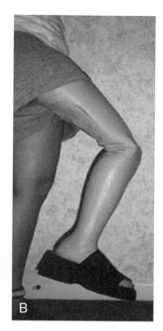
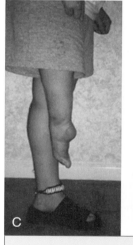
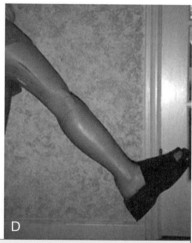

Figure 8 Photographs show the results of a Van Ness rotationplasty in a 17-year-old girl with PFFD. With the ankle rotated 180°, dorsiflexion of the ankle (**A**) results in flexion of the prosthetic knee (**B**), and plantar flexion (**C**) results in extension of the prosthetic knee (**D**). (Reproduced with permission from Morrissy RT, Giavedoni BJ, Coulter-O'Berry C: The child with a limb deficiency, in Morrissy RT, Weinstein SL, eds: *Lovell and Winter's Pediatric Orthopaedics*, ed 6. Philadelphia, PA, Lippincott William and Wilkins, 2006).

b. Surgery is best delayed until the patient is 2.5 to 3.0 years of age.

c. Proximal femoral deformity (varus, pseudarthrosis) and acetabular dysplasia should be addressed before lengthening.

d. Lengthening is indicated if a stable hip, a functional foot, and a projected LLD of less than 20 cm are present.

e. Amputation and prosthetic fitting are indicated if the projected LLD is greater than 20 cm.

f. Van Ness rotationplasty is an option if the projected LLD is greater than 20 cm. This procedure converts the ankle joint into a functional knee joint by rotating the foot 180° (**Figure 8**).

C. Fibular deficiency

1. Overview

a. Previously termed fibular hemimelia

b. Most common long-bone deficiency

2. Pathoanatomy

a. The Achterman and Kalamchi classification system describes the spectrum of deficiency ranging from shortened fibula to complete absence of the fibula

b. Associated anomalies include femoral deficiency, cruciate ligament deficiency, genu valgum secondary to hypoplasia of the lateral femoral condyle, ball-and-socket ankle joint, tarsal coalition, and absent lateral ray(s). (**Figure 9**)

c. The tibia also may be shortened with anteromedial bowing.

3. Evaluation

a. The classic appearance is a short limb with an

equinovalgus foot and skin dimpling over the midanterior tibia (**Figure 10**).

   b. Radiographs

- The fibula is short or absent, and anteromedial bowing of the tibia may be evident.

- The intercondylar notch of the femur is typ-

ically shallow, and the tibial spines are small.

   4. Treatment is guided by the severity of the discrepancy and the functionality of the foot. This is described by the more recent Birch classification system (**Table 7**).

D. Tibial deficiency

   1. Overview

     a. Previously termed tibial hemimelia

     b. Only lower-limb deficiency with a defined inheritance pattern (autosomal dominant)

     c. Other musculoskeletal anomalies occur in 75% of patients.

   2. Pathoanatomy

     a. The Jones classification describes a spectrum of deficiency including complete absence of the tibia, partial absence (either proximal or dis-

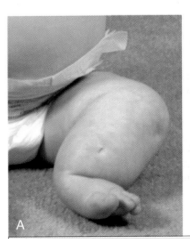

Figure 9   Illustration of a 13-year-old child demonstrating the associated anomalies of congenital fibular deficiency. (Reproduced from Hamdy RC, Makhdom AM, Saran N, Birch J: Congenital fibular deficiency. *J Am Acad Orthop Surg* 2014;22[4]:246-255.)

Table 7

Birch Treatment Guidelines for Fibular Deficiency

Findings	Treatment
Nonfunctional foot	Amputation (Syme or Boyd)
Functional foot plus:	
LLD <10%	Lengthening
LLD 10% to 30%	Lengthening or amputation
LLD >30%	Amputation

LLD = limb-length discrepancy.

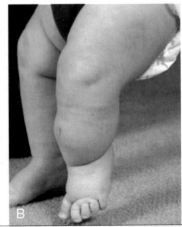
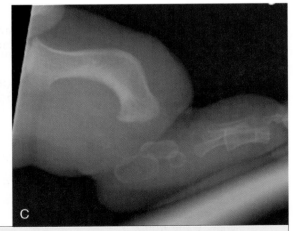

Figure 10   Images depict fibular deficiency. Photographs (**A** and **B**) demonstrate a shortened limb, an equinovalgus foot, and dimpling over the anterior tibia. Lateral radiograph (**C**) reveals the absence of the fibula and bowing of the tibia.

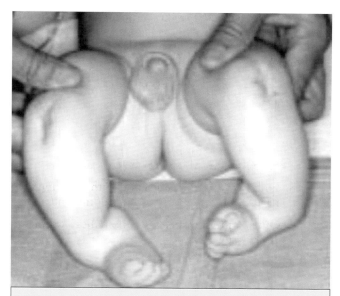

Figure 11 Photograph shows the typical clinical appearance of tibial deficiency. (Reproduced from Krajbich JI: Lower-limb deficiencies and amputations in children. *J Am Acad Orthop Surg* 1998;6[6]:358-367.)

tal), and diastasis of the tibia/fibula.

b. The foot is often in equinovarus.

c. Preaxial polydactyly may be present.

3. Evaluation

a. The typical appearance is a short tibial segment with a flexed knee and a prominent proximal fibula. Commonly, the foot is in rigid equinovarus and supination (**Figure 11**).

b. The presence or absence of active knee extension must be determined.

c. A proximal tibia anlage may be present but not apparent on early radiographs because of delayed ossification. An early clue to the absence of the proximal tibia is a small and minimally ossified distal femoral epiphysis.

d. Associated musculoskeletal anomalies (lobster clawhand associated with tibial deficiency) must be evaluated for.

4. Treatment (**Table 8**)

a. Based on the presence of active knee extension

b. A tibiofibular synostosis is effective at extending a short proximal tibial segment.

c. The Brown procedure (centralization of the fibula under the femur to treat complete tibial absence) has a high failure rate and is not recommended.

Table 8

Treatment Algorithm for Tibial Deficiency

Deformity/Findings	Treatment
No active knee extension	Knee disarticulation
Active knee extension	Synostosis of fibula to partial tibia plus Syme amputation
Ankle diastasis	Syme/Boyd amputation

VI. Congenital Dislocation of the Knee

A. Overview

1. Congenital dislocation of the knee is a rare disorder that is commonly sporadic but occasionally occurs within families.

2. Conditions producing muscle imbalance or laxity (myelodysplasia, arthrogryposis, Larsen syndrome) are associated with congenital dislocation of the knee.

B. Pathoanatomy

1. Fetal positioning, congenital absence of the cruciate ligaments, and fibrosis/contracture of the quadriceps have all been proposed as etiologic factors.

2. The spectrum of deformity ranges from severe genu recurvatum (grade I), through subluxation (grade II), to complete dislocation (grade III).

C. Evaluation

1. The knee can be hyperextended, and the foot is easily placed against the baby's face. Minimal or no flexion of the knee is possible.

2. A dimple or skin crease is seen at the anterior knee.

3. Hip examination is important because an ipsilateral hip dislocation is very common (70% to 100% of cases).

D. Treatment

1. Treatment of a knee dislocation takes priority over treatment of ipsilateral hip dysplasia or clubfoot. The Pavlik harness and clubfoot casts both require knee flexion.

2. Nonsurgical

a. Initial treatment begins with stretching, followed by serial casting.

b. Flexion should be attempted only after the tibia is reduced on the end of the femur (must

5: Pediatrics

confirm with lateral radiograph or ultrasound). Distal femoral physeal separation or plastic deformity of the tibia is possible.

   c. Prognosis is generally excellent if reduction is achieved nonsurgically.

3. Surgical

   a. Surgical treatment is indicated if nonsurgical

treatment fails to reduce the tibia on the end of the femur.

   b. The release always includes quadriceps lengthening.

   c. Best results are seen when surgery is performed in children younger than 6 months.

Top Testing Facts

Limb-Length Discrepancy

1. Estimates of the yearly growth contribution of the distal femur and proximal tibia physes (for example, 9 mm/y for the distal femur) are valid only for the last 4 years of growth.

2. Limb equalization procedures must account for the final projected LLD, not the LLD present at the time of surgery.

3. Undercorrection of an LLD associated with paralysis facilitates the foot clearing the floor during the swing phase of gait and is especially important if the patient walks with a brace in which the knee is locked in extension.

4. A proximal fibular epiphysiodesis should be included with a proximal tibial epiphysiodesis if more than 2 to 3 years of growth remain.

Tibia Vara (Blount Disease)

1. If the MD angle is greater than 16°, there is a 95% chance the bowing will progress. For MD angles between 11° and 16°, monitoring is required.

2. To avoid undercorrection in infantile Blount disease, the distal fragment should be fixed in slight valgus, lateral translation, and external rotation.

3. The risk of postoperative compartment syndrome is reduced if an anterior compartment fasciotomy is performed at the time of surgery.

4. Recurrence is less common when the osteotomy is performed in children younger than 4 years.

Genu Valgum

1. Children age 3 to 4 years typically have up to 20° of genu valgum.

2. Unilateral genu valgum following a Cozen fracture almost always resolves spontaneously.

3. When substantial valgus deformity is present in a growing child, treatment through guided growth (temporary hemiepiphyiodesis) is preferred over an osteotomy.

Rotational Deformities

1. Tibial torsion is best evaluated by measuring the thigh-foot axis in the prone position.

2. Internal torsion is physiologic between 1 and 2 years of age, and typically resolves without treatment.

3. Shoes and orthoses are ineffective treatments for intoeing or outoeing.

Tibial Bowing

1. Anterolateral bowing is typical of congenital tibial pseudarthrosis, which is often associated with neurofibromatosis.

2. Posteromedial bowing is often associated with development of LLD and a calcaneovalgus foot deformity.

3. Anteromedial bowing is associated with fibular deficiency.

Limb Deficiencies

1. The optimal age range to perform amputation and prosthetic fitting for limb deficiency is 10 months to 2 years.

2. Early amputation should be avoided if severe upper extremity deformities may require the use of the feet for activities of daily living.

3. The Syme amputation is simple and accommodates a tapered prosthesis at the ankle for optimal cosmesis. The medial malleolus does not need to be excised in children as is typically done in adults.

4. The Boyd amputation prevents heel pad migration, aids prosthesis suspension, and may provide better end bearing; however, it also may limit prosthetic foot options because of excessive length.

5. The treatment of fibular deficiency is based on the degree of fibular deficiency and the severity of the foot deformity.

6. In tibial deficiency, a good early radiographic clue to the absence of the proximal tibia is a small, minimally ossified distal femoral epiphysis.

7. The Brown procedure has a high failure rate. In contrast, a tibiofibular synostosis is effective at extending a short proximal tibia segment.

Bibliography

Aitken GT: Proximal femoral focal deficiency - definition, classification, and management, in Aitken GT, ed: *Proximal Femoral Focal Deficiency: A Congenital Anomaly*. Washington, DC, National Academy of Sciences, 1969, pp 1-22.

Bowen JR, Leahey JL, Zhang ZH, MacEwen GD: Partial epiphysiodesis at the knee to correct angular deformity. *Clin Orthop Relat Res* 1985;198:184-190.

Brooks WC, Gross RH: Genu varum in children: Diagnosis and treatment. *J Am Acad Orthop Surg* 1995;3(6):326-335.

Crawford AH, Schorry EK: Neurofibromatosis in children: The role of the orthopaedist. *J Am Acad Orthop Surg* 1999; 7(4):217-230.

Dobbs MB, Purcell DB, Nunley R, Morcuende JA: Early results of a new method of treatment for idiopathic congenital vertical talus. *J Bone Joint Surg Am* 2006;88(6):1192-1200.

Krajbich JI: Lower-limb deficiencies and amputations in children. *J Am Acad Orthop Surg* 1998;6(6):358-367.

Lincoln TL, Suen PW: Common rotational variations in children. *J Am Acad Orthop Surg* 2003;11(5):312-320.

Poloushk JD: Congenital deformities of the knee, in Song KM, ed: *Orthopaedic Knowledge Update: Pediatrics, ed 4*. Rosemont, IL, American Academy of Orthopaedic Surgeons, 2011, pp 195-202.

Richards BS, Oetgen ME, Johnston CE: The use of rhBMP-2 for the treatment of congenital pseudarthrosis of the tibia: A case series. *J Bone Joint Surg Am* 2010;92(1):177-185.

Spencer SA, Widmann RF: Limb-length discrepancy and limb lengthening, in Song KM, ed: *Orthopaedic Knowledge Update: Pediatrics*, ed 4. Rosemont, IL, American Academy of Orthopaedic Surgeons, 2011, pp 219-232.

Staheli LT: Motor development in orthopaedics, in Abel MF, ed: *Orthopaedic Knowledge Update: Pediatrics*, ed 3. Rosemont, IL, American Academy of Orthopaedic Surgeons, 2006, pp 3-12.

5: Pediatrics

Chapter 60
Limb Deformity Analysis

David W. Lowenberg, MD

I. General Principles

A. To understand whether a deformity exists, the parameters of a normal limb must be known.

B. If the contralateral limb is unaffected it can be used as a control; with certain conditions, however (for example, metabolic bone disorders), the contralateral limb is usually abnormal.

C. Many nonunions develop a resultant deformity; malunions, by definition, have a deformity.

D. Limb deformity is more of an issue in the lower extremity than in the upper extremity.

E. Normal lower extremity alignment values have been established and are provided in **Figure 1**.

1. The mechanical axis of the lower extremity passes from the center of the hip to the center of the talar dome.

2. Ideal limb alignment occurs when this mechanical axis line passes through the center of the knee.

F. In the pediatric population, a deformity is a dynamic process that can worsen with growth of the limb.

G. Congenital limb-length discrepancy (LLD) may follow five patterns, as defined by Shapiro (**Figure 2**). It is important for the surgeon to realize that not all congenital LLDs follow a linear growth disturbance pattern.

1. Certain types of deformity and growth impairment characterize one pattern of LLD over another.

2. Linear progressive pattern (type I) is the most common in congenital LLD, and all predictor methods (Green-Anderson Growth Remaining Method, Moseley Straight Line Graph, Paley Multiplier Method) apply to this linear pattern only.

3. Growth discrepancy secondary to femoral fracture more commonly follows a type III pattern, whereas type IV is prevalent in Legg-Calvé-Perthes disease.

4. When growth discrepancy does not follow a linear pattern, treatment must be individualized as to the timing of limb equalization. For this reason, it is sometimes more advantageous to perform definitive limb equalization via lengthening of the affected short limb after skeletal maturity

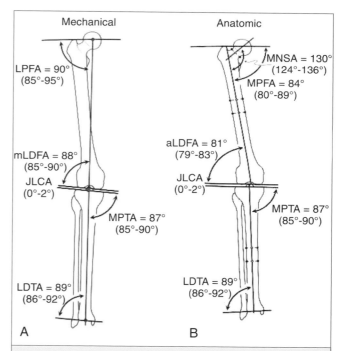

Figure 1   Illustrations show the standard mean values (with ranges) for normal lower extremity limb alignment. **A,** Mechanical alignment values. **B,** Anatomic alignment values. MNSA = medial neck-shaft angle; MPFA = medial proximal femoral angle; aLDFA = anatomic lateral distal femoral angle; JLCA = joint line convergence angle; LDTA = lateral distal tibial angle; MPTA = medial proximal tibial angle; LPFA = lateral proximal femoral angle; mLDFA = mechanical lateral distal femoral angle. (Reproduced with permission from Paley D: *Principles of Deformity Correction.* Berlin, Germany, Springer-Verlag, 2002, pp 1-17.)

5: Pediatrics

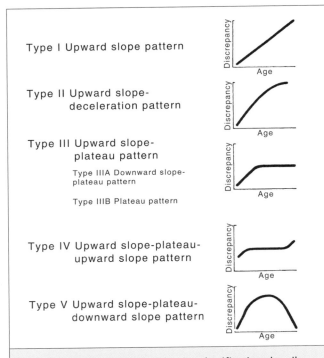

Type I Upward slope pattern

Type II Upward slope-deceleration pattern

Type III Upward slope-plateau pattern

    Type IIIA Downward slope-plateau pattern

    Type IIIB Plateau pattern

Type IV Upward slope-plateau-upward slope pattern

Type V Upward slope-plateau-downward slope pattern

Figure 2   Chart shows the Shapiro classification describing congenital growth disturbance patterns over time. (Adapted with permission from Shapiro F: Developmental patterns in lower extremity length discrepancies. *J Bone Joint Surg Am* 1982;64[5]:639-651.)

is reached, which ensures that proper limb equality is restored.

H. The deformities that one encounters in a limb are angulation, translation, length, and rotation; each can exist independent of the other.

II. Limb Deformity Analysis

A. Mechanical parameters

1. Essential mechanical parameters that must be compared between limbs are the absolute limb segment lengths, the comparative limb segment length, and the total limb rotation.

2. Limb lengths and deformity parameters are independent of each other, as are rotational deformities; all must be measured separately.

3. The nonrotational deformity parameters (**Figure 1, A**) that must be measured and compared with the contralateral limb on appropriate radiographic views include

    a. Lateral proximal femoral angle

    b. Mechanical lateral distal femoral angle

    c. Joint line convergence angle

    d. Medial proximal tibial angle

    e. Lateral distal tibial angle

B. Anatomic parameters

1. Anatomic limb measurement parameters define the alignment of the bones themselves and do not have to mirror the mechanical axis (**Figure 1, B**).

2. In the normal limb, however, the mechanical and anatomic parameters should yield the same measurements at a level from the knee distally.

3. The unique anatomic parameters of the lower extremity are:

    a. Medial neck-shaft angle

    b. Medial proximal femoral angle

    c. Anatomic lateral distal femoral angle

C. Evaluating lower-limb alignment

1. The gold standard for evaluating lower limb alignment include a weight-bearing radiograph of both lower extremities from the hips to the ankles on a 51-inch cassette, as well as true AP and lateral views of the affected limb segment(s) (**Figure 3**).

2. The mechanical and anatomic axis angles described previously are measured on the radiographs. This allows determination of the segment level of deformity (whether it is at the level of the femur, tibia, or joint line due to soft-tissue laxity), the degree of deformity, and the type of deformity.

3. To locate the exact site of the deformity, the mechanical axes and often the anatomic axes of each limb segment must be plotted.

D. Mechanical axis deviation (MAD)

1. The MAD is defined as the distance the mechanical axis has deviated from the normal position through the center of the knee (**Figure 4, A**).

2. This measurement is particularly helpful when treating genu varum and genu valgum.

3. The measurement of the MAD combined with the measurement of the accompanying joint orientation angles is particularly useful in the treatment of any juxta-articular deformity about the knee.

E. Diaphyseal deformities

1. These deformities, especially those that are posttraumatic, often are not simply an angulatory problem. An accompanying translational or rotatory deformity usually is present.

2. Translational deformities can contribute at least as much to mechanical axis deformity as can angulatory deformities (**Figure 4, B**).

3. Translational deformities with accompanying an-

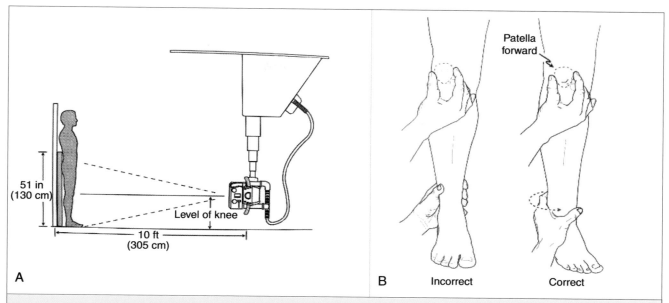

Figure 3   Illustrations show the evaluation of lower limb alignment. **A,** The correct method of obtaining weight-bearing AP radiographs of both lower extremities. **B,** The correct technique for obtaining consistent, true orthogonal views of the leg. (Reproduced with permission from Paley D: *Principles of Deformity Correction.* Berlin, Germany, Springer-Verlag, 2002, pp 1-17.)

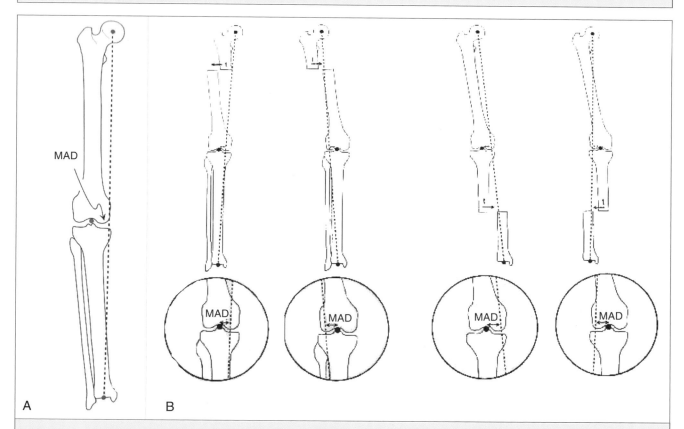

Figure 4   Illustrations depict the mechanical axis deviation (MAD). **A,** The MAD is measured at the level of the knee joint and represents the distance that the mechanical axis is displaced from normal for that limb. "Normal for the limb" is defined as the point that the mechanical axis passes in the contralateral, unaffected limb or a point in a range of 0 to 6 mm medial to the center of the knee, depending on what information is available. **B,** Examples of the effect of femoral and tibial translation on the mechanical axis of the limb. (Reproduced with permission from Paley D: *Principles of Deformity Correction.* Berlin, Germany, Springer-Verlag, 2002, pp 31-60.)

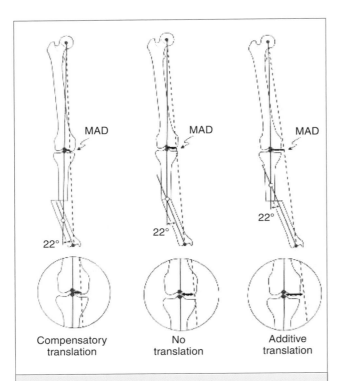

Figure 5 Illustrations show translational limb deformities with accompanying angulatory deformities. Translation of a limb segment can have a compensatory or an additive effect on an angulatory deformity depending on the directional plane of the translation. MAD = mechanical axis deviation. (Reproduced with permission from Paley D: *Principles of Deformity Correction.* Berlin, Germany, Springer-Verlag, 2002, pp 31-60.)

gulatory deformities can be compensatory, in which the translated segment tilts away from the concavity of the deformity, or additive, in which the translated distal segment exists toward the side of the concavity. Hence, a limb having an angulatory deformity with an accompanying compensatory translational component can in effect have no mechanical axis deviation of the overall limb or a negligible one (**Figure 5**).

4. When evaluating posttraumatic deformities, the most common deformity encountered is residual rotational deformity.

F. Center of rotation and angulation (CORA)

1. To determine the true site of deformity, not just the limb segment involved, the CORA must be plotted.

2. The CORA represents both the point in space where the axis of mechanical deformity exists and the virtual point in space where the apex of correction should occur.

3. The CORA is plotted out by drawing the mechanical axes for the limb segments (**Figure 6**).

4. When the affected limb has no translational deformity and no other accompanying juxta-articular deformity or additional site of deformity, then the CORA lies at the site of apparent deformity.

5. If a deformity exists secondary to angulation and translation (for example, malunion), then the CORA will lie at a site other than that of the apparent angulatory deformity. This happens because of the contributory effect (regardless of whether it is a compensatory or additive translational component) of the translated limb segment.

G. Evaluation in the sagittal plane—All the measurements and plotting of limb axes done in the coronal (AP) plane also can be done in the sagittal (lateral) plane, although sagittal plane deformities may be better tolerated in the lower extremity.

H. Upper extremity deformities

1. The same methods of deformity analysis also can be applied to the upper extremity.

2. Common sites of posttraumatic deformity are the elbow, secondary to malreduction of supracondylar fractures, and the wrist, because of shortening and deformity secondary to the malreduction of distal radial fractures.

I. The basic rules that can help the surgeon evaluate orthogonal AP and lateral radiographs to characterize limb deformity are listed in **Table 1**.

1. It is important to understand that radiographs are two-dimensional representations of a three-dimensional entity.

2. Limb deformity often is not present in just a true coronal or sagittal plane, but instead somewhere between these two planes. This is why an angulatory deformity is quite often seen on both true AP and true lateral radiographs.

3. If an AP and/or lateral radiograph shows an angulatory deformity, the actual deformity is always greater than or equal to the greater of the two deformities measured.

III. Treatment

A. General principles

1. Alignment deformities should be corrected in the following order: angulation, translation, length, rotation.

2. Angulatory deformity in skeletally immature patients may be corrected with growth modulation.

a. Hemiepiphysiodesis may be performed using tension-band plating, transphyseal screws, or staples.

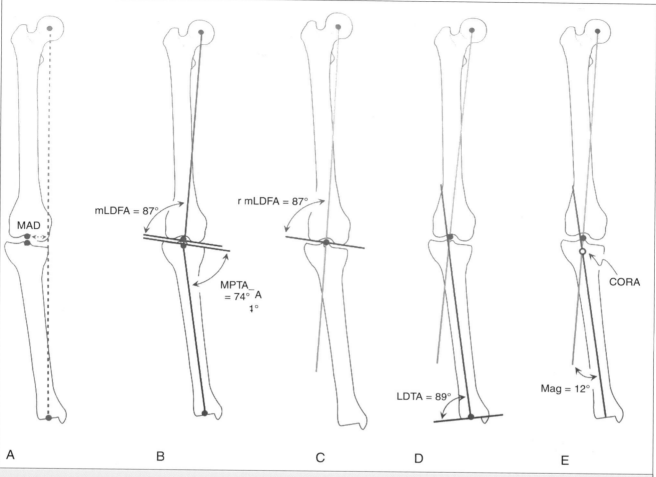

Figure 6 Illustrations depict the determination of the center of rotation of angulation (CORA). **A,** The mechanical axis of the limb is drawn, and the mechanical axis deviation (MAD) is determined. **B,** The mechanical lateral distal femoral angle (mLDFA), joint line convergence angle (JLCA), and medial proximal tibial angle (MPTA) for the limb are determined. Because the mLDFA is in the range of normal, and the JLCA is parallel, then the deformity exists in the tibia, because the MPTA is abnormal at 74°. **C,** Because the mechanical axis of the femur is normal, the mechanical axis line of the femur can then be extended down the limb to represent the mechanical axis of the tibia. **D,** The distal mechanical axis is defined as a line from the center of the ankle and parallel to the shaft of the tibia. The lateral distal tibial angle (LDTA) is found to be normal. **E,** The CORA is now defined as the intersection of the proximal mechanical axis line with the distal mechanical axis line. Imagine translating the distal segment at this level to see how the point of the CORA changes. Mag = magnitude of deformity. (Reproduced with permission from Paley D: *Principles of Deformity Correction.* Berlin, Germany, Springer-Verlag, 2002, pp 195-234.)

   b. Growth modulation requires close follow-up to monitor the correction of the deformity and the resultant changes to the mechanical axis.

3. Rotational malalignment is the most common posttraumatic deformity encountered; however, it is the least precise of the variables that can be measured. It is most often assessed clinically by comparing the affected limb with the contralateral limb.

4. Various values of acceptable lower extremity malalignment have been published, but no definitive value of the maximum acceptable rotatory deformity tolerated in the lower limb has been established. Any rotatory deformity of the leg greater than 10° typically is poorly tolerated, however.

B. Surgical technique

  1. Order of correction

    a. Alignment deformities should be corrected in the following order: angulation, translation, length, rotation. Following this order of correction results in the most predictable restoration of limb alignment.

    b. In correcting the rotation, especially if an external fixator is used, a resultant residual translation can be encountered (**Figure 7**). This translation occurs because of the inevitability of the center of rotational correction not being

5: Pediatrics

Table 1

The Five Rules of Deformity Analysis

1. The true angle of bone deformity is always equal to or greater than the measured angle of deformity on a radiograph.

2. The closer the measured values of deformity on AP and lateral radiographs are to each other, the closer the true plane of deformity is to the 45° axis.

3. Equal angles of deformity on true AP and true lateral radiographs define a true axis of deformity at the 45° axis, with the actual degree of deformity being 1.43 times that measured on the AP or lateral projection.

4. If a measured deformity on an AP view = 0°, then the plane of deformity is 90° to this plane, and the degree of deformity equals that measured on the lateral radiograph; and vice versa.

5. No direct relationship exists between angulation and translation in a deformity, although translation can have an additive or compensatory effect to angulation on limb mechanical axis.

at the exact center of the bone segment being rotated. This residual translation must be corrected.

2. Newer versions of external fixation allow simultaneous correction of all deformity parameters without having to correct the residual translation. The need to follow the classic order of correction remains, however.

3. Simple deformities without clinically substantial limb-length inequality usually can be successfully corrected acutely using locked intramedullary nail or plate and screw osteosynthesis.

4. Regardless of the method of fixation, proper preoperative planning and templating remains important.

5. In correcting a mechanical axis for genu varum, the ideal correction of the mechanical axis has classically been described as a point at the lateral edge of the tibial spine known as the Fujisawa point. Correction to this point generally gives an optimal mechanical axis load distribution for symptomatic medial compartment disease.

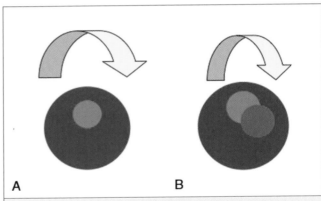

Figure 7 Illustrations depict residual translation. **A**, Initial graphic shows the bone (inner circle) within the soft-tissue envelope (outer circle) before rotational limb correction. **B**, Bone translation following limb rotational correction. Because of the eccentric position of the bone within the rings of the fixator, a resultant translation occurs, which needs subsequent correction.

Top Testing Facts

1. The mechanical axis of the lower extremity passes from the center of the hip to the center of the talar dome. Ideal limb alignment is defined as passage of this mechanical axis line through the center of the knee.

2. If the surgeon suspects a nonlinear congenital growth disturbance, it must be weighed when deciding the timing of definitive limb equalization and deformity correction.

3. The types of deformity that can exist in a limb are angulation, translation, length, and rotation. Rotation is generally measured clinically, whereas the other parameters are measured on appropriate radiographs.

4. It is important to recognize that translation deformities can be compensatory or additive to an angulatory deformity.

5. Because angulation is a phenomenon independent of translation, an apparent site of deformity might not actually be the true CORA. Therefore, this site must be precisely determined by obtaining the measurements on long radiographs.

6. Rotational deformities are the most common posttraumatic deformity encountered.

7. In congenital deformity analysis, limb-length inequality is an important accompanying deformity parameter that must be evaluated and projected over time.

8. The pattern of growth disturbance and resultant deformity is not always linear and can follow certain described growth rate disturbance patterns.

9. The order of correction of deformity is angulation, translation, length, and rotation.

Bibliography

Bowen JR, Leahey JL, Zhang ZH, MacEwen GD: Partial epiphysiodesis at the knee to correct angular deformity. *Clin Orthop Relat Res* 1985;198:184-190.

Green SA, Gibbs P: The relationship of angulation to translation in fracture deformities. *J Bone Joint Surg Am* 1994; 76(3):390-397.

Green SA, Green HD: The influence of radiographic projection on the appearance of deformities. *Orthop Clin North Am* 1994;25(3):467-475.

Handy RC, McCarthy JJ, eds: *Management of Limb-Length Discrepancies*. Rosemont, IL, American Academy of Orthopaedic Surgeons, 2011.

Paley D: *Principles of Deformity Correction*. Berlin, Germany, Springer-Verlag, 2002.

Shapiro F: Developmental patterns in lower-extremity length discrepancies. *J Bone Joint Surg Am* 1982;64(5):639-651.

Stevens PM: Guided growth for angular correction: A preliminary series using a tension band plate. *J Pediatr Orthop* 2007;27(3):253-259.

5: Pediatrics

Chapter 61

Musculoskeletal Conditions and Injuries in the Young Athlete

Jay C. Albright, MD

I. Overview

A. Child athlete versus adult athlete

1. A child athlete is not a small adult.

2. Because children have open physes growing at variable rates, they are susceptible to injury.

3. Children are less coordinated and have poorer mechanics than adults.

4. Children have less efficient thermoregulatory mechanisms than adults, including a less efficient sweating response, and cannot acclimatize as rapidly.

B. Sex-specific considerations

1. The female athlete triad—amenorrhea, disordered eating, osteoporosis—places the female athlete at higher risk of insufficiency or stress fractures, overuse injuries, and recurrent injuries.

2. Knee injuries

   a. The female knee becomes more susceptible to injury at puberty.

   b. Differences in anatomy, sex hormone levels, neuromuscular control, and overall strength and coordination have been implicated in the higher incidence of knee injuries in females than in males in the same sport.

II. Little Leaguer Shoulder

A. Overview and epidemiology

1. Little Leaguer shoulder is an epiphysiolysis, or fracture, through the proximal humeral epiphysis caused by repetitive microtrauma.

2. It occurs most commonly in overhead athletes

such as pitchers and tennis players who are skeletally immature.

3. Mechanism of injury—Results from repeated high loads of torque in a rapidly growing child athlete.

B. Evaluation

1. History and physical examination—Patients present with generalized shoulder pain that is typically at its worst during the late cocking or deceleration phases, pain with resisted elevation of the shoulder and with extremes of motion in any direction, and point tenderness over the physis of the proximal humerus, which is hard to discern from subdeltoid bursal pain.

2. Imaging—Radiographs show a widened proximal humeral physis compared with the opposite side (**Figure 1**).

C. Treatment—Same as for a fracture, nonsurgical, with no throwing for at least 2 to 3 months.

D. Rehabilitation

1. When painless full range of motion (ROM) is achieved, physical therapy for rotator cuff strengthening is initiated.

2. After 2 to 3 months of no throwing, a progressive throwing program is started.

   a. The athlete begins with short tosses at low velocity and gradually progresses to longer tosses; eventually the longer tosses are made with increasing velocity.

   b. After long tosses at higher velocities have been achieved, the patient can fully return to play.

E. Complications

1. Low incidence of premature growth arrest with or without angular deformity

2. Subsequent Salter-Harris fractures also can occur.

F. Prevention—Avoiding overuse by adhering to guidelines set by multiple entities, including the American Academy of Orthopaedic Surgeons, USA Baseball,

Dr. Albright or an immediate family member has received royalties from Biomet and is a member of a speakers' bureau or has made paid presentations on behalf of Arthrex.

5: Pediatrics

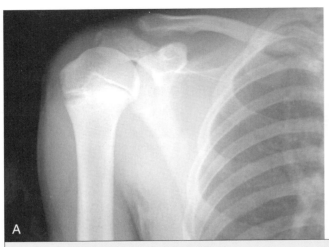
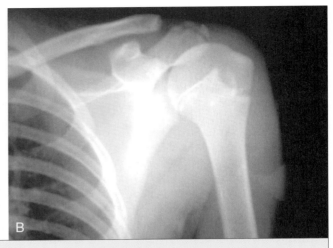

Figure 1 AP radiographs show the shoulders of a 12-year-old child who had right shoulder pain during the deceleration phase of throwing. Compare the physeal widening of the right shoulder (**A**) with the unaffected left shoulder (**B**).

Table 1

Pitching Recommendations for the Young Baseball Player

Age (Years)	Maximum Pitches per Game	Maximum Games per Week
8–10	52 ± 15	2 ± 0.6
11–12	68 ± 18	2 ± 0.6
13–14	76 ± 16	2 ± 0.4
15–16	91 ± 16	2 ± 0.6
17–18	106 ± 16	2 ± 0.6

Reproduced from Pasque CB, McGinnis DW, Griffin LY: Shoulder, in Sullivan JA, Anderson ST, eds: *Care of the Young Athlete.* Rosemont, IL, American Academy of Orthopaedic Surgeons, 2000, p 347.

and the American Orthopaedic Society for Sports Medicine (**Table 1**).

III. Little Leaguer Elbow

A. Overview and epidemiology—Little Leaguer elbow is a generic term for any injury to a child's elbow accompanied by pain along the medial aspect of the proximal forearm or elbow. These injuries are commonly related to the excessive stresses experienced by the immature skeleton during pitching.

B. Pathoanatomy

1. Little Leaguer elbow is a progressive problem resulting from repetitive microtrauma. Therefore, most of the early symptoms are assumed to be a result of soft-tissue strains and sprains.

2. By the time the symptoms are severe enough for

referral to an orthopaedic surgeon, more serious ligament, cartilage, physis, and bone pathology should be assumed to be present.

C. Mechanism of injury

1. The forces are similar to those that occur in the adult elbow—valgus-hyperextension overloading of the elbow during throwing—but the symptoms of each different injury in a child can be much more varied. Children often experience pain on the compressed radial side of the joint and the distracted ulnar side.

2. The syndrome is associated with throwing curveballs and other "junk" pitches or with an infielder bent-elbow throw that involves a whipping mechanism used to gain adequate speed.

D. Evaluation

1. Patients experience pain after, and then during, a game. The pain may be mild at first but eventually inhibits throwing.

2. Patients lose the ability to achieve throwing distance and accuracy early, followed by a loss of velocity. Eventually, persistent pain at rest is noted.

3. The differential diagnosis includes medial epicondylar apophysitis, posterior stress impingement, osteochondritis dissecans (OCD) or Panner disease, and instability with valgus extension overload.

4. Physical examination

   a. The patient is seated, and the arm is observed for deformity. Chronic conditions may produce an increased carrying angle or a flexion contracture.

   b. Sites of maximum point tenderness are sought. Point tenderness over the medial epicondyle

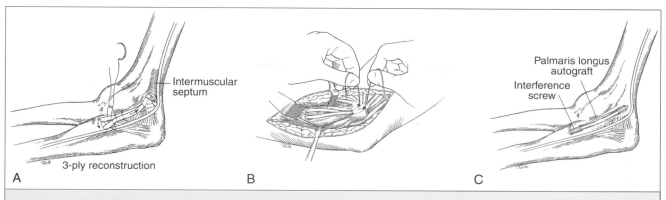

Figure 2 Illustrations show medial ulnar collateral ligament reconstruction techniques. **A,** Tendon graft passed through bone tunnels. **B,** Docking technique. **C,** Anatomic interference technique. (Reproduced with permission from ElAttrache NS, Bast SC, David T: Medial collateral ligament reconstruction. *Tech Shoulder Elbow Surg* 2001;2:38-49.)

and/or flexor mass could be a result of muscle strain, ulnar collateral ligament (UCL) sprain, or medial epicondylitis.

  c. Valgus stress is applied, with the arm in varied degrees of flexion and extension.

- As in a UCL injury, in which the ligament is avulsed at its origin on the apophysis of the medial epicondyle, instability may be present.

- UCL instability is evaluated using the valgus stress test, the milking maneuver, valgus stress radiographs, MRI, and/or magnetic resonance arthrography.

- The younger the patient, the more likely the diagnosis is to be an apophysitis or an avulsion injury, rather than a UCL sprain.

5. Imaging

  a. Bilateral AP, lateral, and oblique radiographs of the elbow should be obtained.

  b. Compare with the unaffected side to determine whether an irregular appearance of the physis is evident. This step also may help determine the degree of displacement. A radiograph of the involved extremity only is sufficient to determine whether the apophysis has closed.

  c. Fragmentation of the medial epicondyle, trochlea, olecranon, or capitellum may be present.

  d. Medial epicondyle hypertrophy or radial head hypertrophy also may be present.

E. Treatment

1. Nonsurgical

  a. Alterations in the athlete's form, motion, and playing habits as well as adherence to recommended pitch and inning counts are advised.

  b. Medial epicondylitis is managed with 4 to 6 weeks of no stress on the physis.

  c. Management of OCD and Panner disease is discussed in section V.

  d. Valgus extension overload and posterior stress syndromes typically can be managed with activity and throwing modifications.

  e. Intra-articular steroids may be used to control inflammation.

2. Surgical

  a. Indications

- Failure to respond to nonsurgical treatment

- Instability of the elbow with avulsion fracture or fragmentation of the medial epicondyle

  b. Contraindications—Uncertain diagnosis with ulnar nerve symptoms

  c. Procedures

- UCL reconstruction of choice when indicated for UCL insufficiency (**Figure 2**)

- Open reduction and internal fixation is recommended by most surgeons for medial epicondyle avulsion fractures in serious, competitive throwers, although definitive research is lacking.

- Arthroscopic débridement of posterolateral synovium and olecranon osteophytes for recalcitrant posterior symptoms; arthroscopic decompression of valgus-extension overload with failed prolonged nonsurgical treatment

  d. Complications

- Ulnar nerve neuropathy

- Loss of motion

- Infection

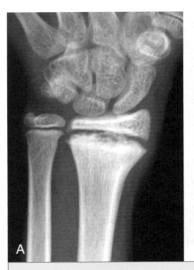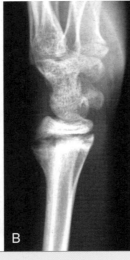

Figure 3 AP (**A**) and lateral (**B**) radiographs of the wrist of a 13-year-old elite-level female gymnast who presented with persistent pain and progressive deformity of the left wrist.

- Continued pain
- Inability to return to play at same level
- Aggressive débridement of the olecranon or osteophytes may result in instability.

F. Rehabilitation

1. Should be tailored according to whether ligament injury is involved

2. For injuries not involving ligaments, minimal immobilization with early ROM, strengthening, and pain modalities

3. For ligament reconstructions, a brief period of immobilization followed by protected ROM

G. Prevention—Educating coaches, parents, and athletes

IV. Distal Radius Epiphysiolysis/Epiphysitis

A. Overview and pathoanatomy

1. Injury to the distal radial epiphysis most commonly occurs in adolescent athletes in sports that require weight bearing on the upper extremities, such as gymnastics or cheerleading.

2. Children aged 10 to 14 years at higher skill levels spend more time in intensive training, so these injuries are more likely to occur in this age group.

B. Mechanism of injury—Overloading of the distal radial epiphysis, causing inflammation and/or fracture of the epiphysis.

C. Evaluation

1. History—Painful wrist with weight-bearing activities.

2. Physical examination consistent with pain and swelling at the joint with or without deformity of the wrist

3. Imaging—Radiographs may show a widened physis, blurred growth plate, metaphyseal changes, and fragmentation of radial and volar aspects of the plate, as shown in **Figure 3**.

D. Treatment

1. Nonsurgical

a. The patient should be allowed to participate in choosing treatment.

b. Relative rest is indicated in mild to moderate cases, complete rest in severe cases. In-season athletes and less severe cases may be managed with relative rest in a splint and physical therapy.

c. Immobilization is always indicated, a splint in mild to moderate cases, and casting in more severe cases. Aggressive immobilization is encouraged.

d. For severe cases, bone stimulation can be used.

2. Surgical—Typically indicated only for the correction of complications.

E. Rehabilitation—Physical therapy is useful for regaining motion after casting and helps control the return to activity.

F. Complications

1. This injury may recur, even with casting for 6 to 8 weeks, particularly if the athlete returns to full activities immediately.

2. Positive ulnar variance is a common eventual outcome in untreated athletes and may result in triangular fibrocartilage complex pathology or ulnar abutment.

V. OCD and Panner Disease

A. Overview

1. OCD occurs in the elbow, knee, and ankle in asymptomatic skeletally immature individuals but may not be detected until early adulthood.

2. No single etiologic theory is uniformly accepted; potential causes include macrotrauma or microtrauma, or vascular, hereditary, or constitutional factors.

B. Elbow OCD

1. Epidemiology

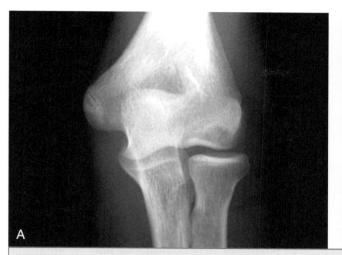
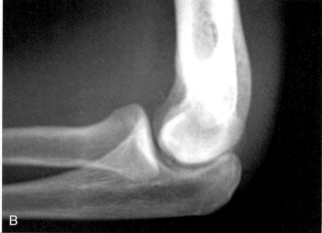

Figure 4 AP (**A**) and lateral (**B**) radiographs show capitellar osteochondritis dissecans in a 14-year-old child who is a gymnast.

a. Osteonecrosis of the capitellum, or Panner disease, has a relatively benign course and typically occurs in the first decade of life.

b. Capitellar OCD typically occurs after 10 years of age. It frequently causes permanent disability.

2. Pathoanatomy

a. Panner disease and capitellar OCD result from repetitive overuse or overload compression-type injuries, resulting in insult to the blood supply of the immature capitellum.

b. Ossification of the capitellum usually is complete by 10 years of age, distinguishing Panner disease from OCD.

3. Staging and classification of OCD—Based on radiographic studies and arthroscopy (**Figure 4**)

a. Type I lesions—Intact cartilage with or without bony stability underneath

b. Type II lesions—Cartilage fracture with bony collapse or displacement

c. Type III lesions—Loose fragments in the joint

4. Evaluation

a. Presentation—An insidious onset of activity-related pain with or without stiffness in the dominant arm of an overhead throwing or weight-bearing athlete

b. A history of locking or catching may be present.

c. Physical examination—Reveals a flexion contracture, point tenderness, and possibly crepitus

d. Radiographs—AP, lateral, and oblique views

5. Nonsurgical treatment

a. Panner disease and type I OCD lesions are best managed nonsurgically, with a success rate greater than 90%.

b. Rest with or without immobilization for 3 to 6 weeks, longer for OCD than Panner disease

c. A slow progression back to activity is allowed over the next 6 to 12 weeks.

6. Surgical treatment

a. Indications

• Failure of nonsurgical management

• Persistent pain

• Symptomatic loose bodies

• Displacement of OCD lesions

b. Contraindications—Patients younger than 10 years without loose bodies, chondral fractures, or displacement of the OCD have Panner disease.

c. Procedures

• Extra-articular or transarticular drilling of type I lesions without bony stability or type II lesions that are stable arthroscopically has good clinical success.

• Fixation of OCD lesions of the capitellum has variable success and should be reserved for large lesions with primary intact fragments that sit well or are not completely displaced.

• Débridement of the base of the lesion with or without drilling of the subchondral bone and loose body excision is frequently

5: Pediatrics

required in unstable type II and type III lesions.

- Cartilage restoration may be necessary if symptoms continue or the lesion is large, starting with a high anteromedial portal.

d. Pearls

- The posterior portals and anconeus portal are used for most of the work; nearly all of the capitellum can be visualized through this approach.

- Excessive cartilage débridement should be avoided; only flaps or loose cartilage should be débrided.

- Extra-articular drilling avoids damaging the cartilage.

- Large lesions may need cartilage restoration initially or if symptoms do not abate after débridement.

7. Complications—Elbow stiffness, infection, progression of arthritis, continued pain, and an inability to return to sports

8. Rehabilitation

a. The rehabilitation protocol depends on the procedure.

- Débridement or loose body excisions call for early ROM with or without an elbow brace. Progression to strengthening can be initiated when painless ROM is achieved, with avoidance of valgus positions, throwing, and weight bearing for 3 to 4 months.

- Elbows that undergo fixation or drilling procedures need more prolonged protection, with protected early ROM followed by strengthening at approximately 2 months, then a slow return to valgus position. Throwing, then weight bearing are begun at 4 to 6 months.

b. Overhead or weight-bearing athletes may not be able to return to the same level of play.

c. Changes in mechanics, position, or sport may be necessary.

C. Knee OCD

1. Overview and epidemiology

a. The knee is the most common site of osteochondrosis in growing children.

b. The actual incidence may be far greater than thought; no studies exist for a general population of asymptomatic children.

c. Often confused with irregularities of epiphyseal ossification, knee OCD does not always improve with benign neglect.

d. Age and level of skeletal maturity at onset are considered prognostic. Generally, children with closed or nearly closed growth plates at the onset have a worse prognosis.

2. Classification—Lesions are classified by evaluating radiographs and MRIs and using arthroscopic evaluation; multiple classifications exist in the literature, including the Guhl classification (**Figure 5**).

3. Evaluation

a. Patients present with generalized, often anterior, knee pain and variable swelling with or without temporally related trauma.

b. Onset may be associated with an increase or change in activity.

c. Careful assessment can clarify whether symptoms include only pain or mechanical popping and locking to determine appropriate treatment.

d. In thin patients, deep pressure over the medial parapatellar area may produce pain when the knee is flexed, but not when it is extended.

e. Application of varus stress throughout a full ROM may produce reports of pain and popping if a fragment is sufficiently loose.

f. Physical examination—A thorough provocative and ligamentous examination is necessary to identify any comorbid conditions, such as meniscal tears, loose bodies, or instability.

g. Imaging—Standard weight-bearing AP, lateral, tunnel, and Merchant radiographic views should be obtained.

- An OCD lesion in the classic position on the lateral aspect of the medial femoral condyle may be overlooked on the AP view in extension because of overriding bone.

- Classic lesions are best visualized on the tunnel view (**Figure 6**).

h. MRIs and bone scans are adjunctive studies that help stage the lesions and predict the prognosis.

4. Nonsurgical treatment

a. Patients of any age with stable lesions are treated with rest, activity restriction, anti-inflammatory medication, and pain modalities as needed.

b. If symptoms persist, 6 weeks of protected weight bearing or immobilization may be needed.

5. Surgical treatment

a. Indications

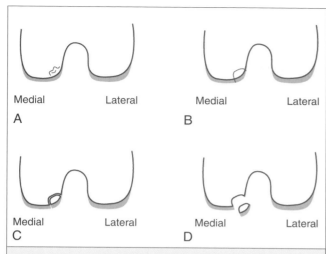

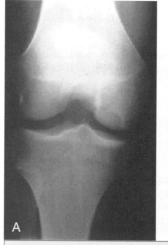

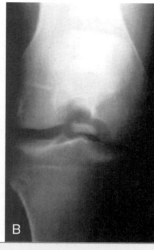

Figure 5 Illustrations show the Guhl classification for osteochondritis dissecans. **A**, Type I: Signal change around the lesion without bright signal. **B**, Type II: High signal intensity surrounding the bone portion of the lesion without signs of cartilage breach. **C**, Type III: High signal intensity around the whole lesion including cartilage (unstable lesion). **D**, Type IV: Empty bed of the lesion with loose body. (Courtesy of Jay Albright, MD, and the Children's Specialists of San Diego, San Diego, CA.)

Figure 6 Tunnel radiographic views of the knee emonstrate the classic location of an osteochondritis dissecans lesion on the lateral aspect of the medial femoral condyle, before (**A**) and after (**B**) displacement. (Reproduced from Crawford DC, Safran MR: Osteochondritis dissecans of the knee. *J Am Acad Orthop Surg* 2006;14[2]: 90-100.)

- Unstable lesions with or without loose bodies

- Older children with persistent pain despite sufficient nonsurgical treatment

- Younger patients with continued pain and swelling with or without loss of motion in whom 3 to 6 months of nonsurgical treatment has failed

b. Contraindications—Very young patients with inconsistent pain in whom a long course of nonsurgical treatment has been successful

c. Procedures

- Stable lesions are amenable to extra-articular or transarticular arthroscopic drilling. When drilling a stable OCD lesion arthroscopically, care must be taken to avoid slipping across the cartilage or producing excessive heat that creates cartilage damage when transarticularly perforating a lesion. Fluoroscopy or an anterior cruciate ligament (ACL) type of drill guide is used to perform extra-articular drilling.

- Unstable lesions are managed with arthroscopic or open débridement with fixation. In young adolescents, fixation of unstable lesions should be attempted; additional procedures may be necessary later. Bioabsorbable pins or screws of appropriate length work

well; they must be cut flush so that no excess protrudes from the cartilage surface.

- A loose body that does not fit or is severely damaged should be removed, followed by arthroplasty or a cartilage restoration procedure; the piece should be saved if possible by trimming it and securing it with pins and/or screws.

6. Complications—Stiffness, infection, failure of fixation, continued pain, and arthrofibrosis

7. Rehabilitation

a. Crutches and touch-down weight bearing are prescribed for 6 weeks.

b. Immediate active-assisted and passive motion is begun, along with quadriceps activation and strengthening.

c. Progression of weight bearing is allowed between 6 and 12 weeks with or without radiographic evidence of healing, as long as no pain or swelling is clinically present.

VI. Knee Ligament Injuries

A. Overview and pathoanatomy

1. Posterior cruciate ligament (PCL) and lateral collateral ligament tears are relatively rare. Medial collateral ligament tears are the most common, but ACL tears in adolescents seem to be increasing in frequency.

5: Pediatrics

2. Ligaments fail when loaded at speeds and forces that result in elongation in excess of 10% of the original length of the ligament.

3. The speed at which the load is applied determines whether the ligament fails or the bone or physis fails.

B. Classification—Ligament injuries are graded according to the severity of injury of each ligament.

C. Evaluation

1. The history can be traumatic—a motor vehicle accident or injury sustained during contact or noncontact sports—or atraumatic. Patients present with acute pain and swelling, with or without instability. Loss of motion is frequent.

2. Physical examination may be difficult in the acute setting. Instability and point tenderness in this setting can be diagnostic. Examination should be repeated in a few days to a week to aid in the diagnosis in lieu of an MRI.

3. Radiographs obtained during the initial examination can rule out physeal or other fractures about the knee. They may demonstrate abnormalities of alignment, such as an anteriorly translated tibia seen on a lateral view, that make diagnosis of a ligament injury possible.

4. MRI is useful for confirming a suspected diagnosis or when an adequate physical examination is not possible.

D. Treatment

1. General principles

a. When determining treatment, factors including the ligament injured and the patient's age, remaining growth, severity of injury, and planned level of activity should be considered.

b. For a patient who is not within 2 years of skeletal maturity, treatment is chosen carefully and all factors are weighed. When in doubt, other pathology is repaired and rehabilitation is initiated, with or without bracing.

c. Although uncommon, physeal injury or arrest can occur no matter what procedure is used.

d. When considering ligament reconstruction, skeletal age should be determined using growth charts, bone age, and Tanner staging.

e. Complete tears

- Complete PCL injuries seem to cause less instability than ACL tears but probably have the same potential for long-term arthritis, although surgical intervention is more easily avoided until skeletal maturity.

- Posterolateral corner injuries rarely occur by themselves. When combined with PCL inju-

ries, a more difficult problem is created.

f. When managing any ligament injury, the surgeon must balance the risk of iatrogenic physeal injury from surgical reconstruction with long-term disability and/or arthritis resulting from nonsurgical treatments. The younger the patient, the greater the risk of deformity if a growth arrest occurs after a reconstructive procedure.

2. Nonsurgical treatment

a. The initial management of all ligament tears should be nonsurgical, unless the tear is associated with meniscal damage, loose bodies, or other urgent surgical indications.

b. Partial tears of the ACL, PCL, medial collateral ligament, or lateral collateral ligament without other intra-articular pathology are amenable to nonsurgical treatment.

- Bracing provides initial stabilization and support for the return to sports.

- Physical therapy, including strength and gait training and pain modalities, helps achieve full ROM.

- Anti-inflammatory medications may be used initially, but uncertainty exists about their effect on the soft-tissue healing process.

- Return to sports is allowed when full motion, strength, and stability have returned with or without a brace.

c. Activity modification, brief immobilization, physical therapy, and pain modalities are all indicated initially.

d. Obtaining full motion and relative stability with bracing and muscle control may obviate the need for surgical intervention in a select group of individuals (copers: those who can perform activities without an ACL and not sustain further pivot shift or buckling events) even when skeletally mature.

3. Surgical treatment

a. Indications

- Failure to maintain stability despite physical therapy and bracing

- Unwillingness to modify activities

- Need to assess other pathology, such as meniscal pathology

b. Procedures

- Ligament repair—Has not been shown to prevent long-term disability or arthritis in skeletally immature or mature patients.

- Physeal sparing—All epiphyseal or extra-articular reconstructions (**Figure 7**).

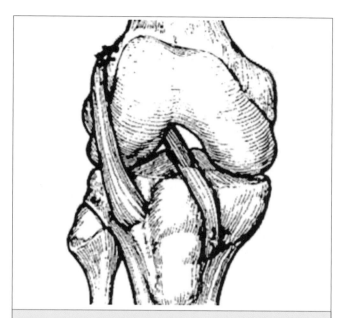

Figure 7 Illustration shows extraphyseal anterior cruciate ligament reconstruction. (Reproduced with permission from Kocher MS, Garg S, Micheli LJ: Physeal sparing reconstruction of the anterior cruciate ligament in skeletally immature prepubescent children and adolescents. *J Bone Joint Surg Am* 2005;87:2371-2379.)

- Transtibial procedures over the top of the femur

- Transphyseal procedures

- Combination procedures

c. Pearls

- Spanning the physis with bone or metal must be avoided.

- Transphyseal tunnels should be kept to a minimum size in a central location.

- Dissection or damage to the perichondral ring should be avoided (do not dissect subperiosteally) when going around the over-the-top position on the femur.

E. Complications—Partial or complete physeal arrest, arthrofibrosis, infection, short-term or long-term ligament failure, arthritis, and atrophy.

F. Rehabilitation

1. Immediate motion, quadriceps activation, swelling, and pain control

2. Prolonged physical therapy

a. Slow, steady progress back to straight line activities at approximately 6 months

b. No start-stop or cutting action for 8 to 12 months

c. Return to sports in 1 year with or without a brace

VII. Patellofemoral Instability

A. Pathoanatomy

1. Of all instability events, more than 90% occur with lateral patellar movement.

2. Common injuries occurring during an event

a. A torn medial patellofemoral ligament (MPFL) and/or medial retinaculum (femoral-, midsubstance-, or patellar-based)

b. Avulsion fracture of the medial patella

c. Osteochondral injuries resulting in loose body formation

d. Bone bruising of the patella and lateral femoral condyle

3. Factors contributing to the risk of sustaining this type of injury

a. Valgus alignment

b. Increased quadriceps angle

c. Excessive femoral anteversion

d. Excessive external tibial torsion

e. Trochlear dysplasia

f. Disorders that affect collagen, such as Ehlers-Danlos syndrome or Down syndrome

B. Classification—Patellofemoral instability is classified descriptively.

1. Subluxation or dislocation

2. Acute (first dislocation) or chronic

C. Mechanism of injury—Patellofemoral subluxation or dislocation can result from a direct blow forcing the patella out of place or from noncontact mechanisms.

D. Evaluation

1. History

a. As with other knee ligament injuries, instability of the patellofemoral joint can occur during innocuous maneuvers such as swinging a bat; it also can occur during direct contact.

b. If a frank dislocation of the patella occurs, it sometimes relocates in the recovery process or when positioning the athlete after the event.

c. The patella also may remain dislocated until the knee is straightened, with or without a reduction maneuver.

2. Physical examination

a. Point tenderness is maximal at the site of the retinacular or ligament tear along the course from the medial epicondyle to the medial patella.

b. An effusion may be subtle or tense.

c. An apprehension test is typically positive.

d. Evaluation of axial and rotational alignment is performed.

e. The quadriceps angle is assessed.

3. Imaging

a. Radiographs show an osteochondral injury.

b. After the first dislocation, ordering an MRI is debatable but is advised if a tense knee effusion is present without radiographic signs of an osteochondral injury.

E. Nonsurgical treatment

1. Initial management includes immobilization for comfort, rest, ice, compression, and elevation.

2. Physical therapy is initiated to strengthen the injured extremity and address core and hip weakness.

3. A patellar stabilizing brace for activities of daily living also can be used after the athlete is ready to return to play

F. Surgical treatment

1. Indications

a. Osteochondral injury with loose body

b. Chronic instability

c. Failure of nonsurgical treatment

2. Contraindications

a. Bony procedures such as tibial tubercle transfer that affect the growth plate in a young athlete

b. First-time dislocation without a loose body or other pathology is a relative contraindication.

3. Procedures

a. Lateral release

b. Medial retinacular or MPFL repair

c. Medial plication

d. Reconstruction of the MPFL

e. Guided growth, hemiepiphysiodesis

f. Rotational osteotomy of the femur and/or tibia

g. Removal or fixation of concomitant injuries, such as osteochondral injuries

h. Treating dysplasia is more controversial in

skeletally immature patients than in adults.

4. Pearls

a. Osteochondral injuries should be fixed whenever possible.

b. Each underlying problem contributing to the dislocation should be addressed when possible.

c. A near-anatomic reconstruction of the MPFL is performed, avoiding injury to the growth plate.

   • The tension of the construct is set at 45° of knee flexion using the retinacular repair; this tension is matched with the ligament tension.

   • The femoral attachment is within 1 to 3 mm from the growth plate. Any femoral drill hole in this area can affect growth.

d. Overconstraining the patella should be avoided. Bending the knee to 90° will be difficult after over tensioning of the repair or reconstruction.

e. Excessive lateral release will result in iatrogenic medial instability or dislocation.

f. Tibial tubercle procedures and other procedures affecting the patellar attachment to the proximal tibia can result in recurvatum deformity.

g. When the surgeon cannot address all underlying factors, recurrent dislocation is more likely.

5. Complications

a. Arthrofibrosis

b. Arthritis

c. Recurrent dislocations

d. Infection

e. Scar widening

f. Premature growth arrest

g. Nerve injury

h. Overcorrection of axial or rotational alignment

i. Iatrogenic medial dislocation

6. Rehabilitation

a. Postoperative bracing for 4 to 6 weeks

b. Immediate weight bearing in a brace

c. Immediate physical therapy to control pain and swelling, quadriceps activation, and ROM, which should be restricted to 0° to 90° for 4 weeks, then progress to full ROM as tolerated.

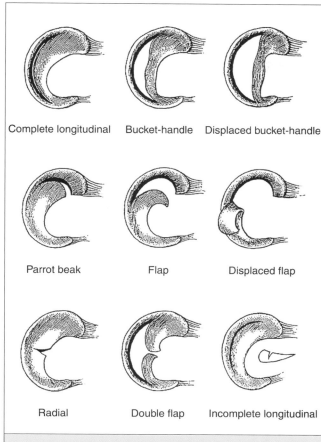

Complete longitudinal   Bucket-handle   Displaced bucket-handle

Parrot beak   Flap   Displaced flap

Radial   Double flap   Incomplete longitudinal

Figure 8   Illustrations show common meniscal tear morphology. (Reproduced with permission from Tria AJ, Klein KS: *An Illustrated Guide to the Knee.* New York, NY, Churchill Livingstone, 1992.)

d. Return to sports or activities may occur at 3 to 4 months postoperatively.

e. A patellar stabilizing brace may be used for return to play.

VIII. Meniscal Injuries and Discoid Meniscus

A. Pathoanatomy

1. Injuries to the meniscus result from twisting events during loading of the knee on a normal or discoid meniscus.

2. Meniscal injuries occur in the vascular and avascular zones.

3. Tear location and pattern have substantial implications for the success of repair attempts; tears occurring close to the vascular zone have higher rates of success than parrot beak and radial tears.

4. Tears in the vascular (red zone) may heal with nonsurgical treatment, unless locking symptoms

exist or symptoms have been present for a prolonged period.

5. Removing any part of the meniscus substantially reduces its effectiveness and function.

B. Classification

1. Meniscal tears are classified descriptively.

a. Location of tear—Red zone, vascular, outer third; red-white zone, middle third; white zone, avascular, inner third.

b. Size

c. Pattern—Horizontal, vertical, radial, bucket-handle, parrot beak, complex, or combination (**Figure 8**).

2. Discoid menisci are classified by shape and stability as complete, incomplete, or Wrisberg ligament (**Figure 9**).

C. Evaluation

1. History

a. As with ligament tears, meniscal tears may follow a traumatic or nontraumatic event such as twisting, turning, or even kneeling.

b. Young children often cannot recall when the pain began and may present with insidious onset.

2. Physical examination

a. Point tenderness at the joint line anterior and posterior to the collateral ligament on the same side is typical.

b. Pain with deep knee flexion, loss of motion, and a positive provocative test also may result.

3. Imaging

a. Radiographs may indicate discoid lateral meniscus with a widened lateral joint line, with or without lateral femoral condyle changes.

b. MRI should be used as a confirmatory test for discoid meniscus, tears of the meniscus, and evaluation of other confounding diagnoses. MRI has a high false-positive rate in children younger than 10 years of age because the vascularity can be misinterpreted.

D. Nonsurgical treatment

1. The management of asymptomatic discoid menisci is observation.

2. Small or peripheral tears may heal or become asymptomatic with nonsurgical care, which may include activity modification, physical therapy, anti-inflammatory medication, and pain modalities.

3. Bracing may help diminish effusion but will not

5: Pediatrics

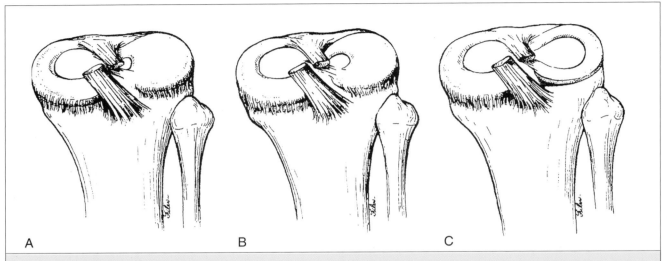

Figure 9 Illustrations show the classification system for lateral discoid menisci. **A,** Type I (complete); **B,** Type II (incomplete); and **C,** Type III (Wrisberg ligament). Type III discoid menisci have no posterior attachment to the tibia. The only posterior attachment is through the ligament of Wrisberg toward the medial femoral condyle. (Reproduced with permission from Neuschwander DC: Discoid lateral meniscus, in Fu FH, Harner CD, Vince KG, eds: *Knee Surgery.* Baltimore, MD, Williams and Wilkins, 1994, p 394.)

prevent incarceration of the tear.

E. Surgical treatment

  1. Indications

    a. True mechanical symptoms, presence of a loose body, and associated ligament tears

    b. Failure of nonsurgical treatment

  2. Contraindications

    a. Peripheral tears in the red-red vascular zone, where the meniscus is more likely to heal without intervention, unless the patient has pain after a prolonged period of activity modification.

    b. Equivocal MRI without locking symptoms

  3. Procedures

    a. Fixation methods

      • Inside-out is the gold standard.

      • All-inside is common for fixation for torn or unstable menisci because it can be used quickly and does not require an extra incision. Meniscal healing using all-inside devices is less reliable than that related to the inside-out technique, particularly in the lateral meniscus. The new lower-profile devices are less likely to damage articular cartilage.

      • Outside-in is used less frequently than the other types but may be useful for anterior horn repair.

    b. Partial meniscectomy

  4. Pearls

    a. It is best to leave only sutures or devices with a closely matched modulus of elasticity in the joint on the surface of the meniscus.

    b. When repairing a large tear, it is important to stabilize the superior and inferior surfaces.

    c. The vertical divergent suture pattern is the strongest.

    d. Partial meniscectomy is reserved only for tears that are irreparable—fix first, remove second.

F. Complications

  1. Arthrofibrosis

  2. Infection

  3. Short-term or long-term repair failure

  4. New tears

  5. Arthritis

  6. Atrophy

G. Rehabilitation

  1. Immediate motion, quadriceps activation, swelling and pain control

  2. For a repaired meniscus, 4 to 6 weeks of touch-down weight bearing, depending on the size and side of the tear

  3. Longer periods of restricted weight bearing are reserved for larger and/or lateral tears.

  4. Three to 4 weeks of restricted ROM at 0° to 90° can be considered.

  5. When repair is not possible, weight bearing is al-

lowed as tolerated and as return of quadriceps strength dictates.

IX. Plica Syndrome

A. Epidemiology

1. Painful plica is a diagnosis of exclusion; its true incidence is difficult to discern.

2. Plicae are medially based parapatellar bands in approximately 90% of symptomatic patients.

B. Pathoanatomy

1. A plica is a remnant of embryologic development; it consists of normal synovial tissue that causes mechanically based synovitis from repetitive motion.

2. Plicae may even cause arthroscopically visible evidence of chondromalacia of the edge of the femoral condyle.

C. Evaluation

1. Plica syndrome is diagnosed by excluding other pathologies.

2. Patients report activity-related anteromedial-to-medial knee pain, sometimes with catching or partial giving way.

3. Physical examination reveals a painful, palpable band of tissue along the medial parapatellar area.

   a. The knee is palpated while the patient performs active motion. If patellar compression is not painful in 45° of knee flexion, but is painful in the parapatellar soft tissue, then plicae may be present.

   b. Examining for an accompanying, highly sensitive lateral suprapatellar soft-tissue mass lying under the vastus lateralis is helpful.

   c. The parapatellar bands also can be palpated lateral and even inferior to the patella.

   d. MRI may not reveal a plica, which is easier to see when knee effusion is present, but usually is difficult to visualize. A high index of suspicion is warranted.

D. Treatment

1. Nonsurgical

   a. Anti-inflammatory medications, ice, activity modification, immobilization

   b. Physical therapy modalities, such as ultrasound and iontophoresis of cortisone solution

   c. Cortisone injections

2. Surgical

   a. Indications

      • Pain not resolved by nonsurgical methods

      • An erroneous diagnosis explained only by an irritated plica

   b. Contraindications—Reflex sympathetic dystrophy, chronic regional pain syndrome, or saphenous neuritis, which can be ruled out before surgery.

   c. Procedure

      • Arthroscopic resection of the plica is performed using a standard two-portal or three-portal approach.

      • The inferomedial parapatellar portal or the medial/lateral suprapatellar portals are sufficient for excision using the shaver, biter, or heat probe of choice.

   d. Pearls

      • The most worrisome pitfall is an overaggressive resection of the plica that includes the retinaculum and not just the abnormal band of synovium.

      • Denudement, irritation, or deformation of the medial condylar articular surface under the contact area of the plica is an indication that the plica should be resected.

      • An arthroscopic punch or heat device can create a working resection edge in the thickened yet smooth plicae that are difficult to treat using a shaver.

E. Complications—Same as those that occur after routine arthroscopy: arthrofibrosis, infection, nerve or vessel injury, patellar instability, unresolved pain.

F. Rehabilitation

1. Immediate motion and quadriceps activation, with quick return to weight bearing as tolerated

2. At 3 to 4 weeks, the patient may be ready to return to full participation, depending on any other pathology present at the time of surgery.

5: Pediatrics

Top Testing Facts

1. Little Leaguer shoulder is an epiphysiolysis, or a fracture through the proximal humeral physis, that causes pain during the late cocking or deceleration phases of pitching.

2. Little League elbow (medial epicondylitis) occurs secondary to valgus loading of the elbow during throwing/pitching. Initial management of this epicondylitis is nonsurgical.

3. The radiographic diagnosis of a capitellar lesion in a child younger than 10 years is Panner disease; in a child older than 10 years, it is OCD.

4. OCD of the knee classically involves the lateral aspect of the medial femoral condyle and is best visualized on a tunnel radiograph. The stability of the lesion influences the treatment.

5. Initial management of OCD of the knee includes activity modification and/or rest with or without immobilization, unless locking symptoms or a loose body is present.

6. Partial ACL tears can be managed nonsurgically with physical therapy, with or without bracing.

7. Partial or complete physeal arrest in the skeletally immature patient is a potential complication of ACL reconstruction.

8. Surgery should be performed for tears of the meniscus in the outer, vascular zone only if locking symptoms exist or if no improvement occurs after prolonged nonsurgical treatment.

Bibliography

Andrish JT: Meniscal injuries in children and adolescents: Diagnosis and management. *J Am Acad Orthop Surg* 1996;4(5):231-237.

Cahill BR: Osteochondritis dissecans of the knee: Treatment of juvenile and adult forms. *J Am Acad Orthop Surg* 1995;3(4):237-247.

Cassas KJ, Cassettari-Wayhs A: Childhood and adolescent sports-related overuse injuries. *Am Fam Physician* 2006;73(6):1014-1022.

Chambers HG, Shea KG, Anderson AF, et al: American Academy of Orthopaedic Surgeons clinical practice guideline on: the diagnosis and treatment of osteochondritis dissecans. *J Bone Joint Surg Am* 2012;94(14):1322-1324.

Chen FS, Diaz VA, Loebenberg M, Rosen JE: Shoulder and elbow injuries in the skeletally immature athlete. *J Am Acad Orthop Surg* 2005;13(3):172-185.

Crawford DC, Safran MR: Osteochondritis dissecans of the knee. *J Am Acad Orthop Surg* 2006;14(2):90-100.

Jackson RW, Marshall DJ, Fujisawa Y: The pathologic medical shelf. *Orthop Clin North Am* 1982;13(2):307-312.

Kobayashi K, Burton KJ, Rodner C, Smith B, Caputo AE: Lateral compression injuries in the pediatric elbow: Panner's disease and osteochondritis dissecans of the capitellum. *J Am Acad Orthop Surg* 2004;12(4):246-254.

Kocher MS, Saxon HS, Hovis WD, Hawkins RJ: Management and complications of anterior cruciate ligament injuries in skeletally immature patients: Survey of the Herodicus Society and The ACL Study Group. *J Pediatr Orthop* 2002;22(4):452-457.

Larsen MW, Garrett WE Jr, Delee JC, Moorman CT III: Surgical management of anterior cruciate ligament injuries in patients with open physes. *J Am Acad Orthop Surg* 2006;14(13):736-744.

Lawrence JT, Argawal N, Ganley TJ: Degeneration of the knee joint in skeletally immature patients with a diagnosis of an anterior cruciate ligament tear: Is there harm in delay of treatment? *Am J Sports Med* 2011;39(12):2582-2587.

Lewallen LW, McIntosh AL, Dahm DL: Predictors of recurrent instability after acute patellofemoral dislocation in pediatric and adolescent patients. *Am J Sports Med* 2013;41(3):575-581.

National Federation of State High School Associations: 2005-2006 High School Athletics Participation Survey. Indianapolis, IN, National Federation of State High School Associations, 2006. www.nfhs.org/participation/sportsearch.aspx. Accessed April 9, 2014.

Noyes FR, Albright JC: Reconstruction of the medial patellofemoral ligament with autologous quadriceps tendon. *Arthroscopy* 2006;22(8):e1-e7.

Stanitski CL: Anterior cruciate ligament injury in the skeletally immature patient: Diagnosis and treatment. *J Am Acad Orthop Surg* 1995;3(3):146-158.

Chapter 62

Pediatric Multiple Trauma and Upper Extremity Fractures

Robert M. Kay, MD

I. Skeletal Differences Between Children and Adults

A. Pediatric bone is more elastic, leading to unique fracture patterns, including torus (buckle) fractures and greenstick fractures.

B. The thicker periosteum generally remains intact on the side of the bone toward which the distal fragment is displaced.

1. This periosteal hinge facilitates reduction.

2. Aggressive reduction attempts can disrupt the hinge, making a satisfactory reduction more difficult.

C. Open physes (growth plates) can allow remodeling and straightening of a malunited fracture; however, with growth disturbance, ongoing growth can result in angular deformity, limb-length discrepancy, or both.

1. Remodeling occurs more rapidly and fully in the plane of joint motion (for example, sagittal malalignment at the wrist remodels more successfully than a coronal plane deformity).

2. In the upper extremity, the fastest growth occurs at the upper and lower ends of the extremity (that is, at the proximal humerus and distal radius and ulna), whereas in the lower extremity, most growth occurs in the middle (that is, at the distal femur and proximal tibia and fibula).

II. Growth Plate (Physeal) Fractures

A. Classification—Most commonly used is the Salter-Harris classification (**Figure 1**).

1. Advantages—Ease of use and prognostic value.

Dr. Kay or an immediate family member has stock or stock options held in Medtronic, Zimmer, Johnson & Johnson, and Pfizer.

2. Disadvantage—Salter-Harris V fractures, which are rare, cannot be distinguished from Salter-Harris I fractures at initial presentation; the differentiation cannot be made until a growth arrest has occurred.

B. Growth arrest following physeal fracture

1. Recognition—Following fracture healing, Park-Harris lines should be moving away from the physis while remaining parallel to the physis (**Figure 2**). If the lines are not moving away from or are not parallel to the physis, then a growth arrest (partial or whole) has occurred (**Figure 3**).

2. Imaging—Advanced imaging, particularly MRI, facilitates the determination of physeal bar size and location. CT is now used less frequently because of radiation exposure.

3. Management—Depends on the size of the physeal bar, its location, and the amount of growth remaining in the affected bone.

a. Upper extremity growth arrests result in fewer functional problems than do lower extremity arrests and less commonly require intervention.

b. Physeal bar excision—Attempts at excision (with interposition of an inert material such as autogenous fat) may be considered for bars less than 33% to 50% of the cross-sectional area of the physis in a physis with more than 2 years of remaining growth. Results of physeal bar excision are best with small bars in younger children.

4. Epiphysiodesis

a. Ipsilateral extremity—The functioning part of the affected physis may be ablated if angular deformity is developing.

b. Contralateral epiphysiodesis is considered if the physeal arrest will result in unacceptable limb-length discrepancy, typically 2 cm or larger, in the legs.

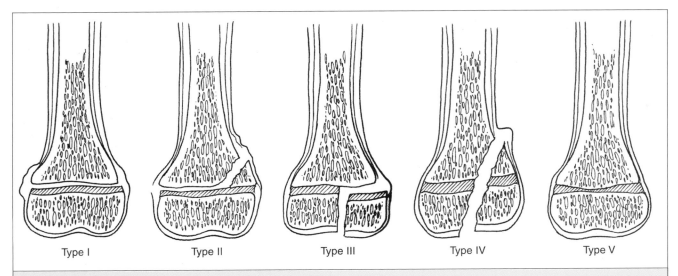

Figure 1   Illustrations show the Salter-Harris classification of physeal fractures. Type I is characterized by a physeal separation; type II by a fracture that traverses the physis and exits through the metaphysis; type III by a fracture that traverses the physis before exiting through the epiphysis; type IV by a fracture that passes through the epiphysis, physis, and metaphysis; and type V by a crush injury to the physis. (Reproduced from Kay RM, Matthys GA: Pediatric ankle fractures: Evaluation and treatment. *J Am Acad Orthop* Surg 2001;9[4]:268-278.)

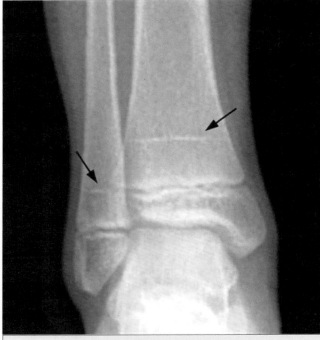

Figure 2   AP radiograph demonstrates growth arrest lines (arrows) following ankle fracture in a pediatric patient. These lines lie parallel to the adjacent physes and thus do not represent asymmetrical growth. (Reproduced from Wuerz TH, Gurd DP: Pediatric physeal ankle fracture. *J Am Acad Orthop Surg* 2013;21[4]:234-244.)

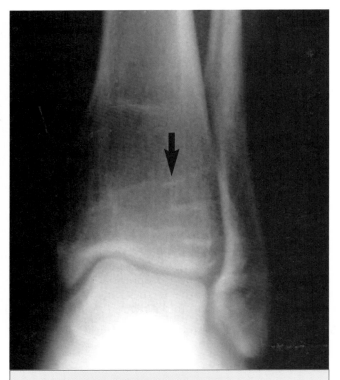

Figure 3   AP radiograph of a 14-year-old girl obtained 4 years after a distal tibial fracture complicated by medial growth arrest shows a 1.7-cm leg-length disparity and a 15° varus deformity of the ankle. Growth-disturbance lines (arrow) converge medially because of the medial growth arrest. (Reproduced from Kay RM, Matthys GA: Pediatric ankle fractures: Evaluation and treatment. *J Am Acad Orthop Surg* 2001;9[4]:268-278.)

Pediatric Glasgow Coma Scale

Score	Age 5 Years and Older	Age 1 to 5 Years	Age 1 Year and Younger
Best Motor Response			
6	Obeys commands	Obeys commands	
5	Localizes pain	Localizes pain	Localizes pain
4	Withdrawal	Withdrawal	Abnormal withdrawal
3	Flexion to pain	Abnormal flexion	Abnormal flexion
2	Extensor rigidity	Extensor rigidity	Abnormal extension
1	None	None	None
Best Verbal Response			
5	Oriented	Approriate words	Smiles/cries appropriately
4	Confused	Inappropriate words	Cries
3	Inappropriate words	Cries/screams	Cries inappropriately
2	Incomprehensible	Grunts	Grunts
1	None	None	None
Eye Opening			
4	Spontaneous	Spontaneous	Spontaneous
3	To speech	To speech	To shout
2	To pain	To pain	To pain
1	None	None	None

Reproduced from Sponseller PD, Paidas C: Management of the pediatric trauma patient, in Sponseller PD, ed: *Orthopaedic Knowledge Update: Pediatrics,* ed 2. Rosemont, IL, American Academy of Orthopaedic Surgeons, 2002, pp 73-79.

III. Multiple Trauma

A. Epidemiology

1. Trauma is the most common cause of death in children older than 1 year.

2. The most common causes are falls and motor vehicle accidents.

   a. Many injuries and deaths could be avoided by appropriate use of child seats and restraints.

   b. Cervical spine injuries following a motor vehicle accident are more common in children younger than 8 years. Two contributing elements are restraints that do not fit young children well, and the disproportionately large size of the head relative to the trunk; deceleration mechanisms lead to distraction injuries.

B. Initial evaluation, resuscitation, and transport

1. Fluid resuscitation

   a. If venous access is difficult, intraosseous infusion with a large-bore needle may be necessary.

   b. Unlike adults, children often remain hemodynamically stable for extended periods of time following substantial blood loss. Hypovolemic shock eventually ensues if fluid resuscitation is inadequate.

2. Because young children have a large head size, a special transport board with an occipital cutout is necessary when transporting children younger than 6 years to the hospital, to prevent cervical spine flexion and potential iatrogenic cervical spinal cord injury.

C. Secondary evaluation

1. The Glasgow Coma Scale (GCS, **Table 1**), scored on a scale of 3 to 15 points, is most commonly used for evaluating head injury.

   a. A GCS score less than 8 at presentation in verbal children indicates a higher risk of mortality.

   b. The GCS motor score at 72 hours postinjury predicts permanent disability following traumatic brain injury.

2. Abdominal bruising (lap belt sign) often indicates abdominal visceral injuries and spine fractures.

3. Up to 10% of injuries are initially missed by the treating team because of head injury and/or severe pain in other locations.

D. CT—Only approximately one half of pelvic fractures identified on CT scans are identified on AP pelvic radiographs.

E. Head and neck injuries

1. Children can make remarkable recoveries following severe traumatic brain injury and should be treated as if such a recovery will occur.

2. Intracranial pressure should be controlled to minimize ongoing brain damage.

5: Pediatrics

Table 2

Antibiotics Used in the Treatment of Pediatric Open Fractures

Antibiotic	Dose	Interval	Maximum Dose	Indications
Cefazolin	100 mg/kg/d	Q8 h	6 g/d	All open fractures
Gentamicin	5-7.5 mg/kg/d	Q8 h	None specified	Severe grade II and III injuries
Penicillin	150,000 units/kg/d	Q6 h	24 million units/d	Farm-type or vascular injuries
Clindamycin	15-40 units/kg/d	Q6-8 h	2.7 g/d	Patients with allergies to cefazolin or penicillin

3. Musculoskeletal manifestations of head injuries

  a. Spasticity begins within days to weeks; splinting helps prevent contractures.

    • Part-time positioning of the hip and knee in flexion can reduce the plantar flexor tone to help prevent equinus contracture.

    • Pharmacologic intervention with botulinum toxin A may help acutely control spasticity and facilitate rehabilitation.

  b. Heterotopic ossification (HO), especially around the elbow, is common following traumatic brain injury.

    • An increase in serum alkaline phosphatase may herald the onset of HO.

    • Treatment is generally observation; early administration of NSAIDs to reduce the likelihood of severe HO is controversial.

  c. Fractures heal more rapidly following traumatic brain injury, but the mechanism is not yet understood.

  d. The timing of surgical intervention for fractures in patients with head injuries should be decided in concert with trauma surgeons and neurosurgeons to minimize secondary injuries to the brain.

F. Treatment of the patient with multiple injuries

1. Surgical fracture treatment is much more common in multiple-trauma patients because it facilitates patient care and mobilization and reduces the risk of pressure sores from immobilization.

2. Open fractures are discussed in section IV.

G. Complications in multiply injured patients

1. Mortality rates can be as high as 20% following pediatric multiple trauma.

2. Long-term morbidity is present in one third to one half of children following multiple trauma. Most long-term morbidity results from head injuries and orthopaedic injuries.

3. Fat embolism syndrome in children is a rare, but life-threatening, complication.

H. Rehabilitation

1. Pediatric patients often improve for 1 year or more following injury; many make dramatic neurologic and functional gains.

2. Splinting and bracing prevent contractures and enhance function.

IV. Open Fractures

A. Epidemiology

1. Open fractures are often high-energy injuries; associated injuries are common.

2. Lawnmower injuries are a common cause of open fractures in children. They are devastating, with high rates of amputation, infection, and growth disturbance.

B. Initial evaluation and management

1. Thorough evaluation for other injuries is essential; many children with open fractures have injuries to the head, abdomen, chest, or multiple extremities.

2. Tetanus status should be confirmed and updated; children with an unknown vaccination history or who have not had a booster within 5 years should receive a dose of tetanus toxoid.

3. Prompt administration of intravenous antibiotics is essential to minimize the risk of infection (**Table 2**).

C. Classification—As in adults, the Gustilo-Anderson classification is used to grade open fractures (**Table 3**).

D. Treatment

1. Prompt administration of intravenous antibiotics is the most important factor in preventing infection following open fractures.

2. Irrigation and débridement should be performed

Table 3

Gustilo-Anderson Classification of Open Fractures

Grade	Contamination	Wound Length	Defining Feature
I	Clean	< 1 cm	
II	Moderate	1-10 cm	
III	Severe	> 10 cm	
IIIA	Severe	> 10 cm	Adequate soft-tissue coverage
IIIB	Severe	> 10 cm	Bone exposure without adequate soft-tissue coverage; soft-tissue coverage often required
IIIC	Severe	Any length	Major vascular injury in injured segment

in all open fractures.

   a. Type I fractures generally need only one instance of irrigation and débridement, whereas grade II and III injuries often need repeat irrigation and débridement every 48 to 72 hours until all remaining tissue appears clean and viable.

   b. The risk of infection following open fractures is no higher if irrigation and débridement are performed 8 to 24 hours postinjury than if performed within 8 hours.

   c. Because of the better soft-tissue envelope and vascularity in children, tissue of apparently marginal viability may be left behind at initial débridement. Tissue viability often declares itself by reexploration time, 2 to 3 days later.

   d. Because of enhanced periosteal new bone formation in children, some bone defects may fill in spontaneously, particularly in young children.

3. Wound cultures

   a. Wound cultures are contraindicated in the absence of clinical signs of infection.

   b. The correlation of predébridement and postdébridement cultures with the development of infection is low; such cultures should not be performed routinely.

4. Fracture fixation (internal or external) is almost universally indicated to stabilize the soft tissues, allow wound access, and maintain alignment.

E. Complications

1. Compartment syndrome is a substantial risk, particularly in children with a head injury or other distracting injuries.

2. Infection risk is minimized with the prompt administration of intravenous antibiotics and appropriate irrigation and débridement.

3. Chronic pain and psychological sequelae are common manifestations following severe trauma.

V. Child Abuse (Nonaccidental Trauma)

A. Evaluation

1. Nonaccidental trauma (NAT) should be suspected in the following circumstances.

   a. Any fracture before walking age

   b. Femur fractures

     • Most femur fractures before walking age result from abuse.

     • Femur fractures up to age 3 years are sometimes related to abuse.

   c. Multiple injuries in a child without a witnessed and reasonable explanation

   d. Multiple injuries in a child younger than 2 years

   e. A child with long-bone and head injuries

2. Corner fractures (seen at the junction of the metaphysis and physis) and posterior rib fractures are essentially pathognomonic for NAT, but isolated, transverse long bone fractures are actually more common following NAT. Corner fractures result from shear forces associated with pulling and twisting an extremity.

3. A skeletal survey must be obtained in all children in whom child abuse is suspected to rule out additional fractures (including skull and rib fractures). Repeat imaging may be necessary in these children because periosteal new bone formation, which often does not appear for 1 week or more after injury, may be the first evidence of fracture.

4. Thorough examination of the child by nonorthopaedists is necessary to rule out other evidence of abuse, including skin bruising (especially bruises

5: Pediatrics

of different ages) or scarring, retinal hemorrhages, intracranial bleeds, or evidence of sexual abuse.

B. Treatment

1. Reporting of suspected child abuse is mandatory.

a. The orthopaedic surgeon is protected from litigation when reporting cases of suspected abuse.

b. Failure to report suspected abuse puts the abused child at a 50% risk of repeat abuse and up to a 10% risk of being killed.

2. Many fractures are sufficiently healed at the time of presentation that they do not require treatment.

VI. Pathologic Fractures

A. General—A pathologic fracture occurs when a low-energy mechanism (not usually sufficient to cause fracture) results in a fracture through a weakened bone (see Chapter 45). Common causes in children include neoplasm, metabolic bone disease, infection, and disuse osteoporosis (especially in children with neuromuscular diseases).

B. Evaluation

1. A high index of suspicion is necessary for a fracture resulting from a low-energy mechanism.

2. Plain radiographs are evaluated for the appearance of bone quality, the presence of osseous lesions, and any evidence (for example, periosteal new bone) of preexisting osseous injury.

3. Lesions are staged before intervention.

C. Treatment

1. Children with potentially malignant lesions are referred to tertiary musculoskeletal oncology centers.

2. For benign lesions, the tumor is treated appropriately; the fracture can typically be treated concomitantly.

VII. Fractures of the Shoulder and Humeral Shaft

A. Clavicle fractures

1. Overview

a. Common in all pediatric age groups; account for 90% of obstetric fractures; often associated with brachial plexus palsy

b. Clavicle fractures may be confused with congenital pseudarthrosis of the clavicle.

• Congenital pseudarthrosis results from a congenital failure of fusion of the medial and lateral ossification centers of the clavicle; may be related to external compression by the subclavian artery against the developing clavicle.

• Typical findings include (1) presence at birth, although prominence of a "bump" often increases with age, (2) right-sidedness, (3) no pain, (4) radiographs showing convexity of the ends of the nonfused portions of the clavicle.

2. Fracture location

a. Medial clavicle fracture

• The medial clavicular physis is the last physis in the body to close, at 23 to 25 years of age.

• Many medial clavicle fractures are physeal fractures; sternoclavicular joint dislocations also can occur.

• Posteriorly displaced fractures or dislocations may impinge on the mediastinum, including the great vessels and trachea.

b. Clavicle shaft fracture—Displaced fractures rarely cause problems, although compression of the subclavian vessels and/or brachial plexus can occur.

c. Lateral clavicle fracture—May be confused with an acromioclavicular joint dislocation, which is rare in children.

3. Treatment

a. Medial clavicle fractures and sternoclavicular dislocations

• Nonsurgical treatment, with a sling for 3 to 4 weeks as needed

• Percutaneous reduction with a towel clip may be indicated for posteriorly displaced fractures or dislocations impinging on the mediastinum. Some authors recommend a vascular surgeon be present because of potential vascular complications.

• Open reduction may be needed for open fractures or if percutaneous reduction fails. Suture fixation generally suffices in such cases.

b. Clavicle shaft fractures

• Nonsurgical treatment with a figure-of-8 harness or sling for 4 to 6 weeks is appropriate. A swathe may be used in infants.

• Open reduction and internal fixation (ORIF); indications may include floating shoulder injuries and multiple trauma; some authors recommend ORIF for substantially shortened fractures in adolescents.

c. Lateral clavicle fractures

- Most are treated symptomatically with a sling.

- For markedly displaced fractures, surgical treatment is controversial.

4. Complications

a. Medial fractures and dislocations—Compression of the mediastinal structures may occur with posterior displacement.

b. Shaft fractures

- Complications are rare with closed treatment; prominence at the fracture site is expected.

- Compression of the subclavian vessels and brachial plexus is rare.

- Surgical treatment increases the risks of infection and delayed union.

c. Lateral fractures—Complications are rare with closed treatment.

B. Proximal humerus fractures

1. General—Because 90% of humeral growth is proximal, these are very forgiving fractures.

2. Evaluation

a. Plain radiographs are almost universally sufficient for evaluating fracture configuration and to rule out associated shoulder dislocation.

b. Thorough neurologic examination is necessary because of the proximity of the brachial plexus.

3. Classification—The Neer and Horwitz classification is used to define the amount of fracture displacement. Grade I fractures are displaced 5 mm or less, grade II fractures one third of the humeral diameter or less, grade III fractures two thirds of the humeral diameter or less, and grade IV fractures greater than two thirds of the humeral diameter.

4. Nonsurgical treatment

a. Most can be treated nonsurgically with a sling and swathe, shoulder immobilizer, or coaptation splint.

b. Reduction may be performed for grade III and IV fractures.

- Reduction is generally obtained by shoulder abduction to 90° and external rotation to 90°.

- Impediments to reduction may include the long head of the biceps or the periosteum.

c. Gentle shoulder range-of-motion (ROM) exercises should begin 1 to 3 weeks after injury.

5. Surgical treatment

a. Surgical treatment is indicated for adolescents with grade III and IV injuries and for open fractures.

b. Closed reduction and percutaneous pinning is used in most surgical cases.

c. Open reduction and pinning is necessary if interposed structures (biceps tendon, periosteum) prevent closed reduction in adolescents with grade III or IV injuries.

6. Complications

a. Malunion, growth arrest, and other complications are rare.

b. Brachial plexus injuries are almost always stretch injuries, which resolve spontaneously.

C. Humeral shaft fractures

1. Evaluation—Radial nerve palsy occurs in less than 5% of humeral shaft fractures and is almost always a neurapraxia following middle or distal third fractures.

2. Nonsurgical treatment

a. Nonsurgical therapy (with sling and swathe, sugar-tong splint, or fracture brace) is the mainstay of treatment.

b. Substantial displacement and angulation up to 30° are acceptable because range of shoulder motion is generally excellent.

c. ROM exercises are started by 2 to 4 weeks postinjury.

3. Surgical treatment

a. Indications for surgical treatment include open fractures, multiple trauma, and floating elbow or shoulder injuries.

b. Procedures

- Intramedullary rod fixation (flexible titanium nails) is preferred for most shaft fractures requiring fixation.

- Plate fixation involves more surgical dissection and puts the radial nerve at risk during surgery.

4. Complications

a. Malunion rarely has functional consequences because normal shoulder ROM can compensate for the humeral malalignment.

b. Radial nerve palsy—Primary radial nerve palsies (present at the time of injury) are almost always caused by neurapraxia, resolve

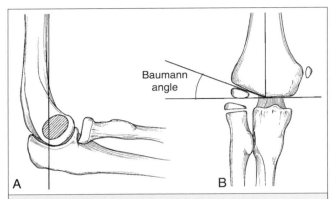

Figure 4 Illustrations show the typical anatomic relationships in the elbow. **A,** The anterior humeral line, shown as would be drawn on a lateral radiograph, should bisect the capitellum. In extension-type supracondylar fractures, the capitellum moves posterior to the anterior humeral line. **B,** The Baumann angle, shown as would be measured on an AP view, is the angle subtended by a line perpendicular to the long axis of the humerus and a line along the lateral condylar physis. The Baumann angle may be used to assess the adequacy of the reduction in the coronal plane and may be compared with the contralateral elbow. (Reproduced from Skaggs DL: Elbow fractures in children: Diagnosis and management. *J Am Acad Orthop Surg* 1997;5[6]:303-312.)

Table 4

Treatment for Vascular Injuries With Supracondylar Humerus Fractures

Vascular Status	Treatment
Pulse lost after reduction and pinning	Explore brachial artery and treat
Pulseless, well-perfused hand	Observe for 24-72 h
Pulseless, cool hand	Explore brachial artery and treat

Table 5

Nerve Injuries With Supracondylar Humerus Fractures

Nerve Injury	Association
Anterior interosseous nerve	Most common nerve injury with supracondylar humerus fracture
Median nerve	Associated with posterolateral fracture displacement
Radial nerve	Seen with posteromedial fracture displacement
Ulnar nerve	Rare traumatic injury; cause is almost always iatrogenic (due to medial pin)

spontaneously, and should be observed.

- If they do not resolve spontaneously by 3 to 5 months, electrophysiologic studies are indicated, and surgical exploration may be needed.

- Secondary nerve palsies (present after intervention) are more complete injuries and typically require exploration acutely.

  c. Stiffness is rare; early ROM minimizes this risk.

  d. Limb-length discrepancy is common but generally mild and of no functional consequence.

VIII. Supracondylar Humerus Fractures

A. Epidemiology

  1. Supracondylar humerus (SCH) fractures account for more than one half of pediatric elbow fractures.

  2. Of the total, 95% to 98% are extension-type injuries.

B. Relevant anatomy

  1. Distal humeral anatomy is shown in **Figure 4**.

  2. The Baumann angle may be measured on AP radiographs of the distal humerus to assess the coronal plane fracture alignment but is used less commonly now because of variability in measurement.

C. Associated injuries

  1. Vascular injuries occur in approximately 1% of SCH fractures. Because of the rich collateral flow at the elbow, distal perfusion may remain good despite a vascular injury (**Table 4**).

  2. Nerve injuries—Described in **Table 5**.

D. Classification—The modified Gartland classification is used to classify SCH fractures (**Figure 5**).

E. Nonsurgical treatment

  1. Type I fractures are treated closed with a long arm cast in approximately 90° of elbow flexion.

  2. Type II fractures may be treated closed only if the following criteria are met.

    a. No substantial swelling is present.

    b. The anterior humeral line intersects the capitellum.

    c. No medial cortical impaction of the distal humerus and/or varus malalignment is present.

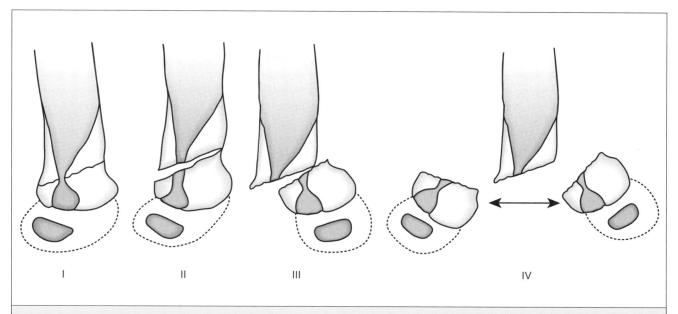

Figure 5 Illustrations depict the Gartland classification of supracondylar fractures. Type I injuries are nondisplaced. Type II injuries are displaced but have an intact hinge of bone (located posteriorly in extension-type fractures). Type III fractures are completely displaced and have no intact hinge. Type IV refers to completely displaced fractures that are unstable in both flexion and extension.

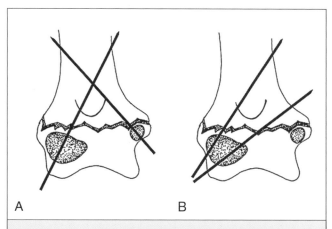

Figure 6 Illustrations show typical pin configurations for crossed pinning (**A**) and lateral-entry pinning (**B**) for supracondylar humerus fractures. Regardless of pin configuration, the medial and lateral columns should be engaged proximal to the fracture site. (Reproduced from Flynn JM, Cornwall R: Elbow: Pediatrics, in Vaccaro AR, ed: *Orthopaedic Knowledge Update*, ed 8. Rosemont, IL, American Academy of Orthopaedic Surgeons, 2005, pp 705-713.)

Table 6

Comparison of Crossed Pins and Lateral-Entry Pins for Supracondylar Humerus Fractures

	Laboratory Testing	Clinical Stability	Iatrogenic Ulnar Nerve Injury
Crossed pins	More stable	Comparable	3%-8%
Lateral-entry pins	Less stable	Comparable	0%

a. Crossed pins

- Crossed pins were found to be more stable biomechanically in laboratory studies than lateral-entry pins.

- Using a medial pin results in a substantial (3% to 8%) risk of iatrogenic ulnar nerve injury, especially if the medial pin is inserted with the elbow fully flexed.

b. Lateral-entry pins

- Lateral-entry pins should be separated sufficiently to engage the medial and lateral columns of the distal humerus at the level of the fracture.

- When inserted with appropriate technique, lateral-entry pins are comparable in maintaining reduction of SCH fractures.

3. The casts are removed after fracture healing at 3 weeks.

F. Surgical treatment

1. Indications—Most type II and all type III and IV fractures are treated with reduction and pinning.

2. Pin configuration (**Figure 6** and **Table 6**)

- Iatrogenic ulnar nerve injury does not occur with lateral-entry pins.

G. Complications

1. Volkmann ischemic contracture is a devastating complication that more commonly results from compression of the brachial artery with casting in greater than 90° of flexion than from arterial injury at the time of fracture.

2. Cubitus varus (gunstock deformity) is a cosmetic deformity with few functional sequelae in childhood, although it may increase the risk of refracture of the lateral condyle. The incidence is much lower with reduction and pinning than with closed reduction and casting.

3. Recurvatum is common following cast treatment of type II and III fractures and remodels poorly because of the limited growth of the distal humerus.

4. Stiffness is rare following casting or reduction and pinning, particularly with cast removal at 3 weeks.

Table 7

Order of Appearance of Ossification Centers of the Elbow on Radiographs[a]

	Age of Appearance in Girls (Years)	Age of Appearance in Boys (Years)
Capitellum	1	1
Radius (proximal)	4-5	5-6
Medial epicondyle	5-6	7-8
Trochlea	8-9	10-11
Olecranon	9	11
Lateral epicondyle	10	11-12

[a]A rough guide is that the capitellum appears at age 1 year, and in girls, 2 years should be added for each additional ossification center (except the proximal radius, which appears in girls at 4 to 5 years). There is a 2-year delay for boys for all centers except the capitellum.

IX. Other Elbow Fractures

A. Relevant anatomy

1. Ossification centers of the elbow (**Table 7**)

2. Distal humerus—Knowledge of the normal alignment (including the anterior humeral line and Baumann angle) is important.

3. Proximal radius

   a. Normally, a 12° valgus angle of the proximal radius exists.

   b. The proximal radius should be directed toward the capitellum on all radiographs.

   c. The relationship between the proximal radius and the capitellum and the relationship between the ulna and the humerus often facilitate fracture identification (**Figure 7**).

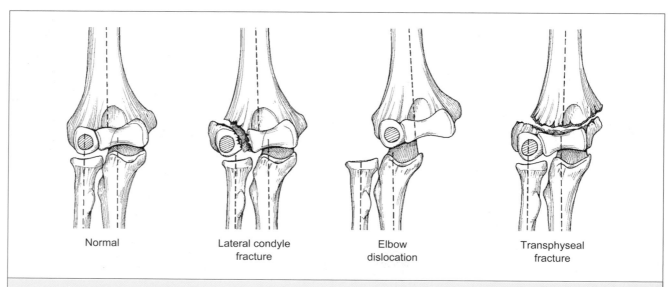

Normal	Lateral condyle fracture	Elbow dislocation	Transphyseal fracture

Figure 7   Illustrations show the osseous relationships about the elbow as seen on AP radiographs. In transphyseal fractures, the radius is directed toward the capitellum; in elbow dislocations, the proximal radius is not directed toward the capitellum. (Reproduced from Skaggs DL: Elbow fractures in children: Diagnosis and management. *J Am Acad Orthop Surg* 1997;5[6]:303-312.)

B. Lateral condyle fractures

1. Classification

a. The most widely used classification is based on the amount of fracture displacement (**Figure 8**). The oblique view may be the only view on which the fracture is visualized (**Figure 9**). Because the oblique view is most sensitive for detecting maximal displacement, it should be obtained if closed treatment is contemplated.

b. The Milch classification is rarely used because it is irrelevant to patient care. Milch I fractures are considered Salter-Harris IV fractures and Milch II fractures are considered Salter-Harris II fractures.

2. Treatment algorithm

a. Type I fractures are treated with casting for 3 to 6 weeks; 2% to 10% of these fractures displace sufficiently in a cast to require reduction and pinning.

b. Type II fractures are treated surgically with closed versus open reduction and percutaneous fixation (generally with smooth pins).

- Closed reduction and pinning is appropriate if, following pinning, no intra-articular incongruity is present on an intraoperative arthrogram.

- Open reduction is required if joint congruity cannot be obtained with closed treatment.

c. Type III fractures—ORIF (with percutaneous pins or screws) is typically indicated; some authors suggest some of these fractures may be amenable to percutaneous reduction and fixation.

3. Surgical technique

a. Pin configuration (**Figure 10**)—The pins must be divergent to minimize fracture displacement, and the distal pin should engage at least a portion of the ossified distal humeral metaphysis.

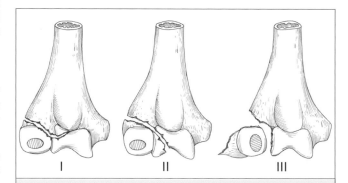

Figure 8   Illustrations show the types of lateral condyle fractures. Type I fractures are displaced < 2 mm and generally have an intact intra-articular surface. Type II fractures are displaced 2 to 4 mm and have a displaced joint surface. Type III injuries are displaced > 4 mm and often are completely displaced and rotated. (Reproduced from Sullivan JA: Fractures of the lateral condyle of the humerus. *J Am Acad Orthop Surg* 2006;14[1]:58-62.)

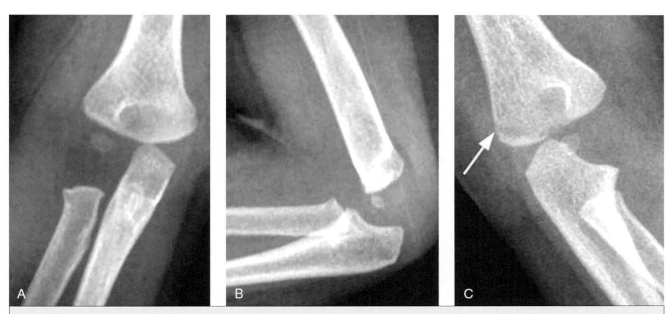

Figure 9   AP (**A**) and lateral (**B**) radiographs show the elbow of a 16-month-old boy with elbow pain after an unwitnessed fall. No fracture lines were visible. **C**, Internal oblique radiograph demonstrates a lateral condylar humeral fracture (arrow). (Reproduced from Tejwani N, Phillips D, Goldstein RY: Management of lateral humeral condylar fracture in children. *J Am Acad Orthop Surg* 2011;19[6]:350-358.)

5: Pediatrics

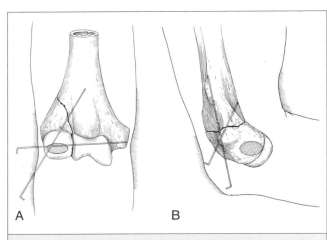

Figure 10 Typical pin configuration for lateral condyle fractures. The pins must be divergent, and the distal pin should engage metaphyseal bone (rather than simply unossified cartilage). (Reproduced from Sullivan JA: Fractures of the lateral condyle of the humerus. *J Am Acad Orthop Surg* 2006;14[1]:58-62.)

b. Open reduction

- The posterior soft tissues should never be dissected off the lateral condyle because the blood supply enters posteriorly, and posterior dissection can result in osteonecrosis.

- The entire length of the fracture, including the joint line, must be visualized to ensure an anatomic reduction.

4. Complications

a. Stiffness is minimized by mobilizing the elbow after complete fracture healing, generally by 4 weeks.

b. Osteonecrosis is minimized by avoiding posterior soft-tissue dissection.

c. Nonunion is rare if the aforementioned protocol is followed.

- If nonunion is evident within 1 year of injury, it may be treated with bone grafting and screw fixation.

- Cubitus valgus is frequent in nonunion.

d. Tardy ulnar nerve palsy may occur following nonunion and cubitus valgus, but typically not until decades after the injury.

C. Medial condyle fractures

1. Classification—Based on the amount of displacement; comparable to that of lateral condyle fractures.

2. Treatment—Same as that described for lateral condyle fractures.

3. Complications—Most common is malunion or nonunion.

D. Medial epicondyle fractures

1. Overview

a. Mechanism of injury—Avulsion of the medial epicondyle apophysis.

b. Half of medial epicondyle fractures are associated with elbow dislocations.

2. Classification—Based on the amount of displacement and whether the medial epicondyle is entrapped in the elbow joint.

3. Nonsurgical treatment

a. Nonsurgical care has been the mainstay of treatment; surgical treatment is increasing in many pediatric centers.

b. Closed attempts to extricate an entrapped medial condyle may be undertaken by supinating the forearm, placing a valgus stress on the elbow, and extending the wrist and fingers.

c. Early motion (within 3 to 5 days) minimizes the risk of elbow stiffness.

4. Surgical treatment

a. Indications

- Absolute—Intra-articular entrapment of the medial epicondyle.

- Relative—Fracture of the dominant arm in a throwing athlete or a weight-bearing extremity in an athlete (such as a gymnast), fracture associated with elbow dislocation, and ulnar nerve dysfunction.

b. Technique—Open reduction with screw fixation is preferred to allow early motion. Kirschner wires (K-wires) may be used in young children.

5. Complications

a. Stiffness is almost universal, but rarely of functional consequence.

b. Ulnar neuropathy is generally a neurapraxia, which spontaneously resolves.

c. Chronic instability is rare but may occur if the fracture was associated with elbow dislocation.

d. Failure to diagnose an incarcerated medial epicondyle may lead to elbow stiffness and degenerative changes.

E. Lateral epicondyle fractures

1. Nonsurgical treatment is indicated for most.

2. Surgery is indicated when the epicondyle has displaced into the elbow joint.

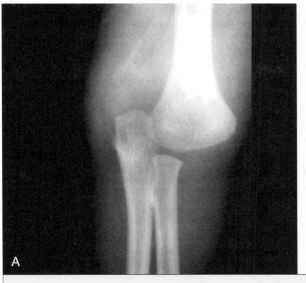
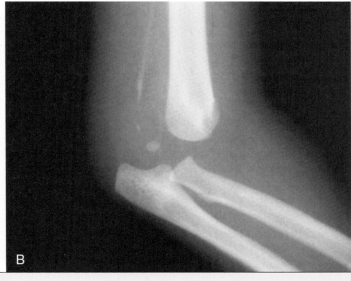

Figure 11   AP (**A**) and lateral (**B**) radiographs of the elbow of an 18-month-old infant show the typical alignment of the elbow following a physeal fracture of the distal humerus. Although the appearance resembles an elbow dislocation, the age of the child is younger than the age at which dislocation typically occurs, and the radius is directed at the capitellum in these radiographs. Most of these injuries are displaced posteromedially. Periosteal new bone is evident in this 2-week-old fracture. (Reproduced from Sponseller PD: Injuries of the arm and elbow, in Sponseller PD, ed: *Orthopaedic Knowledge Update: Pediatrics*, ed 2. Rosemont, IL, American Academy of Orthopaedic Surgeons, 2002, pp 93-107.)

F. Distal humeral physeal fractures

1. Epidemiology—Most common in children younger than 3 years but may occur up to 6 years of age.

2. Evaluation

    a. These fractures almost always displace posteromedially (**Figure 11**); frequently misdiagnosed as elbow dislocations.

    b. Elbow dislocations are very rare in young children, so a physeal fracture should be assumed in young children with displacement of the proximal radius and ulna relative to the distal humerus.

    c. Elbow arthrography or MRI can clarify the diagnosis.

    d. This fracture pattern is often seen in cases of NAT, which should be considered in all cases.

3. Classification—The Salter-Harris classification is used; all fractures are type I or II.

4. Treatment

    a. Closed reduction and percutaneous pinning is the mainstay of treatment.

    b. Pin configuration is comparable to that used for supracondylar fractures.

    c. Closed reduction should not be performed if the injury is diagnosed late (5 to 7 days postinjury), to minimize the risk of iatrogenic physeal injury.

5. Complications are rare following prompt diagnosis and treatment and include malunion or nonunion.

G. Proximal radius fractures

1. Overview

    a. Most fractures are radial neck and/or physeal fractures.

    b. Most are associated with valgus loading of the elbow or elbow dislocation.

2. Classification—Based on the location of the fracture (neck or head) and the angulation and/or displacement.

3. Nonsurgical treatment

    a. Most of these fractures are treated closed.

    b. Manipulative techniques

        • Patterson maneuver—The elbow is held in flexion and varus while direct pressure is applied to the radial head.

        • Israeli technique—Direct pressure is held over the radial head with the elbow flexed 90° while the forearm is pronated and supinated.

        • Elastic bandage—Spontaneous reduction may occur with tight application of an elastic bandage around the forearm and elbow.

    c. Early mobilization (within 3 to 7 days) minimizes stiffness.

4. Surgical treatment

   a. Indications following attempted closed reduction

- More than 30° of residual angulation

- More than 3 to 4 mm of translation

- Less than 45° of pronation and supination

   b. Procedures

- Percutaneous manipulation is attempted using a K-wire, awl, elevator, or other metallic device.

- In the Metaizeau technique, a flexible rod or nail is inserted retrograde, passed across the fracture site, rotated to reduce the fracture, and advanced into the proximal fragment.

- Open reduction via a lateral approach is rarely necessary but may be required for severely displaced fractures.

- Internal fixation is used only for fractures that are unstable following reduction.

5. Complications

   a. Elbow stiffness is extremely common, even after nondisplaced fractures.

   b. Overgrowth of the radial head also is common.

H. Olecranon fractures

1. Evaluation—Palpation over the radial head is necessary to rule out a Monteggia fracture. Tenderness over a reduced radial head indicates a Monteggia fracture with spontaneous reduction of the radial head.

2. Classification—Apophyseal fractures may be the first indication of osteogenesis imperfecta and must be differentiated from the more common metaphyseal fractures.

3. Nonsurgical treatment—Most are treated nonsurgically, with casting in relative extension (usually 10° to 45° of flexion) for 3 weeks.

4. Surgical treatment

   a. Indications—Fractures with intra-articular displacement greater than 2 to 3 mm benefit from surgery.

   b. Fixation—Stabilized using tension-band fixation, often with an absorbable suture as the tension band.

5. Complications are rare and rarely of clinical significance, although failure to diagnose associated injuries (such as radial head dislocation) may result in substantial morbidity.

I. Nursemaid elbow

1. Epidemiology—Occurs with longitudinal traction on the outstretched arm of a child younger than 5 years as the orbicular ligament subluxates over the radial head.

2. Evaluation

   a. The history and physical examination are classic, with the child holding the elbow extended and the forearm pronated.

   b. Radiographs are not needed unless the classic history and arm positioning are absent. If radiographs are obtained, they are normal.

3. Treatment—With one thumb held over the affected radial head (to feel for a "snap" as the orbicular ligament reduces), the forearm is supinated and the elbow is flexed past 90°.

4. Complications—Recurrent nursemaid elbow is relatively common in children younger than 5 years.

X. Fractures of the Forearm, Wrist, and Hand

A. Diaphyseal forearm fractures

1. Evaluation—Open wounds are often punctate and are commonly missed when not evaluated by an orthopaedic surgeon.

2. Classification

   a. Greenstick fractures are incomplete fractures common in children. They should be described as apex volar or apex dorsal to guide reduction.

   b. Complete fractures are categorized as in adults, by fracture location, pattern, angulation, and displacement.

3. Nonsurgical treatment

   a. Most pediatric forearm fractures can be treated nonsurgically.

   b. Greenstick fractures are generally rotational injuries. Apex volar fractures (supination injuries) may be treated by forearm pronation; apex dorsal injuries (pronation injuries) by forearm supination.

   c. Casting for 6 weeks is typical.

4. Surgical treatment

   a. Indications

- Persistent malalignment following closed reduction (angulation > 15° in children younger than 10 years and > 10° in children 10 years or older, and bayonet apposition in children 10 years or older) may necessitate open reduction.

Table 8

Bado Classification of Monteggia Fractures

Bado Type	Apex of Ulnar Fracture	Radial Head Pathology
I	Anterior	Anterior dislocation
II	Posterior	Posterior dislocation
III	Lateral	Lateral dislocation
IV	Any direction (typically anterior)	Proximal radius dislocation and fracture

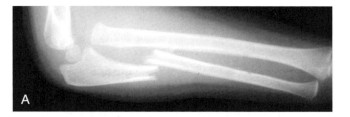

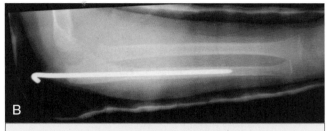

Figure 12 Radiographs show a Bado I Monteggia fracture-dislocation. **A,** Preoperative radiograph shows the injury. **B,** Postoperative radiograph shows the fracture after treatment by closed reduction and intramedullary nail fixation. (Reproduced from Waters PM: Injuries of the shoulder, elbow, and forearm, in Abel MF, ed: *Orthopaedic Knowledge Update: Pediatrics*, ed 3. Rosemont, IL, American Academy of Orthopaedic Surgeons, 2006, pp 303-314.)

- Substantially displaced fractures in adolescents are at high risk for redisplacement and are a relative indication for surgery.
- Open fractures are commonly treated surgically.

  b. Technique

- Internal fixation with intramedullary devices or plates has high rates of success in children.
- Fixation of one bone is often sufficient to stabilize an unstable forearm, particularly in children younger than 10 years.

5. Complications

a. Refracture occurs in 5% to 10% of children following forearm fractures.

b. Malunion is unusual if serial radiographs are obtained in the first 3 weeks following fracture.

c. Compartment syndrome may occur, particularly in high-energy injuries. The rate after intramedullary fixation is high, especially with multiple attempts at reduction and rod passage.

d. Loss of pronation and supination is common, although generally mild.

B. Monteggia fractures

1. Evaluation

a. Palpation over the radial head must be performed for all children with ulnar fractures to rule out Monteggia injuries.

b. Isolated radial head dislocations almost never occur in children. Presumed "isolated" injuries almost universally result from plastic deformation of the ulna with concomitant radial head dislocation.

2. Classification

a. The Bado classification (**Table 8**) is most commonly used.

b. Fractures may be classified as acute or chronic (> 2 to 3 weeks since injury).

3. Nonsurgical treatment

a. Much more common (and successful) in children with Monteggia fractures than in adults

b. Reestablishment of ulnar length is necessary to maintain reduction of the radial head.

c. For Bado I and III fractures, the forearm should be supinated in the cast.

4. Surgical treatment

a. Acute fractures

- Indications for surgery include open and/or unstable fractures.
- Fixation
  - An intramedullary nail is often sufficient to maintain ulnar length (**Figure 12**) in transverse fractures.
  - Plate fixation is needed for comminuted fractures.
- Annular ligament reconstruction is rarely needed for acute fractures.

b. Chronic fractures

- Most should be reduced surgically if symptomatic (preferably within 6 to 12 months following injury).

- Technique—These complex reconstructions require ulnar osteotomy with internal fixation, radial head reduction, and annular ligament reconstruction.

5. Complications

a. Posterior interosseous nerve palsy occurs in up to 10% of acute injuries but almost always resolves spontaneously.

b. Delayed or missed diagnosis of a Monteggia fracture is common when the child is not evaluated by an orthopaedic surgeon.

c. Complication rates and severity are much greater if the diagnosis is delayed more than 2 to 3 weeks.

C. Distal forearm fractures

1. Classification

a. Physeal fractures are categorized using the Salter-Harris classification.

b. For metaphyseal fractures, distinction is made between buckle fractures and complete fractures.

2. Nonsurgical treatment

a. Most are treated by closed means.

- Short arm casts are as effective as long arm casts in maintaining reduction for displaced fractures.

- Buckle fractures may be treated with removable splints or short arm casts.

b. Healing times

- Physeal fractures heal in 3 to 4 weeks.

- Metaphyseal fractures heal in 4 to 6 weeks.

- Buckle fractures heal in 3 weeks.

3. Surgical treatment

a. Indications

- Open fractures are treated surgically with ORIF following irrigation and débridement.

- Unacceptable closed reduction

  ○ Complete metaphyseal fractures—Quoted unacceptable alignment is greater than 20° of angulation in a child of any age and bayonet apposition in children older than 10 years, although the growth potential in this area allows such fractures to remodel successfully.

  ○ Physeal fractures—Residual displacement greater than 50% is unacceptable. Attempting reduction of a physeal fracture more than 5 to 7 days postinjury is dis-

couraged because of the increased risk of iatrogenic physeal injury.

  ○ Floating elbow injuries—Percutaneous pinning of the distal radius results in much lower rates of fracture reduction loss and malunion.

b. Procedures

- Closed reduction successfully reduces most of these fractures.

- Percutaneous pinning (avoiding the superficial radial nerve) is generally sufficient to maintain reduction for very unstable fractures or those with associated injuries.

4. Complications

a. Malunion generally results in cosmetic deformity rather than functional deficits and often remodels spontaneously.

b. Growth arrest occurs in less than 1% to 2% of distal radius physeal fractures and less than 1% of metaphyseal fractures.

c. Compartment syndrome is a substantial risk in children with floating elbow injuries (ipsilateral forearm and humeral fractures).

D. Carpal injuries

1. Nonsurgical treatment

a. Scaphoid fractures are most commonly treated with a short arm or long arm thumb spica cast.

- Distal pole fractures routinely heal with closed treatment.

- Waist fractures have worse results (especially in adolescents) and may result in osteonecrosis and/or nonunion.

b. Triangular fibrocartilage complex (TFCC) tears may accompany distal radial and/or ulnar styloid fractures and are treated closed.

2. Surgical treatment

a. Scaphoid fractures may be treated with ORIF for displaced waist fractures or with ORIF and bone grafting for established nonunions.

b. If ongoing wrist pain occurs following closed treatment of a wrist fracture, TFCC tears may be repaired arthroscopically.

3. Complications

a. Scaphoid waist fractures—Osteonecrosis and nonunion.

b. TFCC tears—Chronic wrist pain.

E. Metacarpal fractures

1. Classification

a. For physeal injuries, the Salter-Harris classification is used.

b. For nonphyseal fractures, classification is based on fracture location, configuration, angulation, and displacement, as in adults.

c. Some of these fractures are "open" injuries ("fight bites" or "clenched-fist" injuries); lacerations over the knuckles should be sought to rule out such an injury.

2. Nonsurgical treatment

a. Most of these fractures are treated closed.

- Rotational alignment must be good for acceptable closed treatment.

- Acceptable sagittal angulation increases from radial to ulnar as in adults, according to these guidelines: Second metacarpal, 10° to 20°; third metacarpal, 20° to 30°; fourth metacarpal, 30° to 40°; and fifth metacarpal, 40° to 50°.

b. Closed treatment is successful for diaphyseal and metaphyseal fractures of the thumb metacarpal.

3. Surgical treatment

a. Indications—Unacceptable rotational, sagittal, and/or coronal alignment.

b. Physeal fractures of the base of the thumb metacarpal often require surgery because of instability and/or intra-articular step-off.

4. Complications—Most common is malalignment (including rotational deformity, which results in overlapping fingers), requiring late osteotomy.

F. Phalangeal fractures

1. Classification

a. Physeal fractures are described using the Salter-Harris classification.

b. Shaft and neck fractures are categorized by fracture type and displacement.

2. Nonsurgical treatment suffices for most fractures, with healing in approximately 3 weeks.

3. Surgical treatment

a. Indications—Most intra-articular phalangeal fractures.

b. Procedures

- Closed reduction and pinning is indicated for most minimally displaced intra-articular fractures.

- Open reduction and pinning is often needed for more displaced unicondylar and bicondylar fractures.

4. Complications—Stiffness, fixation loss, growth disturbance, and malunion are relatively uncommon.

Top Testing Facts

1. The surgeon should assume that complete recovery from other injuries (including head injuries) will occur; many children make excellent recoveries from such injuries.

2. Prompt administration of intravenous antibiotics is the most important factor in reducing the rate of infection following open fractures.

3. A pulseless, well-perfused hand may need only careful observation following SCH fracture because of the excellent collateral circulation around the elbow.

4. Injury to the anterior interosseous nerve is the most common nerve injury associated with SCH fractures.

5. Ulnar nerve injury with extension-type SCH fractures is almost always iatrogenic from medial pin insertion, particularly if the medial pin is inserted with the elbow in a fully flexed position.

6. The oblique radiograph is the most sensitive for detecting maximal displacement of lateral condyle fractures and is required when contemplating closed treatment.

7. Elbow dislocations in children younger than 3 to 6 years are very rare, so transphyseal fractures should be suspected in young patients with displacement of the proximal radius and ulna relative to the humerus.

8. Isolated radial head dislocations almost never occur in children. These presumed "isolated" injuries almost always result from plastic deformation of the ulna with concomitant radial head dislocation (Monteggia fracture).

9. Buckle fractures of the distal radius can be treated with removable wrist splints.

10. Floating elbow injuries have high complication rates, including loss of forearm fracture reduction when internal fixation has not been used and increased risk of compartment syndrome.

Bibliography

Abzug JM, Herman MJ: Management of supracondylar humerus fractures in children: Current concepts. *J Am Acad Orthop Surg* 2012;20(2):69-77.

Kay RM, Skaggs DL: Pediatric polytrauma management. *J Pediatr Orthop* 2006;26(2):268-277.

Price CT: Surgical management of forearm and distal radius fractures in children and adolescents. *Instr Course Lect* 2008; 57:509-514.

Ring D: Monteggia fractures. *Orthop Clin North Am* 2013; 44(1):59-66.

Ring D, Jupiter JB, Waters PM: Monteggia fractures in children and adults. *J Am Acad Orthop Surg* 1998;6(4):215-224.

Sink EL, Hyman JE, Matheny T, Georgopoulos G, Kleinman P: Child abuse: The role of the orthopaedic surgeon in nonaccidental trauma. *Clin Orthop Relat Res* 2011;469(3): 790-797.

Skaggs DL, Cluck MW, Mostofi A, Flynn JM, Kay RM: Lateral-entry pin fixation in the management of supracondylar fractures in children. *J Bone Joint Surg Am* 2004;86(4): 702-707.

Skaggs DL, Friend L, Alman B, et al: The effect of surgical delay on acute infection following 554 open fractures in children. *J Bone Joint Surg Am* 2005;87(1):8-12.

Stewart DG Jr, Kay RM, Skaggs DL: Open fractures in children: Principles of evaluation and management. *J Bone Joint Surg Am* 2005;87(12):2784-2798.

Tejwani N, Phillips D, Goldstein RY: Management of lateral humeral condylar fracture in children. *J Am Acad Orthop Surg* 2011;19(6):350-358.

Weiss JM, Graves S, Yang S, Mendelsohn E, Kay RM, Skaggs DL: A new classification system predictive of complications in surgically treated pediatric humeral lateral condyle fractures. *J Pediatr Orthop* 2009;29(6):602-605.

Chapter 63

Pediatric Pelvic and Lower Extremity Fractures

Robert M. Kay, MD

I. Pelvic Fractures

A. Evaluation—Half of pelvic fractures identified on CT are not identified on plain AP pelvis radiographs.

B. Classification

1. The most common systems are the Tile classification system and the Torode and Zieg classification system.

   a. Tile classification

      • Type A—Stable fractures.

      • Type B—Rotationally unstable but vertically stable.

      • Type C—Rotationally and vertically unstable.

   b. Torode and Zieg classification

      • Type I—Avulsion fractures.

      • Type II—Iliac wing fractures.

      • Type III—Ring fractures without segmental instability.

         ○ Type IIIA—Simple anterior ring fractures.

         ○ Type IIIB—Have anterior and posterior ring disruptions, but are stable.

      • Type IV—Ring disruptions with segmental instability.

2. Regardless of the classification system, it is essential to determine whether the pelvic fracture is stable.

C. Treatment

1. Nonsurgical—Produces good results in almost all pediatric pelvic fractures; bed rest and bed-to-chair transfers for 3 to 4 weeks, followed by progressive weight bearing. Some may need protection and immobilization by a spica cast.

2. Surgical indications

   a. External fixation may be applied rapidly, and is occasionally indicated to stabilize the pelvic ring and/or decrease the volume of the pelvis in open book injuries.

   b. Open reduction and internal fixation (ORIF) is most commonly indicated in adolescents with vertically unstable injuries or substantially displaced acetabular fractures.

D. Complications

1. Malunion and nonunion are uncommon.

2. Limb-length discrepancy (LLD) may occur in vertically unstable fractures.

II. Avulsion Fractures of the Pelvis

A. Epidemiology

1. Typically occur in adolescent athletes involved in explosive-type activities, such as sprinting, jumping, and/or kicking

2. The most common avulsion sites (and the causative muscles) are shown in **Table 1**.

B. Treatment

1. Nonsurgical—Local measures, including rest, ice, and anti-inflammatory medication for 2 to 3 weeks, followed by gradual resumption of activities.

2. Surgical—Almost never indicated for these injuries; surgery may be considered for symptomatic nonunions.

C. Complications—Few, if any, long-term sequelae.

Dr. Kay or an immediate family member has stock or stock options held in Medtronic, Zimmer, Johnson & Johnson, and Pfizer.

5: Pediatrics

Table 1

Pelvic Avulsion Fracture Sites and Causative Muscles

Avulsion Site	Causative Muscles
Ischium	Hamstrings/adductors
Anterior-superior iliac spine	Sartorius
Anterior-inferior iliac spine	Rectus femoris
Iliac crest	Abdominals
Lesser trochanter	Iliopsoas

III. Hip Fractures

A. Classification—The Delbet classification is used for proximal femur fractures (**Figure 1**).

B. Treatment

  1. Nonsurgical—Rarely indicated because of the increased risks of coxa vara and nonunion with closed treatment.

  2. Surgical

    a. When feasible, gentle, closed reduction and internal fixation is preferred.

    b. Decompression of the intracapsular hematoma by arthrotomy (or joint aspiration) appears to reduce the risk of osteonecrosis in intracapsular injuries.

    c. Fixation

      • Fixation is performed with Kirschner wires (K-wires) or cannulated screws for Delbet type I fractures, cannulated screws for type II and III fractures, and a pediatric hip screw, dynamic hip screw, or proximal femoral locking plate for type IV fractures.

      • Stability of fixation is paramount to reduce the chance of nonunion or malunion; fixation should extend across the physis if needed for stability.

C. Complications

  1. Osteonecrosis is the most common, and severe, complication and is related to fracture level. The risk of osteonecrosis is 90% to 100% for type I fractures, 50% for type II, 25% for type III, and 10% for type IV. Femoral head collapse often leads to joint penetration of the previously placed hardware, which may result in chondrolysis and exacerbation of pain.

  2. Coxa vara and nonunion are much more common after nonsurgically treated fractures, particularly Delbet type II and III fractures.

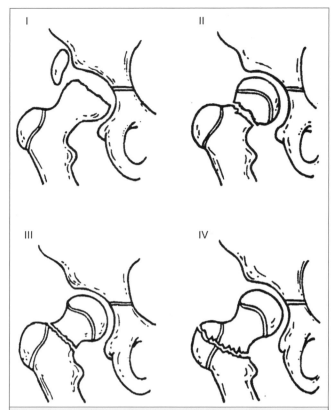

Figure 1 Illustrations depict the Delbet classification of pediatric hip fractures. Type I fractures are physeal; type II, transcervical; type III, cervicotrochanteric; and type IV, intertrochanteric. (Reproduced with permission from Hughes LO, Beaty JH: Fractures of the head and neck of the femur in children. J Bone Joint Surg Am 1994; 76:283-292.)

  3. LLD is common after hip fractures in young children because the proximal femoral physis accounts for about 15% of total leg length.

IV. Femoral Shaft Fractures

A. Epidemiology

  1. Child abuse is the cause of most femur fractures before walking age.

  2. Abuse must be considered in children up to 3 years of age, but it is a less common cause of femur fractures after walking age.

B. Treatment

  1. Nonsurgical

    a. Indications—Spica casting is routine in children younger than 6 years.

    b. Contraindications to immediate spica casting

      • Shortening greater than 2.5 to 3.0 cm is a

relative contraindication.

- Multiple trauma is an absolute contraindication.

c. Complications

- LLD

  ◦ Ipsilateral overgrowth of 7 to 10 mm occurs in children aged 2 to 10 years who sustain a femur fracture.

  ◦ LLD may result from excessive overgrowth or excessive shortening at the time of fracture healing following cast treatment.

- Malunion

  ◦ Angular malunion (usually varus and/or procurvatum) can be minimized with careful technique and cast molding.

  ◦ Torsional malunion is common but mild and rarely of clinical consequence.

2. Surgical treatment

a. Indications—Most children older than 6 years are treated surgically, as are many younger multiple-trauma patients.

b. Procedures

- Flexible intramedullary (IM) rodding

  ◦ Indications—Most pediatric femoral shaft fractures in children aged 6 to 10 years.

  ◦ Relative contraindications—Comminuted or very distal or proximal fractures are harder to control with flexible IM rods.

  ◦ Complication rates (particularly loss of reduction) are higher in children older than 10 years and in those who weigh more than 50 kg.

- Trochanteric entry nails

  ◦ Often used in children older than 8 to 10 years, in those weighing more than 50 kg, and in extremely comminuted fractures.

  ◦ Complications (1) May cause abnormalities of proximal femoral growth resulting in a narrow femoral neck. (2) The risk of osteonecrosis and coxa valga appears to be low.

- Submuscular bridge plating

  ◦ Indications—Submuscular plating may be considered especially for comminuted femoral shaft fractures, although its popularity appears to be waning.

  ◦ Complications (1) Fracture following hardware removal may occur because of numerous stress risers in the femoral shaft following hardware removal. (2) Distal femoral valgus is relatively common following healing. (3) Complications, including malunion, may occur more commonly until the surgeon gains experience with this technique because a substantial learning curve exists.

- Open femoral plating

  ◦ Indications—Rarely used currently but may be used for comminuted fractures, particularly in those with osteoporotic bone.

  ◦ Complications—Numerous stress risers increase the risk of fracture after hardware removal.

- Antegrade rigid femoral nails

  ◦ Indications—Femoral shaft fractures in children at, or nearing, skeletal maturity.

  ◦ Complications—Osteonecrosis occurs in 1% to 2% of children with open physes.

- External fixation

  ◦ Indications—For comminuted or segmental fractures or in "damage control" situations requiring rapid application (sometimes at the bedside).

  ◦ Complications (1) Delayed union and refracture are more frequent than with other forms of fixation. (2) Pin tract infections (usually superficial) are frequent.

V. Distal Femur Fractures

A. Distal femoral metaphyseal fractures

1. Nonsurgical treatment—Casting suffices for most low-energy insufficiency fractures in children with neuromuscular disease.

2. Surgical treatment

a. Indications—Displaced fractures almost always require surgical treatment with closed reduction and pinning.

b. Technique—Hardware should not cross the physis, if possible.

3. Complications—Malunion is the most common complication following displaced fractures because accurate assessment of coronal plane alignment is difficult following casting.

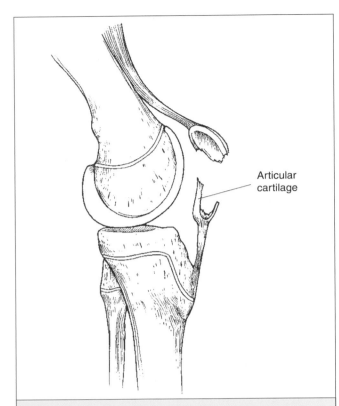

Articular
cartilage

Figure 2   Illustration shows a lateral view of a patellar sleeve fracture. The only sign on plain radiographs may be patella alta. (Adapted with permission from Tolo VT: Fractures and dislocations around the knee, in Green NE, Swiontkowski MF, eds: *Skeletal Trauma in Children*. Philadelphia, PA, WB Saunders, 1994, vol 3, pp 369-395.)

B. Distal femoral physeal fractures

1. Classification—The Salter-Harris classification.

2. Nonsurgical treatment is indicated for nondisplaced Salter-Harris type I and II fractures.

3. Surgical treatment

a. Indications—Displaced fractures of the distal femoral physis.

b. Procedures

- Closed reduction and internal fixation if anatomic reduction is obtainable closed

- ORIF if closed reduction is not satisfactory

- Fixation avoids the physis when possible. When fixation must cross the physis, smooth K-wires are used and should be removed by 3 to 6 weeks after surgery.

- Some surgeons prefer antegrade pin placement to avoid intra-articular pins and reduce the chance of septic arthritis, which is associated with pin tract sepsis.

4. Complications

a. Popliteal artery injury and compartment syndrome are rare but more likely when the epiphysis displaces anteriorly.

b. Growth arrest occurs in 30% to 50% of distal femoral physeal injuries.

- Sequelae of distal femoral physeal fractures include LLD and angular deformity.

- These sequelae are often severe because the distal femur accounts for 70% of femoral growth.

VI. Patellar Fractures

A. Evaluation—Bipartite patella is a normal variant (in ≤5% of knees) and differs from a patellar fracture in two ways.

1. Bipartite patella has rounded borders.

2. Bipartite patella is located superolaterally.

B. Classification

1. Categorized based on location, fracture configuration, and amount of displacement

2. Patellar sleeve fractures are a relatively common type of pediatric patellar fracture, in which a chondral sleeve of the patella separates from the main portion of the patella and ossific nucleus. The only finding on plain radiographs may be apparent patella alta for distal fractures (**Figure 2**) or patella baja for proximal fractures, so these fractures are often missed on initial presentation.

C. Treatment

1. Nonsurgical—Indicated for nondisplaced and minimally displaced fractures in children without an extensor lag.

2. Surgical

a. Indications

- Patella fractures displaced greater than 2 mm at the articular surface should be fixed surgically. The indication for surgery is confirmed by an extensor lag or the inability to actively extend the knee.

- Patellar sleeve fractures require surgery.

b. Procedures

- For osseous fractures, fixation (as in adults) with tension banding; a cerclage wire may be needed for extensively comminuted fractures.

- For patellar sleeve fractures, repair of the torn medial and lateral retinaculum along

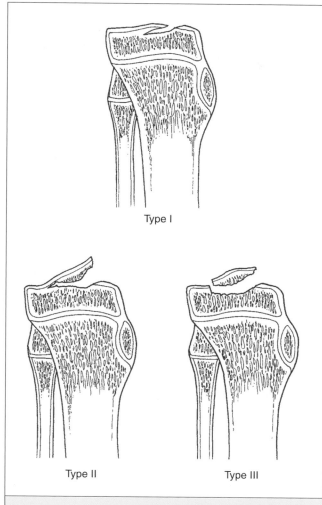

Type I

Type II   Type III

Figure 3   Illustrations depict the Meyers and McKeever classification of tibial spine fractures. (Adapted with permission from Tolo VT: Fractures and dislocations around the knee, in Green NE, Swiontkowski MF, eds: *Skeletal Trauma in Children*. Philadelphia, PA, WB Saunders, 1994, pp 369-395.)

with sutures through the cartilaginous and osseous portions of the patella

VII. Tibia and Fibula Fractures

A. Tibial spine fractures

1. Evaluation

   a. Children with fractures of the tibial spine present with a mechanism consistent with an anterior cruciate ligament (ACL) tear and an acutely unstable knee. Because ligaments are typically stronger than bones in children, pediatric tibial spine fractures occur more frequently than ACL tears.

   b. The physical examination is comparable to that following a ligamentous ACL tear.

2. Classification—The Meyers and McKeever classification (**Figure 3**) is used. Type I are minimally displaced; type II are hinged with displacement of the anterior portion; and type III are completely displaced.

3. Nonsurgical treatment

   a. Indications—Closed reduction and casting suffices for type I and some type II fractures. For type II fractures, the reduction must be within a few millimeters of anatomic to accept closed treatment.

   b. Procedure

   • Arthrocentesis before casting if a large hemarthrosis is present

   • The optimal amount of knee flexion for reduction is controversial but generally recommended to be 0° to 20°.

4. Surgical treatment

   a. Indications—Type II fractures that do not reduce with casting and type III fractures.

   b. Procedures

   • ORIF and arthroscopic reduction and internal fixation are both effective.

   • Type of fixation used (sutures versus screws) is often determined by fracture configuration; comminuted fractures with small fracture fragments typically require suture fixation. Fixation should avoid the physis.

   • The meniscus is often entrapped and must be moved to allow reduction.

5. Complications

   a. Arthrofibrosis is common after surgically and nonsurgically treated tibial spine fractures. Early mobilization following surgical fixation seems to reduce the rate.

   b. ACL laxity is common but generally not clinically significant.

   c. Malunion with persistent elevation of the fracture fragment may result in impingement in the notch.

B. Proximal tibial physeal fractures

1. Classification—The Salter-Harris classification is used (**Figure 4**).

2. Nonsurgical treatment indications— Nondisplaced fractures (which include 30% to 50% of Salter-Harris type I and II fractures) may be treated with cast immobilization.

3. Surgical treatment

5: Pediatrics

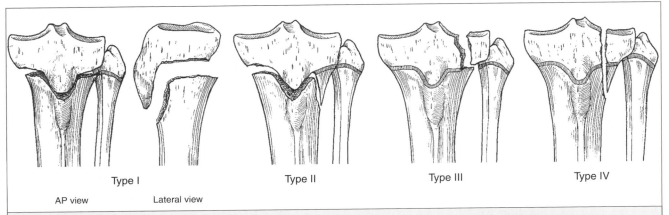

Type I Type II Type III Type IV

AP view Lateral view

Figure 4   Illustrations show Salter-Harris fractures of the proximal tibial physis. (Adapted from Hensinger RN, ed: *Operative Management of Lower Extremity Fractures in Children*. Park Ridge, IL, American Academy of Orthopaedic Surgeons, 1992, p 49.)

a. Indications—Displaced fractures are treated with closed (or open) reduction and internal fixation.

b. Procedures

- Closed reduction typically suffices. If unsuccessful, open reduction is required.

- Fixation devices

  ∘ Crossed smooth K-wires for most Salter-Harris type I and II fractures; they are removed by 3 to 4 weeks after surgery.

  ∘ Cannulated screws (inserted parallel to the physis) for Salter-Harris type III and IV fractures (and type II fractures with large metaphyseal fragments)

4. Complications

a. Neurovascular complications include popliteal artery injuries (5%), compartment syndrome (3% to 4%), and peroneal nerve injury (5%). Vascular complications are particularly common with hyperextension injuries (**Figure 5**).

b. Redisplacement of the fracture is common in displaced fractures treated without internal fixation.

c. Growth arrest occurs in 25% of patients and can result in LLD and/or angular deformity.

C. Proximal tibial metaphyseal fractures

1. Classification—No specific classification is used.

2. Nonsurgical treatment with a long leg cast is the mainstay treatment of low-energy injuries in children younger than 10 years.

3. Surgical treatment—Generally necessary for high-energy proximal tibial fractures in older children because these fractures are often substantially dis-

placed and unstable.

4. Complications

a. Genu valgum is common following low-energy injuries (so-called Cozen fractures). No treatment is needed acutely because these deformities often improve spontaneously.

b. Neurovascular damage, compartment syndrome, and malunion may occur after high-energy fractures.

D. Tibial tubercle fractures

1. Classification—The classification has evolved since Watson-Jones first described three types of fractures (**Figure 6**).

2. Nonsurgical treatment is rarely indicated but may be used in children with minimally displaced fractures (< 2 mm) and no extensor lag.

3. Surgical treatment

a. Indications—Recommended for children with fractures having greater than 2 mm of displacement and/or an extensor lag.

b. Procedures

- ORIF with screws for fracture types I through IV. For type III fractures, the joint must be visualized to accurately reduce the joint surface and to assess for meniscal injury.

- Suture reattachment (which may be supplemented with small screws) of the periosteal sleeve is the technique of choice for type V fractures.

4. Complications—Compartment syndrome and genu recurvatum are rare.

E. Tibial shaft fractures

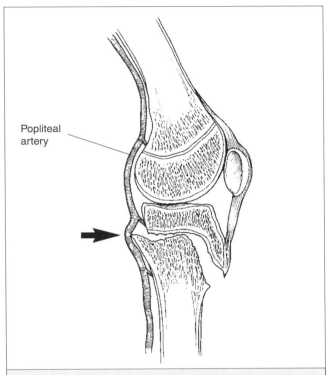

Figure 5 Lateral illustration of the knee depicts the potential for popliteal artery injury from proximal tibial physeal fracture. Arrow indicates the point at which the fractured bone can injure the artery. (Adapted with permission from Tolo VT: Fractures and dislocations around the knee, in Green NE, Swiontkowski MF, eds: *Skeletal Trauma in Children*. Philadelphia, PA, WB Saunders, 1994, pp 369-395.)

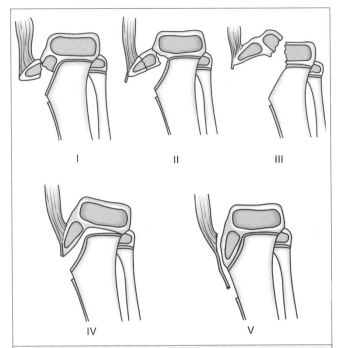

Figure 6 Illustrations show the classification of tibial tubercle injuries. Types I through IV are true fractures, whereas type V is actually a soft-tissue injury with detachment of the periosteal sleeve.

1. Nonsurgical treatment

   a. Most tibial fractures in children can be treated with reduction and casting.

   b. Healing takes 3 to 4 weeks for toddler fractures and 6 to 8 weeks for other tibial fractures.

2. Surgical treatment

   a. Indications include open fractures, marked soft-tissue injury, unstable fractures, multiple trauma, more than 1 cm of shortening, and unacceptable closed reduction (> 10° of angulation).

   b. Fixation options include IM rod fixation, external fixation, or percutaneous pins or plates.

3. Complications

   a. When closed reduction is lost, isolated tibial fractures typically drift into varus, and combined tibia and fibula fractures drift into valgus.

   b. Delayed union and nonunion are almost never

seen in closed fractures but are more common following external fixation.

   c. Compartment syndrome can occur with open or closed fractures.

VIII. Ankle Fractures

A. Classification

1. An anatomic classification system is typically used for ankle fractures. The Salter-Harris classification is commonly used for physeal fractures.

2. A mechanistic classification system such as the Dias-Tachdjian classification may be used. This classification is patterned after the Lauge-Hansen categorization of adult fractures and describes four main mechanisms: supination-inversion, supination–plantar flexion, supination–external rotation, and pronation/eversion–external rotation.

B. Special considerations

1. Inversion ankle injuries in children typically result in distal fibular physeal fractures (almost exclusively Salter-Harris type I or II).

   a. These fractures are believed to be more common than ankle sprains following an ankle inversion injury in a child, but recent MRI studies do not show physeal injuries of the distal

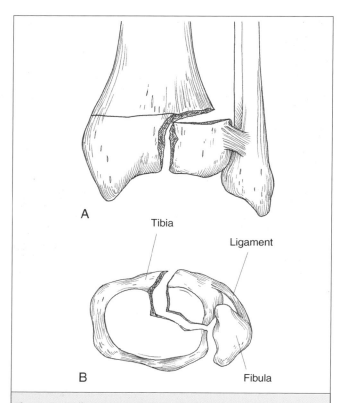

Figure 7 Illustrations depict a Tillaux fracture as seen from the anterior (**A**) and inferior (**B**) views. The anterolateral fragment is avulsed by the anterior inferior tibiofibular ligament. (Part A adapted with permission from Weber BG, Sussenbach F: Malleolar fractures, in Weber BG, Brunner C, Freuler F, eds: *Treatment of Fractures in Children and Adolescents*. New York, NY, Springer-Verlag, 1980.)

fibula and question this dogma.

    b. Salter type I fractures are diagnosed clinically by tenderness at the level of the physis and radiographs that show no malalignment of the physis and soft-tissue swelling over the distal fibula.

2. Transitional fractures occur as the distal tibial physis is closing.

    a. These fractures involve the anterolateral distal tibial epiphysis because the distal tibial physis closes centrally first, then medially, and finally laterally.

    b. Tillaux fractures (**Figure 7**) are Salter-Harris type III fractures of the anterolateral tibial epiphysis that occur with supination–external rotation injuries.

    c. Triplane fractures (**Figures 8** and **9**) are Salter-Harris type IV fractures that include an anterolateral fragment of the distal tibial epiphysis (as in a Tillaux fracture) in conjunction with a metaphyseal fracture. They may be two-part or three-part fractures.

C. Nonsurgical treatment

1. Distal tibial physeal fracture indications

    a. Most distal tibial Salter-Harris type I, II, and III fractures; closed reduction is acceptable if postreduction radiographs show less than 2 to 3 mm of displacement and up to 10° of angulation for Salter-Harris type I and II fractures and postreduction CT shows less than 2 to

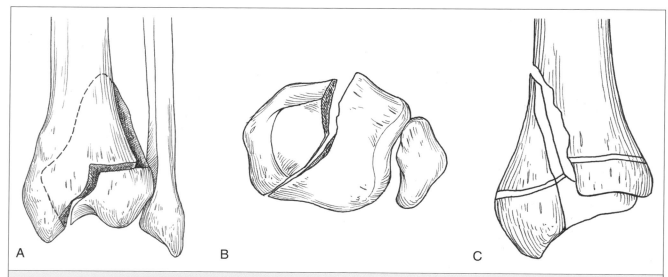

Figure 8 Illustrations show a two-part lateral triplane fracture as seen from the anterior (**A**) and inferior (**B**) aspects of the ankle. **C,** A two-part medial triplane fracture. (Panels A and B adapted with permission from Jarvis JG: Tibial triplane fractures, in Letts RM, ed: *Management of Pediatric Fractures*. Philadelphia, PA, Churchill Livingstone, 1994, p 739. Panel C, adapted with permission from Rockwood CA Jr, Wilkins KE, King RE: *Fractures in Children*. Philadelphia, PA, JB Lippincott, 1984, p 933.)

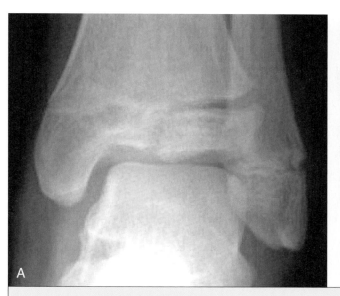
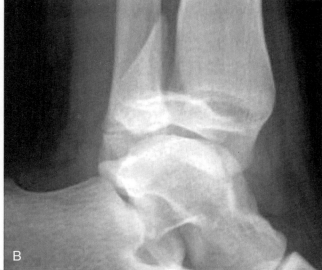

Figure 9   Anteroposterior (**A**) and lateral (**B**) radiographs show a classic triplane fracture. (Reproduced from Schnetzler KA, Hoernschemeyer D: The pediatric triplane ankle fracture. *J Am Acad Orthop Surg* 2007;15[12]:738-747.)

3 mm of displacement (fracture diastasis or articular step-off) for type III fractures.

b. Nondisplaced or minimally displaced Salter-Harris type IV fractures (medial malleolus or triplane) can be treated closed. CT should be obtained after casting for triplane fractures to confirm that reduction is satisfactory (< 2 to 3 mm of fracture diastasis and articular step-off).

2. Distal fibular fractures

a. Isolated injuries—Almost always Salter-Harris type I and II fractures; typically treated closed with a short leg walking cast or fracture boot for 3 weeks.

b. Closed treatment suffices for almost all distal fibula fractures associated with distal tibia fractures, unless the fibula fracture is "high" and/or comminuted in a child nearing skeletal maturity.

D. Surgical treatment

1. Distal tibial physeal fracture indications

a. Salter-Harris type I and II fractures with greater than 2 to 3 mm of displacement or greater than 10° of angulation

b. Salter-Harris type III fractures with greater than 2 to 3 mm articular displacement (diastasis or step-off) on postreduction CT

c. Salter-Harris type IV fractures with greater than 2 to 3 mm of displacement postreduction

2. Distal fibular fractures

a. Isolated injuries—Surgery may be necessary

for the unusual Salter-Harris type III or IV fracture that is displaced.

b. Distal fibula fractures associated with distal tibia fractures—ORIF may be needed for a "high" and/or comminuted fibula fracture in a child nearing skeletal maturity.

E. Complications

1. Growth arrest with angular deformity and/or LLD is minimized by reduction within 2 mm of anatomic. Medial malleolar Salter-Harris type IV shear ankle fractures have the highest risk of growth arrest.

2. Joint incongruity and late osteoarthritis are risks with distal tibial Salter-Harris type III and IV fractures.

3. Complex regional pain syndrome is relatively common in children following ankle fractures and should be suspected in children who do not show prompt resolution of pain following immobilization.

IX. Foot Fractures

A. Pathoanatomy—Accessory ossicles in the foot (**Figure 10**) are common and must be differentiated from acute injuries.

B. Talar fractures and dislocations

1. Overview

a. Most talar fractures are avulsion fractures.

b. Talar neck and body fractures are generally

5: Pediatrics

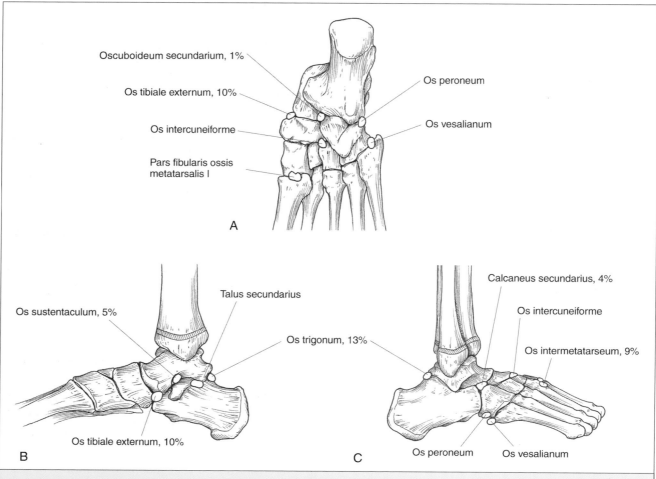

Oscuboideum secundarium, 1%

Os tibiale externum, 10%

Os intercuneiforme

Pars fibularis ossis metatarsalis I

Os peroneum

Os vesalianum

A

Os sustentaculum, 5%

Talus secundarius

Os trigonum, 13%

Os tibiale externum, 10%

B

Calcaneus secundarius, 4%

Os intercuneiforme

Os intermetatarseum, 9%

Os peroneum

Os vesalianum

C

Figure 10   Illustrations show accessory ossicles of the foot and their frequency of occurrence (when data are available) as viewed from the plantar (**A**), medial (**B**), and lateral (**C**) aspects of the foot. (Adapted with permission from Tachdjian MO, ed: *Pediatric Orthopaedics*, ed 2. Philadelphia, PA, WB Saunders, 1990, p 471.)

high-energy injuries; falls from a height and motor vehicle accidents account for 70% to 90%.

2. Classification

   a. Categorized as avulsion fractures, talar neck fractures, or talar body fractures

   b. Classified by the Hawkins classification (as are adult fractures) (**Table 2**).

3. Nonsurgical treatment is indicated for nondisplaced talar neck and body fractures; closed reduction should be attempted for displaced fractures. Because talar neck fractures are dorsiflexion injuries, they are most stable in plantar flexion.

4. Surgical treatment—Surgical indications are not well defined; surgery should be considered for displaced talar neck and body fractures.

5. Complications

   a. Chronic pain is common following talar neck and body fractures.

   b. Osteonecrosis also is common after such fractures; incidence is highest for Hawkins type III and IV injuries.

C. Calcaneal fractures

1. Classification—A variety of classifications have been described; the most important distinctions are whether the fracture is intra-articular or extra-articular and whether the fracture is displaced.

2. Nonsurgical treatment is the mainstay for pediatric calcaneal fractures because of its favorable results and potential calcaneal remodeling.

3. Surgical treatment is often indicated in adolescent children with displaced intra-articular calcaneal fractures.

4. Complications are rare because of potential calcaneal remodeling in pre-adolescents.

Table 2		
Hawkins Classification of Talar Neck Fractures		
Hawkins Type	**Talar Fracture**	**Subluxated or Dislocated Joint(s)**
I	Nondisplaced	None
II	Displaced	Subtalar
III	Displaced	Subtalar and tibiotalar
IV	Displaced	Talonavicular and subtalar and/or tibiotalar

D. Other tarsal fractures

1. Avulsion fractures of the navicular, cuneiforms, and cuboid are the most common type and are generally low-energy injuries. Treatment includes a walking cast for 2 to 3 weeks; results are excellent.

2. Displaced fractures of the navicular, cuneiforms, and cuboid are generally high-energy injuries, with high rates of associated injuries and compartment syndrome. ORIF is generally required.

E. Lisfranc injuries

1. Treatment

   a. Closed treatment is indicated for nondisplaced fractures and is attempted for displaced fractures.

   b. Fixation in adolescents is performed with cannulated screws, in younger children with smooth K-wires.

2. Complications— Chronic pain can occur and results in poor outcomes.

F. Metatarsal fractures

1. Classification—No specific classification system exists.

2. Treatment

   a. Nonsurgical—Suffices for most metatarsal fractures. Weight bearing is allowed for almost all such fractures; one exception is a fifth metatarsal base fracture at or distal to the metaphyseal-diaphyseal junction.

   b. Surgical—The rare indications for surgical intervention include

   • Marked displacement of the metatarsal head in the sagittal plane

   • Fractures of the fifth metatarsal distal to the metaphyseal-diaphyseal junction that do not unite with closed treatment

3. Complications

a. Most pediatric metatarsal fractures heal uneventfully.

b. Delayed union or nonunion are relatively common for fifth metatarsal base fractures distal to the metaphyseal-diaphyseal junction.

G. Phalangeal fractures

1. Treatment

   a. Nonsurgical treatment suffices for almost all phalangeal fractures.

   b. Surgical—The few indications for surgical intervention include

   • Open fractures

   • Substantially displaced intra-articular fractures

2. Complications—Rare, although growth arrest may occasionally occur following a physeal fracture of the great toe.

H. Occult foot fractures

1. Overview

   a. Occult foot fractures are a common cause of limp in preschool-age children.

   b. If a child crawls without difficulty but limps or refuses to bear weight when standing, the pathology is distal to the knee.

2. Evaluation

   a. Radiographs are typically negative.

   b. Bone scans (although rarely necessary) show increased uptake in the affected tarsal bones.

3. Treatment includes a short leg walking cast for 2 to 3 weeks. If the child does not feel better within days of cast application, another source of pain should be sought.

Top Testing Facts

1. Plain AP pelvis radiographs fail to identify about half of all pediatric pelvic fractures found on CT.

2. The rate of osteonecrosis of the hip is inversely related to the Delbet fracture category (90% to 100% for type I fractures, 50% for type II, 25% for type III, and 10% for type IV).

3. Femoral overgrowth of 7 to 10 mm is typical in children who sustain a femoral shaft fracture between the ages of 2 and 10 years.

4. Distal femoral physeal fractures have a worse prognosis than other physeal fractures because of the high rate of growth arrest (up to 50%) and the rapid growth of the distal femur.

5. Because ligaments in children are typically stronger than bone in children, pediatric tibial spine fracture are more frequent than ACL tears.

6. Vascular injury and/or compartment syndrome occurs in nearly 10% of patients with fractures of the proximal tibial physis; the risk is highest with hyperextension injury.

7. Proximal tibial metaphyseal fractures in children younger than 6 years typically grow into valgus after injury (the so-called Cozen fracture). Observation is indicated in these cases because the genu valgum often resolves spontaneously.

8. Tillaux fractures and triplane fractures both occur in the anterolateral distal tibial physis because of the order of distal tibial physeal closure (the central portion closes first, followed by the medial, and then the lateral).

9. Medial malleolar Salter-Harris type IV fractures have the highest rate of growth arrest for pediatric ankle fractures and often result in varus deformity and LLD.

10. Calcaneal fractures can remodel in children and generally have favorable long-term outcomes, although ORIF may be indicated in adolescents with substantially displaced intra-articular calcaneal fractures.

Bibliography

Boardman MJ, Herman MJ, Buck B, Pizzutillo PD: Hip fractures in children. *J Am Acad Orthop Surg* 2009;17(3): 162-173.

Flynn JM, Schwend RM: Management of pediatric femoral shaft fractures. *J Am Acad Orthop Surg* 2004;12(5):347-359.

Flynn JM, Skaggs DL, Sponseller PD, Ganley TJ, Kay RM, Leitch KK: The surgical management of pediatric fractures of the lower extremity. *Instr Course Lect* 2003;52:647-659.

Holden CP, Holman J, Herman MJ: Pediatric pelvic fractures. *J Am Acad Orthop Surg* 2007;15(3):172-177.

Hosalkar HS, Pandya NK, Cho RH, Glaser DA, Moor MA, Herman MJ: Intramedullary nailing of pediatric femoral shaft fracture. *J Am Acad Orthop Surg* 2011;19(8):472-481.

Kay RM, Matthys GA: Pediatric ankle fractures: Evaluation and treatment. *J Am Acad Orthop Surg* 2001;9(4):268-278.

Kay RM, Tang CW: Pediatric foot fractures: Evaluation and treatment. *J Am Acad Orthop Surg* 2001;9(5):308-319.

Kuremsky MA, Frick SL: Advances in the surgical management of pediatric femoral shaft fractures. *Curr Opin Pediatr* 2007;19(1):51-57.

Lafrance RM, Giordano B, Goldblatt J, Voloshin I, Maloney M: Pediatric tibial eminence fractures: Evaluation and management. *J Am Acad Orthop Surg* 2010;18(7):395-405.

Li Y, Hedequist DJ: Submuscular plating of pediatric femur fracture. *J Am Acad Orthop Surg* 2012;20(9):596-603.

Wuerz TH, Gurd DP: Pediatric physeal ankle fracture. *J Am Acad Orthop Surg* 2013;21(4):234-244.

Zionts LE: Fractures around the knee in children. *J Am Acad Orthop Surg* 2002;10(5):345-355.

Index